Management of Breast Diseases

Ismail Jatoi · Achim Rody
Editors

Management of Breast Diseases

Second Edition

Springer

Editors
Ismail Jatoi
Department of Surgery
University of Texas Health Science Center
San Antonio, TX
USA

Achim Rody
Obstetrics and Gynecology
University Medical Center
Schleswig-Holstein
Lübeck
Germany

ISBN 978-3-319-46354-4 ISBN 978-3-319-46356-8 (eBook)
DOI 10.1007/978-3-319-46356-8

Library of Congress Control Number: 2016951967

Printed on acid-free paper

This Springer imprint is published by Springer Nature
The registered company is Springer International Publishing AG
The registered company address is: Gewerbestrasse 11, 6330 Cham, Switzerland

Preface

In 2002, Lippincott published the Manual of Breast Diseases, edited by Prof. Ismail Jatoi. That book was expanded and a larger text entitled Management of Breast Diseases was published by Springer in 2010, edited by Prof. Jatoi and Prof. Manfred Kaufmann of the Goethe-University of Frankfurt. Professor Kaufmann subsequently retired, and the current text is the second edition of the Springer text, with Prof. Achim Rody of the University Hospital Schleswig-Holstein in Lübeck, Germany now serving as co-editor. Many of the chapters have been extensively revised and numerous other authors have been added to the second edition of this text. We hope that this updated text will continue to serve as a useful guide to the wide spectrum of clinicians who treat benign and malignant diseases of the breast: surgeons, gynecologists, medical oncologists, radiation oncologists, internists, and general practitioners.

Today, the management of breast diseases, and particularly breast cancer, is predicated upon the results of large randomized prospective trials. The authors of the various chapters in this text have highlighted the major trials that have contributed to our improved understanding and treatment of breast diseases. Many of these trials have, in particular, revolutionized the treatment of breast cancer. Indeed, there has been a very rapid decline in breast cancer mortality throughout the industrialized world since 1990, due largely to the implementation of the results of landmark randomized trials. For this progress to continue, we will need to design innovative trials in the future, and recruit large numbers of women into those trials. We should always be grateful to the thousands of women throughout the world who have participated in clinical trials, and thereby enabled progress in the treatment of breast cancer.

We are deeply indebted to all the investigators who have contributed chapters to this text. They have diverse interests, but all share the common goal of reducing the burden of breast diseases. We would also like to thank the editorial staff of the Springer publishing company for their continued assistance with updating this text. In particular, we are most grateful to Portia Levasseur of the Springer publishing company. Without Portia's persistence and diligence, this second edition would not have been possible. We hope that clinicians will continue to find this text to be an informative guide to the management of breast diseases.

San Antonio, USA — Ismail Jatoi
Lübeck, Germany — Achim Rody

Contents

Contributors

Lisa H. Amir Judith Lumley Centre, La Trobe University, Melbourne, VIC, Australia; Breastfeeding service, Royal Women's Hospital, Melbourne, Australia

Yash J. Avashia Surgery, Duke University Medical Center, Durham, NC, USA

Kristin Baumann Clinic for Gynaecology and Obstetrics, University Medical Centre Schleswig-Holstein Campus Lübeck, Lübeck, Schleswig-Holstein, Germany

John R. Benson Cambridge Breast Unit, Addenbrooke's Hospital, Cambridge University Hospitals NHS Trust, Cambridge, UK

Alicia Brunßen Department of Surgery, University of Texas Health Science Center at San Antonio, San Antonio, TX, USA

Carissia Calvo Department of Surgery, University of Texas Health Science Center, San Antonio, TX, USA

David A. Cameron Edinburgh Cancer Research Centre, Western General Hospital, University of Edinburgh, Edinburgh, UK

Fátima Cardoso Breast Unit, Champalimaud Clinical Center, Lisbon, Portugal

Monica Castiglione Coordinating Center, International Breast Cancer Study Group (IBCSG), Berne, Switzerland

Sarah Colonna Oncology, Huntsman Cancer Institute, Salt Lake City, UT, USA

Rosaria Condorelli Department of Medical Oncology, Institute of Oncology of Southern Switzerland, Bellinzona, Switzerland

Mary L. Cutler Department of Pathology, Uniformed Services University, Bethesda, MD, USA

Jack Cuzick Wolfson Institute of Preventive Medicine, Queen Mary University of London, Centre for Cancer Prevention, London, UK

Jill R. Dietz Surgery, University Hospitals Seidman Cancer Center, Bentleyville, OH, USA

Phuong Dinh Westmead Hospital, Westmead, NSW, Australia

Detlev Erdmann Surgery, Duke University Medical Center, Durham, NC, USA

Andrew Evans Division of Imaging and Technology, University of Dundee, Dundee, Scotland, UK

Tamer M. Fouad Department of Breast Medical Oncology, The University of Texas MD Anderson Cancer Center, Houston, TX, USA

Amanda Gammon High Risk Cancer Research, Huntsman Cancer Institute, Salt Lake City, UT, USA

Amit Goyal Royal Derby Hospital, Derby, UK

Donna B. Greenberg Department of Psychiatry, Harvard Medical School, Massachusetts General Hospital, MGH Cancer Center, Boston, MA, USA

Emily J. Guerard Medicine, Division of Hematology Oncology, University of North Carolina, Chapel Hill, NC, USA

Nadia Harbeck Breast Center, University of Munich, Munich, Germany

Ruth Heimann Department of Radiation Oncology, University of Vermont Medical Center, Burlington, VT, USA

Gabriel N. Hortobagyi Department of Breast Medical Oncology, The University of Texas MD Anderson Cancer Center, Houston, TX, USA

Anne C. Hoyt Department of Radiological Sciences, UCLA, Los Angeles, CA, USA

Joachim Hübner Institute for Social Medicine and Epidemiology, University of Luebeck, Luebeck, Schleswig-Holstein, Germany

Ismail Jatoi Division of Surgical Oncology and Endocrine Surgery, University of Texas Health Science Center, San Antonio, TX, USA

Jong-Hyeon Jeong Department of Biostatistics, University of Pittsburgh, Pittsburgh, PA, USA

Martha C. Johnson Department of Anatomy, Physiology and Genetics, Uniformed Services University, Bethesda, MD, USA

Alexander Katalinic Institute for Social Medicine and Epidemiology, University of Luebeck, Luebeck, Schleswig-Holstein, Germany

Ian H. Kunkler Institute of Genetics and Molecular Medicine (IGMM), University of Edinburgh, Edinburgh, Scotland, UK

Cornelia Liedtke Department of Obstetrics and Gynecology, University Hospital Schleswig-Holstein/Campus Lübeck, Luebeck, Schleswig-Holstein, Germany

Verity H. Livingstone Department of Family Practice, The Vancouver Breastfeeding Centre, University of British Columbia, Vancouver, BC, Canada

Robert E. Mansel Cardiff University, Monmouth, UK

Frederik Marmé Department of Gynecologic Oncology, National Center of Tumor Diseases, Heidelberg University Hospital, Heidelberg, Germany

Hyman B. Muss Medicine, Division of Hematology Oncology, University of North Carolina, Chapel Hill, NC, USA

Rachel Nirsimloo Edinburgh Cancer Centre, NHS LOTHIAN, Edinburgh, UK

Maria R. Noftz Institute for Social Medicine and Epidemiology, University of Luebeck, Luebeck, Schleswig-Holstein, Germany

Olivia Pagani Institute of Oncology and Breast Unit of Southern Switzerland, Ospedale San Giovanni, Bellinzona, Ticino, Switzerland

Laia Paré Translational Genomics and Targeted Therapeutics in Solid Tumors Lab, August Pi I Sunyer Biomedical Research Institute (IDIBAPS), Barcelon, Spain

Martine J. Piccart Medicine Department, Institut Jules Bordet, Bruxelles, Belgium

Vassilis Pitsinis Breast Unit, Ninewells Hospital and Medical School, NHS Tayside, Dundee, UK

Aleix Prat Medical Oncology, Hospital Clinic of Barcelona, Barcelona, Spain

Telja Pursche Clinic for Gynaecology and Obstetrics, University Medical Centre Schleswig-Holstein Campus Lübeck, Lübeck, Schleswig-Holstein, Germany

Manuela Rabaglio Department of Medical Oncology, University Hospital/Inselspital and IBCSG Coordinating Center, Berne, Switzerland

Joseph Ragaz School of Population and Public Health, University of British Columbia, North Vancouver, BC, Canada

Carol K. Redmond Department of Biostatistics, University of Pittsburgh, Pittsburgh, PA, USA

Joana M. Ribeiro Breast Unit, Champalimaud Clinical Center, Lisbon, Portugal

Domen Ribnikar Medical Oncology Department, Institute of Oncology Ljubljana, Ljubljana, Slovenia

Achim Rody Department of Obstetrics and Gynecology, University Hospital Schleswig-Holstein/Campus Lübeck, Luebeck, Schleswig-Holstein, Germany

Mutlay Sayan Department of Radiation Oncology, University of Vermont Medical Center, Burlington, VT, USA

Darryl Schuitevoerder Department of Surgery, Oregon Health & Science University, Portland, OR, USA

Shayan Shakeraneh Infection Prevention and Control, Providence Health Care, Vancouver, BC, Canada; School of Population and Public Health, University of British Columbia, Vancouver, BC, Canada

Hans-Peter Sinn Department of Pathology, University of Heidelberg, Heidelberg, Baden-Württemberg, Germany

Berta Sousa Breast Unit, Champalimaud Clinical Center, Lisbon, Portugal

Amir Tahernia Plastic and Reconstructive Surgery, Beverly Hills, CA, USA

Alastair M. Thompson Department of Breast Surgical Oncology, University of Texas MD Anderson Cancer Center, Houston, TX, USA

Irene Tsai Department of Radiological Sciences, UCLA, Los Angeles, CA, USA

Naoto T. Ueno Department of Breast Medical Oncology, The University of Texas MD Anderson Cancer Center, Houston, TX, USA

John T. Vetto Department of Surgery, Division of Surgical Oncology, Oregon Health & Science University, Portland, OR, USA

Maria Vidal Medical Oncology, Hospital Clinic of Barcelona, Barcelona, Spain

Madhuri V. Vithala Duke University, Durham Veteran Affairs, Durham, NC, USA

Annika Waldmann Institute for Social Medicine and Epidemiology, University of Luebeck, Luebeck, Schleswig-Holstein, Germany

David P. Winchester American College of Surgeons, Chicago, IL, USA

Michael R. Zenn Surgery, Duke University Medical Center, Durham, NC, USA

Anatomy and Physiology of the Breast

1

Martha C. Johnson and Mary L. Cutler

Abbreviations

BCL-2	B-cell CLL/lymphoma 2
BRCA1	Breast cancer 1
BM	Basement membrane
BrdU	Bromodeoxyuridine
CD	Cluster of differentiation
CSF	Colony-stimulating factor
CTGF	Connective tissue growth factor
DES	Diethylstilbestrol
ECM	Extracellular matrix
EGF	Epidermal growth factor
EGFR	Epidermal growth factor receptor
ER	Estrogen receptor
FGF	Fibroblast growth factor
FSH	Follicle-stimulating hormone
GH	Growth hormone
GnRH	Gonadotropin-releasing hormone
hCG	Human chorionic gonadotropin
HGF	Hepatocyte growth factor
HIF	Hypoxia-inducible factor
HPG	Hypothalamic–pituitary–gonadal
hPL	Human placental lactogen
ICC	Interstitial cell of Cajal
IgA	Immunoglobulin A
IGF	Insulin-like growth factor
IGFBP	IGF-binding protein
IgM	Immunoglobulin M
IR	Insulin receptor
Jak	Janus kinase

M.C. Johnson
Department of Anatomy, Physiology and Genetics, Uniformed Services University, 4301 Jones Bridge Road, Bethesda, MD 20814, USA
e-mail: a1gingy@gmail.com

M.L. Cutler (✉)
Department of Pathology, Uniformed Services University, 4301 Jones Bridge Road, Bethesda, MD 20814, USA
e-mail: mary.cutler@usuhs.edu

I. Jatoi and A. Rody (eds.), *Management of Breast Diseases*, DOI 10.1007/978-3-319-46356-8_1

Ki67	A nuclear antigen in cycling cells
LH	Luteinizing hormone
MMPs	Matrix metalloproteinases
OXT	Oxytocin
PR	Progesterone receptor
PRL	Prolactin
PRLR	Prolactin receptor
PTH	Parathyroid hormone
PTHrP	Parathyroid hormone-related peptide
Sca	Stem cell antigen
SP	Side population
Stat	Signal transducer and activator of transcription
TDLU	Terminal ductal lobular unit
TEB	Terminal end bud

This chapter is a review of the development, structure, and function of the normal human breast. It is meant to serve as a backdrop and reference for the chapters that follow on pathologies and treatment. It presents an overview of normal gross anatomy, histology, and hormonal regulation of the breast followed by a discussion of its structural and functional changes from embryonic development through postmenopausal involution. This section includes recent information on some of the hormones, receptors, growth factors, transcription factors, and genes that regulate this amazing nutritive organ.

From the outset, it is important to keep in mind that information in any discussion of human structure and function is hampered by the limited methods of study available. Observations can be made, but experimental studies are limited. Therefore, much of what is discussed in terms of the regulation of function has, of necessity, been based on animal studies, primarily the mouse, and/or studies of cells in culture. Significant differences between human and mouse mammary glands are summarized at the end of the chapter.

The number of genes and molecules that have been investigated as to their role in the breast is immense. In discussing each stage of breast physiology, we have included a summary of the important hormones and factors involved. Some of the additional factors that have received less attention in the literature are included in Table 1.1 in the appendix. Table 1.2 in the appendix is a list of important mouse gene knockouts and their effects on the mammary gland.

1.1 Gross Anatomy of the Breast

Milk-secreting glands for nourishing offspring are present only in mammals and are a defining feature of the class Mammalia [1]. In humans, mammary glands are present in both females and males, but typically are functional only in the postpartum female. In rare circumstances, men have been reported to lactate [2]. In humans, the breasts are rounded eminences that contain the mammary glands as well as an abundance of adipose tissue (the main determinant of size) and dense connective tissue. The glands are located in the subcutaneous layer of the anterior and a portion of the lateral thoracic wall. Each breast contains 15–20 lobes that each consist of many lobules (Fig. 1.1). At the apex of the breast is a pigmented area, the areola, surrounding a central elevation, the nipple. The course of the nerves and vessels to the nipple runs along the suspensory apparatus consisting of a horizontal fibrous septum that originates at the pectoral fascia along the fifth rib and vertical septa along the sternum and the lateral border of the pectoralis minor [3].

1.1.1 Relationships and Quadrants

The breast is anterior to the deep pectoral fascia and is normally separated from it by the retromammary (submammary) space (Fig. 1.1). The presence of this space allows for a breast mobility relative to the underlying musculature: portions of the pectoralis major, serratus anterior, and external oblique muscles. The breast extends laterally from the lateral

Table 1.1 Additional factors that have been studied in the breast

Factor	Experimental model	Function	References
Jak/Stat	Various	Signaling pathway used by PRL and other hormones	Review [323]
Leptin	Cell culture	Promotes mammary epithelial cell proliferation	[324]
Hypoxia-inducible factor (HIF) 1	Mice null for HIF 1	Required for secretory differentiation and activation and production and secretion of milk of normal volume and composition	[146]
Notch signaling pathway	Human epithelial cell mammospheres in culture	Promotes proliferation of progenitor cells and promotes myoepithelial cell fate commitment and branching morphogenesis	[325]
Wnt signaling pathway	Human epithelial cell mammospheres in culture	(May) play role in human mammary stem cell self-renewal, differentiation, and survival	[326]
" "	Rodents	Mammary rudiment development, ductal branching, and alveolar morphogenesis	[327]
GATA-3	Genetically altered mice	Promotes stem cell differentiation into luminal cells and maintains the luminal cell type and is required for lactational sufficiency	[175, 176]
Msx2	Genetically altered mice	Transcription factor that promotes duct branching	[131]
Tbx3	Humans with ulnar mammary syndrome and genetically altered mice	Required for normal mammary development	[327]
Hedgehog signaling pathway	Mice	Involved in every stage of mammary gland development	[328]
Hedgehog signaling pathway	Genetically altered mice	Repression is required for mammary bud formation	[329]
Stat5	Humans and genetically altered mice	Present in luminal cells and not myoepithelial cells. Regulates PRLR expression. Promotes growth and alveolar differentiation during pregnancy and cell survival during lactation	[256, 330]
Elf5	Mice	Required for growth and differentiation of alveolar epithelial cells in pregnancy and lactation	[331]
HEX, a homeobox gene	Normal human breast and normal and tumor cell lines	Amount in nucleus much higher during lactation. May play role in lactational differentiation	[332]

Table 1.2 Selected mammary gland-related mouse gene knockouts

Gene knocked out	Stage	Effect of knockout	Reference
LEF-1	Embryo	Fails to form first mammary buds	[333]
Tbx3	Embryo	Fails to form first mammary buds	[334]
Msx2	Embryo	Arrests at mammary sprout stage	[335]
PTHrP	Embryo	Failure of branching morphogenesis	[336]
c-Src	Puberty	Fewer TEBs and decreased ductal outgrowth	[337]
ERα	Puberty	Failed expansion of ductal tree	[214]
PR	Puberty	Failed lobuloalveolar development	[338]
PRL	Virgin adult	No lobular decorations	[339]
Stat5	Pregnancy	Incomplete mammary epithelial differentiation	[340]
Jak2	Pregnancy	Impaired alveologenesis and failure to lactate	[341]
α-lactalbumin	Lactation	Viscous milk	[342]
Whey acidic protein	Lactation	Pups die	[343]
OXT	Lactation	Inability to eject milk	[344]
CSF 1	Pregnancy	Incomplete ducts with precocious lobuloalveolar development	[345]
Cyclin D1	Pregnancy	Reduced acinar development and failure to lactate	[346]

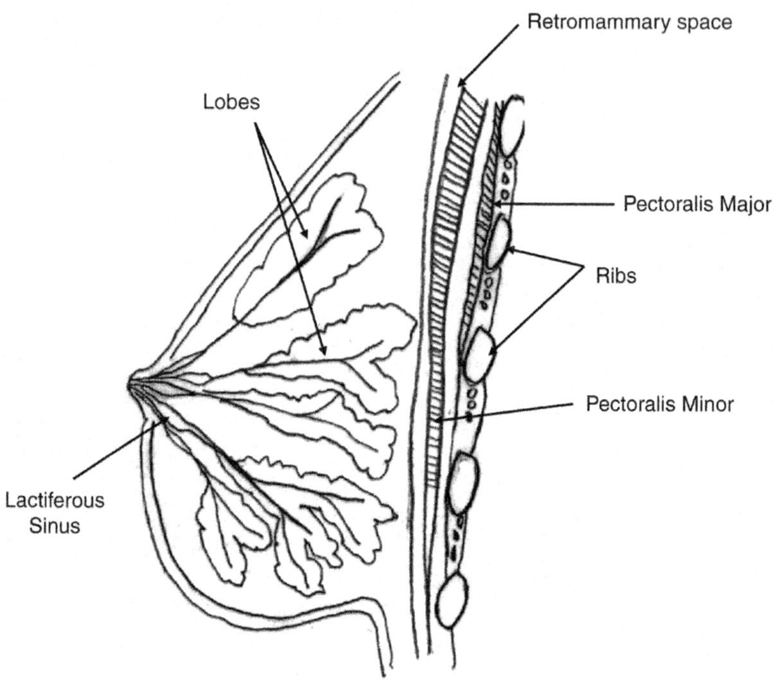

Fig. 1.1 Sagittal section through the lactating breast

edge of the sternum to the mid-axillary line and from the second rib superiorly to the sixth rib inferiorly. An axillary tail (of Spence) extends toward the axilla, or armpit.

For clinical convenience, the breast is divided into quadrants by a vertical line and a horizontal line intersecting at the nipple. The highest concentration of glandular tissue is found in the upper outer quadrant. A separate central portion includes the nipple and areola (Fig. 1.2). Positions on the breast are indicated by numbers based on a clock face [4, 5].

1.1.2 Nerve Supply

Innervation of the breast is classically described as being derived from anterior and lateral cutaneous branches of intercostal nerves four through six, with the fourth nerve the primary supply to the nipple [6]. The lateral and anterior cutaneous branches of the second, third, and sixth intercostal nerves, as well as the supraclavicular nerves (from C3 and C4), can also contribute to breast innervation [6]. Most of

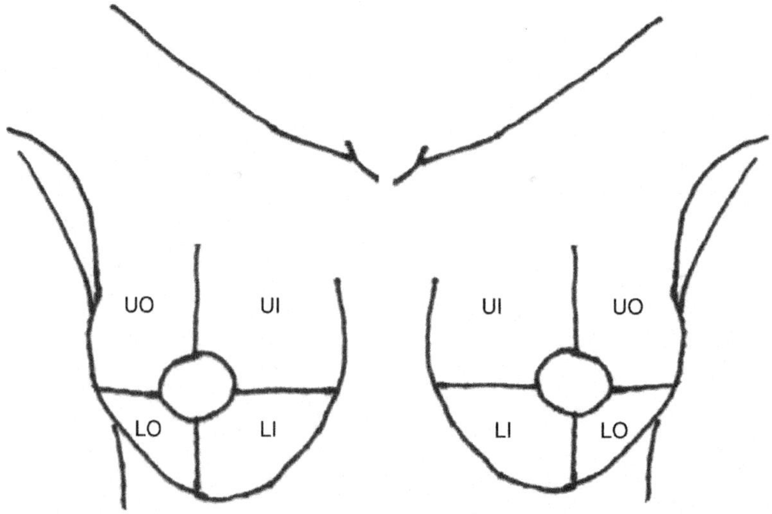

Fig. 1.2 Breast quadrants: *UO* upper outer, *UI* upper inner, *LO* lower outer and *LI* lower inner

the cutaneous nerves extend into a plexus deep to the areola. The extent to which each intercostal nerve supplies the breast varies among individuals and even between breasts in the same individual. In many women, branches of the first and/or the seventh intercostal nerves supply the breast. Fibers from the third (most women [7]) and fifth intercostal nerves may augment the fourth in supplying the nipple [8].

Sensory fibers from the breast relay tactile and thermal information to the central nervous system. Cutaneous sensitivity over the breast varies among women, but is consistently greater above the nipple than below it. The areola and nipple are the most sensitive and are important for sexual arousal in many women [9]. This likely reflects the high density of nerve endings in the nipples [10]. Small breasts are more sensitive than large breasts [11], and women with macromastia report relatively little sensation in the nipple–areola complex [12].

While the apical surface of the nipple has abundant sensory nerve endings, including free nerve endings and Meissner's corpuscles, the sides of the nipple and the areola are less highly innervated. The dermis of the nipple is supplied by branched free nerve endings sensitive to multiple types of input. Nipple innervation is critical since normal lactation requires stimulation from infant suckling [13]. The peripheral skin receptors are specialized for stretch and pressure.

Efferent nerve fibers supplying the breast are primarily postganglionic sympathetic fibers that innervate smooth muscle in the blood vessels of the skin and subcutaneous tissues. Neuropeptides regulate mammary gland secretion indirectly by regulating vascular diameter. Sympathetic fibers also innervate the circular smooth muscle of the nipple (causing nipple erection), smooth muscle surrounding the lactiferous ducts and the arrector pili muscles [14]. The abundance of sympathetic innervation in the breast is evident following mammoplasty, when postsurgical complex regional pain syndrome (an abnormal sympathetic reflex) is relieved by sympathetic blockade of the stellate ganglion [15].

When milk is ejected by myoepithelial cell contraction, the normally collapsed large milk ducts that end on the nipple surface must open up to allow milk to exit. The opening of these ducts is likely to be mediated by neurotransmitters that are released antidromically from axon collaterals in response to stimulation of nerve endings in the nipple. This local reflex may also promote myoepithelial contraction. In stressful situations, neuropeptide Y released from sympathetic fibers may counteract this local reflex, resulting in a diminished volume of milk available to the infant [16].

1.1.3 Vascular Supply

Arteries contributing to the blood supply of the breast include branches of the axillary artery, the internal thoracic artery (via anterior intercostal branches), and certain posterior intercostal arteries (Fig. 1.3). Of the anterior intercostal arteries, the second is usually the largest and, along with numbers three through five, supplies the upper breast, nipple, and areola. The branches of the axillary artery supplying breast tissue include the highest thoracic, lateral thoracic and subscapular and the pectoral branches of the thoracoacromial trunk [4]. Venous drainage of the breast begins in a plexus around the areola and continues from there and from the parenchyma into veins that accompany the arteries listed above, but includes an additional superficial venous plexus [17]. The arterial supply and venous drainage of the breast are both variable. The microvasculature within lobules differs from that found in the denser interlobular tissue, with vascular density (but not total vascular area) being higher in the interlobular region than within the lobules [18]. Vascularity of the breast, as measured by ultrasound Doppler, changes during the menstrual cycle and is greatest close to the time of ovulation [19].

1.1.4 Lymphatic Drainage

Lymphatics of the breast drain primarily to the axillary nodes, but also to non-axillary nodes, especially internal mammary (aka parasternal) nodes located along the internal mammary artery and vein. Some lymphatics travel around the lateral edge of pectoralis major to reach the pectoral group of axillary nodes, some travel through or between pectoral muscles directly to the apical axillary nodes, and others follow blood vessels through pectoralis major to the internal mammary nodes. Internal mammary nodes are located anterior to the parietal pleura in the intercostal spaces. Connections between lymphatic vessels can cross the median plane to the contralateral breast [20].

There are 20–40 axillary nodes that are classified into groups based on their location relative to the pectoralis minor. From inferior to superior, (a) the nodes below and lateral to pectoralis minor comprise the low (level I) nodes, (b) those behind the pectoralis minor make up the middle (level II) nodes, and (c) those above the upper border of pectoralis minor constitute the upper (level III) nodes (Fig. 1.4). Lymphatic plexuses are found in the subareolar region of the breast, the interlobular connective tissue, and the walls of lactiferous ducts. Vessels from the subareolar lymphatic plexus drain to the contralateral breast, the internal lymph node chain, and the axillary nodes [4]. Both dermal and parenchymal lymphatics drain to the same axillary lymph nodes irrespective of quadrant, with lymph from the entire breast often draining through a small number of lymphatic trunks to one or two axillary lymph nodes [21].

Sentinel lymph nodes are those that are the first stop along the route of lymphatic drainage from a primary tumor

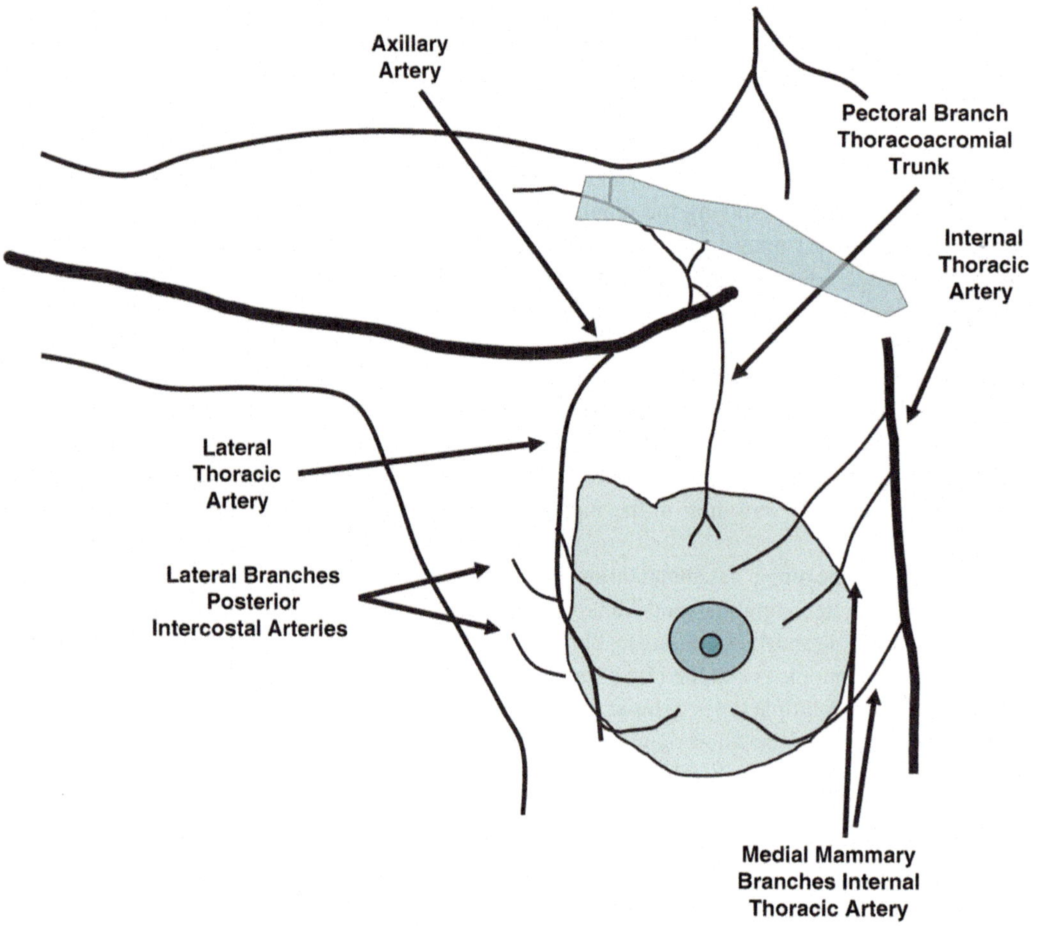

Fig. 1.3 Vascular supply of the breast. Arterial blood is supplied by branches of the axillary artery (Lateral Thoracicand Pectoral Branch of the Thoracoacromial Trunk). Additional blood supply is from Medial Mammary Branches ofthe Internal Thoracic (Internal Mammary) artery and from Lateral Branches of the Posterior Intercostal Arteries.Venous drainage is via veins that parallel the arteries with the addition of a superficial plexus (not shown)

[22]. Much of the information about breast lymphatic drainage has been derived from clinical studies aimed at identifying sentinel nodes and determining likely sites of metastases (a topic beyond the scope of this chapter). These studies often use the injection of radioactive tracer into a lesion, but techniques vary as do results. It is generally accepted that most breast tumors metastasize via lymphatics to axillary lymph nodes. The degree to which metastasis involves internal mammary nodes is debated. One study [23] states that the rate of metastasis to internal mammary nodes is less than 5 %, while another claims that over 20 % of tumors drain at least in part to internal mammary nodes [24].

In women volunteers with normal breast tissue, isotope injected into parenchyma or into subareolar tissue drained, at least in part, into internal mammary nodes in 20–86 % of cases [25]. Microinjection of dye directly into lymph vessels of normal cadavers revealed that all superficial lymph vessels, including those in the nipple and areolar regions, enter a lymph node in the axilla close to the lateral edge of the pectoralis minor (group I). Superficial vessels run between the dermis and the parenchyma, but some run through the breast tissue itself to deeper nodes and into the internal mammary system [26]. Drainage to internal mammary nodes from small breasts (especially in thin and/or young women) is more likely to pass into internal mammary nodes than is drainage from large breasts [27].

1.1.5 Gross Anatomic Changes Throughout the Life span

The breast of the newborn human is a transient slight elevation that may exude small amounts of colostrum-like fluid known colloquially as “witch’s milk.” Human female and male breasts are indistinguishable until puberty [28]. Puberty begins with thelarche, the beginning of adult breast development. The age of thelarche is getting younger. Among whites in 1970, the mean age was 11.5 years of age, but in

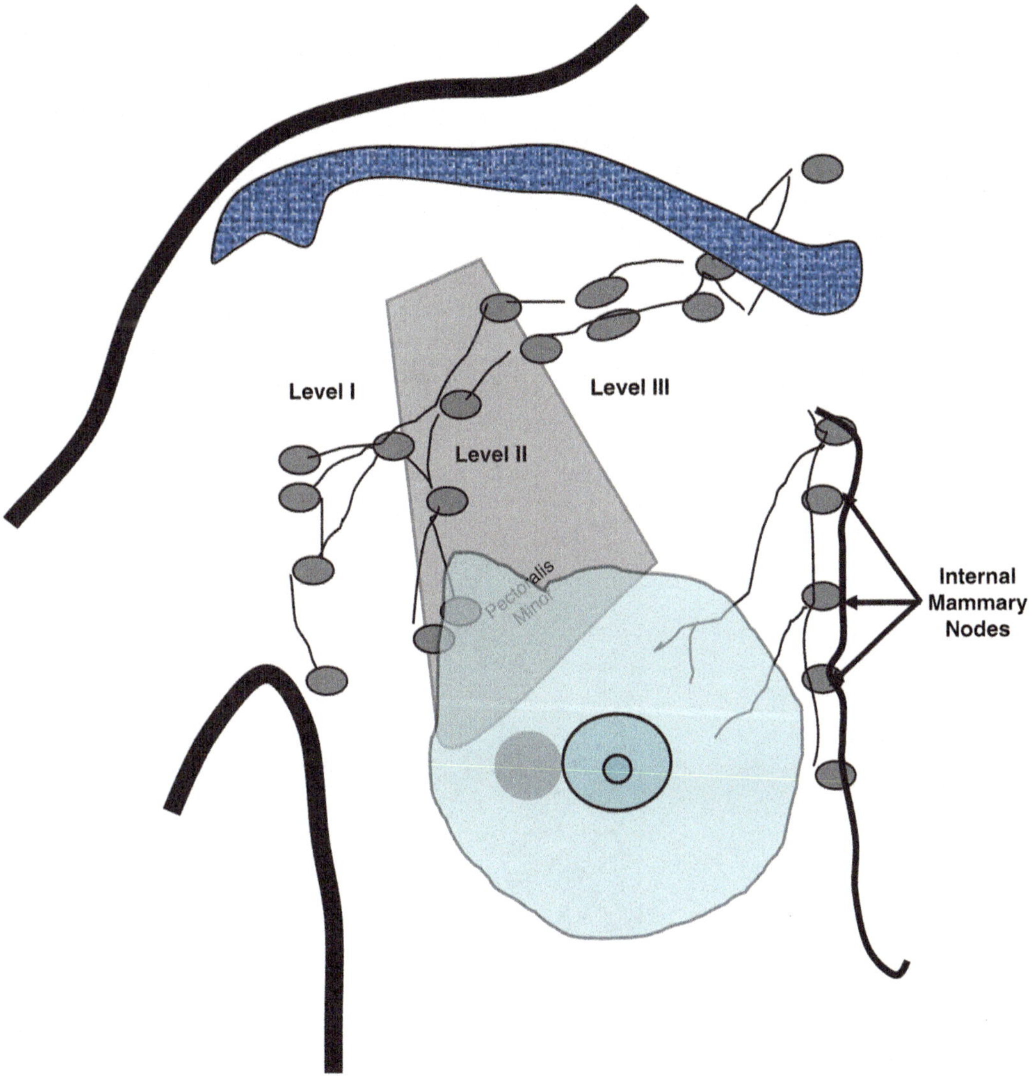

Fig. 1.4 Lymphatic drainage of the breast. Most drainage is into the axillary nodes indicated as Level I, Level II and Level III, based on their relationship to the Pectoralis Minor muscle. Level I nodes are lateral to the muscle, LevelI I are behind it and Level III are medial to it. Also note the Internal Mammary Nodes located just lateral to the edge of the sternum and deep to the thoracic wall musculature

1997, it was 10 years of age. Among blacks, thelarche occurs about one year earlier than in whites [29]. The first indication of thelarche is the appearance of a firm palpable lump deep to the nipple, the breast bud. It corresponds to stage II of the Tanner [30] staging system. (Stage I is prepubertal; stage III exhibits obvious enlargement and elevation of the entire breast; stage IV, very transient, is the phase of areolar mounding and it contains periareolar fibroglandular tissue; stage V exhibits a mature contour and increased subcutaneous adipose tissue). The human breast achieves its final external appearance 3–4 years after the beginning of puberty [31].

Following puberty, the breast undergoes less dramatic changes during each menstrual cycle (discussed in detail later). The texture of the breast is least nodular just before ovulation; therefore, clinical breast examinations are best done at this time. In addition, the breast is less dense on mammogram during the follicular phase. The volume of each breast varies 30–100 mL over the course of the menstrual cycle. It is greatest just prior to menses and minimal on day 11 [32]. The breast enlarges during pregnancy and lactation, and the postlactational breast may exhibit stria (stretch marks) and sag. The postmenopausal breast is often pendulous.

1.2 Histology

1.2.1 Overview

The adult human breast is an area of skin and underlying connective tissue containing a group of 15–20 large modified sweat glands [referred to as lobes (Fig. 1.1)] that collectively make up the mammary gland. The most striking thing about breast morphology is its remarkable heterogeneity among normal breasts, both within a single breast and between breasts [33]. The glands that collectively make up the breast are embedded in extensive amounts of adipose tissue and are separated by bands of dense connective tissue (Fig. 1.5) (suspensory or Cooper's ligaments [6]) that divide it into lobes [34] and extend from the dermis to the deep fascia.

The lobules within each lobe drain into a series of intralobular ducts that, in turn, drain into a single lactiferous duct (Fig. 1.6) that opens onto the surface of the nipple. The part of each lactiferous duct closest to the surface of the nipple is lined by squamous epithelium [35] that becomes more stratified as it nears its orifice. In a non-lactating breast, the opening of the lactiferous duct is often plugged with keratin [4, 36]. Deep to the areola, the lactiferous ducts expand slightly into a sinus that acts as a small reservoir (Fig. 1.1).

The mammary gland is classified as branched tubuloalveolar, although true alveoli do not typically develop until pregnancy. Individual lobules are embedded in a loose connective tissue stroma that is highly cellular and responds to several hormones [35]. Terminal ductal lobular units

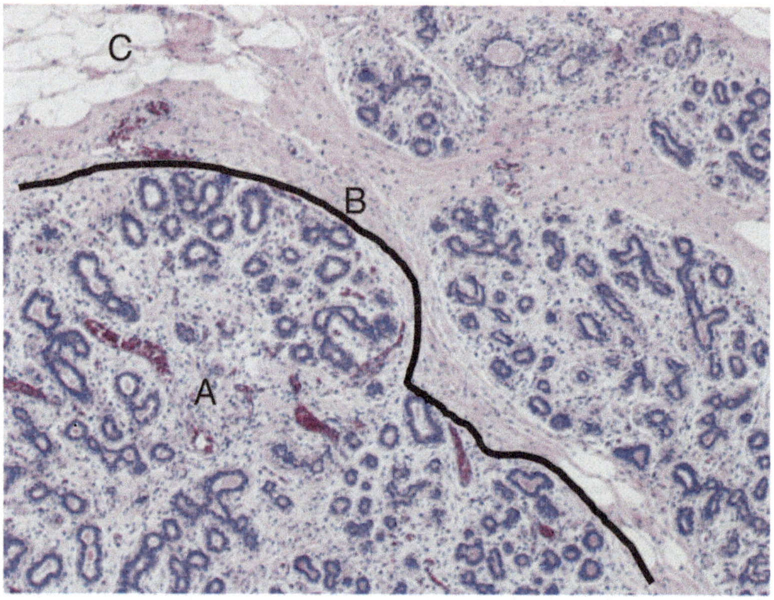

Fig. 1.5 Low power micrograph (50×) of an active (but not lactating) human breast. The dark line outlines a portion of a lobule. Note *A* the areolar connective tissue within the lobule and between the ductules, *B* the dense connective tissue between lobules and *C* adipose tissue. Some secretory product has accumulated within the ductules of the lobule

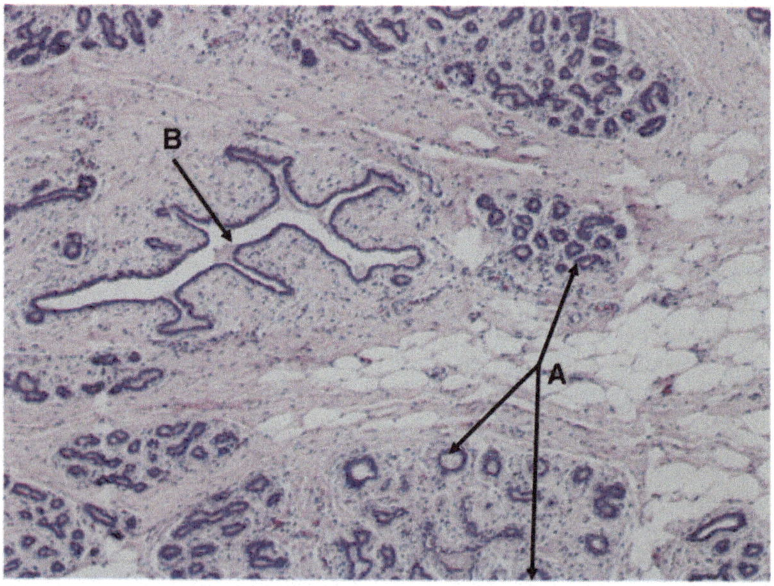

Fig. 1.6 Low power micrograph (50×) of an active (but not lactating) human breast. Arrows at *A* indicate intralobular ducts (ductules) within lobules. True acini are not present at this stage. The arrow at *B* indicates the lumen of a lactiferous (interlobular) duct

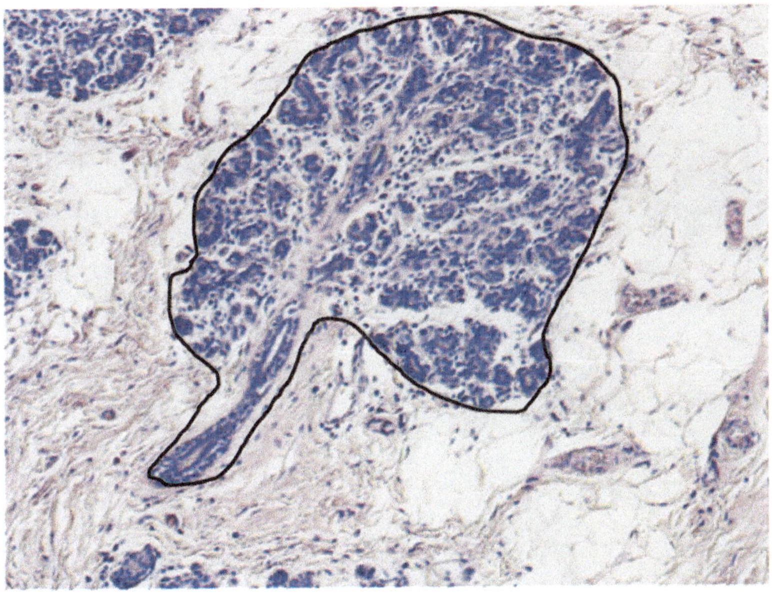

Fig. 1.7 Intermediate power micrograph (100×) of an active (but not lactating) human breast. A Terminal Ductal Lobular Unit (TDLU) and its duct are outlined. Note the abundant adipose tissue and dense irregular connective tissue surrounding the TDLU

(TDLUs) are considered to be the functional units of the human mammary gland. Each TDLU consists of an intralobular duct and its associated saccules (also called ductules). These saccules differentiate into the secretory units referred to as acini or alveoli [37]. The alveoli are outpocketings along the length of the duct and at its terminus. A TDLU resembles a bunch of grapes [38] (Fig. 1.7).

Three-dimensional reconstruction of the parenchyma from serial sections of human breast tissue [39] revealed no overlap in territories drained by adjacent ducts. However, a recent computer-generated 3-D model based on a single human breast found that anastomoses do exist between branching trees of adjacent ducts [40].

The ductwork of the breast has progressively thicker epithelium as its tributaries converge toward the nipple. The smallest ducts are lined with simple cuboidal epithelium, while the largest are lined with stratified columnar epithelium [41]. The epithelial cells have little cytoplasm, oval central nuclei with one or more nucleoli, and scattered or peripheral chromatin [36].

The entire tubuloalveolar system, including each saccule, is surrounded by a basement membrane (BM) (Fig. 1.8). Between the luminal epithelial cells and the BM is interposed an incomplete layer of stellate myoepithelial cells. The myoepithelial layer is more attenuated in the smaller branches of the ductwork and in the alveoli. Macrophages and lymphocytes are found migrating through the epithelium toward the lumen [42].

1.2.2 Nipple and Areola

The nipple and the areola are hairless [36]. Nipple epidermis is very thin and sensitive to estrogen. Sweat glands and small sebaceous glands (of Montgomery) are found in the areola and produce small elevations on its surface. The skin of the adult nipple and areola is wrinkled due to the presence of abundant elastic fibers [4] and contains long dermal papillae. Lactiferous ducts open on the surface of the nipple, and parenchymal tissue radiates from it into the underlying connective tissue. The stroma of the nipple is dense irregular connective tissue that contains both radial and circumferential smooth muscle fibers. Contraction of the smooth muscle fibers results in erection of the nipple and further wrinkling of the areola [4]. Nipple erection can occur in response to cold, touch, or psychic stimuli. Smaller bundles of smooth muscle fibers are located along the lactiferous ducts [43].

1.2.3 Parenchyma

1.2.3.1 Luminal Epithelial Cells

Luminal epithelial cells carry out the main function of the breast: milk production. The secretory prowess of the luminal epithelial cells is impressive. They can produce three times their own volume per day. Luminal epithelial cells have scant cytoplasm and a central, oval nucleus with marginal heterochromatin. They are cuboidal to columnar, and

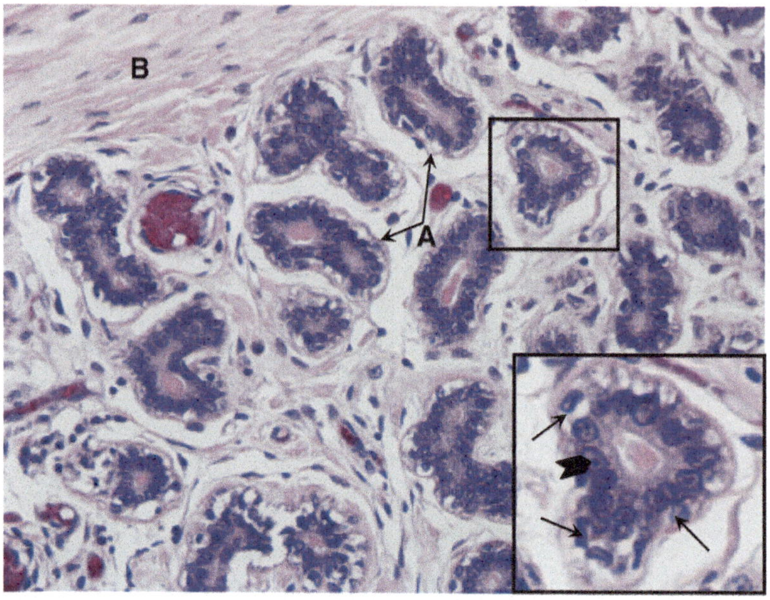

Fig. 1.8 Intermediate power micrograph (200×) of an active (but not lactating) human breast. The arrows labeled *A* indicate basement membranes (BM) surrounding individual ductules. The letter *B* is in the dense irregular connective tissue surrounding this lobule. Note the pale elongated nuclei of fibroblasts and the collagen fibers surrounding the letter *B*. The inset indicated by the rectangle is enlarged in the lower right corner. Arrows in theinset indicate myoepithelial cells and the chevron indicates a luminal epithelial cell

each cell has a complete lateral belt of occluding (tight) junctions near its apex and E-cadherin (a transmembrane protein found in epithelial adherens junctions) on its lateral surfaces [44]. During lactation, luminal cells contain the organelles typical of cells secreting protein, as well as many lipid droplets for release into milk [36].

1.2.3.2 Myoepithelial Cells

Myoepithelial cells surround the luminal cell layer (inset, Fig. 1.8) and are located between it and the BM, which they secrete [45]. In the ducts and ductules, myoepithelial cells are so numerous that they form a relatively complete layer [4, 46]. In alveoli, the myoepithelial cells form a network of slender processes that collectively look like an open-weave basket [35]. Myoepithelial cell processes indent the basal surface of nearly every secretory cell [36] and contain parallel arrays of myofilaments and dense body features commonly found in smooth muscle cells. They also contain smooth muscle-specific proteins and form gap junctions with each other [47].

While myoepithelial cells exhibit many features of smooth muscle cells, they are true epithelial cells. They contain cytokeratins 5 and 14, exhibit desmosomes and hemidesmosomes [48], and are separated from connective tissue by a BM. Compared to luminal cells, they contain higher concentrations of β-integrins (receptors that attach to extracellular matrix (ECM) elements and mediate intracellular signals) [49, 50].

Myoepithelial cells utilize the adhesion molecule P-cadherin [44] (a transmembrane protein), the knockout of which results in precocious and hyperplastic mammary gland development in mice [51]. They also express growth factor receptors and produce matrix metalloproteinases (MMPs) and MMP inhibitors that modify ECM composition. Cell–cell contacts between the myoepithelial cells and their luminal cell neighbors allow for direct signaling [52] between the two cell types, and their basal location positions them to mediate interactions between the luminal cells and the ECM.

In addition to contracting to express milk toward the nipple, myoepithelial cells establish epithelial cell polarity by synthesizing the BM. Specifically, they deposit fibronectin (a large glycoprotein that mediates adhesion), laminin (a BM component that has many biologic activities), collagen IV, and nidogen (a glycoprotein that binds laminin and type IV collagen). Human luminal cells cultured in a type I collagen matrix form cell clusters with reversed polarity and no BM [50]. Introducing myoepithelial cells corrects the polarity and leads to the formation of double-layered acini with central lumina. Laminin [53] is unique in its ability to substitute for the myoepithelial cells in polarity reversal [50].

Other roles of the myoepithelial cell in the breast include lineage segregation during development and promoting luminal cell growth and differentiation [45, 54]. They also play an active role in branching morphogenesis [55] and even exhibit a few secretory droplets during pregnancy and lactation [31]. The myoepithelial cell rarely gives rise to tumors itself [56] and is thought to act as a natural tumor suppressor [45].

1.2.3.3 Stem Cells

Definitions and Terms

The idea of a population of mammary gland stem cells [57] has existed since the 1950s. These cells would give rise either to two daughter cells or to one stem cell and one lineage-specific progenitor cell that would, in turn, give rise to either luminal cells or myoepithelial cells [58].

A rigorous definition of a tissue-specific stem cell requires that it meets five criteria [59]. It must (1) be multipotential, (2) self-renew, (3) lack mature cell lineage markers, (4) be relatively quiescent, and (5) effect the long-term regeneration of its "home" tissue in its entirety. Much of the mammary cell literature takes liberty with these criteria, often applying the term "stem cell" to cells that can give rise to either (but not both) of the two parenchymal cell types. Some still argue [60] that the existence of true human mammary epithelial stem cells in adults has not been unequivocally demonstrated.

Structure and Function of Mammary Stem Cells

A cell that stains poorly with osmium [61] in mouse mammary epithelium has been equated to the mammary gland stem cell. These cells are present at all stages of differentiation and undergo cell division shortly after being placed in culture, even in the presence of DNA synthesis inhibitors. They do not synthesize DNA in situ or in vitro, but do incorporate the nucleotide precursors needed for RNA synthesis. In mice, stem cell daughter cells functionally differentiate in explant cultures in the presence of lactogenic hormones [62].

Stem cells are distinguishable phenotypically from mammary epithelial progenitor cells. The progenitor cells produce adherent colonies in vitro, are a rapidly cycling population in the normal adult, and have molecular features indicating a basal position. Stem cells have none of those properties, and in serial culture studies, murine stem cells disappear when growth stops [63]. Murine mammary gland cells transplanted into host tissue will reconstitute a functional mammary ductal tree that is morphologically indistinguishable from the normal gland [64]. Furthermore, a fully differentiated mammary gland can be derived from a single murine stem cell clone [65, 66].

Identification of Mammary Stem Cells

If mature luminal human cells express certain markers and myoepithelial cells express others, then epithelial cells with little or none of either set of markers are likely to be more primitive. If mammary gland cells are separated by flow cytometry and subpopulations are plated on collagen matrices, a subpopulation can be identified that produces colonies containing both luminal and myoepithelial cells [67].

Human mammary stem cells are positive for both keratins 19 and 14 and are capable of forming TDLU-like structures in 3-D gel cultures. They can give rise to K19/K14 +/−, −/− (both are luminal), and −/+ (myoepithelial) cells, each of which are lineage-restricted progenitors [68]. The embryonic marker CD133 is detected in the mammary gland also serving as a marker of mammary stem cells [69].

The ability of certain cells to pump out loaded Hoechst 33342 dye allows them to be separated by flow cytometry into a "side population" (SP), claimed by some to be a population of stem cells. However, in the mammary gland, the evidence that the SP is enriched for stem cells is only correlative. Cells have been identified as quiescent stem cells based on their retention of BrdU incorporated during a prior period of proliferation plus their lack of both luminal and myoepithelial cell markers. Using this method, 5 % of the cells in the mouse mammary gland are quiescent stem cells. They express Sca-1 (a stem cell marker), are progesterone receptor (PR) negative, and are located within the luminal cell layer [70].

Lineage-tracing experiments can follow stem and progenitor cell fate during development and tissue reorganization in mice using promoters of genes linked to a specific lineage ex: Elf5, the gene linked to luminal progenitors driving visual markers. The results obtained with this approach called into question the existence of bipotent mammary stem cells, given the apparent disparity between results obtained with transplantation versus lineage-tracing assays. This suggested that tissue disruption and sorting of cells prior to implantation may activate them or contribute to their "stemness." While it has been postulated that bipotent stem cells detected in the embryo no longer function in the postnatal animal, recent evidence detected bipotent stem cells participating in epithelial differentiation in the adult mammary gland [71].

Examples of Cells Referred to as Mammary Stem Cells:

- Human mammary epithelial cells with neither luminal cell nor myoepithelial cell markers.

- Subpopulations of mammary gland cells separated by flow cytometry that produce colonies containing both luminal and myoepithelial cells [67].
- Human mammary stem cells that are capable of forming TDLU-like structures in 3-D gel cultures. They can give rise to K19/K14 +/−, −/− (both are luminal), and −/+ (myoepithelial) cells, each of which are lineage-restricted progenitors [68].
- Mammary cells that pump out loaded Hoechst 33342 dye and separate by flow cytometry into a "side population" (SP). However, in the mammary gland, the evidence that the SP is enriched for stem cells is only correlative.
- Mammary cells that are quiescent, based on their retention of BrdU that was incorporated during a prior period of proliferation, that also lack both luminal and myoepithelial cell markers. By this method, 5 % of mouse mammary epithelial cells are quiescent stem cells. They also express Sca-1 (a stem cell marker), are progesterone receptor (PR) negative, and are located within the luminal cell layer [69].
- Cell fate mapping studies in mice using multicolor reporters indicated the presence of bipotent stem cells that coordinate remodeling in the adult mammary gland but demonstrate that both stem and progenitor cells drive morphogenesis during puberty [71].
- Breast cancer stem cells (BCSCs) are defined as a subset (1–5 %) of CD44+/CD24-/lin- cells from primary human tumors that can form tumors in athymic mice [72]. These cells typically express aldehyde dehydrogenase (ALDH) which correlates with level of HER2 [73].
- CD133 is detected on stem cells in the mammary gland [69]. It is identified as stem cell marker in multiple tumor types including triple-negative breast cancer [74, 75], often correlating with the level of vascular mimicry [76].

Location of Mammary Stem Cells

The concentration of stem cells in the human is highest in ducts [68]. They tend to be quiescent and surrounded by patches of proliferating cells and differentiated progeny [77]. Stem cells are believed to be the pale cells intermediate in position between the basal and the luminal compartments of the mammary epithelium. However, a cell line has been isolated from the luminal compartment in humans that can generate itself, secretory cells, and myoepithelial cells [55].

Classification of Mammary Stem Cells

Human stem cells and progenitors are classified into several ways. One classification system is based on steroid hormone receptors: Estrogen receptor (ER)α/PR-negative stem cells function during early development, and ERα/PR-positive stem cells are required for homeostasis during menstrual cycling [77]. The existence of receptor (ER)α/PR- stem cells suggests the need for paracrine mechanisms for regulation by hormones, and in fact, ERα/PR + act as sensors to relay hormonal cues to the (ER)α/PR- cells [78, 79]. In another scheme, stem cells in nulliparous women are classified as type one, while stem cells found in parous women are classified as type two. Parity-induced (type two) murine mammary epithelial cells are able to form mammospheres in culture and, when transplanted, establish a fully functional mammary gland [80]. These cells reside in the luminal layer of the ducts and contribute to secretory alveoli that appear in pregnancy [81]. The nulliparous type is more vulnerable to carcinogenesis [82]. A third scheme [83] classifies the mammary progenitors into three types: (1) a luminal-restricted progenitor that produces only daughter cells with luminal cell markers, (2) a bipotent progenitor (the "stem cell" described by other investigators) that produces colonies with a core of luminal cells surrounded by cells with the morphology and markers typical of myoepithelial cells, and (3) a progenitor that generates only myoepithelial cells.

A special stem cell (like) type has been identified in multiparous human females. It is pregnancy-induced, does not undergo apoptosis following lactation, and is capable of both self-renewal and production of progeny with diverse cellular fates [84]. This cell type increases to constitute as much as 60 % of the epithelial cell population in multiparous women and may be related to the parity-related resistance to breast cancer [82].

Factors Regulating Stem Cells

The development of suspension cultures in which human stem cells form "mammospheres" [85] has facilitated the study of the various pathways regulating the self-renewal and differentiation of normal mammary stem and progenitor cells [86]. A specific cell's "stemness" decreases as that cell becomes more differentiated. Stem cells can self-renew and proliferate within their niche, where they are maintained in their undifferentiated state by cell–ECM and cell–cell interactions. These interactions involve integrins and cadherins, respectively. Wnt/β-catenin signaling is a regulator of self-renewal in stem cells [87, 88]. Wnt4 is a regulator of stem cell proliferation downstream of progesterone as is RANKL, which has been implicated as a paracrine mediator [89–91]. Chromatin regulators can also affect the balance between self-renewal and differentiation. For example, the histone methylation reader Pygo2 is a Wnt pathway coactivator that facilitates binding of β-catenin to Notch3 to suppress luminal and alveolar differentiation by coordinating these pathways [92]. Lineage-tracing experiments determined that the Notch pathway is critical in the luminal lineage. Notch3-expressing cells are luminal progenitors that give rise to ER+ and ER- ductal progeny [93], which exhibit functional similarity to parity-induced cells that contribute to secretory alveoli.

HER2 is required for early stages of mammary development [94, 95] and it is an important regulator of CSCs [96]. It can be targeted by trastuzumab, and the success of trastuzumab therapy in tumors where HER2 is not amplified is thought to occur through targeting CSCs [97, 98].

Hormones and cytokines stimulate proliferation of stem cells and this has implications for the development of breast cancer [90]. Obesity is associated with the incidence and mortality of breast cancer [99, 100], and cytokine-mediated increase in stem cell number may be mechanistically involved. Pituitary growth hormone, acting via IGF-1 as well as through receptor-mediated JAK-Stat signaling, is required for mammary development as is IGF-1 [101, 102]. IGF-1 treatment increases the number of mammary stem cells in rodents, and IGF-1R expression correlates with the risk of breast cancer in humans [103]. Leptin increases mammary stem cell self-renewal, and its level in human serum correlates with obesity [104]. An increase in the number of cycling cells in normal breast tissue in premenopausal women is associated with an increased risk of developing breast cancer [105], suggesting that environmental stimulation of human mammary progenitor cells may contribute to the subsequent development of breast cancer.

1.2.4 Basement Membrane

The luminal cells of the mammary gland rest on a BM (except where myoepithelial cell processes intervene). Components of the mammary gland BM include collagen type IV, laminin, nidogens 1 and 2, perlecan, and fibronectin [106–108]. All of these components are found within the BMs of ducts, lobules, and alveoli in both the human and the mouse.

Many mammary epithelial cell functions require a BM including milk production [109], suppression of programmed cell death [110], interaction with prolactin (PRL) [111], and the expression of ERα needed to respond to estrogen. Reconstituted BM (or collagen type IV or laminin I) and lactogenic hormones can substitute for the BM requirement for ER expression [112]. Precise contact between epithelial cells and their underlying BM is critical for the maintenance of tissue architecture and function. For example, cultured mammary epithelial cells unable to anchor normally to the laminin in their BM have disrupted polarity and are unable to secrete β-casein, the most abundant milk protein [113]. Laminin activates expression of the β-casein gene [114]. In tissue culture, mammary epithelial cells require laminin and specific β1-integrins for survival [107, 115]. Nidogen-1 connects laminin and collagen networks to each other, is essential for BM structural integrity [107], and promotes lactational differentiation [116]. Integrins are essential for cell–BM interactions that are required for lactogenic cellular differentiation [117]. β1-integrin is required for alveolar organization and optimal luminal cell proliferation [118] and, along with laminin, is required for end bud growth during puberty [119]. The fibronectin-specific integrin is localized to myoepithelial cells and is thought to be required for hormone-dependent cell proliferation [120].

The ability to culture cells in 3-D using synthetic BM culture systems, such as Matrigel™, has opened the door to investigations of normal, as well as cancerous breast physiology [121]. Normal mammary epithelial cells seeded into Matrigel™ form small cell masses, develop apicobasal polarity, secrete ECM components basally, and develop apical Golgi and junctional complexes. The cell masses form a lumen by cavitation involving the removal of central cells by programmed cell death [122] and, in the process of becoming differentiated, form tight junctions prior to secreting milk [123].

1.2.5 Stroma

There are three types of connective tissue in the breast: loose connective tissue within lobules (intralobular), dense irregular connective tissue between lobules (interlobular), and adipose tissue (also interlobular) (Fig. 1.5). The dense connective tissue contains thick bundles of collagen and elastic fibers that surround the individual lobular units. Breast stroma is not a passive structural support; epithelial–stromal interactions play key roles in development and differentiation. The intralobular loose connective tissue is in close relationship to the ductules and alveoli of the mammary gland and is responsive to hormones.

1.2.5.1 Cells in Breast Stroma

While cells found in the interlobular connective tissue are primarily fibroblasts or adipocytes, the intralobular connective tissue also contains macrophages, eosinophils, lymphocytes, plasma cells, and mast cells.

Fibroblasts form a basket-like layer around the human TDLU external to its BM [124] (Fig. 1.9). In the intralobular connective tissue, fibroblasts have attenuated cytoplasmic processes that form a network via cell–cell connections [33]. The connections serve to link the fibroblasts adjacent to the BM with those found within the lobular stroma. Mammary gland fibroblasts have ultrastructural features typical of synthetically active cells. Other cells in the intralobular connective tissue are interspersed within the fibroblast network such that cell–cell interaction is facilitated. Intralobular fibroblasts are CD34 (a marker for early stem-like cells) positive [35].

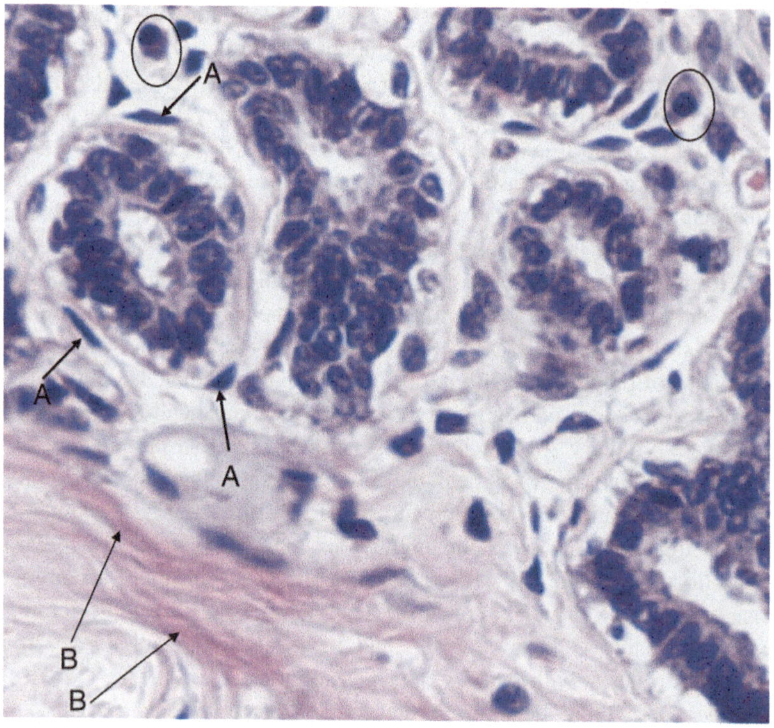

Fig. 1.9 High power micrograph (400×) of an active (but not lactating) human breast. Arrows labeled *A* indicate nuclei of fibro blasts surrounding a ductule. Arrows labeled *B* indicate collagen fiber bundles and the ovals surround plasma cells

Two populations of human mammary gland fibroblasts can be distinguished based on staining for the cell surface enzyme dipeptidyl peptidase IV, an enzyme implicated in breast cancer metastasis. Intralobular fibroblasts are negative for this enzyme, but interlobular fibroblasts are positive [125]. Human breast fibroblasts have the ability to inhibit the growth of epithelial cells. If the ratio of fibroblasts to epithelial cells is high, however, the fibroblasts enhance epithelial proliferation [126, 127].

Adipocytes (Fig. 1.5) are common in the breast. High breast density on mammogram (negatively correlated with fat) is a risk factor for breast cancer [102]. In pregnant women, the adipocytes are closer to the epithelium and the number of fat-filled cells is markedly reduced throughout pregnancy and lactation. Adding adipocytes to murine epithelial cells in vitro enhances mammary cell growth and seems to be required for the synthesis of casein.

Macrophages are localized near the epithelium during certain stages of breast development and have been shown to be critical for proper duct elongation. The macrophage growth factor, CSF1, promotes murine mammary gland development from branching morphogenesis to lactation [128]. Macrophages may play a role in both angiogenesis and the ECM remodeling required during morphogenesis [129]. They are localized in close proximity to developing alveoli during pregnancy and are present during involution, where they likely help clear out milk lipid droplets and/or apoptotic debris [130]. Eosinophils are present during postnatal development, where they are believed to interact with macrophages to induce proper branching morphogenesis [131].

Lymphocyte migration into the mammary gland during lactation is facilitated by specific adhesion molecules located on the endothelial cells. Lymphocytes themselves can be found in milk. Plasma cells derived from B lymphocytes are abundant in the stroma before and during lactation when they secrete antibodies that are taken up by the epithelial cells and secreted into milk [132].

Mast cells contain several potent mediators of inflammation including histamine, proteinases, and several cytokines. Nevertheless, the precise functions of mast cells are still unknown [133]. Since mast cells are associated with bundles of collagen in human breast stroma, they may play a role in collagen deposition [134].

Recently, two additional stromal cell types have been identified: the interstitial cell of Cajal (ICC) and the ICC-like cell. These cells have two or three long, thin moniliform processes [135] and establish close contacts with various immunoreactive cells, including lymphocytes, plasma cells, macrophages, and mast cells [136]. ICCs from the breast form "intercellular bridges" in vitro [137]. They have caveolae, overlapping processes, stromal synapses (close contacts), and gap junctions. They also exhibit dichotomous branching. Collectively, the ICCs make up a labyrinthine system that may play a pivotal role in integrating stromal cells into a functional assembly with a defined 3-D structure [138].

1.2.5.2 Extracellular Matrix

The 3-D organization of the ECM affects many aspects of cell behavior: shape, proliferation, survival, migration, differentiation, polarity, organization, branching, and lumen formation [131]. Two principal ways that the ECM can affect cell behavior are to (1) harbor various factors and/or their binding proteins to be released when needed and (2) directly regulate cell behavior via cell–ECM interactions [111].

Stromal fibronectin and its receptor, $\alpha_5\beta_1$-integrin, play an important role in ovarian hormone-dependent regulation of murine epithelial cell proliferation. The fibronectin receptor is more closely correlated with proliferation and more rapidly regulated by estrogen and progesterone than is fibronectin itself. Thus, it is likely that the receptor, rather than fibronectin, is hormonally regulated. Mouse fibronectin levels increase threefold between puberty and sexual maturity and remain high during pregnancy and lactation [139].

Integrins, the major ECM receptors, link the ECM to the actin cytoskeleton and to signal transduction pathways [140] involved in directing cell survival, proliferation, differentiation, and migration. They mediate interactions between stroma and parenchyma. Specific integrin functions in the human mammary gland have been reviewed elsewhere [141].

Proteoglycans, large heavily glycosylated glycoproteins, are abundant in breast ECM and correlate with increased mammographic density, a risk factor for breast cancer [142]. They are also important in coordinating stromal and epithelial development and mediating cell–cell and cell–matrix interactions. Several regulatory proteins in the mammary gland bind to proteoglycan glycosaminoglycans, including fibroblast growth factors (FGFs), epidermal growth factors (EGFs), and hepatocyte growth factor (HGF) [143].

1.3 Synopsis of Hormones and Other Factors that Regulate Breast Structure and Function

1.3.1 Hormones

This segment is a brief overview of reproductive hormonal events in the female, particularly as they affect the breast. Details of endocrine involvement in each phase of breast development and function are discussed in Sect. 1.4.

The hormonal control of human reproduction involves a hierarchy consisting of the hypothalamus, the anterior pituitary gland and the gonads: the hypothalamic–pituitary–gonadal (HPG) axis. In the female, the main hormones involved are (1) gonadotropin-releasing hormone (GnRH) from the hypothalamus, (2) luteinizing hormone (LH) and follicle-stimulating hormone (FSH) from the pituitary, and (3) estrogen and progesterone, steroid hormones derived from cholesterol and made in the ovary (Fig. 1.10). The levels of these hormones vary dramatically throughout each menstrual cycle (Fig. 1.11), as well as during the various stages of a woman's lifetime.

GnRH causes the anterior pituitary gland to secrete LH and FSH. The hypothalamus releases GnRH in a pulsatile manner from axon terminals of neurons in the medial basal hypothalamus [144]. Pulsatile release of GnRH into the hypothalamo-hypophyseal portal system, which carries it directly to the pituitary gland, is essential to its function.

LH and FSH promote new ovarian follicle growth during the first 11–12 days of the menstrual cycle. The follicle, in turn, secretes both steroid hormones, estrogen and progesterone. Estrogen and progesterone are transported in the blood bound to proteins, primarily albumin and specific hormone binding globulins [145]. Just before ovulation, there is a sudden marked increase in both LH and FSH, a surge that leads to ovulation and the subsequent formation of the corpus luteum from the follicle.

Between ovulation and the beginning of menstruation, the corpus luteum secretes large amounts of estrogen and progesterone. These hormones have a negative feedback effect on secretion of LH and FSH in the pituitary gland, as well as GnRH secretion in the hypothalamus (Fig. 1.11). Estrogen primarily promotes the development of female secondary sex characteristics, including the breast. Progesterone mainly prepares the uterus for the receipt and nurture of the embryo and fetus and prepares the breast for lactation. During pregnancy, estrogen and progesterone are secreted primarily by the placenta. The main effects of estrogen on the breast are (1) stromal tissue development, (2) growth of breast ductwork, and (3) fat deposition [145]. Progesterone is required for lobuloalveolar differentiation of the breast [146].

These steroid hormones bind to receptors that belong to a superfamily of related receptors. The ER is an intracellular receptor that functions as a DNA-binding transcription factor [147, 148]. There are two forms of ER: ERα and ERβ that are coded on different genes [149]. Estrogen-binding affinity is high at both receptors and both are expressed in the breast. In the normal human breast, ERα is expressed in approximately 15–30 % of luminal epithelial cells [150], whereas ERβ is found in myoepithelial cells and stromal cells [147]. Estrogen binds to the ER and the ER–estrogen complex translocates to the nucleus of the cell, where it binds to DNA and effects transcriptional changes leading to alterations in cell function. ER signaling can also act in a non-classical pathway by interacting with other transcription factors bound to promoters of responsive genes [151]. ERα–estrogen complexes activate gene transcription, while ERβ–estrogen complexes can either activate or inhibit transcription [147, 152]. In mice, binding of estrogen to ERα stimulates mammary cell

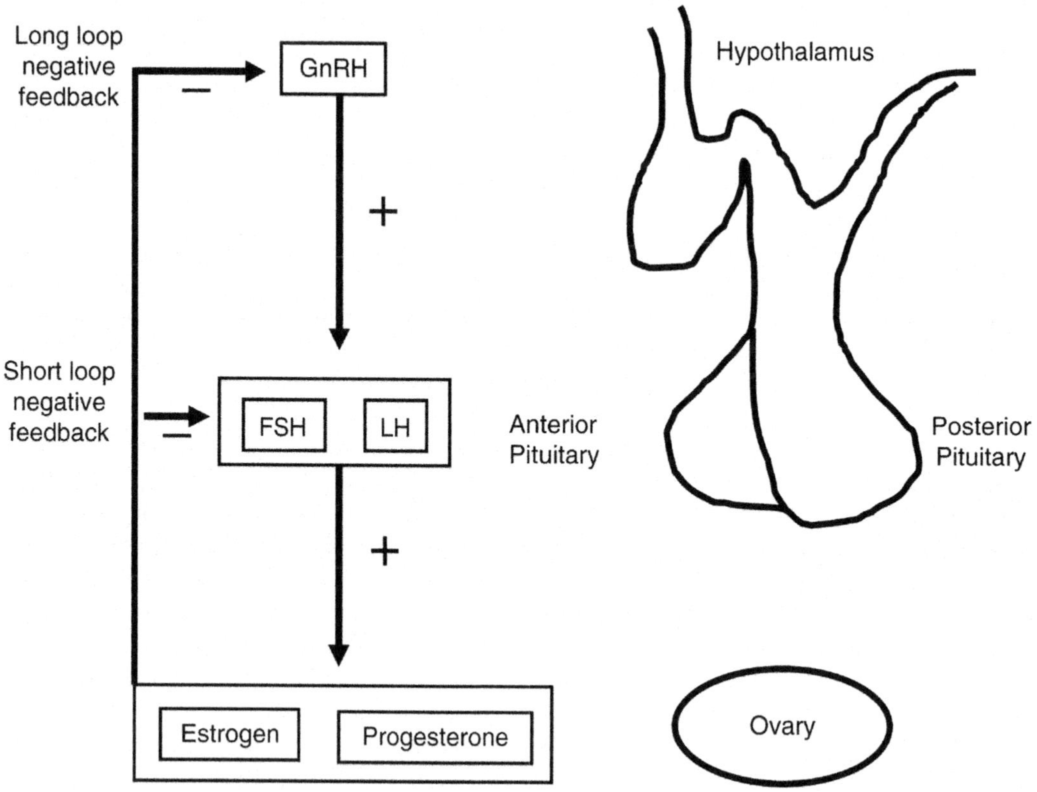

Fig. 1.10 Endocrine feedback loops in the hypothalamo-hypophyseal-gonadal axis

Fig. 1.11 Graph of hormonal levels in the menstrual cycle. The upper panel of the graph indicates levels of ovarian steroid hormones. The lower panel indicates levels of pituitary gonadotropins

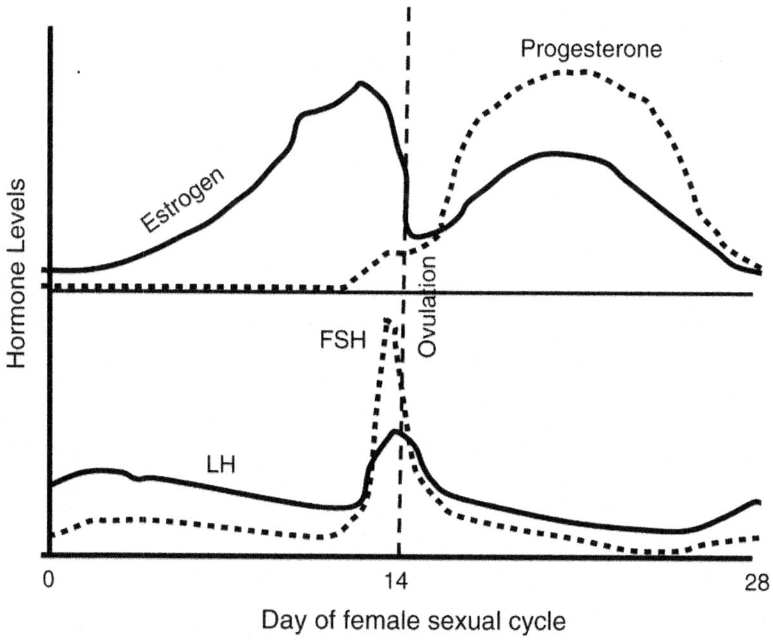

proliferation in nearby cells, but ERα-positive cells themselves do not seem to proliferate and stem cells are ERα [153, 154]. However, in humans, some quiescent ERα- and PR-positive cells are believed to be stem cells that act as steroid sensors and stimulate proliferation in neighboring ERα- and PR-negative cells [155]. It is also possible, however, that estrogen downregulates ERα in mammary epithelial cells and that ERα-positive cells divide later, when they are no longer identifiable as ERα-positive [156, 157]. The dissociation of ER-positive cells and proliferating cells implies that paracrine factors mediate the mitogenic activity of estrogen [78, 150]. ERβ is important in alveolar differentiation, specifically for the development of adhesion molecules and zonulae occludentes required for lactation [158].

The PR (see review by Seagroves and Rosen [159]) comes in two isoforms, PRA and PRB, that arise from a single gene. PR knockout mice have demonstrated the critical role of progesterone in both pregnancy-associated ductal branching and lobuloalveolar development [160]. Estrogen induces the expression of PRs [155], and 96–100 % of cells expressing steroid receptors express both ER and PR [150, 155]. Progesterone bound to its receptor enters the nucleus where the PR–progesterone complex binds to DNA [161]. In mice, PRA expression is associated with progesterone-induced lateral branching, whereas PRB is associated with alveologenesis [162]. PRA expression is found in cells adjacent to the ones that respond to progesterone by increased proliferation and/or differentiation. Thus, the actions of progesterone are also likely to be mediated by paracrine factors [163–165]. Neuregulin, a member of the EGF family of proteins and known for its role in neural development, promotes lobuloalveolar development and may be one such paracrine factor [166]. Both luminal and myoepithelial cells express PRB, and PRB-positive cells may be directly stimulated to proliferate [167] by progesterone. When human postmenopausal breast tissue is treated with estrogen, progesterone, or both, epithelial cells proliferate, apoptosis declines, and expression of ERα, ERβ, and PR decreases [168].

Hormones not made in the ovary are also important to breast function, especially the neuroendocrine hormones PRL and oxytocin (OXT). PRL, named for its ability to promote lactation, is a polypeptide secreted in the anterior pituitary gland. The hypothalamus-derived PRL inhibitory hormone (dopamine) inhibits PRL secretion. PRL's actions are diverse, but it is an absolute requirement for normal lactation. It promotes mammary gland growth and development, as well as synthesis and secretion of milk [169, 170]. PRL signal transduction involves the PRL receptor (PRLR, a transmembrane cytokine receptor whose expression is induced by estrogen [171]) and requires Jak2 and the transcription factor Stat5 for developmental activity. Signal transduction leading to the Stat protein activation is essential in mammary morphogenesis as well as lactation. Stat5a and Stat5b are essential mediators of lobular alveolar development [172, 173]. Their loss does not affect ductal morphogenesis, but the expression of Elf5, the regulator of the luminal lineage, is greatly inhibited [174]. The cytokines IL4 and IL13 activate Stat6 signaling in the mammary gland contributing to the development of alveoli. Defects in this pathway can be rescued in late pregnancy by elevated GATA-3 [175, 176]. LIF activates Stat3 signaling required for apoptosis during involution [177, 178], and other contributors to Stat3 in involution include TGF-β3 [179] and oncostatin M [180].

OXT is a peptide synthesized by neurons in the supraoptic and paraventricular nuclei of the hypothalamus [181]. It travels along the axons of these neurons to be stored in the posterior pituitary, where it is released directly into blood. OXT stimulates uterine contraction during labor and parturition and acts on myoepithelial cells in the breast to eject milk from alveoli into lactiferous ducts. Both PRL and OXT releases are stimulated by the suckling reflex. The OXT receptor is a G-protein-coupled receptor and has been localized to human myoepithelial cells, even in non-lactating glands [182]. Mammary gland OXT receptors increase near parturition [10]. OXT has also been implicated in breast development, mating, and maternal behavior. However, OXT-deficient female rodents are fertile, mate normally, conceive and deliver offspring, and appear to show normal maternal behavior. Nevertheless, their pups die within 24 h because the mothers are unable to nurse them [183].

Many other hormones are important to the breast development and function, but their roles are less well understood, including growth hormone (GH) [101]; androgens [184]; and thyroid hormone.

1.3.2 Other Regulators of Breast Development

Amphiregulin, HGF, EGF, IGF, and FGF3 have all been proposed as paracrine mediator(s) of estrogen effects [185, 186]. For example, amphiregulin is upregulated during ductal elongation [187] and amphiregulin and HGF promote ductal branching [166, 188–191]. EGF, a potent mitogen, is expressed on human breast stromal fibroblasts, and EGF receptors (EGFRs[1]) are found on epithelial cells [166]. EGF is a potent mitogen that binds to its plasma membrane receptor, and then, the EGFR–EGF complex is internalized [192]. EGF is essential for mammary ductal growth and branching (193 Kamalati, 1999 #374). Both EGF and HGF work with transforming growth factor alpha (TGF-α), another mitogen [194], to promote lobuloalveolar development

IGF-I is important in pubertal ductal morphogenesis in rodents, where it is believed to mediate the actions of GH [195] and estrogen [196]. IGF-I and IGF-II can bind to

[1]EGFRs belong to the ErbB family of receptors, a group of receptors that are interdependent from the binding of their ligands to the activation of downstream pathways. Some ErbB-targeted therapies are aimed at inhibiting multiple ErbB receptors and interfering with the cooperation that exists between receptors. Members of the ErbB family accept cues from multiple ligands, including EGF, TGF-α, amphiregulin, and several neuregulins [157].

several different receptors including IGF-IR, the insulin receptor (IR), and EGFR. In fact, the mitogenic action of IGF-I may require EGFR [197]. Both IFG-I and IGF-II bind to IGF-binding proteins (IGFBPs) that modulate their actions. The binding proteins bind the IGFs to matrix proteins and to cell membranes, providing a local pool that enhances their availability. Within the breast, IGFs are believed to function both as endocrine and as autocrine/paracrine factors [196].

A recent addition to the list of growth factors important in breast development is connective tissue growth factor (CTGF). CTGF promotes lactational differentiation and its expression can be induced by glucocorticoids in the murine breast cell line HC11, a cell line established from a mid-pregnant mouse mammary gland. Neither estrogen nor progesterone regulates CTGF expression, but it is expressed in the mouse mammary gland during pregnancy and lactation [198]. CTGF is also present in normal human breast epithelial cells and stromal cells [199].

1.4 Mammary Gland Structure and Function Throughout Life

1.4.1 Prenatal Development of the Breast

1.4.1.1 Events of Prenatal Breast Development

It is especially important to understand the prenatal development of the breast, since initial carcinogenic events may occur in this period [200–202]. Studies of prenatal human breast development have, of necessity, been observational and not experimental. They are based on postmortem analyses of difficult-to-obtain human specimens. Mechanisms of differentiation have largely been inferred from studies on animals, primarily the mouse. Very early development of the mouse mammary gland and the factors that regulate it [including Wnt, FGF, TBX3, and parathyroid hormone-related protein (PTHrP)] have been recently reviewed [203], but the initial cues that induce the formation of the human breast remain unknown [58].

Complicating matters in the study of human breast development is the heterogeneity of staging systems. Some are based on physical measurements and others on the date of last known menses. This heterogeneity makes interstudy comparisons difficult, at best. In addition, there is dramatic intrabreast variability at any given time with respect to developmental progress [204]. Stages of human breast development include (dates are approximate, overlapping, and highly variable) the following: ridge, 4 weeks—proliferation of epithelial cells [127], disk, 6 weeks—globular thickening, cone, 7 weeks, bud, 8 weeks, branching, 10–12 weeks, canalization, 16 weeks, vesicle, 20–32 weeks, and newborn [205, 206].

Typically, the first indications of human mammary glands are two parallel band-like thickenings of ectodermally derived epidermis: the mammary line or ridge that in the [35] 5–7 weeks old [207] embryo extends from axilla to groin. The most convincing evidence that this ridge is actually the precursor to the human breast is the fact that supernumerary nipples and breasts locate along that line [33]. Only part of the thoracic region of each ridge normally persists and forms a nodule [33]. This epithelial nodule penetrates the underlying mesenchyme and gives off 15–24 sprouts, each of which, in turn, gives rise to small side branches [207]. Epithelial–mesenchymal tissue interaction involves extensive cross talk between parenchyma and stroma and is requisite for normal breast development [208]. The epithelial ingrowth is made up of solid cords of primitive glycogen-rich cells surrounded by a basal lamina. Each sprout will later canalize to form a lactiferous duct. The primary bud is initially about the size of a hair follicle and contains two distinct epithelial cell populations, central and peripheral. Concentric layers of supporting mesenchyme surround the bud. Hair follicles do not form in the area near the breast bud, possibly due to lateral inhibition [33].

As secondary outgrowths vertically penetrate the mesenchyme [33], each projection has a slender stalk with a bulbous end and is covered by a continuous BM [194]. The papillary layer of the dermis encases the growing cords and gives rise to the vascularized fibrous tissue around ducts and within the lobules. The deeper reticular layer becomes interlobular connective tissue and suspensory ligaments [35].

The cellular constituents of the secondary outgrowths are morphologically similar, but immunologically diverse. Immunohistochemical staining for luminal and myoepithelial cell markers reveals a gradual progression to the adult phenotypes [204]. At 28 weeks, the primordial breast cells still stain positively for both luminal and myoepithelial markers [209]. Between 20 and 32 weeks, differentiation of mesenchyme into fat within the dense connective tissue stroma occurs.

Prenatal branching morphogenesis is accompanied by canalization via apoptosis of centrally located cells [210]. By the end of the fetal period, the secondary outgrowths are canalized and distinct luminal and myoepithelial cell populations are present (Fig. 1.12).

Late in the fetal period, the original invagination site of the primary bud evaginates to form the nipple [35]. Prior to parturition, the lumens of the mammary gland ductal tree are distended with secretory products of the epithelial cells, but the extent of this activity varies greatly from individual to individual as well as from lobule to lobule within a single breast. Typically, luminal cells already contain fat droplets, rough endoplasmic reticulum, and apical membranes with blebs and pits characteristic of secretory cells. Underlying myoepithelial cells are structurally mature with numerous

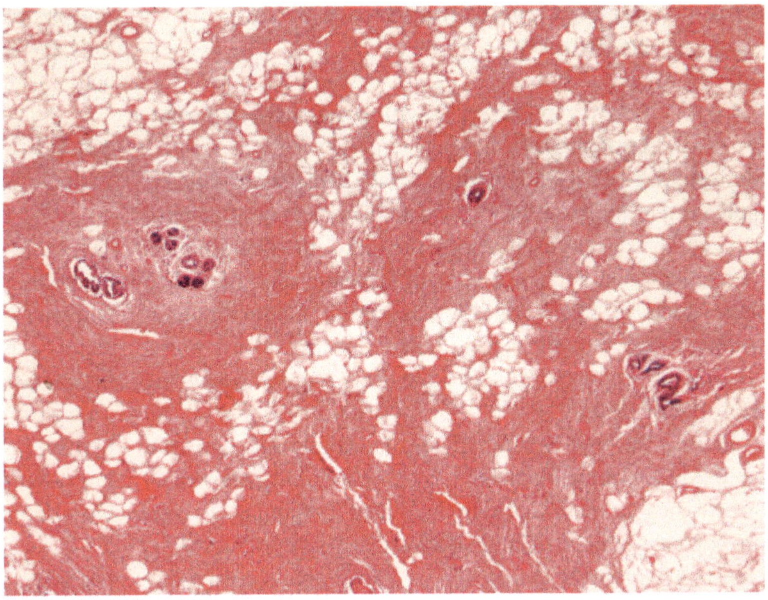

Fig. 1.12 Low power micrograph (50×) of a fetal human breast. A few ducts are present, but adipose and dense irregular connective tissues predominate

hemidesmosomes anchored to a tortuous BM. Their orientation, in contrast to the luminal cells, is parallel to the BM [211]. Myoepithelial cells late in gestation contain typical smooth muscle markers and are positive for Ki-67, a nuclear marker that indicates proliferation [204].

1.4.1.2 Hormonal Regulation of Prenatal Breast Development

Human female and male mammary glands develop similarly in utero (not so in some animals [212, 213]) and this phase of breast development is thought to be autonomous, in the sense that it does not require hormonal input [208]. This statement is based partly on the observation that fetal mice lacking receptors for estrogen, progesterone, GH, or PRL exhibit normal prenatal mammary gland development [131, 214].

However, several observations point to an endocrine input in prenatal breast development. Toward the end of gestation, the alveolar epithelium becomes active and it makes the "witch's milk" seen in newborn infants. This event is attributed to the release of fetal pituitary PRL from maternal and placental steroid inhibition. Also, human fetal serum PRL rises in late gestation and peaks at term [215], and the PRLR is present in fetal breast tissue [210]. ERα is present in human mammary epithelial cells beginning in the 30th week of gestation [216], a time of high mammary epithelial cell proliferative activity. PR expression is also present in the fetus, but both ER and PR expressions are highly variable during this period [217]. ERα and PR are both upregulated shortly before birth [216]. In addition, some claim that after week 15, human breast development is influenced by testosterone [35]. Near term, the breast can respond to maternal and placental steroids and to PRL.

1.4.1.3 Genes, Transcription Factors, and Growth Factors During Prenatal Breast Development

BCL-2, an inhibitor of apoptosis, is expressed maximally in fetal breast and absent in the epithelium of the normal adult breast. At week 18 of gestation, BCL-2 is highly expressed in the basal epithelial cell layer and surrounding mesenchyme and is thought to play a role in preventing apoptosis and allowing for cell population expansion [218]. *BRCA1*, a tumor suppressor gene, is expressed at a high level in human fetal breasts between week 21 and 26 of gestation and is closely associated with differentiation [219].

TGF-α is expressed in the developing breast where it promotes both proliferation and differentiation [194]. It is localized to the developing stroma and the epithelial bud. TGF-β is seen in the ECM throughout prenatal development and modulates cell–ECM interaction [35], inhibiting cell proliferation [131, 194, 220, 221]. BM inhibits the expression of TGF-β [222]. Tenascin-C, known to regulate rodent mammary cell differentiation in culture [223] and promotes growth in fetal tissues, is present around the neck of the human breast bud (a highly proliferative region) [35]. During the prenatal period, as in other life stages, EGF and its receptor may mediate estrogen effects. PTHrP is required for the formation of mammary specific mesenchyme [131] and appears to modulate stromal function during fetal branching morphogenesis [224].

1.4.2 Breast Development from Birth to Puberty

1.4.2.1 Events in Breast Development from Birth to Puberty

Studies [225, 226] of newborn infants and young children indicate that the mammary gland remains active after birth and even produces casein during the first 2 months. Lobules are well formed and some contain secretions. Ducts end in short ductules lined with two layers of cells: an inner epithelial and an outer myoepithelial. Specialized intra- and interlobular connective tissues are similar to those in the adult breast [33].

During the first 2 years of life, branching and terminal lobule development continues. By 2 years of age, however, the lobules have completely involuted (although myoepithelial cells remain) [209]. Between 2 years and puberty, breast development essentially just keeps pace with body growth [206], and during this time, epithelial proliferation is consistently low [217].

There are four stages of lobule development in the human mammary gland [227]. Type 1 lobules consist of clusters of 6–11 ductules and are present prior to puberty; type 2 lobules have more ductules, develop during puberty, and are characteristic of the inactive breasts of nulliparous women; type 3 lobules have still more ductules (up to 80) and develop during pregnancy; and type 4 lobules are characteristic of lactating breasts and are never found in nulliparous women. Women at various life stages have different percentages of each lobule type and each type is thought to give rise to specific kinds of pathologies [228].

1.4.2.2 Hormones in Breast Development from Birth to Puberty

During fetal life, although the breast does not require hormones to develop, it is exposed to placental hormones, especially estrogen and progesterone. These hormones promote growth, but inhibit PRL, which is required for the mammary gland to become functional. At birth, the release of infant PRL from the inhibitory maternal and placental hormones frees PRL to promote milk secretion. As a result, 80–90 % of infants (female and male) secrete "witch's milk."

Breast size in infants is related to circulating PRL levels [229]. Preterm infants have higher PRL levels between weeks two and six after birth than during the first week [229]. Between eight and 16 weeks of age, children of both genders have a surge of reproductive hormones, including estrogen. Three-month-old girls have higher estrogen levels than boys, and the amount of breast tissue is positively correlated with estrogen levels [230]. PRs are expressed in 5–60 % of mammary epithelial cells for up to 3 months postpartum [216]. Collectively, these observations seem to indicate that the child's own gonadal secretions may be active in the breast in early postnatal life.

1.4.2.3 Other Regulatory Factors in Breast Development from Birth to Puberty

TGF-α is present in the infant breast in both the luminal epithelium and interlobular stroma. It is concentrated in epithelia of terminal buds and lobular buds. TGF-α disappears from the breasts of male newborn infants after 4 days, but persists in females for up to 25 days postpartum [194]. The proliferation marker, Ki-67, is present in infant breast bud epithelium, predominantly in the neck region of terminal buds, but not in infants older than 25 days (coinciding with the disappearance of TGF-α). TGF-β (the growth inhibitor) [231] localizes to the stromal tissue near the epithelium in neonates. It declines after three months of age [194]. BCL-2 is found in luminal cells, but no longer is found in myoepithelial cells or fibroblasts, from 28 weeks of gestation through puberty [217].

1.4.3 Puberty

1.4.3.1 Events in the Breast During Puberty

The mammary gland is unique among glands in that it undergoes most of its branching during adolescent rather than fetal development. Branching in puberty, as in the fetus, involves cross talk between epithelium and stroma during which patterns of side branching are determined by stromal cues [131]. The mammary gland duct system develops into its mature lobuloalveolar arrangement in a sequential manner. Ducts elongate, their epithelia thicken, and the adjacent connective tissue increases in volume. In mice, club-shaped structures called terminal end buds (TEBs) form at the end of the ducts. They are formed by stem cells and have the greatest proliferation rates [232]. Each TEB is the leading edge of a growing duct, as it advances, branches, and then forms alveolar buds.

The TEB is made up of a single outer layer of undifferentiated cap cells and multiple inner layers of "body" cells. Cells in the trailing edge of the cap cell layer differentiate into myoepithelial cells. Lumen formation in the segment trailing the TEB involves apoptosis [233], with as much as 14 % of internally located cells undergoing apoptosis concurrently. Subsequent branching is both via TEB bifurcation and more proximal lateral branching [234].

Branching during puberty is highly variable. The previously blunt-ended ductal termini undergo dichotomous branching, while lateral buds form more proximally. The primary ducts extend into underlying tissue from the nipple, giving rise to segmental ducts, subsegmental ducts, and terminal ducts (in order). The terminal ducts give rise to acini. The acini arising from one human terminal duct and surrounded by intralobular connective tissue collectively make up a TDLU [33]. During puberty, stem cell numbers increase [235]. By age 15, human breast structure is established centrally, but continues to expand peripherally. By age 18, parenchymal architecture is typical of the nulliparous adult [33].

Within the stroma, undifferentiated mesenchymal cells attach to the under surface of the basal lamina in the mid-section of each end bud and form a monolayer outside of the myoepithelial cell layer. The mesenchymal cells will eventually become fibrocytes synthesizing collagen and other ECM molecules [236]. Large quantities of adipose tissue are deposited within the dense inter- and intralobular connective tissue during this time, although dense irregular connective tissue remains the predominant tissue type at the end of puberty in humans.

While significant glandular differentiation occurs in puberty, the process continues for at least another 10 years [35], but the most dramatic phases of parenchymal breast development must await pregnancy. Between puberty and the first pregnancy, the mammary gland is resting or inactive (Fig. 1.13). There is some debate as to whether any true secretory units develop prior to pregnancy. There is, however, agreement that the lobules of the resting breast consist essentially of ducts and that a few alveoli may be present during the late luteal (postovulatory) phase of menstrual cycles. It is an issue that is moot, since ducts, as well as alveoli, are capable of secretion. Over the next few years, clusters of 8–11 alveolar buds are found within each TDLU. Later cyclic hormonal variations result in smaller, but more numerous alveolar buds.

1.4.3.2 Hormonal Regulation of the Breast During Puberty

Puberty is initiated by the maturation of the HPG axis and results in the hormonally driven outgrowth of the mammary epithelial tree [234]. A gradual increase in GnRH secretion by the hypothalamus, which does not secrete it in significant amounts during childhood [145], promotes ovarian steroid production by the way of LH and FSH. Changes during puberty result from the surges of both pituitary and ovarian hormonal activities.

During the first 1–2 years following menarche, when cycles are often anovulatory, the breast is exposed to the unopposed actions of estrogen. This period is a window during which ductal growth occurs [237]. Estrogen responsiveness and control are essential for normal pubertal breast development [238], and serum estrogen levels parallel breast development during this period [210]. Duct epithelial thickening, elongation, and branching are all promoted by estrogen. So are the expansion and differentiation of stromal and adipose tissue [131, 237]. Not surprisingly, ERs are found in both epithelium and stroma. Estrogen is so potent that women with the gonadal dysgenesis of Turner's syndrome, who normally do not develop breasts, will do so if treated with estrogen [239].

During puberty (as is true in all life stages), the lobules with the greatest degree of proliferation consistently have the highest numbers of both ER- and PR-positive cells and the highest proliferation rates. There is a progressive decrease in both proliferation and steroid receptor expression as lobules (and their cells) become more differentiated [240]. GH and its receptor are essential for mammary gland development during puberty in the rodent [101, 241]. In fact, GH may be the pituitary hormone most central to mammary

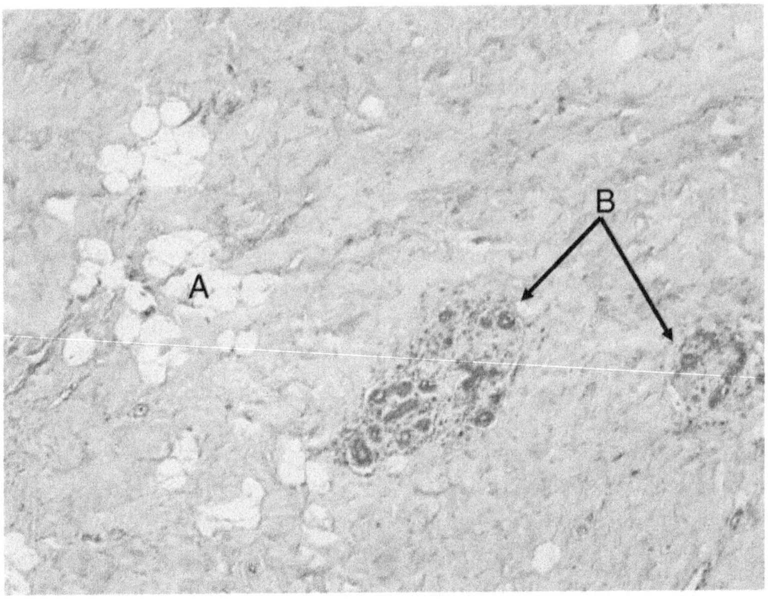

Fig. 1.13 Low power micrograph (50×) of an inactive human breast. The letter A indicates adipose tissue. The arrows at B indicate lobules. Note the low number of ductules in each lobule, as compared to the lobules in the active breast at the same magnification in Fig 1.5, and the lobules of the pregnant breast, also at the same magnification in Fig 1.15

development at this time and probably acts by the way of stromal IGF-I [241]. Two other hormones participating in pubertal breast development are glucocorticoids and vitamin D3.

1.4.3.3 Other Regulatory Factors in the Breast During Puberty

Factors important to breast development during puberty include transcriptional target genes and locally produced factors that mediate the effects of the major mammogens. IGFs are important to the survival of mammary gland cells during puberty and are known to suppress apoptosis [242]. Other factors include immune mediators, such as CSF-1 and eotaxin (important in the recruitment or production of macrophages and eosinophils, respectively), cell adhesion and axonal guidance proteins, ECM-remodeling enzymes (e.g., MMPs and their inhibitors), and TGF-βs (inhibitors of duct development) [243].

1.4.4 The Adult Premenopausal Breast

1.4.4.1 Cyclic Events in the Premenopausal Adult Breast

Early in each menstrual cycle, ducts are cord-like with little or no lumen. The midcycle increase of estrogen causes luminal cells to get taller, lumens to form, and secretions to accumulate in ducts and alveoli. Ductule cells undergo secretory differentiation during the luteal phase [36], while the stroma becomes more vascular [13] and accumulates fluid. Premenstrual enlargement and discomfort are attributed to this hyperemia and edema.

Mammary proliferative rates are higher in the luteal phase as measured by thymidine labeling [244], number of mitotic figures [245], and the percentage of cells that stain for Ki-67. When samples are controlled for both menstrual dates and progesterone levels, the proliferative index is found to be more than twice as high in the luteal phase than in the follicular phase. The apoptosis index does not differ significantly between phases of the cycle [246].

Morphological changes [245] divide the menstrual cycle into four phases. In stage 1 (days 0–5), it is difficult to distinguish between the luminal and myoepithelial layers. Both cell types have round nuclei and minimal amounts of pale cytoplasm. Sharp luminal borders with eosinophilic intraluminal secretions are common, but apoptosis and mitosis are mostly absent. The stroma is slightly edematous. In stage 2 (days 6–15), it is easier to distinguish epithelial and myoepithelial layers and many lobules show myoepithelial cell vacuolation. There are no mitoses or apoptotic bodies, and there is no stromal edema or infiltrate. In stage 3 (days 16–24), lobules are larger and each lobule contains more ductular units. Two distinct layers of epithelial cells are easily distinguished. Myoepithelial cells are more vacuolated, and luminal cells are more oval and basophilic. Mitotic and apoptotic cells are both detected, and edema and infiltrate are again found in the interlobular stroma. In the last stage (days 25–28), vacuolization is extensive and luminal cells have cytoplasmic basophilia and prominent nuclei with large nucleoli. The most characteristic features of this final stage are frequent mitotic figures and increased apoptotic activity. While this phase of the cycle demonstrates more apoptosis, there are still only a small number of scattered cells undergoing the process [247]. Stromal edema is extensive, and there are more inflammatory cells.

During the preovulatory period (days 0–14; stages 1 and 2), epithelial cells exhibit few microvilli and sparse secretory organelles. In the postovulatory phase (days 15–28; stages 3 and 4), luminal cells have prominent microvilli and more rough endoplasmic reticulum, secretory vacuoles, and glycogen [248]. Several BM components vary in amount during the menstrual cycle, including laminin, fibronectin, collagen types IV and V, and proteoglycans, all of which are lowest in mid-cycle. Collagen types I, III, VI, and VII do not exhibit cyclic variation [249]. Immunoglobulin secretion within the human mammary gland exhibits cyclic fluctuations [250], specifically levels of IgA and the secretory component; both are highest in the preovulatory phase of the menstrual cycle. However, there is conflicting evidence that immunoglobulin levels may be constant throughout the cycle [244].

Mammary gland development in each cycle never fully regresses to the starting point of the preceding cycle. Each cycle results in slightly more development and new budding until about the age of 35. The progressive increase in the number of lobules is accompanied by an increase in the size of each lobule and a reduction in the size of individual ductules and alveoli within the lobules.

1.4.4.2 Hormones Regulating the Adult Premenopausal Breast

The part of the menstrual cycle exhibiting the highest rate of epithelial proliferation in the breast is the luteal phase. The luteal phase is also the period during which both estrogen and progesterone levels are highest [155, 210] (Fig. 1.11). When breast tissue from non-pregnant women is xenografted into mice, treatment with estrogen (at high, i.e., luteal, levels) is the best inducer of epithelial proliferation [155]. Estrogen stimulates both DNA synthesis and bud formation [206].

Proliferation is highest during the luteal phase and, hence, the hormonal milieu at this time favors proliferation in the breast. The ERs and PRs in the human breast vary with the stage of the menstrual cycle, but there is disagreement as to when, in the cycle, levels for each receptor are high and low [251]. One study states that ER-positive cells are most abundant during day 3 through day 7 and PR-positive cells are most abundant during the following week (days 8–14) [252], while another study found both ER- and PR-positive cells most abundant in the second week (days 8–14) of the cycle [253].

Estrogen at low (i.e., follicular) concentrations induces PR expression, and cells expressing ERα are also PR-positive. ERα/PR-positive cells may act as steroid sensors, secreting paracrine factors that, in turn, regulate the proliferative activity of adjacent ERα/PR-negative cells [155]. Local levels of estradiol in the normal human breast are highest during the luteal phase when plasma progesterone levels are also high. Progesterone may promote the local conversion of estrogen precursors into potent estradiol in normal breast tissue [254]. EGFR is also maximally expressed in the luteal phase and is found primarily in stromal and myoepithelial cells [255].

1.4.4.3 Other Factors Regulating the Adult Premenopausal Breast

Stat5 is activated at a basal level in non-pregnant human breast epithelial cells and is specific to luminal cells and absent in myoepithelial cells. It regulates PRLR expression and may prevent apoptosis in differentiated epithelial cells. It is maintained in a state of activation by PRL [256].

1.4.5 Pregnancy

1.4.5.1 Events in the Breast During Pregnancy

In pregnancy, as in other phases of breast structure and function, there is remarkable heterogeneity among lobules; some are quiescent, while others proliferate. During early pregnancy, distal ducts branch and create both more lobules and more alveoli within each lobule [251]. During the first trimester, there can be as much as a 10-fold increase in the number of alveoli/lobule. Breast enlargement in this phase of pregnancy is due to both cellular hypertrophy and hyperplasia [257] (Fig. 1.14). Luminal epithelial cells differentiate into cells with typical secretory cell morphology. At the same time, the epithelial and adipose compartments of the mammary gland shift their lipid metabolism in a concerted way, such that fatty acid availability to the epithelial cell is increased [258]. Some adipocytes may actually transdifferentiate into epithelial cells.

By mid-pregnancy, lobuloalveolar structure is established and ductules differentiate into alveoli. Each lobule contains a mixture of alveolar and tubular end pieces that have budded off from the terminal portion of the duct system, and many of these end pieces are still solid knots of cells [259]. The lobules now include some that can be classified as type 3 (described earlier) [227].

In the last trimester, epithelial cells are full of lipid droplets and adipophilin (lipid droplet-associated protein) expression is increased. Luminal cells also have prominent endoplasmic reticulum, hypertrophied Golgi, and swollen mitochondria. Enzymes characteristic of lactation are present [257]. Although luminal cell differentiation into secretory cells is advanced, it is not yet maximal. The secretory product (colostrum) filling the lumens has a high antibody content and is more similar in composition to blood plasma than to milk [36]. Breast enlargement in the third trimester is both due to this distention of acini by colostrum and due to an increase in stromal vascularity. Fat and connective tissues at this stage have now largely been replaced by parenchyma [251]. The remaining fibrous connective tissue has been

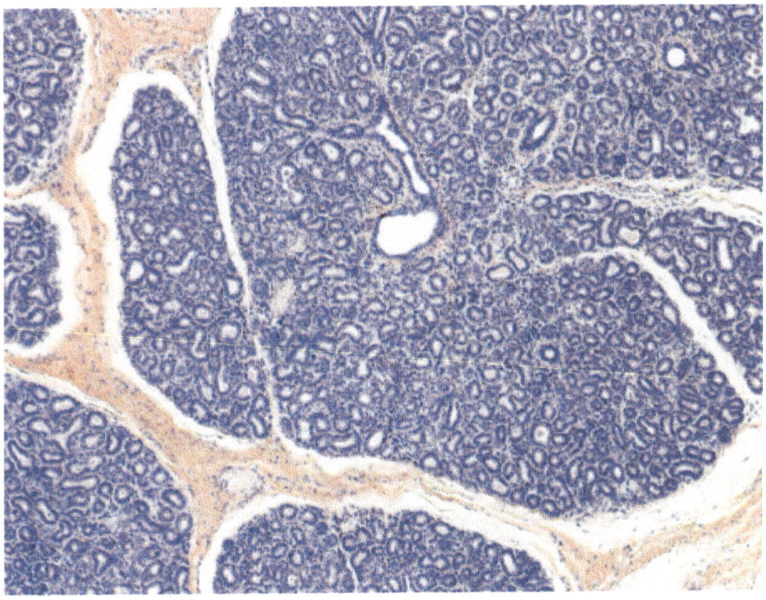

Fig. 1.14 Low power micrograph (50×) of a pregnant human breast. Note the huge number of ductules in each lobule and the dense irregular connective tissue separating the lobules. There is little adipose tissue

infiltrated with plasma cells, lymphocytes, and eosinophils [43].

Nulliparous women have lobules that are less differentiated than those of parous women. Among parous women, those who were pregnant before the age of 20 have a greater persistence of the more differentiated lobule type [206]. Changes in the breast that occur during pregnancy, specifically the complete differentiation of type 3 lobules, are permanent, and each subsequent pregnancy results in the accumulation of additional differentiated lobules [227]. In animal models, exposures to the high levels of estrogen and progesterone typical of pregnancy induce long-term alterations in gene expression in mammary epithelial cells. These alterations may induce a decrease in growth factors and an increase in apoptosis [260] and may contribute to the widespread phenomenon of pregnancy-induced protection against cancer. Breast tissues of postmenopausal parous women express numerous genes in both parenchyma and stroma that differ from those expressed in postmenopausal nulliparous women [261].

1.4.5.2 Hormones in the Breast During Pregnancy (Fig. 1.15)

The placenta secretes estrogen and progesterone and takes over this function from the corpus luteum as pregnancy continues into the second and third trimesters. Near the end of pregnancy, maternal estrogen levels are as much as 30-fold greater than before conception. Progesterone levels increase about tenfold during pregnancy [145]. Estrogen, with the help of progesterone, prepares the mother's breasts for lactation by promoting breast enlargement and growth of the duct system. Progesterone also promotes lobuloalveolar differentiation at this time [163]. However, estrogen and progesterone both inhibit the actual secretion of milk by the breast during pregnancy.

The xenograft model in which human mammary epithelial cells are seeded into collagen gels containing fibroblasts, and then placed under the renal capsule of athymic nude mice, has been a fruitful tool for examining hormonal regulation of human mammary gland development [127]. Normal human ductal structure develops in the graft. Treatment of host mice with diethylstilbestrol (DES), a synthetic estrogen, increases the number of ducts per unit area. Continuous treatment with DES induces expression of PR in luminal cells and downregulates epithelial ERα. Estrogen plus progesterone treatment induces epithelial PR, and then, progesterone downregulates its own receptor.

When the host mice become pregnant, mammary epithelial cells proliferate, the human ducts become distended with secretions, and the apical cytoplasm of luminal cells is vacuolated. Both β-casein and fat globule protein are increased [127]. PR knockout mice have shown that pregnancy-associated ductal side branching and lobuloalveolar development require PRB expression [160].

During pregnancy, the trophoblast also secretes human chorionic gonadotropin (hCG). Levels of this hormone rise dramatically in early pregnancy, peak in the eighth to tenth week after fertilization, and then fall to a constant level that is maintained until parturition (Fig. 1.15). hCG causes the corpus luteum to secrete massive quantities of estrogen and

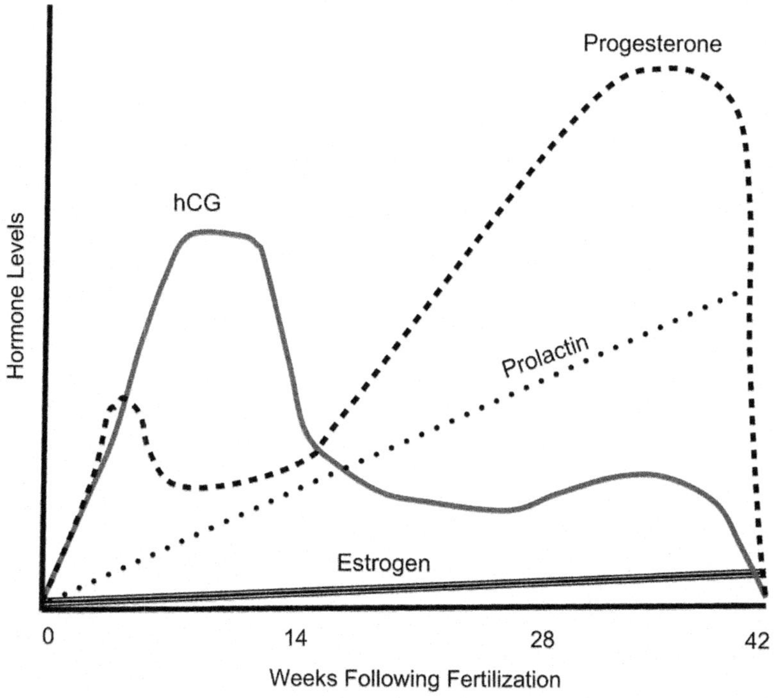

Fig. 1.15 Graph of hormonal levels during pregnancy

progesterone that are required to maintain the endometrium. Peak levels of hCG coincide with the highest levels of proliferation in the mother's breast. Human breast tissue implanted into nude mice that were then impregnated shows the same concurrence of proliferation and hCG levels. Implants in non-pregnant mice can be stimulated to proliferate in a dose-dependent manner by exogenous hCG, but only if ovaries are intact, implying that hCG acts indirectly by increasing ovarian steroid production [262].

Even a single pregnancy carried to term (especially by a young mother) can protect against breast cancer. Pregnancy exposes the breast to a unique hormone profile including prolonged progesterone elevation, human placental lactogen (hPL, aka human chorionic somatomammotropin), altered glucocorticoid secretion, and increased levels of estrogen and PRL [263]. There are multiple pregnancy-induced permanent changes in the breasts of parous women, including lower levels of PRL [264], a more differentiated gland with greater complexity of secretory lobules and less proliferative activity [227], an altered gene expression profile involving over 70 genes (in rodents) [265], and increased innate immune response proteins and DNA repair proteins [261]. In rats, it has been shown that hCG can substitute for pregnancy in its protective benefit. Furthermore, both pregnancy and treatment with hCG create the same (protective) genomic signature [266]. Some believe that this transformation occurs in the stem cell population, changing stem cells from a less differentiated "stem cell 1" to a more differentiated, less vulnerable "stem cell 2" [267]. hPL is a general metabolic hormone that is made by the placenta in quantities several times greater than the other placental hormones combined. Secretion of hPL begins about three weeks after fertilization and continues to rise throughout the rest of pregnancy. It enhances the effect of estrogen [127].

As is true in other life stages, several additional hormones are important to breast development in pregnancy. PRL from the mother's anterior pituitary rises from the fifth week of pregnancy until birth, at which time the levels of PRL are 10–20-fold higher than before conception. Estrogen, progesterone, PRL, GH, and thyroid hormones are all essential to duct elongation and branching, as well as to alveolar budding [210].

1.4.5.3 Other Regulatory Factors in the Breast During Pregnancy

FGFs [268] promote growth and alveolar differentiation during pregnancy, and CTGF/CCN2 is expressed during this time, possibly promoting lactational differentiation just as it does in epithelial cells in culture [198]. BRCA1 protects genomic stability and is expressed in rapidly proliferating tissues such as the mammary epithelium during pregnancy [269], where it favors differentiation at the expense of proliferation [270].

1.4.6 Lactation

1.4.6.1 Events in the Lactating Breast

During lactation, mammary lobules enlarge further and acinar lumens dilate, filled with a granular material and fat globules. Lobule size still varies significantly within the gland, at this time probably reflecting variations in milk secretory activity. The lactating breast is very similar to the breast of a pregnant woman, except that secretory products have markedly distended the ducts and acini [43] (Fig. 1.16).

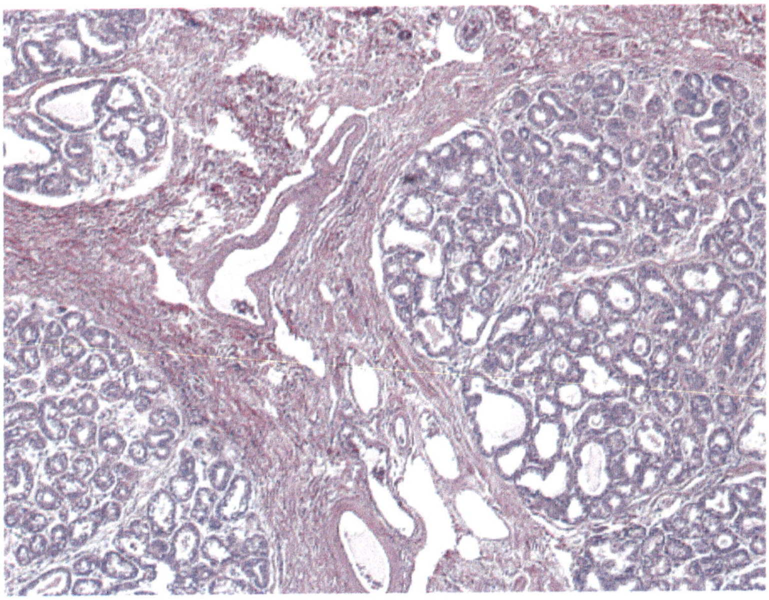

Fig. 1.16 Low power micrograph (50×) of a lactating human breast. Note the dilated ductules (now acini), many of which are filled with milk. The vasculature is abundant in the interlobular connective tissue

Myoepithelial cells increase in number during pregnancy, but their differentiation is not complete until the onset of lactation when the number of myofilaments increases dramatically and contractile activity begins [10].

The luminal epithelium in the lactating breast has the expected secretory machinery: rough endoplasmic reticulum, a moderate number of rod-shaped mitochondria, and Golgi complexes lateral and apical to the nucleus [36]. The membrane-bounded secretory vesicles contain extremely electron-dense protein granules (casein) suspended in a less dense fluid, presumably containing lactose and non-casein whey proteins [36, 271]. Endocytic vesicles seen throughout the luminal cell are thought to be involved in transcellular transport of immunoglobulins and other substances. Abundant lipid droplets are not membrane-bounded, occur in a variety of sizes, and contain fatty acids from the blood as well as some synthesized within mammary cells [36].

The lactating breast has increased density on MRI, consistent with increased glandular volume. There is diffuse high signal intensity on T2-weighted images, reflecting the high water fraction within milk [272].

1.4.6.2 The Process of Lactation

Placental hormones hPL, estrogen, and progesterone are withdrawn at parturition, and maternal PRL, like fetal PRL, is freed of their inhibitory effects allowing the functional differentiation of the mammary gland to proceed. A 2–3-week period of secretion ensues before the appearance of fully mature milk.

In humans, transplacental transport of immunoglobulins provides humoral immunity to the newborn for the first weeks of life. This protection is complemented by IgA and lactoferrin, a protein with antimicrobial properties, in the colostrum. These proteins are able to cross the epithelium lining the infant digestive tract intact [273].

Beginning about 36 h after parturition, milk volume increases more than tenfold [274]. Tight junctions in the breast are tightly closed during lactation [123], and this decrease in permeability is accompanied by an increase in milk secretion. In the transition to mature milk, concentrations of sodium and chloride fall and lactose concentration increases, changes dependent on the closure of mammary epithelial tight junctions [275].

Milk composition varies during lactation and even between suckling episodes. Usually, milk is about 88 % water, 7 % carbohydrate (mainly lactose), 3.5 % lipid (mainly triglycerides), and 1.5 % protein (mainly lactalbumin and casein). Milk also contains important ions (sodium, potassium, chloride, calcium, and phosphate), vitamins, and IgA antibodies [276], as well as other antimicrobial substances such as cytokines and complement [277]. Human milk has several components not found in cow's milk, including lactoferrin, growth factors, long-chain polyunsaturated fatty acids, and glycoconjugates. The advantages of breast milk over formula feeding are many, including immune benefits and better mental development [278]. Formula-fed infants have a different growth pattern and a greater risk of obesity than do breast-fed infants [279]. However, the touted advantages of lower cancer risk and lower blood pressure later in life, as well as the claim that over half of the infant deaths in North America are due to a failure to fully breast-feed, may be exaggerated [280–282].

The lactating breast can be viewed as a lipid-synthesizing machine. In mice, lipid secretion over a 20-day period is equal in weight to the entire lactating mouse [283]. In humans, maternal body fat and milk fat concentration are positively related. Low milk fat is correlated with increased milk volume, perhaps because infant demand is higher [284].

Secretory processes in the mammary gland involve five mechanisms: merocrine secretion, apocrine secretion, transport across the apical membrane, transcytosis of interstitial molecules, and paracellular transit [274]. The two main mechanisms utilized by the luminal epithelial cells during lactation are merocrine and apocrine secretion.

Proteinaceous material is secreted by the merocrine method. Proteins destined for release into the lumen are synthesized in the rough endoplasmic reticulum, shuttled through the Golgi apparatus, and carried by secretory vesicles to the surface membrane with which they fuse, emptying only their contents into the lumen. Protein secretion in the breast is primarily constitutive [274]. Most of the calcium in milk is also likely released via exocytosis of Golgi-derived secretory vesicles. Additional transport from the cytoplasm to the surface is mediated by a calcium ATPase [285].

Lipid droplets are released from the cell by apocrine secretion, even though the loss of cytoplasm is slight [43]. The total amount of membrane lost over time, however, is extensive [36] and must be replaced by the endoplasmic reticulum—Golgi system [286]. The membrane released into the milk has two functions: It is the main source of phospholipids and cholesterol for the infant, and it prevents released fat globules from coalescing into larger globules that might be difficult to secrete [274].

Specific transport mechanisms for sodium, potassium, chloride, calcium, and phosphate ions are all present in the breast. Sodium, potassium, chloride, and water directly permeate the cell membrane [287]. There is a glucose pathway across the apical membrane [288], and apical pathways also provide a means for the direct transfer of therapeutic drugs into milk [289]. Lactose secretion is primarily responsible for the osmotic movement of water into milk.

Transcytosis of interstitial molecules is one means whereby intact proteins can cross the mammary epithelium.

Immunoglobulins enter milk via this mechanism [290]. IgA is synthesized by plasma cells and binds to receptors on the basal surface of the mammary alveolar cell. The IgA–receptor complex is endocytosed and transported to the apical surface where the receptor is cleaved, and the cleaved portion is secreted along with the IgA. Other proteins, hormones, and growth factors are thought to be secreted by similar mechanisms [274]. Once the IgA enters the newborn gut, it is also transcytosed across that epithelium [290].

The paracellular pathway allows the passage of substances between epithelial cells. During lactation, however, the passage of even small molecular weight substances between epithelial cells is blocked by the very tight junctions mentioned earlier. Neutrophils, however, can apparently diapedese between epithelial cells to reach the milk after which the tight junctions reform behind them. It is important that the tight junctions are leaky both during pregnancy and following involution. This allows secretory products to leave the gland (presumably preventing distention) and protective molecules to enter the milk space in the former case and products of mammary cell dissolution to be cleared from the breast in the latter [274].

1.4.6.3 Hormones During Lactation and Nursing

As mentioned earlier, progesterone promotes the functional differentiation of the breasts: budding of alveoli and transition of luminal epithelial cells into cells capable of milk secretion. PRL is essential for the functional differentiation of the breast following parturition, and pulsatile release of PRL is essential for successful lactation [58]. During labor, the levels of β-endorphins increase and stimulate the release of PRL [291]. PRL enhances the development of tight junctions [275] and is one of several hormones important for lactation that are secreted in the breast itself [292] (GH is another [293]). After birth, maternal PRL levels fall, but a surge of PRL secretion occurs during each nursing episode. Unlike OXT release, which can occur in response to a baby's cry, the burst in PRL secretion requires the suckling stimulus [294]. Women with low levels of PRL during pregnancy have difficulty lactating [295]. GH, parathyroid hormone, and insulin also promote lactation.

Each time the baby nurses, neural impulses transmitted to the hypothalamus result in the release of OXT. OXT, in turn, causes myoepithelial cells to contract and express milk from the alveoli into the lactiferous ducts, a process known as milk "letdown." However, psychogenic factors can inhibit the "letdown" reflex [145, 294] since the hypothalamic neurons that synthesize OXT receive inputs from higher brain centers and afferent somatic signals from the breast.

The short-term regulation of milk synthesis is related to the degree to which the breast is emptied in each feeding and perhaps to the frequency of feeding; thus, it is coupled closely to infant appetite [296]. After several months of breast-feeding, especially if the infant is also being fed solid foods, FSH and LH levels will rise and reestablish the menstrual cycle. However, prior to that time, PRL inhibits LH and FSH secretion, preventing ovulation and mediating the contraceptive effect of breast-feeding [145]. Even if nursing remains the sole source of infant nutrients, the secretory capacity of the breast eventually diminishes. Theories abound as to why this occurs, including secretory cell aging or a programmed developmental response related to maternal endocrine changes and/or target cell adaptations [297].

1.4.6.4 Other Regulatory Factors During Lactation

Clusterin, a glycoprotein involved in epithelial differentiation and morphogenesis, is upregulated at the end of pregnancy. Blocking clusterin production in mice results in a decrease in the levels of milk production [298]. Alcohol consumption, often recommended to mothers with lactational difficulty, has been shown to increase PRL, but it decreases OXT, with the net effect of reducing milk yield [299].

1.4.6.5 Effects of Lactation on the Nursing Mother

While the breast and its hormonal milieu are important in the production of milk, lactation, in turn, has effects on the mother's body. These effects are highly variable. Most reports indicate that postpartum weight loss does not differ between lactating and non-lactating women, nor does regional weight distribution. Pregnancy promotes fat deposition in a gynoid subcutaneous distribution (buttocks and thighs), and postpartum weight loss is from the same regions, returning proportions to pre-pregnancy ratios [300].

PRL inhibits GnRH secretion and it also inhibits the action of GnRH on the pituitary and antagonizes the action of gonadotropins on the ovaries. As a result of these interactions, ovulation is inhibited. Thus, ovaries are inactive and estrogen and progesterone outputs fall. Nearly half of the menstrual cycles after menses resume are still anovulatory. Nevertheless, 5–10 % of women who are breast-feeding become pregnant [301].

New mothers are often anxious to lose the weight gained during pregnancy. Slow weight loss (about 1 lb/week) does not have an adverse effect on milk volume or composition if proper nutrition is maintained and nursing is on demand. Maternal plasma PRL concentration generally increases under conditions of negative energy balance and may protect lactation [302].

1.4.6.6 Calcium Metabolism During Lactation

Since milk is rich in calcium, the mammary gland needs a steady supply of calcium and mechanisms to secrete and concentrate it in milk. Mothers are in negative calcium balance during lactation. In spite of the fact that calcium is toxic to cells, mammary epithelial cells must transport large amounts of it from extracellular fluid, through their cytoplasm into milk. The huge amount of calcium leaving the mother results in the mobilization of skeletal calcium and a reduction in her bone mass. The increased bone resorption has been attributed to falling estrogen levels and increased PTHrP levels during lactation. Mammary epithelial cells secrete PTHrP into the circulation, directly participating in the dissolution of bones [303]. Amazingly, the calcium lost during breast-feeding is fully restored within a few months of weaning and women who breast-feed do not have long-term deficits in bone calcium [304].

1.4.7 Postlactational Involution

There are three overlapping stages to postlactational involution [130]. The first phase is reversible (by suckling [305]) and includes secretion cessation and loss of alveolar cell phenotype. The second involves alveolar cell apoptosis and phagocytosis, and the third is characterized by the regrowth of stromal adipose tissue.

While the size and secretory activity of the human mammary gland decline slowly as the infant begins to eat other foods, scientific understanding of postlactational involution is based primarily on laboratory animal studies where weaning is artificially abrupt and early (however, apoptosis also occurs in gradual weaning [305]). In these animals, secretion continues for a day or so and glands become so distended with milk that cells and alveolar walls rupture. Milk accumulation in the lumens of ducts and alveoli, as well as within the luminal epithelium itself, inhibits milk synthesis. A reduction in the volume of secretory cells and further inhibition of secretion ensue [206]. Immediately before postweaning apoptosis, the conformation of β1-integrin changes to a non-binding state [107], disrupting the cell–ECM interaction and leading to a loss of the differentiated lactational phenotype [306]. Lactation-associated genes are inactivated (e.g., for β-casein), and involution-associated genes (e.g., for stromelysin) are activated [307]. This phase ultimately involves hundreds of genes [308, 309].

Dedifferentiation and apoptosis will occur even if the animal becomes pregnant, suggesting that tissue remodeling is necessary for subsequent lactation [305]. Apoptosis, the actual death process, involves a loss of cell junctions and microvilli, nuclear chromatin condensation, and margination, nucleolar dispersion, folding of nuclear membrane, and nuclear fragmentation [310]. As much as 80 % of mammary epithelial cells undergo apoptosis [311].

Autophagy, a mechanism whereby a cell destroys its own organelles [312], is intense in the luminal epithelium during involution. Lysosomal enzymes increase and remain high, while other enzymes decline. Vacuoles contain organelles in various stages of degradation [36]. Cell autolysis, collapse of acini, and narrowing of tubules, as well as macrophage infiltration, occur in parallel with the regeneration of connective tissue [206]. Degenerating cells and debris are likely removed by the macrophages [313], although viable alveolar epithelial cells also phagocytose their apoptotic neighbors [314]. The large number of apoptotic cells is cleared quickly and efficiently [311]. Myoepithelial cells generally persist [36].

During postlactational involution, inflammatory processes are suppressed and ECM-degrading MMPs increase, as does the ratio of metalloproteinases to their inhibitors [130, 306, 315]. Both the BM and the stromal matrices are degraded [316, 317] in rodents, but BMs remain intact in cows and goats [305].

Although breast vascularity increases throughout life in nulliparous women, it is reset at a level below baseline subsequent to lactation [318] in women who have given birth. But, from the end of lactation to the onset of menopause, breasts of parous women contain more glandular tissue than those of nulliparous women [206].

IGFBP may initiate apoptosis by sequestering IGF-I, an important cell survival factor in the mammary gland [242, 319, 320]. TGF-β_3 also may be an apoptosis initiator for alveolar cells [190] and is upregulated by milk stasis at the beginning of weaning [311].

1.4.8 Postmenopausal Involution

The permanent cessation of the menstrual cycle, menopause, occurs naturally with the decline of hormonal production between the ages of 35 and 60. Ovarian steroid production ceases almost completely. Following menopause, the breast regresses, with a decline in the number of more highly differentiated lobules and an increase in the number of less differentiated lobules (Figs. 1.17 and 1.18). Since parous women begin menopause with a higher number and percentage of the more differentiated lobule type, the postmenopausal events in the two groups differ in extent [33].

In postmenopausal involution, in contrast to postlactational involution, lobules and ducts are both reduced in number. Intralobular stroma (loose connective tissue) is replaced by collagen, while glandular epithelium and interlobular connective tissue regress and are replaced by fat. Periductal macrophages containing lipofuscin are often seen in postmenopausal breast. Eventually, all that remains are a few acini and ducts embedded in a fatty stroma containing scattered wisps of collagen. Fibroblasts and elastic fibers

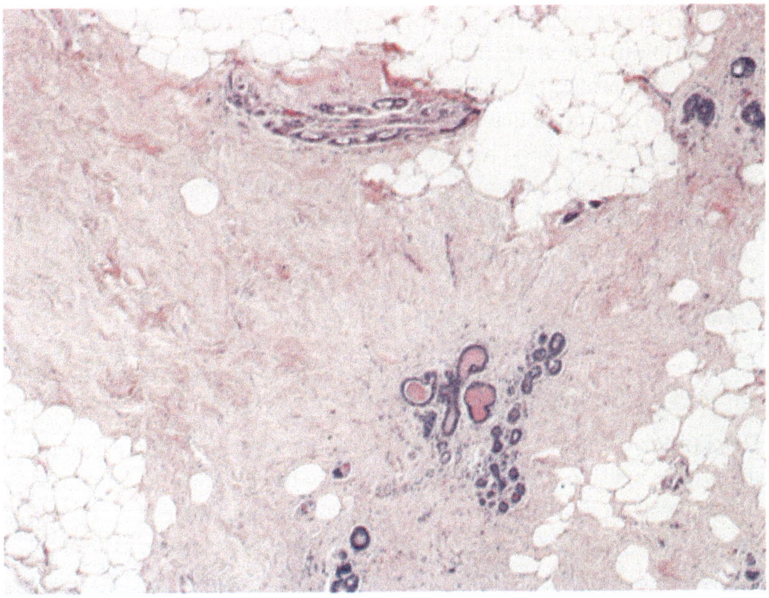

Fig. 1.17 Low power micrograph (50×) of a postmenopausal involuting human breast. As in the fetal breast (Fig 1.12) there are few ductules, abundant adipose tissue and dense irregular connective tissue

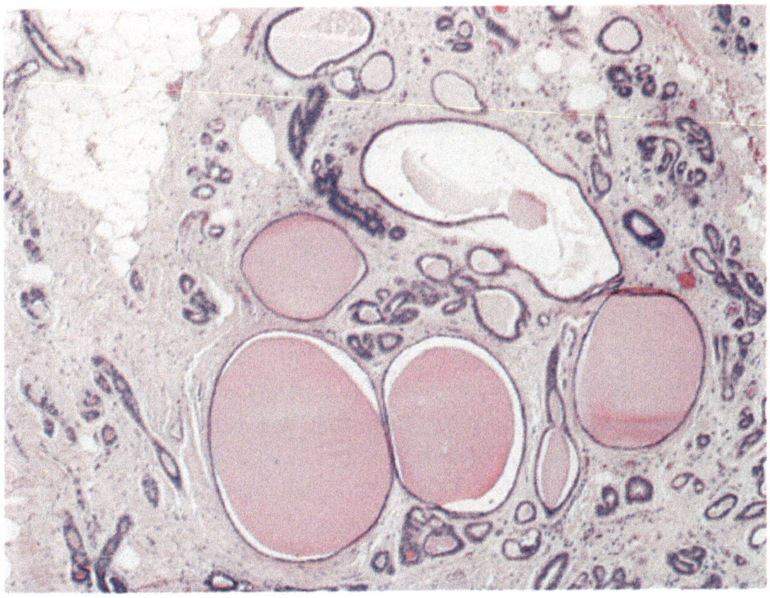

Fig. 1.18 Low power micrograph (50×) of a postmenopausal involuting human breast. Note the large cysts common in involuted breasts

decline in number [43]. A positive side effect of the replacement of dense stroma with fat is the more effective use of mammographic screening in postmenopausal women, since the dense tumors contrast to the fat [33]. The epithelium of some ducts may proliferate, and that of others may secrete and convert interrupted ducts into cysts [257] (Fig. 1.18).

1.4.9 Concluding Comments

The breast is studied by clinicians primarily due to its pathologies, especially cancer, and these will be addressed in the remainder of this text. In this chapter, we have attempted to provide a synopsis of current understanding of its normal structure and function. It is a unique and fascinating organ. It is the only gland that completes the majority of its development after birth as it undergoes dramatic, complex and hormonally regulated changes during puberty. It varies moderately during each menstrual cycle, prepares for its primary function during pregnancy, and reaches its most differentiated status only following parturition. Involution ensues following each cycle of pregnancy, parturition, and lactation, though permanent changes occur after the birth of even a single child that can be protective against cancer. The breast regresses after lactation to a much less differentiated state and may repeat this cycle over several more pregnancies and births. Once the ovary ceases to produce adequate estrogen and progesterone, the breast involutes, reverting to a structure not unlike that of a prepubertal child. We hope that this rather cursory review of normal breast biology serves as adequate foundation for the subsequent chapters and a reminder that the normal human breast is truly a fascinating and wonderful organ[2,3] (Table 1.1).

Acknowledgments We remain extremely grateful to colleagues for their critical reading of the original chapter, and we again thank Richard Conran, M.D. Ph.D., J.D., and Stephen Rothwell, Ph.D., for providing specimens for the micrographs included herein.

Disclaimer The opinions or assertions contained herein are the private ones of the authors and are not to be construed as official or reflecting the views of the Department of Defense or the Uniformed Services University of the Health Sciences.

Appendix

A Brief Comparison of Murine and Human Breast

Differences between human and murine breasts include the following: (1) The mouse has a well-defined "fat pad" stroma into which its ductwork grows. Human stroma is much more fibrous. (2) The functional unit of the human is the terminal ductal lobular unit (TDLU), which has the appearance of a bunch of grapes arising from a stem (duct) and is embedded in loose connective tissue. The comparable mouse structure is the lobuloalveolar unit. It also contains alveoli and ductwork. However, during murine development, the terminal end bud (TEB), a solid bulbous structure, is most often referred to in the literature. (3) Male mouse mammary glands regress prenatally under the influence of androgens, but infant human breasts are indistinguishable by gender. (4) Estrogen receptor alpha (ERα) is found in epithelia and stroma in the mouse, but while expressed in human breast epithelial cells, it has not been documented in human breast stroma. (5) The mouse has five pairs of mammary glands, each pair regulated by slightly different factors, while the human has just one pair (Table 1.2).

[2]Much more extensive list of factors and the effects of their mutations in mouse mammary gland development can be found in the Mikkola and Millar review comparing mammary gland development with that of other skin appendages [321]. Their applicability to the human has not been documented, and the failure of gene deletion experiments addressing most of these factors to result in mammary gland abnormalities may indicate a high degree of functional redundancy [322].

[3]Many descriptions of "embryonic" development in the literature on human breast development are better referred to as prenatal, since the embryonic period extends only from the end of the second to the end of the eighth postfertilization week. The more inclusive term, prenatal, is used here.

References

1. Romer AS. The vertebrate body. 4th ed. Philadelphia: W. B. Saunders Company; 1970.
2. Swaminathan N. Strange but true: males can lactate. Sci Am. 2007. Available from: www.sciam.com.
3. Wuringer E, Mader N, Posch E, Holle J. Nerve and vessel supplying ligamentous suspension of the mammary gland. Plast Reconstr Surg. 1998;101(6):1486–93.
4. Stranding S, editor. Gray's anatomy: the anatomical basis of clinical practice. 39th ed. Elsevier, Churchill, Livingstone: Edinburgh; 2005.
5. Moore KA. Clinically oriented anatomy. 5th ed. Baltimore: Lipincott Williams and Wilkins; 2006.
6. Sarhadi NS, Shaw-Dunn J, Soutar DS. Nerve supply of the breast with special reference to the nipple and areola: Sir Astley Cooper revisited. Clin Anat. 1997;10(4):283–8.
7. Schlenz I, Kuzbari R, Gruber H, Holle J. The sensitivity of the nipple-areola complex: an anatomic study. Plast Reconstr Surg. 2000;105(3):905–9.
8. Jaspars JJ, Posma AN, van Immerseel AA, Gittenberger-de Groot AC. The cutaneous innervation of the female breast and nipple-areola complex: implications for surgery. Br J Plast Surg. 1997;50(4):249–59.
9. Schlenz I, Rigel S, Schemper M, Kuzbari R. Alteration of nipple and areola sensitivity by reduction mammaplasty: a prospective comparison of five techniques. Plast reconstructive surgery. 2005;115(3):743–51; discussion 52–4.
10. Wakerley JB. Milk ejection and its control. In: Neill JD, editor. Knobil and Neill's physiology. 3 ed. Amsterdam: Elsevier; 2006. p. 3129–90.
11. DelVecchyo C, Caloca J Jr, Caloca J, Gomez-Jauregui J. Evaluation of breast sensibility using dermatomal somatosensory evoked potentials. Plast Reconstr Surg. 2004;113(7):1975–83.
12. Godwin Y, Valassiadou K, Lewis S, Denley H. Investigation into the possible cause of subjective decreased sensory perception in the nipple-areola complex of women with macromastia. Plast Reconstr Surg. 2004;113(6):1598–606.
13. Bloom WD. A textbook of histology. 10th ed. Philadelphia: W. B. Saunders Company; 1975.
14. Franke-Radowiecka A, Wasowicz K. Adrenergic and cholinergic innervation of the mammary gland in the pig. Anat Histol Embryol. 2002;31(1):3–7.
15. Papay FA, Verghese A, Stanton-Hicks M, Zins J. Complex regional pain syndrome of the breast in a patient after breast reduction. Ann Plast Surg. 1997;39(4):347–52.
16. Eriksson M, Lindh B, Uvnas-Moberg K, Hokfelt T. Distribution and origin of peptide-containing nerve fibres in the rat and human mammary gland. Neuroscience. 1996;70(1):227–45.
17. Ricbourg B. [Applied anatomy of the breast: blood supply and innervation]. Annales de chirurgie plastique et esthetique. 1992;37(6):603–20. Anatomie appliquee du sein. Vascularisation et innervation.
18. Naccarato AG, Viacava P, Bocci G, Fanelli G, Aretini P, Lonobile A, et al. Definition of the microvascular pattern of the normal human adult mammary gland. J Anat. 2003;203(6):599–603.

19. Weinstein SP, Conant EF, Sehgal CM, Woo IP, Patton JA. Hormonal variations in the vascularity of breast tissue. J Ultrasound Med. 2005;24(1):67–72; quiz 4.
20. O'Rahilly M, Mueller F, Carpenter S, Swenson R. Vessels, lymphatic drainage and the breast. Hanover, NH: Dartmouth Medical School Publ; 2004.
21. Nathanson SD, Wachna DL, Gilman D, Karvelis K, Havstad S, Ferrara J. Pathways of lymphatic drainage from the breast. Ann Surg Oncol. 2001;8(10):837–43.
22. Braithwaite LR. The flow of lymph from the ileocaecal angel, and its possible bearing on the cause of duodenal and gastric ulcer. Br J Surg. 1923;11:7–26.
23. Krag D, Weaver D, Ashikaga T, Moffat F, Klimberg VS, Shriver C, et al. The sentinel node in breast cancer–a multicenter validation study. N Engl J Med. 1998;339(14):941–6.
24. Estourgie SH, Nieweg OE, Olmos RA, Rutgers EJ, Kroon BB. Lymphatic drainage patterns from the breast. Ann Surg. 2004;239 (2):232–7.
25. Vendrell-Torne E, Setoain-Quinquer J, Domenech-Torne FM. Study of normal mammary lymphatic drainage using radioactive isotopes. J Nuclear Med. 1971;13(11):801–5.
26. Suami H, Pan WR, Mann GB, Taylor GI. The lymphatic anatomy of the breast and its implications for sentinel lymph node biopsy: a human cadaver study. Ann Surg Oncol. 2008;15(3):863–71.
27. Krynyckyi BR, Shim J, Kim CK. Internal mammary chain drainage of breast cancer. Ann Surg. 2004;240(3):557; author reply 8.
28. Kellokumpu-Lehtinen P, Johansson RM, Pelliniemi LJ. Ultrastructure of human fetal mammary gland. Anat Rec. 1987;218(1):66–72.
29. Herman-Giddens ME, Slora EJ, Wasserman RC, Bourdony CJ, Bhapkar MV, Koch GG, et al. Secondary sexual characteristics and menses in young girls seen in office practice: a study from the Pediatric Research in Office Settings network. Pediatrics. 1997;99 (4):505–12.
30. Tanner J. Growth at adolescence. 2nd ed. Oxford: Blackwell Scientific Publications; 1962.
31. Tavassoli FA. Pathology of the breast. 2nd ed. Stamford, CT: Appleton & Lange; 1999.
32. Hussain Z, Roberts N, Whitehouse GH, Garcia-Finana M, Percy D. Estimation of breast volume and its variation during the menstrual cycle using MRI and stereology. Br J Radiol. 1999;72(855):236–45.
33. Howard BA, Gusterson BA. Human breast development. J Mammary Gland Biol Neoplasia. 2000;5(2):119–37.
34. Nelson CM, Bissell MJ. Modeling dynamic reciprocity: engineering three-dimensional culture models of breast architecture, function, and neoplastic transformation. Semin Cancer Biol. 2005;15(5):342–52.
35. Rosen PR. Rosen's breast pathology. 2nd ed. Philadelphia: Lippincott williams & Wilkins; 2001.
36. Pitelka DR. The mammary gland. In: Weiss L, editor. Cell and tissue biology: a textbook of histology. 6th ed. New York: Elsevier Biomedical; 1988. p. 880–98.
37. Pathology UoVDo. I. Gross anatomy and histology. Charlottesville 1998–2007; Available from: www.med-ed.virginia.edu/courses/path/gyn/breast1.cfm.
38. Cardiff RD. Are the TDLU of the human the same as the LA of mice? J Mammary Gland Biol Neoplasia. 1998;3(1):3–5.
39. Moffat DF, Going JJ. Three dimensional anatomy of complete duct systems in human breast: pathological and developmental implications. J Clin Pathol. 1996;49(1):48–52.
40. Ohtake T, Kimijima I, Fukushima T, Yasuda M, Sekikawa K, Takenoshita S, et al. Computer-assisted complete three-dimensional reconstruction of the mammary ductal/lobular systems: implications of ductal anastomoses for breast-conserving surgery. Cancer. 2001;91(12):2263–72.
41. Junqueira LJ. Basic histology text and atlas. 10th ed. New York: Lange Medical Books McGraw-Hill; 2003.
42. Ferguson DJ. Intraepithelial lymphocytes and macrophages in the normal breast. Virchows Arch. 1985;407(4):369–78.
43. Ross M, Pawlina W. Histology, a text and atlas. 5th ed. Baltimore: Lippincott Williams & Wilkins; 2006.
44. Daniel CW, Strickland P, Friedmann Y. Expression and functional role of E- and P-cadherins in mouse mammary ductal morphogenesis and growth. Dev Biol. 1995;169(2):511–9.
45. Deugnier MA, Teuliere J, Faraldo MM, Thiery JP, Glukhova MA. The importance of being a myoepithelial cell. Breast Cancer Res. 2002;4(6):224–30.
46. Woodward WA, Chen MS, Behbod F, Rosen JM. On mammary stem cells. J Cell Sci. 2005;118(Pt 16):3585–94.
47. Monaghan P, Moss D. Connexin expression and gap junctions in the mammary gland. Cell Biol Int. 1996;20(2):121–5.
48. Schmeichel KL, Weaver VM, Bissell MJ. Structural cues from the tissue microenvironment are essential determinants of the human mammary epithelial cell phenotype. J Mammary Gland Biol Neoplasia. 1998;3(2):201–13.
49. Glukhova M, Koteliansky V, Sastre X, Thiery JP. Adhesion systems in normal breast and in invasive breast carcinoma. Am J Pathol. 1995;146(3):706–16.
50. Gudjonsson T, Ronnov-Jessen L, Villadsen R, Rank F, Bissell MJ, Petersen OW. Normal and tumor-derived myoepithelial cells differ in their ability to interact with luminal breast epithelial cells for polarity and basement membrane deposition. J Cell Sci. 2002;115(Pt 1):39–50.
51. Radice GL, Ferreira-Cornwell MC, Robinson SD, Rayburn H, Chodosh LA, Takeichi M, et al. Precocious mammary gland development in P-cadherin-deficient mice. J Cell Biol. 1997;139 (4):1025–32.
52. Faraldo MM, Teuliere J, Deugnier MA, Taddei-De La Hosseraye I, Thiery JP, Glukhova MA. Myoepithelial cells in the control of mammary development and tumorigenesis: data from genetically modified mice. J Mammary Gland Biol Neoplasia. 2005;10 (3):211–9.
53. Adriance MC, Inman JL, Petersen OW, Bissell MJ. Myoepithelial cells: good fences make good neighbors. Breast Cancer Res. 2005;7(5):190–7.
54. El-Sabban ME, Abi-Mosleh LF, Talhouk RS. Developmental regulation of gap junctions and their role in mammary epithelial cell differentiation. J Mammary Gland Biol Neoplasia. 2003;8 (4):463–73.
55. Gudjonsson T, Adriance MC, Sternlicht MD, Petersen OW, Bissell MJ. Myoepithelial cells: their origin and function in breast morphogenesis and neoplasia. J Mammary Gland Biol Neoplasia. 2005;10(3):261–72.
56. Lakhani SR, O'Hare MJ. The mammary myoepithelial cell–Cinderella or ugly sister? Breast Cancer Res. 2001;3(1):1–4.
57. Liu S, Dontu G, Mantle ID, Patel S, Ahn NS, Jackson KW, et al. Hedgehog signaling and Bmi-1 regulate self-renewal of normal and malignant human mammary stem cells. Cancer Res. 2006;66 (12):6063–71.
58. Hennighausen L, Robinson GW. Information networks in the mammary gland. Nat Rev. 2005;6(9):715–25.
59. Savarese TM, Low HP, Baik I, Strohsnitter WC, Hsieh CC. Normal breast stem cells, malignant breast stem cells, and the perinatal origin of breast cancer. Stem cell reviews. 2006;2 (2):103–10.
60. Smalley M, Ashworth A. Stem cells and breast cancer: a field in transit. Nat Rev Cancer. 2003;3(11):832–44.

61. Chepko G, Smith GH. Three division-competent, structurally-distinct cell populations contribute to murine mammary epithelial renewal. Tissue Cell. 1997;29(2):239–53.
62. Smith GH, Medina D. A morphologically distinct candidate for an epithelial stem cell in mouse mammary gland. J Cell Sci. 1988;90(Pt 1):173–83.
63. Smith GH, Strickland P, Daniel CW. Putative epithelial stem cell loss corresponds with mammary growth senescence. Cell Tissue Res. 2002;310(3):313–20.
64. Daniel CW, De Ome KB, Young JT, Blair PB, Faulkin LJ Jr. The in vivo life span of normal and preneoplastic mouse mammary glands: a serial transplantation study. Proc Natl Acad Sci USA. 1968;61(1):53–60.
65. Kordon EC, Smith GH. An entire functional mammary gland may comprise the progeny from a single cell. Development. 1998;125(10):1921–30.
66. Shackleton M, Vaillant F, Simpson KJ, Stingl J, Smyth GK, Asselin-Labat ML, et al. Generation of a functional mammary gland from a single stem cell. Nature. 2006;439(7072):84–8.
67. Stingl J, Eaves CJ, Kuusk U, Emerman JT. Phenotypic and functional characterization in vitro of a multipotent epithelial cell present in the normal adult human breast. Differentiation (research in biological diversity). 1998;63(4):201–13.
68. Villadsen R, Fridriksdottir AJ, Ronnov-Jessen L, Gudjonsson T, Rank F, LaBarge MA, et al. Evidence for a stem cell hierarchy in the adult human breast. J Cell Biol. 2007;177(1):87–101.
69. Florek M, Haase M, Marzesco AM, Freund D, Ehninger G, Huttner WB, et al. Prominin-1/CD133, a neural and hematopoietic stem cell marker, is expressed in adult human differentiated cells and certain types of kidney cancer. Cell Tissue Res. 2005;319(1):15–26 Epub 2004/11/24.
70. Welm BE, Tepera SB, Venezia T, Graubert TA, Rosen JM, Goodell MA. Sca-1(pos) cells in the mouse mammary gland represent an enriched progenitor cell population. Dev Biol. 2002;245(1):42–56.
71. Rios AC, Fu NY, Lindeman GJ, Visvader JE. In situ identification of bipotent stem cells in the mammary gland. Nature. 2014;506(7488):322–7 Epub 2014/01/28.
72. Al-Hajj M, Wicha MS, Benito-Hernandez A, Morrison SJ, Clarke MF. Prospective identification of tumorigenic breast cancer cells. Proc Natl Acad Sci USA. 2003;100(7):3983–8 Epub 2003/03/12.
73. Ginestier C, Wicha MS. Mammary stem cell number as a determinate of breast cancer risk. Breast Cancer Res. 2007;9 (4):109.
74. Storci G, Sansone P, Trere D, Tavolari S, Taffurelli M, Ceccarelli C, et al. The basal-like breast carcinoma phenotype is regulated by SLUG gene expression. J Pathol. 2008;214(1):25–37 Epub 2007/11/02.
75. Wright MH, Calcagno AM, Salcido CD, Carlson MD, Ambudkar SV, Varticovski L. Brca1 breast tumors contain distinct CD44 +/CD24- and CD133+ cells with cancer stem cell characteristics. Breast Cancer Res. 2008;10(1):R10. Epub 2008/02/05.
76. Liu TJ, Sun BC, Zhao XL, Zhao XM, Sun T, Gu Q, et al. CD133 + cells with cancer stem cell characteristics associates with vasculogenic mimicry in triple-negative breast cancer. Oncogene. 2013;32(5):544–53 Epub 2012/04/04.
77. Clarke RB. Isolation and characterization of human mammary stem cells. Cell Prolif. 2005;38(6):375–86.
78. Mallepell S, Krust A, Chambon P, Brisken C. Paracrine signaling through the epithelial estrogen receptor alpha is required for proliferation and morphogenesis in the mammary gland. Proc Natl Acad Sci USA. 2006;103(7):2196–201.
79. Beleut M, Rajaram RD, Caikovski M, Ayyanan A, Germano D, Choi Y, et al. Two distinct mechanisms underlie progesterone-induced proliferation in the mammary gland. Proc Natl Acad Sci USA. 2010;107(7):2989–94 Epub 2010/02/06.
80. Matulka LA, Triplett AA, Wagner KU. Parity-induced mammary epithelial cells are multipotent and express cell surface markers associated with stem cells. Dev Biol. 2007;303(1):29–44.
81. Chang TH, Kunasegaran K, Tarulli GA, De Silva D, Voorhoeve PM, Pietersen AM. New insights into lineage restriction of mammary gland epithelium using parity-identified mammary epithelial cells. Breast Cancer Res. 2014;16(1):R1. Epub 2014/01/09.
82. Russo J, Balogh GA, Chen J, Fernandez SV, Fernbaugh R, Heulings R, et al. The concept of stem cell in the mammary gland and its implication in morphogenesis, cancer and prevention. Front Biosci. 2006;11:151–72.
83. Stingl J, Raouf A, Emerman JT, Eaves CJ. Epithelial progenitors in the normal human mammary gland. J Mammary Gland Biol Neoplasia. 2005;10(1):49–59.
84. Wagner KU, Smith GH. Pregnancy and stem cell behavior. J Mammary Gland Biol Neoplasia. 2005;10(1):25–36.
85. Dontu G, Abdallah WM, Foley JM, Jackson KW, Clarke MF, Kawamura MJ, et al. In vitro propagation and transcriptional profiling of human mammary stem/progenitor cells. Genes Dev. 2003;17(10):1253–70.
86. Liu S, Dontu G, Wicha MS. Mammary stem cells, self-renewal pathways, and carcinogenesis. Breast Cancer Res. 2005;7(3):86–95.
87. Kouros-Mehr H, Werb Z. Candidate regulators of mammary branching morphogenesis identified by genome-wide transcript analysis. Dev Dyn. 2006;235(12):3404–12 Epub 2006/10/14.
88. Incassati A, Chandramouli A, Eelkema R, Cowin P. Key signaling nodes in mammary gland development and cancer: beta-catenin. Breast Cancer Res. 2010;12(6):213. Epub 2010/11/12.
89. Joshi PA, Jackson HW, Beristain AG, Di Grappa MA, Mote PA, Clarke CL, et al. Progesterone induces adult mammary stem cell expansion. Nature. 2010;465(7299):803–7 Epub 2010/05/07.
90. Asselin-Labat ML, Vaillant F, Sheridan JM, Pal B, Wu D, Simpson ER, et al. Control of mammary stem cell function by steroid hormone signalling. Nature. 2010;465(7299):798–802 Epub 2010/04/13.
91. Gonzalez-Suarez E, Jacob AP, Jones J, Miller R, Roudier-Meyer MP, Erwert R, et al. RANK ligand mediates progestin-induced mammary epithelial proliferation and carcinogenesis. Nature. 2010;468(7320):103–7 Epub 2010/10/01.
92. Gu B, Watanabe K, Sun P, Fallahi M, Dai X. Chromatin effector Pygo2 mediates Wnt-notch crosstalk to suppress luminal/alveolar potential of mammary stem and basal cells. Cell Stem Cell. 2013;13(1):48–61 Epub 2013/05/21.
93. Lafkas D, Rodilla V, Huyghe M, Mourao L, Kiaris H, Fre S. Notch3 marks clonogenic mammary luminal progenitor cells in vivo. J Cell Biol. 2013;203(1):47–56 Epub 2013/10/09.
94. Andrechek ER, White D, Muller WJ. Targeted disruption of ErbB2/Neu in the mammary epithelium results in impaired ductal outgrowth. Oncogene. 2005;24(5):932–7 Epub 2004/12/08.
95. Jackson-Fisher AJ, Bellinger G, Ramabhadran R, Morris JK, Lee KF, Stern DF. ErbB2 is required for ductal morphogenesis of the mammary gland. Proc Natl Acad Sci USA. 2004;101 (49):17138–43 Epub 2004/12/01.
96. Korkaya H, Paulson A, Iovino F, Wicha MS. HER2 regulates the mammary stem/progenitor cell population driving tumorigenesis and invasion. Oncogene. 2008;27(47):6120–30 Epub 2008/07/02.
97. Paik S, Kim C, Wolmark N. HER2 status and benefit from adjuvant trastuzumab in breast cancer. N Engl J Med. 2008;358 (13):1409–11 Epub 2008/03/28.

98. Perez EA, Reinholz MM, Hillman DW, Tenner KS, Schroeder MJ, Davidson NE, et al. HER2 and chromosome 17 effect on patient outcome in the N9831 adjuvant trastuzumab trial. J Clin Oncol. 2010;28(28):4307–15.
99. Bianchini F, Kaaks R, Vainio H. Overweight, obesity, and cancer risk. Lancet Oncol. 2002;3(9):565–74 Epub 2002/09/10.
100. Calle EE, Rodriguez C, Walker-Thurmond K, Thun MJ. Overweight, obesity, and mortality from cancer in a prospectively studied cohort of U.S. adults. N Engl J Med. 2003;348(17):1625–38 Epub 2003/04/25.
101. Kleinberg DL, Feldman M, Ruan W. IGF-I: an essential factor in terminal end bud formation and ductal morphogenesis. J Mammary Gland Biol Neoplasia. 2000;5(1):7–17.
102. Kleinberg DL, Ruan W. IGF-I, GH, and sex steroid effects in normal mammary gland development. J Mammary Gland Biol Neoplasia. 2008;13(4):353–60 Epub 2008/11/27.
103. Tamimi RM, Colditz GA, Wang Y, Collins LC, Hu R, Rosner B, et al. Expression of IGF1R in normal breast tissue and subsequent risk of breast cancer. Breast Cancer Res Treat. 2011;128(1):243–50 Epub 2011/01/05.
104. Esper RM, Dame M, McClintock S, Holt PR, Dannenberg AJ, Wicha MS, et al. Leptin and adiponectin modulate the self-renewal of normal human breast epithelial stem cells. Cancer Prev Res (Phila). 2015;8(12):1174–83 Epub 2015/10/22.
105. Huh SJ, Oh H, Peterson MA, Almendro V, Hu R, Bowden M, et al. The proliferative activity of mammary epithelial cells in normal tissue predicts breast cancer risk in premenopausal women. Cancer Res. 2016;76(7):1926–34 Epub 2016/03/05.
106. Guelstein VI, Tchypysheva TA, Ermilova VD, Ljubimov AV. Myoepithelial and basement membrane antigens in benign and malignant human breast tumors. Int J Cancer. 1993;53(2):269–77.
107. Prince JM, Klinowska TC, Marshman E, Lowe ET, Mayer U, Miner J, et al. Cell-matrix interactions during development and apoptosis of the mouse mammary gland in vivo. Dev Dyn. 2002;223(4):497–516.
108. Woodward TL, Mienaltowski AS, Modi RR, Bennett JM, Haslam SZ. Fibronectin and the alpha(5)beta(1) integrin are under developmental and ovarian steroid regulation in the normal mouse mammary gland. Endocrinology. 2001;142(7):3214–22.
109. Streuli CH, Bissell MJ. Expression of extracellular matrix components is regulated by substratum. J Cell Biol. 1990;110(4):1405–15.
110. Pullan S, Wilson J, Metcalfe A, Edwards GM, Goberdhan N, Tilly J, et al. Requirement of basement membrane for the suppression of programmed cell death in mammary epithelium. J Cell Sci. 1996;109(Pt 3):631–42.
111. Streuli C. Extracellular matrix remodelling and cellular differentiation. Curr Opin Cell Biol. 1999;11(5):634–40.
112. Novaro V, Roskelley CD, Bissell MJ. Collagen-IV and laminin-1 regulate estrogen receptor alpha expression and function in mouse mammary epithelial cells. J Cell Sci. 2003;116(Pt 14):2975–86.
113. Weir ML, Oppizzi ML, Henry MD, Onishi A, Campbell KP, Bissell MJ, et al. Dystroglycan loss disrupts polarity and beta-casein induction in mammary epithelial cells by perturbing laminin anchoring. J Cell Sci. 2006;119(Pt 19):4047–58.
114. Streuli CH, Schmidhauser C, Bailey N, Yurchenco P, Skubitz AP, Roskelley C, et al. Laminin mediates tissue-specific gene expression in mammary epithelia. J Cell Biol. 1995;129(3):591–603.
115. Farrelly N, Lee YJ, Oliver J, Dive C, Streuli CH. Extracellular matrix regulates apoptosis in mammary epithelium through a control on insulin signaling. J Cell Biol. 1999;144(6):1337–48.
116. Pujuguet P, Simian M, Liaw J, Timpl R, Werb Z, Bissell MJ. Nidogen-1 regulates laminin-1-dependent mammary-specific gene expression. J Cell Sci. 2000;113(Pt 5):849–58.
117. Streuli CH, Edwards GM. Control of normal mammary epithelial phenotype by integrins. J Mammary Gland Biol Neoplasia. 1998;3(2):151–63.
118. Li N, Zhang Y, Naylor MJ, Schatzmann F, Maurer F, Wintermantel T, et al. Beta1 integrins regulate mammary gland proliferation and maintain the integrity of mammary alveoli. EMBO J. 2005;24(11):1942–53.
119. Klinowska TC, Soriano JV, Edwards GM, Oliver JM, Valentijn AJ, Montesano R, et al. Laminin and beta1 integrins are crucial for normal mammary gland development in the mouse. Dev Biol. 1999;215(1):13–32.
120. Naylor MJ, Li N, Cheung J, Lowe ET, Lambert E, Marlow R, et al. Ablation of beta1 integrin in mammary epithelium reveals a key role for integrin in glandular morphogenesis and differentiation. J Cell Biol. 2005;171(4):717–28.
121. Barcellos-Hoff MH, Aggeler J, Ram TG, Bissell MJ. Functional differentiation and alveolar morphogenesis of primary mammary cultures on reconstituted basement membrane. Development. 1989;105(2):223–35.
122. Blatchford DR, Quarrie LH, Tonner E, McCarthy C, Flint DJ, Wilde CJ. Influence of microenvironment on mammary epithelial cell survival in primary culture. J Cell Physiol. 1999;181(2):304–11.
123. Neville MC. Lactation and its hormonal control. In: Neill JD, editor. Knobil and Neill's physiology of reproduction. 3rd ed. Amsterdam: Elsevier; 2006. p. 2993–3054.
124. Eyden BP, Watson RJ, Harris M, Howell A. Intralobular stromal fibroblasts in the resting human mammary gland: ultrastructural properties and intercellular relationships. J Submicrosc Cytol. 1986;18(2):397–408.
125. Atherton AJ, Monaghan P, Warburton MJ, Robertson D, Kenny AJ, Gusterson BA. Dipeptidyl peptidase IV expression identifies a functional sub-population of breast fibroblasts. Int J Cancer. 1992;50(1):15–9.
126. Sadlonova A, Novak Z, Johnson MR, Bowe DB, Gault SR, Page GP, et al. Breast fibroblasts modulate epithelial cell proliferation in three-dimensional in vitro co-culture. Breast Cancer Res. 2005;7(1):R46–59.
127. Parmar H, Cunha GR. Epithelial-stromal interactions in the mouse and human mammary gland in vivo. Endocr Relat Cancer. 2004;11(3):437–58.
128. Gouon-Evans V, Lin EY, Pollard JW. Requirement of macrophages and eosinophils and their cytokines/chemokines for mammary gland development. Breast Cancer Res. 2002;4(4):155–64.
129. Schwertfeger KL, Rosen JM, Cohen DA. Mammary gland macrophages: pleiotropic functions in mammary development. J Mammary Gland Biol Neoplasia. 2006;11(3–4):229–38.
130. Monks J, Geske FJ, Lehman L, Fadok VA. Do inflammatory cells participate in mammary gland involution? J Mammary Gland Biol Neoplasia. 2002;7(2):163–76.
131. Sternlicht MD. Key stages in mammary gland development: the cues that regulate ductal branching morphogenesis. Breast Cancer Res. 2006;8(1):201.
132. Nishimura T. Expression of potential lymphocyte trafficking mediator molecules in the mammary gland. Vet Res. 2003;34(1):3–10.
133. Dabiri S, Huntsman D, Makretsov N, Cheang M, Gilks B, Bajdik C, et al. The presence of stromal mast cells identifies a subset of invasive breast cancers with a favorable prognosis. Mod Pathol. 2004;17(6):690–5.

134. Hartveit F. Mast cell association with collagen fibres in human breast stroma. Eur J Morphol. 1993;31(3):209–18.
135. Popescu LM, Andrei F, Hinescu ME. Snapshots of mammary gland interstitial cells: methylene-blue vital staining and c-kit immunopositivity. J Cell Mol Med. 2005;9(2):476–7.
136. Popescu LM, Gherghiceanu M, Cretoiu D, Radu E. The connective connection: interstitial cells of Cajal (ICC) and ICC-like cells establish synapses with immunoreactive cells. Electron microscope study in situ. J Cell Mol Med. 2005;9(3):714–30.
137. Radu E, Regalia T, Ceafalan L, Andrei F, Cretoiu D, Popescu LM. Cajal-type cells from human mammary gland stroma: phenotype characteristics in cell culture. J Cell Mol Med. 2005;9(3):748–52.
138. Gherghiceanu M, Popescu LM. Interstitial Cajal-like cells (ICLC) in human resting mammary gland stroma. Transmission electron microscope (TEM) identification. J Cell Mol Med. 2005;9(4):893–910.
139. Haslam SZ, Woodward TL. Host microenvironment in breast cancer development: epithelial-cell-stromal-cell interactions and steroid hormone action in normal and cancerous mammary gland. Breast Cancer Res. 2003;5(4):208–15.
140. Hynes RO. Integrins: bidirectional, allosteric signaling machines. Cell. 2002;110(6):673–87.
141. Schatzmann F, Marlow R, Streuli CH. Integrin signaling and mammary cell function. J Mammary Gland Biol Neoplasia. 2003;8(4):395–408.
142. Alowami S, Troup S, Al-Haddad S, Kirkpatrick I, Watson PH. Mammographic density is related to stroma and stromal proteoglycan expression. Breast Cancer Res. 2003;5(5):R129–35.
143. Delehedde M, Lyon M, Sergeant N, Rahmoune H, Fernig DG. Proteoglycans: pericellular and cell surface multireceptors that integrate external stimuli in the mammary gland. J Mammary Gland Biol Neoplasia. 2001;6(3):253–73.
144. Silverman AJ, Livne I, Witkin JW. The gonadotropin-releasing hormone (GnRH), neuronal systems: immunocytochemistry and *in situ* hybridisation. In: Knobil E, Neill JD, editors. Physiol · Reprod. New York: Raven Press Ltd.; 1994. p. 1683–709.
145. Guyton AJ. Textbook of medical hysiology. 11th ed. Philadelphia: Elsevier Saunders.
146. Seagroves TN, Hadsell D, McManaman J, Palmer C, Liao D, McNulty W, et al. HIF1alpha is a critical regulator of secretory differentiation and activation, but not vascular expansion, in the mouse mammary gland. Development. 2003;130(8):1713–24.
147. Speirs V, Skliris GP, Burdall SE, Carder PJ. Distinct expression patterns of ER alpha and ER beta in normal human mammary gland. J Clin Pathol. 2002;55(5):371–4.
148. Levin ER. Integration of the extranuclear and nuclear actions of estrogen. Mol Endocrinol. 2005;19(8):1951–9.
149. Li X, Huang J, Yi P, Bambara RA, Hilf R, Muyan M. Single-chain estrogen receptors (ERs) reveal that the ERalpha/beta heterodimer emulates functions of the ERalpha dimer in genomic estrogen signaling pathways. Mol Cell Biol. 2004;24(17):7681–94.
150. Clarke RB, Howell A, Potten CS, Anderson E. Dissociation between steroid receptor expression and cell proliferation in the human breast. Cancer Res. 1997;57(22):4987–91.
151. Howell A. Pure oestrogen antagonists for the treatment of advanced breast cancer. Endocr Relat Cancer. 2006;13(3):689–706.
152. Hall JM, McDonnell DP. The estrogen receptor beta-isoform (ERbeta) of the human estrogen receptor modulates ERalpha transcriptional activity and is a key regulator of the cellular response to estrogens and antiestrogens. Endocrinology. 1999;140(12):5566–78.
153. Asselin-Labat ML, Shackleton M, Stingl J, Vaillant F, Forrest NC, Eaves CJ, et al. Steroid hormone receptor status of mouse mammary stem cells. J Natl Cancer Inst. 2006;98(14):1011–4.
154. Sleeman KE, Kendrick H, Robertson D, Isacke CM, Ashworth A, Smalley MJ. Dissociation of estrogen receptor expression and in vivo stem cell activity in the mammary gland. J Cell Biol. 2007;176(1):19–26.
155. Clarke RB. Ovarian steroids and the human breast: regulation of stem cells and cell proliferation. Maturitas. 2006;54(4):327–34.
156. Cheng G, Weihua Z, Warner M, Gustafsson JA. Estrogen receptors ER alpha and ER beta in proliferation in the rodent mammary gland. Proc Natl Acad Sci USA. 2004;101(11):3739–46.
157. Khan SA, Bhandare D, Chatterton RT Jr. The local hormonal environment and related biomarkers in the normal breast. Endocr Relat Cancer. 2005;12(3):497–510.
158. Forster C, Makela S, Warri A, Kietz S, Becker D, Hultenby K, et al. Involvement of estrogen receptor beta in terminal differentiation of mammary gland epithelium. Proc Natl Acad Sci USA. 2002;99(24):15578–83.
159. Seagroves TN, Rosen JM. Control of mammary epithelial cell proliferation: the unique role of the progesterone receptor. In: Burnstein K, editor. Sex hormones and cell cycle regulation: Alphen aan den Rijn: Kluwer Press; 2002. p. 33–55.
160. Conneely OM, Jericevic BM, Lydon JP. Progesterone receptors in mammary gland development and tumorigenesis. J Mammary Gland Biol Neoplasia. 2003;8(2):205–14.
161. Leonhardt SA, Boonyaratanakornkit V, Edwards DP. Progesterone receptor transcription and non-transcription signaling mechanisms. Steroids. 2003;68(10–13):761–70.
162. Aupperlee MD, Haslam SZ. Differential hormonal regulation and function of progesterone receptor isoforms in normal adult mouse mammary gland. Endocrinology. 2007;148(5):2290–300.
163. Lydon JP, Sivaraman L, Conneely OM. A reappraisal of progesterone action in the mammary gland. J Mammary Gland Biol Neoplasia. 2000;5(3):325–38.
164. Cunha GR, Young P, Hom YK, Cooke PS, Taylor JA, Lubahn DB. Elucidation of a role for stromal steroid hormone receptors in mammary gland growth and development using tissue recombinants. J Mammary Gland Biol Neoplasia. 1997;2(4):393–402.
165. Brisken C, Rajaram RD. Alveolar and lactogenic differentiation. J Mammary Gland Biol Neoplasia. 2006;11(3–4):239–48.
166. Yang Y, Spitzer E, Meyer D, Sachs M, Niemann C, Hartmann G, et al. Sequential requirement of hepatocyte growth factor and neuregulin in the morphogenesis and differentiation of the mammary gland. J Cell Biol. 1995;131(1):215–26.
167. Kariagina A, Aupperlee MD, Haslam SZ. Progesterone receptor isoforms and proliferation in the rat mammary gland during development. Endocrinology. 2007;148(6):2723–36.
168. Eigeliene N, Harkonen P, Erkkola R. Effects of estradiol and medroxyprogesterone acetate on morphology, proliferation and apoptosis of human breast tissue in organ cultures. BMC Cancer. 2006;6:246.
169. Freeman ME, Kanyicska B, Lerant A, Nagy G. Prolactin: structure, function, and regulation of secretion. Physiol Rev. 2000;80(4):1523–631.
170. Horseman ND. Prolactin and mammary gland development. J Mammary Gland Biol Neoplasia. 1999;4(1):79–88.
171. Dong J, Tsai-Morris CH, Dufau ML. A novel estradiol/estrogen receptor alpha-dependent transcriptional mechanism controls expression of the human prolactin receptor. J Biol Chem. 2006;281(27):18825–36.

172. Miyoshi K, Shillingford JM, Smith GH, Grimm SL, Wagner KU, Oka T, et al. Signal transducer and activator of transcription (Stat) 5 controls the proliferation and differentiation of mammary alveolar epithelium. J Cell Biol. 2001;155(4):531–42 Epub 2001/11/14.
173. Cui Y, Riedlinger G, Miyoshi K, Tang W, Li C, Deng CX, et al. Inactivation of Stat5 in mouse mammary epithelium during pregnancy reveals distinct functions in cell proliferation, survival, and differentiation. Mol Cell Biol. 2004;24(18):8037–47 Epub 2004/09/02.
174. Yamaji D, Na R, Feuermann Y, Pechhold S, Chen W, Robinson GW, et al. Development of mammary luminal progenitor cells is controlled by the transcription factor STAT5A. Genes Dev. 2009;23(20):2382–7 Epub 2009/10/17.
175. Asselin-Labat ML, Sutherland KD, Barker H, Thomas R, Shackleton M, Forrest NC, et al. Gata-3 is an essential regulator of mammary-gland morphogenesis and luminal-cell differentiation. Nat Cell Biol. 2007;9(2):201–9.
176. Kouros-Mehr H, Slorach EM, Sternlicht MD, Werb Z. GATA-3 maintains the differentiation of the luminal cell fate in the mammary gland. Cell. 2006;127(5):1041–55.
177. Chapman RS, Lourenco PC, Tonner E, Flint DJ, Selbert S, Takeda K, et al. Suppression of epithelial apoptosis and delayed mammary gland involution in mice with a conditional knockout of Stat3. Genes Dev. 1999;13(19):2604–16 Epub 1999/10/16.
178. Kritikou EA, Sharkey A, Abell K, Came PJ, Anderson E, Clarkson RW, et al. A dual, non-redundant, role for LIF as a regulator of development and STAT3-mediated cell death in mammary gland. Development. 2003;130(15):3459–68. Epub 2003/06/18.
179. Nguyen AV, Pollard JW. Transforming growth factor beta3 induces cell death during the first stage of mammary gland involution. Development. 2000;127(14):3107–18. Epub 2000/06/23.
180. Tiffen PG, Omidvar N, Marquez-Almuina N, Croston D, Watson CJ, Clarkson RW. A dual role for oncostatin M signaling in the differentiation and death of mammary epithelial cells in vivo. Molecular endocrinology. 2008;22(12):2677–88. Epub 2008/10/18.
181. Honda K, Kazumi N, Murata T, Higuchi T. Prolactin releasing peptides modulate background firing rate and milk-ejection related burst of oxytocin cells in the supraoptic nucleus. Brain Res Bull. 2004;63:315–9.
182. Bussolati G, Cassoni P, Ghisolfi G, Negro F, Sapino A. Immunolocalization and gene expression of oxytocin receptors in carcinomas and non-neoplastic tissues of the breast. Am J Pathol. 1996;148(6):1895–903.
183. Reversi A, Cassoni P, Chini B. Oxytocin receptor signaling in myoepithelial and cancer cells. J Mammary Gland Biol Neoplasia. 2005;10(3):221–9.
184. Labrie F. Dehydroepiandrosterone, androgens and the mammary gland. Gynecol Endocrinol. 2006;22(3):118–30.
185. Wilson CL, Sims AH, Howell A, Miller CJ, Clarke RB. Effects of oestrogen on gene expression in epithelium and stroma of normal human breast tissue. Endocr Relat Cancer. 2006;13(2):617–28.
186. Woodward TL, Xie JW, Haslam SZ. The role of mammary stroma in modulating the proliferative response to ovarian hormones in the normal mammary gland. J Mammary Gland Biol Neoplasia. 1998;3(2):117–31.
187. Lamarca HL, Rosen JM. Estrogen regulation of mammary gland development and breast cancer: amphiregulin takes center stage. Breast Cancer Res. 2007;9(4):304.
188. Zhang HZ, Bennett JM, Smith KT, Sunil N, Haslam SZ. Estrogen mediates mammary epithelial cell proliferation in serum-free culture indirectly via mammary stroma-derived hepatocyte growth factor. Endocrinology. 2002;143(9):3427–34.
189. Soriano JV, Pepper MS, Orci L, Montesano R. Roles of hepatocyte growth factor/scatter factor and transforming growth factor-beta1 in mammary gland ductal morphogenesis. J Mammary Gland Biol Neoplasia. 1998;3(2):133–50.
190. Pollard JW. Tumour-stromal interactions. Transforming growth factor-beta isoforms and hepatocyte growth factor/scatter factor in mammary gland ductal morphogenesis. Breast Cancer Res. 2001;3(4):230–7.
191. Kamalati T, Niranjan B, Yant J, Buluwela L. HGF/SF in mammary epithelial growth and morphogenesis: in vitro and in vivo models. J Mammary Gland Biol Neoplasia. 1999;4(1):69–77.
192. Cohen S. EGF and its receptor: historical perspective. Introduction. J Mammary Gland Biol Neoplasia. 1997;2(2):93–6.
193. Wiesen JF, Young P, Werb Z, Cunha GR. Signaling through the stromal epidermal growth factor receptor is necessary for mammary ductal development. Development. 1999;126(2):335–44.
194. Osin PP, Anbazhagan R, Bartkova J, Nathan B, Gusterson BA. Breast development gives insights into breast disease. Histopathology. 1998;33(3):275–83.
195. Ruan W, Kleinberg DL. Insulin-like growth factor I is essential for terminal end bud formation and ductal morphogenesis during mammary development. Endocrinology. 1999;140(11):5075–81.
196. Wood TL, Yee D. Introduction: IGFs and IGFBPs in the normal mammary gland and in breast cancer. J Mammary Gland Biol Neoplasia. 2000;5(1):1–5.
197. Ahmad T, Farnie G, Bundred NJ, Anderson NG. The mitogenic action of insulin-like growth factor I in normal human mammary epithelial cells requires the epidermal growth factor receptor tyrosine kinase. J Biol Chem. 2004;279(3):1713–9.
198. Wang W, Morrison B, Galbaugh T, Jose CC, Kenney N, Cutler ML. Glucocorticoid induced expression of connective tissue growth factor contributes to lactogenic differentiation of mouse mammary epithelial cells. J Cell Physiol. 2008;214(1):38–46.
199. Jiang WG, Watkins G, Fodstad O, Douglas-Jones A, Mokbel K, Mansel RE. Differential expression of the CCN family members Cyr61, CTGF and Nov in human breast cancer. Endocr Relat Cancer. 2004;11(4):781–91.
200. Anbazhagan R, Gusterson BA. Prenatal factors may influence predisposition to breast cancer. Eur J Cancer. 1994;30A(1):1–3.
201. Hilakivi-Clarke L, de Assis S. Fetal origins of breast cancer. Trends Endocrinol Metab: TEM. 2006;17(9):340–8.
202. Trichopoulos D, Lagiou P, Adami HO. Towards an integrated model for breast cancer etiology: the crucial role of the number of mammary tissue-specific stem cells. Breast Cancer Res. 2005;7(1):13–7.
203. Hens JR, Wysolmerski JJ. Key stages of mammary gland development: molecular mechanisms involved in the formation of the embryonic mammary gland. Breast Cancer Res. 2005;7(5):220–4.
204. Jolicoeur F. Intrauterine breast development and the mammary myoepithelial lineage. J Mammary Gland Biol Neoplasia. 2005;10(3):199–210.
205. Arey L. Developmental anatomy: a textbook adn laboratory manual of embryology. Revised 7th ed. Philadelphia: W. B. Saunders; 1974.
206. Russo J, Russo IH. Mammary gland development. In: Knobil E, Neill, JD, editors. Encyclopedia of reproduction; 1999.
207. Sadler TW. Langman's medical embryolgy. 9th ed. Baltimore: Lippincott Williams & Wilkins; 2003.
208. Robinson GW, Karpf AB, Kratochwil K. Regulation of mammary gland development by tissue interaction. J Mammary Gland Biol Neoplasia. 1999;4(1):9–19.

209. Anbazhagan R, Osin PP, Bartkova J, Nathan B, Lane EB, Gusterson BA. The development of epithelial phenotypes in the human fetal and infant breast. J Pathol. 1998;184(2):197–206.
210. Hovey RC, Trott JF, Vonderhaar BK. Establishing a framework for the functional mammary gland: from endocrinology to morphology. J Mammary Gland Biol Neoplasia. 2002;7(1):17–38.
211. Tobon H, Slazar H. Ultrastructure of the human mammary gland. I. Development of the fetal gland throughout gestation. J Clin Endocrinol Metab. 1974;39(3):443–56.
212. Kratochwil K, Schwartz P. Tissue interaction in androgen response of embryonic mammary rudiment of mouse: identification of target tissue for testosterone. Proc Natl Acad Sci USA. 1976;73(11):4041–4.
213. Turner CW. The anatomy of the mammary gland in cattle. II. Fetal development. Missouri Agric Exp Sta Res Bull. 1930;160:5–39.
214. Bocchinfuso WP, Lindzey JK, Hewitt SC, Clark JA, Myers PH, Cooper R, et al. Induction of mammary gland development in estrogen receptor-alpha knockout mice. Endocrinology. 2000;141(8):2982–94.
215. Aubert MJ, Grumbach MM, Kaplan SL. The ontogenesis of human fetal hormones. III. Prolactin. J Clin Investig. 1975;56(1):155–64.
216. Keeling JW, Ozer E, King G, Walker F. Oestrogen receptor alpha in female fetal, infant, and child mammary tissue. J Pathol. 2000;191(4):449–51.
217. Naccarato AG, Viacava P, Vignati S, Fanelli G, Bonadio AG, Montruccoli G, et al. Bio-morphological events in the development of the human female mammary gland from fetal age to puberty. Virchows Arch. 2000;436(5):431–8.
218. Nathan B, Anbazhagan R, Clarkson P, Bartkova J. Expression of BCL-2 in the developing human fetal and infant breast. Histopathology. 1994;24:73–6.
219. Magdinier F, Dalla Venezia N, Lenoir GM, Frappart L, Dante R. BRCA1 expression during prenatal development of the human mammary gland. Oncogene. 1999;18(27):4039–43.
220. Casey TM, Mulvey TM, Patnode TA, Dean A, Zakrzewska E, Plaut K. Mammary epithelial cells treated concurrently with TGF-alpha and TGF-beta exhibit enhanced proliferation and death. Exp Biol Med. 2007;232(8):1027–40.
221. Stull MA, Rowzee AM, Loladze AV, Wood TL. Growth factor regulation of cell cycle progression in mammary epithelial cells. J Mammary Gland Biol Neoplasia. 2004;9(1):15–26.
222. Streuli CH, Schmidhauser C, Kobrin M, Bissell MJ, Derynck R. Extracellular matrix regulates expression of the TGF-beta 1 gene. J Cell Biol. 1993;120(1):253–60.
223. Chammas R, Taverna D, Cella N, Santos C, Hynes NE. Laminin and tenascin assembly and expression regulate HC11 mouse mammary cell differentiation. J Cell Sci. 1994;107(Pt 4):1031–40.
224. Dunbar ME, Wysolmerski JJ. The role of parathyroid hormone-related protein (PTHrP) in mammary development, lactation, and breast cancer. 1996; Available from: http://mammary.nih.gov/reviews/development/Wyso1001/slides/introduction.html.
225. McKiernan J, Coyne J, Cahalane S. Histology of breast development in early life. Arch Dis Child. 1988;63(2):136–9.
226. McKiernan JF, Hull D. Breast development in the newborn. Arch Dis Child. 1981;56:525–9.
227. Russo J, Russo IH. Toward a physiological approach to breast cancer prevention. Cancer Epidemiol Biomark Prev. 1994;3(4):353–64.
228. Russo J, Russ IH. Development of the human mammary gland. In: Neville MD, Daniel C, editors. The mammary gland: development, regulation and function. New York: Plenum Press; 1987.
229. McKiernan JF, Hull D. Prolactin, maternal oestrogens, and breast development in the newborn. Arch Dis Child. 1981;56(10):770–4.
230. Schmidt IM, Chellarkooty M, Haavisto A, Boisen KA, Damgaard IN, Steendahl U, et al. Gender difference in breast tissue size in infancy: correlation with serum estradiol. Pediatr Res. 2002;52(5):682–6.
231. Pierce DF Jr, Johnson MD, Matsui Y, Robinson SD, Gold LI, Purchio AF, et al. Inhibition of mammary duct development but not alveolar outgrowth during pregnancy in transgenic mice expressing active TGF-beta 1. Genes Dev. 1993;7(12A):2308–17.
232. Russo I, Medado J, Russo J. Endocrine influences on the mammary gland. In: Jones T, Mohr U, Hunt E, editors. Integument and mammary glands. Berlin: Springer; 1989.
233. Humphreys RC. Programmed cell death in the terminal endbud. J Mammary Gland Biol Neoplasia. 1999;4(2):213–20.
234. Humphreys RC, Krajewska M, Krnacik S, Jaeger R, Weiher H, Krajewski S, et al. Apoptosis in the terminal endbud of the murine mammary gland: a mechanism of ductal morphogenesis. Development. 1996;122(12):4013–22.
235. Britt K, Ashworth A, Smalley M. Pregnancy and the risk of breast cancer. Endocr Relat Cancer. 2007;14(4):907–33.
236. Williams JM, Daniel CW. Mammary ductal elongation: differentiation of myoepithelium and basal lamina during branching morphogenesis. Dev Biol. 1983;97(2):274–90.
237. Topper YJ, Freeman CS. Multiple hormone interactions in the developmental biology of the mammary gland. Physiol Rev. 1980;60(4):1049–106.
238. Anderson E, Clarke RB, Howell A. Estrogen responsiveness and control of normal human breast proliferation. J Mammary Gland Biol Neoplasia. 1998;3(1):23–35.
239. Laurence DJ, Monaghan P, Gusterson BA. The development of the normal human breast. Oxf Rev Reprod Biol. 1991;13:149–74.
240. Russo J, Hu YF, Silva ID, Russo IH. Cancer risk related to mammary gland structure and development. Microsc Res Tech. 2001;52(2):204–23.
241. Feldman M, Ruan W, Cunningham BC, Wells JA, Kleinberg DL. Evidence that the growth hormone receptor mediates differentiation and development of the mammary gland. Endocrinology. 1993;133(4):1602–8.
242. Marshman E, Streuli CH. Insulin-like growth factors and insulin-like growth factor binding proteins in mammary gland function. Breast Cancer Res. 2002;4(6):231–9.
243. Howlin J, McBryan J, Martin F. Pubertal mammary gland development: insights from mouse models. J Mammary Gland Biol Neoplasia. 2006;11(3–4):283–97.
244. Going JJ, Anderson TJ, Battersby S, MacIntyre CC. Proliferative and secretory activity in human breast during natural and artificial menstrual cycles. Am J Pathol. 1988;130(1):193–204.
245. Ramakrishnan R, Khan SA, Badve S. Morphological changes in breast tissue with menstrual cycle. Mod Pathol. 2002;15(12):1348–56.
246. Navarrete MA, Maier CM, Falzoni R, Quadros LG, Lima GR, Baracat EC, et al. Assessment of the proliferative, apoptotic and cellular renovation indices of the human mammary epithelium during the follicular and luteal phases of the menstrual cycle. Breast Cancer Res. 2005;7(3):R306–13.
247. Andres AC, Strange R. Apoptosis in the estrous and menstrual cycles. J Mammary Gland Biol Neoplasia. 1999;4(2):221–8.
248. Fanager H, Ree HJ. Cyclic changes of human mammary gland epithelium inrelation to the menstrual cycle–an ultrastructural study. Cancer. 1974;34:574–85.

249. Ferguson JE, Schor AM, Howell A, Ferguson MW. Changes in the extracellular matrix of the normal human breast during the menstrual cycle. Cell Tissue Res. 1992;268(1):167–77.
250. McCarty KS Jr, Sasso R, Budwit D, Georgiade GS, Seigler HF. Immunoglobulin localization in the normal human mammary gland: variation with the menstrual cycle. Am J Pathol. 1982;107(3):322–6.
251. Kass R, Mancino AT, Rosenbloom A L, Klimberg VS, Bland KI. Breast physiology: normal and abnormal development and function. In: Bland KI, Copeland III EM, editors. The breast: comprehensive management of benign and malignant disorders. 3rd ed. St. Louis, Missouri: Saunders; 2004.
252. Silva JS, Georgiade GS, Dilley WG, McCarty KS Sr, Wells SA Jr, McCarty KS Jr. Menstrual cycle-dependent variations of breast cyst fluid proteins and sex steroid receptors in the normal human breast. Cancer. 1983;51(7):1297–302.
253. Fabris G, Marchetti E, Marzola A, Bagni A, Guerzoli P, Nenci I. Pathophysiology of estrogen receptors in mammary tissue by monoclonal antibodies. J Steroid Biochem. 1987;27:171–6.
254. Dabrosin C. Increased extracellular local levels of estradiol in normal breast in vivo during the luteal phase of the menstrual cycle. J Endocrinol. 2005;187(1):103–8.
255. Gompel A, Martin A, Simon P, Schoevaert D, Plu-Bureau G, Hugol D, et al. Epidermal growth factor receptor and c-erbB-2 expression in normal breast tissue during the menstrual cycle. Breast Cancer Res Treat. 1996;38(2):227–35.
256. Nevalainen MT, Xie J, Bubendorf L, Wagner KU, Rui H. Basal activation of transcription factor signal transducer and activator of transcription (Stat5) in nonpregnant mouse and human breast epithelium. Mol Endocrinol. 2002;16(5):1108–24.
257. Ham AW. Histology. 6th ed. Philadelphia: J.B. Lippincott Company; 1969.
258. Russell TD, Palmer CA, Orlicky DJ, Fischer A, Rudolph MC, Neville MC, et al. Cytoplasmic lipid droplet accumulation in developing mammary epithelial cells: roles of adipophilin and lipid metabolism. J Lipid Res. 2007;48(7):1463–75.
259. Piliero SJ, Jacobs MS, Wischnitzer S. Atlas of histology. Philadelphia: J.B. Lippincott Company; 1965.
260. Medina D. Mammary developmental fate and breast cancer risk. Endocr Relat Cancer. 2005;12(3):483–95.
261. Balogh GA, Heulings R, Mailo DA, Russo PA, Sheriff F, Russo IH, et al. Genomic signature induced by pregnancy in the human breast. Int J Oncol. 2006;28(2):399–410.
262. Popnikolov N, Yang J, Liu A, Guzman R, Nandi S. Reconstituted normal human breast in nude mice: effect of host pregnancy environment and human chorionic gonadotropin on proliferation. J Endocrinol. 2001;168(3):487–96.
263. Numan M. Maternal behavior. In: Knobil E, Neill JD, editors. The physiology of reproduction. New York: Raven Press; 1994. p. 221–302.
264. Eliassen AH, Tworoger SS, Hankinson SE. Reproductive factors and family history of breast cancer in relation to plasma prolactin levels in premenopausal and postmenopausal women. Int J Cancer. 2007;120(7):1536–41.
265. Blakely CM, Stoddard AJ, Belka GK, Dugan KD, Notarfrancesco KL, Moody SE, et al. Hormone-induced protection against mammary tumorigenesis is conserved in multiple rat strains and identifies a core gene expression signature induced by pregnancy. Cancer Res. 2006;66(12):6421–31.
266. Russo J, Mailo D, Hu YF, Balogh G, Sheriff F, Russo IH. Breast differentiation and its implication in cancer prevention. Clin Cancer Res. 2005;11(2 Pt 2):931s–6s.
267. Russo J, Moral R, Balogh GA, Mailo D, Russo IH. The protective role of pregnancy in breast cancer. Breast Cancer Res. 2005;7(3):131–42.
268. Jackson D, Bresnick J, Dickson C. A role for fibroblast growth factor signaling in the lobuloalveolar development of the mammary gland. J Mammary Gland Biol Neoplasia. 1997;2(4):385–92.
269. Laud K, Hornez L, Gourdou I, Belair L, Arnold A, Peyrat JP, et al. Expression of BRCA1 gene in ewe mammary epithelial cells during pregnancy: regulation by growth hormone and steroid hormones. Eur J Endocrinol/Eur Fed Endocr Soc. 2001;145(6):763–70.
270. Furuta S, Jiang X, Gu B, Cheng E, Chen PL, Lee WH. Depletion of BRCA1 impairs differentiation but enhances proliferation of mammary epithelial cells. Proc Natl Acad Sci USA. 2005;102(26):9176–81.
271. Burkitt HG, Young B, Heathe JW. Wheater's functional histology, a text and coulour atlas. 3rd ed. Edinburgh: Churchill Livingstone; 1993.
272. Espinosa LA, Daniel BL, Vidarsson L, Zakhour M, Ikeda DM, Herfkens RJ. The lactating breast: contrast-enhanced MR imaging of normal tissue and cancer. Radiology. 2005;237(2):429–36.
273. Forsyth I. Mammary gland, overview. In: Knobil E, Neill JD, editors. Encyclopedia of reproduction. 1999: Cambridge: Academic Press; 1999. p. 81–8.
274. Neville MC. Milk secretion: an overview. Denver, CO1998 [updated 199807/31/2007]; Available from: http://mammary.nih.gov/Reviews/lactation/Neville001/index.html.
275. Itoh M, Bissell MJ. The organization of tight junctions in epithelia: implications for mammary gland biology and breast tumorigenesis. J Mammary Gland Biol Neoplasia. 2003;8(4):449–62.
276. Young B, Wheater PR. Wheater's functional histology: a text and colour atlas. 5th ed. Oxford: Churchill Livingstone Elsevier; 2006. x, 437p.
277. Kolb AF. Engineering immunity in the mammary gland. J Mammary Gland Biol Neoplasia. 2002;7(2):123–34.
278. Uauy R, De Andraca I. Human milk and breast feeding for optimal mental development. J Nutr. 1995;125(8 Suppl):2278S–80S.
279. Lawson M. Contemporary aspects of infant feeding. Paediatr Nurs. 2007;19(2):39–46.
280. Owen CG, Whincup PH, Gilg JA, Cook DG. Effect of breast feeding in infancy on blood pressure in later life: systematic review and meta-analysis. BMJ. 2003;327(7425):1189–95.
281. Martin RM, Middleton N, Gunnell D, Owen CG, Smith GD. Breast-feeding and cancer: the Boyd Orr cohort and a systematic review with meta-analysis. J Natl Cancer Inst. 2005;97(19):1446–57.
282. Frank JW, Newman J. Breast-feeding in a polluted world: uncertain risks, clear benefits. CMAJ. 1993;149(1):33–7.
283. Rudolph MC, McManaman JL, Phang T, Russell T, Kominsky DJ, Serkova NJ, et al. Metabolic regulation in the lactating mammary gland: a lipid synthesizing machine. Physiol Genomics. 2007;28(3):323–36.
284. Villalpando S, del Prado M. Interrelation among dietary energy and fat intakes, maternal body fatness, and milk total lipid in humans. J Mammary Gland Biol Neoplasia. 1999;4(3):285–95.
285. Neville MC. Calcium secretion into milk. J Mammary Gland Biol Neoplasia. 2005;10(2):119–28.
286. Keenan TS, Franke WW, Mather IH, Morre DJ. Endomembrane composition and function in milk formation. In: Larson BL, editor. Lactation. New York: Academic Press, Inc.; 1978. p. 105.
287. Linzell JL, Peaker M. Mechanism of milk secretion. Physiol Rev. 1971;51(3):564–97.
288. Neville MC. The physiological basis of milk secretion. Ann NY Acad Sci. 1990;586:1–11.

289. Fleishaker JC, McNamara PJ. In vivo evaluation in the lactating rabbit of a model for xenobiotic distribution into breast milk. J Pharmacol Exp Ther. 1988;244(3):919–24.
290. Hunziker W, Kraehenbuhl JP. Epithelial transcytosis of immunoglobulins. J Mammary Gland Biol Neoplasia. 1998;3 (3):287–302.
291. Csontos K, Rust M, Hollt V, Mahr W, Kromer W, Teschemacher HJ. Elevated plasma beta-endorphin levels in pregnant women and their neonates. Life Sci. 1979;25(10):835–44.
292. Clevenger CV, Plank TL. Prolactin as an autocrine/paracrine factor in breast tissue. J Mammary Gland Biol Neoplasia. 1997;2 (1):59–68.
293. Mol JA, Lantinga-van Leeuwen I, van Garderen E, Rijnberk A. Progestin-induced mammary growth hormone (GH) production. Adv Exp Med Biol. 2000;480:71–6.
294. McNeilly AS, Robinson IC, Houston MJ, Howie PW. Release of oxytocin and prolactin in response to suckling. Br Med J. 1983;286(6361):257–9.
295. Martin RH, Oakey RE. The role of antenatal oestrogen in post-partum human lactogenesis: evidence from oestrogen-deficient pregnancies. Clin Endocrinol. 1982;17 (4):403–8.
296. Daly SE, Kent JC, Owens RA, Hartmann PE. Frequency and degree of milk removal and the short-term control of human milk synthesis. Exp Physiol. 1996;81(5):861–75.
297. Hadsell D, George J, Torres D. The declining phase of lactation: peripheral or central, programmed or pathological? J Mammary Gland Biol Neoplasia. 2007;12(1):59–70.
298. Itahana Y, Piens M, Sumida T, Fong S, Muschler J, Desprez PY. Regulation of clusterin expression in mammary epithelial cells. Exp Cell Res. 2007;313(5):943–51.
299. Mennella JA, Pepino MY, Teff KL. Acute alcohol consumption disrupts the hormonal milieu of lactating women. J Clin Endocrinol Metab. 2005;90(4):1979–85.
300. Butte NF, Hopkinson JM. Body composition changes during lactation are highly variable among women. J Nutr. 1998;128(2 Suppl):381S–5S.
301. Ganong W. Review of medical physiology. 22nd ed: New York: Lange; 2005.
302. Dewey KG. Effects of maternal caloric restriction and exercise during lactation. J Nutr. 1998;128(2 Suppl):386S–9S.
303. Wysolmerski J. Calcium handling by the lactating breast and its relationship to calcium-related complications of breast cancer. J Mammary Gland Biol Neoplasia. 2005;10(2):101–3.
304. Kovacs CS. Calcium and bone metabolism during pregnancy and lactation. J Mammary Gland Biol Neoplasia. 2005;10(2):105–18.
305. Wilde CJ, Knight CH, Flint DJ. Control of milk secretion and apoptosis during mammary involution. J Mammary Gland Biol Neoplasia. 1999;4(2):129–36.
306. Talhouk RS, Bissell MJ, Werb Z. Coordinated expression of extracellular matrix-degrading proteinases and their inhibitors regulates mammary epithelial function during involution. J Cell Biol. 1992;118(5):1271–82.
307. Marti A, Lazar H, Ritter P, Jaggi R. Transcription factor activities and gene expression during mouse mammary gland involution. J Mammary Gland Biol Neoplasia. 1999;4(2):145–52.
308. Stein T, Salomonis N, Gusterson BA. Mammary gland involution as a multi-step process. J Mammary Gland Biol Neoplasia. 2007;12(1):25–35.
309. Watson CJ, Kreuzaler PA. Remodeling mechanisms of the mammary gland during involution. Int J Dev Biol. 2011;55(7–9):757–62 Epub 2011/12/14.
310. Jaggi R. Morphological changes during programmed cell death (PCD) in the involuting mouse mammary gland. 1996; Available from: http://mammary.nih.gov/reviews/development/Jaggi001/index.html.
311. Baxter FO, Neoh K, Tevendale MC. The beginning of the end: death signaling in early involution. J Mammary Gland Biol Neoplasia. 2007;12(1):3–13.
312. Thorburn A. Apoptosis and autophagy: regulatory connections between two supposedly different processes. Apoptosis. 2007; online first.
313. Atabai K, Sheppard D, Werb Z. Roles of the innate immune system in mammary gland remodeling during involution. J Mammary Gland Biol Neoplasia. 2007;12(1):37–45.
314. Fadok VA. Clearance: the last and often forgotten stage of apoptosis. J Mammary Gland Biol Neoplasia. 1999;4(2):203–11.
315. Watson CJ. Involution: apoptosis and tissue remodelling that convert the mammary gland from milk factory to a quiescent organ. Breast Cancer Res. 2006;8(2):203.
316. Streuli CH, Gilmore AP. Adhesion-mediated signaling in the regulation of mammary epithelial cell survival. J Mammary Gland Biol Neoplasia. 1999;4(2):183–91.
317. Martinez-Hernandez A, Fink LM, Pierce GB. Removal of basement membrane in the involuting breast. Lab Invest; a journal of technical methods and pathology. 1976;34(5):455–62.
318. Simpson HW, McArdle CS, George WD, Griffiths K, Turkes A, Pauson AW. Pregnancy postponement and childlessness leads to chronic hypervascularity of the breasts and cancer risk. Br J Cancer. 2002;87(11):1246–52.
319. Flint DJ, Tonner E, Allan GJ. Insulin-like growth factor binding proteins: IGF-dependent and -independent effects in the mammary gland. J Mammary Gland Biol Neoplasia. 2000;5(1):65–73.
320. Lochrie JD, Phillips K, Tonner E, Flint DJ, Allan GJ, Price NC, et al. Insulin-like growth factor binding protein (IGFBP)-5 is upregulated during both differentiation and apoptosis in primary cultures of mouse mammary epithelial cells. J Cell Physiol. 2006;207(2):471–9.
321. Mikkola ML, Millar SE. The mammary bud as a skin appendage: unique and shared aspects of development. J Mammary Gland Biol Neoplasia. 2006;11(3–4):187–203.
322. Dillon C, Spencer-Dene B, Dickson C. A crucial role for fibroblast growth factor signaling in embryonic mammary gland development. J Mammary Gland Biol Neoplasia. 2004;9(2):207–15.
323. Watson CJ, Burdon TG. Prolactin signal transduction mechanisms in the mammary gland: the role of the Jak/Stat pathway. Rev Reprod. 1996;1(1):1–5.
324. Hu X, Juneja SC, Maihle NJ, Cleary MP. Leptin–a growth factor in normal and malignant breast cells and for normal mammary gland development. J Natl Cancer Inst. 2002;94(22):1704–11.
325. Dontu G, Jackson KW, McNicholas E, Kawamura MJ, Abdallah WM, Wicha MS. Role of Notch signaling in cell-fate determination of human mammary stem/progenitor cells. Breast Cancer Res. 2004;6(6):R605–15.
326. Dontu G, Wicha MS. Survival of mammary stem cells in suspension culture: implications for stem cell biology and neoplasia. J Mammary Gland Biol Neoplasia. 2005;10(1):75–86.
327. Rowley M, Grothey E, Couch FJ. The role of Tbx2 and Tbx3 in mammary development and tumorigenesis. J Mammary Gland Biol Neoplasia. 2004;9(2):109–18.
328. Lewis MT, Veltmaat JM. Next stop, the twilight zone: hedgehog network regulation of mammary gland development. J Mammary Gland Biol Neoplasia. 2004;9(2):165–81.
329. Hatsell S, Frost AR. Hedgehog signaling in mammary gland development and breast cancer. J Mammary Gland Biol Neoplasia. 2007;12(2–3):163–73.
330. Groner B. Transcription factor regulation in mammary epithelial cells. Domest Anim Endocrinol. 2002;23(1–2):25–32.

331. Zhou J, Chehab R, Tkalcevic J, Naylor MJ, Harris J, Wilson TJ, et al. Elf5 is essential for early embryogenesis and mammary gland development during pregnancy and lactation. EMBO J. 2005;24(3):635–44.
332. Puppin C, Puglisi F, Pellizzari L, Manfioletti G, Pestrin M, Pandolfi M, et al. HEX expression and localization in normal mammary gland and breast carcinoma. BMC Cancer. 2006;6:192.
333. van Genderen C, Okamura RM, Farinas I, Quo RG, Parslow TG, Bruhn L, et al. Development of several organs that require inductive epithelial-mesenchymal interactions is impaired in LEF-1-deficient mice. Genes Dev. 1994;8(22):2691–703 Epub 1994/11/15.
334. Davenport TG, Jerome-Majewska LA, Papaioannou VE. Mammary gland, limb and yolk sac defects in mice lacking Tbx3, the gene mutated in human ulnar mammary syndrome. Development. 2003;130(10):2263–73. Epub 2003/04/02.
335. Satokata I, Ma L, Ohshima H, Bei M, Woo I, Nishizawa K, et al. Msx2 deficiency in mice causes pleiotropic defects in bone growth and ectodermal organ formation. Nat Genet. 2000;24(4):391–5 Epub 2000/03/31.
336. Dunbar ME, Wysolmerski JJ. Parathyroid hormone-related protein: a developmental regulatory molecule necessary for mammary gland development. J Mammary Gland Biol Neoplasia. 1999;4(1):21–34 Epub 1999/04/29.
337. Kim H, Laing M, Muller W. c-Src-null mice exhibit defects in normal mammary gland development and ERalpha signaling. Oncogene. 2005;24(36):5629–36 Epub 2005/07/12.
338. Lydon JP, DeMayo FJ, Funk CR, Mani SK, Hughes AR, Montgomery CA Jr, et al. Mice lacking progesterone receptor exhibit pleiotropic reproductive abnormalities. Genes Dev. 1995;9(18):2266–78 Epub 1995/09/15.
339. Horseman ND, Zhao W, Montecino-Rodriguez E, Tanaka M, Nakashima K, Engle SJ, et al. Defective mammopoiesis, but normal hematopoiesis, in mice with a targeted disruption of the prolactin gene. EMBO J. 1997;16(23):6926–35 Epub 1998/01/31.
340. Liu X, Robinson GW, Wagner KU, Garrett L, Wynshaw-Boris A, Hennighausen L. Stat5a is mandatory for adult mammary gland development and lactogenesis. Genes Dev. 1997;11(2):179–86 Epub 1997/01/15.
341. Wagner KU, Krempler A, Triplett AA, Qi Y, George NM, Zhu J, et al. Impaired alveologenesis and maintenance of secretory mammary epithelial cells in Jak2 conditional knockout mice. Mol Cell Biol. 2004;24(12):5510–20 Epub 2004/06/01.
342. Stinnakre MG, Vilotte JL, Soulier S, Mercier JC. Creation and phenotypic analysis of alpha-lactalbumin-deficient mice. Proc Natl Acad Sci USA. 1994;91(14):6544–8 Epub 1994/07/05.
343. Triplett AA, Sakamoto K, Matulka LA, Shen L, Smith GH, Wagner KU. Expression of the whey acidic protein (Wap) is necessary for adequate nourishment of the offspring but not functional differentiation of mammary epithelial cells. Genesis. 2005;43(1):1–11 Epub 2005/08/18.
344. Wagner KU, Young WS 3rd, Liu X, Ginns EI, Li M, Furth PA, et al. Oxytocin and milk removal are required for post-partum mammary-gland development. Genes Funct. 1997;1(4):233–44 Epub 1998/07/25.
345. Pollard JW, Hennighausen L. Colony stimulating factor 1 is required for mammary gland development during pregnancy. Proc Natl Acad Sci USA. 1994;91(20):9312–6 Epub 1994/09/27.
346. Fantl V, Stamp G, Andrews A, Rosewell I, Dickson C. Mice lacking cyclin D1 are small and show defects in eye and mammary gland development. Genes Dev. 1995;9(19):2364–72 Epub 1995/10/01.

Congenital and Developmental Abnormalities of the Breast

2

Kristin Baumann and Telja Pursche

2.1 Embryology

Development in the prenatal breast is characterized by two main processes: formation of a primary mammary bud and development of a rudimentary mammary gland [1]. Formation of the glands in the embryo starts independent of gender in an identical way. Embryogenesis in the first trimester runs largely hormone independent [2, 3], whereas in the second trimester regulatory factors are important for development [4].

During the 4th and 6th week of gestation, two ridges called the mammary crests or milk lines are formed out of a pair of epidermal ectoderm. The ridges extend in a line between the fetal axilla and inguinal region, but rapidly regress except in the thorax. The primary bud forms by penetration in the chest wall mesenchyme. Out of this, diverse secondary buds rise and develop into lactiferous ducts and their branches. The fibrous stroma and fat of the mammary gland develop out of the surrounding mesenchyme. The small ducts and alveoli are formed out of the lactiferous ducts.

At the beginning of the second trimester, the nipple–areolar complex (NAC) starts to form out of differentiated mesenchymal cells. Hair follicles and sweat glands differentiate. By 20 and 30 weeks, canalization of the branched epithelial tissues is induced by placental sex hormones. Between 32 and 40 weeks, differentiation of the parenchyma into alveolar and lobular structures takes place. A shallow mammary pit is formed by depression of the epidermis, becoming the NAC onto which the lactiferous ducts open. At 34 weeks, the breast bud becomes palpable, sized approximately 3 mm at 36 weeks of age and 4–10 mm by 40 weeks.

In exploring data concerning breast development, most sources agree that the secondary processes end in rudimentary lobular structures or end buds [1, 5, 6]. Contrary to this, some assume that there cannot be found any evidence of lobules breast at birth, only ductal structures with surrounding stroma [7].

2.2 Early Development of the Mammary Gland

In the neonate, the breast is usually palpable with variation in amount of tissue and no significant difference between the genders [8]. From four to seven days, postpartum neonates may show a unilateral or bilateral breast enlargement and/or transient secretion of colostral milk under the influence of maternal estrogens, also known as witch's milk [9].

The nipples evert soon after birth by proliferation of the underlying mesoderm and the pigmentation of the areolae increases [10]. Until puberty, the breast remains largely quiescent, independent of gender.

Nodular growth of one or both breasts in either gender before puberty is quite usual; up to 90 % of neonates may have palpable breast tissue that typically resolves spontaneously within few months [11]. Tumors of the infantile breast are benign in most cases. Nevertheless, observation is recommended due to rarely malignant occurrence [12].

One has to consider that biopsy of the pre-pubertal breast may irreversibly cause disruption of breast development [13], and therefore, application should be used with restrictions.

2.3 Thelarche

The physiological breast development in females is called thelarche, normally occurring at the age of eight years as a result of rising levels of estradiol. Estrogen stimulates ductal growth and branching, whereas progesterone influences lobular and alveolar development. Androgens as testosterone and

K. Baumann (✉) · T. Pursche
Clinic for Gynaecology and Obstetrics, University Medical Centre Schleswig-Holstein Campus Lübeck, Ratzeburger Allee 160, 23538 Lübeck, Schleswig-Holstein, Germany
e-mail: Kristin.baumann@uksh.de

T. Pursche
e-mail: telja.pursche@uksh.de

I. Jatoi and A. Rody (eds.), *Management of Breast Diseases*, DOI 10.1007/978-3-319-46356-8_2

dihydrotestosterone limit breast development [11]. Prolactin stimulates the alveolar buds. Increase of volume and elasticity of the connective tissues, vascularity, and fat deposition occurs resulting in progressive enlargement of the breasts.

The breast expansion normally lasts approximately until 25 years of age. This should be taken into consideration concerning interventional options including neoplasms and malformations. It has to be pointed out that every breast trauma (including iatrogenic intervention) before completed development can lead to developmental disorders.

2.4 Anatomy of the Breast

Superficial to the pectoralis major muscle on the anterior chest wall, the human breast is vertically located between the second anterior rib to the sixth anterior rib and horizontally between the lateral edge of the sternum and the mid-axillary line.

The breast tissue is formed by mammary gland, fat tissue, blood vessels, lymphatics, and nerves. The surface of the breast is attached by suspensory fibrous ligaments, called Cooper's ligament. These ligaments pass through the mammary gland from the superficial fascia to the deep fascia overlying the pectoralis major muscle. The extension of the breast varies in females, lasting from the midline to the near the mid-axillary line. Based on the embryological development, the maximum percentage of mammary gland is situated in the upper outer quadrant of the breast. Characteristically, the breast shows an elliptical base and a hemispheric shape.

The architecture of the breast is built by lactiferous ducts and lobes which are arranged radially around the nipple–areolar complex (NAC), opening on the nipple.

Functionally, the milk production takes place in the lobes, whereas the transport of the lactation products occurs by the ducts. Anatomically, each lobe consists of 20–40 lobules, containing 10–100 alveoli. During the lactation period, milk accumulates in the so-called lactiferous sinus, representing the excretory duct of each lactiferous duct. Breast parenchyma consists of connective tissue, including lymphatic and vascular components as well as fat.

Vascular supply of the breast is performed by the internal mammary and lateral thoracic arteries supplemented by lateral and anterior cutaneous branches of the intercostal arteries and subdermal vessels. The venous drainage primarily leads into the axilla and then further flows into the internal thoracic, lateral thoracic, and intercostal veins.

The lymphatic drain of the breast ends up in the regional lymph nodes, composed of axillary, supra-, and infraclavicular lymph nodes as well as the internal mammary lymph node chain, intrathoracic located in the parasternal space.

Innervation of the breast gland and overlying skin is performed mainly by the fourth lateral intercostal nerve.

2.5 Premature Thelarche

Premature thelarche is defined as premature breast tissue development unilaterally or bilaterally without other signs of sexual maturation. Common premature thelarche occurs between 6 and 24 months of age [14]. Most girls undergo puberty appropriately. Premature thelarche is in approximately 18 % of girls, the first manifestation sign of central precocious puberty [15]. Continued clinical observation every six months is recommended to distinguish from that differential diagnosis.

Higher levels of estrogen were found in girls with premature thelarche, measured by ultrasensitive bioassays compared to controls [16].

The etiology of premature thelarche is multifactorial. Endocrine disruptors, genetic, and nutritional factors can be proofed. It has been shown that some girls with exaggerated or fluctuating thelarche show an activating mutation in the GNAS gene, codifying for alpha subunit of G stimulating protein (Gsalpha) [16, 17].

Typical benign idiopathic thelarche is a self-limiting condition without need for treatment. If a precocious puberty is suspected, the referral to a pediatric endocrinologist is strongly recommended.

2.6 Accessory Breast Tissue: Polymastia/Polythelia

Based on the embryological development, accessory breast tissue can occur in the realm of the former embryonic milk line (Fig. 2.1). Occurrence is most often sporadic with an average in the general population between 0.22 and 6 % and a higher rate in women compared to men [18].

A distinction is drawn between polythelia, the most common type of accessory breast tissue and polymastia.

Polythelia describes the existence of supernumerary nipples or nipple–areolar complexes. It can be found in both males and females and may occur at any point along the embryonic milk line between axilla and groin. An association with nephrourologic abnormalities exists in sporadic cases [18, 19]. High blood pressure and conductive or rhythm disturbances represent cardiovascular problems which are associated with polythelia [19]. Surgery is requested for esthetic reasons or due to discomfort.

Polymastia describes the presence of supernumerary breasts along the former milk line which may appear with or

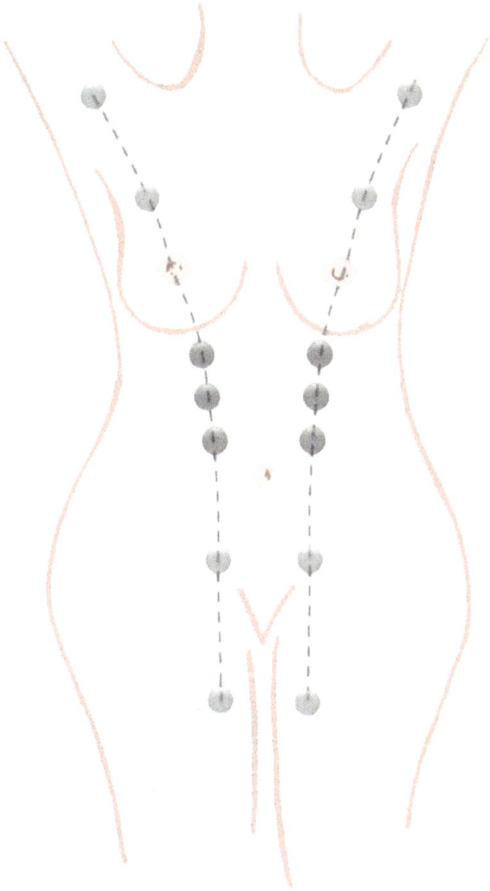

Fig. 2.1 Schematic illustration of the former embryonic milk line, where accessory breast tissue may appear

without nipples or areolae. The axilla is a common site of ectopic breast tissue [19] (Fig. 2.2); rarely, aberrant breast tissue can also be found at face, neck, torso, vulva, and lower extremities [18].

Symptomatic manifestation often occurs during menstrual periods or pregnancy when the breast tissue becomes tender, enlarged, or lactates. Reasons for surgical excision would include discomfort due to tenderness, milk secretion [19], or perhaps purely for esthetics.

2.7 Underdevelopment of the Mammary Corpus

Female breasts are typically not equal in size, especially during development, for unknown reasons. The left breast is statistically more often larger [20].

Depending on the underlying developmental disturbance, several forms can be discriminated [21]. The various developmental forms are addressed below.

2.7.1 Breast Hypoplasia

Hypoplasia can occur unilaterally, causing an asymmetric body image or bilateral. In some cases, it is associated with complex developmental syndromes such as the Poland syndrome, which is described later in this text.

Besides congenital causes, a variety of acquired reasons can lead to breast hypoplasia such as hormonal disorders or tumors. Iatrogenic causes, including medication, operations, radiation, and trauma, can also lead to hypoplasia [22, 23].

Depending on severity, breast hypoplasia may cause physical discomfort and significant psychological burden, especially in adolescence.

For the treating physicians, it is a huge challenge to determine the optimal timing for surgical intervention. The wishes of the adolescent girl for early adjustment must be considered in contrast to the risk of postoperative

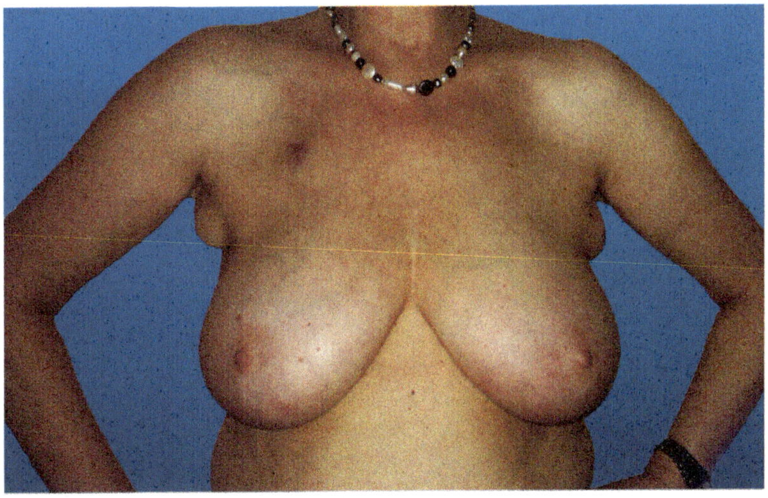

Fig. 2.2 Woman with polymastia with accessory axillary breast tissue

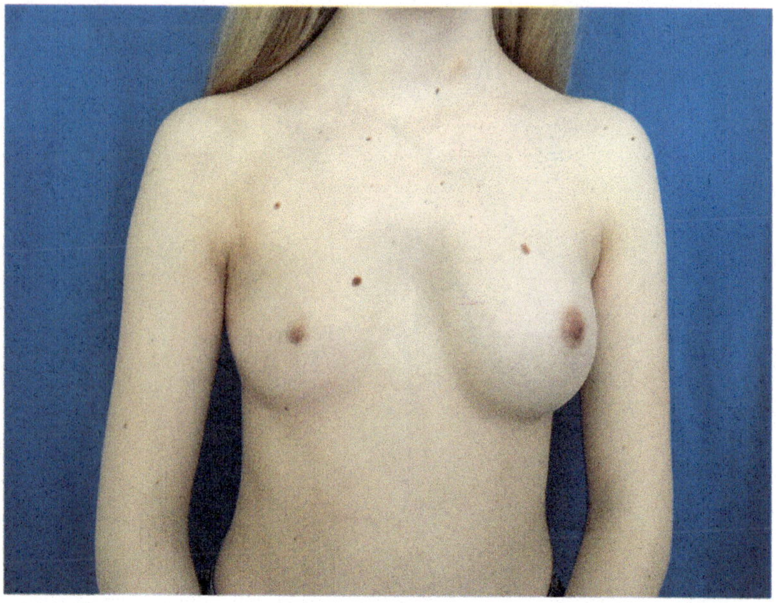

Fig. 2.3 Young woman with right breast micromastia

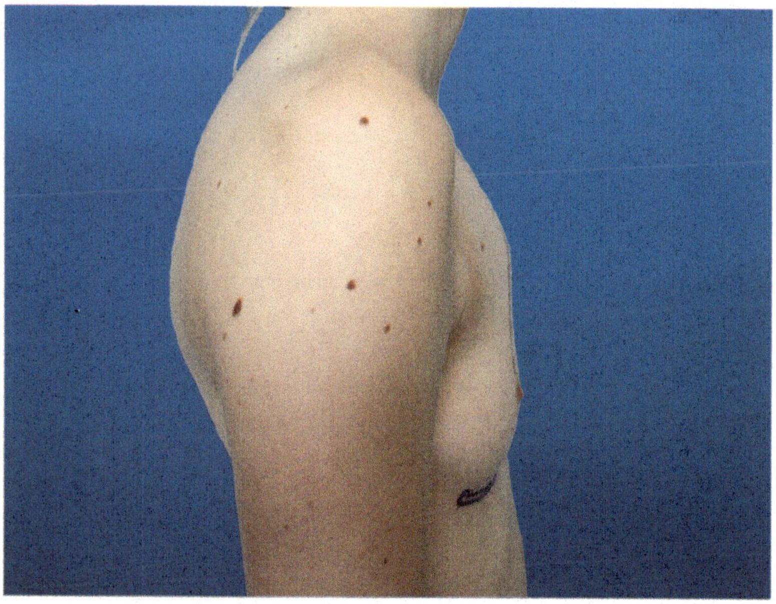

Fig. 2.4 Young woman with right breast micromastia

asymmetrical growth that may necessitate additional surgery and increase the risk of morbidity.

Still, many surgeons recommend protracting treatment until the breast development has finished or at least the patient shows stable adult weight and breast volume for one year [24, 25].

Generally, treatment of unilateral breast hypoplasia contains augmentation of the affected breast but remains a reconstructive challenge. Autologous versus heterologous techniques as one- and two-stage procedures with prior expansion of the overlying skin envelope should be carefully weighed against each other. The advantage of autologous reconstruction contains better long-term results but acceptance of longer operation time and additional donor site morbidity (Figs. 2.3, 2.4, 2.5 and 2.6).

2.7.2 Amastia/Athelia

Once the mammary ridges fail to develop or disappear completely [26], hypoplasia of mammary tissue results in varying specificity. Congenital disorders concerning breast development can be discriminated into amastia, amazia, and athelia.

- *Amastia* describes the complete absence of breast tissue, nipple, and areola.

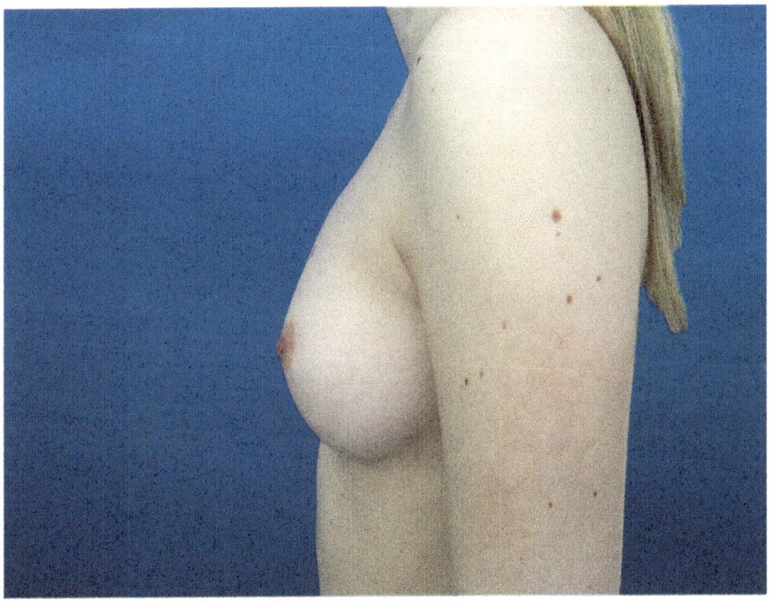

Fig. 2.5 Young woman with right breast micromastia

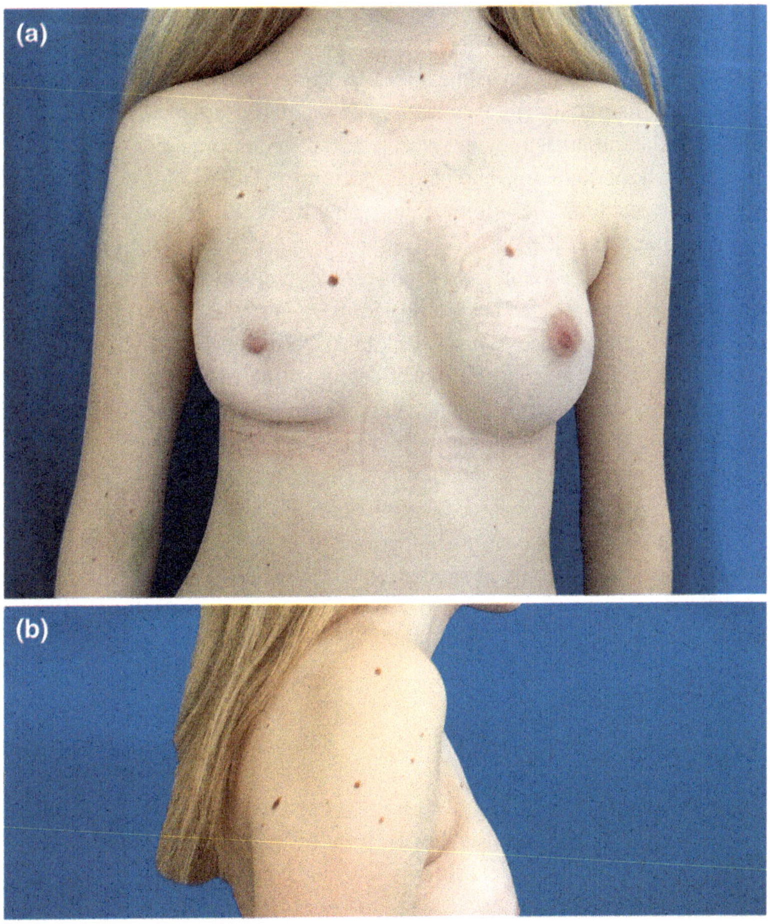

Fig. 2.6 **a** Young woman with *right* breast micromastia. **b** Postoperative result after performing *right* breast augmentation

Table 2.1 Classification of Poland syndrome

	Class I	Class II	Class III
Hypoplastic breast	√		
Hypoplastic NAC	√		
Hypoplastic pectoralis muscle	√		
Hypoplastic breast or absence of breast		√	√
Hypoplastic NAC or absence of NAC		√	√
Absence of pectoralis muscle (sternocostal portion)		√	√
Thoracic skeleton abnormalities minimal		√	
Thoracic skeleton abnormalities distinct			√
Others			√

Source Data from Hartrampf [37]

- *Amazia* is defined as the absence of one or both of the mammary glands without impairment of nipple and areola [27].
- *Athelia* is the congenital lack of one or both nipples.

Causes can be congenital as well as iatrogenic. The first case of amastia was reported in 1939 by Froriep. Because of the rare occurrence, data refer to only few cases. There are three subgroups of amastia. (1) congenital ectodermal defects leading to bilateral amastia; (2) unilateral amastia; and (3) bilateral amastia with variable associated anomalies, including hypertelorism, anomalous pectoral muscles, cleft palate, upper limb deformities, and abnormalities of the genitourinary tract [28].

Associations between special congenital syndromes and amastia or athelia have been reported. This includes ectodermal dysplasia, the Mayer–Rokitansky–Kuster–Hauser syndrome, where a failure of development of the Müllerian duct leads to accompanying vaginal-uterine agenesis [29, 30], as well as the Poland Syndrome (see Sect. 2.7.3). Exclusive occurrence of athelia is extremely rare. It is described in some various congenital syndromes.

Surgical correction is normally performed in several steps, for instance, the procedure commences with tissue expansion and finishing with placing the definitive implant or use of autogenous tissue such as abdominals or gluteal flaps.

2.7.3 Poland Syndrome

In 1841, Alfred Poland described a rare congenital anomaly characterized by unilateral underdevelopment or absence of the pectoralis major muscle. It was first named in 1962 by Clarkson [31]. It may occur with different gravity, with range from mild to severe which makes the classification difficult. Ribs, sternum, other muscles of thorax and abdomen, skin, breast, and nipple can all be abnormal, missing, or underdeveloped [32–35].

Most often, occurrence is sporadic with an incidence ranging from one in 20,000–30,000 live births [12, 35]. Males and the right side are more often affected with a ratio of 3:1 [32, 36].

One possible classification was described by Hartrampf, who defined three classes occurring since the 1980s (Table 2.1).

The cause of Poland syndrome is unknown. Etiology is hypothesized to be related to an intrauterine interruption of the embryonic blood supply to the subclavian arteries at about the 46th day of embryonic development, disrupting normal development of the chest wall and upper limb [35, 38]. The range of signs and symptoms that occur in Poland syndrome may be explained by variations in the site and extent of the disruption.

Another theory postulates an abnormal migration of embryonic tissues. Development of the primitive limb bud that later forms the pectoralis muscle takes place in the 9-mm embryo; later, the bud splits into clavicular, pectoral, and sternal components in the 15-mm embryo. An explanation for Poland deformity could be defective attachment or failure of attachment of that bud to the upper rib cage and sternum [39, 40].

The aim of surgical reconstruction treatment is to conceal the deformity and create an esthetic, natural appearing décolleté and breast according to the unaffected opposite side.

Possible techniques include the use of breast implants, tissue expanders, and autologous tissue (pedicled or free). While planning the reconstruction, one ought to consider that volume discrepancies might lead to displacement of the NAC and a new symmetric inframammary fold has to be formed. If necessary, a contralateral adjustment of breast might be indicated to achieve an esthetic and satisfactory goal.

2.7.4 Tubular/Tuberous Breast

Rees and Aston [41] first shaped the term tuberous breast, describing a hypoplastic breast deformity with a narrowed breast base diameter, malposition of the constricted inframammary fold, and herniation of breast tissue through the areola (Fig. 2.7).

Due to the reduced transverse breast diameter and base constriction, the breast seems to herniate into the NUC. This unique appearance caused the descriptive term "*Snoopy-nose deformity*" [42].

The condition may be unilateral or bilateral. In many cases, there exists a significant asymmetry between both breasts. Exact incidence and etiology remains unknown.

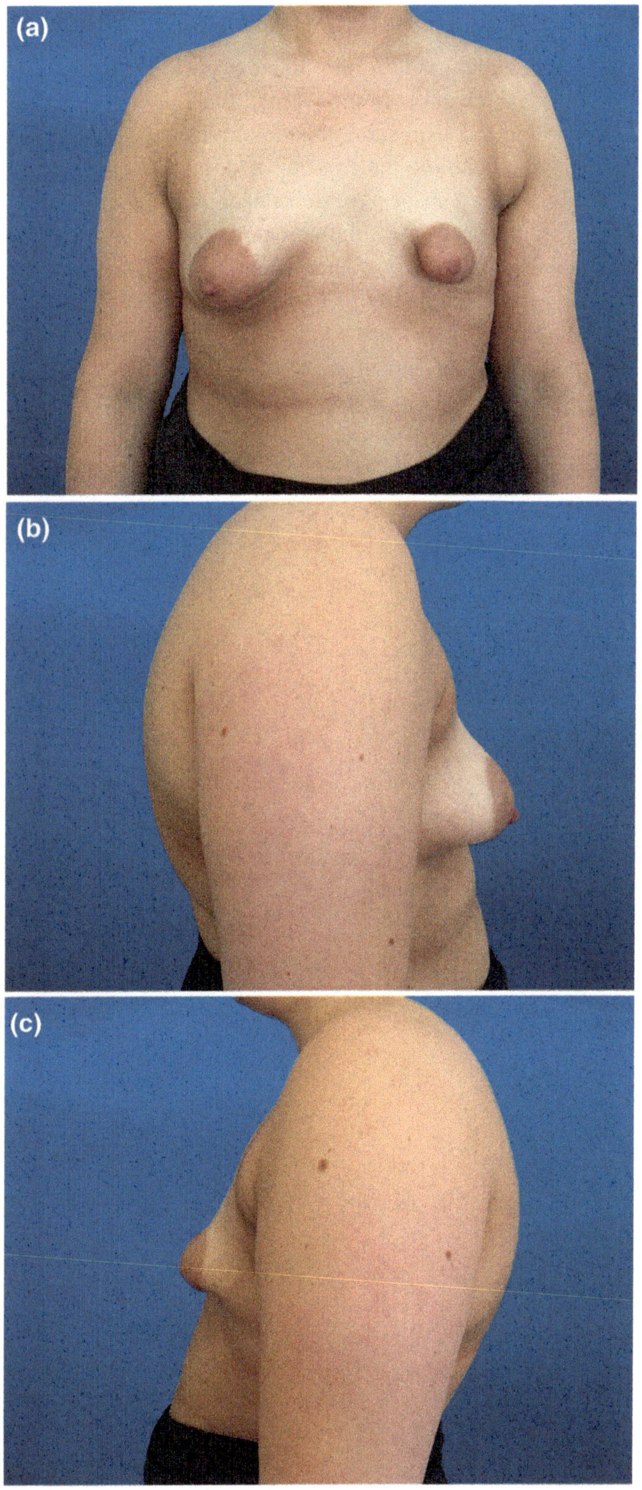

Fig. 2.7 Young woman with tubular breast deformity, characterized by a narrowed base diameter and pseudo-herniated breast tissue through the enlarged nipple–areolar complex (NAC). **a** anterior view, **b** right, and **c** left facing lateral view

Table 2.2 Classification of tuberous breast

Type I	Hypoplasia of the lower medial quadrant
Type II	Hypoplasia of the lower medial and lateral quadrants sufficient skin in the subareolar region
Type III	Hypoplasia of the lower medial and lateral quadrants deficiency of skin in the subareolar region
Type IV	Severe breast constriction with minimal breast base

Source Data from von Heimburg [43]

Classifications graduate the different occurrence of malformation. An example is shown in Table 2.2.

Regarding reconstruction, this deformity remains a challenge. While planning the concept of surgery, all abnormal elements in breast shape have to be taken into consideration.

Depending on tissue volume, autologous reconstruction with internal flaps or combinations with heterologous materials such as implants or expanders are used.

Furthermore, the ideal timing for surgery should be identified and the possible advantage of a two-stage reconstructive approach should be debated for gradually expanding the skin envelope.

In order to correct the tuberous breast deformity, surgical objectives include remodeling of the existing breast tissue to expand the base circumference and when indicated, also the skin. Incision of the tethering bands releases the constriction through the base of the breast, allowing the breast to re-expand. Conclusively, the inframammary fold has to be reformed at a lower, anatomically correct position [44, 45]. Taking a peri-areolar access allows modification of the

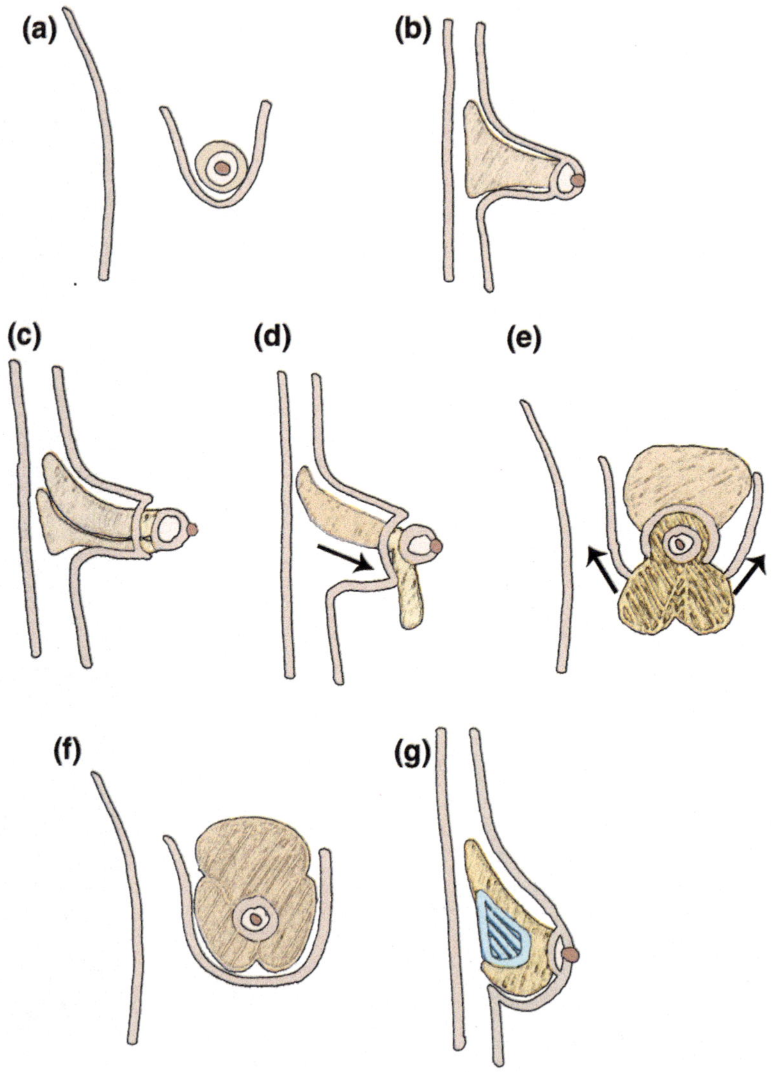

Fig. 2.8 Schematic illustration of the operational technique of tubular breast (modified according to Puckett and Mandrekas [46, 49]). **a** Tubular breast frontal, peri-areolar approach. **b** Tubular breast side view. **c** Tissue flap from the deep superior portion of the breast. **d** Elevation of glandular flap tissue and forming a new inframammary fold by extending the skin envelope. **e** Glandular flap tissue divided vertically to dispense the constriction and fill out the lower pole. **f** Reduction of the areola. **g** Breast contouring, e.g., by using an implant if needed

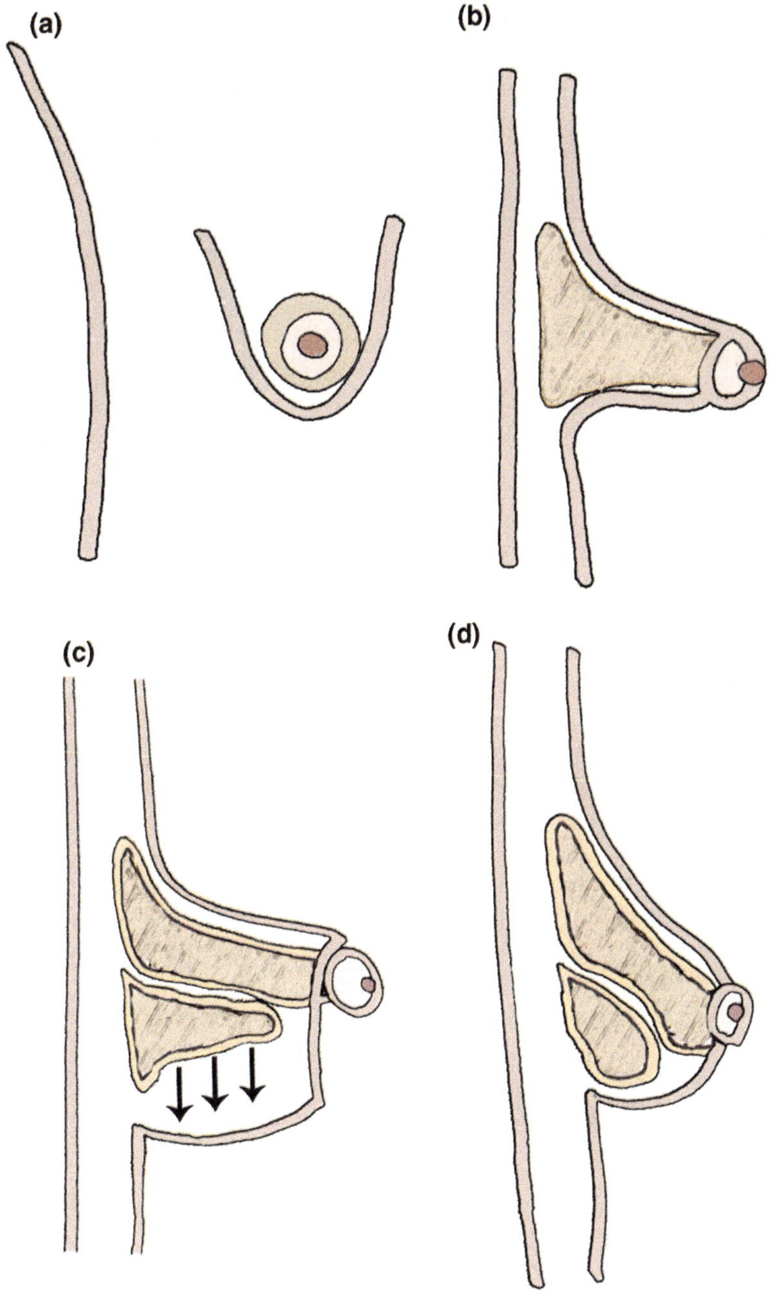

Fig. 2.9 Schematic illustration of the operational technique of tubular breast (modified according to Ribeiro [47]). **a** Tubular breast frontal, peri-areolar approach. **b** Tubular breast side view. **c** Forming a tissue flap petiolate to the pectoralis muscle and forming a new inframammary fold by extending the skin envelope. **d** Breast contouring by turning over the tissue flap

areolar diameter as well as expansion and dilatation of breast tissue for increased breast base diameter.

For compensation of deficient breast volume, a tissue expander or implant can be placed under the divided breast tissue [43, 48–50] (Figs. 2.8 and 2.9).

2.8 Inverted Nipples

An inverted nipple is defined as a condition where a part or the complete nipple is covered below the level of the areola. In some cases, the nipple might temporarily protrude after stimulation, whereas in others the retraction persists. Depending on the constellation of how easily the nipple can be pulled out, the grade of breast fibrosis, and the degree of damage caused to the milk ducts, severity codes can be defined.

This state was primarily described in 1840 by Cooper. Nipple inversion appears with a reported prevalence ranging from 1.8 to 3.3 % quite frequently [51, 52] and occurrence is most frequently bilateral [52, 53]. The cause is congenital in most cases or can be caused by, e.g., repeated inflammation and breast surgery or can occur after sudden and major weight loss. Some syndromes such as Robinow syndrome

Fig. 2.10 Woman with inverted nipple

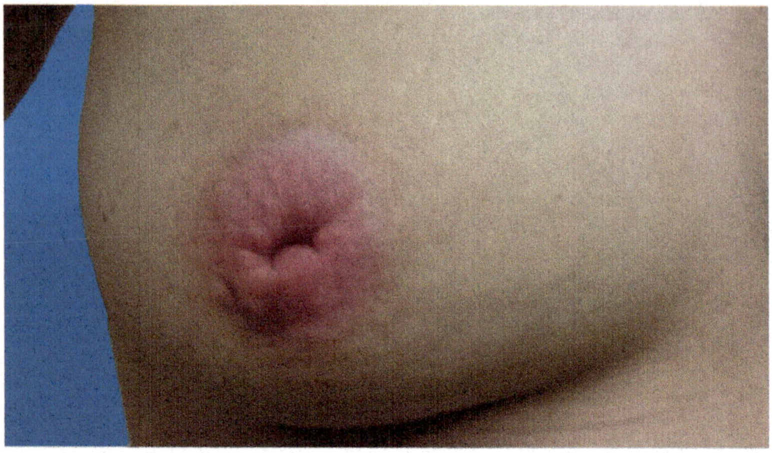

and carbohydrate-deficient glycoprotein syndrome go along with inverted nipples [54, 55].

The clinical presentation of patients with inverted nipples (Fig. 2.10) is characterized by a relatively short lactiferous duct which is attached to the nipple via dense and highly inelastic connective fibers [51, 56]. That condition may result in psychological, esthetic, and functional problems such as inconvenience with breast-feeding.

The first adjusting operation was reported by Kehrer in 1879. Over time, numerous methods have been proposed to correct this deformity. Commonly, techniques forming bilateral triangular dermal flaps crossing under the nipple in modified forms are used [57–60]. Figure 2.11 illustrates the use of subcutaneous turnover flaps for creation of a tent suspension-like effect [61]. Nevertheless, a remaining problem portrays the postoperative incomplete correction as well as a high rate of recurrence. Further problems can include change in nipple sensory, vascular compromise, scarring, and obliterated ducts with defective lactation.

2.9 Hyperplasia of the Breast

Hyperplasia of the breast, also called macromastia or gigantomastia, describes a rare medical condition with growing of excessive breast tissue (Fig. 2.12).

Breast hypertrophy might be caused by abnormally elevated hormone levels or increased end organ hypersensitivity toward female sex hormones, growth factors or prolactin, or a combination of both [62]. Histologically, hypertrophy of breast tissue represents a benign situation, which can occur unilaterally or bilaterally. Depending on etiology and chronological occurrence, different subgroups can be described.

Associated symptoms contain bra grooving, pain of shoulder, neck and back, postural problems, breathing difficulties while in supine position, and skin necrosis [63].

Juvenile (or *virginal*) *hypertrophy* describes a rare condition of an atypical and rapid breast growth during puberty often defined as a 6-month period of extreme breast

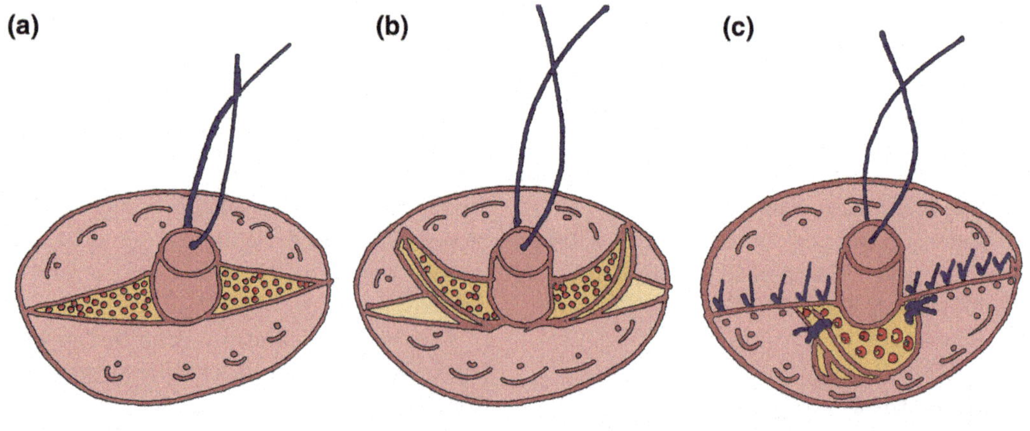

Fig. 2.11 Schematic illustration of an operative technique, showing the use of subcutaneous turnover flaps to create a tent suspension-like effect [61]. **a** Two bilateral de-epithelized subcutaneous triangular flaps are formed. Subcutaneous tunneling below the areolar level by vertical blunt dissection is performed. **b** The triangular flaps are rotated about 90° and then crossed through the vertical slit. **c** Postoperative view. The space under the nipple is filled by reposition of the flaps in the vertical direction and fixation. Finally, nipple skin and surrounding areolar skin is re-draped

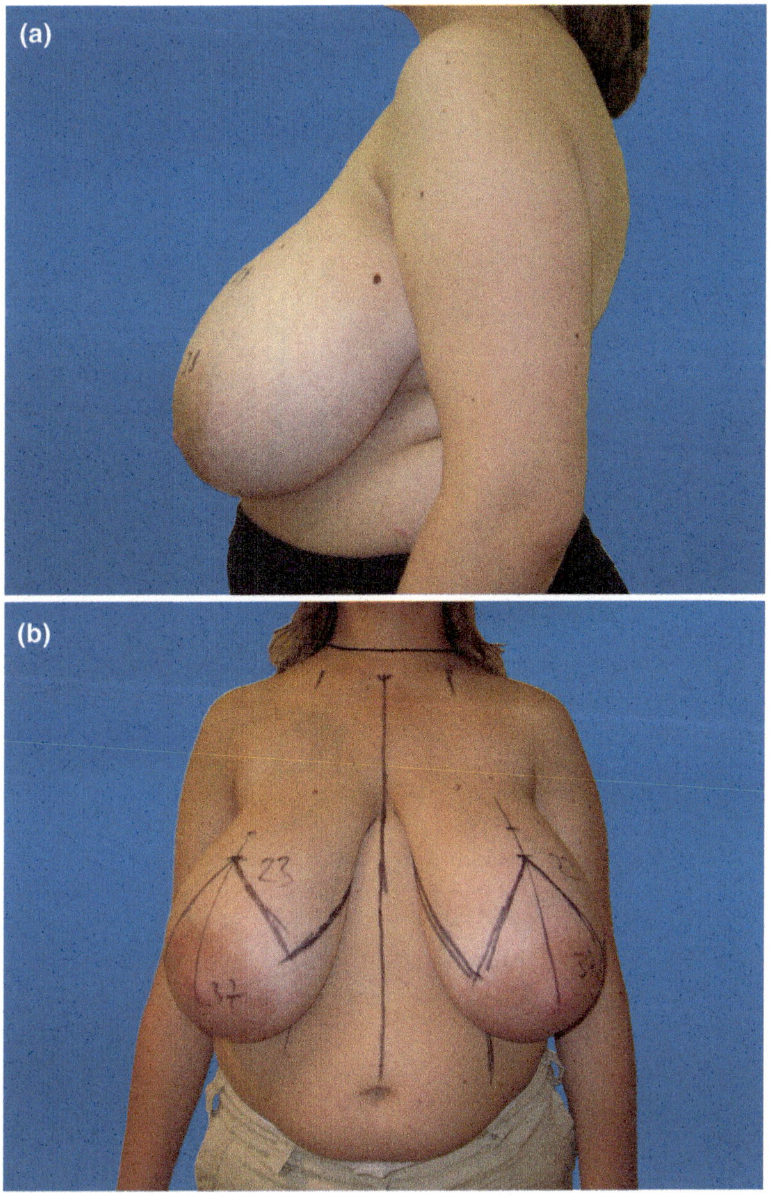

Fig. 2.12 Two women with bilateral gigantomastia from **a** lateral view and **b** anterior view

enlargement, followed by a longer period of slower, but lasting breast growth [63, 64]. Occurrence can be unilateral or bilateral. Serum levels of estrogen, progesterone, gonadotropins, and growth hormone are normal in previous studies [65]. Pharmacotherapeutic attempts include drugs such as tamoxifen, danazol, or bromocriptine to control this condition [66, 67]—safety and efficacy still unknown [68]. More common is to perform volume reduction mammoplasty as soon as the breast growth is completed (Fig. 2.13).

Cause of *adolescent macromastia* is multifactorial and usually idiopathic. It is normally associated with hormonal imbalances or obesity and develops throughout puberty with steadily ongoing breast growth. It can have significant long-term medical and psychological impacts.

Gravid-induced gigantomastia describes a very rare condition that is similar to virginal hypertrophy, where excessive breast growth occurs during pregnancy [69, 70]. It is related to breast hypersensitivity to elevated circulating hormone levels such as estrogen and prolactin. Bromocriptine can be used as a therapeutic option after delivery to induce breast involution by lowering secretion of prolactin [71].

Drug-induced gigantomastia can occur after taking several medications or drugs such as hormonal therapy, corticosteroids, marijuana, D-penicillamine, cimetidine, and the antiepileptic sulpiride. It can result in unilateral or bilateral hyperplasia. An optional treatment for D-penicillamine-induced gigantomastia has been reported with danazol [72]. Medications either stimulate hormones or act locally. If

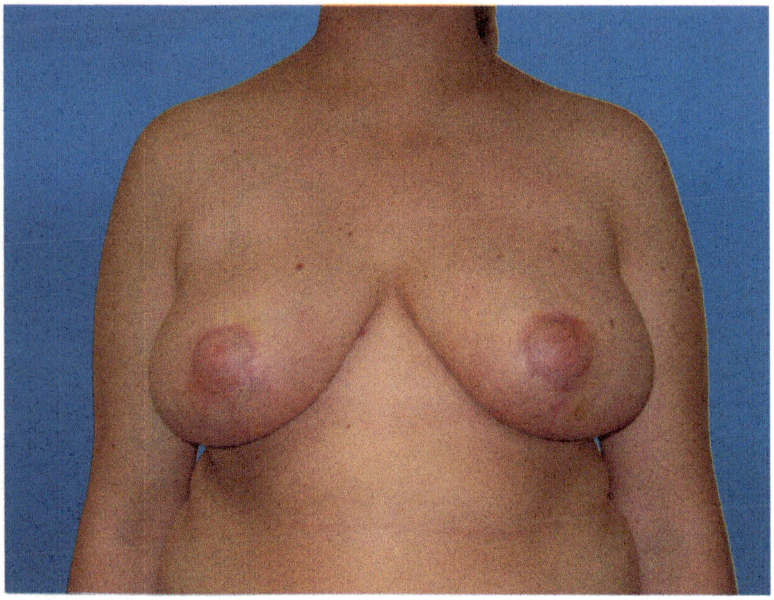

Fig. 2.13 Postoperative result of bilateral reduction mammoplasty

possible, the first attempt should cease the potentially triggering medication to reverse gigantomastia.

2.10 Gynecomastia

The excessive development of male breast tissue is a common phenomenon and appears in 32–65 % of healthy men [73–75] (Fig. 2.14).

Deriving from the Greek, the term gynecomastia combines gyne (woman) and mastos (breast), describing a female-like enlargement of the male breast which leads to glandular proliferation [11].

Gynecomastia appears in 75 % of all cases bilateral and asymmetric [76]. It is often clinical asymptomatically but may also cause local pain or psychical disturbance.

The classification of gynecomastia is based on the amount of glandular tissue. Division has to be made between the glandular, true gynecomastia, and simple fatty gynecomastia which is often found in obese man, also known as pseudo-gynecomastia. In true gynecomastia, glandular tissue can be palpated and verified via ultrasound.

The pathological process involves a relative increase in the ratio of free estrogen to androgen locally in the breast [74, 77]. Etiological factors can range from physiologic to pathologic conditions; several illnesses (e.g., hyperthyroidism; benign Leydig cell tumor, liver, and renal failure) or medication (e.g., spironolactone and drugs) could be causal. Possible causes of gynecomastia are shown in Table 2.3.

In newborns, bilateral proliferation of breast tissue is induced by maternal and placental estrogens, resolving within a few weeks after birth.

During adolescence—usually at 13 or 14 years of age—a physiological pubertal gynecomastia appears, lasting up to 6 months. Causal is a relative increase in estrogens derived mostly from peripheral aromatization of testicular and adrenal androgens. In late puberty, testicular testosterone production increases, resulting in spontaneous regression [78].

In any case, careful taking of a patient's history, as well as physical examination, should be utilized to evaluate and define the cause. The differential diagnosis of breast cancer should always be taken into consideration. If suspected, mammography, mamma sonography, and diagnostic fine needle or core biopsy should be performed, showing a 90 % sensitivity and specificity for distinguishing benign from malignant [79].

Laboratory diagnostics should include hCG (human chorionic gonadotropin), luteinizing hormone (LH), testosterone, and estradiol [75]. Due to the circadian rhythm of hormone secretion, measurement is recommended in the morning at time of the maximum release.

As soon as hypogonadism—which is increasing in elderly patients—is detected, a symptomatic therapy with testosterone should be performed.

Without question, if drug-induced gynecomastia is suspected medication should be stopped or adapted if possible.

A therapeutic approach is the use of tamoxifen, a selective estrogen receptor modulator. A daily orally dose of 20 mg tamoxifen for up to 3 months shows good results in randomized and not randomized trials. Regression of gynecomastia is shown in up to 80 % of patients. It has to be qualified that data on tamoxifen therapy are limited due to small cohorts. Adverse side effects, including epigastric

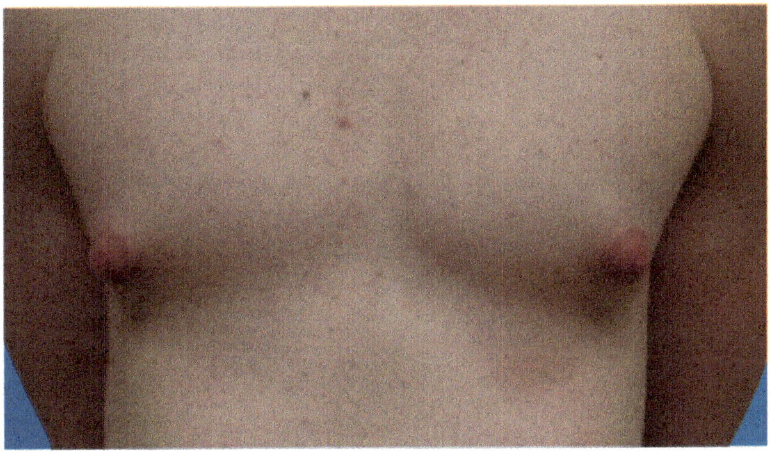

Fig. 2.14 Adolescent male presenting with bilateral gynecomastia

Table 2.3 Causes of gynecomastia

Physiologic	• Antiandrogens • Antibiotics • Antihypertensive agents • Gastrointestinal (GI) agents • Hormones • Illicit drugs • Psychiatric drugs
Decreased androgen production	• Primary (testicular) hypogonadism • Secondary (central) hypogonadism
Decreased androgen effect or synthesis	• Androgen insensitivity syndrome • 5α-reductase deficiency • 17-β-hydroxysteroid dehydrogenase deficiency
Increased estrogen production	• Adrenal tumor • Testicular tumor • hCG-secreting tumor • Familial aromatase excess syndrome
Other	• Liver disease • Thyrotoxicosis • Obesity • Renal disease • Malnutrition

Source Data from Morcos and Kizy [77]

distress and a post-traumatic deep-vein thrombosis, are rarely reported [80, 81].

Use of anastrozole, an aromatase inhibitor did not show more effectiveness than placebo in boys with pubertal gynecomastia [82].

If gynecomastia persists more than 12 months, a fibrosis remodeling takes place. Therefore, the effect of endogen treatment by testosterone or tamoxifen is limited.

Indications for surgical intervention include psychosocial stress and pain as well as cosmetic discomfort. Therapeutic interventions include liposuction, breast tissue resection, and reduction mammoplasty considering size of hypertrophic tissue and expertise of the surgeon. Aim is to remove the hypertrophic glandular tissue and not only fat. Sometimes a combination of methods can be effective. In particular, liposuction can be used after open excisional surgery for contouring the chest wall to achieve a nice shape [83, 84].

2.11 Conclusion

In their entirety, breast deformities or developmental breast disorders represent a small group of patients. Nevertheless, people affected by these body shape malformations often suffer from relevant psychological strain, which can cause isolation and withdrawal from social situations. In our increasingly sexualized society, idealized archetypes gain progressive influence. Therefore, an obstacle for receiving support may be the avoidance of consulting a physician due to embarrassment.

Plenty of these deformities are congenital and result from false processes in development. Therefore, underlying systemic disorders or syndromes should be excluded. Other breast deformities are iatrogenic, so the potential damage of surgery to the developing breast must be considered when contemplating an intervention on the chest of an infantile or adolescent patient.

The aim of the reconstructive breast surgeon includes preservation of breast structures while achieving improved symmetry for better appearance. Even if exact symmetry cannot be achieved, self-esteem is often much improved after accomplished surgery. At the present time, plenty of therapeutic options exist. Individualized counseling has to be achieved, leading to a unique concept for all patients.

Knowing all that one should, however, keep in mind: breasts are sisters, not twins!

References

1. Hughes ESR. The development of the mammary gland. Ann R Coll Surg Eng. 1949;6:99–119.
2. Sternlicht MD. Key stages in mammary gland development: the cues that regulate ductal branching morphogenesis. Breast Cancer Res. 2006;8(1):201.
3. Robinson GW, Karpf AB, Kratochwil K. Regulation of mammary gland development by tissue interaction. J Mammary Gland Biol Neoplasia. 1999;4(1):9–19.
4. Turashvili GBJ, Bouchal J, Burkadze G, Kolar Z. Mammary gland development and cancer. Cesk Patol. 2005;41(3):94–101.
5. Tobon H, Salazar H. Ultrastructure of the human mammary gland. I. Development of the fetal gland throughout gestation. J Clin Endocrinol Metab. 1974;39(3):443–56.
6. Osin PP, Anbazhagan R, Bartkova J, Nathan B, Gusterson BA. Breast development gives insights into breast disease. Histopathology. 1998;33(3):275–83.
7. Naccarato AG, Viacava P, Vignati S, Fanelli G, Bonadio AG, Montruccoli G, Bevilacqua G. Bio-morphological events in the development of the human female mammary gland from fetal age to puberty. Virchows Arch. 2000;436(5):431–8.
8. Jayasinghe YCR, Cha R, Horn-Ommen J, O'Brien P, Simmons PS. Establishment of normative data for the amount of breast tissue present in healthy children up to two years of age. J Pediatr Adolesc Gynecol. 2010;23(5):305–11.
9. McKiernan JF, Hull D. Breast development in the newborn. Arch Dis Child. 1981;56(7):525–9.
10. Howard BA, Gusterson BA. Human breast development. J Mammary Gland Biol Neoplasia. 2000;5.
11. Diamantopoulos S, Bao Y. Gynecomastia and premature thelarche: a guide for practitioners. Pediatr Rev. 2007;28:e57–68.
12. Sadove AM, van Aalst JA. Congenital and acquired pediatric breast anomalies: a review of 20 years' experience. Plast Reconstr Surg. 2005;115(4):1039–50.
13. West KW, Rescoria FJ, Scherer LR, Grosfeld JL. Diagnosis and treatment of symptomatic breast masses in the pediatric population. J Pediatr Surg. 1995;30:182–7.
14. Volta C, Bernasconi S, Cisternino M, et al. Isolated premature thelarche and thelarche variant: clinical and auxological follow-up of 119 girls. J Endocrinol Invest. 1998;21:180–3.
15. Verrotti A, Ferrari M, Morgese G, Chiarelli F. Premature thelarche: a long-term follow-up. Gynecol Endocrinol. 1996;10:241–7.
16. Codner E, Román R. Premature thelarche from phenotype to genotype. Pediatr Endocrinol Rev. 2008;5(3):760–5.
17. Wiseman BS, Werb Z. Stromal effects on mammary gland development and breast cancer. Science. 2002;296:1046–9.
18. Loukas M, Clarke P, Tubbs RS. Accessory breasts: a historical and current perspective. Am Surg. 2007;73:525–8.
19. Grossl NA. Supernumerary breast tissue: historical perspectives and clinical features. Southern Med J. 2000;93:29–32.
20. Loughry CW, et al. Breast volume measurement of 598 women using biostereometric analysis. Ann Plast Surg. 1989;22(5):380–5.
21. Rosen P. Abnormalities of mammary growth and development. Philadelphia, PA: Lippincott Williams & Wilkins; 2009, pp. 23–7.
22. Argenta LC, VanderKolk C, Friedman RJ, et al. Refinements in reconstruction of congenital breast deformities. Plast Reconstr Surg. 1985;76:73–80.
23. Smith KJ, Palin WE, Katch V, et al. Surgical treatment of congenital breast asymmetry. Ann Plast Surg. 1986;17:92–101.
24. Oakes MB, Quint EH, Smith YR, Cederna PS. Early, staged reconstruction in young women with severe breast asymmetry. J Pediatr Adolesc Gynecol. 2009;22(4):223–8.
25. Caouette-Laberge L, Bortoluzzi PA. Correction of breast asymmetry in teenagers. Philadelphia, PA: Saunders; 2010, pp. 601–30.
26. Arca MJ, Caniano DA. Breast disorders in the adolescent patient. Adolesc Med. 2004;15:473–85.
27. Ozsoy Z, Gozu A, Ozyigit MT, Genc B. Amazia with midface anomaly: case report. Aesthetic Plast Surg. 2007;31(4):392–4.
28. Trier WC. Complete breast absence. Plast Reconstr Surg. 1965;36:431–9.
29. Amesse L, Yen FF, Weisskopf B, Hertweck SP. Vaginal uterine agenesis associated with amastia in a phenotypic female with a de novo 46, XX, t(8;13) (q22.1;q32.1) translocation. Clin Genet. 1999;55:493–5.
30. Breslau-Siderius EJ, Toonstra J, Baart JA, Koppeschaar HP, Maassen JA, Beemer FA. Ectodermal dysplasia, lipoatrophy, diabetes mellitus, and amastia: a second case of the AREDYLD syndrome. Am J Med Genet. 1992;44:374–7.
31. Clarkson P. Poland's syndactyly. Guys Hosp Rep. 1962;111: 335–46.
32. da Silva Freitas R, Tolazzi ARD, Martins VDM, et al. Poland's syndrome: different clinical presentations and surgical reconstructions in 18 cases. Aesth Plast Surg. 2007;31:140–6.
33. Marks MW, Argenta LC, Izenberg PH, et al. Management of the chest wall deformity in male patients with Poland's syndrome. Plast Reconstr Surg. 1991;87:674–81.
34. Poland A. Deficiency of the pectoral muscles. Guys Hosp Rep. 1841;6:191.
35. Borschel GH, Costantin DA, Cederna PS. Individualized implant-based reconstruction of Poland syndrome breast and soft tissue deformities. Ann Plast Surg. 2007;59:507–14.
36. Fraser FC, Teebi AS, Walsh S, Pinky L. Poland sequence with dextrocardia: which comes first? Am J Med Genet. 1997;73: 194–6.
37. Spear SL, Namnoum JD et al. Breast reconstruction in patients with poland's syndrom (Chapter 99). In: Surgery of the breast. 2nd ed. 2006, p. 1384.
38. Poullin P, Toussirot E, Schiano A, Serratrice G. Complete and dissociated forms of Poland's syndrome (5 cases). Rev Rhum Mal Osteoartic. 1992;59(2):114–20.
39. Urschel HC, Byrd S, Sethi SM, et al. Poland's syndrome: improved surgical management. Ann Thorac Surg. 1984;37: 204–11.

40. Pinsolle V, Chichery A, Grolleau J-L, Chavoin JP. Autologous fat injection in Poland's syndrome. J Plast Reconstr Aesthetic Surg. 2008;61:784–91.
41. Rees TD, Aston S. The tuberous breast. Clin Plast Surg. 1976;49:339–47.
42. Teimourian B, Adham MN. Surgical correction of the tuberous breast. Ann Plast Surg. 1983;10:190–3.
43. von Heimburg D, Exner K, Kruft S, Lemperle G. The tuberous breast deformity: classification and treatment. Br J Plast Surg. 1996;49(6):339–45.
44. Dinner MI, Dowden RV. The tubular/tuberous breast syndrome. Ann Plast Surg. 1987;19:414–20.
45. Elliott MP. A musculocutaneous transposition flap mammaplasty for correction of the tuberous breast. Ann Plast Surg. 1988;1987 (201):53–7.
46. Puckett CL, Concannon MJ. Augmenting the narrow-based breast: the unfurling technique to prevent the double-bubble deformity. Aesthetic Plast Surg. 1990 Winter;14(1):15–9.
47. Ribeiro L, Canzi W, Buss A Jr, Accorsi A Jr. Tuberous breast: a new approach. Plast Reconstr Surg. 1998;101(1):42–50.
48. Foustanos A, Zavrides H. Surgical reconstruction of tuberous breasts. Aesthetic Plast Surg. 2006;30:294–300.
49. Mandrekas AD, Zambacos GJ, Anastasopoulos A, et al. Aesthetic reconstruction of the tuberous breast deformity. Plast Reconstr Surg. 2003;112:1099–108.
50. Toranto IR. Two-stage correction of tuberous breasts. Plast Reconstr Surg. 1981;67:642–6.
51. Schwager RG, Smith JW, Gray GF, Goulian D. Inversion of the human female nipple, with a simple method of treatment. Plast Reconstr Surg. 1974;54:564–9.
52. Park HS, Yoon CH, Kim HJ. The prevalence of congenital inverted nipple. Aesthetic Plast Surg. 1999;23:144–6.
53. Lee HB, Roh TS, Chung YK, et al. Correction of inverted nipple using strut reinforcement with deepithelialized triangular flaps. Plast Reconstr Surg. 1998;102:1253–8.
54. Lorenzetti MH, Fryns JP. Inverted nipples in Robinow syndrome. Genet Couns. 1996;7:67–9.
55. Young G, Driscoll MC. Coagulation abnormalities in the carbohydrate-deficient glycoprotein syndrome: case report and review of the literature. Am J Hematol. 1999;60:66–9.
56. Crestinu J. The inverted nipple: a blind method of correction. Plast Reconstr Surg. 1987;79:127–30.
57. Elsahy NI. An alternative operation for inverted nipple. Plast Reconstr Surg. 1976;57:438–91.
58. Elsahy N. Correction of inverted nipples by strong suspension with areola based dermal flaps. Plast Reconstr Surg. 2009;123:1131–2.
59. Teimourian B, Adham MN. Simple technique for correction of inverted nipple. Plast Reconstr Surg. 1980;65:504–6.
60. Lee KY, Cho BC. Surgical correction of inverted nipples using the modified Namba or Teimourian technique. Plast Reconstr Surg. 2004;113:328–36 (discussion 337–28).
61. Jeong H-S, Lee H-K. Correction of inverted nipple using subcutaneous turn-over flaps to create a tent suspension-like effect (Rubino C, ed.). PLoS ONE. 2015;10(7):e0133588.
62. Ohlsén L, Ericsson O, Beausang-Linder M. Rapid, massive and unphysiological breast enlargement. Eur J Plast Surg 1996;19 (6):307–13.
63. Baker SB, Burkey BA, Thronton P, LaRossa D. Juvenile gigantomastia: presentation of four cases and review of the literature. Ann Plast Surg. 2001;46:517–25.
64. Barreto AU. Juvenile mammary hypertrophy. Plast Reconstr Surg. 1991;87(3):583–4.
65. Kupfer D, Dingman D, Broadbent R. Juvenile breast hypertrophy: report of a familial pattern and review of the literature. Plast Reconstr Surg. 1992;90(2):303–9.
66. Sperling RL, Gold JJ. Use of an anti-estrogen after a reduction mammaplasty to prevent recurrence of virginal hypertrophy of breasts. Case report. Plast Reconstr Surg. 1973;52(4):439–42.
67. Arscott GD, Craig HR, Gabay L. Failure of bromocriptine therapy to control juvenile mammary hypertrophy. Br J Plast Surg. 2001;54(8):720–3.
68. Wolfswinkel EM, Lemaine V, Weathers WM, Chike-Obi CJ, Xue AS, Heller L. Hyperplastic breast anomalies in the female adolescent breast. Semin Plast Surg. 2013;27(1):49–55.
69. Kullander S. Effect of 2 br-alpha-ergocryptin (CB 154) on serum prolactin and the clinical picture in a case of progressive gigantomastia in pregnancy. Ann Chir Gynaecol. 1976;65:227–33.
70. Swelstad MR, Swelstad BB, Rao VK, Gutowski KA. Management of gestational gigantomastia. Plast Reconstr Surg. 2006;118: 840–8.
71. Gargan TJ, Goldwyn RM. Gigantomastia complicating pregnancy. Plast Reconstr Surg. 1987;80:121–4.
72. Taylor PJ, Cumming DC, Corenblum B. Successful treatment of D-penicillamine-induced breast gigantism with danazol. Br Med J (Clin Res Ed). 1981;282:362–3.
73. Narula HS, Carlson HE. Gynaecomastia–pathophysiology, diagnosis and treatment. Nat Rev Endocrinol. 2014;10(11):684–98.
74. Lanitis S, Starren E, Read J. Surgical management of gynaecomastia: outcomes from our experience. The Breast. 2008;17 (6):596–603.
75. Braunstein G. Gynecomastia. N Engl J Med. 2007;357:1229–37.
76. Böcker W, Denk H, Heitz PhU. Pathologie, 2. Auflage, 2001, 925.
77. Morcos RN, Kizy T. Gynecomastia. When is treatment indicated? J Fam Pract. 2012;61(12):719–25.
78. Nordt C, Divanta A. Gynecomastia in adolescents. Curr Opin Pediatr. 2008;20:375–82.
79. Evans GF, Anthony T, Turnage RH, et al. The diagnostic accuracy of mammography in the evaluation of male breast disease. Am J Surg. 2001;181:96–100.
80. Ting ACW, Chow LWC, Leung YF. Comparison of tamoxifen with danazol in the management of idiopathic gynecomastia. Am Surg. 2000;66:38–40.
81. Hanavadi S, Banerjee D, Monypenny IJ, Mansel RE. The role of tamoxifen in the management of gynaecomastia. Breast. 2006;15:276–80.
82. Plourde PV, Reiter EO, Jou HC, et al. Safety and efficacy of anastrozole for the treatment of pubertal gynecomastia: a randomized, double-blind, placebo-controlled trial. J Clin Endocrinol Metab. 2004;89:4428–33.
83. Rosenberg GJ. Gynecomastia: suction lipectomy as a contemporary solution. Plast Reconstr Surg. 1987;80(3):379–86.
84. Voigt M, Walgenbach KJ, Andree C, Bannasch H, Looden Z, Stark GB. Minimally invasive surgical therapy of gynecomastia: liposuction and exeresis technique. Chirurg. 2001;72(10):1190–5.

3 Nipple Discharge

Jill R. Dietz

3.1 Introduction

Nipple discharge is the presenting complaint of approximately 5% of women seeking medical care for a breast problem [1, 2]. While the majority of these patients will have a benign process, nipple discharge can be the sole presenting sign of cancer in 1 % of patients [3]. Historical reports suggest malignancy rates up to 24 % [4] in these patients, but with improved imaging and overall earlier detection, current rates are 3–7 % [5]. The evaluation and treatment of nipple discharge vary greatly in practice and in the literature, causing confusion for both patients and physicians. Differentiating between physiologic and pathologic nipple discharge is critical in order to identify patients in need of a diagnostic work-up and treatment plan.

3.2 Anatomy and Physiology

A review of the anatomy and physiology of the human mammary ductal system and nipple anatomy is helpful in understanding the etiology of nipple discharge. There has been a resurgence of attention to nipple anatomy secondary to the popularity of nipple-sparing mastectomy. There are rarely terminal ductal lobular units (TDLUs) in the nipple itself so it is more often a conduit for discharge than the source of primary cancer [6].

The female breast has approximately 15–20 lobes that radiate from the nipple. Each lobe is comprised of glands (lobules) and branching milk ducts. The breast milk is produced in the TDLUs, which empty into a branching ductal network that leads to the proximal duct. The proximal ducts converge toward the areola and empty into the nipple. The mammary ducts are lined by actively dividing epithelial cells that slough on a regular basis. The nipple orifices of non-lactating women are usually blocked by a keratin plug that prevents the leakage of normal ductal secretions.

During pregnancy, the ductal system proliferates and secretions are produced in response to large increases in estrogen, progesterone, and prolactin (which is released by the anterior pituitary gland). After parturition, lactation is promoted by persistently elevated levels of prolactin, and rapidly declining levels of estrogen and progesterone. The nursing infant causes further release of prolactin via the suckling reflex, thus stimulating milk production. These same hormones that promote and sustain breast-feeding can also contribute to physiologic nipple discharge in nonlactating women. Pathologic discharge is caused by a growth or proliferation of the mammary ductal epithelial lining.

3.3 Definition

Nipple discharge is fluid that flows or is expressed from the mammary ducts and is present in a small percentage of women. Nipple secretions are found within the ductal system and are by-products of the epithelial cells that are undergoing cellular turnover. These physiologic secretions are generally not evident to most women because they are blocked by the keratin plug and eventually reabsorbed. Goodson and King found secretions, or nipple aspirate fluid (NAF), in up to 81.2 % of asymptomatic women by using a suction aspirating device [7]. Studies have confirmed that the ability to aspirate nipple secretions is influenced by age, race, parity, and hormonal status but is successful in the majority of patients [8, 9]. Although nipple secretions are considered normal, the mammary ducts are the origin of most breast cancers, making the fluid secreted by the ducts a point of interest for researchers.

Many studies have been done on aspirated nipple secretions examining cellular changes and biochemical composition [8, 10–12]. NAF contains cholesterol and other steroids, estrogens and other hormones, immunoglobulin,

J.R. Dietz (✉)
Surgery, University Hospitals Seidman Cancer Center, 3909 Orange Place, Suite 4400, Beachwood, Bentleyville, OH 44122, USA
e-mail: jill.dietz@uhhospitals.org

I. Jatoi and A. Rody (eds.), *Management of Breast Diseases*, DOI 10.1007/978-3-319-46356-8_3

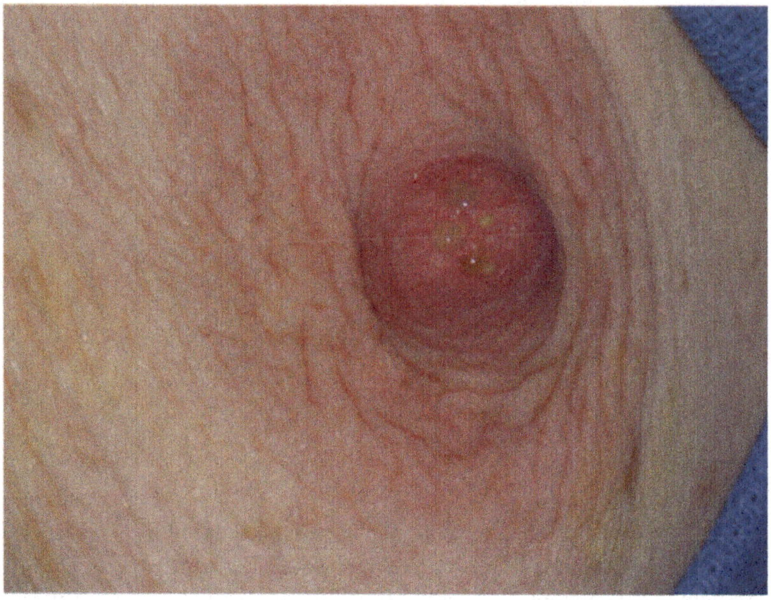

Fig. 3.1 Classic presentation of physiologic nipple discharge

lactose, fatty acids, and alpha-lactalbumin. Exogenous compounds such as caffeine, nicotine, pesticides, and other drugs are also found in nipple secretions. Lang and Kuerer have compiled an extensive list of compounds found intraductally by various studies [13]. The color of NAF, which can vary from white to dark green, is related to the cholesterol, lipid peroxide, and estrogen content [14]. The normal cellular make up of NAF consists of foam cells, a few epithelial cells, and other cells of hematogenous origin [15].

When secretions become abundant or persistent enough that they discharge spontaneously from the duct orifice, they are known as nipple discharge. Nipple discharge is generally categorized as "physiologic" or "pathologic" discharge. Physiologic discharge can be caused by exogenous or endogenous hormones, medications, direct stimulation, stress, or endocrine abnormalities. Although the cause of the hormonal influence may be pathologic, as is the case with prolactinoma, the ductal system itself has no abnormality, so the resultant discharge is classified as physiologic. Most physiologic discharge is bilateral, nonspontaneous, and involves multiple ducts. These characteristics result from the central effect of an outside influence on the breast. The color of the discharge can vary from milky to yellow, gray, brown, or dark green depending on the composition and cause of the physiologic discharge. As with NAF, darker-colored discharges are associated with higher levels of estrogens and cholesterol [16] (Fig. 3.1). Because there is rarely an intraductal pathologic abnormality involved with this type of discharge, localization procedures, breast biopsies, or surgeries are not necessary.

Pathologic nipple discharge or PND is caused by an abnormality of the duct epithelium. It is typically unilateral and from a single duct. The discharge is spontaneous or at least easily expressible. The patient often notices the discharge after a warm shower that likely removes the keratin plug. The pathologic lesion often causes ductal obstruction and dilatation so that the fluid which collects in the duct is subsequently released when the plug is removed or the duct is expressed. The color of the discharge is usually clear, serous, or bloody, although pathologic nipple discharge can present as other colors (Fig. 3.2). This type of discharge tends not to be affected by the menstrual cycle or hormonal status. While some women seek care when they first notice the discharge, many will delay until the discharge becomes socially embarrassing or bloody. Although the majority of these women will have a benign etiology for their nipple discharge, all patients with PND need a thorough evaluation to rule out malignancy as the source.

3.4 Incidence

Approximately, 5 % of women presenting for breast care have a complaint of nipple discharge [17, 18]. The incidence is likely underreported since many women do not seek medical care for this symptom. Women who have physiologic discharge, an otherwise normal exam and normal imaging, have a very low chance of having a malignancy [19, 20].

Patients with nipple discharge have a higher relative risk for cancer than the asymptomatic population. While the vast majority of patients with pathologic nipple discharge have benign proliferative lesions as the etiology, breast cancer is found to be the cause of the nipple discharge in 4–21 % of cases [1, 3, 21–27]. Those patients with nipple discharge associated with a mass or skin change have an even higher

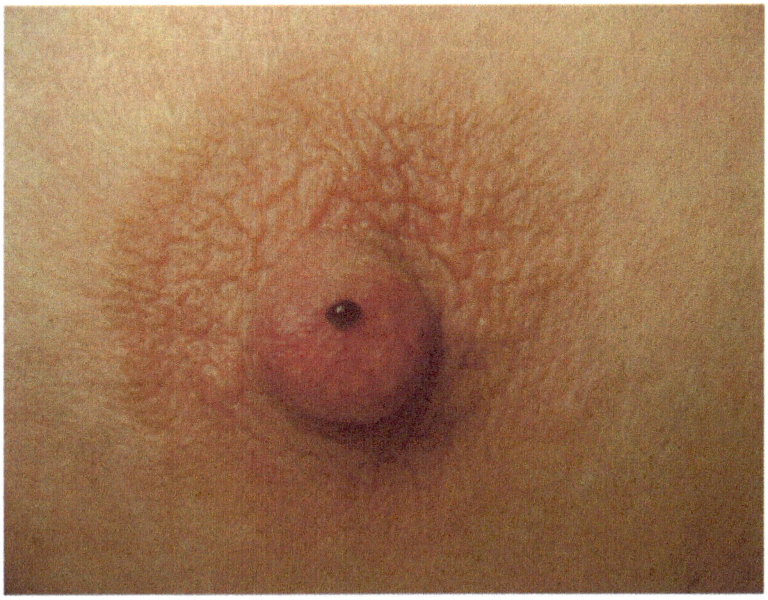

Fig. 3.2 Classic presentation of pathologic nipple discharge

relative risk of cancer. One study showed that the incidence of carcinoma for patients with discharge and a mass was 61.5 % as compared to 6.1 % for patients with discharge alone [2].

While most patients with pathologic nipple discharge have normal mammograms, many studies have shown that an abnormal mammogram in patients with pathologic nipple discharge is associated with an increased risk for cancer [21, 27–30]. As should palpable masses, suspicious radiologic findings should be evaluated by stereotactic or core needle biopsy prior to duct excision. This will diagnose a malignancy in some patients, allowing for definitive surgical treatment. If minimally invasive biopsy is not available, then the mammographic abnormality will need to be evaluated at the time of duct excision.

Bloody or guaiac positive discharge also increases a person's risk of cancer, although most cases of bloody nipple discharge are benign, and cancer has been found to be the cause of discharge of milky and serous fluid [3]. A recent report showed that the malignancy rate for bloody PND was 14 % compared to 6 % for nonbloody discharge [31]. Advanced age or postmenopausal status, imaging abnormality, and mass have also been shown to increase the risk of breast cancer being the cause of the pathologic discharge [25].

The number of breast cancer cases presenting as nipple discharge has dropped over the last few decades. Copeland's series of patients in the 1950s reported that 25 out of 67 (37 %) patients with nipple discharge had breast cancer [32] whereas more recent studies of patients undergoing duct excision for pathologic nipple discharge tend to have cancer rates between 5 and 10 % [19, 25, 26]. The decrease in the incidence of cancer presenting in this way is likely due to the earlier detection of breast cancer with improved imaging techniques and increased screening, which shifts diagnosis to earlier stage disease. Another possibility is that minimally invasive biopsy of imaging and clinical abnormalities is being performed to establish a preoperative cancer diagnosis, thus moving these patients out of the category of women undergoing surgical biopsy for the diagnosis of nipple discharge.

Even though the most significant cause of nipple discharge is cancer, most cases have a benign etiology. Many studies do not differentiate the exact histology of benign lesions, although it is clear that papillomas or papillomatosis are responsible for a large percentage of pathologic nipple discharge. Other reported causes are duct ectasia, epithelial hyperplasia, and fibrocystic changes [3, 21, 28]. Localizing techniques increase the diagnostic yield of duct excision: The percentage of proliferative lesions increases, while fewer cases of duct ectasia and fibrocystic changes are found. This suggests that there is a proliferative ductal process accounting for most, if not all, cases of pathologic nipple discharge [25, 26, 29].

3.5 Characteristics and Etiology

Discharge from the nipple can present as a spectrum of signs, from a tiny opaque drop during breast examination to alarming bloody discharge that stains the patients clothing. The presentation and history are important in categorizing the discharge as either "physiologic" or "pathologic." Even though some causes of bilateral multiduct discharge are from a pathologic source, such as a pituitary adenoma, the effect is central and not the result of a ductal abnormality. These

Table 3.1 Characteristics of pathologic and physiologic nipple discharge

Characteristic	Physiologic	Pathologic
Laterality	Bilateral	Unilateral
#Ducts	Multiple	One
Spontaneity	Expressed	Spontaneous
Color	Multicolored, milky, gray, green, brown, yellow	Bloody, serous, clear
Consistency	Sticky, thick	Watery, copious

Table 3.2 Causes of nonpathologic nipple discharge

Hormonal
Pregnancy/postlactational
Mechanical stimulation
Galactorrhea
Duct ectasia
Bloody discharge of pregnancy
Infection (Zuska's disease)
Montgomery gland discharge
Fibrocystic change

discharges are better categorized as physiologic or "nonpathologic" discharge. This grouping system is helpful in determining both the evaluation and treatment necessary for that patient. Table 3.1 shows the classic presentation of each type of nipple discharge.

Physiologic nipple discharge has various presentations and etiologies. Table 3.2 reviews the most common causes of nonpathologic nipple discharge. Over 75 % of nipple discharges are physiologic in nature and do not require surgical intervention [1]. The evaluation and treatment of physiologic nipple discharge should be focused on identifying the external factor that is stimulating the breasts.

Galactorrhea is physiologic discharge from the nipple that resembles breast milk but occurs in a patient who is not lactating. The discharge is a thin, watery milk-like substance that usually arises from both breasts. The most common scenario is a postpartum woman who continues to discharge from one or both breasts long after she has stopped breast-feeding. She may have some concern regarding the discharge and may attempt to repeatedly express the fluid. The continued stimulation of the nipple causes further discharge perpetuating the cycle. Other sources of nipple stimulation such as the friction of clothing, or nipple involvement during intimacy, can also aggravate the symptom. Again, explaining to the patient the likely etiology of the discharge and reassurance is usually sufficient.

Thin, milky discharge can occur around menarche and menopause when the breasts are exposed to extreme hormonal variation. The discharge is self-limited and simply requires reassuring the patient. Nipple discharge can also be seen in newborns as a result of maternal hormones that cross the placental barrier prior to parturition. After delivery, the precipitous drop in estrogen and progesterone levels associated with the high neonatal prolactin levels causes stimulation of the infant's breast tissue. This discharge, commonly referred to as "witches' milk," lasts only a few weeks [33].

Galactorrhea can result from an increase in prolactin levels. Most often, the levels are elevated due to medication, although the most significant cause is a pituitary adenoma that secretes prolactin. Prolactinoma should be expected if the patient has the classic triad of symptoms: amenorrhea, galactorrhea, and infertility. The tumor arises from the anterior pituitary gland and can become quite large causing symptoms of diplopia from compression of the optic chiasm. If a prolactinoma is suspected, a prolactin level should be drawn, which will be abnormal (>30 ng/mL). Screening nipple discharge patients with prolactin levels is not cost-effective, considering fewer than one in one thousand cases are due to a pituitary adenoma [34]. If a tumor is found, it can be successfully treated with a dopamine agonist, which will also eliminate the discharge. Occasionally, surgical excision of the tumor may be necessary.

Other rare causes of galactorrhea are listed in Table 3.3 along with the categories of medications that have been known to cause nipple discharge [35]. Thoracic surgery or chest trauma has been reported to cause nipple discharge. The injury stimulates the afferent thoracic nerves and the hypothalamic-pituitary axis resulting in increased prolactin release, which in turn stimulates nipple discharge [36].

Opalescent physiologic discharges, which are multicolored and nonserous, emanate from one or both breasts and usually from multiple ducts. The discharge may only be evident with vigorous expression by the patient, or may be very easily expressed and copious. Creamy white, tan, or yellow discharge may present next to a duct producing a brown, dark green, or blackish discharge. Although this type of discharge is often alarming to the patient because the dark color is assumed to be blood, it is quite unlikely for it to be associated with an intraductal lesion. A tissue test, where the discharge is placed on a thin white tissue, often results in absorption of the drop, which then proves the discharge is green. It can be difficult to differentiate green discharge from guaiac positive discharge on hemoccult testing. When duct excision is done for this type of discharge, histology often shows normal breast tissue, duct ectasia, or fibrocystic changes. Most patients with physiologic discharge are willing to be followed after being reassured of its benign

Table 3.3 Causes of galactorrhea (hyperprolactinemia)

Physiologic:
Postlactational
Mechanical stimulation
Chest wall abnormalities
Chest trauma or surgery
Burns
Herpes zoster
Spinal cord injury
Tumors
Pituitary
Hypothalamic tumors
Craniopharyngiomas, meningioma
Ectopic prolactin (bronchogenic carcinoma)
Acromegaly
Metabolic
Chronic renal failure
Hypothyroidism
Cushing's disease
Idiopathic
Medication induced
Lactogenic drugs
Estrogens, progestins, androgens
Long-term opiate use (e.g., morphine, cocaine)
Anesthetics
Phenothiazines (e.g., Compazine®, Thorazine®)
Antidepressants (e.g., Elavil®, Prozac®, Paxil®)
Monoamine oxidase inhibitors (e.g., Nardil®, Parmate®)
Antipsychotics (e.g., Clozaril®)
Antihypertensives (e.g., Aldomet®, Calan®)
Butyrophenones (e.g., Haldol®)
Thioxanthenes (e.g., Navane®)
Benzodiazepines (e.g., Valium®)
Other prescribed drugs (e.g., Tagamet®, INH, Danocrine, Reglan®)

nature. On a rare occasion, the patient may request surgery to eliminate copious discharge. If the discharge is associated with pain and fibrocystic changes, the patient should be informed that it is not likely that the surgery will decrease her pain. It may also result in decreased nipple sensation and the inability to breast-feed, particularly if bilateral excisions are performed. If an underlying cause for the nipple discharge can be identified, then it can be addressed, such as a medication change or cessation of hormones.

Communication of cysts with ductal structures appears to be responsible for nipple discharge in some instances. In these situations, the cyst, often presenting as a mass, may disappear with the onset of discharge. Whenever a patient presents with nipple discharge and an associated mass, the mass must be evaluated. In this case, aspirated cyst fluid characteristics will likely correlate to the nipple discharge, and no further evaluation is necessary. A ductogram may show communication with the cyst. Although this is an interesting finding, a ductogram is not necessary if there is clinical evidence that the cyst is related to the discharge. If the problem persists, many patients prefer excision to control the discharge.

Some breast infections present with purulent and malodorous nipple discharge. This condition is treated like other breast infections. Large abscess cavities may be apparent and should be drained. Cellulitis in association with nipple discharge may be indicative of a deep abscess cavity. If it is unclear whether an abscess has formed, an ultrasound may be useful. Otherwise, conservative treatment with an antibiotic that has adequate gram-positive coverage is an appropriate initial therapy. The discharge itself may be a useful source to test for microbiology and sensitivities. Zuska's disease is a condition of chronic periareolar abscess with sinus formation and can result in intermittent nipple discharge and infection. Excision of the entire ductal system on the effected side, including the sinus tract, is often associated with the fewest recurrences [37]. Because this problem occurs almost exclusively in smokers, major duct excision in this setting is also associated with a higher incidence of ischemic necrosis and other complications. A smoking cessation program may reverse this cycle of chronic infection or at least decrease the complications if duct excision is performed.

Duct ectasia is a condition, which results in poor emptying of ductal secretions, stagnation, and inflammation of the ducts. The associated nipple discharge can present spontaneously or require vigorous expression to elicit a thick, white discharge. Bilateral, multiduct involvement varying in color is the most common presentation. The drainage is thought to be secondary to increased glandular secretions due to chronic inflammation [38].

Fibrocystic disease: Several series report that fibrocystic disease is a common histologic finding in many duct excision specimens from patients with pathologic nipple discharge. Series using localization techniques have very high proliferative lesion retrieval rates, which suggest that most cases of pathologic discharge are caused by intraductal abnormalities and not fibrocystic change [25, 29, 39]. In cases where fibrocystic change or normal breast tissue is reported, it is important to ensure that all the excised tissues are analyzed or that the correct tissue was excised. Some papillomas are only 1–2 mm in size and could easily be missed with the sampling error of serial sectioning. A high suspicion for a missed proliferative lesion should remain when the histologic diagnosis of fibrocystic change is reported for duct excision specimens.

Occasionally, women who are in their third trimester of pregnancy or who are postpartum will experience bloody nipple discharge. While it is common to have a milky discharge at this time, bloody discharge is rare, often unilateral, and may be expressible from multiple ducts. The bloody discharge is often noted after an abrupt increase in breast size associated with the pregnancy. In women, who have asymmetrical breast growth during pregnancy, bloody nipple discharge is more often associated with the larger breast [40]. The bloody discharge can accompany normal lactation and is often found during pumping. She may be concerned about breast cancer or the blood harming her nursing infant. The bleeding is usually minimal and self-limited and is unlikely to cause a problem for the nursing infant. The majority of case reports describe resolution of bleeding by the third month after delivery. Cytologic evaluation of nipple discharge in pregnant or postpartum patients often reveals abnormal appearing cells that are the result of normal epithelial changes during lactation. These cells may be falsely interpreted as arising from cancer; therefore, cytologic examination of this discharge must be interpreted with caution. This bloody discharge during pregnancy and lactation is an unusual circumstance in which it may be reasonable to postpone or at least delay further evaluation. It must be appreciated that if the discharge is associated with a mass or persists as a unilateral, single duct discharge, then further evaluation is needed.

Montgomery gland discharge presents from the large areolar sebaceous glands known as Montgomery's tubercles and is not truly the nipple discharge. This type of discharge usually occurs at times of extreme changes in hormonal status such as menarche or menopause. The discharge has characteristics of physiologic discharge as it is commonly found coming from many glands and is either serous or opaque in nature. This type of discharge requires reassurance unless infection occurs. In this case, antibiotic therapy and, occasionally, excision of the infected gland are indicated. There are rare reports of duct communication to the Montgomery glands causing nipple discharge. This presents as pathologic discharge from the tubercle of the areola [41].

Nipple discharge in the male patient is treated similar to that in females. Puberty in adolescents, and the same drugs and medical conditions that stimulate gynecomastia in men can cause nipple discharge. The evaluation should include mammography in addition to careful history and physical examination. Any suspicious mass or mammographic abnormality should be biopsied. In one study of 6200 patients, Leis found that 5 out of 24 (20.8 %) men diagnosed with cancer had nipple discharge as the presenting symptom. Evaluation is mandatory for male patients with PND, especially when associated with a mass, because of the increased risk of cancer and decreased survival rate of male patients with invasive breast cancer [21].

Table 3.4 Causes of pathologic nipple discharge

Papilloma
Papillomatosis
Papillary cancer
Ductal carcinoma in situ
Invasive ductal carcinoma
Ductal epithelial hyperplasia
(?) Cysts/fibrocystic disease/duct ectasia

Pathologic nipple discharge is caused by an intraductal abnormality and is therefore typically a unilateral finding. Although it is possible for the pathology to involve more than one ductal system, the typical presentation is consistent discharge from a single duct orifice. The discharge can be watery clear, serosanguinous, dark brown old blood, or bright blood. Occasionally, reports of carcinoma with other types of discharge, such as milky, have been reported, but this is distinctly unusual [20, 42]. Table 3.4 reviews the common etiologies of pathologic nipple discharge.

Papilloma: (Fig. 3.3) A large percentage of pathologic nipple discharge is attributed to papillomas or papillomatosis. Papillomas are often found centrally in the subareolar region. Solitary papillomas arise from the larger ducts compared to the smaller, often multiple papillomas, which are more peripherally located and arise from the TDLUs. Peripheral papillomas can occur bilaterally and have a higher recurrence rate after excision than the solitary central variety. Multiple, peripheral papillomas present with pathologic nipple discharge less frequently than central papillomas [36, 43].

In the past, there has been much controversy over whether papillomas are premalignant. It is generally accepted that central, solitary papillomas have little malignant potential although they should be completely excised to avoid recurrence [44]. In contrast, papillomas arising in small, more peripheral ducts can be associated with cancer. Ohuchi reconstructed ductal excision specimens from patients with pathologic nipple discharge and found that cancer was associated with 37.5 % of peripheral papillomas but not with central papillomas [45]. Hou et al. showed that 70 % of malignancies found on duct excision for nipple discharge were located over 2 cm from the nipple [46]. Patients with nipple discharge, who are found to have peripheral lesions on ductography, should be considered for a preoperative localizing procedure to guide the surgeon during surgical biopsy. These patients should also have careful follow-up since the risk of recurrence or development of cancer is higher than that for central lesions [4].

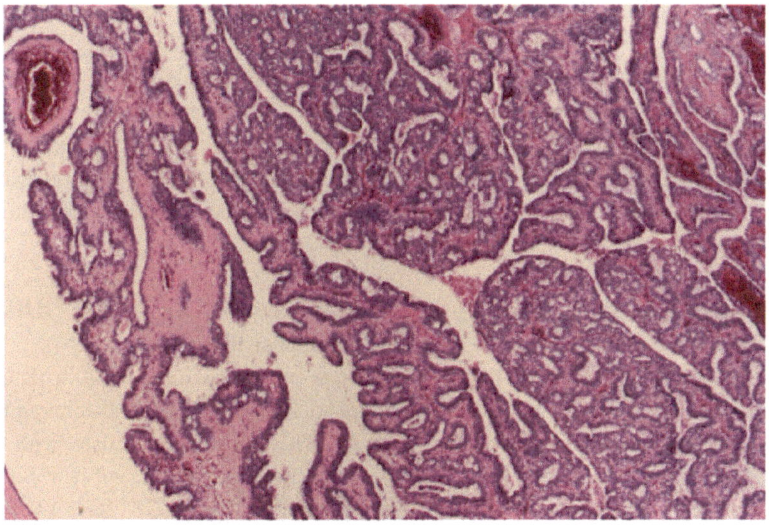

Fig. 3.3 Histologic section through an intraductal papilloma showing the vascular stroma with epithelial lining

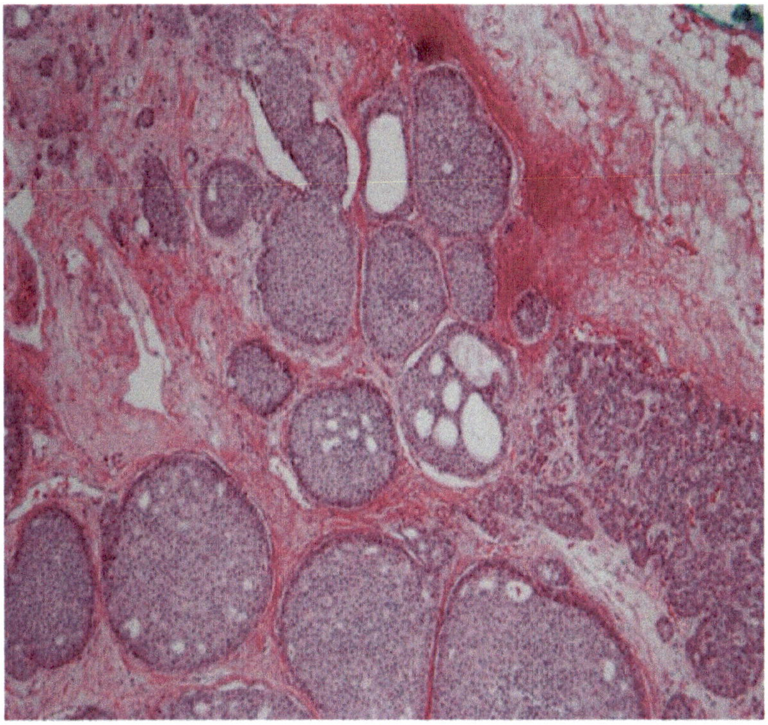

Fig. 3.4 Histologic representation of ductal carcinoma in situ

Carcinoma: (Fig. 3.4) One percent of all breast cancers present with nipple discharge as the only symptom [3]. Approximately, one in ten cases of pathologic nipple discharge will have cancer as the etiology and the incidence increases if the discharge is bloody. The rationale for investigation in patients with pathologic nipple discharge is to rule out cancer as the source. While there are a number of diagnostic tests available that correlate with the malignant potential of a lesion, no single test can rule out carcinoma, so duct excision is recommended. Imaging abnormalities or suspicious clinical findings should be worked up and biopsied to assist in establishing a diagnosis.

3.6 Diagnostic Evaluation

Many diagnostic tests are available to evaluate patients with nipple discharge. Before embarking on any of these, a full history must first be taken, including the patient's age, gynecologic and sexual history, and use of medication and hormones. Pertinent medical history such as previous endocrine problems or chest trauma should also be ascertained. The characteristics of the discharge must be noted, including laterality, spontaneity, number of ducts involved, color, and consistency. PND is a clinical diagnosis based on presentation. Physical exam should include a breast exam, assessing for palpable masses, lymphadenopathy, skin changes, and nipple inversion or lesions. The information obtained from a careful history and a confirming physical exam will frequently lead to a diagnosis and limit the tests needed prior to duct excision.

3.7 Mammography

If it is determined that the patient has physiologic nipple discharge, no additional procedures are needed. Mammography is reserved for patients in the appropriate age group and risk categories if physiologic discharge is the presenting symptom. All patients with pathologic nipple discharge should undergo mammographic evaluation regardless of age. Still, mammography is often normal in cases of discharge associated with cancer. Fung found that only 2 out of 15 patients with cancer causing nipple discharge had mammograms suggestive of malignancy [47]. Mammography might identify a separate or associated lesion that may alter the course of management. Mammographic abnormalities associated with nipple discharge increase the likelihood of a malignancy [28]. If a mammographic abnormality is visualized, this finding takes precedence and a stereotactic or ultrasound-guided core biopsy should be performed. If a minimally invasive biopsy is not done, then a needle localization excisional biopsy should be performed at the duct excision to include the imaging abnormality.

3.8 Ultrasound

Ultrasound has been used for patients with pathologic nipple discharge to view dilated ducts. This technique has also been used with saline lavage of the discharging duct to dilate and obtain cytology from the duct under echographic guidance [48, 49]. Chung compared ultrasound to ductography and found that ultrasound is superior for defining small 0.5 cm lesions and to evaluate multiple ductal systems. Ultrasound-guided localization of the lesion is particularly helpful in cases of failed cannulation during ductography. Ductography remains superior to ultrasound for visualizing the extent of abnormality within a ductal system and for detection of microcalcifications [50, 51]. The addition of US to ductography has the highest sensitivity and specificity; however, even if both of these tests are negative, malignancy cannot be excluded [52].

High-resolution ultrasound is performed at 13–15 MHz and has a higher sensitivity for the diagnosis of intraductal pathology than conventional ultrasound (75 vs. 30 %). Although it has a lower specificity than conventional ultrasound performed at 7.5 MHz, high-resolution ultrasound appears to be better for evaluating proximal ducts [53, 54] (Fig. 3.5). If an identified peripheral lesion can be visualized

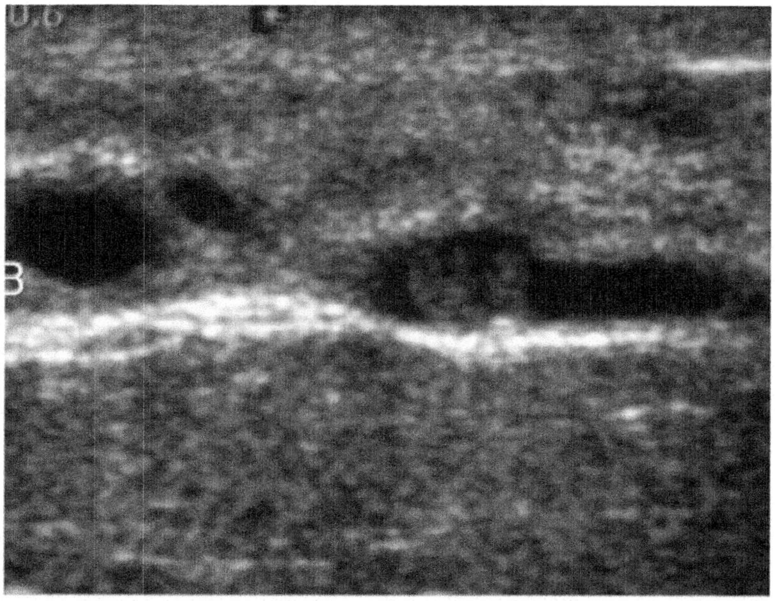

Fig. 3.5 Ultrasound of a dilated duct showing an intraductal lesion

by ultrasound, needle localization or ultrasound-guided fine needle aspiration (FNA) may be performed. The sensitivity of cytologic examination of ultrasound-guided FNA is only 50 %; however, duct excision is warranted to remove the lesion [55]. Two recently published studies looked at patients with nipple discharge who underwent ultrasound-guided percutaneous Mammotome excision of their intraductal abnormalities. Both of these studies report that 95 % of patients were discharge free after the procedure. Thorough pre-biopsy work-up and patient selection are critical for this procedure to be successful [56, 57].

3.9 MRI

Magnetic resonance imaging is being used more often as an additional diagnostic tool for breast diseases. It is particularly useful in young women with dense breast tissue where more conventional tests such as mammography and ultrasound have a lower sensitivity. MRI has a higher sensitivity than standard ductography but still cannot reliably differentiate benign from malignant disease [58–60]. MR can be helpful if other localizing techniques such as ductoscopy or ductography are not available [61]. MR ductography has been developed as an additional tool for patients with pathologic nipple discharge and can be useful for identifying the extent of the disease. While expense is an issue, it is not as invasive as conventional ductography and does not have the problem of failed cannulation. Fusion imaging of MR ductography and contrast-enhanced MR mammography can provide useful information on the extent of disease, and size and shape of the lesion. This is helpful for resection planning and in suspected cancer cases where breast conservation will be attempted [62–64].

3.10 Occult Blood

Testing nipple discharge for occult blood has been evaluated in many studies. Bloody or heme-positive discharge has been associated with an increased incidence of cancer. In one large series, discharge was tested for occult blood using a Bililabstix reagent strip. All patients with the eventual diagnosis of cancer tested positive even though less than half were grossly bloody [3]. Since there are reports of cancers identified in nonbloody discharge, if the discharge is characteristically pathologic, it should be evaluated even if it is hemoccult negative.

3.11 Cytology

Many physicians will send nipple discharge for cytologic evaluation. In a large screening study where cytology was performed on over 20,000 patients with nipple discharge, only 0.2 % patients were either positive or suspicious for malignancy. In this same series, 61 of 404 detected cancers had nipple discharge. In these 61 cases, cytology findings were as follows: 24 negative, 18 positive, 7 suspicious, and 12 atypical for a sensitivity of 60.7 % [65]. The ability to detect malignancy by cytologic examination of nipple discharge ranges from 45 to 82 % [20, 21, 66–68]. Nipple discharge cytology has a 0.9–2.6 % false-positive rate [21, 68] (Fig. 3.6).

A recent study from the CAP Interlaboratory Comparison Program queried pathologists with a brief history and slides of nipple discharge. The results indicated a high 12.8 % false-positive rate and a 3.4 % false-negative rate, confirming the difficulties in relying on cytologic results in this condition [69]. Cytology alone should not be used to

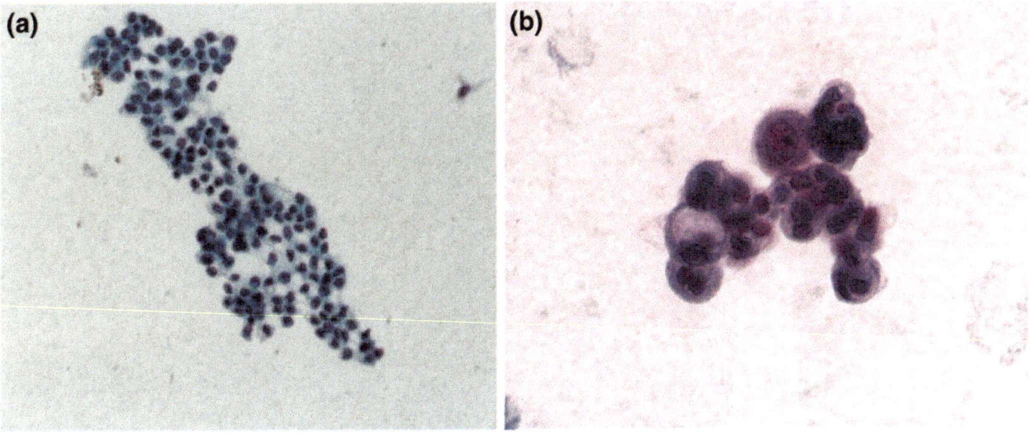

Fig. 3.6 **a** Nipple discharge cytology showing benign ductal cells and proteinaceous material. **b** Nipple discharge cytology showing malignant cells

determine if surgical excision is necessary because of the high false-negative and false-positive rates. In cases of positive nipple cytology and mammographic changes suggestive of malignancy, a diagnostic surgical procedure may be justified [70]. If the mammographic abnormality is biopsied preoperatively and a cancer diagnosis is established, then a thorough work-up and definitive diagnosis can be performed. For patients with pathologic nipple discharge and no mass or mammographic abnormality, a biopsy should be done regardless of cytologic findings.

Cytology examination is not recommended for pregnant patients due to the difficulty in differentiating normal from abnormal proliferative changes. Positive cytology in cases of pathologic nipple discharge or nipple lesions can be helpful, but in cases in which the clinical evaluation is suspicious without positive cytology or if cytology is positive without a corresponding high level of clinical suspicion, tissue biopsy is required. A negative cytology report in the setting of clinical nipple discharge could erroneously reassure the patient who still needs further evaluation.

3.12 Biochemical Markers

Several researchers have addressed the role of biochemical markers in nipple discharge in an attempt to diagnose breast cancer. Certain LDH isoenzyme levels have been found to be elevated in the nipple discharge of patients with breast cancer. The test is relatively simple and inexpensive but is associated with a false-negative rate in cases where a cancer is in another area of the breast and not associated with the discharge [71]. Immunoassays for CEA have been done using small nitrocellulose-backed disks placed on the nipples of cancer patients. Nipple secretions from 94 % of the patients with cancer had significantly higher levels of CEA than from those without cancer. This difference was not apparent in healthy controls [72]. Several studies of NAF and abnormal discharge using immunoassays for CEA show similar trends whereas others show no difference [73–75]. Using a modified breast pump to obtain NAF, Sauter found that decreased levels of prostatic specific antigen (PSA) were associated with an increased breast cancer risk [9]. In a recent study, Liu found that basic fibroblast growth factor (bFGF) from nipple fluid was significantly increased in breast cancer patients over controls [76]. Sauter's group has also looked at proteomic analysis of ductal fluids using SELDI-TOF mass spectrometry showing differential expression between women with and without breast cancer [77]. These tests using nipple discharge or secretions may aid in the diagnosis of breast cancer and are promising for future screening and diagnosis but are currently not accurate enough to rule out carcinoma or negate the need for biopsy in patients with nipple discharge.

3.13 Ductal Imaging

Ductography or galactography has proven useful for preoperative localization of intraductal lesions [78, 79] (Fig. 3.7). Due to the significant false-negative rate, however, the decision to operate should not be based solely on the ductogram results [23]. The ability of ductography to distinguish between benign and malignant disease remains limited [51, 80]. A recent study reported an increase in the

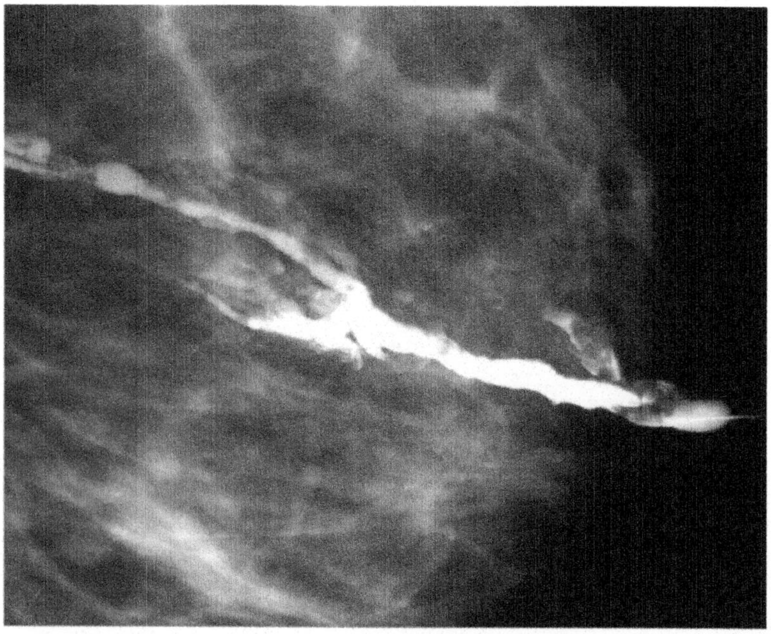

Fig. 3.7 Ductogram showing the typical lobulated appearance of a benign intraductal papilloma

duct excision yield of neoplastic growths from 67 to 100 % by using preoperative ductography [79]. This procedure is easily performed by inserting a 30-gauge blunt-tip needle into the discharging duct orifice and instilling 0.1–1.5 mL of water-soluble contrast. Mammograms are taken in two views and will show a filling defect or duct cutoff in most circumstances [22]. In cases where the ductal lesion is far from the nipple, ductography can be combined with preoperative needle localization to assist the surgeon with the excision [79, 81]. Other techniques combine preoperative ductography with methylene blue dye injection to assist the surgeon in removing the lesion [79, 82].

Standard ductography via the nipple is not possible in many patients who have had previous duct surgery with retained or new duct lesions or for patients who have dilated ducts that cannot be accessed through the nipple. In these cases, percutaneous ductography has been described using ultrasound guidance. This procedure allows for identification and localization of the lesion to assist with surgical excision [83].

3.14 Surgical Evaluation and Treatment

Surgery for pathologic nipple discharge can be less than satisfying procedure. Duct excision is typically performed blindly because the intraluminal pathology cannot be visualized directly during surgery. Duct excision can cause decreased sensation to the nipple and prevent the ability to breast-feed depending on the extent of dissection. The surgeon must judge the amount of tissue to be excised so as to assure adequate removal of the lesion without unnecessary destruction of normal breast tissue. Benign or normal pathology findings could result from not excising the lesion, from the pathologist not identifying the lesion within the specimen, or possibly from a truly negative pathology.

Various techniques for surgical removal of the mammary ducts have been described. A major duct excision removes all or most of the subareolar ductal tissue through either a circumareolar or radial incision [21, 84]. Traditionally, this approach was used for pathologic nipple discharge prior to the availability of localizing procedures. It is still useful in cases of copious physiologic discharge for which the patient requests surgery or for cases where localizing attempts are unsuccessful or show multiple duct involvement. After the incision is made, the ducts are encircled and tied off as they enter the nipple. The subareolar tissue is coned out for several centimeters to remove all apparent ductal tissues. The recurrence rate of nipple discharge after this procedure is very low, although the proliferative lesion retrieval rate is less than for more directed techniques [19]. The circumareolar incision and more extensive subareolar tissue resection necessary to perform a major duct excision may disrupt the nerve supply to the nipple and leave the patient with numbness, nipple retraction, and the inability to nurse on that side. Care must be taken to avoid cautery burn to the undersurface of the nipple to limit the possibility of nipple necrosis [84].

A more limited or segmental duct resection can be performed by cannulating the discharging duct with a probe. The tissue is removed from around the probe deep within the breast. The goal is to remove an entire ductal system from the nipple to the terminal duct-lobular unit. This is useful in cases where localizing attempts have failed and the location of the lesion is unknown or for deep lesions. A circumareolar incision is commonly made in the quadrant of the discharging duct [85]. A flap is created undermining to the nipple, and the dilated or blue duct is encircled. It is important to dissect into the nipple to remove the proximal duct tissue to prevent recurrent discharge [84]. A useful adjunct to this procedure is preoperative ductography combined, if necessary, with needle localization for a deep abnormality. The proximal duct is removed with the assistance of a probe or blue dye while the deep lesion is identified by excising the tissue around the localizing wire [81]. Duct excision using a lacrimal probe guide has the advantage of identifying the proximal portion of the discharging duct. The probe may, however, enter the wrong duct at a bifurcation or be unable to be advanced to the level of pathology.

Microdochectomy is a procedure, which removes the abnormal duct while preserving surrounding normal breast tissue [25, 86]. The technique involves identifying and cannulating the discharging duct preoperatively by ductography. Blue dye is then injected into the abnormal ductal system through the cannula placed during the preoperative ductogram. The duct is dissected from the nipple toward the deeper ducts removing only the blue-stained duct tissue. This technique is described with a transareolar incision, which is a radial incision through the nipple, or a small curvilinear incision within the areola or at the areolar edge can be used as well [78, 87]. This technique has the benefit of removing the discharging duct while preserving the normal ducts in an effort to limit sensation loss and retain the ability to breast-feed.

3.15 Mammary Ductoscopy

Mammary ductoscopy allows for direct visualization of the intraductal lesion by passing a small endoscope through the nipple into the ductal system after the duct orifice is dilated. This technique is becoming more widely used especially in cases of pathologic nipple discharge and reports the highest proliferative lesion rates of all localizing techniques [29, 88–91]. The visual component alone of ductoscopy cannot

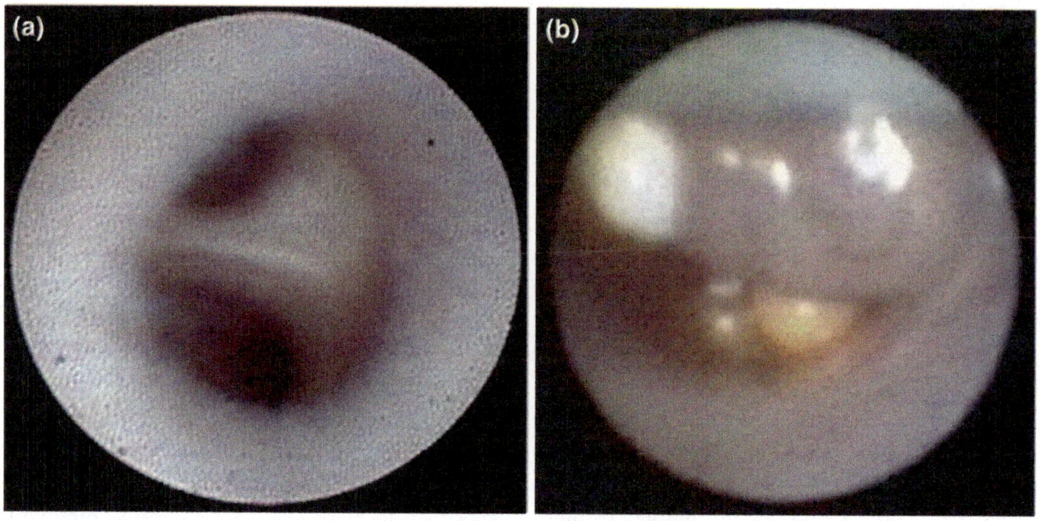

Fig. 3.8 Intraductal images through the mammary ductoscope. **a** Normal duct bifurcation. **b** Intraductal papilloma

adequately differentiate benign from malignant lesions [92]. Other studies show excellent sensitivity (98 and 96 %) with ductoscopy and cytology or intraductal biopsy, which can help with planning resection [39, 93].

The ability to enter the ductal system and directly visualize ductal abnormalities has distinct advantages. The intraductal pathology can be visualized during the time of surgical excision and the scope itself can direct the surgeon to the lesion (Fig. 3.8). Intraoperative visualization of the lesion enables adequate removal of the abnormality while preserving surrounding normal tissue. Ductoscopy enables the surgeon to identify the abnormality within the specimen and assists the pathologist in locating the lesion [94]. Mammary ductoscopy may limit the extent of surgery necessary to excise intraductal pathology, as well as help in identifying the lesions to be removed including lesions within the nipple itself, which can be left behind, and multiple deeper lesions, which occur in 25 % of cases, more accurately [29]. Intraductal biopsy tools are becoming available, which will provide histology samples of intraductal pathology [95]. A recent study used such tools to successfully remove 22 of 26 intraductal papillary lesions in an office setting. Short-term follow-up showed no recurrent discharge in these patients. [96] A recent Japanese study successfully removed 24 lesions in 75 patients with PND (29.3 %) negating surgical excision. One patient is subsequently developing DCIS and one developed recurrent discharge from multiple papillomas [97].

3.16 Follow-up

Anywhere from 5 to 20 % of duct excision cases will turn out to be malignant. As preoperative evaluation becomes more thorough, and malignant cases are identified preoperatively, this number declines. The treatment of breast cancer presenting as nipple discharge has traditionally been mastectomy. Many series suggest that intraductal cancer presenting as nipple discharge is more extensive and has a higher recurrence rate than DCIS in other areas of the breast [46, 98–100]. Ito found that in 26 patients with nonpalpable breast cancer associated with nipple discharge that were treated with duct-lobular segmentectomy, only one patient had microscopic residual disease found in the follow-up mastectomy specimen. These findings suggest that segmental duct resection is an adequate surgery for nonpalpable cancers presenting with nipple discharge [101]. If cancer is found at the time of duct excision for PND, then MRI may be useful for determining the extent of disease. Reexcision, which is often needed to obtain clear margins, will also help determine residual disease.

Carcinoma of the ipsilateral breast following duct excision has been reported in a number of series [3, 28, 46]. Many of these patients were found to have benign disease or no pathologic diagnosis at the original surgery. In these cases, it is likely that the lesion causing the discharge was not removed during the first procedure. These cancers typically present as masses rather than recurrent nipple discharge

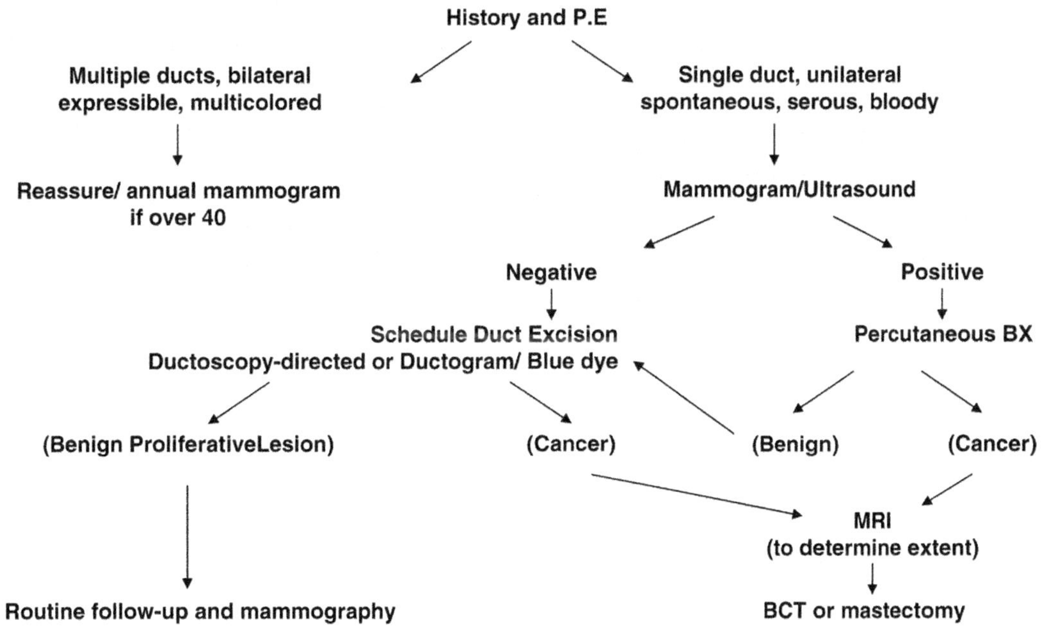

Fig. 3.9 Algorithm

because of the interruption of the ductal system at the time of the original duct excision. Close follow-up is essential for patients with nipple discharge in which no proliferative lesion was seen on analysis of the specimen, and for patients with peripheral papillomas. Patients undergoing breast conservation who have in situ carcinomas as the cause of their nipple discharge should also have postoperative radiation therapy and close mammographic and clinical follow-up [46].

Nipple discharge, in the majority of patients, is physiologic and usually does not require further evaluation. Spontaneous, clear or bloody, single duct discharge should be worked up with imaging modalities and most of these patients need excision to rule out carcinoma. While technology is rapidly advancing and we have many options available for ductal evaluation, none of these can satisfactorily rule out malignancy as the cause of the discharge. There are a few reports that suggest surveillance in patients with PND and negative extensive work-up is feasible; however, most studies advocate for excision [102–105]. Therefore, at this time, excision of the affected duct is still considered standard of care. The preoperative and excisional techniques you will utilize in this patient population will depend somewhat on the availability of equipment and expertise at your institution. It is clear, however, that localized excisions result in a greater lesion identification rate. Figure 3.9 illustrates the algorithm used at University Hospitals Seidman Cancer Center for the evaluation of nipple discharge. As imaging and biopsy techniques become more advanced, many nipple discharge patients will be able to forgo surgical excision altogether without compromising their diagnosis.

References

1. Devitt JE. Management of nipple discharge by clinical findings. Am J Surg. 1985;149:789.
2. Gulay H, Bora S, Kilicturgay S, Hamaloglu E, Goskel HA. Management of nipple discharge. J Am Coll Surg. 1994;178:471–4.
3. Chaudary M, Millis R, Davies G, et al. Nipple discharge: the diagnostic value of testing for occult blood. Ann Surg. 1982;196:651.
4. Van Zee K, Ortega P, Minnard E, Cohen M. Preoperative galactography increases the diagnostic yield of major duct excision for pathologic nipple discharge. Cancer. 1988;82 (10):1874–80.
5. Waaijer L, Simons J, Borel Rinkes H, et al. Systematic review and meta-analysis of the diagnostic accuracy of ductoscopy in patients with pathologic nipple discharge. BJS. 2016;103:632–43.
6. Zucca-Matthes G, Urban C, Vallejo A. Anatomy of the nipple and breast ducts. Gland Surgery. 2016;5(1):32–6.
7. Goodson WH, King EB. Discharges and secretions of the nipple. In: Bland KI, Copeland EM, editors. The breast: comprehensive management of benign and malignant diseases. 2nd ed. Philadelphia: WB Saunders; 1998. p. 51–74.
8. Sartorius OW, Smith HS, Morris P, et al. Cytological evaluation of breast fluid in the detection of breast diseases. J Natl Cancer Inst. 1977;59:1073–80.
9. Sauter ER, Daly M, Linahan K, et al. Prostate-specific antigen levels in nipple aspirate fluid correlate with breast cancer risk. Cancer Epidemiol Biomark Prev. 1996;5(120):967–70.
10. Petrakis NL, Mason L, Lee R. Association of race, age, menopausal status, and cerumen type with breast fluid secretion in nonlactating women as determined by nipple aspiration. J Natl Cancer Inst. 1975;54:829–34.
11. Sauter E, Wagner-Mann C, Ehya H, et al. Biologic markers of breast cancer in nipple aspirate fluid and nipple discharge are associated with clinical findings. Cancer Detect Prev. 2007;31 (1):50–8.

12. Wrensch MR, Petrakis NL, Gruenke LD, et al. Factors associated with obtaining nipple aspirate fluid: analysis of 1,428 women and literature review. Breast Cancer Res Treat. 1990;15(1):39–51.
13. Lang J, Kuerer H. Breast ductal secretions: clinical features, potential uses, and possible applications. Cancer Control. 2007;14(4):350–9.
14. Petrakis NL. Physiologic, biochemical, and cytologic aspects of nipple aspirate fluid. Breast Cancer Res Treat. 1986;8:7–19.
15. Papanicolaou GN, Bader GM, Holmquist DG. Exfoliative cytology of the human mammary gland and its value in the diagnosis of cancer and other diseases of the breast. Cancer. 1958;11:337–409.
16. Petrakis NL, Lee RE, Miike R, et al. Coloration of breast fluid related to concentration of cholesterol, cholesterol epoxides, estrogens and lipid peroxides. Am J Clin Pathol. 1988;89:117–20.
17. Santen RJ, Mansel R. Benign Breast disorders. N Engl J Med. 2005;353(3):275–85.
18. Seltzer MH. Breast complaints, biopsies, and cancer correlated with age in 10,000 consecutive new surgical referrals. Breast J. 2004;10:111–7.
19. Dillon M, NaMohd Nazri S, Nasir S, et al. The role of major duct excision and microdochectomy in the detection of breast carcinoma. BMC Cancer. 2006;6:164.
20. Ciatto S, Bravetti P, Cariaggi P. Significance of nipple discharge clinical patterns in selection of cases for cytologic examination. Acta Cytol. 1986;30(1):17–20.
21. Leis HP Jr. Management of nipple discharge. World J Surg. 1989;13(6):736–42.
22. Tabar L, Dean PB, Pentek Z. Galactography: the diagnostic procedure of choice for nipple discharge. Radiology. 1983;149:31–8.
23. Dawes LG, Bowen C, Luz VA, Morrow M. Ductography for nipple discharge: no replacement for ductal excision. Surgery. 1998;124(4):685–91.
24. Paterok EM, Rosenthal H, Sabel M. Nipple discharge and abnormal galactogram. Results of a long-term study (1964–1990). Eur J Obstet Gynecol Reprod Biol. 1993;50:227–34.
25. Lau S, Kuchenmeister I, Stachs A, et al. Pathologic nipple discharge: surgery is imperative in postmenopausal women. Ann Surg Oncol. 2005;12(7):246–51.
26. Vargas H, Perla Vargas M, Eldrageely K, et al. Outcomes of clinical and surgical assessment of women with pathological nipple discharge. Am Surg. 2006;72:124–8.
27. Cabioglu N, Hunt KK, Singletary SE, et al. Surgical decision-making and factors determining a diagnosis of breast carcinoma in women presenting with nipple discharge. Am Coll Surg. 2003;196(3):354–64.
28. Carty NJ, Mudan SS, Ravichandran D, Royle GT, Taylor I. Prospective study of outcome in women presenting with nipple discharge. Ann R Coll Surg Engl. 1994;76:387–9.
29. Dietz JR, Crowe JP, Grundfest S, et al. Directed duct excision by using mammary ductoscopy in patients with pathologic nipple discharge. Surgery. 2002;132:582–7.
30. Johnson TL, Kini SR. Cytologic and Clinicopathologic features of abnormal nipple secretions: 225 cases. Diagn Cytopathol. 1991;7:17–22.
31. Wong Chung J, Jeuriens-van de Ven J, Helmond N, et al. Does nipple discharge color predict (pre-) malignant breast pathology? Breast J. (2016);22(2):202–8.
32. Copeland M, Higgins T. Significance of discharge from the nipple in nonpuerperal mammary conditions. Ann Surg. 1960;151(5):638–48.
33. Arnold G, Neiheisel M. A comprehensive approach to evaluating nipple discharge. Nurse Pract. 1997;22(7):96–111.
34. Newman HF, Klein M, Northrup JD, et al. Nipple discharge: frequency and pathogenesis in an ambulatory population. NY St J Med. 1983;83:928.
35. Huang W, Molitch M. Evaluation and management of galactorrhea. Am Fam Physician. 2012;85(11):1073–80.
36. Haagensen DD (1971) Diseases of the breast., 2nd edn. WB. Saunders, Philadelphia.
37. Zuska JJ, Crile G Jr, Ayres NW. Fistulas of lactiferous ducts. Am J Surg. 1951;81:312–7.
38. Fiorica JV. Nipple discharge. Obstet Gynecol Clin North Am. 1994;21:453–60.
39. Liu GY, Lu JS, Shen KW, Wu J, Chen CM, et al. Fiberoptic ductoscopy combined with cytology testing in the patients of spontaneous nipple discharge. Breast Cancer Res Treat. 2008;108:271–7.
40. Lafreniere R. Bloody nipple discharge during pregnancy and/or lactation: a rational for conservative treatment. J Surg Oncol. 1990;43:228–30.
41. Sakai T, Makita M, Akiyama F, Uehara K, et al. Intraductal papilloma with bloody discharge from Montgomery's areolar tubercle examined by ductoscopy from the areola. Breast Cancer. 2006;13(1):104–6.
42. Bauer RL, Eckhert KH Jr, Nemoto T. Ductal carcinoma in situ-associated nipple discharge: a clinical marker for locally extensive disease. Ann Surg Oncol. 1998;5(5):452–5.
43. Cardenosa G, Eklund GW. Benign papillary neoplasms of the breast: mammographic findings. Radiology. 1991;181:751–5.
44. Carter D. Intraductal papillary tumors of the breast. Cancer. 1977;39:1689–92.
45. Ohuchi N, Abe R, Kasai M. Possible cancerous change of intraductal papilloma of the breast. Cancer. 1984;54:605–11.
46. Hou MF, Huang TJ, Liu GC. The diagnostic value of galactography in patients with nipple discharge. Clin Imaging. 2001;25:75–81.
47. Fung A, Rayter Z, Fisher C, et al. Preoperative cytology and mammography in patients with single-duct nipple discharge treated by surgery. Br J Surg. 1990;77(11):1211–2.
48. Teboul M. A new concept in breast investigation: echo-histological acino-ductal analysis or analytic echography. Biomed Pharmacoth. 1988;42:289–96.
49. Feige C. Dynamic morpho-cyto-echography and the echographic galactoscopy endoductal sample; intrinsic and extrinsic markers in the detection of breast cancers. Ultrasound Med and Biol. 1988;14(1):97–108.
50. Rissanen T, Reinikainen H, Apaja-Sarkkinen M. Breast sonography in localizing the cause of nipple discharge. J Ultrasound Med. 2007;26:1031–9.
51. Chung SY, Lee K, Park KS, Lee Y, Bae SH. Breast tumors associated with nipple discharge: correlation of findings on galactography and sonography. Clin Imaging. 1995;9(3):165–71.
52. Blum K, Rubbert C, Antoch G, et al. Diagnostic accuracy of abnormal galactographic and sonoraphic findings in the diagnosis of intraductal pathology in patients with abnormal nipple discharge. Clin Imaging. 2015;39:587–91.
53. Cilotti A, Campassi C, Bagnlesi P, et al. Pathologic nipple discharge. High resolution versus conventional ultrasound in the evaluation of ductal disease. Breast Dis. 1996;9:1–13.
54. Ballesio L, Maggi C, Savelli S, et al. Adjunctive diagnostic value of ultrasonography evaluation in patients with suspected ductal breast disease. Radiol Med. 2007;112:354–65.
55. Sardanelli F, Imperiale A, Zandrino F, et al. Breast intraductal masses. Ultrasound-guided fine needle aspiration after galactography. Radiology. 1997;204:143–8.
56. Govindarajulu S, Narreddy SR, Shere MH, et al. Sonographically guided mammotome excision of ducts in the diagnosis and

management of single duct nipple discharge. EJSO. 2006;32:725–8.
57. Torres-Tabanera M, Alonso-Bartolome P, Vega-Bolivar A, Sanchez-Gomez SM, et al. Percutaneous microductectomy with directional vacuum-assisted system guided by ultrasonography for the treatment of breast discharge: experience in 63 cases. Acta Radiol. 2008;49(3):271–6.
58. Yoshimoto M, Kasumi F, Iwase T, Takahashi K, Tada T, Uchida Y. Magnetic resonance galactography for a patient with nipple discharge. Breast Cancer Res Treat. 1997;42:87–90.
59. Ballesio L, Maggi C, Savelli S, et al. Role of breast magnetic resonance imaging (MRI) in patients with unilateral nipple discharge: preliminary study. Radiol med. 2008;113:249–64.
60. Morrogh M, Morris E, Liberman L, et al. The predictive value of ductography and magnetic resonance imaging in the management of nipple discharge. Ann Surg Oncol. 2007;14(12):3369–77.
61. Bahl M, Baker J, Greenup R, et al. Evaluation of pathologic nipple discharge: What is the added diagnostic value of MRI? Ann Surg Oncol. 2015;22:S435–41.
62. Hirose M, Nobusawa H, Gokan T. MR ductography: comparison with conventional ductography as a diagnostic method in patients with nipple discharge. Radiographics. 2007;27:S183–96.
63. Hirose M, Otsuki N, Hayano D, Shinjo H, Gokan T, et al. Multi-volume fusion imaging of MR ductography and MR mammography for patients with nipple discharge. Magn Reson Med Sci. 2006;5(2):105–12.
64. Nicholson B, Harvey J, Patrie J, Mugler J. 3D-MR Ductography and contrast-enhanced MR mammography in patients with suspicious nipple discharge; a feasibility study. Breast J. 2015;21(4):352–62.
65. Takeda T, Matsui A, Sato Y, et al. Nipple discharge cytology in mass screening for breast cancer. Acta Cytol. 1990;34(2):161–4.
66. Dunn JM, Lucarotti E, Wood SJ, et al. Exfoliative cytology in the diagnosis of breast disease. Br J Surg. 1995;82:789–91.
67. Florio M, Manganaro T, Pollicino A, et al. Surgical approach to nipple discharge: a ten-year experience. J Surg Oncol. 1999;71:235–8.
68. Knight DC, Lowell D, Heimann A, Dunn E. Aspiration of the breast and nipple discharge cytology. Surg Gynecol Obstet. 1986;163:415–20.
69. Moriarty A, Schwartz M, Laucirica R, et al. Cytology of spontaneous nipple discharge- is it worth it? Performance of nipple discharge preparations in the college of American pathologists interlaboratory comparison progrogram in nongynecologic cytopathology. Arch Pathol Lab Med. 2013;137: 1039–42.
70. Ranieri E, Virno F, D'Andrea M, et al. The role of cytology in differentiation of breast lesions. Anticancer Res. 1955;15:607–12.
71. Kawamoto M. Breast cancer diagnosis by lactate dehydrogenase isoenzymes in nipple discharge. Cancer. 1994;73:1836–41.
72. Imayama IS, Mori M, Ueo H, et al. Presence of elevated carcinoembryonic antigen on absorbent disks applied to nipple area of breast cancer patients. Cancer. 1996;78(6):12229–34.
73. Inaji H, Yayoi E, Maeura Y, Matsuura N, Tominaga S, Koyama H, et al. Carcinoembryonic antigen estimation in nipple discharge an adjunctive tool in the diagnosis of early breast cancer. Cancer. 1987;60:3008–13.
74. Nishiguchi T, Hishimoto T, Funahashi S, et al. Clinical usefulness of carcinoembryonic antigen measurement in nipple discharge as an adjunctive tool for diagnosis of breast cancer. Jpn J Clin Path. 1992;40(1):67–72.
75. Fortova L, Garber JE, Sadowsky NL, et al. Carcinoembryonic antigen in breast nipple aspirate fluid. Cancer Epidemiol Biomark Prev. 1998;7(3):195–8.
76. Liu Y, Wang JL, Chang H, et al. Breast-cancer diagnosis with nipple fluid bFGF (letter). Lancet. 2000;356(9229):567.
77. Sauter E, Shan S, Hewett J, et al. Proteomic analysis of nipple aspirate fluid using SELDI-TOF-MS. Int J Cancer. 2005;114:791–6.
78. Baker KS, Davey DD, Stelling CB. Ductal abnormalities detected with galactography: frequency of adequate excisional biopsy. Am J Roentgenol. 1994;162:821–4.
79. Van Zee KJ, Perez GO, Minnard E, Cohen M. Preoperative ductography increases the diagnostic yield of major duct excision for nipple discharge. Cancer. 1998;82(10):1874–80.
80. Rongione AJ, Evans BD, Kling KM, McFadden DW. Ductography is a useful technique in evaluation of abnormal nipple discharge. Am Surg. 1996;62:785–8.
81. Cardenosa G, Doudna C, Eklund GW. Ductography of the breast: techniques and findings. Am J Roentgenol. 1994;162:1081–7.
82. Saarela AO, Kiviniemi HO, Rissanen TJ. Preoperative methylene blue staining of galactographically suspicious breast lesions. Int Surg. 1997;82(4):403–5.
83. Hussain S, Lui DM. Ultrasound-guided percutaneous galactography. Eur J Radiol. 1997;24:163–5.
84. Urban JA. Excision of the major duct system of the breast. Cancer. 1963;16:516–20.
85. Jardines L. Management of nipple discharge. Am Surg. 1996;62:119–22.
86. Tan W, Lim TC. Transareolar dye-injection microdochectomy. Am Surg. 1992;58(7):404–8.
87. Sharma N, Huston T, Simmons R. Intraoperative intraductal injection of methylene blue dye to assist in major duct excision. Am J Surg. 2006;191:553–4.
88. Matsunaga T, Ohta D, Misaka T, et al. Mammary ductoscopy for diagnosis and treatment of intraductal lesions of the breast. Breast Cancer. 2001;8:213–21.
89. Shen KW, Wu J, Lu J, Han Q, Shen Z, Nguyen M, et al. Fiberoptic ductoscopy for patients with nipple discharge. Cancer. 2000;89:1512–9.
90. Escobar PF, Crowe JP, Matsunaga T, Mokbel K. The clinical applications of mammary ductoscopy. Am J Surg. 2006;191 (2):211–5.
91. Al Sarakbi W, Salhab M, Mokbel K. Does mammary ductoscopy have a role in clinical practice? Int Semin Surg Oncol. 2006;3:16.
92. Louie LD, Crowe JP, Dawson AE, Lee KB, et al. Identification of breast cancer in patients with pathologic nipple discharge: does ductoscopy predict malignancy? Am J Surg. 2006;192:530–3.
93. Hunerbein M, Dubowy A, Raubach M, Gebauer B, Topalidis T, Schlag P. Gradient index ductoscopy and intraductal biopsy of intraductal breast lesions. Am J Surg. 2007;194:511–4.
94. Pereira B, Mokbel K. Mammary ductoscopy: past, present, and future. Int J Clin Oncol. 2005;10:112–6.
95. Hunerbein M, Raubach M, Gebauer B, Wolfgang S, Schlag P. Ductoscopy and intraductal vacuum-assisted biopsy in women with pathologic nipple discharge. Breast Cancer Res Treat. 2006;99:301.
96. Balci F, Feldman S. Interventional ductoscopy for pathologic nipple discharge. Ann Surg Oncol. 2013;20:3352–4.
97. Kamali S, Bender O, Harman Kamali G, et al. Diagnostic and therapeutic value of ductoscopy in nipple discharge and intraductal proliferations compared with standard methods. Breast Cancer. 2014;21:154–61.
98. Solin LJ, Recht A, Fourquet A, et al. Ten-year results of breast-conserving surgery and definitive irradiation for intraductal carcinoma of the breast. Cancer. 1991;68:2337–44.
99. Fowable BL, Solin LJ, Goodman RL. Results of conservative surgery and radiation for intraductal noninvasive breast cancer. Am J Clin Oncol. 1987;10:110–1.

100. Recht A, Danoff B, Solin LJ, et al. Intraductal carcinoma of the breast: results of treatment with excisional biopsy and radiation. J Clin Oncol. 1985;3:1339–43.
101. Ito Y, Tamaki Y, Nakano Y, et al. Nonpalpable breast cancer with nipple discharge: how should it be treated? Anticancer Res. 1997;17(1B):791–4.
102. Dupont S, Boughey J, Jimenez R, et al. Surgery. 2015;158 (4):988–95.
103. Foulkes R, Heard G, Boyce T, et. al. (2011) Int J Br Cancer 2011; article ID 495315.
104. Sabel M, Helvie M, Breslin T, et al. Is duct excision still necessary for all cases of suspicious nipple discharge? Breast J. 2011;18(2):157–62.
105. Ashfaq A, Senior D, Pockaj B, et al. Validation study of a modern treatment algorithm for nipple discharge. The Am J Surgery. 2014;208:222–7.

Mastalgia

4

Amit Goyal and Robert E. Mansel

Mastalgia is a common breast symptom that may affect up to 70 % of women in their lifetime [1]. It is most common in women aged 30–50 years. Breast pain may be bilateral, unilateral, or in part of one breast. While most patients experience mastalgia of mild or moderate severity and accept this as a part of the normal changes that occur in relation to the menstrual cycle, a proportion (10–20 %) experience severe pain that causes distress, affects their daily lives, and leads them to seek treatment [2]. The severity of pain associated with cyclical mastalgia can be substantial, similar in magnitude to chronic cancer pain and slightly less than that associated with rheumatoid arthritis [3].

In a study of 1171 premenopausal women attending a gynecology clinic, 69 % reported regular premenstrual discomfort, 11 % had moderate-to-severe cyclic mastalgia, and 36 % had consulted a doctor about the symptoms. Breast pain interfered with usual sexual activities (48 %), physical activities (37 %), social activities (12 %), and school activities (8 %) [4].

4.1 Etiology

The etiology of cyclical mastalgia has not been established. Some evidence has implicated elevated estrogen levels, low progesterone levels, or an abnormal estrogen/progesterone ratio [5]. The cyclical nature of pain, swelling, tenderness, and nodularity together with postmenopausal cessation suggests a relationship between the symptoms and estrogen effects [6, 7]. However, measurement of estrogen, progesterone, and prolactin levels has not shown consistent abnormalities. There is no correlation of water retention, psychological factors, or caffeine intake with mastalgia. The role of iodine deficiency, alterations in levels of fatty acid in the breast, and fat intake in the diet remains unclear.

4.2 Classification

Mastalgia can be separated into four main groups, cyclical mastalgia, non-cyclical mastalgia, chest wall pain, and non-chest wall pain [8] (Table 4.1). History will often reveal the temporal association of cyclical mastalgia with the menstrual cycle, but the best way to assess whether pain is cyclical is to ask the patient to complete a breast pain chart (Fig. 4.1). This is especially useful in patients who have had a hysterectomy. A pain chart quantifies patient's symptoms and has the added advantage of assessing effectiveness of therapy. Two-thirds of women have cyclical pain, and the remaining third have non-cyclical pain.

4.3 Cyclical Mastalgia

Cyclical breast pain usually occurs during the late luteal phase of the menstrual cycle and resolves at the onset of menses (Table 4.1). Patients with cyclical pain are by definition premenopausal and most often in their thirties. Many women normally experience premenstrual discomfort, fullness, tenderness, or heaviness of the breast 3–7 days before each period in relation to the menstrual cycle. Tender lumpiness in breasts and increased breast size at this time, which regresses postmenstrually, are equally normal. Patients with cyclical mastalgia typically suffer increasing severity of pain from mid-cycle onward, with the pain improving at menstruation. The pain is usually bilateral, described as heaviness with the breast being tender to touch, and it commonly affects the upper outer quadrant of the

A. Goyal (✉)
Royal Derby Hospital, Uttoxeter Road, Derby, DE22 3NE, UK
e-mail: amit.goyal@nhs.net

R.E. Mansel
Cardiff University, The Gables, The Parade, Monmouth, NP25 3PA, UK
e-mail: ManselRE@cardiff.ac.uk

I. Jatoi and A. Rody (eds.), *Management of Breast Diseases*, DOI 10.1007/978-3-319-46356-8_4

Table 4.1 Classification of mastalgia

Breast pain	Cause
Cyclical pain	Hormonal stimulation of normal breast lobules before menses
Non-cyclical pain	Stretching of Cooper's ligaments Pressure from brassiere Fat necrosis from trauma Hidradenitis suppurativa Focal mastitis Periductal mastitis Cyst Mondor's disease (sclerosing periphlebitis of breast veins)
Non-breast pain	
Chest wall pain	Tietze's syndrome (costochondritis) Localized lateral chest wall pain Diffuse lateral chest wall pain Radicular pain from cervical arthritis
Non-chest wall pain	Gallbladder disease Ischemic heart disease

Source From The New England Journal of Medicine, Santen RJ, Mansel R, Benign breast disorders, Vol. 353, pp. 275–85 [8] © 2005 Massachusetts Medical Society. Reprinted with permission from Massachusetts Medical Society

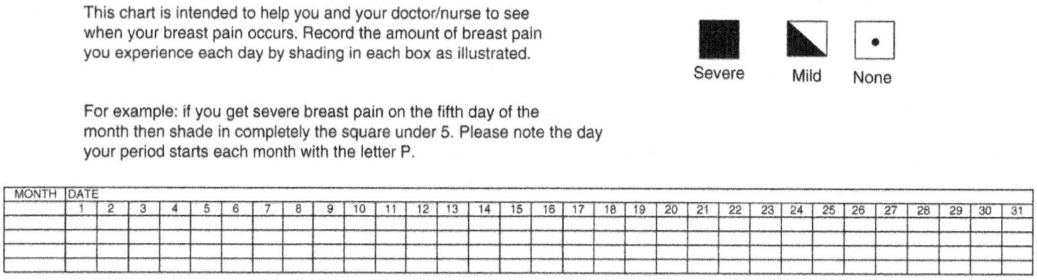

Fig. 4.1 Cardiff breast pain chart

breast. The pain may radiate to the axilla and down the medial aspect of the upper arm. The pain varies in severity from cycle to cycle but can persist for many years. Cyclical mastalgia is relieved by menopause. Physical activity can increase the pain; this is particularly relevant for women whose occupations include lifting and prolonged use of the arms. The impact of mastalgia on quality of life is often underestimated. Cyclical mastalgia is distinct from premenstrual syndrome (PMS), which is characterized by physical, psychological, and emotional symptoms associated with the menstrual cycle. The two may occur together or independently. Although mastalgia is a well-documented symptom in PMS, PMS is not necessarily present in women with cyclical mastalgia [9].

4.4 Non-cyclical Mastalgia

Non-cyclical breast pain is unrelated to the menstrual cycle and occurs in both pre- and postmenopausal women. Patients are usually in their forties. Pain may be continuous but is usually described as having a random time pattern. The pain is often localized and described as "burning" or "drawing." The pain may be due to a tender cyst, periductal mastitis, stretching of Cooper's ligaments, trauma (including breast biopsy or surgery), sclerosing adenosis, Mondor's disease, and cancer [8]. The majority of patients, however, are found to have no cause to explain their mastalgia despite thorough investigations.

4.5 Chest Wall Pain

Musculoskeletal pain is almost always unilateral, brought on by activity, and can be reproduced by pressure on specific area of the chest wall. Women known to have spondylosis or osteoarthritis are more likely to have musculoskeletal pain rather than true breast pain. Pain arising from the chest wall may be mistakenly attributed to the breast. Pain that is limited to a particular area and characterized as burning or knifelike in nature may arise from the chest wall. Several distinct types of pain can be distinguished, including localized or diffuse lateral chest wall pain, radicular pain from cervical arthritis, and pain from Tietze's syndrome (costochondritis). In Tietze's syndrome, the pain is often felt in the medial quadrants of the breast overlying the costal cartilages, which are the source of the pain. It has a chronic time course, and on examination, one or several costal cartilages are tender and feel enlarged.

4.6 Non-chest Wall Pain

This group consists of patients who have pain due to a non-breast cause, such as gallstones and angina.

4.7 Mastalgia and Breast Cancer

Cancer is an uncommon cause of breast pain. Breast pain associated with cancer is non-cyclical, unilateral, and well localized. Breast cancer is found in 2–7 % of patients presenting with pain as the primary symptom [10–14]. It is not clear whether breast pain increases the risk of subsequent breast cancer. Two case–control studies and one cohort study [15–17] have shown a significant increase in breast cancer risk in women with cyclical mastalgia. Plu-Bureau et al. [17] studied 210 premenopausal women diagnosed to have breast cancer who were matched with 210 controls from the same geographic area on age, education level, and age at first full-term pregnancy. The previous history of cyclical mastalgia was found to be associated with an increased risk of breast cancer (relative risk adjusted for family history of breast cancer, prior benign breast disease, age at menarche, oral contraceptive use >2.12). Similar findings were reported by the authors in a cohort study of 247 premenopausal women diagnosed to have benign breast disease [15]. They showed that the breast cancer risk increased with increasing duration of cyclical mastalgia. Goodwin et al. [16] studied 192 premenopausal women with a node-negative breast cancer and 192 age-matched premenopausal controls. Breast tenderness scores were significantly higher premenstrually in patients with breast cancer. The odds ratio of breast cancer for severe tenderness was 3.32. However, it is documented that women presenting to physicians with symptoms have higher mammographic and biopsy interventions, which may lead to a diagnosis bias in these studies.

In contrast, Khan et al. [18] found that women who experienced breast pain were less likely to have breast cancer. They analyzed data of 5463 women attending a breast care center in New York. Eight hundred and sixty-one of thousand five hundred and thirty-two women who reported breast pain at their initial visit were diagnosed with breast cancer. Odds ratio after adjustment for age and additional risk factors was 0.63.

Further evidence is needed to define the association between mastalgia and breast cancer. Clinical examination of the breasts and assessment of the patient's individual risk of breast cancer should be the main determinants of offering diagnostic breast imaging to patients with mastalgia.

4.8 Psychosocial Factors

Traditional surgical view that pain in the breast is largely an expression of psychoneurosis was challenged by Preece et al. [19] who found that women with mastalgia had similar anxiety, and depression and phobia to women with varicose veins. The psychological morbidity in varicose vein and mastalgia patients was significantly lower than that of psychiatric patients, except for few patients with breast pain who failed to respond to treatment.

Other studies have found that women with mastalgia have increased anxiety and depression compared with asymptomatic women [20]. It is not clear whether psychological distress contributes to or is a consequence of mastalgia. The emotional symptoms are significantly higher in women with severe mastalgia. The anxiety and depression in women with severe mastalgia are comparable with those of women with newly diagnosed breast cancer on the morning of their surgery [21]. Those who respond to treatment have a significant improvement in psychosocial function, but patients refractory to treatment continue to have high levels of distress [21].

More recently, Colegrave et al. [22] found that women with breast pain had increased anxiety, depression, somatization, and history of emotional abuse compared to women with breast lumps alone, suggesting psychosocial factors contribute to mastalgia. Relaxation therapy by listening to relaxation audio tape can improve symptoms of mastalgia [23].

4.9 Clinical Assessment and Investigations

A careful history is necessary to exclude non-breast conditions. Clinical examination must be performed to exclude a mass lesion in the breast and define breast tenderness and chest wall tenderness. Breast lump should be evaluated by "triple assessment," which includes palpation, imaging, and percutaneous core needle biopsy or fine-needle aspiration cytology. Chest wall should be examined by lifting the breast with one hand while palpating the underlying muscles and ribs with the other hand (Fig. 4.2). Lateral and medial chest wall tenderness can be elicited by rolling the patient to her side, allowing the breast to fall away from the chest wall (Fig. 4.2). If no mass is identified, further investigation is not indicated and the patient should be reassured that there is no sinister cause for her symptoms. The impact of the pain on the patient's quality of life should then be determined. Severe mastalgia tends to interfere with work, hugging children, and sexual relationships. If treatment is being considered, patients should be asked to complete a pain chart (Fig. 4.1) for at least 2 months to allow identification of the pattern of pain and to assess the number of days of pain in each menstrual cycle.

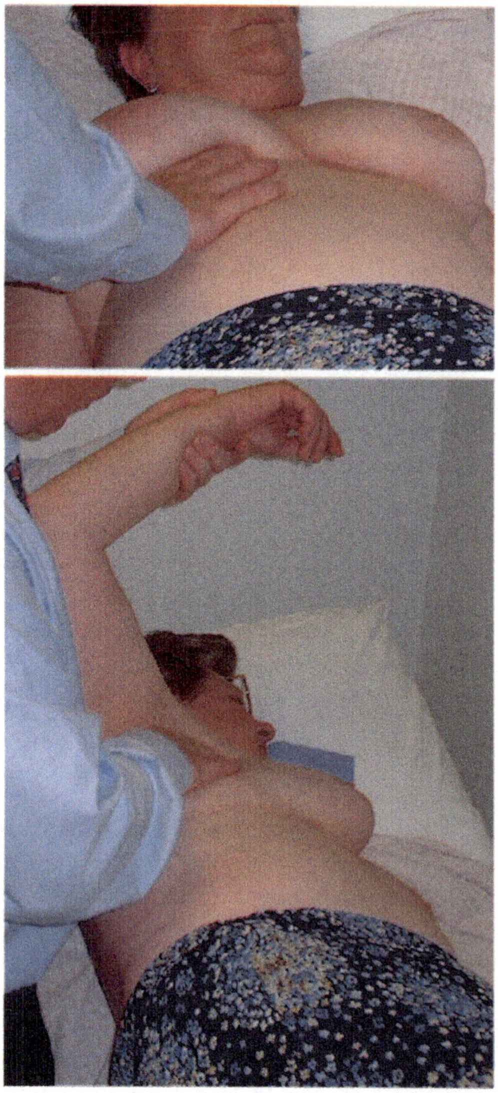

Fig. 4.2 Examination techniques to elicit chest wall tenderness

4.10 Treatment

4.10.1 Cyclical Mastalgia

The primary indication for treatment is pain, which interferes with everyday activities. Many women who present to hospital do so because they are worried that mastalgia may indicate breast cancer. Reassurance that cancer is not responsible for their symptoms is the only treatment necessary in up to 85 % of women with cyclical mastalgia [24]. The key to effective management of patients with mastalgia is a "listening physician" who can express empathy and understanding for the impact that breast pain has on women's lifestyle. Some women can improve their pain with simple measures such as wearing a well-fitting bra to support the pendulous breasts. Antibiotics are ineffective for mastalgia and should be used only when a specific diagnosis of periductal mastitis or lactational infection has been made. Diuretics, vitamin E, vitamin B6, caffeine reduction, and progestogens (oral or topical) have not been shown to be of value in cyclical mastalgia [25–31]. Women who start oral contraceptive or hormone replacement therapy may report breast pain, which usually settles with continued therapy. Some patients who are taking an oral contraceptive find that their breast pain improves after stopping the pill and changing to mechanical contraception, but no individual oral contraceptive has been shown to specifically cause mastalgia. The use of oral contraceptives and hormone replacement therapy has not been systematically studied, but for persistent symptoms, the use of alternative preparations, preparations that contain low-dose estrogen or stopping medication, may produce relief.

Evening primrose oil has been used, at oral doses of 1–3 g daily; however, two recent randomized trials have found that its efficacy does not differ from that of placebo [31, 32]. Evening primrose oil's prescription license in the UK was revoked in October 2002 due to lack of efficacy over placebo. One small randomized trial found improvement in premenstrual breast swelling and tenderness with low-fat (15 % of total calories) and high-carbohydrate diet [33]. This diet may be difficult to sustain, and further research is needed before low-fat diet can be recommended to reduce breast pain. There has been a growing interest in phytoestrogens, herbal agents, and nutritional supplements for the treatment of breast pain. Isoflavones were found to be effective in cyclical mastalgia in a small randomized trial [34]. *Agnus castus* was well tolerated and was effective in controlling the symptoms of cyclical mastalgia in a placebo-controlled, randomized trial of 97 women suffering from cyclical mastalgia [35]. These studies need to be repeated in larger numbers to clarify the therapeutic value of these alternative approaches in breast pain.

Topical non-steroidal anti-inflammatory drugs (NSAIDs) are well tolerated and effective in treating breast pain and should be considered for pain control in those who prefer topical therapy. In a randomized controlled trial, diclofenac gel was found to be superior to placebo in premenopausal women with cyclical or non-cyclical mastalgia [36].

The efficacy of bromocriptine (dopamine agonist) has been confirmed in randomized trials and in a recent meta-analysis [37], but it is not used these days because of frequent and intolerable side effects (nausea, dizziness, headache, and postural hypotension).

Goserelin (Zoladex®), a potent synthetic analog of luteinizing hormone-releasing hormone (LHRH), induces reversible ovarian suppression with castrate levels of ovarian hormones being attained within 72 h [38–40]. In a randomized controlled trial, we found that goserelin injection was superior to sham injection in treating severe mastalgia [41]. However, side effects (vaginal dryness, hot flushes, decreased libido, oily skin or hair, and decrease in breast size) are common, and thus, goserelin should be kept in reserve for patients who are refractory to other forms of treatment. Goserelin can be used to induce a rapid relief of symptoms in patients with severe mastalgia, and the response can be maintained with alternative therapies.

Danazol is a synthetic androgen that has antigonadotrophic effects on the pituitary. It prevents luteinizing hormone surge and inhibits ovarian steroid formation. Danazol relieves breast pain and tenderness, and the response is usually seen within 3 months [42, 43]. However, side effects occur in 30 % of patients and result in discontinuation of treatment in a significant number of patients [44]. Danazol has superior efficacy compared with bromocriptine [45]. The side effects of danazol treatment (weight gain, deepening of the voice, menstrual irregularity or amenorrhea, hot flashes, depression, headaches, and muscle cramps) can be limited by reducing the dose once the response has been achieved. The response can be maintained with doses as low as 100 mg daily, given on days 14–28 of the menstrual cycle [42].

Tamoxifen has proven to be effective in the treatment of both cyclical and non-cyclical mastalgia in randomized controlled trials [46, 47]. Tamoxifen 10 mg daily has equal efficacy but fewer adverse effects compared with 20 mg daily [48]. Its use is limited to no more than 6 months under specialist supervision as tamoxifen is not licensed for mastalgia in the USA or the UK. Common side effects with 10-mg daily regimen are menstrual irregularities, hot flashes, weight gain, vaginal dryness, and bloating. The incidence of thromboembolic events, endometrial cancer, and cataracts with short-term treatment for mastalgia is unknown. Tamoxifen is cheaper and has higher response rates and less side effects compared with danazol [49].

4-hydroxytamoxifen (4-OHT) is a potent antiestrogenic metabolite of tamoxifen with much higher affinity for estrogen receptors than tamoxifen. A percutaneous gel formulation of 4-hydroxytamoxifen (Afimoxifene®) has been found to be superior to placebo in the treatment of cyclical mastalgia in a phase II randomized trial [50]. Topical application avoids high systemic exposure to 4-OHT compared with oral tamoxifen, thus potentially reducing the risk of systemic side effects. Further studies are needed before Afimoxifene® can be recommended for mastalgia.

There is insufficient evidence on the role of surgery in the treatment of mastalgia, and surgical intervention should be approached with great caution. Retrospective data from Cardiff found that mastectomy in contrast to localized excision needs to be performed for symptom relief [51]. Surgery should be reserved for a minority of women who suffer from intractable symptoms and in whom non-breast causes of pain have been excluded. A multidisciplinary team approach involving the surgeon, psychologist, and breast care nurse is required when offering surgery to these women. The women should be counseled to inform them of the potential complications and the risk of persistence of symptoms.

4.10.2 Non-cyclical Mastalgia

When pain is truly arising from the breast, the approach outlined for cyclical pain is used. Musculoskeletal pain often responds to oral or topical NSAIDs. Patients with persistent localized chest wall symptoms can be effectively treated by injection of a combination of local anesthetic and steroid into the tender site. Injection of local anesthetic confirms the correct identification of the painful area by producing complete disappearance of the pain.

4.11 Management Algorithm

The protocol followed in Cardiff Breast Unit is outlined in Fig. 4.3. Most patients can be reassured and discharged from the clinic if breast examination is normal. Imaging (mammogram/ultrasonography) is only done based on the patient's breast cancer risk and examination findings. Patients requesting treatment are given lifestyle advice (e.g., wear well-fitted bra) and asked to record their pain in the Cardiff Breast Pain Chart and return to the clinic in 3 months. First-line treatment includes the use of topical or oral mild analgesic agents such as paracetamol and NSAIDs. Patients with persistent symptoms after 3 months of treatment are started on tamoxifen, at a dose of 10 mg daily for three to 6 months. Treatment failures are started on danazol, at a dose of 200 mg daily (reduced to 100 mg a day after

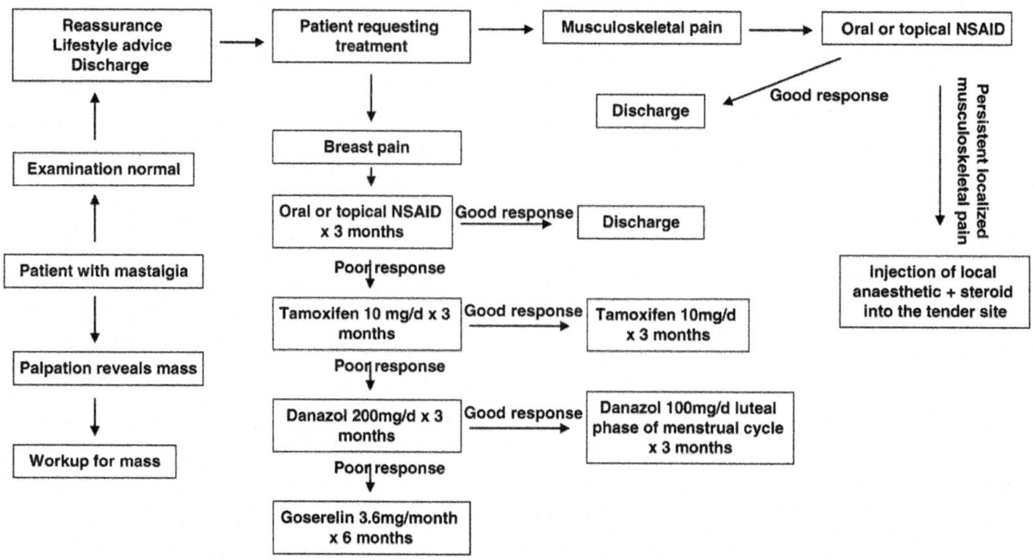

Fig. 4.3 Algorithm for the management of mastalgia

relief of symptoms) or only during the luteal phase of the menstrual cycle. Non-responders with severe pain are started on goserelin depot injection, 3.6 mg/month for 6 months. If the outlined treatment plan is followed, about 70–80 % of patients should experience substantial relief of symptoms. Non-hormonal contraception is essential with tamoxifen and danazol because both have deleterious effects on the fetus.

References

1. Ader DN, South-Paul J, Adera T, Deuster PA. Cyclical mastalgia: prevalence and associated health and behavioral factors. J Psychosom Obstet Gynaecol. 2001;22:71–6.
2. Cyclical breast pain–what works and what doesn't. Drug Ther Bull. 1992;30:1–3.
3. Khan SA, Apkarian AV. The characteristics of cyclical and non-cyclical mastalgia: a prospective study using a modified McGill Pain Questionnaire. Breast Cancer Res Treat. 2002;75:147–57.
4. Ader DN, Shriver CD. Cyclical mastalgia: prevalence and impact in an outpatient breast clinic sample. J Am Coll Surg. 1997;185:466–70.
5. Rose DP, Boyar AP, Cohen C, Strong LE. Effect of a low-fat diet on hormone levels in women with cystic breast disease. I. Serum steroids and gonadotropins. J Natl Cancer Inst. 1987;78:623–6.
6. Wang DY, Fentiman IS. Epidemiology and endocrinology of benign breast disease. Breast Cancer Res Treat. 1985;6:5–36.
7. Wisbey JR, Kumar S, Mansel RE, Peece PE, Pye JK, Hughes LE. Natural history of breast pain. Lancet. 1983;2:672–4.
8. Santen RJ, Mansel R. Benign breast disorders. N Engl J Med. 2005;353:275–85.
9. Ader DN, Shriver CD, Browne MW. Cyclical mastalgia: premenstrual syndrome or recurrent pain disorder? J Psychosom Obstet Gynaecol. 1999;20:198–202.
10. Barton MB, Elmore JG, Fletcher SW. Breast symptoms among women enrolled in a health maintenance organization: frequency, evaluation, and outcome. Ann Intern Med. 1999;130:651–7.
11. Lumachi F, Ermani M, Brandes AA, Boccagni P, Polistina F, Basso SM, Favia G, D'Amico DF. Breast complaints and risk of breast cancer. Population-based study of 2,879 self-selected women and long-term follow-up. Biomed Pharmacother. 2002;56:88–92.
12. Fariselli G, Lepera P, Viganotti G, Martelli G, Bandieramonte G, Di Pietro S. Localized mastalgia as presenting symptom in breast cancer. Eur J Surg Oncol. 1988;14:213–5.
13. Smallwood JA, Kye DA, Taylor I. Mastalgia; is this commonly associated with operable breast cancer? Ann R Coll Surg Engl. 1986;68:262–3.
14. Preece PE, Baum M, Mansel RE, Webster DJ, Fortt RW, Gravelle IH, Hughes LE. Importance of mastalgia in operable breast cancer. Br Med J (Clin Res Ed). 1982;284:1299–300.
15. Plu-Bureau G, Le MG, Sitruk-Ware R, Thalabard JC. Cyclical mastalgia and breast cancer risk: results of a French cohort study. Cancer Epidemiol Biomarkers Prev. 2006;15:1229–31.
16. Goodwin PJ, DeBoer G, Clark RM, Catton P, Redwood S, Hood N, Boyd NF. Cyclical mastopathy and premenopausal breast cancer risk. Results of a case-control study. Breast Cancer Res Treat. 1995;33:63–73.
17. Plu-Bureau TJC, Sitruk-Ware R, Asselain B, Mauvais-Jarvis P. Cyclical mastalgia as a marker of breast cancer susceptibility: results of a case-control study among French women. Br J Cancer. 1992;65:945–9.
18. Khan SA, Apkarian AV. Mastalgia and breast cancer: a protective association? Cancer Detect Prev. 2002;26:192–6.
19. Preece PE, Mansel RE, Hughes LE. Mastalgia: psychoneurosis or organic disease? Br Med J. 1978;1:29–30.
20. Jenkins PL, Jamil N, Gateley C, Mansel RE. Psychiatric illness in patients with severe treatment-resistant mastalgia. Gen Hosp Psychiatry. 1993;15:55–7.
21. Ramirez AJ, Jarrett SR, Hamed H, Smith P, Fentiman IS. Psychosocial adjustment of women with mastalgia. Breast. 1995;4:48–51.
22. Colegrave S, Holcombe C, Salmon P. Psychological characteristics of women presenting with breast pain. J Psychosom Res. 2001;50:303–7.
23. Fox H, Walker LG, Heys SD, Ah-See AK, Eremin O. Are patients with mastalgia anxious, or does relaxation therapy help? Breast. 2009;6:138–42.

24. Barros AC, Mottola J, Ruiz CA, Borges MN, Pinotti JA. Reassurance in the treatment of mastalgia. Breast J. 1999;5:162–5.
25. Smallwood J, Ah-Kye D, Taylor I. Vitamin B6 in the treatment of pre-menstrual mastalgia. Br J Clin Pract. 1986;40:532–3.
26. Ernster VL, Goodson WH III, Hunt TK, Petrakis NL, Sickles EA, Miike R. Vitamin E and benign breast "disease": a double-blind, randomized clinical trial. Surgery. 1985;97:490–4.
27. Parazzini F, La Vecchia C, Riundi R, Pampallona S, Regallo M, Scanni A. Methylxanthine, alcohol-free diet and fibrocystic breast disease: a factorial clinical trial. Surgery. 1986;99:576–81.
28. Allen SS, Froberg DG. The effect of decreased caffeine consumption on benign proliferative breast disease: a randomized clinical trial. Surgery. 1987;101:720–30.
29. McFadyen IJ, Raab GM, Macintyre CC, Forrest AP. Progesterone cream for cyclic breast pain. BMJ. 1989;298:931.
30. Maddox PR, Harrison BJ, Horobin JM, Walker K, Mansel RE, Preece PE, Nicholson RI. A randomised controlled trial of medroxyprogesterone acetate in mastalgia. Ann R Coll Surg Engl. 1990;72:71–6.
31. Goyal A, Mansel RE. A randomized multicenter study of gamolenic acid (Efamast) with and without antioxidant vitamins and minerals in the management of mastalgia. Breast J. 2005;11:41–7.
32. Blommers J, de Lange-De Klerk ES, Kuik DJ, Bezemer PD, Meijer S. Evening primrose oil and fish oil for severe chronic mastalgia: a randomized, double-blind, controlled trial. Am J Obstet Gynecol. 2002;187:1389–94.
33. Boyd NF, McGuire V, Shannon P, Cousins M, Kriukov V, Mahoney L, Fish E, Lickley L, Lockwood G, Tritchler D. Effect of a low-fat, high-carbohydrate diet on symptoms of cyclical mastopathy. Lancet. 1988;2:128–32.
34. Ingram DM, Hickling C, West L, Mahe LJ, Dunbar PM. A double-blind, randomized controlled trial of isoflavones in the treatment of cyclical mastalgia. Breast. 2002;11:170–4.
35. Halaska M, Beles P, Gorkow C, Sieder C. Treatment of cyclical mastalgia with a solution containing a Vitex agnus castus extract: results of a placebo-controlled double-blind study. Breast. 1999;8:175–81.
36. Colak T, Ipek T, Kanik A, Ogetman Z, Aydin S. Efficacy of topical nonsteroidal anti-inflammatory drugs in mastalgia treatment. J Am Coll Surg. 2003;196:525–30.
37. Srivastava A, Mansel RE, Arvind N, Prasad K, Dhar A, Chabra A. Evidence-based management of mastalgia: a meta-analysis of randomised trials. Breast. 2007;16:503–12.
38. Thomas EJ, Jenkins J, Lenton EA, Cooke ID. Endocrine effects of goserelin, a new depot luteinising hormone releasing hormone agonist. Br Med J (Clin Res Ed). 1986;293:1407–8.
39. Shaw RW. An open randomized, comparative study of the effect of goserelin depot and danazol in the treatment of endometriosis. Zoladex endometriosis study team. Fertil Steril. 1992;58:265–72.
40. Fraser HM, Sandow J. Suppression of follicular maturation by infusion of a luteinizing hormone-releasing hormone agonist starting during the late luteal phase in the stumptailed macaque monkey. J Clin Endocrinol Metab. 1985;60:579–84.
41. Mansel RE, Goyal A, Preece P, Leinster S, Maddox PR, Gateley C, Kubista E, von Fournier D. European randomized, multicenter study of goserelin (Zoladex) in the management of mastalgia. Am J Obstet Gynecol. 2004;191:1942–9.
42. O'Brien PM, Abukhalil IE. Randomized controlled trial of the management of premenstrual syndrome and premenstrual mastalgia using luteal phase-only danazol. Am J Obstet Gynecol. 1999;180:18–23.
43. Mansel RE, Wisbey JR, Hughes LE. Controlled trial of the antigonadotropin danazol in painful nodular benign breast disease. Lancet. 1982;1:928–30.
44. Gateley CA, Miers M, Mansel RE, Hughes LE. Drug treatments for mastalgia: 17 years experience in the Cardiff mastalgia clinic. J R Soc Med. 1992;85:12–5.
45. Hinton CP, Bishop HM, Holliday HW, Doyle PJ, Blamey RW. A double-blind controlled trial of danazol and bromocriptine in the management of severe cyclical breast pain. Br J Clin Pract. 1986;40:326–30.
46. Fentiman IS, Caleffi M, Brame K, Chaudary MA, Hayward JL. Double-blind controlled trial of tamoxifen therapy for mastalgia. Lancet. 1986;1:287–8.
47. Messinis IE, Lolis D. Treatment of premenstrual mastalgia with tamoxifen. Acta Obstet Gynecol Scand. 1988;67:307–9.
48. Fentiman IS, Caleffi M, Hamed H, Chaudary MA. Dosage and duration of tamoxifen treatment for mastalgia: a controlled trial. Br J Surg. 1988;75:845–6.
49. Kontostolis E, Stefanidis K, Navrozoglou I, Lolis D. Comparison of tamoxifen with danazol for treatment of cyclical mastalgia. Gynecol Endocrinol. 1997;11:393–7.
50. Mansel R, Goyal A, Nestour EL, Masini-Eteve V, O'Connell K. A phase II trial of Afimoxifene (4-hydroxytamoxifen gel) for cyclical mastalgia in premenopausal women. Breast Cancer Res Treat. 2007;106:389–97.
51. Davies EL, Cochrane RA, Stansfield K, Sweetland HM, Mansel RE. Is there a role for surgery in the treatment of mastalgia? Breast. 1999;8:285–8.

5 Management of Common Lactation and Breastfeeding Problems

Lisa H. Amir and Verity H. Livingstone

Lactation is a physiologic process under neuroendocrine control; breastfeeding is a technical process by which milk is transferred from the maternal breast to the infant. Success depends on maternal health, adequate mammogenesis, unimpeded lactogenesis, successful galactopoiesis, effective milk transfer, and appropriate quality and quantity of daily milk intake. Each phase of lactation and breastfeeding is influenced by multiple predisposing, facilitating, or impeding biopsychosocial factors: puberty, pregnancy, childbirth, breast stimulation and drainage, maternal milk ejection reflex, maternal and infant breastfeeding technique, frequency and duration of suckling, and the pattern of breast use. All these factors are influenced by other factors such as maternal knowledge, attitude, motivation, mood, and health; infant health and behavior; and support from family, friends, and healthcare professionals.

The concept of breastfeeding kinetics as developed by Livingstone conveys the idea that there is a dynamic interaction between a breastfeeding mother and her infant over time [1]. Most disorders of lactation are iatrogenic due to impeded establishment of lactation or inadequate ongoing stimulation and drainage of the breast. Most breastfeeding difficulties are due to the lack of knowledge, poor technical skills, or lack of support. Almost all problems are reversible. Prevention, early detection, and management should become a routine part of the maternal and child health care.

L.H. Amir (✉)
Judith Lumley Centre, La Trobe University, 215 Franklin St, Melbourne, VIC 3000, Australia
e-mail: L.Amir@latrobe.edu.au

V.H. Livingstone
Department of Family Practice, The Vancouver Breastfeeding Centre, University of British Columbia, Canada Suite 340-943 West Broadway, Vancouver, BC V5Z 4E1, Canada

L.H. Amir
Breastfeeding service, Royal Women's Hospital, Melbourne, Australia

5.1 Prenatal Period

Prenatal breastfeeding goals are to assist families to make an informed choice about infant feeding, prepare women cognitively and emotionally for breastfeeding, identify and modify risk factors to lactation and breastfeeding, and offer anticipatory guidance. These goals can be achieved by providing prenatal breastfeeding education and by performing a prenatal lactation assessment [2, 3].

5.1.1 Informed Choice

Health professionals must assist families in making an informed decision by discussing the recommended infant feeding guidelines, including the benefits of breastfeeding and the risks of breast milk substitutes [4–6]. The World Health Organization recommends exclusive breastfeeding for the first 6 months, with the introduction of complementary foods and continued breastfeeding for up to 2 years or beyond [7, 8]. Dettwyler [9] has examined the relationships between age at weaning and life history variables, such as length of gestation, body weight, and eruption of molars, among nonhuman primates. She estimates that if humans followed primate patterns rather than cultural customs, children would continued to be breastfed for somewhere between 2.5 and 7 years [9].

5.1.2 Benefits of Breastfeeding

To the Infant

- Human milk is species-specific; it is the ideal nutrition because the protein and fat contents are uniquely suited to the needs of the infant. It also provides protection against iron and vitamin deficiencies [10].

I. Jatoi and A. Rody (eds.), *Management of Breast Diseases*, DOI 10.1007/978-3-319-46356-8_5

- Breast milk contains more than 100 biologically active ingredients. It offers immunologic protection to an otherwise immunodeficient neonate [11]. The entero-mammary immune cycle provides specific maternal antibodies to infant antigens [12]. It protects against otitis media, gastroenteritis, respiratory tract infections, urinary tract infections, other bacterial and viral diseases, and necrotizing enterocolitis [13–20].
- Breastfeeding provides a close interaction between mother and infant and helps the two develop a strong, positive, emotional bond, which has long-term psychological advantages [21].
- The action of breastfeeding facilitates correct jaw and dental development [22].
- Breastfeeding may prevent overweight and obesity in children and adults [19, 23, 24] and is associated with lower blood pressure [25].

To the Mother

- Breastfeeding provides psychological satisfaction and close maternal bonding between mother and infant [26]. It offers a regular opportunity to sit and relax during the often exhausting early parenting period [27].
- Women who do not breast-feed are at increased risk of developing premenopausal breast cancer [28] and possibly ovarian cancer [29].
- Using breastfeeding as the sole nourishment activity causes lactation amenorrhea, which is an effective and reliable method of contraception and child spacing [30].
- It reduces postpartum anemia.

To Society

- Breast milk is a natural resource that is replenished and does not leave waste.
- The future of a society depends on the health of its children.
- Breastfeeding is the most health-promoting, disease-preventing, and cost-effective activity mothers can do.

5.1.3 The Hazards of Infant Formula

Inadequate nutrition: Infant formula may contain inadequate or excessive micronutrients. They lack essential fatty acids known to be vital for myelination and proper brain and retinal development. Some brands of formula contain excess vitamin D [31].

Bacterial contaminants: Powdered infant formula is not a sterile product [32, 33]. The most serious bacterial contaminant, *Enterobacter sakazakii*, can cause rare, but life-threatening neonatal meningitis, bacteremia, and necrotizing enterocolitis [32, 34].

Contaminants: A variety of other contaminants—including excessive aluminum, lead, and iodine—have been identified, and many brands of formula have been withdrawn due to these discoveries [35–37].

Impaired cognitive development: Several well-controlled studies have reported significantly lower intelligence quotient scores and poorer development in children who lack breast milk in their diet [38–41].

Allergies: More formula-fed infants develop atopic dermatitis [42].

Morbidity and mortality: The added risk of bottle-feeding can account for 7 % of infants hospitalized for respiratory infections, and in the USA, formula-fed infants have a tenfold risk of being hospitalized for any bacterial infection. They have more than double the risk of contracting lower respiratory tract infections, and otitis media is up to 3–4 times more prevalent [43, 44]. Formula-fed infants have a higher incidence of childhood cancers and inflammatory bowel diseases in adulthood [45–47]. Formula feeding accounts for 2–26 % of insulin-dependent diabetes mellitus in children [48, 49].

Costs: It costs approximately $1000–$2300 to formula feed an infant for 12 months (depending on the type of formula used) [50]; therefore, many infants in low-income families are at risk for receiving low-cost and inappropriate alternative fluids and the early introduction of table foods. It is also time-consuming to purchase and prepare formula. Lack of breastfeeding results in increased healthcare costs [51, 52].

5.1.4 Prenatal Education

Breastfeeding is a learned skill that should be taught prenatally; physicians can use models in their offices to help reinforce the learning process [53]. Industry-developed literature on infant feeding should not be distributed because it gives mixed messages to breastfeeding families [54].

5.1.5 Prenatal Lactation Assessment

Lactation is essential for the survival of most mammalian species and can be considered the final stage of the reproductive cycle. Mammogenesis begins in the embryo and continues throughout life, with active growth phases during puberty and pregnancy. It is controlled by a complex hormonal milieu. Clinical signs of successful mammogenesis are breast growth, increased breast sensitivity, and the excretion of a colostrum-like fluid by the end of pregnancy (lactogenesis I [55]). Failure of mammogenesis presents clinically as a lack of, or an abnormality, in breast growth and development during puberty or pregnancy.

5.1.6 Screening for Risk Factors

During the prenatal period, physicians have an opportunity to screen women for certain biological, psychological, and social risk factors that might interfere with mammogenesis, successful lactation, or breastfeeding. A formal *prenatal lactation assessment* should be performed in the third trimester as a routine component of antenatal care for all women.

5.1.6.1 Maternal Biological Risk Factors for Successful Lactation

- Anatomically abnormal breasts, including hypoplastic or conical breasts, may never lactate adequately because of insufficient glandular development associated with the failure of mammogenesis [56, 57].
- Breast surgery, in particular reduction mammoplasty, may interfere with glandular or lactiferous duct function [58, 59].
- Certain endocrinopathies, including thyroid, pituitary and ovarian dysfunction, and relative infertility, may interfere with lactation [60, 61].
- Chronic maternal illnesses, such as diabetes mellitus, systemic lupus erythematosus, and hypertension, may cause maternal fatigue but usually do not affect lactation.
- Women with physical disabilities usually can breastfeed, but they may have to be given guidance and assistance with regard to safe, alternative nursing positions.
- Complications of pregnancy such as gestational diabetes, pregnancy-induced hypertension, and preterm labor may result in early maternal infant separation, which can interfere with the initiation of lactation. Antenatal expression of colostrum may be useful when potential neonatal hypoglycemia is anticipated [62].
- Maternal infections such as hepatitis B and C, human immunodeficiency virus (HIV), or cytomegalovirus may be transmitted to the infant in utero, but the added viral load through breast milk is probably clinically insignificant [63]. In industrial countries, it would seem prudent to advise HIV-positive women not to breast-feed [64].
- Women who use illicit drugs, such as amphetamines, cocaine, or heroin, should be informed about the risks and counseled about abstinence [65]. If the use continues, the women should be advised not to breastfeed. Maternal smoking is not advisable; however, the risks of smoking and artificial feeding are greater than the risks of smoking and breastfeeding [66, 67]. Breastfeeding should therefore be recommended in spite of smoking. Moderate use of alcohol should not be a contraindication to breastfeeding [65].
- A previous unsuccessful breastfeeding experience may herald future problems.
- Previous or chronic psychiatric disorders, including depression, may recur in the postpartum period and interfere with maternal parenting abilities. These mothers need extra help during the early postpartum period.

5.1.6.2 Infant Biological Risk Factors for Successful Lactation

Several infant factors interfere with the establishment of lactation and breastfeeding. These include neonatal illness, which necessitates early maternal/infant separation and sucking, swallowing, or breathing disorders. Some factors can be identified or predicted prenatally.

5.1.6.3 Psychological Risk Factors

There is interplay between the many forces that influence a woman's choice of feeding methods [68–70].

Beliefs: Many women have preconceived ideas about feeding their infants. They may have anxieties and concerns over their ability to breastfeed, they may believe their breasts are too small or their nipples too large, or they may fear the consequences of altered breast appearance. They may have had previous unsuccessful breastfeeding experiences or family members who offer negative advice. It is important to clarify beliefs surrounding breastfeeding.

Attitudes: The physician should explore the woman's attitudes toward breastfeeding, returning to work, and breastfeeding in public. Prenatal exploration of these areas helps families start addressing their own attitudes.

Knowledge and skills: The physician should explore the woman's knowledge by asking what she knows about infant feeding and how she is planning to feed her infant.

5.1.6.4 Social Risk Factors

Women are more likely to succeed in breastfeeding if they have support from their family and friends. In the prenatal phase, the goal is to help to foster a positive emotional environment among family, friends, and community.

Family support: Throughout history, women have been supported in their decision to breast-feed by grandmothers, sisters, close friends, or doulas. Nowadays, with the disintegration of the traditional family, lack of support often culminates in abandonment of breastfeeding [71, 72].

Peer support: Single teenaged mothers experience considerable peer pressure to continue the carefree life of youth, and they may opt for the perceived freedom of bottle-feeding rather than the commitment to breastfeeding. Peer support programs have been shown to be an effective way of helping to increase the duration of breastfeeding [73].

Community support: Many women are embarrassed about breastfeeding in public. A prenatal discussion around the issue of breastfeeding in public may help. Employment outside the home need not be a reason for stopping breastfeeding; planning, flexibility, and good childcare can support a mother to maintain lactation during prolonged hours of separation.

5.1.7 Prenatal Breast Examination

After reviewing the woman's history, a careful breast examination should be performed.

5.1.7.1 Size and Symmetry

It is not until pregnancy that the full maturation of the mammary glands occurs. Lactogenic hormones, including estrogen, progesterone, prolactin, insulin, thyroid, and growth hormones, trigger the development of the mammary epithelial cells, acinar glands, and lactiferous ducts. By 16 weeks of gestation, lactation can occur. The breasts usually enlarge by at least one bra cup size or about 200 mL during pregnancy or in the first month postpartum [74, 75]. Variations in breast appearance or asymmetry may indicate lactation insufficiency and therefore should be noted; future milk synthesis should be closely monitored. Scars give clues to potential glandular, ductal, or nerve disruption.

5.1.7.2 Nipple Graspability

For infants to latch and suckle effectively, they should be able to grasp the nipple and areola tissue and form a teat. The areola can be gently pinched to assess its elasticity and graspability. Nipples may protrude, pseudoprotrude, remain flat, pseudoinvert, or truly invert. They may be large or small. There is no evidence to support nipple preparation such as nipple stretching exercises or the use of nipple shells because the anatomy of the nipple and areola is not altered by prenatal exercises [76]. The action of sucking by the infant helps to thaw out the nipple and form a teat during the process of breastfeeding. It is only true inverted nipples that may impede correct latching and suckling. The Niplette (Avent, Suffolk, England) was designed to help correct inverted nipples prenatally [77]. Cutting off the needle end of a 20-mL syringe and reversing the plunger can make a simplified version [78]. The flange end of the syringe can be placed over the nipple and gentle suction applied to draw out the nipple slowly. There are no data to confirm that the syringe works, but clinical experience suggests that it may be useful in helping to make the nipple area more graspable [78]. There is no need to apply lotions or oils to the breasts to soften the skin, and normal daily bathing with soap is recommended.

5.1.8 Anticipatory Guidance

After completing a careful history and physical examination, the following anticipatory guidance should be offered.

- Avoid medicated or interventional labor. Soon after natural childbirth, infants exhibit an instinctive rooting behavior to locate and latch onto the breast. Medications and complications of childbirth may interfere with this neurodevelopmental behavior [79, 80].
- Initiate breastfeeding or breast pumping as soon as possible following complete delivery of the placenta because it is thought that early breast stimulation initiates lactation [27, 81], although evidence is conflicting [75].
- Breast-feed or pump on demand, every 2–3 h because regular breast drainage and breast stimulation facilitate lactogenesis [82, 83].
- Practice rooming and bedding in for 24 h per day. Maternal–infant separation impedes regular breast drainage and stimulation [84–86].
- Combined mother and infant nursing care facilitates patient-centered teaching [87].
- Relieve engorgement early to prevent involutional atrophy of lactocytes [88].
- Avoid routine supplementation because it causes "breast confusion" by removing an infant's hunger drive, thereby decreasing breast stimulation and drainage [89, 90].
- Avoid rubber nipples and pacifiers. If infants are demonstrating hunger cues by sucking, they are hungry. Offering a pacifier is not an appropriate maternal response to these infants' cues. The infant should suckle on the breast frequently to establish successful lactation [81, 91].
- Exclusive breastfeeding ensures that the infant receives adequate colostrum, including secretary immunoglobulin A (IgA) and other unique hormonal factors that contribute to the infant's health, growth, and development [12].
- Avoid formula because it predisposes the neonate to potential allergies and other risk factors associated with artificial foods. The immature gut is not designed to digest cow milk or soya milk [92].

- Review the availability of community resources postpartum; close follow-up in the postpartum period is crucial for successful breastfeeding [4].

5.2 Intrapartum Period

5.2.1 Establishing Lactation

Breastfeeding should be considered the fourth stage of labor; childbirth is not complete until the infant is latched on to the breast and suckling, thus triggering lactogenesis. Soon after delivery, neonates exhibit a natural locating reflex and can find the nipple themselves, if permitted. Once the nipple is located, they root, latch onto it, and suckle instinctively. Studies have shown that this process may take 60–120 min and that the locating and suckling instinct can be impaired if foreign objects are inserted into neonate's mouths soon after birth or if the infant is sedated secondarily to maternal medication [93, 94].

Early suckling is crucial for four reasons. Firstly, it allows an imprinting to occur as the neonate learns to grasp and shape a teat and suckle effectively while the nipple and areola are still soft and easily grasped. Secondly, the neonate ingests a small amount of colostrum, which has a high content of maternal secretary IgA, which acts as the first immunization to the immunoimmature neonate. Thirdly, following parturition and the delivery of an intact placenta, the inhibitory effects of the hormones of pregnancy are removed, and the prolactin receptors in the mammary gland become responsive. Lastly, early suckling stimulates the release of lactotrophs, including prolactins, which trigger the onset of milk synthesis. Frequent episodes of breast stimulation cause surges of prolactin, which maintain lactogenesis. Clinical signs of successful lactogenesis are fullness of the breasts postpartum with the production of colostrum initially and then a gradual change to transitional milk and mature milk within about 36–48 h [95].

Galactopoiesis is the process of ongoing milk synthesis. It follows successful mammogenesis and unimpeded lactogenesis. The rate of milk synthesis varies throughout the day and between mothers. It is controlled by regular and complete drainage and is primarily an autocrine (i.e., local) action. Recent studies suggest that ongoing milk synthesis is inhibited by the buildup of local suppressor peptide called feedback inhibitor of lactation (FIL) [96]; regular suckling removes this inhibition [97, 98]. Prolactin surges stimulate the breast alveoli to actively secrete milk, and oxytocin causes the myoepithelial cells surrounding the glands and the ductules to contract and eject milk down the ducts to the nipples. These contractions effectively squeeze the fat globules across the cell membrane into the ducts. As a feed progresses, the quality and quantity of milk produced change. The fore milk, at the beginning of the feed, is composed mainly of milk that has collected between feeds, and it has lower fat and higher whey content than hind milk. The fat content increases as the "degree of breast fullness" decreases [99]. Serum prolactin levels should increase several-fold following suckling; lack of a prolactin response may be significant. Prolactin levels fall over the first 4–6 weeks, and the suckling-induced prolactin surges are markedly reduced by 3 months, virtually disappearing by 6 months, and yet lactation can continue [100, 101]. Current understanding is that the requirement of blood prolactin for lactation is permissive rather than regulatory [102].

5.2.2 Factors that Help to Establish Lactation

Following childbirth, mothers and neonates should remain together, skin to skin, to allow the process of breastfeeding to begin. Neonates instinctively know how to locate the breast and suckle, but mothers must be taught.

The World Health Organization and the United Nations Children's Fund recognized the importance of successful establishment of breastfeeding in the hospital, and they launched the global Baby Friendly Hospital Initiative in 1992. This is an educational quality assurance program for hospitals based on the joint statement "Protecting, Supporting and Promoting Breastfeeding—The Special Role of Maternity Services," which outlines ten simple steps designed to protect these delicate physiologic processes [103] (Fig. 5.1).

5.2.3 Factors that Interfere with Lactation

Insufficient maternal milk is the most common reason given for stopping breastfeeding in the early weeks. The cause is often iatrogenic resulting from mismanagement during the critical early phase. Many maternal and infant factors contribute to lactation failure, including premammary gland, mammary gland, and postmammary gland causes.

5.2.3.1 Failure of Mammogenesis

In the normal course of events, mammogenesis begins in the embryo and continues throughout life with active growth phases during puberty and pregnancy. Mammogenesis is controlled by a complex hormonal milieu that cannot be covered in depth in this chapter. The hormones involved include the pituitary hormones: prolactin, adrenocorticotropic hormone, growth hormone, thyrotropin, follicle-stimulating hormone, and luteinizing hormone. In addition, steroid hormones from the ovary, adrenal glands, and placenta, plus thyroid hormones and insulin, contribute to

Every facility providing maternity services and care for newborn infants should:

1. Have a written breastfeeding policy that is routinely communicated to all health care staff
2. Train all health care staff in skills necessary to implement this policy.
3. Inform all pregnant women about the benefits and management of breastfeeding.
4. Help mothers initiate breastfeeding within a half hour of birth.
5. Show mothers how to breastfeed and how to maintain lactation even if they should be separated from their infants.
6. Give newborn infants no food or drink other than breast milk, unless medically indicated.
7. Practice rooming in - allow mothers and infants to remain together 24 hours a day.
8. Encourage breastfeeding on demand.
9. Give no artificial teats or pacifiers (also called dummies or soothers) to breastfeeding infants.
10. Foster the establishment of breastfeeding support groups and refer mothers to them on discharge from the hospital or clinic.

Fig. 5.1 Ten steps to successful breastfeeding

mammary growth and function either directly or indirectly [75].

Failure of mammogenesis presents clinically as a lack of, or an abnormality in, breast growth and development during puberty, adulthood, or pregnancy and may be due to any or a combination of the following factors:

Preglandular Failure

The most common cause of premammary glandular failure is a deficiency of mammary growth-stimulating hormones, but other possibilities include the presence of biologically inactive hormones or antibodies to the hormones preventing their normal action [104]. Pathological conditions associated with disrupted production can be hypothalamic or pituitary in origin. Destruction of the hypothalamus can occur as a result of encephalitis, infiltration of tumor following lymphocytic hypophysitis, or idiopathic causes [105]. Pituitary causes include space-occupying lesions, hyperplasia, empty sella syndrome, acromegaly, pituitary stalk section, and Sheehan syndrome [106]. A pregnancy-specific mammary nuclear factor (PMF) has been identified, which is stimulated by progesterone. PMF may suppress genes involved in mammary gland development [107].

Glandular Failure

Glandular failure is defined as lack of mammary gland response to normal lactogens during pregnancy. A PMF imbalance or end-organ receptor failure, such as estrogen or prolactin mammary gland receptor deficits, may occur. The regulatory factors involved in the development of the myoepithelial cells prior to lactation are not well understood.

5.2.3.2 Failure of Lactogenesis

Lactogenesis II, or the onset of copious milk secretion, occurs close to parturition. It is under endocrine control of the pituitary gland via prolactin and other lactogenic hormones. The decline of placental hormones, particularly progesterone, following delivery of an intact placenta, associated with early and frequent suckling, is the major triggers to establishing milk synthesis. Clinical evidence of lactogenesis II is an increase in breast size, which occurs about 60 h postpartum, but can range between 24 and 102 h after birth [108]. Failure of lactogenesis presents clinically as a lack of breast engorgement and lack of colostrum production.

Preglandular

Preglandular causes of failure of lactogenesis include an intrinsic lack of lactogenic hormones, biologically inactive lactogens or lactogenic antibodies [109]. In addition to the pituitary and hypothalamic pathologies, factors predisposing to a reduction in pituitary hormone production in the postpartum period, in particular prolactin, include drugs such as bromocriptine and retained placental fragments [110]. The latter demonstrates the inhibitory effect of estrogen and progesterone on the initiation of lactogenesis.

Glandular

Glandular causes include a lack of mammary gland responsiveness to lactogenic hormones, including plasma membrane receptor deficits or faulty gene transcription [111].

Postglandular

Postglandular causes relate to a delay in the initiation of breastfeeding. The length of delay that becomes significant has not been clarified, but it undoubtedly plays a role. Unlimited access to the breast increases milk intake and infant growth in the first 2 weeks [112]. The use of supplementary feeding with formula, which is routine in some hospitals, may have a detrimental effect on milk synthesis in a mother who planned exclusively to breast-feed after hospital discharge [113]. Unrelieved engorgement is also recognized as having a negative feedback effect on milk synthesis. This condition may be due to the buildup of inhibitor factors in the milk or to pressure effects by the milk volume.

5.2.3.3 Failure of Galactopoiesis

The action of many hormones is involved in the maintenance of lactation. Failure of galactopoiesis presents clinically as lack of copious milk production. Causes of failure of galactopoiesis include the following:

Preglandular

An intrinsic lack of lactogenic hormones is one cause. Contributing factors to reduced milk synthesis include certain drugs (e.g., estrogen-containing contraceptives, pseudoephedrine [114]), heavy smoking, or superimposed pregnancy.

Glandular

Glandular causes include unresponsiveness to lactogenic hormones or secondary to failure of mammogenesis or lactogenesis.

Postglandular

The most common cause of lactation failure is a delay in early and frequent breast simulation and inadequate drainage, which commonly occurs when mothers and infants are separated because of existing or anticipated health problems. Newborns usually suckle effectively when they are positioned appropriately at the breast; however, the maternal physiological ability to lactate rapidly declines if both breasts are not stimulated quickly following parturition and drained every 2 or 3 h. There is a window for the initiation of lactation, and studies have shown that the duration of lactation correlates inversely with the time of the first breast stimulation. The extrinsic lack of prolactin surges fails to trigger and maintain lactation [115].

Inadequate drainage as a result of infrequent suckling or ineffective breastfeeding techniques leads to the lack of removal of the milk and a buildup of local inhibitor factors in the retained milk, which shuts down ongoing milk synthesis. Involution of the glands commences, leading to premature weaning. After delivery, there is considerable vascular and lymphatic congestion in the breast tissue, leading to a rise in intraductal pressure. If unrelieved, the engorgement impedes the intraductal flow of milk and reduces circulation, rapidly causing pressure atrophy at the alveoli and inhibiting the establishment of a good milk supply. Impairment to milk drainage as a result of lactiferous duct outlet obstruction also may occur following mammoplasty or surgical reconstruction of the breast, although newer surgical techniques attempt to maintain the integrity of the lactiferous ducts [59, 116, 117]. Neifert et al. [58] found a threefold increase in the risk of lactation insufficiency in women who had undergone breast surgery compared to women without surgery. Where there was a periareolar incision, the risk was five times greater than when there was no history of breast surgery [58].

Breast fullness or engorgement may prevent infants from latching effectively. This leads to sore nipples, caused by tongue trauma, inadequate breast stimulation and drainage, and insufficient milk intake by the infant. If the breast milk intake is low, the infant remains hungry and may receive formula supplement and become satiated. The net result is milk retention, impeded lactogenesis, and maternal unhappiness. Hot compresses and manual expression of milk before latching help to improve the attachment, and cold compresses reduce swelling after feeds [118, 119].

The fluid requirements of healthy newborn infants are minimal for the first few days. Neonates drink 7–20 mL of colostrum per feed initially, and they do not require extra fluids. Prelacteal and complementary feeds may upset the process of lactogenesis by removing the neonate's hunger drive and decreasing the frequency of breast stimulation and drainage [90, 120]. Night sedation may offer a temporary respite, but the lack of breastfeeding at night can impede lactogenesis because of irregular breast stimulation and drainage.

If frequent efficient breastfeeding is not possible, for example, if a mother is separated from her sick infant, she should be shown how to express her milk regularly, either by hand or by using a breast pump, to ensure complete breast drainage and prevent milk stasis. Contrary to popular belief, this does not lead to an excessive milk synthesis but prevents early and irreversible involution. Mothers should pump at least six times daily [121].

5.2.4 Milk Transfer

Milk is transferred from the breast by the infant during breastfeeding, in combination with the maternal milk ejection reflex. The rate of transfer of milk from the breast to the infant depends on various factors, including milk synthesis and the volume of pooled milk, the strength and frequency of the milk ejection reflex, and the technical process of breastfeeding [122]. The milk ejection reflex, or letdown, is stimulated by oxytocin released from the posterior pituitary following direct nipple stimulation and via hypothalamic triggering. It causes smooth muscle contractions and propels milk through the ducts and out of the nipple pores. The character of the reflex varies between women and over time; some mothers have a well-developed letdown, whereas others have a slow, irregular reflex. With conditioning, oxytocin release occurs in response to infant crying or as the mother prepares to feed [100]. Confidence facilitates the ejection reflex, and anxiety may impede it [123, 124].

5.2.4.1 Factors that Help Milk Transfer

Basic Breastfeeding Skills

Breastfeeding is a technical process of transferring milk from the breast. It depends on careful positioning and attachment of the infant to the breast and on an intact suckling ability of the infant. Parenting starts at birth; therefore, hospital staff should encourage mothers to assume this role as soon as possible. Mothers should be shown how to breast-feed [87, 125].

Positioning: The mother should be sitting comfortably with her arms and back supported and her feet raised on a small stool. The infant should be placed on her lap, facing the uncovered breast; a pillow may help raise up the baby. The infant's body should be well supported and straight, with the infant snug against her body [126] (Fig. 5.2). Breastfeeding is easier if two hands are used to start with. The breast should be cupped with one hand underneath using the thumb and fingers to shape the breast to form an oval that matches the shape of the mouth, lifting the breast up slightly while directing the nipple toward the infant's mouth. The other hand is used to support the infant's back and shoulders. The infant's arms should be free to embrace the breast and the body held very close to the mother, stomach to stomach.

Attachment: The latching technique involves brushing the nipple against the infant's upper lip and waiting until the infant roots, lifting his or her head and opening the mouth wide. This often requires "teasing the baby" and encouraging the mouth to open wider than before. When the mother can see the gaping mouth, she should quickly draw the baby forward over the nipple and onto areola tissue. The baby's bottom lip, jaw, and chin sink into the breast first, so that he takes a good mouthful of breast [126]. The amount of areola available to the mouth depends on the size of the areola and on the neonate's gape. It is incorrect to assume that all the areola tissue should be covered. The lips should be everted or flanged and placed well behind the nipple base. The chin is extended into the breast, and the nose is adjacent to it. Young infants do not have the ability to maintain their position at the breast alone, and so the mother must continue to sandwich her breast and support the infant's back and shoulders throughout the duration of the feed. Older infants are able to latch and maintain themselves more easily and suckle comfortably in an elbow crook.

Suckling: An infant who is correctly latched and has a mouthful of soft breast tissue will draw the nipple and the areola tissue to the junction of the hard and soft palate to form a teat and then will initiate suckling. The more elastic and extensible the breast tissue, the easier it is for the young infant. A fixed, retracted, or engorged nipple and areola tissue make it harder for this to occur. The jaw is raised, and the gums compress the breast tissue; the tongue protrudes over the lower gums and grooves and undulates in a coordinated manner. The cheeks and tongue help to form a bolus of milk. The jaw lowers, and the soft palate elevates to close the nasopharynx; a slight negative pressure is created, and the milk is effectively transferred and swallowed in a coordinated manner [127, 128] (Fig. 5.3).

5.2.4.2 Factors Impeding Milk Transfer

The milk ejection reflex is a primitive one and is not easily blocked. The effects of adrenaline can reduce it temporarily if the mother is subjected to sudden unpleasant or extremely painful physical or psychological stimuli. This could include embarrassment or fear, inducing a stress reaction with the release of adrenaline, which can cause vasoconstriction and impede the action of oxytocin. Over time, however, this inhibition seems to be overcome. The strength and frequency of the ejection reflex depend on hypophysial stimulation of the posterior pituitary and suckling pressure on the lactiferous ducts, causing oxytocin release. The more the milk that has pooled between feeds, the more is ejected with the initial let down [100, 123].

Inefficient milk transfer may be the result of poor maternal breastfeeding technique in positioning the infant at the breast or in facilitating his or her attachment because of a lack of knowledge or maternal or infant physical disabilities. In addition, improper positioning and attachment lead to

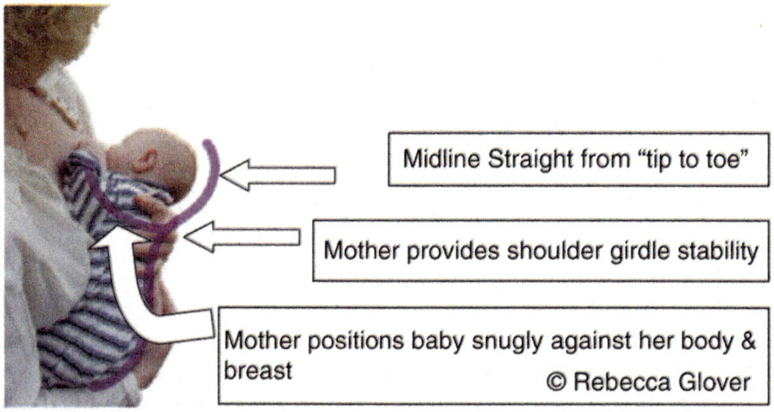
Midline Straight from "tip to toe"
Mother provides shoulder girdle stability
Mother positions baby snugly against her body & breast
© Rebecca Glover

Fig. 5.2 A positionally stable baby (© Rebecca Glover, reprinted with permission)

Fig. 5.3 The essential mouthful

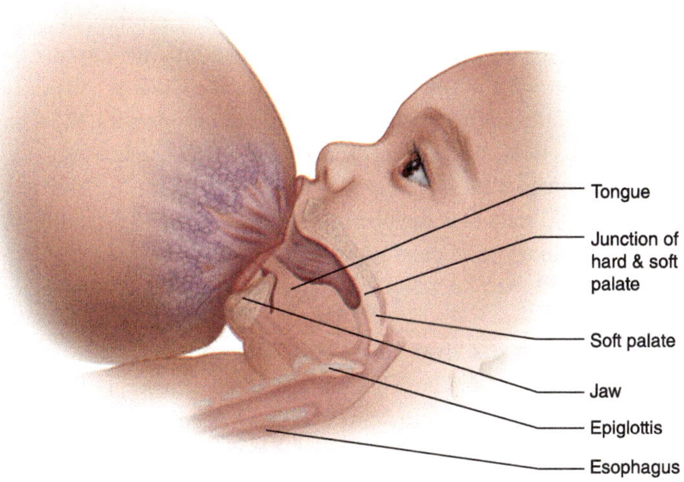

decreased breast stimulation and inadequate drainage, which result in decreased milk production and decreased milk intake. Simple correction of the position and latch is often the only remedy needed to improve the quality of the feed.

Inefficient milk transfer also may result from poor neonate suckling technique either because of an inability to grasp the nipple correctly or because of a suck, swallow, or breath disorder. Large, well-defined nipples may entice the neonate to suckle directly on the nipple, resulting in sore nipples and ineffective milk transfer. Retrognathia, cleft lip or palate, and an uncoordinated, weak, flutter, or bunched-up tongue may interfere with effective sucking dynamics, often because the jaw fails to compress the breast or the tongue and cheeks are unable to create the necessary negative pressure to draw in the milk [129]. These infants may benefit from suck training, but clinical experience suggests that as the mandible elongates and facial muscles strengthen, the dynamics of sucking improve naturally [130]. *Ankyloglossia* (tongue-tie) is an important cause of suckling difficulties. The tethered tongue is unable to protrude over the gum and cannot move upward; the teat is not stripped correctly, and less milk is transferred. The nipple often becomes traumatized and sore. The infant may not thrive, and milk production decreases because of inadequate drainage. A simple surgical release of the frenulum is required and should be done as soon as possible when clinically indicated; after a few weeks, it is often difficult to alter the way these infants suckle [131–133]. Recently, a posterior tongue-tie has been recognized as a cause of nipple pain [134]. In addition to restricted tongue movement and elevation, palpation of resistance at the base of the tongue indicates a posterior tongue-tie [135].

5.2.5 Milk Intake

Over the first few days, the infant drinks small volumes of colostrum of 7–20 mL per feed. This rapidly increases to approximately 760–840 mL/day, with approximately seven or eight feeding episodes. The milk intake per feed is about 80–120 mL. Breasts have a great capacity to yield milk and can produce double this amount. If necessary, a woman can feed from one breast exclusively [136].

5.2.5.1 Frequency

Infants are able to recognize hunger and should be fed according to their cues. Most newborns breast-feed every 2–3 h, causing frequent surges of prolactin, which help to ensure full lactation. Mothers who have a low milk supply should be encouraged to breast-feed frequently to ensure good drainage and stimulation.

5.2.5.2 Duration

Studies show that the duration of a breastfeed varies between mother–infant pairs [137]. The rate of milk transfer is not uniform. Some breastfeeding pairs have a rapid milk transfer and, hence, a very short feed. This is because of the large amount of milk that has collected in the breasts since the previous feed and the well-established milk ejection reflex. Others have long feeds because milk ejection is poor, the breastfeeding technique is relatively ineffective, or milk production is slow, and the pooled milk volume is low, which consequently leads to a slowed milk transfer. Previously held beliefs that most of the feed is taken in the first few minutes or that both breasts should be used at each feed fail to recognize the uniqueness of each nursing pair.

5.2.5.3 Pattern of Breast Use

The quality and quantity of milk intake depend on the pattern of breast use. Between feeds, milk is synthesized and collects in the lactiferous ducts. This low-fat milk is readily available at the start of each feed. As the feed progresses, the volume of milk the infant drinks will decrease, but the quality increases as more fat is passed into the milk. The infant should remain at the first breast until the rate of flow of milk is no longer sufficient to satisfy the infant. The second breast should then be offered.

5.2.5.4 Factors that Help Milk Intake

To establish lactation, both breasts should be offered at each feed. The removal of colostrum facilitates ongoing lactogenesis. When lactation is well established, the first breast should be comfortably drained before switching to the second. This will prevent milk stasis and results in a balanced milk production and optimum infant growth. Mothers with a high milk yield may feed unilaterally, whereas mothers with a slow rate of milk synthesis should feed bilaterally. When the rate of milk transfer is rapid, the infant may gag, choke, and pull away from the breast; frequent burping is recommended in this situation, as is manual expression of some milk before attaching the infant.

5.2.5.5 Factors that Impair Milk Intake

A "happy to starve" infant that sleeps for long periods may fail to thrive because of inadequate daily milk intake. A pause in feeding after a few minutes of sucking may be interpreted incorrectly as the infant having had enough, leading to early termination of the feed. A crying, discontented infant may be given a pacifier to prolong the time between feeds. A mother also may be under the impression that only one breast should be used at each feed and choose not to feed off the second side even though the neonate is still hungry. Newborns frequently pause while feeding, and these episodes may last several minutes. Problems arise when a mother terminates a feed or switches to the other side prematurely because this alters the quality and quantity of the milk consumed.

5.2.6 Maternal Psychosocial Health

The psychological and social health of the mother is crucial throughout all stages of breastfeeding. A mother who is ambivalent about breastfeeding and who lacks support may allow her infant fewer chances to suckle, thereby inhibiting lactogenesis and galactopoiesis. A mother who lacks confidence or knowledge may interpret any breastfeeding infant problem as being due to insufficient milk; a consequent move to bottle-feeding compounds the problem. Lack of support from family and friends can negatively influence her endeavors [72, 138].

5.2.7 In-Hospital Risk Assessment

Some mothers and infants are at high risk for lactation and breastfeeding difficulties. As discussed previously, several biopsychosocial risk factors can be identified prenatally, and this information should be readily available in hospitals. A routine in-hospital breastfeeding risk assessment should be performed [139] (Fig. 5.4).

Newborns often lose weight within the first few days as the result of normal physiologic fluid losses [140]. If breastfeeding is successfully established, this weight loss should be no greater than about 7 %. Excessive weight loss may imply inadequate food intake and deserves a detailed clinical breastfeeding assessment. The underlying cause is usually easy to elucidate, and management can be directed toward either increasing the rate of maternal milk synthesis, improving milk transfer, or increasing the daily quantity or quality of milk intake [1, 141].

If the neonate's weight continues to fall, additional calories must be provided either as the mother's own breast milk, pasteurized donor breast milk, or formula. Some neonates have preexisting difficulties grasping and suckling at the breast. In these situations, width-based rubber nipples and thin silicone nipple shields are useful suck training devices that encourage normal biomechanical jaw excursions.

5.2.8 Hospital Discharge Planning

Hospital stays are short. Discharge planning enables a physician to review the stages of lactation and breastfeeding and allows early identification of potential or actual problems. All mothers should be taught the signs that their baby is breast-feeding well and instructed to call for advice if they have concerns (Fig. 5.5). If an infant has lost more than 7 % of his or her birthweight at the scheduled hospital discharge, or if the mother–infant pair has known risk factors for breastfeeding difficulties, a delayed discharge or early community follow-up for breastfeeding assistance would be appropriate. All other mothers and infants should be reassessed within 1 week of birth [142].

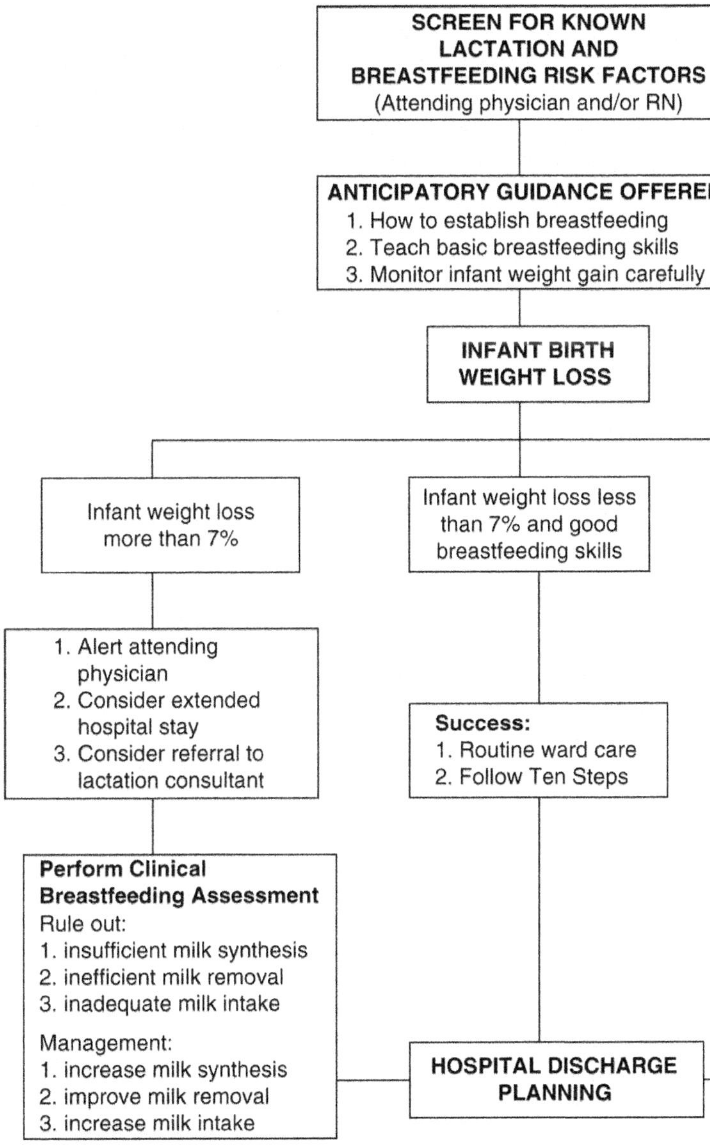

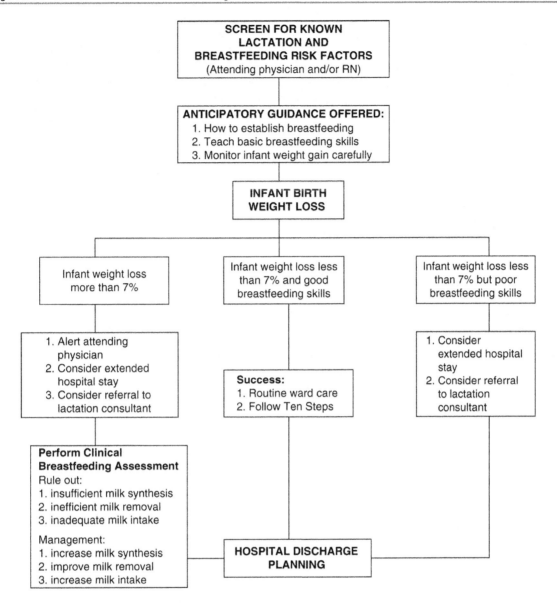

Fig. 5.4 In-hospital breastfeeding assessment

5.3 Postpartum Period

5.3.1 Clinical Breastfeeding Assessment

Lactation and breastfeeding difficulties manifest in many ways, including infant problems such as failure to thrive, colic, fussiness, early introduction of supplements, or maternal concerns such as breast discomfort, sore cracked nipples, engorgement mastitis, or postpartum depression. Different clinical complexes of symptoms and signs or syndromes reflect the normal variations in maternal lactation ability and infant breastfeeding ability. These symptoms and signs are not diagnostic. Diagnosis and problem solving start with a detailed history and physical examination of both mother and infant, including breastfeeding history and observation. Once the etiology and pathophysiology have been elucidated, successful management depends on sound knowledge of the anatomy of the breast, the physiology of lactation, and the mechanics of infant suckle combined with a clear understanding of breastfeeding kinetics [126, 143].

The rate of breast milk synthesis varies throughout the day and between mothers. It depends on a variety of central and local factors, including direct breast stimulation and breast drainage [95, 144]. In clinical practice, approximately 15 % of mothers have a high rate of milk synthesis of 60 mL/h or more (hyperlactation), and about 15 % of mothers have a low rate of synthesis of 10 mL/h or less (hypolactation) (Fig. 5.6).

By three or four days of age, your baby:

- has wet diapers: at least 4-5 noticeable times (looks or feels wet) in twenty-four hours (pale and odorless urine)
- has at least 2-3 bowel movements in twenty-four hours (color progressing from brownish to seedy mustard yellow).
- breastfeeds at least 8 times in twenty-four hours.
- is content after most feedings.

Other signs that suggest your baby is breastfeeding well are:

- You can hear your baby swallowing during feeding.
- Your breasts are full before feedings and soft after feedings.
- Your baby is only drinking breast milk.

If any one of these signs is not present after your baby is 3 or 4 days old or if you are having problems, please call for help.
Physician/Midwife:____________________ Community Health Nurse:

If your baby is breastfeeding well, make an appointment within the first week for you and your baby to see either your Family Physician, Midwife, or Community Health Nurse.

Birth Weight:____________________Discharge Weight:__________________

Weight at One Week:______________________________________

Fig. 5.5 Signs your baby is breastfeeding well

Fig. 5.6 Maternal milk synthesis

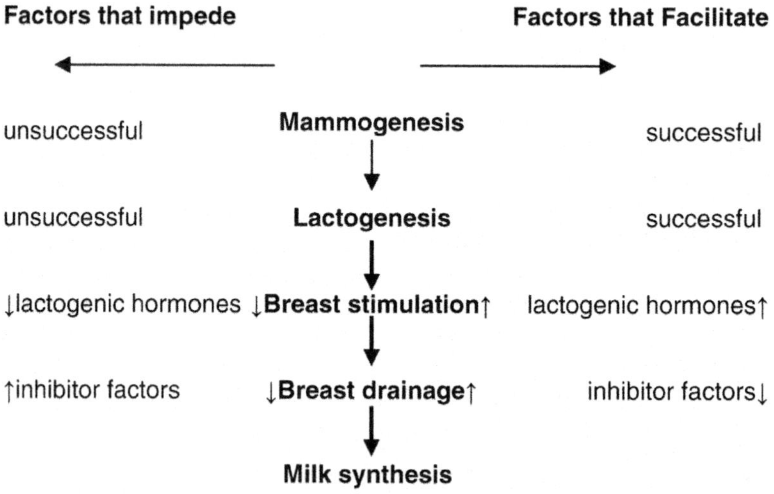

5.3.2 Insufficient Milk Syndrome

The most common reason given for abandoning breastfeeding in the early postpartum period is insufficient milk. The etiology is multifactorial, but most causes are reversible if the mother receives accurate breastfeeding management advice early in the postpartum period. A small percentage is irreversible (Fig. 5.7).

If the mother is having difficulties breastfeeding or if the infant's weight is continuing to fall or is more than 7 %

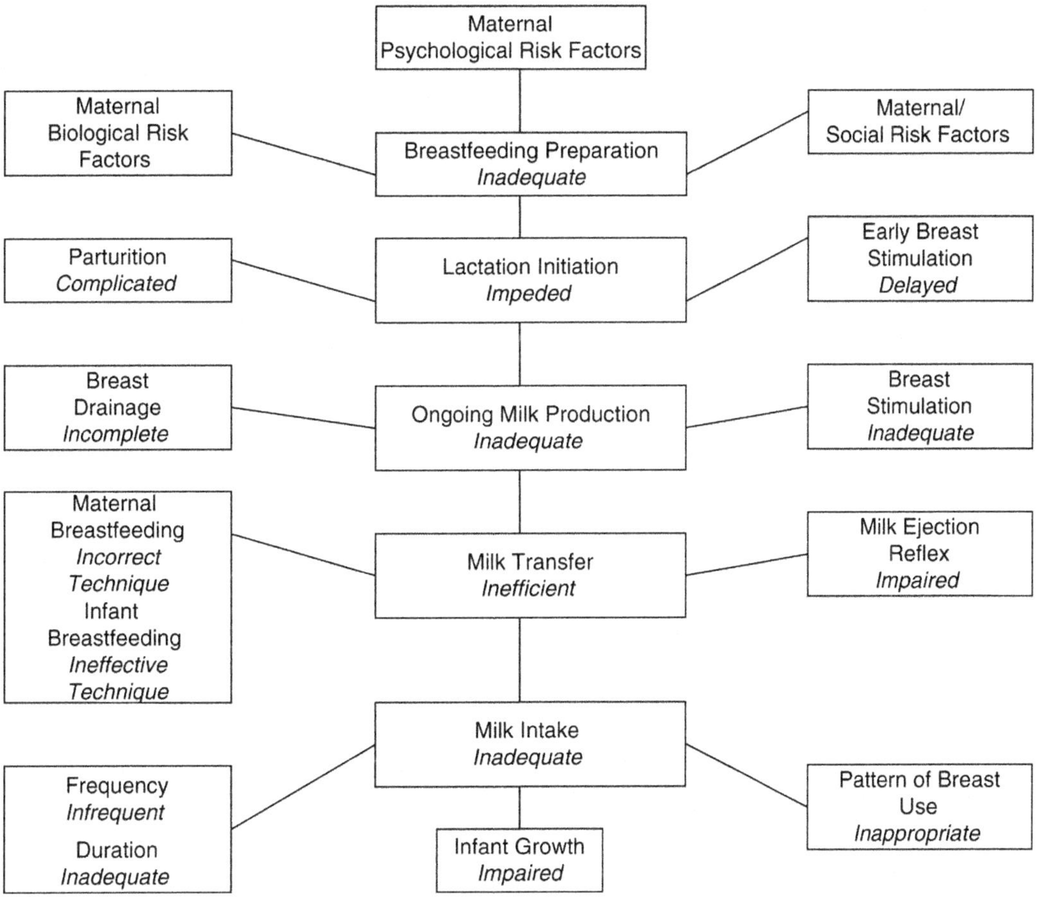

Fig. 5.7 Neonatal insufficient milk syndrome

below birthweight, a careful evaluation is required. This involves a detailed clinical breastfeeding assessment incorporating maternal and infant history and breastfeeding history and includes a careful maternal and infant examination. Observation of breastfeeding is required to assess positioning, latching, suckling, and swallowing. An accurate test feed followed by estimating residual milk in the breasts by pumping is helpful measurements when assessing maternal milk yield and infant milk intake. Caution must be taken when using standard office scales due to their unreliability in measuring small volume changes [145]. Other causes of infant failure to thrive, such as cardiac or respiratory problems, should always be considered.

In broad terms, management includes avoiding the precipitating factors, improving maternal milk synthesis by increasing breast stimulation and drainage, improving milk removal by correcting the breastfeeding technique, and increasing the infant's daily milk intake by increasing the frequency and duration of breastfeeding. A small percentage of neonates will require complementary feeds. Metoclopramide (10 mg three times a day) and domperidone (20 mg three times a day) are effective galactogogues when increased prolactin stimulation is required [146, 147]. Mothers may need support and reassurance that partial breastfeeding or mixed feeding is still beneficial.

5.3.3 Maternal Hyperlactation Syndrome

Hyperlactation may result in a characteristic clustering of maternal and infant symptoms and signs. Milk stasis, blocked ducts, deep radiating breast pain, lactiferous ductal colic, inflammatory mastitis, infectious mastitis, and breast abscess are common problems. Clinical experience has shown that most mothers experiencing any or all these symptoms have a high rate of milk synthesis and have large, thriving infants, or else they have started to wean and are not draining their breasts regularly. These symptoms and signs are all consequences of a rapid rate of milk synthesis combined with milk retention resulting from incomplete breast drainage. They represent the clinical spectrum of the maternal hyperlactation syndrome [148, 149] (Fig. 5.8). The pathophysiology is analogous to the renal system; retention of urine, due to incomplete bladder emptying, may result in

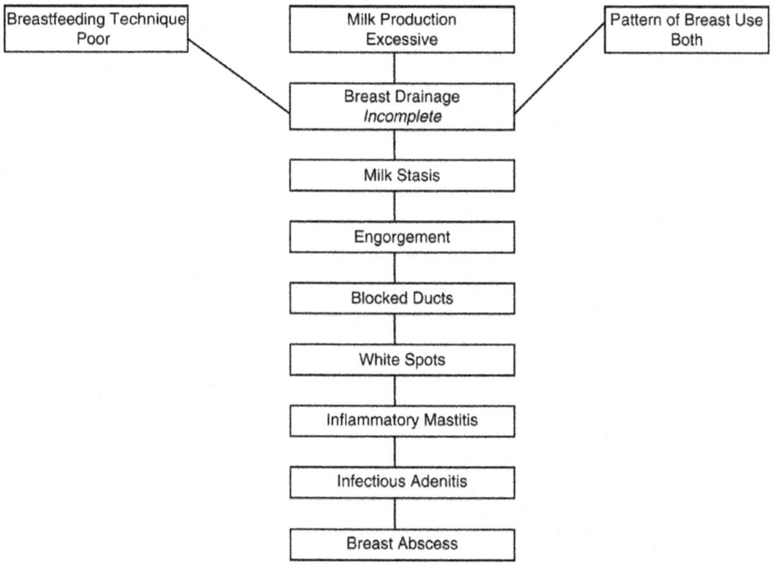

Fig. 5.8 Maternal hyperlactation

lower and upper urinary tract disease, including bladder distension, spasms, ureteric colic, and hydronephrosis. This problem may become complicated with ascending urinary tract infections, including trigonitis, urethritis, cystitis, pyelonephritis, and renal abscess.

Lactation problems occur when a mother with a high milk output switches her infant from one breast to the other before the first side has been adequately drained. A strong milk ejection reflex causes a rapid letdown of a large volume of pooled milk, and the infant quickly becomes satiated before all the lactiferous ducts are drained. Incomplete drainage may be aggravated by poor position and latch or by impaired infant suckling [150]. When this occurs repeatedly, some of the ducts and lobules constantly remain full.

5.3.3.1 White Spot

A small white spot may be visible on the nipple; such a spot represents edematous epithelium blocking the nipple pore and milk flow. In some situations, duct obstruction is due to a small granule of casein milk precipitate [151]. Lactiferous duct outlet obstruction can cause increased retrograde pressure. Mothers may complain of sharp, "knifelike" cramps or shooting pains deep in the breast, often between feeds, because of ductal cramping or colic because of myoepithelial smooth muscle contractions.

5.3.3.2 Milk Stasis

A firm, lumpy, slightly tender quadrant in the breast may be felt because of milk stasis. Over time, if this area is not drained, cytokines from the milk may seep into the interstitial tissue, causing it to become inflamed and erythematous, signifying an inflammatory mastitis [152, 153].

5.3.3.3 Acute Mastitis

It was recognized in 1940 that when a breach occurs in the mucous membrane, such as a cracked nipple, superficial skin infections could lead to a deeper cellulitis, adenitis, and mastitis [154]. Livingstone et al. [155] found that 50–60 % of sore, cracked nipples were contaminated with *Staphylococcus aureus* or other microorganisms. Subsequent study showed that 25 % of mothers with infected, sore nipples developed mastitis if they were not treated aggressively with systemic antibiotic [156]. A high rate of milk synthesis combined with continuous poor drainage of a segment of the breast may result in the stagnant milk becoming secondarily infected with common skin pathogens via an ascending lactiferous duct infection and leads to acute mastitis. Infectious mastitis also may be caused by a blood-borne infection; however, that is uncommon and more likely in nonpuerperal mastitis [157]. Puerperal mastitis has been found to affect 17 % of breastfeeding women who present with breast pain, redness, lumps, general malaise, chills or sweats, and fever [158].

5.3.3.4 Chronic Mastitis

Chronic mastitis, as in chronic urinary tract infections, may be due to reinfection or a relapsed infection. Reinfection occurs sporadically because of exposure to a new pathogen, commonly transmitted from the infant. A relapsed infection occurs shortly after completion of therapy; it signifies inadequate primary treatment and failed eradication of the pathogen. An underlying cause, such as a nidus of infection deep in the breast tissue, should be considered. It is hypothesized that lactiferous duct infections may lead to stricture formation, duct dilation, and impaired drainage. The residual milk remains infected.

5.3.3.5 Breast Abscess

Inadequately treated mastitis and ongoing milk retention can develop into a breast abscess. A high fever with chills and general malaise, associated with a firm, well-demarcated, tender, fluctuating mass, usually with erythema of the skin, indicates abscess formation, although, in some instances, systemic symptoms may be absent. Ultrasonography of the breast and needle aspiration under local anesthesia is useful diagnostic techniques for identifying collections of fluid or pus and distinguishing mastitis from a galactocele or inflammatory breast cancer [159–161].

5.3.3.6 Management Goals

Maternal hyperlactation syndrome can be prevented by decreasing the rate of milk synthesis and preventing milk retention by improving milk removal and breast drainage.

Decreased Rate of Milk Synthesis

Reducing breast stimulation and drainage can decrease the rate of milk synthesis. Decreasing the frequency and duration of breastfeeding reduces prolactin surges, and milk synthesis remains blocked via central inhibitory factors. Decreasing the frequency of breast drainage results in milk retention in the lactiferous ducts, and inhibitor peptides collect and block ongoing milk production via a local negative feedback mechanism. In practical terms, the infant should remain at one breast per feed until he or she is full and spontaneously releases the breast. In this way, the volume of milk ingested is less, but the fat content and calorific value increase as the feed progresses [162]. A higher fat intake often satiates the infant for a longer period and decreases the hunger drive. The interval between feeds is lengthened and milk synthesis declines, whereas the second breast remains full longer, and local inhibitor further reduces milk synthesis in that breast. In a small number of mothers, unilateral breastfeeding may result in overdrainage and can contribute to the ongoing high rate of milk synthesis. In these cases, bilateral breastfeeding and incomplete drainage may result in a decline in overall milk synthesis (e.g., 2–3 min on the first side followed by a good burp and then 3–5 min on the second side). If milk supply does not become manageable with one-sided feeding, the mother can completely express both breasts on one occasion and then feed from one breast for a block of time (e.g., 4–6 h) before switching breasts [163].

Decreased Milk Retention

Regular breastfeeding facilitates milk removal and breast drainage. When positioned and latched correctly, the infant is usually effective at removing milk and draining each segment. The modified cradle position allows the mother to cup the breast with her hand and apply firm pressure over the outer quadrant and compress retained milk toward the nipple while the infant suckles. If the milk is flowing rapidly, the mother should stop compressing the breast. Switching breastfeeding positions and using the under-the-arm hold allow thorough drainage of all segments and prevent milk stasis. Breastfeeding should start on the fullest breast, and the infant should remain on this breast until all areas feel soft. As the pressure in the duct is relieved, breast pain and discomfort lessen.

Removal of Obstruction

If a small white dot on the nipple becomes visible, indicating a blocked nipple pore and outlet obstruction, gentle abrasion or a sterile needle can be used to remove the epithelial skin and relieve the obstruction. Occasionally, a small calculus or granule will pop out suddenly, relieving the obstruction. On firm compression, a thick stream of milk will often gush out, indicating patency. Occasionally, breastfeeding is ineffective at removing the thickened inspissated milk, and manual or mechanical expression may therefore be necessary. The mother should be shown how to compress her breast firmly using a cupped hand, squeezing gently toward the nipple while pumping to dislodge the milk or calculus. It may be helpful to try massaging in front of the lump toward the nipple, as if "trying to clear a pathway" (Smillie CM cited by [164]). If the breast expression fails to relieve the obstructed segment, a technique known as *manual stripping can* be used [165]. This involves cupping the breast between the finger and thumb and applying firm, steady pressure over the tender section, starting from the periphery over the rib cage and drawing the fingers and thumb slowly together toward the nipple, and stripping out thickened milk or pus. This procedure should be repeated several times. The skin must be well lubricated before attempting to do this. Analgesia may be necessary, but even with mastitis, the discomfort lessens as the procedure continues. The intraductal pressure is relieved as milk or pus is slowly extruded. Mothers must be taught this technique and instructed to repeat the procedure every few hours, standing in the shower, using soapy fingers, until the breast feels softer and milk is flowing freely.

If a breast abscess has formed, needle aspiration is preferred to incision and drainage under local or general anesthesia [160, 161]. Repeat needle aspiration may be required [166]. In very large or loculated abscesses, incision may be necessary. The incision should be radial, not circumferential, to minimize duct severance. A large drain should be inserted, and daily irrigations continued until the cavity closes. It is important that the dressings be applied in a manner such that the infant can continue to breast-feed or the mother should use an efficient breast pump. Regular drainage prevents further milk stasis and maintains lactation.

Treating Infection

Correct breastfeeding techniques and improved drainage of milk are the *sine qua non* of treatment, but antibiotic therapy may be necessary. Inflammatory mastitis occurs within 12–24 h of milk blockage, leading to an infectious mastitis within 24–48 h. Under normal conditions, the milk leukocyte count is less than 10^6 mL of milk, and the bacterial count is less than 10^3 bacteria per milliliter. Within 48 h of breast symptoms, the leukocyte count increases to more than 10^6 mL of milk, but the bacterial count remains low. This is considered noninfectious inflammation of the breast, and improved milk drainage will resolve the situation quickly [152]. Infectious mastitis is defined as having a bacterial count of more than 10^6 mL of milk. In clinical practice, treatment is empirical. Breast pain and erythema associated with flu-like systemic symptoms and a fever are highly suggestive of infectious mastitis and require antibiotic therapy if not resolving within 24 h [167]. Common bacterial pathogens include *S. aureus*, *Escherichia coli*, *group A β-hemolytic Streptococcus* with occasional *Streptococcus faecalis,* and *Klebsiella pneumonia.* In contrast, nonpuerperal breast infections are mixed infections with a major anaerobic component. Antibiotics of choice include penicillinase-resistant penicillins such as dicloxacillin or flucloxacillin, cephalosporins, sulfonamides, and clindamycin. A 10–14-day course may be required. The breast milk excretion of these antibiotics is minimal, and continuation of breastfeeding is considered safe. Clinical improvement is usually seen within 24–48 h, the erythema subsides, the fever decreases, and breast pain improves [167]. A persistent fluctuant mass may indicate abscess formation.

Prevention of Recurrence

Excessive milk retention can be prevented by correct breastfeeding techniques, ensuring a proper latch, regular drainage, and not skipping feeds. Mothers should avoid pressure on the breast (e.g., from their finger on the breast, or a seat belt, or tight clothing) as the milk ducts are easily compressed [168]. Sleeping through the night, returning to work, the introduction of breast milk substitutes such as bottles of formula, the introduction of table foods, and weaning are all typical periods when breastfeeds may be missed. The resultant "breast confusion" can lead to inadequate drainage and milk retention. Mothers with a high milk output should become skilled at palpating their breasts for lumps, and the bra should be removed before feeding if it is practical to do so. Areas of breast lumpiness or caking that persist after breastfeeding may indicate milk stasis or a blocked duct. Thorough expression of this residual milk should relieve the situation and prevent secondary complications.

Supportive Measures

Mastitis is an inflammatory process that can be complicated by infection and produce systemic symptoms in an already exhausted mother. Home help and bed rest are advisable, and analgesia such as ibuprofen or acetaminophen may be necessary. Hot compresses applied to the breast, before breastfeeding or milk expression, encourage blood flow and smooth muscle relaxation, which in turn helps milk transfer. Cold compresses after feeds may decrease inflammation and edema.

Anecdotal cases of maternal toxic shock syndrome have been reported, and in rare circumstances, *Staphylococcus* toxins can be ingested by the infant [169]. Continuation of breastfeeding is always recommended. Weaning may lead to increased milk stasis and abscess formation. If a mother chooses to wean abruptly or if clinically indicated, a lactation suppressant such as cabergoline may be used (0.25 mg twice daily for 2 days) [114, 170].

5.3.4 Sore Nipples

Sore nipples, particularly during the first few days of breastfeeding, are a common symptom experienced by an estimated 80 % of breastfeeding mothers. It is generally accepted that transient nipple soreness is within normal limits. Factors such as frequency and duration of breastfeeding, skin or hair color, and nipple preparation do not seem to make a difference in preventing tenderness. Increasing or persistent discomfort is pathological and requires careful evaluation. Detailed studies of infant suckling at the breast have illustrated how tongue friction or gum compression, resulting from inappropriate latch, can cause trauma and result in superficial skin abrasions and painful nipples [171, 172]. In many cases, repositioning can have a dramatic effect and instantaneously remove the pain and discomfort [173, 174]. However, recent research suggests that some infants exert higher than normal intraoral vacuums causing pain to their mothers [175].

A small percentage of women have naturally sensitive nipples, which remain uncomfortable throughout the duration of breastfeeding, despite careful technique. They experience sensitive nipples, even in their nonlactating state. When nipple pain, excoriations, dermatitis, or ulceration continues despite careful maternal breastfeeding technique, a detailed history and physical examination are required to elucidate secondary causes of sore nipples.

5.3.4.1 Nipple Trauma

To suckle correctly, an infant must grasp sufficient breast tissue to form a teat, draw it to the back of the pharynx, and initiate suckling in a coordinated manner using rhythmic jaw compressions and a grooved, undulating tongue. Many maternal nipple and infant oral anatomic anomalies can interfere with effective latch and suckle, resulting in nipple trauma and pain. Clinical findings such as maternal inelastic, flat, pseudoinverted, or inverted nipples and infant cleft lip and palate are easily identified. More subtle findings may include infant retrognathia, which refers to a small or posterior positioned mandible, or the Pierre Robin malformation, which combines severe micrognathia, or a posterior tongue with a relative ineffective activity of the muscles that protract the tongue and ankyloglossia [129, 176].

Management includes using a semi-upright breastfeeding position, which allows gravity to aid in jaw extension and minimizes the degree of overbite and friction. Continuous support and shaping of the breast throughout the feed with hand support of the infant's head and shoulders stabilize the neck and jaw muscles. Heat and gentle manipulation of the nipple may elongate it sufficiently to enable a correct latch. If clinically indicated, frenotomy can release a tethered tongue [177]. Over a period of a few weeks, a hypoplastic mandible rapidly elongates, the facial muscles strengthen, the nipple tissue becomes more distensible, the latch improves, and nipple trauma and pain resolve.

5.3.4.2 Chapped Nipples

Dry, cracked nipples may be chapped due to loss of moisture barrier in the stratum corneum because of constant wet and dry exposure combined with nipple friction. Management goals include avoiding further trauma by modifying breastfeeding technique, avoiding excessive drying, and restoring the moisture barrier. Moist wound healing allows the epithelial cells to migrate inward and heal the cracks and ulcers [178]. Moisturizers and emollients such as USP-modified anhydrous lanolin applied to the nipples and areolae after each feed are cheap and effective. In most situations, breastfeeding should continue during therapy; if repositioning fails to modify or relieve the pain and discomfort, it may be advisable to stop breastfeeding for 48–72 h to allow healing to occur. The breasts should be emptied every 3–4 h, and an alternative feeding method should be used. It is inappropriate to try to mask the pain by numbing with ice or using strong analgesia or nipple shields because this will fail to correct the underlying cause and may lead to further nipple trauma.

5.3.4.3 Bacterial Infection of the Nipple

S. aureus is frequently found distributed over the skin. Natural barriers, such as the stratum corneum, skin dryness, rapid cell turnover, and acid pH of 5–6, of the infant's skin usually prevent infection. For disease to result, preexisting tissue injury or inflammation is of major importance in pathogenesis. As in other clinical situations, when there is a break in the integument of the skin surface, there is a predisposition to a secondary infection because of bacterial or fungal contamination, which may lead to a delay in wound healing. Sore nipples associated with skin breakage, including cracks, fissures, and ulceration, have a high chance of being contaminated with microorganisms. The clinical findings on the nipple and areola of local erythema, excoriations, purulent exudates, and tenderness are suggestive of colonization with coagulase-positive *S. aureus*. Livingstone et al. [155] showed that mothers with young infants who complained of moderate-to-severe nipple pain and who had cracks, fissures, ulcers, or exudates had a 54 % chance of isolation of *S. aureus*. In some clinical situations, a blocked nipple pore appears white and on culturing is found to be contaminated with *S. aureus*. Most cases of cellulitis, mastitis, and breast abscess involve an ascending lactiferous duct infection with *S. aureus* or β-hemolytic streptococcus. Management includes careful washing with soap and water of the nipples to remove crusting and the use of appropriate antibiotics. Topical antibiotic ointments such as fusidic acid (Fuccidin) or mupirocin (Bactroban) may be effective in conjunction with systemic penicillinase-resistant antibiotics, such as dicloxacillin, cephalosporin, or erythromycin in penicillin-allergic patients [156]. Treatment should continue for 7–10 days until the skin is fully healed. The source of the infection is often from the infant's oropharyngeal or ophthalmic flora. In persistent or recurrent infections, it may be necessary to treat the infant as well [179].

5.3.4.4 Candidiasis

Candidiasis is commonly caused by *Candida albicans* and less frequently by other Candida species. It may be a primary or secondary skin infection. *C. albicans* is endogenous to the gastrointestinal tract and mucocutaneous areas. Normal skin does not harbor *C. albicans*; however, almost any skin damage caused by trauma or environmental changes may lead to rapid colonization by *C. albicans*. Isolation of the organism from a diseased skin may not be the cause of the disease but may be coincidental. *C. albicans* can be a secondary invader in preexisting pathological conditions and may give rise to further pathology. Candidiasis should be suspected when persistent nipple symptoms, such as a burning sensation on light touch and severe nipple pain during feeds, are combined with minimal objective findings on the nipple [180]. Typical signs include a shiny or flaky appearance of the nipple and areola associated with nipple and breast pain [181]; the breast appears normal without the inflammation and fullness associated with mastitis. A high incidence of oral mucocutaneous candidiasis has been noted in the newborn following vaginal delivery in the presence of maternal candidal vulvovaginitis. Typical symptoms of nipple/breast candidiasis often develop following maternal antibiotic use [182, 183]. Clinical examination of the infant is mandatory because *C. albicans* is passed from the infant's oral pharynx to the mother's nipple, which, being a warm, moist, frequently macerated epidermis, is easily colonized and possibly infected when the integument is broken. Diagnosis is based on clinical signs and symptoms [184, 185].

The treatment of cutaneous candidiasis includes careful hygiene, removal of excessive moisture, and topical therapy with broad-spectrum antifungal agents such as nystatin, clotrimazole, miconazole, or 2 % ketoconazole. The creams should be applied to the nipple and areola after each breastfeed for 10–14 days. In addition, other sites of candidiasis in both mother and infant, including maternal vulvovaginitis, intertrigo, or infant diaper dermatitis, should be treated simultaneously with a topical antifungal cream. Oral thrush in the infant should be treated aggressively with an oral antifungal solution such as nystatin suspension 100,000 U/g. After each feed, the oral cavity should be carefully painted and then 0.5 mL of nystatin suspension inserted into the mouth by dropper for 14 days. In countries where oral miconazole gel is available, this is used in the infant's mouth and on the mother's nipples [186]. Oral fluconazole 3 mg/kg daily for 14 days or oral ketoconazole 5 mg/kg daily for 7 days may be used for the treatment of oropharyngeal candidiasis in newborns. Gentian violet 0.5–1 % aqueous solution is cheap and effective if used sparingly under medical supervision. Daily painting of the infant's mouth and mother's nipples for about 5–7 days is usually sufficient. Excessive use may cause oral ulceration [187]. Failure to eradicate fungal infections is usually due to user, not medication failure. Occasionally, more serious underlying medical conditions such as diabetes or immunodeficiencies may exist. Systemic antifungal agents may be required; regimes vary from fluconazole 150 mg every second day for three dose [186] to 200 mg loading dose, followed by 100 mg daily for 14 days [143] (p. 282). In addition, topical corticosteroids may reduce nipple pruritus and erythema [188]. Foreign objects contaminated with yeast, including soothers and rubber nipples, should be avoided or sterilized, if possible, to prevent reinfection. Lay literature is full of nonpharmacologic treatments for candidiasis with little evidence to support them. The healthcare provider is cautioned against recommending regimens that are complicated. In an otherwise healthy person, the immune defense mechanism can control the growth of candida, assuming the skin integument is intact and remains dry.

5.3.4.5 Dermatitis

Dermatitis of the nipple may be endogenous atopic eczema, irritant contact, or allergic contact dermatitis [189, 190]. Contact dermatitis in the nipple is an eczematous reaction to an external material applied, worn, or inadvertently transferred to the skin. It may be an allergic or an irritant response. Patients may complain of dry, pruritic, or burning nipples with signs of inflammation, erythema, and edema, or excoriations, desquamation, or chronic plaque formation. The typical description is of an itching, spreading rash. Management includes careful avoidance of all irritants such as creams, preservatives, detergents, and fragrances. Irritation from frequent expressing can be reduced by using a lubricant, such as purified lanolin, on the nipples and areolae prior to pumping. A potent topical corticosteroid such as mometasone furoate can be applied thinly to the nipple and areola after a feed once a day for up to 10 days [189, 190]. Regular use of emollients may prevent recurrence. Chronic dermatitis is often colonized with *S. aureus*, which may require topical or oral antibiotic therapy.

5.3.4.6 Paget's Disease

Paget's disease is an intraepidermal carcinoma for which the most common site is the nipple and areola. It usually presents as unilateral erythema and scaling of the nipple and areola and looks eczematous [191]. Unfortunately, the condition is usually part of an intraductal carcinoma, and treatment necessitates cessation of breastfeeding.

5.3.4.7 Vasospasm or Raynaud's Phenomenon

Vasospasm, or Raynaud's phenomenon, of the nipple manifests as a blanching of the nipple tip with pain and discomfort radiating through the breast after and between feeds [192]. It may be associated with excoriated and infected nipples. There may be a history of cold-induced vasospasm of the fingers (Raynaud's phenomenon). Repetitive trauma to the nipple from incorrect latch or retrognathia, combined with local inflammation or infection and air cooling, can trigger a characteristic painful vasospastic response. Correcting the latch and alternating breastfeeding positions throughout the feed will prevent ongoing nipple trauma. Avoiding air exposure and applying warm dry heat to the nipples after feeds may help. Standard pharmacologic therapy for Raynaud's phenomenon can be effective in reducing the vasospasms; oral magnesium supplements and nifedipine are usually helpful [193, 194]. Local infections should be treated aggressively, and breastfeeding stopped for several days if necessary to allow healing to occur.

5.3.4.8 Psoriasis

Psoriasis may present as a pink, flaky plaque over the areola as a result of skin trauma. There is usually an existing psoriatic history. Standard treatment includes fluorinated steroid ointments and keratolytic agents, which should be applied after feeds and then washed off carefully before feedings.

For many years, the medical and nursing literature has recommended a variety of management approaches for sore nipples, ranging from topical application of cold tea bags, carrots, and vitamin E to lanolin, masse cream, antiseptics, alcohol preparations, and air drying [195]. The efficacy of each of these modalities has not been proven, however; in fact, the latter is now thought to be detrimental by abstracting water from the skin and precipitating protein, which leaves the skin less pliable and more prone to fissuring. Healthcare professionals are cautioned against using nontraditional adjunct management modalities for sore nipples because of the risk of iatrogenic disease.

Reference Books

- Briggs GG, Freeman RK, Yaffe SJ. *Drugs in Pregnancy and Lactation*, 9th ed. Philadelphia: Lippincott Williams & Wilkins, 2011.
- Hale TW, Rowe HE. *Medication and Mothers' Milk*, 16th ed. Texas: Pharmasoft Medical Publishing, 2014. Available from http://neonatal.ttuhsc.edu/lact/

Websites

- A searchable website (LactMed) is available via the US National Library of Medicine at: http://toxnet.nlm/nih.gov/cgi-bin/sis/htmlgen?LACT
- World Health Organization. Breastfeeding and maternal medication http://www.who.int/child-adolescent-health/New_Publications/NUTRITION/BF_Maternal_Medication.pdf

Telephone advice

- Pharmacy departments of tertiary maternity hospitals

Fig. 5.9 Sources of information on medicines for breastfeeding women

5.3.5 Induced Lactation and Relactation

Given the growing understanding of the value of breastfeeding in terms of nutrition and nurturing, women are seeking information about breastfeeding and adoption [26]. Induced lactation in the nonpregnant woman has been described for many years in both scientific and lay publications and includes the first reports by Hippocrates [196]. Auerbach and Avery reported on 240 women who attempted to breast-feed adopted children [197]. There are several anecdotally described methods of inducing lactation and preparing for breastfeeding, some of which can be started before the arrival of the infant. Direct nipple stimulation has been described as the most important component of inducing lactation and preparing to breast-feed [197]. Nipple stimulation can be performed by hand or by such mechanical means as an electric breast pump. Hand stimulation has the advantage of being easy and portable, but mechanical pumping stimulates greater milk production in lactating women [198].

A variety of pharmacological lactotrophs and galactogogues have been used to induce lactation [199, 200]. Estrogen and progesterone are used to promote mammogenesis by stimulating alveoli and lactiferous duct proliferation. They inhibit milk synthesis by blocking the action of prolactin on the mammary glands and therefore are used in preparation for breastfeeding. Galactogogues such as phenothiazine, sulpiride, and domperidone also have been described [114]. They are dopamine antagonists and block the inhibition of prolactin, which is a potent lactotroph. Metoclopramide and chlorpromazine are commonly used galactogogues but have many potential side effects, including sedation, extrapyramidal symptoms, and tardive dyskinesia [201]. Domperidone has little effect on the central nervous system and has fewer side effects [146]. Drug excretion in breast milk is very limited and in combination with low milk production probably does not pose a risk to the infant. Relactation is often more successful than induced lactation [202].

5.3.6 Medicines and Breastfeeding

Most drugs transfer into breast milk, but generally at low, subclinical doses [203]. In general, if the medication is safe to use in infants, it will be safe for the breastfeeding mother [204]. Only a small number of medications are contraindicated during breastfeeding: These include antineoplastic agents, ergotamine, methotrexate, cyclosporine, and radiopharmaceuticals [205]. Physicians and mothers need to consider the risks and benefits of any medicine. General advice is to use topical/local medicines where possible, choose drugs with shorter half-lives, and use drugs where there is previous experience in lactating women. Information is available about safe use of medicines while breastfeeding (see Fig. 5.9 for list of resources).

5.4 Conclusion

As the prevalence of breastfeeding continues to increase, health professionals will be expected to take a leadership role in the promotion, protection, and support of breastfeeding by providing appropriate guidance, diagnosis, and breastfeeding management throughout the full course of lactation. Information on medicines for breastfeeding women is available [206]. See Fig. 5.9 for a list of resources.

References

1. Livingstone V. Breastfeeding kinetics: a problem solving approach to breastfeeding difficulties. World Rev Nutr Diet. 1995;78:28–54.
2. Livingstone V. Prenatal lactation assessment. J SOGC. 1994;16:2351–9.
3. O'Campo P, Faden RR, Gielen AC, et al. Prenatal factors associated with breastfeeding duration: recommendations for prenatal interventions. Birth. 1992;19:195–201.

4. Britton C, McCormick FM, Renfrew MJ, et al. Support for breastfeeding mothers. Cochrane Collab. 2007; CD001141.
5. Miracle DJ, Fredland V. Provider encouragement of breastfeeding: efficacy and ethics. J Midwifery Womens Health. 2007;52:545–8.
6. Berry NJ, Gribble KD. Breast is no longer best: promoting normal infant feeding. Matern Child Health. 2008;4:74–9.
7. World Health Organization. Expert consultation on the optimal duration of exclusive breastfeeding. Conclusions and recommendations. 2001 [cited; Available from: http://www.who.int/inf-pr-2001/en/note2001-07.html.
8. World Health Organization. Global strategy for infant and young child feeding. 2003 [cited; Available from: http://www.who.int/child-adolescent-health/NUTRITION/global_strategy.html.
9. Dettwyler KA. When to wean: biological versus cultural perspectives. Clin Obstet Gynecol. 2004;47:712–23.
10. Pisacane A, De Vizia B, Valiante A, et al. Iron status in breast-fed infants. J Pediatr. 1995;127:429–31.
11. Newburg DS. Innate immunity and human milk. J Nutr. 2005;135:1308–12.
12. Hanson LA. Session 1: feeding and infant development breast-feeding and immune function. Proc Nutr Soc. 2007;66:384–96.
13. Kramer MS, Chalmers B, Hodnett ED, et al. Promotion of breastfeeding intervention trial (PROBIT): a randomized trial in the republic of Belarus. JAMA. 2001;285:413–20.
14. Kramer MS, Guo T, Platt RW, et al. Infant growth and health outcomes associated with 3 compared with 6 months of exclusive breastfeeding. Am J Clin Nutr. 2003;78:291–5.
15. Quigley MA, Cumberland P, Cowden JM, et al. How protective is breast feeding against diarrhoeal disease in infants in 1990s England? A case-control study. Arch Dis Child. 2006;91:245–50.
16. Dewey KG, Heinig MJ, Nommsen-Rivers LA. Differences in morbidity between breast-fed and formula-fed infants. J Pediatr. 1995;126:696–702.
17. Oddy WH, Sly PD, de Klerk NH, et al. Breast feeding and respiratory morbidity in infancy: a birth cohort study. Arch Dis Child. 2003;88:224–8.
18. Marild S, Hansson S, Jodal U, et al. Protective effect of breastfeeding against urinary tract infection. Acta Pediatr. 2004;93:164–8.
19. Horta BL, Bahl R, Martines JC, et al. Evidence on the long-term effects of breastfeeding: systematic reviews and meta-analyses. Geneva: World Health Organization; 2007.
20. McGuire W, Anthony MY. Donor human milk versus formula for preventing necrotising enterocolitis in preterm infants: systematic review. Arch Dis Child Fetal Neonatal Ed. 2003;21:249–54.
21. Baumgartner C. Psychomotor and social development of breast-fed and bottle-fed babies during their first year of life. Acta Paediatr Hung. 1984;25:409–17.
22. Davis DW, Bell PA. Infant feeding practices and occlusal outcomes: a longitudinal study. J Can Dent Assoc. 1991;57:593–4.
23. Owen CG, Martin RM, Whincup PH, et al. Effect of infant feeding on the risk of obesity across the life course: a quantitative review of published evidence. Pediatrics. 2005;115:1367–77.
24. Harder T, Bergmann R, Kallischnigg G, et al. Duration of breastfeeding and risk of overweight: a meta-analysis. Am J Epidemiol. 2005;162:397–403.
25. Martin RM, Gunnell D, Davey Smith G. Breastfeeding in infancy and blood pressure in later life: systematic review and meta-analysis. Am J Epidemiol. 2005;161:15–26.
26. Gribble KD. Mental health, attachment and breastfeeding: implications for adopted children and their mothers. Int Breastfeed J. 2006;1:5.
27. Widstrom AM, Wahlberg V, Matthiesen AS, et al. Short-term effects of suckling and touch of the nipple on maternal behavior. Early Hum Dev. 1990;21:153–63.
28. Collaborative Group on Hormonal Factors in Breast Cancer. Breast cancer and breastfeeding: collaborative reanalysis of individual data from 47 epidemiological studies in 30 countries, including 50,302 women with breast cancer and 96,973 women without the disease. Lancet. 2002;360:187–95.
29. Ip S, Chung M, Raman G, et al. Breastfeeding and maternal and infant health outcomes in developed countries, in evidence report/technology assessment No. 153. Prepared by Tufts-New England Medical Center Evidence-based Practice Center, under Contract No. 290-02-0022. AHRQ Publication No. 07-E007. Rockville, MD: Agency for Healthcare Research and Quality; 2007.
30. Kennedy KI, Visness CM. Contraceptive efficacy of lactational amenorrhoea. Lancet. 1992;339:227–30.
31. Walker M. A fresh look at the risks of artificial infant feeding. J Hum Lact. 1993;9:97–107.
32. Forsythe SJ. *Enterobacter sakazakii* and other bacteria in powdered infant milk formula. Matern Child Nutr. 2005;1:44–50.
33. Morais TB, Sigulem DM, Maranhao HS, et al. Bacterial contamination and nutrient content of home-prepared milk feeding bottles of infants attending a public outpatient clinic. J Trop Pediatr. 2005;51:87–92.
34. FAO/WHO. Expert meeting, *Enterobacter sakazakii* and other microorganisms in powdered infant formula: meeting report, in Microbiological Risk Assessment Series 10; 2006.
35. Frank JW, Newman J. Breast-feeding in a polluted world: uncertain risks, clear benefits. Can Med Assoc J. 1993;149:33–7.
36. Walker M. Summary of the hazards of infant formula: part 2. International Lactation Consultant Association; 1998.
37. Walker M. Summary of the hazards of infant formula: monograph 3. International Lactation Consultant Association; 2004.
38. Lucas A, Morley R, Cole T, et al. Breast milk and subsequent intelligence quotient in children born preterm. Lancet. 1992;339:261–4.
39. Pollock JI. Long-term associations with infant feeding in a clinically advantaged population of babies. Develop Med Child Neurol. 1994;36:429–40.
40. Lanting CI, Fidler V, Huisman M, et al. Neurological differences between 9-year-old children fed breast-milk or formula-milk as babies. Lancet. 1994;344:1319–22.
41. Elwood PC, Pickering J, Gallacher JE, et al. Long term effect of breast feeding: cognitive function in the Caerphilly cohort. J Epidemiol Commun Health. 2005;59:130–3.
42. Gdalevich M, Mimouni D, David M, et al. Breastfeeding and the onset of atopic dermatitis in childhood: a systematic review and meta-analysis of prospective studies. J Am Acad Dermatol. 2001;45:520–7.
43. Howie PW, Forsyth JS, Ogston SA, et al. Protective effect of breast feeding against infection. Br Med J. 1990;300:11–6.
44. Quigley MA, Kelly YJ, Sacker A. Breastfeeding and hospitalization for diarrheal and respiratory infection in the United Kingdom millennium cohort study. Pediatrics. 2007;119: e837–42.
45. Martin RM, Gunnell D, Owen CG, et al. Breastfeeding and childhood cancer: a systematic review with meta-analysis. Int J Cancer. 2005;117:1020–31.
46. Klement E, Cohen RV, Boxman J, et al. Breastfeeding and risk of inflammatory bowel disease: a systematic review with meta-analysis. Am J Clin Nutr. 2004;80:1342–52.
47. Akobeng AK, Ramanan AV, Buchan I, et al. Effect of breastfeeding on risk of coeliac disease: a systematic review

and meta-analysis of observational studies. Arch Dis Child. 2006;91:39–43.
48. Taylor JS, Kacmar JE, Nothnagle M, et al. A systematic review of the literature associating breastfeeding with type 2 diabetes and gestational diabetes. J Am Coll Nutr. 2005;24:320–6.
49. Owen CG, Martin RM, Whincup PH, et al. Does breastfeeding influence risk of type 2 diabetes in later life? A quantitative analysis of published evidence. Am J Clin Nutr. 2006;85: 1043–54.
50. The Breastfeeding Center or Ann Arbor. Cost of formula feeding. c2009–2013 [cited 2015 May 16]. Available from: http://bfcaa.com/cost-of-formula-feeding/.
51. Cattaneo A, Ronfani L, Burmaz T, et al. Infant feeding and cost of health care: a cohort study. Acta Paediatr. 2006;95:540–6.
52. Smith JP, Thompson JF, Ellwood DA. Hospital system costs of artificial infant feeding: estimates for the Australian capital territory. Aust NZ J Public Health. 2002;26:543–51.
53. Su LL, Chong YS, Chan YH, et al. Antenatal education and postnatal support strategies for improving rates of exclusive breastfeeding: randomised controlled trial. Br Med J. 2007;335:596.
54. Minchin MK. Who is responsible for breastfeeding failure? Breastfeeding matters: what we need to know about infant feeding. Melbourne: Alma; 1998. p. 45–79.
55. Kulski JK, Hartmann PE. Changes in human milk composition during the initiation of lactation. Aust J Exp Biol Med Sci. 1981;59:101–14.
56. Neifert M, Seacat J, Jobe WE. Lactation failure due to insufficient glandular development of the breast. Pediatrics. 1985;76:823–8.
57. Huggins KE, Petok ES, Mireles O. Markers of lactation insufficiency: a study of 34 mothers. In: Auerbach K, editor. Current issues in clinical lactation. MA: Jones and Bartlett; 2000. p. 25–35.
58. Neifert M, DeMarzo S, Seacat J, et al. The influence of breast surgery, breast appearance and pregnancy-induced breast changes on lactation sufficiency as measured by infant weight gain. Birth. 1990;17:31–8.
59. Johansson AS, Wennborg H, Blomquist L, et al. Breastfeeding after mammaplasty and augmentation mammaplasty. Epidemiology. 2003;14:127–9.
60. Marasco L, Marmet C, Shell E. Polycystic ovary syndrome: a connection to insufficient milk supply? J Hum Lact. 2000;16:143–8.
61. Buhimschi CS. Endocrinology of lactation. Obstet Gynecol Clin N Am. 2004;31:963–79.
62. Cox SG. Expressing and storing colostrum antenatally for use in the newborn period. Breastfeed Rev. 2006;14:11–6.
63. ACOG committee opinion. Breastfeeding and the risk of hepatitis C virus transmission. Int J Gynecol Obstet. 1999;66:307–8.
64. WHO HIV and Infant Feeding Technical Consultation. Held on behalf of the Inter-agency Task Team (IATT) on prevention of HIV infections in pregnant women, mothers and their infants, Geneva, consensus statement; 2006 Oct 25–27.
65. Howard C, Lawrence RA. Breast-feeding and drug exposure. Obstet Gynecol Clin N Am. 1998;25:195–216.
66. Woodward A, Douglas RM, Graham NMH, et al. Acute respiratory illness in Adelaide children: breastfeeding modifies the effect of passive smoking. J Epidemiol Commun Health. 1990;44:224–30.
67. Nafstad P, Jaakola JJK, Hagen JA, et al. Breastfeeding, maternal smoking and lower respiratory tract infections. Eur Respir J. 1996;9:2623–9.
68. Bottorff JL, Morse JM. Mothers' perceptions of breast milk. J Obstet Gynecol Neonatal Nurs. 1990;19:518–27.
69. Sheehan A, Schmied V, Cooke M. Australian women's stories of their baby-feeding decisions in pregnancy. Midwifery. 2003;19:259–66.
70. Wells KJ, Thompson NJ, Kloeben-Tarver AS. Intrinsic and extrinsic motivation and intention to breastfeed. Am J Health Behav. 2002;26:111–20.
71. Bryant CA. The impact of kin, friend and neighbor networks on infant feeding practices. Cuban, Puerto Rican and Anglo families in Florida. Soc Sci Med. 1982;16(20):1757–65.
72. Baranowski T, Bee D, Rassin DK, et al. Social support, social influence, ethnicity and the breastfeeding decision. Soc Sci Med. 1983;17:1599–611.
73. Rossman B. Breastfeeding peer counselors in the United States: helping to build a culture and tradition of breastfeeding. J Midwifery Womens Health. 2007;52:631–7.
74. Kent JC, Mitoulas L, Cox DB, et al. Breast volume and milk production during extended lactation in women. Exp Physiol. 1999;84:435–47.
75. Czank C, Henderson JJ, et al. Hormonal control of the lactation cycle. In: Hale TW, Hartmann P, editors. Textbook of human lactation. Amarillo, TX: Hale, L.P.; 2007. p. 89–111.
76. Alexander JM, Grant AM, Campbell MJ. Randomised controlled trial of breast shells and Hoffman's exercises for inverted and non-protractile nipples. Br Med J. 1992;304:1030–2.
77. McGeorge DD. The "Niplette": an instrument for the non-surgical correction of inverted nipples. Br J Plast Surg. 1994;47:46–9.
78. Kesaree N, Banapurmath CR, Banapurmath S, et al. Treatment of inverted nipples using a disposable syringe. J Hum Lact. 1993;9:27–9.
79. Righard L, Alade MO. Effect of delivery room routines on success of first breast-feed. Lancet. 1990;336:1105–7.
80. Smith LJ. Impact of birthing practices on the breastfeeding dyad. J Midwifery Womens Health. 2007;52:621–30.
81. Murray EK, Ricketts S, Dellaport J. Hospital practices that increase breastfeeding duration: results from a population-based study. Birth. 2007;34:202–11.
82. Klaus MH. The frequency of suckling. Obstet Gynecol Clin N Am. 1987;14:623–33.
83. Yamauchi Y, Yamanouchi I. Breastfeeding frequency during the first 24 hours after birth in full-term neonates. Pediatrics. 1990;86:171–5.
84. Yamauchi Y, Yamanouchi I. The relationship between rooming-in/not rooming-in and breastfeeding variables. Acta Paediatr Scand. 1990;79:1017–22.
85. Elander G, Lindberg T. Short mother-infant separation during first week of life influences the duration of breastfeeding. Acta Paediatr Scand. 1984;73:237–40.
86. Ball HL, Ward-Platt MP, Heslop E, et al. Randomised trial of infant sleep location on the postnatal ward. Arch Dis Child. 2006;91:1005–10.
87. Royal College of Midwives. Successful breastfeeding. New York: Churchill Livingstone; 1991. p. 25–33.
88. Moon JL, Humenick SS. Breast engorgement: contributing variables and variables amenable to nursing intervention. J Obstet Gynecol Neonatal Nurs. 1989;18:309–15.
89. Newman J. Breastfeeding problems associated with the early introduction of bottle and pacifiers. J Hum Lact. 1990;6:59–63.
90. Shrago L. Glucose water supplementation of the breastfed infant during the first three days of life. J Hum Lact. 1987;3:82–6.
91. Woolridge MW. Baby-controlled breastfeeding: biocultural implications in breastfeeding. In: Stuart-Macadam P, Dettwyler KA, editors. Breastfeeding: biocultural perspectives. New York: Aldine de Gruyter; 1995. p. 217–42.

92. Newburg DS, Walker WA. Protection of the neonate by the innate immune system of developing gut and of human milk. Pediatr Res. 2007;61:2–8.
93. Widström AM, Ransjö-Arvidson AB, Christensson K, et al. Gastric suction in healthy newborn infants. Effects on circulation and developing feeding behaviour. Acta Paediatr Scand. 1987;76:566–72.
94. Nissen E, Lilja G, Matthiesen AS, et al. Effects of maternal pethidine on infants' developing breastfeeding behaviour. Acta Paediatr. 1995;84(2):140–5.
95. Hartmann PE, Prosser CG. Physiological basis of longitudinal changes in human milk yield and composition. Fed Proc. 1984;43:2448–53.
96. Wilde CJ, Addey CV, Boddy LM, et al. Autocrine regulation of milk secretion by a protein in milk. Biochem J. 1995;305:51–8.
97. Prentice A, Addey CVP, Wilde CJ. Evidence for local feedback control of human milk secretion. Biochem Soc Trans. 1989;17:122–4.
98. Wilde CJ, Addey CV, Bryson JM, et al. Autocrine regulation of milk secretion. Biochem Soc Symp. 1998;63:81–90.
99. Czank C, Mitoulas LR, Hartmann PE. Human milk composition —fat. In: Hale TW, Hartmann P, editors. Textbook of human lactation. Amarillo, TX: Hale, L.P.; 2007. p. 49–67.
100. McNeilly AS, Robinson IC, Houston MJ, et al. Release of oxytocin and prolactin in response to suckling. Br Med J. 1983;286:257–9.
101. Cox DB, Owens RA, Hartmann PE. Blood and milk prolactin and the rate of milk synthesis in women. Exp Physiol. 1996;81: 1007–20.
102. Cregan MD, Hartmann PE. Computerized breast measurement from conception to weaning: clinical implications. J Hum Lact. 1999;15:89–96.
103. WHO/UNICEF. Protecting, promoting and supporting breast-feeding: the special role of maternity services. Geneva: World Health Organization; 1989.
104. Djiane J, Houdebine LM, Kelly P. Prolactin-like activity of anti-prolactin receptor antibodies on casein and DNA synthesis in the mammary gland. Proc Natl Acad Sci. 1981;78:7445–8.
105. Pestell RG, Best JD, Alford F. Lymphocytic hypophysitis: the clinical spectrum of the disorder and evidence for an autoimmune pathogenesis. Clin Endocrinol. 1990;33:457–66.
106. Imura H. The pituitary gland. New York: Raven; 1994. p. 1–28.
107. Rillema JA. Development of the mammary gland and lactation. Trends Endocrinol Metab. 1994;5:1469–540.
108. Kent JC. How breastfeeding works. J Midwifery Womens Health. 2007;52:564–70.
109. Livingstone VH, Gout PW, Crickmer SD, et al. Serum lactogens possessed normal bioactivity in patients with lactation insufficiency. Clin Endocrinol. 1994;41:193–8.
110. Neifert MR, McDonough SL, Neville MC. Failure of lactogenesis associated with placental retention. Am J Obstet Gynecol. 1981;140:477–8.
111. Kelly PA, Djiane J, Pastel-Vinay MC, et al. The prolactin/growth hormone receptor family. Endocr Rev. 1991;12:235–51.
112. De Carvalho M, Robertson S, Friedman A, et al. Effect of frequent breastfeeding on early milk production and infant weight gain. Pediatrics. 1983;72:307–11.
113. Forster D, McLachlan H, Lumley J. Factors associated with continuing to feed any breast milk at six months postpartum in a group of Australian women. Int Breastfeed J. 2006;1:18.
114. Hale TW. Medications that alter milk production. In: Hale TW, Hartmann P, editors. Textbook of human lactation. Amarillo, TX: Hale, L.P.; 2007. p. 479–89.
115. Aono T, Shioji T, Shoda T, et al. The initiation of human lactation and prolactin response to suckling. J Clin Endocrinol Metab. 1977;44:1101–6.
116. Widdice L. The effects of breast reduction and breast augmentation surgery on lactation: an annotated bibliography. J Hum Lact. 1993;9:161–7.
117. Ramsay DT. The anatomy of the lactating breast: latest research and clinical implications. Infant. 2007;3:59–63.
118. Newton M, Newton NR. Postpartum engorgement of the breast. Am J Obstet Gynecol. 1951;61:664–7.
119. Shrago LC. Engorgement reconsidered. Breastfeed Abstr. 1991;11:1–2.
120. Lennon I, Lewis BR. Effect of early complementary feeds on lactation failure. Breastfeed Rev. 1987;11:24–6.
121. Hill PD, Aldag JC, Chatterton RT. Effects of pumping style on milk production in mothers of non-nursing preterm infants. J Hum Lact. 1999;15:209–16.
122. Drewett RF, Woolridge MW. Milk taken by human babies from the first and second breast. Physiol Behav. 1981;26:327–9.
123. Newton M, Newton NR. The let-down reflex in human lactation. J Pediatr. 1948;33:698–704.
124. Prime DK, Geddes DT, Hartmann PE. Oxytocin: milk ejection and maternal-infant well-being. In: Hale TW, Hartmann P, editors. Textbook of human lactation. Amarillo, TX: Hale, L.P.; 2007. p. 141–55.
125. Neifert MR. Breastmilk transfer: positioning, latch-on, and screening for problems in milk transfer. Clin Obstet Gynecol. 2004;47:656–75.
126. Glover R, Wiessinger D. The infant-maternal breastfeeding conversation: helping when they lose the thread. In: Watson Genna C, editor. Supporting sucking skills in breastfeeding infants. Sudbury: Jones and Bartlett; 2008. p. 97–129.
127. Woolridge MW. The 'anatomy' of infant sucking. Midwifery. 1986;2:164–71.
128. Righard L, Alade MO. Sucking technique and its effect on success of breastfeeding. Birth. 1992;19:185–9.
129. Watson Genna C. The influence of anatomical and structural issues on sucking skills. In: Watson Genna C, editor. Supporting sucking skills in breastfeeding infants. Sudbury: Jones and Bartlett; 2008. p. 181–226.
130. McBride MC, Danner SC. Sucking disorders in neurologically impaired infants: assessment and facilitation of breastfeeding. Clin Perinatol. 1987;14:109–31.
131. Hogan M, Westcott C, Griffiths M. Randomized, controlled trial of division of tongue-tie in infants with feeding problems. J Paediatr Child Health. 2005;41:246–50.
132. Amir LH, James JP, Beatty J. Review of tongue-tie release at a tertiary maternity hospital. J Paediatr Child Health. 2005;41:243–5.
133. Dollberg S, Botzer E, Grunis E, et al. Immediate nipple pain relief after frenotomy in breast-fed infants with ankyloglossia: a randomized, prospective study. J Pediatr Surg. 2006;41:1598–600.
134. Coryllos E, Genna CW. Congenital tongue-tie and its impact on breastfeeding. Elk Grove Village: American Academy of Pediatrics: Section on Breastfeeding; 2004. p. 1–6.
135. Coryllos EV, Watson Genna C, Fram JLV. Minimally invasive treatment for posterior tongue-tie (the hidden tongue-tie). In: Watson Genna C, editor. Supporting sucking skills in breastfeeding infants. Sudbury: Jones and Bartlett; 2008. p. 227–34.
136. Daly SEJ, Di Rosso A, Owens RA, et al. Degree of breast emptying explains changes in the fat content, but not fatty acid composition, of human milk. Exp Physiol. 1993;78:741–55.
137. Woolridge MW, Baum JD, Drewett RF. Individual patterns of milk intake during breastfeeding. Early Hum Dev. 1982;7:265–72.

138. Anderson AK, Damio G, Himmelgreen DA, et al. Social capital, acculturation, and breastfeeding initiation among Puerto Rican women in the United States. J Hum Lact. 2004;20:39–45.
139. Livingstone V. In-hospital lactation assessment. J SOGC. 1996;18:19–28.
140. Dewey KG, Heinig MJ, Nommsen LA, et al. Growth of breast-fed and formula-fed infants from 0 to 18 months: the DARLING study. Pediatrics. 1992;89:1035–41.
141. Livingstone VH. Problem-solving formula for failure to thrive in breast-fed infants. Can Fam Physician. 1990;36:1541–5.
142. Evans A, Marinelli KA, Taylor JS, The Academy of Breastfeeding Medicine Protocol Committee. ABM clinical protocol #2: guidelines for hospital discharge of the breastfeeding term newborn and mother: "the going home protocol," revised 2014. Breastfeed Med. 2014;9:3–8.
143. Lawrence RA, Lawrence RM. Breastfeeding: a guide for the medical profession, vol. 6. St Louis: Mosby; 2005.
144. Daly SE, Owens RA, Hartmann PE. The short-term synthesis and infant-regulated removal of milk in lactating women. Exp Physiol. 1993;78:209–20.
145. Meier PP. The accuracy of test weighing for preterm infants. J Pediatr Gastroenterol Nutr. 1990;10:62–5.
146. Da Silva OP, Knoppert DC, Angelini MM, et al. Effect of domperidone on milk production in mothers of premature newborns: a randomized, double-blind, placebo-controlled trial. CMAJ. 2001;164:17–21.
147. The Academy of Breastfeeding Medicine Protocol Committee. ABM clinical protocol #9: use of galactogogues in initiating or augmenting the rate of maternal milk secretion (First Revision January 2011). Breastfeed Med. 2011;6:41–9.
148. Livingstone V. Too much of a good thing: maternal and infant hyperlactation syndromes. Can Fam Physician. 1996;42:89–99.
149. Daly S. The short-term synthesis and infant regulated removal of milk in lactating women. Exp Physiol. 1986;78:208–20.
150. Fetherston C. Risk factors for lactation mastitis. J Hum Lact. 1998;14:101–9.
151. Inch S. Breastfeeding problems: prevention and management. Commun Pract. 2006;79:165–7.
152. Thomsen AC, Espersen T, Maigaard S. Course and treatment of milk stasis, noninfectious inflammation of the breast, and infectious mastitis in nursing women. Am J Obstet Gynecol. 1984;149:492–5.
153. Fetherston C. Mastitis in lactating women: physiology or pathology? Breastfeed Rev. 2001;9:5–12.
154. Walsh A. Acute mastitis. Lancet. 1949;2:635–9.
155. Livingstone VH, Willis CE, Berkowitz J. *Staphylococcus aureus* and sore nipples. Can Fam Physician. 1996;42:654–9.
156. Livingstone V, Stringer LJ. The treatment of *Staphylococcus aureus* infected sore nipples: a randomized comparative study. J Hum Lact. 1999;15:241–6.
157. Hughes LE, Mansel RE, Webster DJT. Infection of the breast. In: Hughes LE, Mansel RE, Webster DJT, editors. Benign disorders and diseases of the breast: concepts and clinical management. London: Bailliere Tindall; 1989. p. 143–50.
158. Amir LH, Forster DA, Lumley J, et al. A descriptive study of mastitis in Australian breastfeeding women: incidence and determinants. BMC Public Health. 2007;7:62.
159. Hayes R, Michell M, Nunnerley HB. Acute inflammation of the breast—the role of breast ultrasound in diagnosis and management. Clin Radiol. 1991;44:253–6.
160. Christensen AF, Al-Suliman N, Nielson KR, et al. Ultrasound-guided drainage of breast abscesses: results in 151 patients. Br J Radiol. 2005;78:186–8.
161. Ulitzsch D, Nyman MKG, Carlson RA. Breast abscess in lactating women: US-guided treatment. Radiology. 2004;232: 904–9.
162. Woolridge MW, Ingram JC, Baum JD. Do changes in pattern of breast usage alter the baby's nutrient intake? Lancet. 1990;336:395–7.
163. van Veldhuizen CGA. Overabundant milk supply: an alternative way to intervene by full drainage and block feeding. Int Breastfeed J. 2007;2:11.
164. Campbell SH. Recurrent plugged ducts. J Hum Lact. 2006;22:340–3.
165. Bertrand H, Rosenblood LK. Stripping out pus in lactational mastitis: a means of preventing breast abscess. Can Med Assoc J. 1991;145:299–306.
166. Dixon JM. Repeated aspiration of breast abscesses in lactating women. Br Med J. 1988;297:1517–8.
167. World Health Organization. Mastitis: causes and management. Geneva: WHO/FCH/CAH/00.13; 2000.
168. Ramsay DT, Kent JC, Owens RA, et al. Ultrasound imaging of milk ejection in the breast of lactating women. Pediatrics. 2004;113:361–7.
169. Arsenault G. Toxic shock syndrome associated with mastitis. Can Fam Physician. 1992;38:399, 401, 456.
170. Ferrari C, Piscitelli G, Crosignani PG. Cabergoline: a new drug for the treatment of hyperprolactinaemia. Hum Reprod. 1995;10:1647–52.
171. Langton D, Ramsay D, Jacobs S, et al. Efficacy of frenulotomy for ankyloglossia in breast-fed infants. Perinatal Society of Australia and New Zealand 8th annual congress. Sydney, Australia; 2004. p. 44.
172. Watson Genna C, Sandora L. Normal sucking and swallowing. In: Watson Genna C, editor. Supporting sucking skills in breastfeeding infants. Sudbury: Jones and Bartlett; 2008. p. 1–41.
173. Woolridge MW. Aetiology of sore nipples. Midwifery. 1986;2:172–6.
174. Gunther M. Sore nipples: causes and prevention. Lancet. 1945;2:590–3.
175. McClellan H, Geddes D, Kent J, et al. Infants of mothers with persistent nipple pain exert strong sucking vacuums. Acta Paediatr. 2008;97(9):1205–9.
176. Danner SC. Breastfeeding the infant with a cleft defect. NAACOGS Clin Issu Perinat Womens Health Nurs. 1992;3:634–9.
177. Lalakea ML, Messner AH. Ankyloglossia: does it matter? Pediatr Clin N Am. 2003;50:381–97.
178. Sharp DA. Moist wound healing for sore or cracked nipples. Breastfeed Abstr. 1992;12:1.
179. Amir L. Breastfeeding and *Staphylococcus aureus*: three case reports. Breastfeed Rev. 2002;10:15–8.
180. Amir LH, Pakula S. Nipple pain, mastalgia and candidiasis in the lactating breast. Aust NZ J Obstet Gynaecol. 1991;31:378–80.
181. Francis-Morrill J, Heinig MJ, Pappagianis D, et al. Diagnostic value of signs and symptoms of mammary candidosis among lactating women. J Hum Lact. 2004;20:288–95.
182. Morrill JF, Heinig MJ, Pappagianis D, et al. Risk factors for mammary Candidosis among lactating women. JOGNN. 2005;34:37–45.
183. Dinsmoor MJ, Viloria R, Lief L, et al. Use of intrapartum antibiotics and the incidence of postnatal maternal and neonatal yeast infections. Obstet Gynecol. 2005;106:19–22.
184. Amir LH, Garland SM, Dennerstein L, et al. *Candida albicans*: is it associated with nipple pain in lactating women? Gynecol Obstet Invest. 1996;41:30–4.
185. Brent NB. Thrush in the breastfeeding dyad: results of a survey on diagnosis and treatment. Clin Pediatr (Phila). 2001;40:503–6.

186. The Royal Women's Hospital. Clinical guideline, breast and nipple thrush. c2013 [cited 2016 May 16]. Available from: https://www.thewomens.org.au/health-professionals/clinical-resources/clinical-guidelines-gps/.
187. Utter AR. Gentian violet treatment for thrush: can its use cause breastfeeding problems. J Hum Lact. 1990;6:178–80.
188. Huggins KE, Billon SF. Twenty cases of persistent sore nipples: collaboration between lactation consultant and dermatologist. J Hum Lact. 1993;9:155–60.
189. Amir LH. Eczema of the nipple and breast: a case report. J Hum Lact. 1993;9:173–5.
190. Whitaker-Worth DL, Carlone V, Susser WS, et al. Dermatologic diseases of the breast and nipple. J Am Acad Dermatol. 2000;43:733–51.
191. Webster DJT. Disorders of the nipple and areola. In: Hughes LE, Mansel RE, Webster DJT, editors. Benign disorders and diseases of the breast. Concepts and clinical management. London: WB Saunders; 2000. p. 199–208.
192. Lawlor-Smith L, Lawlor-Smith C. Raynaud's phenomenon of the nipple: a preventable cause of breastfeeding failure? Med J Aust. 1996;166:448.
193. Anderson JE, Held N, Wright K. Raynaud's phenomenon of the nipple: a treatable cause of painful breastfeeding. Pediatrics. 2004;113:e360–4.
194. Garrison CP. Nipple vasospasms, Raynaud's syndrome, and nifedipine. J Hum Lact. 2002;18:382–5.
195. Riordan J, Auerbach KG. Breastfeeding and human lactation, 2nd edn. Boston: Jones and Bartlett; 1999.
196. Jelliffe DB, Jelliffe EFP. Non-puerperal induced lactation (Letter). Pediatrics. 1972;50:170–1.
197. Auerbach KG, Avery JL. Inducted lactation: a study of adoptive nursing by 240 women. Am J Dis Child. 1981;135:340–3.
198. Walker M, Auerbach KG. Breast pumps and other technologies. In: Riordan J, Auerbach KG, editors. Breastfeeding and human lactation. Boston: Jones and Bartlett; 1999. p. 279–332.
199. Goldfarb L. Induced lactation and the Newman-Goldfarb protocols for induced lactation [Internet]. c2002–2015 [cited 2016 May 16]. Available from: http://www.asklenore.info/breastfeeding/induced_lactation/gn_protocols.shtml.
200. Newman J, Goldfarb L. Newman-Goldfarb protocols for induced lactation: decision tool (Poster). Perth, Australia: International Society for Research in Human Milk and Lactation; 2008.
201. Jiménez-Jiménez JR, García-Ruiz PJ, Molina JA. Drug-induced movement disorders. Drug Saf. 1997;16:180–204.
202. Phillips V. Relactation in mothers of children over 12 months. J Trop Pediatr. 1993;39:45–8.
203. Hale TW, Kristensen JH, Ilett KF. The transfer of medications into human milk. In: Hale TW, Hartmann P, editors. Textbook of human lactation. Amarillo, TX: Hale, L.P.; 2007. p. 465–77.
204. Spencer JP, Gonzalez LSI, Barnhart DJ. Medications in the breast-feeding mother. Am Fam Physician. 2001;64:119–26.
205. American Academy of Pediatrics Committee on Drugs. Transfer of drugs and other chemicals into human milk. Pediatrics. 2001;108:776–89.
206. Amir LH, Pirotta MV, Raval M. Breastfeeding—evidence based guidelines for the use of medicines. Aust Fam Physician. 2011;40:684–90.

Evaluation of a Breast Mass

6

Alastair M. Thompson and Andrew Evans

6.1 Introduction

Breast lumps are common in women of all ages and may present clinically through a range of routes including the following:

- A symptomatic breast lump detected by the patient or her partner;
- A breast mass detected on incidental examination by a clinical practitioner;
- Breast screening.

A breast mass in a man, gynaecomastia, is secondary to systemic disturbance or medication or, rarely, male breast cancer [1].

The breast is an adapted sweat gland. In the adult female, the breast responds to cyclical changes under the influence of oestrogen, progesterone and other hormones; thus, the breast changes over a woman's lifetime and on a monthly basis during the reproductive years. The internal architecture of the breast comprises glandular, stromal (collagen, fibroblasts and infiltrating myeloid cells) and adipose tissues based on the anterior chest wall. The arterial blood supply is from the axillary vessels, the internal mammary artery and intercostal perforating vessels with lymphatic drainage predominantly to the axillary lymph nodes.

The diagnosis of a breast mass should be termed ***triple assessment***, namely clinical (history and examination), imaging (usually mammography and/or ultrasound) and histopathological diagnosis (core biopsy or vacuum biopsy). Applying the use of triple assessment aims to minimise the impact of any one modality of diagnosis being less than 100 % sensitive and 100 % specific to diagnose or exclude breast cancer; combining the three modalities means that only 1 in 500 cancers may be initially missed.

This chapter focuses on the evaluation of a breast mass in women from the perspective that a woman with a breast lump will usually consider the lump to be a cancer until proven otherwise. In well-organised health care settings, full assessment and confident diagnosis can be achieved as a single "one-stop" service. The approach presented therefore aims to establish or exclude the presence of breast cancer and thereafter define the nature of a breast mass and treat, if required, any benign lesion identified. This model of assessment of a breast mass requires multidisciplinary input from breast clinicians, radiologists, pathologists and technical/administrative staff working as a team.

6.2 Routes of Presentation

6.2.1 Symptomatic breast mass

Most commonly, a female patient or her partner has found a new lump in one or both breasts. Due to the high level of publicity about breast lumps, the patient will often be concerned that she has breast cancer and therefore seeks rapid review: in some healthcare settings, this will be to a qualified doctor and in others an appropriately trained clinical specialist. However, whatever the route of self-presentation, timely review in order to minimise the duration of anxiety is desirable. In some countries, there are official targets which stipulate that women should visit a specialist breast clinic, for example within two weeks of presenting to a healthcare professional. The efficacy of this approach is unproven and indeed may skew the service provision. Similarly, encouraging regular breast self-examination may not improve early detection of breast cancers but continues to be promoted in much of the Western media. Instead, many organisations promote breast awareness among women with the hope that

A.M. Thompson (✉)
Department of Breast Surgical Oncology, University of Texas MD Anderson Cancer Center, Houston, TX 77030, USA
e-mail: athompson1@mdanderson.org

A. Evans
Division of Imaging and Technology, University of Dundee, Dundee, Scotland DD1 9SY, UK
e-mail: a.z.evans@dundee.ac.uk

I. Jatoi and A. Rody (eds.), *Management of Breast Diseases*, DOI 10.1007/978-3-319-46356-8_6

breast cancer will be detected as a change in the appearance, feel or perception of the breast at an early stage.

6.2.2 Screening

Building on three decades of experience in the Europe and in North America, a number of countries currently have screening programmes for breast cancer, usually in the form of mammographic screening. National screening programmes may be based on balancing efficacy and financial considerations. In general, imaging comprises digital two-view mammography every 1–2 years, with the target group for national breast screening programmes starting for women aged 40–50 and continuing to the age of 70–74 years or more. However, for mammographic screening, there remains debate around the risks versus the benefits. The benefits are a reduction in breast cancer mortality of at least 20 % for women invited and at least 30 % for women who attend regularly. This has to be balanced against the harms of the over diagnosis and over treatment of indolent ductal lesions unlikely to impact on the patient's lifespan [2].

In young women with a family history putting them at high risk or known gene carriers, magnetic resonance imaging (MRI) is increasingly being used and now has an evidence base for detecting breast cancers at an early stage. However, there is no good evidence of mortality reduction, especially in BRCA1 mutations carriers who have aggressive triple negative cancers where early diagnosis may not impact on mortality.

6.2.3 Incidental Detection of the Breast Mass on Clinical Examination

This is more frequently a route of presentation in the older women. Thus, it may be considered good practice that women over the age of 50 undergoing general physical examination should have a routine breast examination as part of an annual healthcare assessment. Certainly, on admission to hospital, all women should undergo clinical breast examination, as this may detect an incidental breast cancer and potentially the cause of symptoms elsewhere in the body.

6.3 History of Presentation

The single best predictor of the probable underlying pathology of a breast mass or breast lump is the age of the patient (Table 6.1). Benign causes of a breast mass are most common at a young age, and breast cancer is increasingly common with age, particularly over the age of 65 years.

The presenting features of a lump (Table 6.2), as noted by the woman or her medical examiner, should include a number of key features which may give some hints as to the underlying pathology. These include whether the lump is single or multiple, any changes in the lump since first noticed (for example with the menses) and any history of trauma/bruising.

While associated features should be sought (Table 6.3), if present, they often reflect a larger and or more advanced breast cancer. Bleeding from the nipple (Fig. 6.1), skin tethering of the cancer on the ligaments of Cooper, reflected by indrawing of the nipple (Fig. 6.2), eczema of the nipple or areolar (which may be eczema or intraepithelial malignancy—Paget's disease of the nipple) (Fig. 6.2), changes in the skin (erythema, peau d'orange—the appearance of the breast skin like that of an orange due to skin oedema). Skin nodules (Fig. 6.3) and enlarged axillary lymph nodes (Fig. 6.3) may be less common in an era of breast screening, but it is important that these features are sought to guide the clinical diagnosis, stage and future therapy.

Other relevant findings include an endocrine history, including hormone replacement therapy or contraceptive usage, gynaecological history, family history and other medical/surgical history. The relevant features of the patient's history may be best recorded using a set proforma in the clinic (for example Fig. 6.4) where the key features of the patient's present history and past medical history can be readily reviewed.

Table 6.1 Patient age and likely diagnosis of a breast mass

Age (Years)	Features	Diagnosis	Management
15–70	Poorly defined lumpiness; may change with menses (often bilateral)	Benign changes "fibrocystic"	Reassurance
15–30	Smooth mobile lump: usually single	Fibroadenoma	Excision if patient requests
35–55	Well-circumscribed lump(s) usually multiple, may be bilateral	Cyst(s)	Aspiration if symptomatic
20–55	Painful, red, hot lump	Abscess	Drainage/antibiotics
40–90	Ill-defined craggy lump	Cancer	Dependent on staging

Table 6.2 Presenting features of a breast lump—questions to ask

One lump or more than one lump? Where is the lump? How big is the lump? Is it sore/tender/painful? Is the lump hard or soft?
Does the lump change with the menses?
Are there any other features of the lump: Skin changes Nipple indrawing Nipple discharge—one or multiple ducts; – Axilla colour of discharge – Axilla blood-stained or not Is it mobile in the breast? Is the lump fixed to the skin or chest wall?
Are there problems in the other breast? Have you had a breast lump before? Are there lumps elsewhere in the body?

Table 6.3 Associated features of a breast lump

Skin changes: erythema Peau d'orange Skin tethering/puckering Eczematous appearance Ulceration
Nipple discharge Nipple retraction/flattening Pain (on palpation, all the time) Palpable axillary lymph nodes—axilla – Infraclavicular – Supraclavicular – Cervical

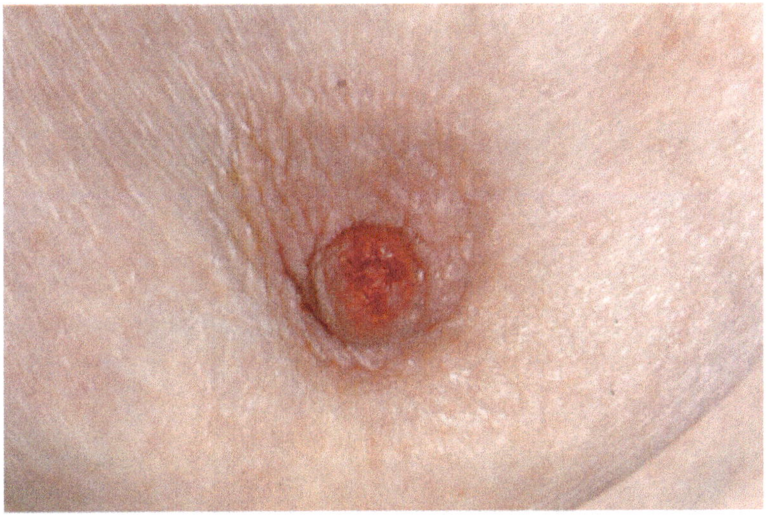

Fig. 6.1 Bleeding nipple discharge. The discharge should be examined for the number of ducts from which it emanates, and the discharge assessed for cytology or the presence of blood as appropriate

6.4 Clinical Examination

Clinical examination should aim to discern how many lumps there are, the nature of the mass and any associated features (Table 6.3). It is important for the practitioner to seek permission from the woman to conduct a bilateral breast examination and, particularly for male practitioners, to have a female chaperone available. Breast examination is considered by some authorities to be an intimate physical examination, and each woman should be accorded due

Fig. 6.2 Nipple retraction due to cancer with areolar Paget's disease; note the small core needle biopsy scar to the right of the areolar

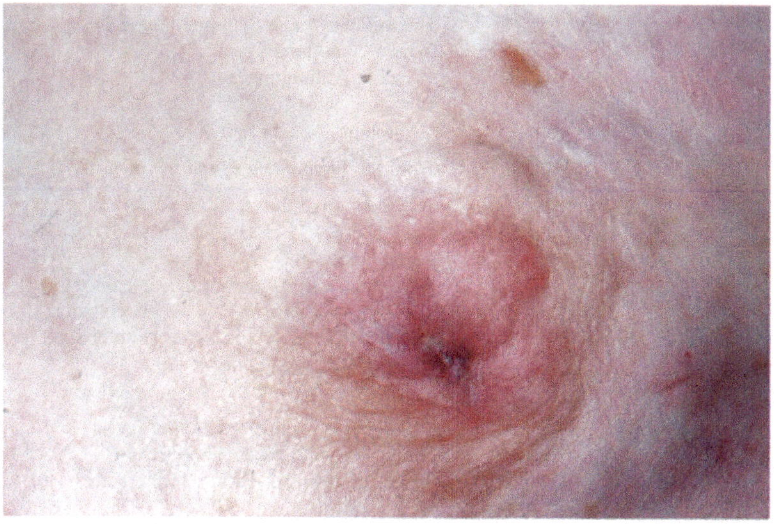

respect. The manner in which the breast examination is conducted is important in optimising the detection of abnormalities in the breast [3].

The patient should be naked to the waist in a warm, private, room. Breast examination should be conducted in a logical and sequential fashion so that both the patient and the practitioner are comfortable and any abnormalities will be detected. Care must be taken to examine each breast in succession, noting differences in symmetry between the two. Usually, the normal breast is best examined first as the appearance and texture of each individual woman's breast can be quite different from other women but is quite likely to be similar to the contra-lateral side. Initial inspection to look for skin dimpling or changes in the shape of the breast may detect benign lesions such as a fibroadenoma, a cyst or a breast cancer. If no immediately apparent abnormality is detected, it may be appropriate to ask the woman to point to the mass she feels.

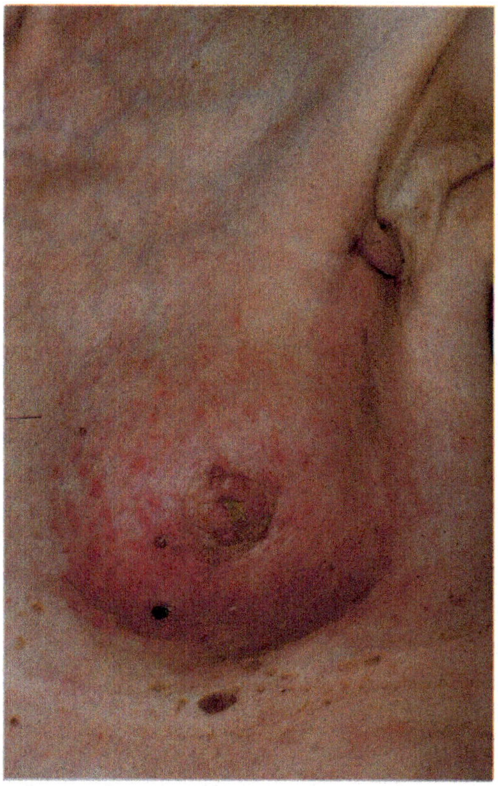

Fig. 6.3 Skin nodules from advanced breast cancer overlying a breast mass; a nodal mass is also visible in the axilla

Initial inspection may be with the patient sitting in an upright position hands by her sides (Fig. 6.5). By asking her to raise her hands, clinical abnormalities such as indrawing of skin tethered to a cancer or nipple indrawing may be accentuated (Fig. 6.6). Next, asking the woman to place her hands on her hips and press in (contracting the pectoralis muscles) may accentuate a deeply tethered cancer and hence draw the eye to a tumour.

While obvious abnormalities (Figs. 6.2, 6.3 and 6.5) merit further inspection and palpation with the patient in the upright position, more detailed palpation may be best carried out with the patient lying flat, with one pillow for comfort, on an examination couch. The patient should be asked to raise her arm behind her head to fix the breast in a relatively static position. By palpation using a gentle rotating movement with the flat of the fingers even small lumps may be detected, using varying degrees of pressure to detect lumps that are lying at different depths in the breast tissue [4]. Using the flattened fingers of one hand and a gentle rotating movement, the whole breast on the normal side (including the retroareolar tissues) may be palpated before moving to the side with a clinical abnormality. Care should be taken to record the position, shape and calliper measurement of the size of the lesion(s) together with any other features (tender,

BREAST CLINIC INITIAL INVESTIGATION FORM
Page 1 of 4

NHS Tayside

PERSONAL DETAILS

Name & Address

CHI

Referring Hospital:
Ninewells ☐ PRI ☐ Well Woman ☐ Screening ☐
Consultant .... Seen by ....
Referring GP/Clinician ....
Screening Patient: YES/NO Date of Referral .... / .... / ....
Date of Last Breast Screen .... / .... / .... Date of Clinic .... / .... / ....

COMPLAINTS

	RIGHT	LEFT	OTHER
Duration:			
Cyclical:			
Other Features:			

PREVIOUS DISEASE

Previous Breast Disease? YES / NO
Diagnosis ....
Previous Breast Clinic Patient: YES / NO Date .... / .... / ....

Previous Open Breast Surgery	Previous Breast Aspiration
NO ☐	NO ☐
RIGHT ☐	RIGHT ☐
LEFT ☐	LEFT ☐
BOTH ☐	BOTH ☐
MULTIPLE ☐	MULTIPLE ☐

PAST MEDICAL HISTORY

Other Cancer YES / NO Site: ....
Illnesses YES / NO What: ....
....
Current Medications YES / NO
What: ....
....
Drug Allergies YES / NO What ....
Smoker / Ex Smoker YES / NO

FAMILY HISTORY

Family History of Breast Cancer YES / NO

If YES,	Age at onset		Age at onset
MOTHER	☐	MATERNAL AUNT	☐
SISTER 1	☐	MATERNAL GRAN	☐
SISTER 2	☐	PATERNAL AUNT	☐
OTHER ✚	☐	PATERNAL GRAN	☐

✚ Specify
....

MENSTRUAL HISTORY

Menopausal Status:		Pregnant	☐
Pre-Menopausal*	☐	Oral Contraceptive Pill	☐
Post-Menopausal*	☐		
Peri-Menopausal*	☐	Hormone Replacement Therapy	☐

SURGERY

Hysterectomy YES / NO Why ....
Bilateral Oopherectomy YES / NO
Unilateral Oopherectomy YES / NO
Other Operations YES / NO What ....
....

*for definitions, see page 4

Fig. 6.4 Proforma for recording the relevant clinical history used in everyday practice. Note the CHI (Community Health Index) is the unique patient identifier from which the patient's age can be deduced

red, single or multiple). Clinical examination has a 54 % sensitivity to detect (rule out) breast cancer and a 94 % specificity to rule in breast cancer [4].

In patients with a history of nipple discharge, the patient may be asked to elicit the discharge by pressing on the nipple or areolar, thus avoiding the practitioner hurting the

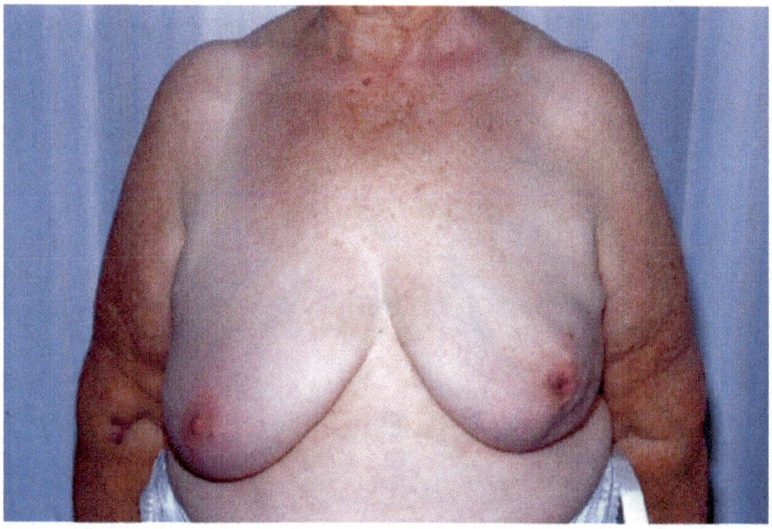

Fig. 6.5 Left breast cancer: nipple retraction and skin tethering

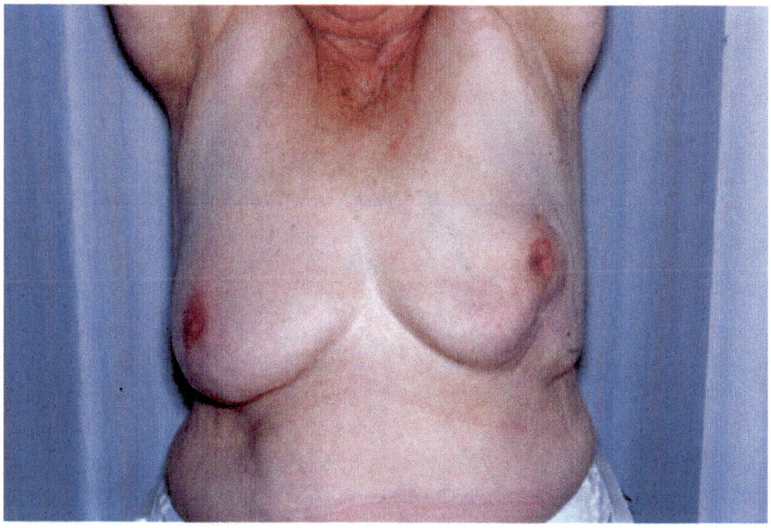

Fig. 6.6 Left breast cancer: skin effects seen in Fig. 6.5 are more prominent as the arms are raised

patient. The number of ducts producing a discharge (single or multiple?), the colour of the discharge (is it milky?, is it obviously blood-stained? Figure 6.1) and testing for blood using urinary dip sticks can be noted.

Following breast examination, bilateral axillary examination should be performed on each side in turn. This may be most readily accomplished by asking the patient to sit up, and for the examination of the right axilla, the practitioner takes the patient's right forearm, supporting the weight of the forearm to relax the axilla. Using the fingers of the practitioner's left hand, the walls of the axilla and the apex of the axilla can be gently palpated, and any lumps and their consistency are noted. Thereafter, a similar arrangement can be used for the left axilla (the practitioner taking the patients' left forearm in his or her left hand and examining the axilla with the fingers of the right hand). Thereafter, the infraclavicular, supraclavicular and cervical lymph nodes should be examined for lymphadenopathy often most comfortably performed (for both patient and clinician) and any findings recorded on the clinical examination sheet (Fig. 6.7).

6.5 Investigation

Investigation of a breast mass is conducted and recorded (Fig. 6.7) following clinical history and examination using imaging before core biopsy or vacuum biopsy as these latter interventions may cause bruising which, in turn, makes it more difficult to interpret the clinical and imaging appearances. For example, post-biopsy discomfort, haematoma and skin oedema can suggest an inflammatory breast cancer but may be due to post-biopsy changes.

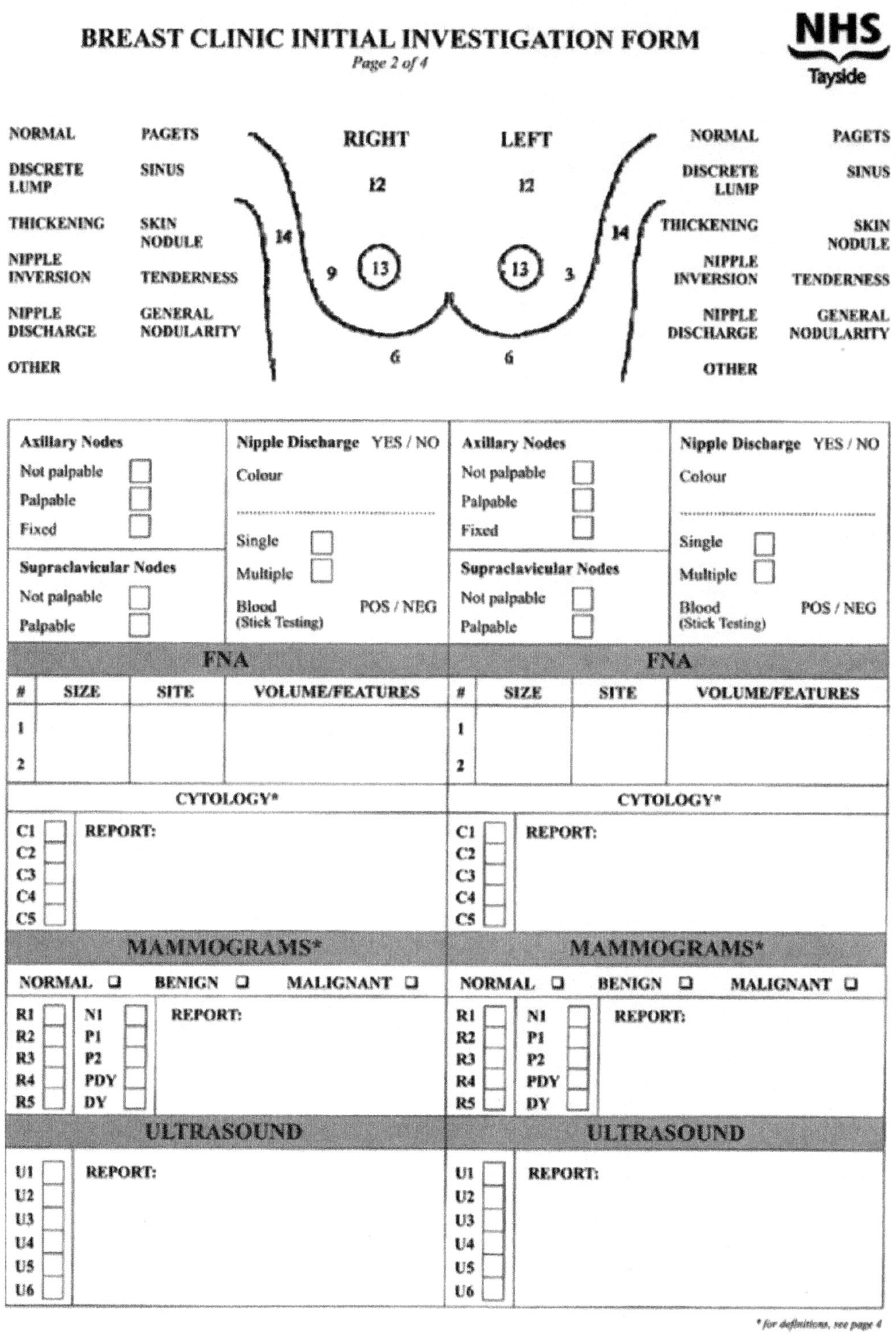

BREAST CLINIC INITIAL INVESTIGATION FORM
Page 2 of 4

NHS Tayside

RIGHT		LEFT	
NORMAL	PAGETS	NORMAL	PAGETS
DISCRETE LUMP	SINUS	DISCRETE LUMP	SINUS
THICKENING	SKIN NODULE	THICKENING	SKIN NODULE
NIPPLE INVERSION	TENDERNESS	NIPPLE INVERSION	TENDERNESS
NIPPLE DISCHARGE	GENERAL NODULARITY	NIPPLE DISCHARGE	GENERAL NODULARITY
OTHER		OTHER	

Axillary Nodes Not palpable ☐ Palpable ☐ Fixed ☐	**Nipple Discharge** YES / NO Colour .... Single ☐ Multiple ☐ Blood (Stick Testing) POS / NEG	**Axillary Nodes** Not palpable ☐ Palpable ☐ Fixed ☐	**Nipple Discharge** YES / NO Colour .... Single ☐ Multiple ☐ Blood (Stick Testing) POS / NEG
Supraclavicular Nodes Not palpable ☐ Palpable ☐		**Supraclavicular Nodes** Not palpable ☐ Palpable ☐	

FNA (Right) / **FNA** (Left)

#	SIZE	SITE	VOLUME/FEATURES	#	SIZE	SITE	VOLUME/FEATURES
1				1			
2				2			

CYTOLOGY*		CYTOLOGY*	
C1 ☐ C2 ☐ C3 ☐ C4 ☐ C5 ☐	REPORT:	C1 ☐ C2 ☐ C3 ☐ C4 ☐ C5 ☐	REPORT:

MAMMOGRAMS* / **MAMMOGRAMS***

NORMAL ☐ BENIGN ☐ MALIGNANT ☐			NORMAL ☐ BENIGN ☐ MALIGNANT ☐		
R1 ☐ R2 ☐ R3 ☐ R4 ☐ R5 ☐	N1 ☐ P1 ☐ P2 ☐ PDY ☐ DY ☐	REPORT:	R1 ☐ R2 ☐ R3 ☐ R4 ☐ R5 ☐	N1 ☐ P1 ☐ P2 ☐ PDY ☐ DY ☐	REPORT:

ULTRASOUND / **ULTRASOUND**

U1 ☐ U2 ☐ U3 ☐ U4 ☐ U5 ☐ U6 ☐	REPORT:	U1 ☐ U2 ☐ U3 ☐ U4 ☐ U5 ☐ U6 ☐	REPORT:

** for definitions, see page 4*

Fig. 6.7 Proforma for recording the relevant examination findings and investigations (continuation of the proforma shown in Fig. 6.4)

6.6 Imaging

Standard initial imaging is to use bilateral two-view digital mammography (craniocaudal (Fig. 6.8) and medio-lateral oblique (Fig. 6.9) views), with additional coned or magnified views (Fig. 6.10) of abnormalities as appropriate, for women aged 35 years and older and ultrasound as the primary imaging modality for women younger than 35 years. This somewhat arbitrary cut-off (some health care systems use 40 years) is based on the higher breast density

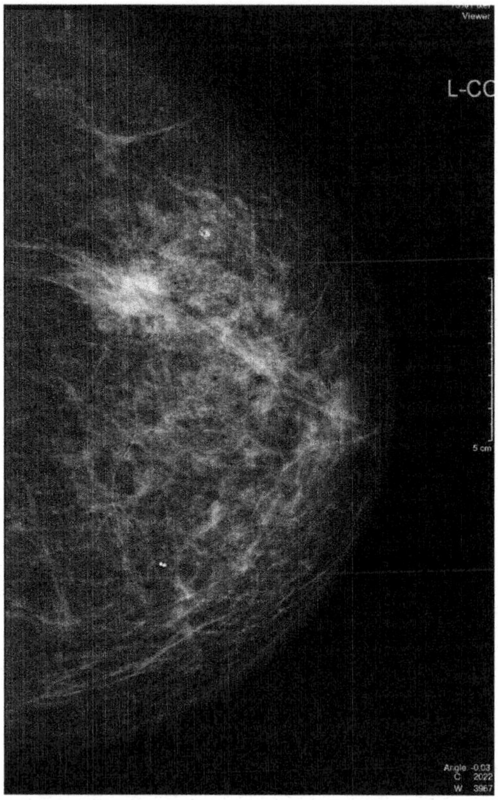

Fig. 6.8 Craniocaudal mammograms showing a left breast cancer as a stellate lesion which was clinically palpable. The horizontal guideline allows ready comparison between the two breasts

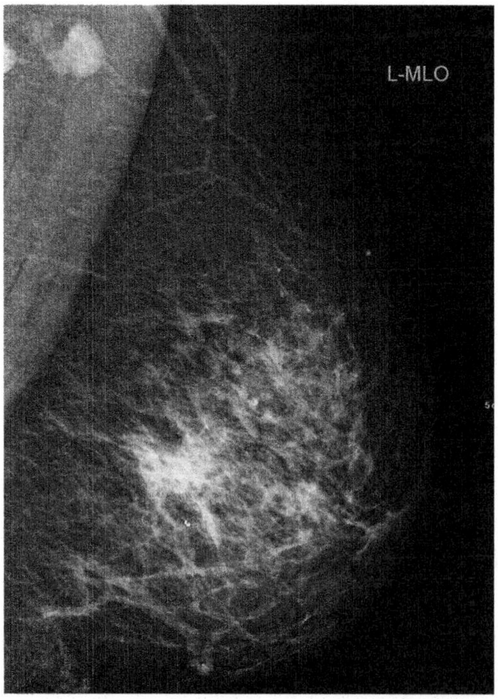

Fig. 6.9 Medio-lateral oblique views of the same patient as in Fig. 6.8

in younger women which may make it difficult to detect even quite a large cancer. With increasing age, the breast parenchyma is replaced by fatty tissue and breast cancer becomes easier to detect in the older breast. Premenopausal women should confirm they are not pregnant before undergoing mammography, although the likelihood to cause harm to a foetus is low. Ultrasound should always be used in addition to mammography in the older age group and, similarly, if ultrasound detects what appears to be a malignant lesion in a younger women, or clinical suspicion persists, then mammography should be performed. On average, ultrasound is more likely to definitively characterise a palpable mass than mammography. Mammography has the advantage of picking up associated DCIS in women with breast cancer. It is important that the clinician marks on the skin, the site of the palpable abnormality to enable the sonographer to be sure that that any ultrasound lesion spatially correlates with the palpable abnormality.

6.7 Breast Ultrasound

Ultrasound is performed using warmed gel to ensure contact and good transmission between the probe and the patient's breast and may accurately measure a breast mass in multiple dimensions. Ultrasound can identify whether a breast mass is cystic (Fig. 6.11) or solid (Fig. 6.12), may identify multiple pathologies (e.g. an intracystic cancer, Fig. 6.13) and can also be used to demonstrate blood flow (using Doppler) and stiffness (using elastography) in and around a breast mass (Fig. 6.14). The ultrasound appearances can be categorised for reporting (Table 6.4).

Ultrasound is particularly useful to delineate cysts (Fig. 6.11) and to subsequently direct and confirm drainage of a cyst. Ultrasound is also extremely useful to delineate a fibroadenoma (Fig. 6.15). The typical picture of a carcinoma with an irregular border and casting an acoustic shadow (Fig. 6.12) is usually quite different to a fibroadenoma (Fig. 6.15) and cysts (Fig. 6.11), and makes ultrasound particularly useful in the clinic to indicate the likely pathology of a lump. However, distinguishing between a carcinoma and a fibroadenoma usually requires needle sampling of such lesions.

Ultrasound is routinely used to examine the axilla and regional nodal basins in women with a suspicious breast mass (Fig. 6.16), and in combination with fine needle aspiration cytology or core biopsy (see below) can diagnose axillary metastases in up to 90 % of positive nodes and most patients with a high axillary disease burden [5]. Women with markedly abnormal nodes in their axilla should have the infraclavicular and supraclavicular nodes examined and biopsied if required.

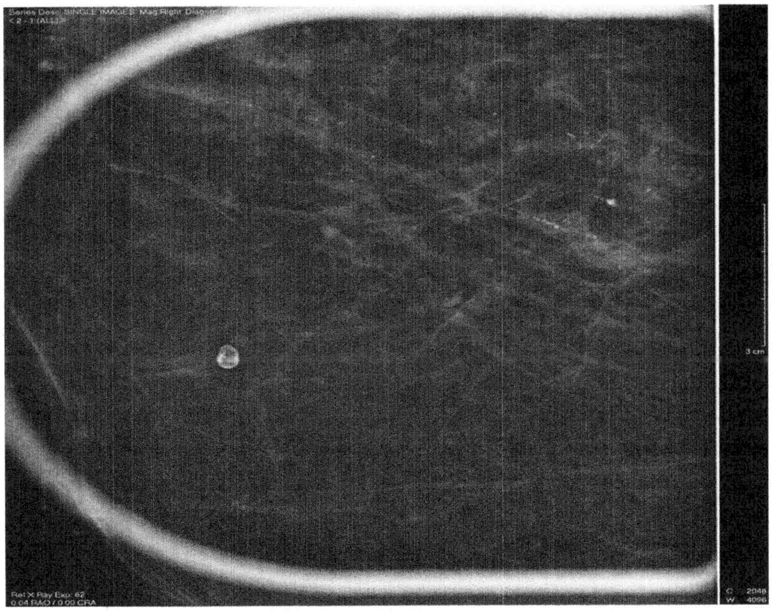

Fig. 6.10 Magnification views of a breast mass showing the fine microcalcifications associated with ductal carcinoma in situ; an additional coarse calcified area is non-malignant

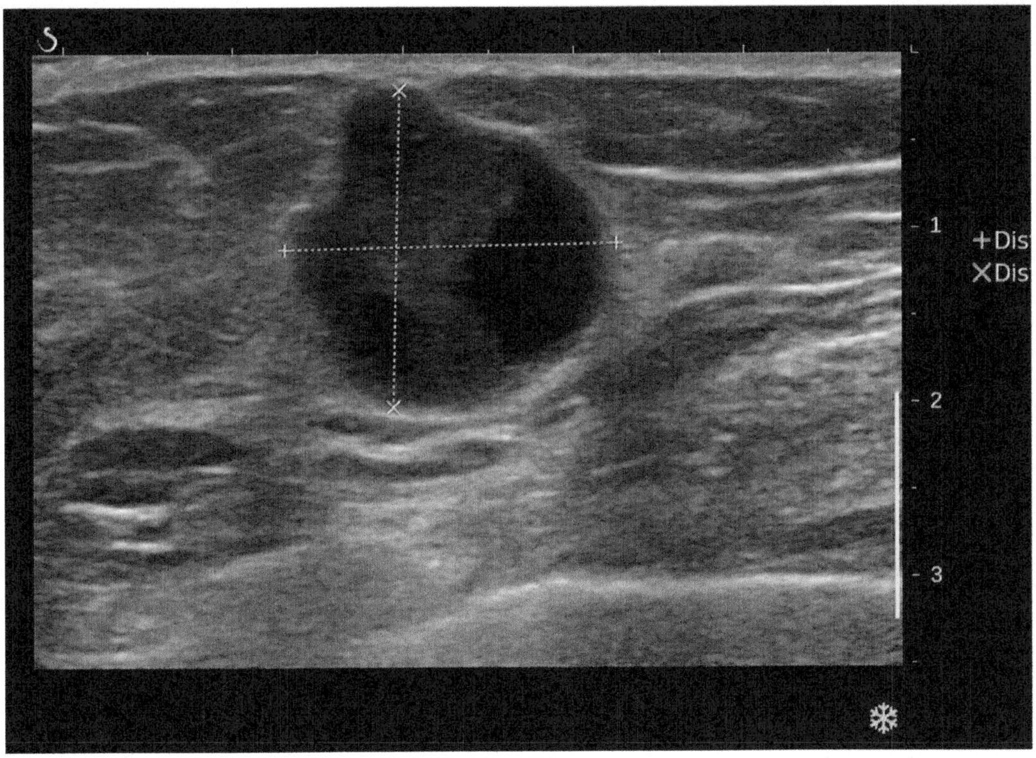

Fig. 6.11 Ultrasound of a breast cyst: note the smooth outline, fluid-filled lesion

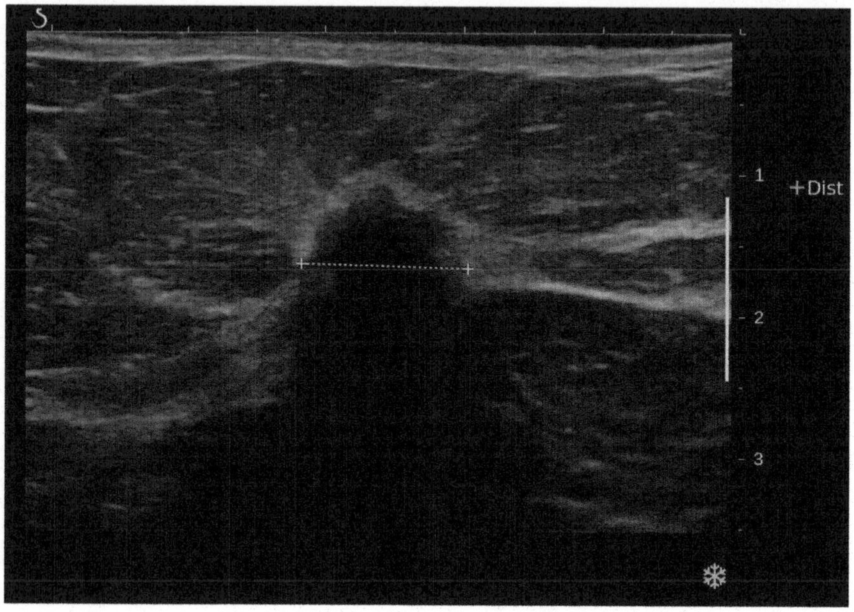

Fig. 6.12 Ultrasound of a breast cancer: note the irregular margin and dense acoustic shadow in contrast to Fig. 6.11 and Fig. 6.15

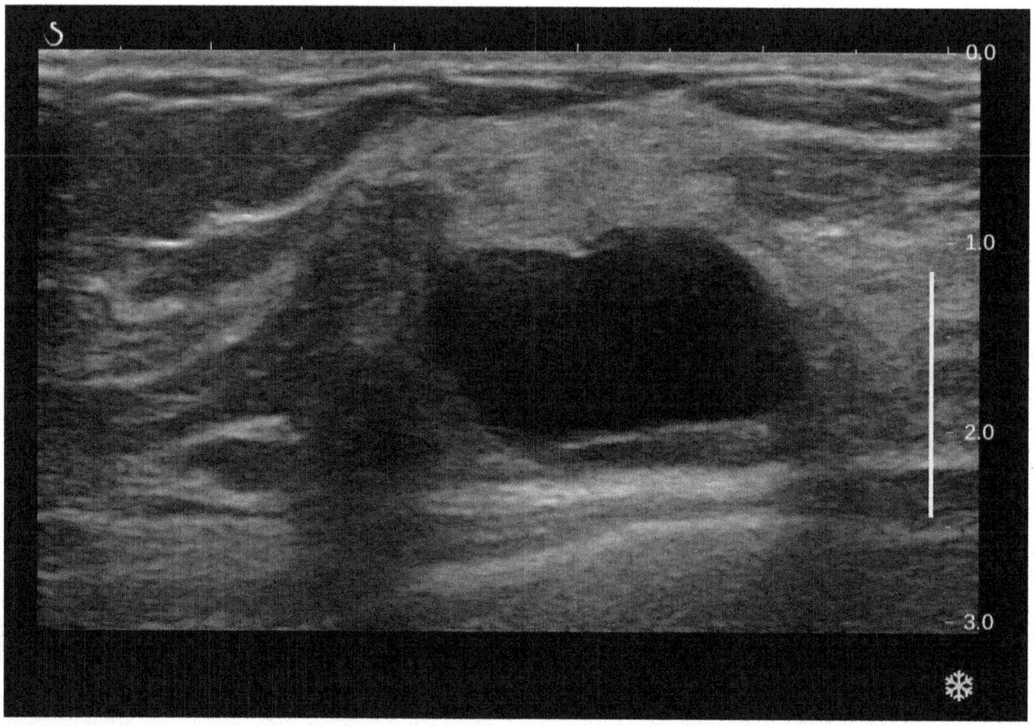

Fig. 6.13 Ultrasound of a breast cyst within which there is an intracystic tumour

6.8 Mammography

Mammography may suggest the nature of a breast mass as benign (e.g. breast cysts: smooth outlines with multiple masses visible; Fig. 6.17) or malignant (stellate mass with irregular outline; Figs. 6.8 and 6.9). Mammography is more sensitive with increasing age as the breast density declines and breast adipose tissue increases.

An abnormality on the mammograms is often visible on two-view mammography (Figs. 6.8 and 6.9), but finer

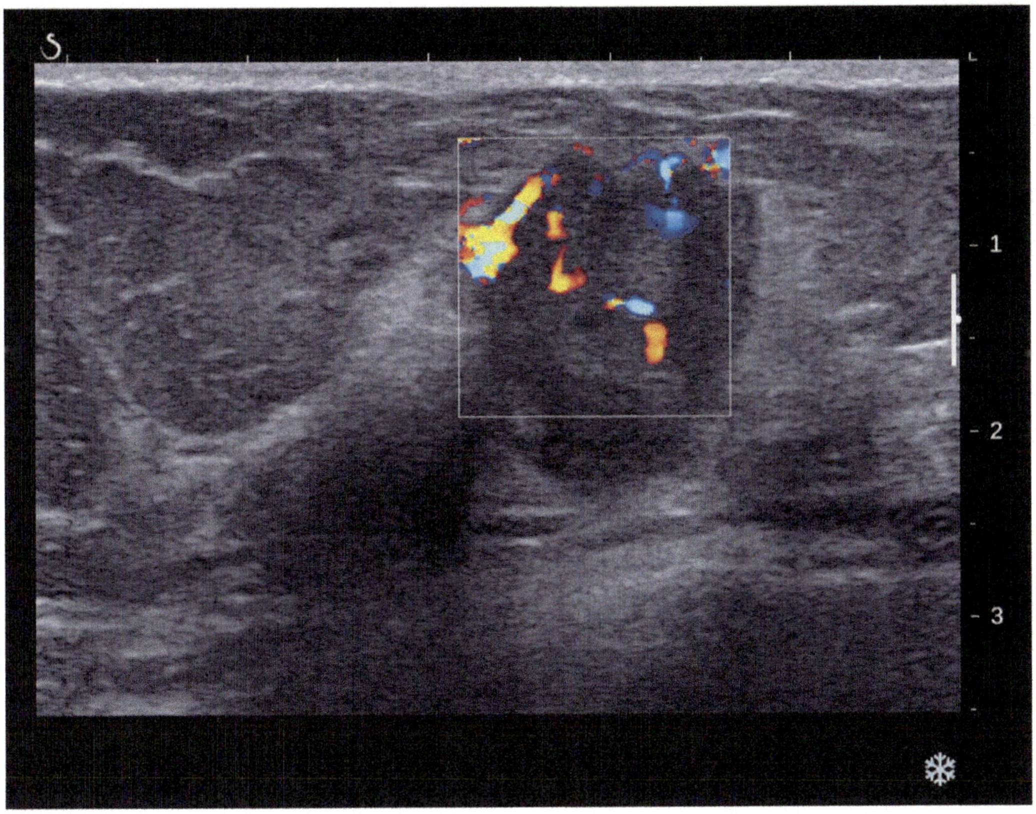

Fig. 6.14 Ultrasound of a breast cancer demonstrating the vascularity of the cancer

Table 6.4 Ultrasound classification for breast masses

Code	Description
U1	Normal diffuse benign
U2	Single cyst
U3	Solid benign
U4	Suspicious of malignancy
U5	Malignant
U6	Multiple cysts

details such as microcalcification may require magnification views (Fig. 6.10) and may or may not correspond to a palpable abnormality. While such fine details may indicate a benign or malignant (DCIS) (Fig. 6.10) pathology, further localisation and investigation will be required. Calcifications are best biopsied using a vacuum-assisted biopsy device. Whatever the findings, they can be annotated for future reference and reporting (Table 6.5). Digital breast tomosynthesis offers a computer-generated 3-D reconstruction of the breast and may have a particular role in detecting small low-grade spiculated cancers otherwise obscured on two-view mammography in a dense breast. The value of such detection with regard to breast cancer mortality is unknown.

Breast ultrasound and mammography are the mainstays of radiological evaluation of a breast mass and may be conducted at the time of clinical history and examination to allow progress to needle biopsy of a lesion as part of a one-stop diagnostic breast clinic.

6.9 Magnetic Resonance Imaging (MRI)

Magnetic resonance imaging (MRI) has been increasingly adopted [6] particularly to image the breast in the presence of silicone implants, screening women with a strong family history or genetic-tested high risk of breast cancer and monitoring women receiving neo-adjuvant chemotherapy.

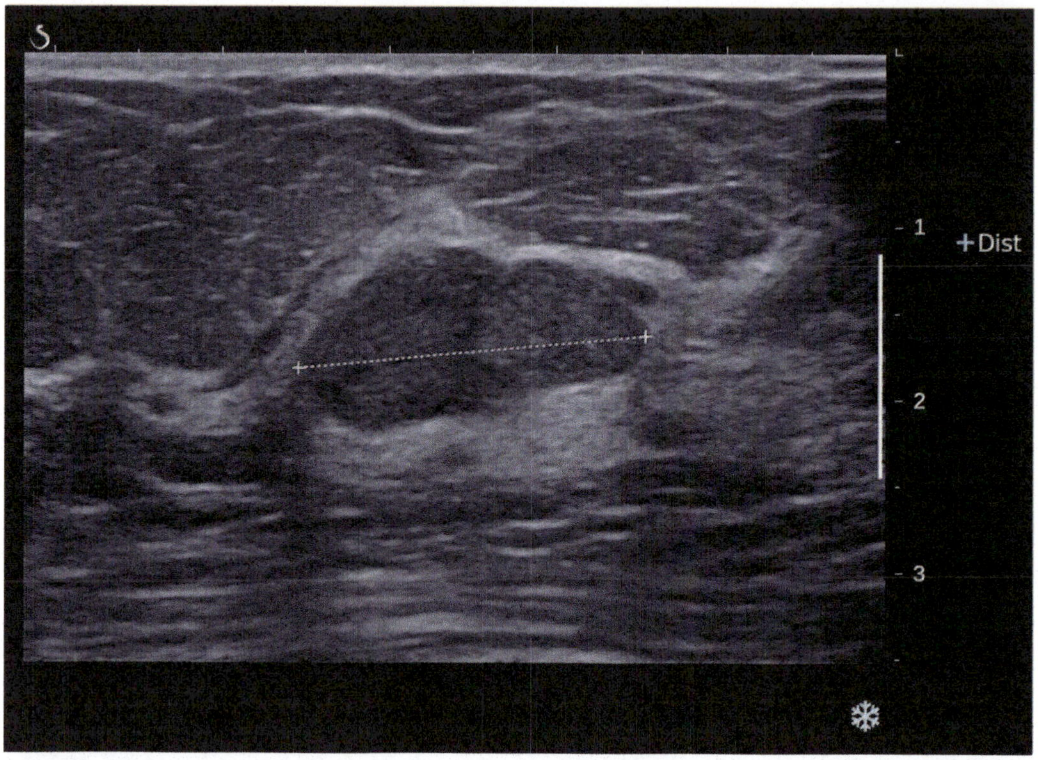

Fig. 6.15 Ultrasound of a fibroadenoma; note the ovoid appearance with the long axis parallel to the skin surface and the well-defined edges of the lesion. Contrast the appearances to those of Fig. 6.12

Fig. 6.16 Ultrasound of a malignant axillary lymph node

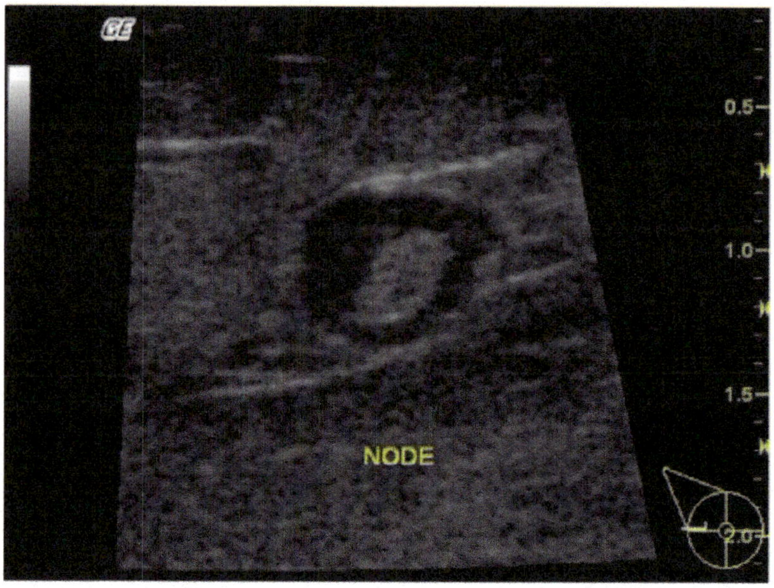

MRI can also be used to assess size and focality in women with breast cancer looking towards breast conservation particularly in women with a lobular cancer; MRI can also detect DCIS not visible on mammography (Figures 6.18, 6.19 and 6.20).

6.10 Other Imaging Techniques

Positron emission tomography combined with computerised tomography (PET/CT) or MRI (PET/MRI) may be performed as an investigation for breast cancer either to obtain

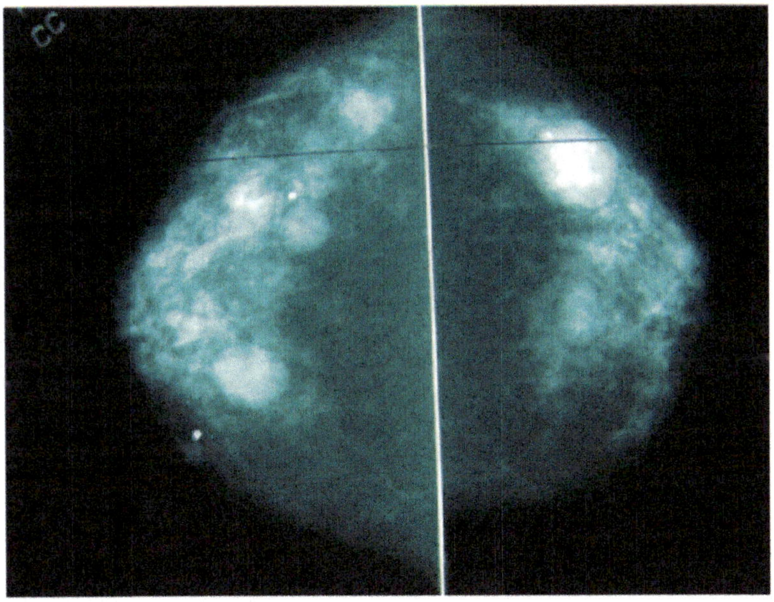

Fig. 6.17 Bilateral cysts on craniocaudal mammograms

Table 6.5 Mammographic appearances of the breast

Code	Description
R1	Normal
R2	Benign
R3	Indeterminate
R4	Probably malignant
R5	Malignant

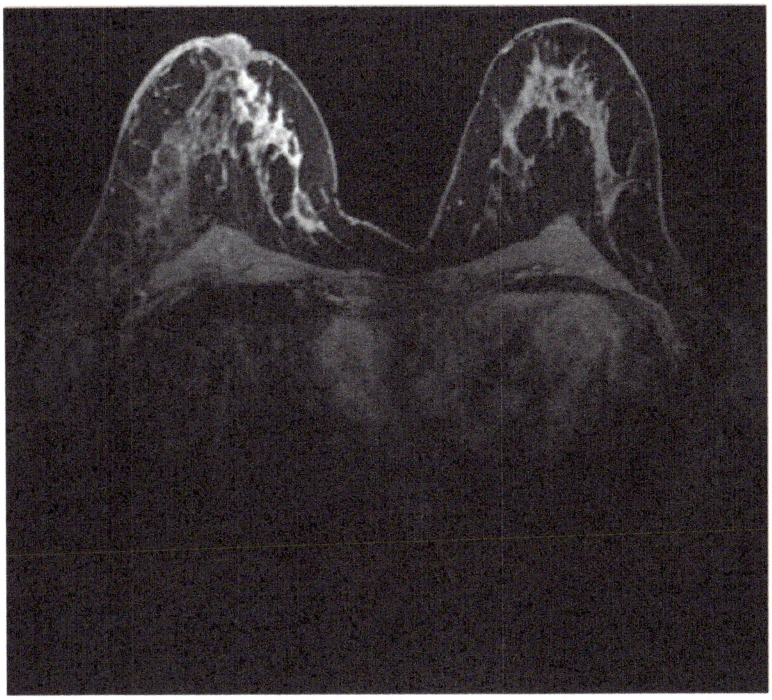

Fig. 6.18 MRI demonstrating mass secondary to DCIS (*left* half of figure)

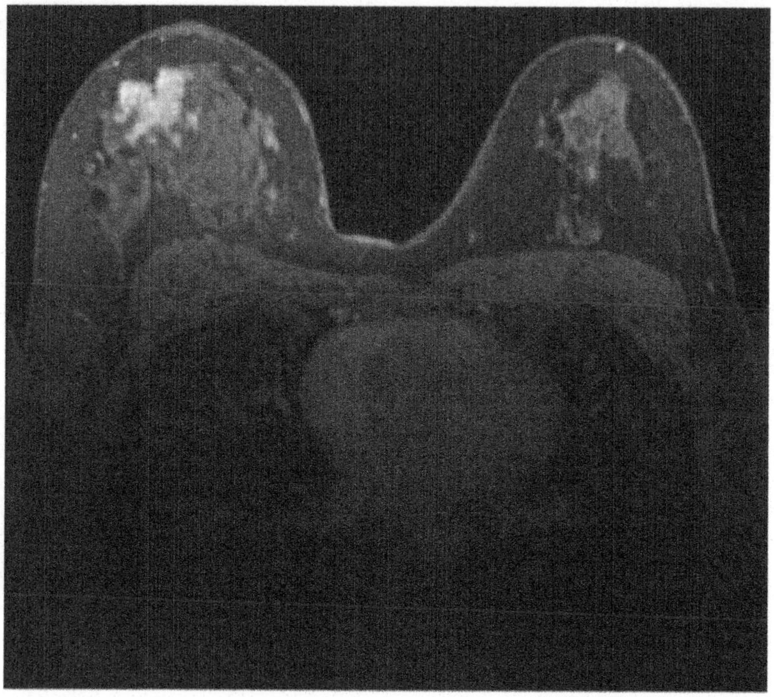

Fig. 6.19 MRI of invasive breast cancer (*left* half of figure)

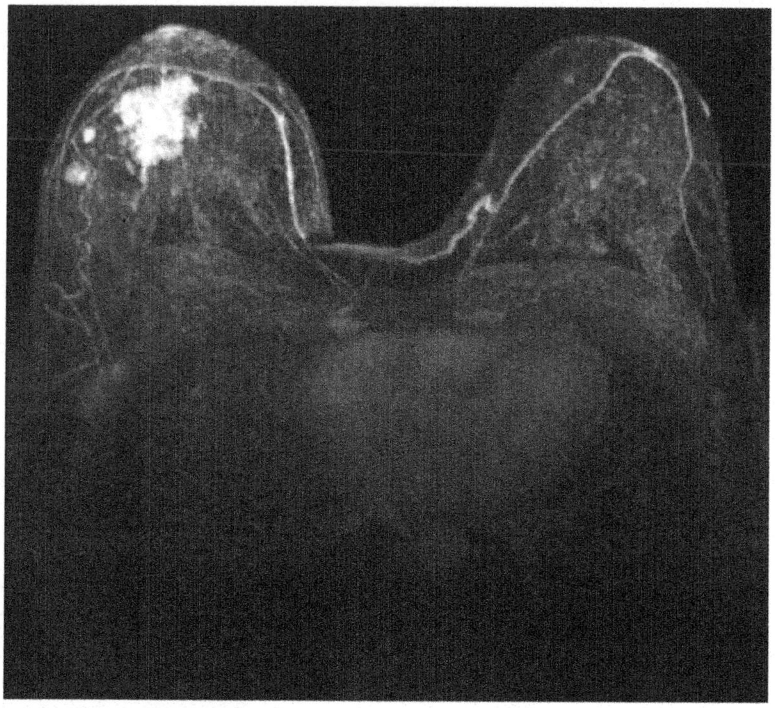

Fig. 6.20 Early enhancement of MRI of patient in Fig. 6.19 demonstrating multifocality

functional imaging as a baseline for subsequent therapy or as part of whole body imaging for metastatic disease. Although the radiation dosages (for PET) or access to such facilities at present may limit their use, PET may play a role in future in the evaluation of locally advanced breast cancer or in the evaluation of regional lymph nodes (including internal mammary and mediastinal nodes) for metastatic disease.

6.11 Pathology Diagnosis

The third component of triple assessment after clinical history/examination and imaging is histopathological diagnosis. Cytology is inferior to core biopsy in the diagnosis of breast lesions and should not be used. Until recently, it was used widely in the assessment of abnormal axillary nodes, but recent comparisons with core biopsy have confirmed the superiority of core biopsy in this clinical setting also [5].

While a palpable solid mass may be core biopsied "free hand," ultrasound guidance is preferable as accuracy is greater. Biopsy using a 14-gauge needle following infiltration with local anaesthetic should be used to confirm the diagnosis of a benign lesion such as a fibroadenoma (Fig. 6.21) in women over 25 years and thus prevents the need for excisional biopsy. Stereotactically guided core biopsies can take an extremely accurate core sample from lesions with radiological features such as microcalcification, and subsequent specimen X-rays can confirm that the microcalcification has been adequately sampled (Fig. 6.22). Core biopsy also has the virtue of demonstrating tissue architecture and thus distinguishing between DCIS and invasive breast cancer.

More recently, vacuum-assisted biopsies (VAB) taken under radiological guidance have the advantage of multiple relatively large cores of tissue from the same small area and may, under some circumstances, actually be able to excise a lesion completely. Eleven- or nine-gauge VAB is the method of choice for diagnosing microcalcification. Seven- or

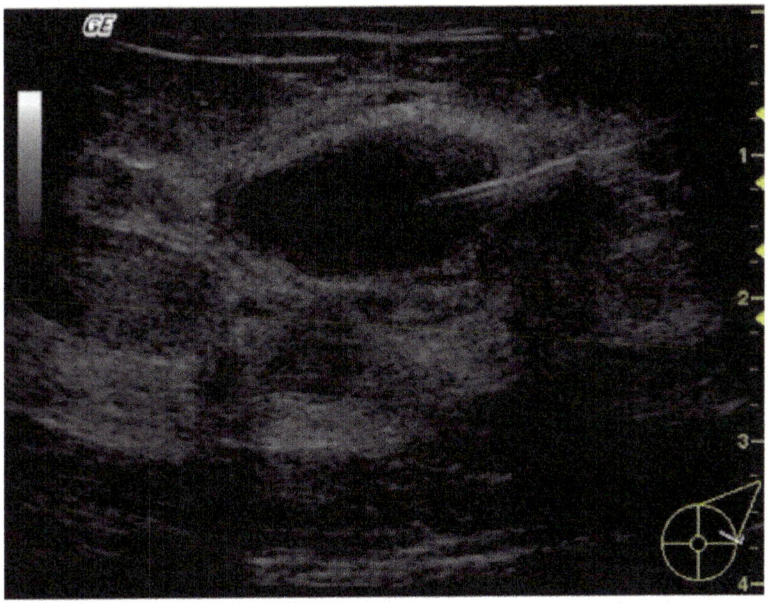

Fig. 6.21 Core needle inserted under ultrasound guidance into a fibroadenoma for histological confirmation of the diagnosis

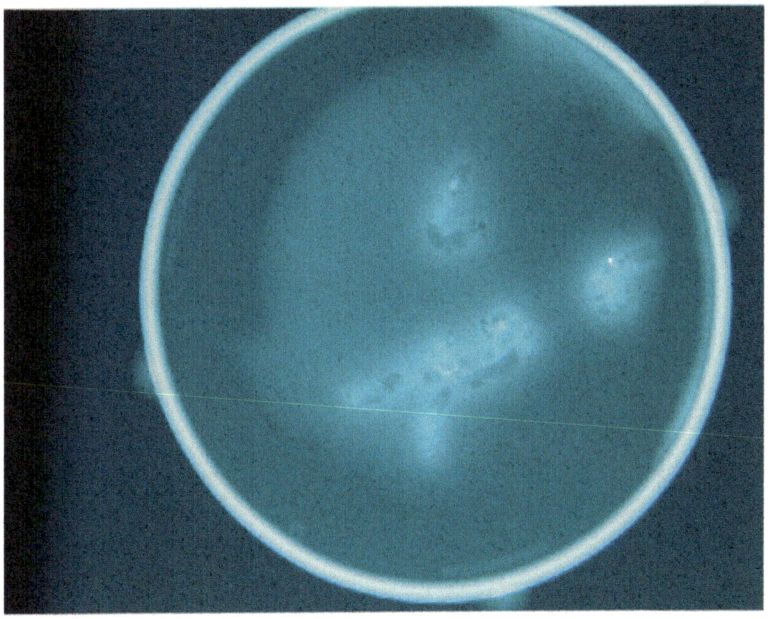

Fig. 6.22 X-ray image of cores from a core biopsy confirming the calcification present in the targeted mass is represented in the cores

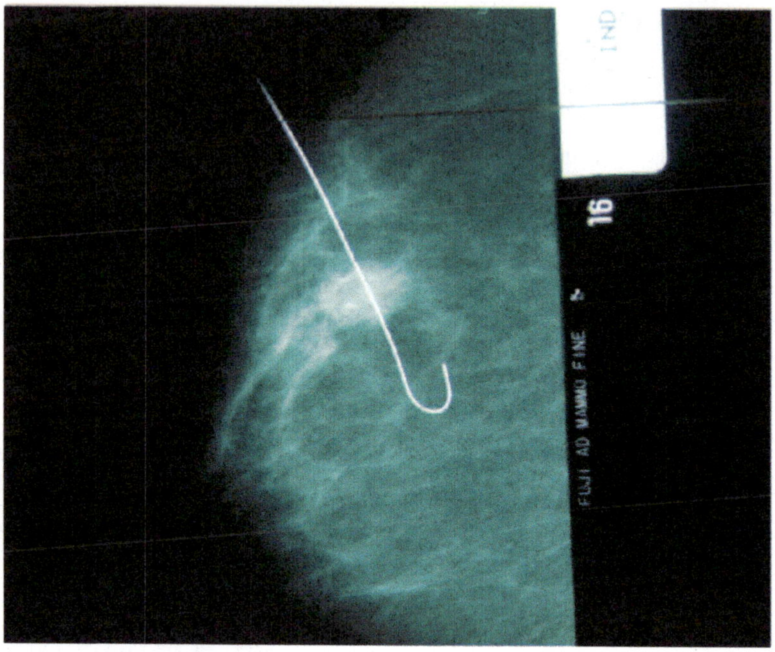

Fig. 6.23 Needle localisation of a breast mass to ensure the correct mass is excised at the time of surgery

nine-gauge VAB, usually under US control, should be used for the percutaneous excision of papillomas, radials scars and fibroadenomas if the patient requests removal. A marker clip is often deployed to allow localisation if malignant pathology is found.

Very rarely, it is impossible to establish a diagnosis even with repeated core biopsy or VAB. In such circumstances, a diagnostic excisional biopsy of the lump may be considered. This will require image-guided localisation, particularly on the background of a lumpy breast, to ensure that the correct breast mass is excised (Fig. 6.23) so that the diagnosis can be established. However, routine use of excisional (and often incomplete) surgical open biopsy of a palpable mass should no longer be standard practice.

6.12 Patient Plan

Following triple assessment, it is thereafter important to discuss with the patient whether any lump can be left alone, should be excised or whether—if a diagnosis of cancer has been made—staging tests should be performed prior to definitive treatment. These decisions should be formally recorded in the case record (Fig. 6.24).

6.13 Benign Breast Masses

The focus of this chapter on malignant breast masses reflects the concerns of patients to exclude cancer and that of clinicians not to miss diagnosis of cancer. However, benign

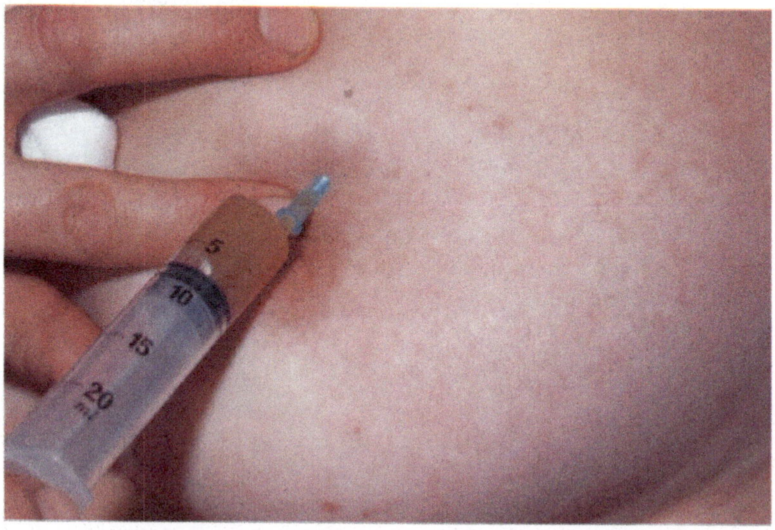

Fig. 6.24 Needle aspiration of a breast cyst yielding typical breast cyst fluid

breast changes and lumps are more common than breast cancer. Only approximately one in twenty women attending a symptomatic breast clinic will have a mass that turns out to be malignant, and the management of benign breast masses is thus an important component of clinical practice.

The same principles of triple assessment apply to all benign breast masses as apply to a lump which turns out to be malignant. The features of a benign breast lump can also be described in a similar fashion with associated features noted (Tables 6.1, 6.2 and 6.3). Following the diagnosis of a benign breast mass, if no further intervention is required, a written information booklet describing the benign findings in the breast may be helpful to reinforce verbal reassurance. Women should still be encouraged to seek re-evaluation if any new mass or breast symptom appears in future—it is not unknown for a woman to have sought and obtained appropriate reassurance for benign breast changes then at a later date to find a new mass which turns out to be malignant.

6.13.1 Benign Nodularity

Many women notice changes in their breasts on a monthly cycle, but may become worried if lumpiness or a breast mass persists beyond 2 menstrual cycles (6–8 weeks), particularly if associated with asymmetry between the two sides, even if there is some cyclical change. The history and clinical examination will often point to this variation in normal breast which is in accordance with the expected responses to endocrine fluctuations on a monthly basis in premenopausal women. Premenstrual discomfort or pain may also highlight the "normality" of this change. However, even with a low clinical concern on history and examination, imaging (ultrasound or mammography as first line, dependent on the age of the patient), if necessary, supplemented by core biopsy may be required for reassurance of the patient and clinician. This may be particularly useful if there is a family history of breast cancer or if the patient is anxious about the changes she has noted.

6.13.2 Changes Associated with Pregnancy and Lactation

The breasts undergo enormous physiological and morphological changes during the early stages of pregnancy (and indeed are one of the first symptoms a woman may note when pregnant) which develop as pregnancy continues and evolve during the post-partum period into the lactating breast. Benign lumpiness is a common feature of the breasts in pregnant women and when breast feeding. However, pathological changes can occur, and breast cancer, which may present as inflammatory breast cancer mimicking an abscess (see below) while rare, should be considered and new, focal breast lumps investigated by triple assessment (using ultrasound rather than mammography due to the pregnancy). Lactational cysts are not uncommon; aspiration should lead to resolution though may need to be repeated if the cyst refills.

6.13.3 Fibroadenoma

An aberration of normal development and involution (ANDI), this smooth, non-tender mobile lump may be single, lobulated or occasionally multiple. Ultrasound as part of triple assessment may identify a typical appearance (Fig. 6.15). Under the age of 25, typical ultrasound appearances may provide sufficient reassurance that some practices do not require needle sampling. In women over 25 years, core biopsy is the preferred diagnostic method and avoids the need for excision. Excision (by surgery or vacuum device) or cryoablation may be performed if the patient wishes.

6.13.4 Phyllodes Tumour

Phyllodes tumour (a biphasic stromal and epithelial lesion) may appear on clinical and imaging evidence to be very similar to a fibroadenoma. However, histology (core biopsy) will demonstrate features (number of mitoses per high powered field; morphological appearances) ranging from benign, through borderline histology, to frankly sarcomatous (hence the former term cystosarcoma phyllodes) or alternatively classed as high- or low-grade variants. Excision with a margin of normal tissue and follow-up for local recurrence for 5 years thereafter is required.

6.13.5 Cysts

One in twelve women develops a symptomatic cyst in their lifetime. A cyst may be single or multiple, and both mammography (Fig. 6.17) and ultrasound (Fig. 6.11) are diagnostically useful. Aspiration both establishes the diagnosis and treats the cyst. However, blood in the cyst aspirates or a residual mass may be due to an intracystic cancer (Fig. 6.13), so the remaining lesion requires core biopsy. Cysts may refill, particularly if not completely aspirated, and require repeated aspiration or, rarely, if large and recurring after repeated aspiration, excision.

6.13.6 Breast Sepsis

A breast abscess develops from tender, erythematous cellulitis (mastitis) to present as a painful red, mass warm to the touch which may occupy part or the entire breast. An abscess occurs in two groups of women. In young, breast-feeding mothers, Staphylococcus aureus is the usual organism; the abscess usually sits adjacent to the areolar, and early intervention with amoxycillin (or erythromycin if penicillin allergic) at the cellulitic stage may prevent the formation of an abscess. The differential diagnosis includes inflammatory breast cancer, and so ultrasound evaluation is useful to identify focal pus. Once formed, an abscess may be drained under local anaesthesia using aspiration through a wide-bore needle under ultrasound guidance and antibiotic cover or, more rarely, by formal incision and drainage particularly if loculated. A subsequent mammary duct fistula may emerge at the junction of the areolar and breast skin and requires surgical excision. If possible, the mother should be encouraged to continue breast feeding to reduce breast engorgement.

In women aged 35–55, often smokers, multiple abscess formation may occur throughout both breasts (Fig. 6.25) and may not be confined to the nipple areolar area. The process of duct ectasia with enlarged ectatic ducts surrounded by an inflammatory infiltrate may lead to a slit-like nipple retraction (in contrast to the retraction seen with a cancer) and creamy nipple discharge which may be blood-stained. Subsequent inflammatory episodes with periductal mastitis may progress to abscess formation. While the anaerobic bacteria may respond to amoxycillin (or erythromycin and metronidazole) if treatment is commenced early, the repeated development of abscesses which may require formal drainage leaves a scarred, often discoloured breast (Fig. 6.25)

6.13.7 Intraduct Papilloma

Intraduct papilloma may imitate breast cancer by presenting as a blood-stained nipple discharge from a single duct (Fig. 6.1). Triple assessment should exclude other pathologies, and the papilloma may be visible on ultrasound. If so, this should undergo core biopsy. If core biopsy shows a papilloma with no atypia, VAB biopsy is a good alternative to surgical excision and usually results in cure of the discharge. Cytology of the nipple discharge may reveal papillary clusters of epithelial cells, and although ductoscopy has some advocates, excision of the relevant duct under general anaesthesia is advocated to establish the diagnosis and exclude any evidence of malignancy which may be focal within a papilloma.

6.13.8 Skin Lesions

Skin lesions may occur on the breast as elsewhere in the body. An epidermoid cyst (formerly referred to as sebaceous cyst) may give the impression of a small (usually < 1 cm) breast mass; it is usually possible to demonstrate the intradermal location, a visible punctum and may produce creamy material. Epidermoid cysts are usually located adjacent to the sternum or in the inframammary fold. In contrast, a lipoma is usually 1–4 cm in size, deep to the skin and may require triple assessment to distinguish it from other breast masses. Additional breast tissue in the form of an accessory breast tissue can present as a mass in the axilla or subcutaneous mass just inferior to the breast in the midclavicular line. Assessment with ultrasound may establish the diagnosis. Accessory breast tissue rarely requires intervention unless symptomatic.

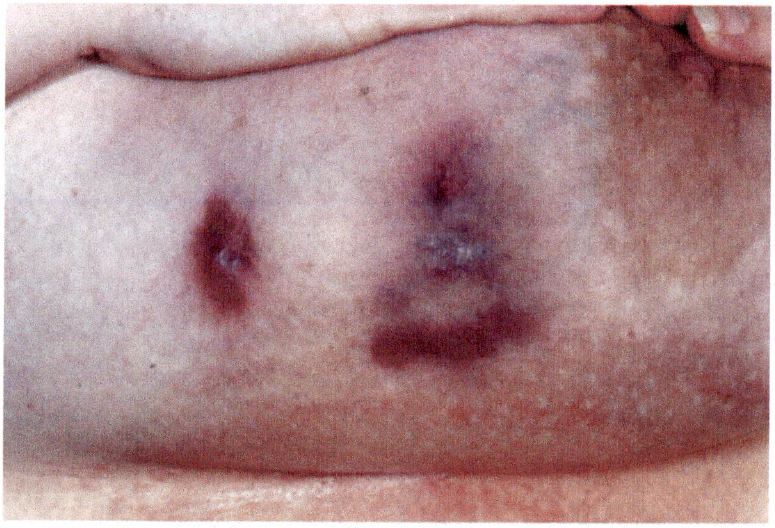

Fig. 6.25 Multiple abscesses and scars in a 50-year-old smoker with periductal mastitis for 5 years

6.13.9 Fat Necrosis

A woman presenting with a breast mass secondary to fat necrosis is usually suggested by a history of trauma and bruising post-injury with a palpable lump which takes several weeks to resolve. On mammography, fat necrosis, if it is longstanding, may have similar features to a breast cancer with a stellate appearance. Most women with fat necrosis have normal mammography. Ultrasound often shows characteristic subcutaneous hyperechogenicity with central oil cysts. Aspiration of oil from an oil cyst confirms the diagnosis and, if required, core biopsy can also be performed.

6.13.10 Other Lesions

Other breast lesions, usually detected by breast screening, such as sclerosing adenosis or a radial scar, may mimic small breast cancers on imaging but rarely present as a palpable breast mass.

In general, surgical excision of benign lumps, if required, should try to use approaches which minimise scarring to the breast, whether conducted under local anaesthetic or general anaesthesia. This includes using a circumareolar incision (with tunnelling to the lesion if required), submammary or axillary approaches. In a larger breast, it may be necessary to cut directly into the breast skin overlying a breast mass, and then the skin tension lines of the breast should be used to ensure scars heal with minimal cosmetic deficit.

References

1. Niewoehner CB, Schorer AE. Gynaecomastia and breast cancer in men. Brit Med J. 2008;336:709–13.
2. Independent UK Panel on Breast Cancer Screening. The benefits and harms of breast cancer screening: an independent review. Lancet. 2012;380(9855):1778–86. doi:10.1016/S0140-6736(12) 61611-0 PMID:23117178.
3. Saslow D, Hannan J, Osuch J, et al. Clinical breast examination: practical recommendations for optimising performance and reporting. CA Cancer J Clincians. 2004;54:327–44.
4. Barton MB, Harris R, Fletcher SW. Does this patient have breast cancer?: the screening clinical examination: should it be done? How? JAMA. 1999;282:1270–80.
5. Rautiainen S, Masarwah A, Sudah M, Sutela A, Pelkonen O, Joukainen S, Sironen R, Kärjä V, Vanninen R. Axillary lymph node biopsy in newly diagnosed invasive breast cancer: comparative accuracy of fine-needle aspiration biopsy versus core-needle biopsy. Radiology. 2013;269(1):54–60. doi:10.1148/radiol.13122637 Epub 2013 Jun 14.
6. Bluemke DA, Gatsonis CA, Chen MH, et al. Magnetic resonance imaging of the breast prior to biopsy. JAMA. 2004;292:2735–42.

Breast Cancer Epidemiology

7

Alicia Brunßen, Joachim Hübner, Alexander Katalinic, Maria R. Noftz, and Annika Waldmann

7.1 Descriptive Epidemiology

Breast cancer affects women all over the world, but the burden of disease is not equally distributed. Which countries have a high burden of breast cancer? How many women per year develop breast cancer and how many die from it? How do incidence and mortality rates change over time and how many women living today had breast cancer in the past 5 years? Answers to these questions are given in the following subsections on incidence, mortality and prevalence of breast cancer.

7.1.1 Incidence

The World Health Organization estimates that 1.7 million breast cancer cases occurred in 2012 among women worldwide [1]. Breast cancer accounts for 25 % of all cancer cases in women and is therefore the most frequent cancer[1] in women worldwide as well as in 140 countries [2]. Among men and women overall, breast cancer is the second most common cancer; only lung cancer has a higher incidence [1].

[1]Excluding non-melanoma skin cancer.

A. Brunßen
Department of Surgery, University of Texas Health Science Center at San Antonio, San Antonio, TX 78229, USA
e-mail: calvoc@uthscsa.edu

J. Hübner · A. Katalinic (✉) · M.R. Noftz · A. Waldmann
Institute for Social Medicine and Epidemiology, University of Luebeck, Ratzeburger Allee 160 (Hs. 50), Luebeck, 23562, Schleswig-Holstein, Germany
e-mail: alexander.katalinic@uksh.de

J. Hübner
e-mail: Joachim.Huebner@uksh.de

M.R. Noftz
e-mail: Maria.Noftz@uksh.de

A. Waldmann
e-mail: Annika.Waldmann@uksh.de

Breast cancer is more common in highly developed countries. The global distribution of incidence rates is shown in Fig. 7.1a. In more developed regions, the age-standardized (world standard) incidence rate per 100,000 women (WASR) is 73.4 in contrast to 31.3 in less developed regions. The incidence rate in women all over the world is 43.1 (WASR). Highest incidence rates (WASR) are observed in Northern America (91.6), Western Europe (91.1) and Northern Europe (89.4), whereas lowest incidence rates occur in Middle Africa (26.8), Eastern Asia (27.0) and South-Central Asia (28.2) [1]. Among the countries of Eastern Asia, Korea and Japan have increased incidence rates (WASR) of 52.1 and 51.5 per 100,000 women, respectively. Around 43 % of new breast cancer cases are diagnosed in Europe and Northern America and about 39 % in Asia (see Fig. 7.2a) [1].

As outlined in Fig. 7.3a, in most areas of the world, incidence rates have been increasing, but in some high developed countries, incidence had reached a peak and decreased in the past decade [2]. Based on population forecasts, it is predicted that the estimated number of new breast cancer cases will increase by the demographic effect from 1.7 million cases worldwide (2012) to 2.6 million cases in the year 2035 [1].

Breast cancer incidence increases with age. Whereas the worldwide incidence is 14.0 per 100,000 women who are 15–39 years old, breast cancer is much more common in the age of 65–69 (159.1/100,000) [1]. In the United States of America (USA), the median age of breast cancer patients at diagnosis is 61. A median age at diagnosis of 55–60 years is typical in most Western countries [3, 4]. In contrast, breast cancer patients in China show a lower median age at diagnosis of 50–54 years [5].

Breast cancer occurs in men as well, but male breast cancer is a rare disease and accounts for about 1 % of all cases of breast cancer cases in Europe and the USA [6–10]. For one male breast cancer, there are nearly 100–140 female breast cancer cases [8, 10, 11].

I. Jatoi and A. Rody (eds.), *Management of Breast Diseases*, DOI 10.1007/978-3-319-46356-8_7

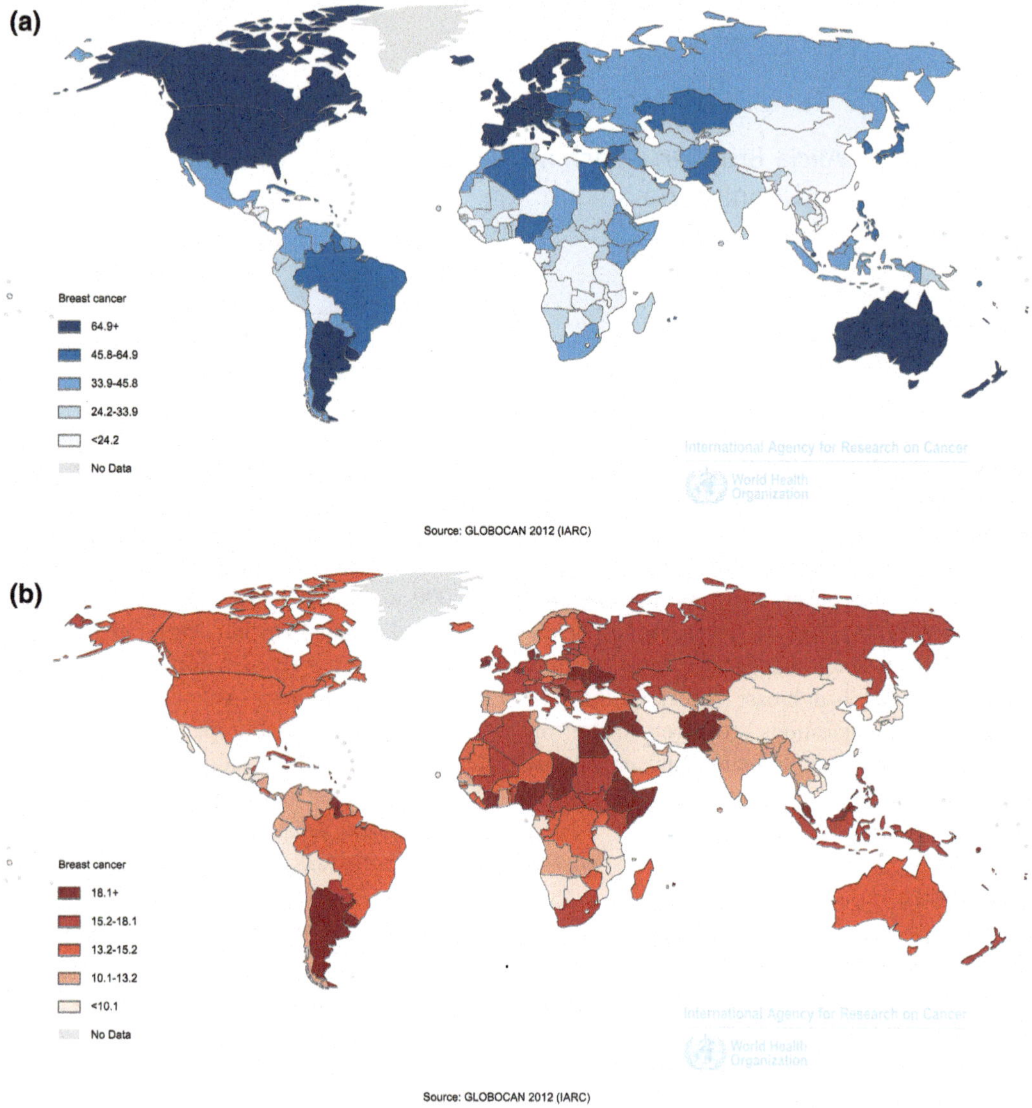

Fig. 7.1 Global distribution of estimated age-standardized breast cancer incidence (**a**) and mortality rates (**b**) per 100,000 women (world standard population) in 2012. (Reproduced and modified with permission from Ferlay J, Soerjomataram I, Ervik M, Dikshit R, Eser S, Mathers C, Rebelo M, Parkin DM, Forman D, Bray, F. GLOBOCAN 2012 v1.0, Cancer Incidence and Mortality Worldwide: IARC CancerBase No. 11 [Internet]. Lyon, France: International Agency for Research on Cancer; 2013. Available from: http://globocan.iarc.fr, accessed on 19 February 2016. [1])

7.1.2 Mortality

Worldwide breast cancer is not only the most frequent cancer, but also the most common cause of cancer-related death among women just as in 101 single countries [2]. It is estimated that 522,000 women died from breast cancer in 2012 worldwide. This equals a proportion of 15 % of all cancer deaths in women [1, 2].

Age-standardized mortality rates (WASR) are higher for breast cancer than for all other causes of cancer in both more developed and less developed regions (breast cancer mortality rates are 14.9 and 11.5/100,000, respectively). In more developed regions though, the absolute number and proportion of all cancer deaths are higher for lung cancer (210,000 deaths, 16.3 %) than for breast cancer (198,000 deaths, 15.4 %). Considering both men and women together, breast cancer is the fifth most common cause of cancer-related deaths [1].

Disparities in the global distribution of breast cancer mortality rates are not as big as differences in incidence rates (see Fig. 7.4). Mortality rates (WASR) are lowest in Eastern Asia (6.1) and Central America (9.5), while the highest mortality rate occurs in Western Africa (20.1) [1]. A twofold to fivefold variation of mortality rates is observed between the countries worldwide [2].

About 35 % of breast cancer deaths occur in Europe and North America and round 44 % in Asia (see Fig. 7.2b).

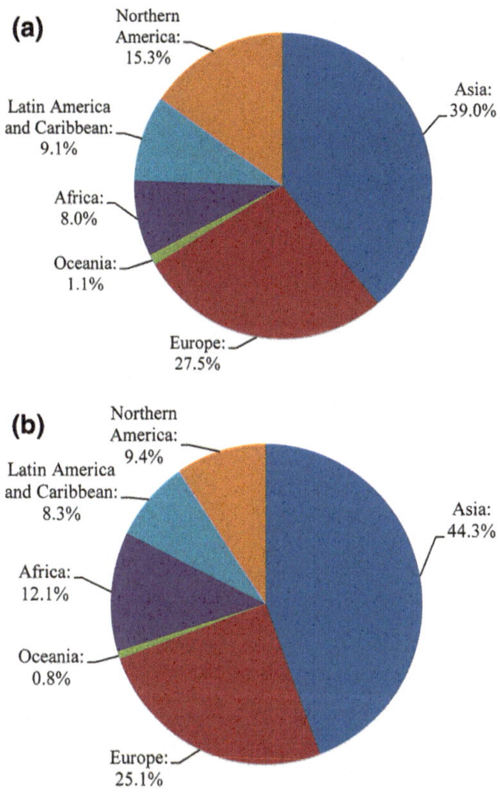

Fig. 7.2 Proportions of 1.7 million estimated incident breast cases (**a**) and of 522.000 estimated breast cancer deaths (**b**) in women by major world regions in 2012 (Reproduced and modified with permission from Ferlay J, Soerjomataram I, Ervik M, Dikshit R, Eser S, Mathers C, Rebelo M, Parkin DM, Forman D, Bray, F. GLOBOCAN 2012 v1.0, Cancer Incidence and Mortality Worldwide: IARC CancerBase No. 11 [Internet]. Lyon, France: International Agency for Research on Cancer; 2013. Available from: http://globocan.iarc.fr, accessed on 19 February 2016. [1])

While the age-standardized mortality rate (WASR) in Africa (17.3) is higher than in Europe (16.1) and Northern America (14.8), the crude mortality rate (CR) is much lower in Africa (11.8) than in Europe (34.2) and Northern America (27.5). Africa accounts for only 12 % of all breast cancer deaths worldwide [1].

As shown in Fig. 7.3b, mortality rates declined in some highly developed countries over the last two and a half decades. This decline has been ascribed to improved detection and early diagnosis by population-based screening as well as better treatment of breast cancer [2]. It is predicted that in the year 2035, about 847,000 women will die from breast cancer worldwide [1].

For an adequate understanding of the relative magnitude of competing health risks, it is important to put the risk of death from breast cancer into context with other leading causes of death. Stroke and ischaemic heart disease account together for about 26 % of all deaths in women worldwide compared to 2 % of deaths caused by breast cancer [12]. This amounts to about 44,000 deaths from breast cancer in the USA in 2012 [1]. In the United Kingdom (UK), relative proportion of deaths attributable to breast cancer is highest in women 25–49 years of age [13].

Breast cancer mortality rates rise highly with age. Most women die from breast cancer in the age of 55–59 and in the age of 75 or above. Median age at death from breast cancer is 60–64 years in women worldwide [1]. While the median age at death from breast cancer is higher in the USA (68 years), breast cancer patients in China die in a younger age (median = 55–59 years) [1, 3].

7.1.3 Prevalence

An estimated number of 6.2 million adult women (at the age of 15 or older) who had breast cancer diagnosed in the previous five years were alive in the year 2012. Worldwide, 1-year, 3-year and 5-year prevalence rates per 100,000 women are 56.3, 154.8 and 239.9, respectively. In more developed regions, the 5-year prevalence rate is four times higher compared to less developed regions (593.6 vs. 147.3) and the highest 5-year prevalence rates are observed in Western Europe (767.1) and Northern America (744.5). About 46 % of 5-year prevalent breast cancer cases live in Europe and Northern America and almost 37 % live in Asia. Latin America and Caribbean (9 %) as well as Africa (7 %) and Oceania (1 %) account for a much lower proportion of the 5-year prevalent cases [1].

7.2 Risk Factors

Intense research into the risk factors of breast cancers has been done for more than 100 years. Yields of that work improve the understanding of breast cancer biology and help to design optimal prevention and screening strategies. In the following the most relevant factors are described, amended by a broader overview of possible risk factors.

7.2.1 Sex and Age

While breast cancer affects both men and women, it is basically a gynaecological disease (see Sect. 7.1.1) and female sex is the major risk factor. According to its overwhelming epidemiological relevance, the following overview focuses solely on female breast cancer.

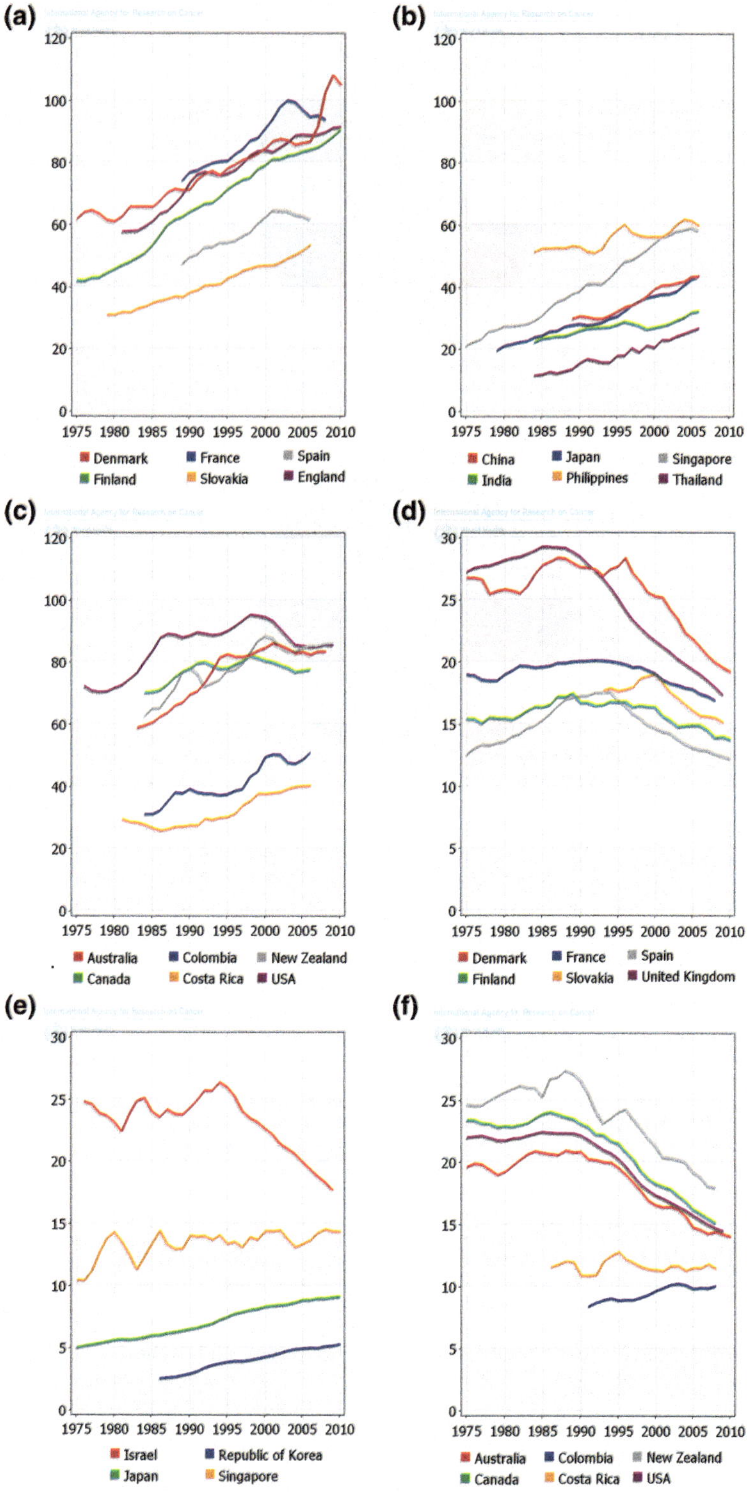

Fig. 7.3 Trends of age-standardized breast cancer incidence (**a–c**) and mortality (**d–f**) rates (world standard population) per 100,000 women in selected countries (Reproduced and modified with permission from Ferlay J, Soerjomataram I, Ervik M, Dikshit R, Eser S, Mathers C, Rebelo M, Parkin DM, Forman D, Bray, F. GLOBOCAN 2012 v1.0, Cancer Incidence and Mortality Worldwide: IARC CancerBase No. 11 [Internet]. Lyon, France: International Agency for Research on Cancer; 2013. Available from: http://globocan.iarc.fr, accessed on 19 February 2016. [1])

Considering the whole life span of a woman, age is the second most important risk factor for breast cancer. Breast cancer is exceptional in premenopausal women and rare before the age of 25. Incidence rises by age. Women aged 65 and older are at sixfold higher risk than younger women [14].

7.2.2 Genetic Predispositions

7.2.2.1 Family History

Familial clustering of female breast cancer has long been thought to indicate the presence of inherited genetic conditions that predispose to the disease. A large meta-analysis

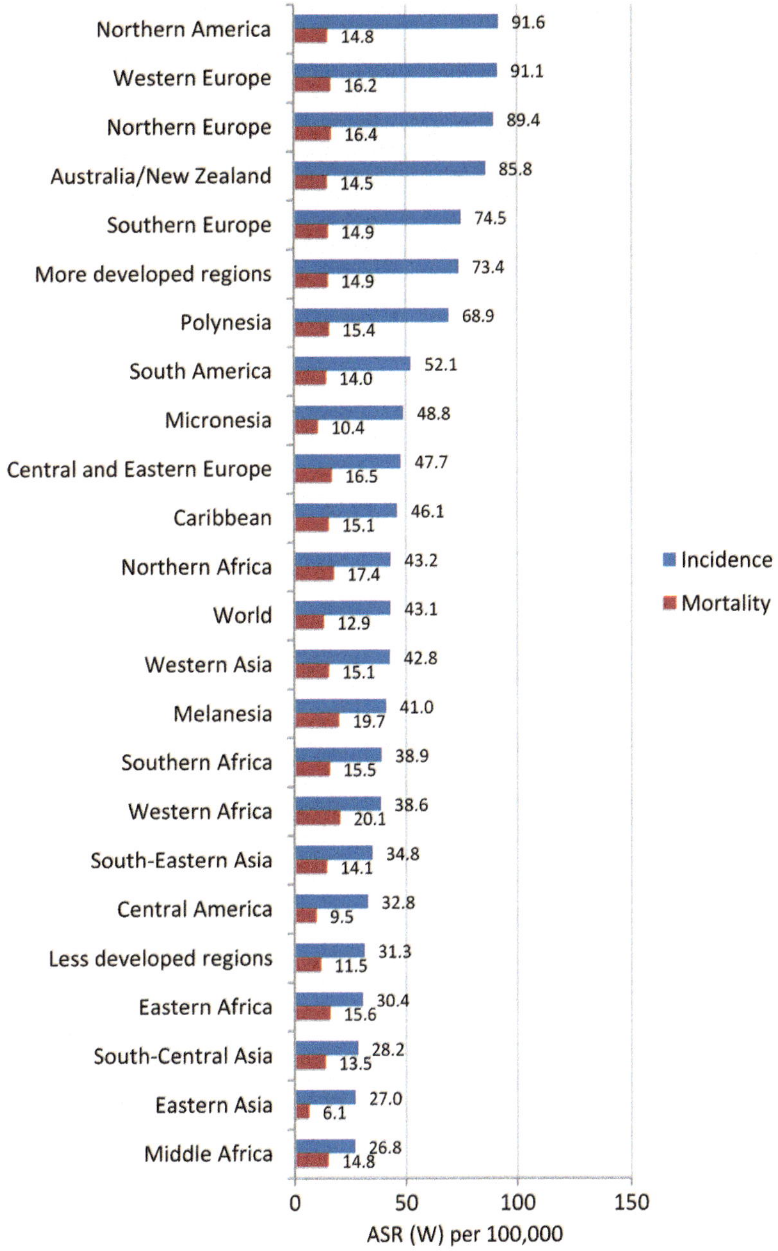

Fig. 7.4 Bar chart of age-standardized breast cancer incidence and mortality rates (world standard population) per 100,000 women for WHO regions in 2012 (Reproduced and modified with permission from Ferlay J, Soerjomataram I, Ervik M, Dikshit R, Eser S, Mathers C, Rebelo M, Parkin DM, Forman D, Bray, F. GLOBOCAN 2012 v1.0, Cancer Incidence and Mortality Worldwide: IARC CancerBase No. 11 [Internet]. Lyon, France: International Agency for Research on Cancer; 2013. Available from: http://globocan.iarc.fr, accessed on 19 February 2016. [1])

estimated the relative risk of women with at least one affected first-degree relative (mother, daughter, sister) to be 2.1 (95 % CI, 2.0–2.2) [15]. The risk ratio increases with increasing numbers of affected first-degree relatives. Compared with women who had no affected relative, the ratios are 1.80 (99 % CI, 1.69–1.91), 2.93 (CI, 2.36–3.64) and 3.90 (CI, 2.03–7.49), respectively, for one, two and three or more affected first-degree relatives [16]. The strengths of the risks vary according to both the age of the woman and the age of the relative. The risk ratios are greatest at young ages, and for women of a given age, are greater the younger the relative was at diagnosis. The respective relative risks range from 5.7 (99 % CI, 2.7–11.8), when both are aged < 40 years to 1.4 (CI, 1.2–1.7) and when both are aged ≥ 60 years [16]. Breast cancer in more distant relatives also increases the risk. If the nearest affected relative is a second- or third-degree relative, the estimated RR is 1.82 (95 % CI, 1.39–2.24) and 1.35 (CI, 1.07–1.64), respectively [17].

7.2.2.2 Molecular Genetic Substrates

In the last two decades, much research has been done to identify the molecular genetic substrates of hereditary factors. Until now, about 90 genes or genetic loci have been found to be involved in breast cancer susceptibility [18]. While most of genetic variants confer a low risk of breast cancer, there is a small group of high-penetrance genes, which are clinically relevant. Although pathogenic mutations in these genes are rare, testing for them has proved its worth in genetic counselling, determining eligibility for enhanced screening and prevention strategies and as markers for targeted therapy. Best known and most important high-risk genes are BRCA1 and BRCA2, both involved in maintaining DNA integrity. Pathologic mutations in them are prevalent in only about 0.1 % of the population and increase the risk of breast cancer by 10- to 20-fold, resulting in a lifetime risk in women of 60–85 % and 40–85 %, respectively [19]. Other germline mutations are even rarer. The lifetime risk of cancer for TP53 mutation carriers is estimated to be 73 % for males and nearly 100 % for females with a high risk of breast cancer [20]. Other genes that confer a moderate-to-high risk and therefore deserve attention in the clinical management of familial breast cancer cases are CDH1, STK11 and PTEN. For these and other—clinically less important—breast cancer susceptibility genes, see Couch et al. [21].

However, taking these genes into account, a part of heritability remains unexplained. Nowadays, it is recognized that breast cancer susceptibility is largely 'polygenic', that is susceptibility is conferred by a large number of loci, each with a small effect on breast cancer risk [22]. By use of genome-wide association studies (GWAS), nearly 80 common genetic variants (single nucleotide polymorphisms, or SNPs) associated with breast cancer risk have been identified to date [21, 23]. Current research aims at the revelation of overlaps between phenotypic risk factor that are under genetic control and SNPs associated with breast cancer risk.

7.2.3 Anthropometric Measures

7.2.3.1 Adult Height

Adult height has been found to be positively related to breast cancer risk in many epidemiological studies. In a recent meta-analysis of prospective studies, the pooled relative risk of breast cancer was 1.17 (95 % CI, 1.15–1.19) per 10 cm increase in height [24]. The association has been related to shared underlying genetic pathways, to environmental factors (e.g. energy intake and socio-economic status during childhood and adolescence), to hormonal activity during puberty and to the number of cells at risk of becoming cancerous.

7.2.3.2 BMI and Body Fat Distribution

The relation between body mass index (BMI) and breast cancer risk is complex and differs by menopausal status. A pooled analysis of data from seven cohort studies found an inverse nonlinear association between BMI and breast cancer risk in premenopausal women. Compared with women with a BMI of less than 21 kg/m^2, women with a BMI exceeding 31 kg/m^2 had a relative risk of 0.54 (95 % CI, 0.34–0.85). In postmenopausal women, the breast cancer risk increased with increasing BMI, but no further increase was found, when BMI exceeded 28 kg/m^2; the relative risk for these women was 1.26 (95 % CI: 1.09, 1.46) [25]. The influence of fat distribution on breast cancer risk has been investigated in several studies using different measures. Most consistent results had been found in cohort studies for postmenopausal women. Central body fat distribution has been associated with an approximately twofold risk of breast cancer compared with a more peripheral distribution of body fat, independent of BMI [26].

7.2.4 Reproductive Factors

The risk of breast cancer is largely influenced by endocrine factors. Early menarche and late menopause prolong a woman's exposure to oestrogens and other female hormones. In accordance with this, it has been found that breast cancer risk increases by a factor of 1.050 (95 % CI: 1.044–1.057) for every year younger at menarche and independently by a factor of 1.029 (95 % CI: 1.025–1.032) for every year older at menopause [27].

Parity and breastfeeding lower the risk of breast cancer. Parous women, i.e. women who gave birth to at least one child, have an approximately 30 % lower risk of breast cancer than nulliparous women [28]. The risk decreases with the number of children. A reanalysis of individual data from 47 epidemiological studies in 30 countries demonstrated that relative risk of breast cancer decreases by 4.3 % (95 % CI: 2.9–5.8) for every 12 months of breastfeeding in addition to a decrease of 7.0 % (5.0–9.0) for each birth. Young woman's age at first birth is another protective factor, independent of breastfeeding. The relative risk declines by 3.0 % for each year younger that women were when their first child was born [29].

7.2.5 Hormones

7.2.5.1 Endogenous Hormones

Compared to the strong body of evidence relating to reproductive, largely hormone-related factors and breast cancer risk, knowledge on direct associations between specific endogenous hormone levels and breast cancer is limited. Complex studies have found that high levels of both oestrogens and androgens approximately double the risk, when comparing the top quintile with the lowest quintile [28]. Similar effects have been reported for insulin-like growth factor 1 in premenopausal women [30]. The relevance of other endogenous hormone levels, e.g. prolactin and progesterone, is unclear.

7.2.5.2 Exogenous Hormones

A meta-analysis of 44 breast cancer studies found that a history of oral contraceptive use slightly but significantly increases breast cancer risk compared with never oral contraceptive use (odds ratio (OR) 1.08; 95 % CI: 1.00–1.17). There is a higher risk associated with more recent or current use; the odds ratio for the use within the last 0–5 years is 1.21 (95 % CI: 1.04–1.41) [31].

The influence of hormone replacement therapy (HRT) on breast cancer risk has been evaluated in a large number of studies. The extensive body of evidence suggests that current users of combined (oestrogen–progesterone) HRT have a higher risk than never users, particularly when started close to menopause. The risk excess increases with the duration of use and dissipates within 2 years of cessation of treatment [32]. The estimates of the increase in risk associated with HRT vary across studies and could range from less than 1.2-fold to twofold [28]. For oestrogen-only therapy, the evidence is inconsistent [33].

7.2.6 Breast Density and Benign Breast Disease

Mammographic density, defined as per cent breast density (mammary gland mass as a fraction of the total breast area), is one of the strongest risk factors for breast cancer. Women with a breast density of ≥75 % have an approximately fivefold risk compared to women with little gland mass (<5 %) [34]. History of benign breast disease is another organ-related risk factor. Compared to women without history of benign breast disease, those with the history of proliferative breast diseases with or without atypia have an increased risk of developing breast cancer by factor approximately 4 or 2, respectively. The risk conferred by non-proliferative breast disease is small, if any [35].

7.2.7 Ionizing Radiation

Exposure to ionizing radiation may cause somatic DNA mutations and, in succession, breast cancer. Epidemiologic evidence is largely based on studies in women who were exposed to atomic bomb explosions and women who received obsolete diagnostic measures and treatments. The magnitude of the effect strongly increases with radiation dose and decreases with age at exposure. Although advanced medical technologies result in lower exposure to ionizing radiation, restrained use, especially in children and adolescents, is necessary.

7.2.8 Diet and Lifestyle

There is consistent evidence for a positive dose–risk relation between alcohol drinking and breast cancer. The increase in risk for additional 10 g/day of alcohol amounts to approximately 10 % [36]. With regard to other dietary factors, the evidence is limited. Meta-analyses reported that higher intake of fruits [37] and dietary marine n-3 polyunsaturated fatty acids (n-3 PUFA) [38] are associated with a lower risk of breast cancer. A slight protective effect of carotenoid intake is likely [39]. The effect of folate has not been finally clarified yet. A higher folate intake is likely to decrease the breast cancer risk in women who regularly drink alcohol [40].

There is substantial evidence that physical activity decreases the risk of postmenopausal breast cancer. A systematic review of 48 cohort and case–control studies reported an inverse association between physical activity and postmenopausal breast cancer with risk reductions ranging from 20 to 80 %. For premenopausal breast cancer, the evidence was much weaker [41].

7.2.9 Overview

An overview of the aforementioned and additional factors is given in Table 7.1.

7.3 Prevention

7.3.1 Primary Prevention

The main strategies in primary prevention for breast cancer include the modification, ideally the avoidance of the risk factors (see Chap. 2). Lifestyle changes (weight control, maintenance of physical activity and reduced intake of alcohol) play a decisive role [42, 43]. As lifestyle changes can be recommended to all women, other preventive interventions such as chemoprevention with selective oestrogen receptor modulators (SERMs) or aromatase inhibitors (AIs) are only suggested for women at high risk of breast cancer (strong family history, BRCA1/2 gene, increased risk through risk assessment models) [44]. The effect of chemoprevention with SERMs and AIs for primary prevention has been investigated in several randomized controlled trials with the result of a significant decrease of the incidence of invasive breast cancer (50 %) in high-risk women [45, 46]. Still, the chemoprevention is not without risk as SERMs like tamoxifen are associated with an

Table 7.1 Summary of risk and protective factors for female breast cancer

Risk factor	Direction and strength of effect*
Well-confirmed risk factors	
Age (65+ vs. <65 years)	↑↑
Family history ≥1 affected first-degree relative (mother, daughter, sister) ≥1 affected second- or third-degree relative	↑↑ ↑
High-penetrance gene mutations	↑↑
Height	↑
High body mass index (premenopausal)	↓
High body mass index (postmenopausal)	↑
Younger age at menarche	↑
Older age at menopause	↑
Parity (vs. nulliparity)	↓
Young age at first birth	↓
Breastfeeding	↓
High endogenous hormone levels of oestrogens and androgens (top quintile vs. the lowest quintile)	↑↑
Current or recent combined hormone replacement therapy (HRT)	↑
Mammographic breast density (of ≥75 % vs. <5 %)	↑↑
History of proliferative benign breast disease with atypia	↑↑
History of proliferative benign breast disease without atypia	↑
Ionizing radiation, especially before age 20	↑↑
Alcohol use (≥10 g/day)	↑
Physical activity (postmenopausal breast cancer)	↓
Probable relationship exists, based on substantial data	
Endogenous hormone levels of insulin-like growth factor 1 (75th vs. 25th percentile)	↑
Current or recent oral contraceptive use	↑
High intake of carotenoids, marine n−3 polyunsaturated fatty acids and fruits	↓
High folate intake in women, who regularly drink alcohol	↓
Weak, if any relationship, based on substantial data	
History of non-proliferative breast disease	
Cigarette smoking	
Coffee and caffeine intake	
Past oral contraceptive use and past hormone replacement therapy (HRT; >2 years)	
Inconsistent findings or limited study today	
High folate intake in women who do not drink alcohol	
Oestrogen-only HRT	
High endogenous hormone levels of prolactin and progesterone	
Nightshift work	

Source Modified from Hankinson et al. [82] by permission of Oxford University Press, USA
Arrows indicate the approximate magnitude of relation: ↑, slight to moderate increase in risk (relative risk (RR): 1.01-1.99); ↑↑, moderate to large increase in risk (RR: ≥ 2.00); ↓, decrease in risk (RR: < 1.00)

increased chance of developing endometrial cancer, thromboembolic events and cataract, next to potential impacts on quality of life [45].

The concept of risk-reduction surgery should only be considered in women with high-inherited susceptibility for breast/ovarian cancer especially in women with

BRCA-1/BRCA-2 mutation. Even though studies report a significant risk reduction in breast cancer incidence [43, 47, 48], the decision to undergo such an aggressive surgical procedure remains complex and requires an extensive and detailed counselling [48].

Risk assessment models for a women's individual risk for the disease are regularly used in the clinical setting, such as the Gail model, Claus model and Tyrer–Cuzick model [49–51]. Additionally to any risk assessment, a comprehensive counselling on the individual preventive possibilities for women at risk should be vital.

7.3.2 Secondary Prevention

Secondary prevention measures for breast cancer include mammography screening, clinical breast examination (CBE) and breast self-examination (BSE). Of these measures, only mammography screening has proven an effect on breast cancer mortality [52].

Correctly applied clinical breast examination is an easily applied and inexpensive method for breast cancer screening. There is sufficient evidence for an association of CBE and detection of smaller and earlier stage tumours, but no sufficient data on the impact on breast cancer mortality [53]. A reduction in breast cancer mortality for BSE is only reported in observational studies, as data from randomized controlled trials are still insufficient [54]. Nevertheless, training in BSE can lead to detection of smaller tumours and thus to a possible impact on prolonged survival [55].

Breast cancer screening programs (BSC) exist worldwide in an organized or opportunistic setting mainly for the age group of women 50–69 years. Several expert groups such as Cochrane Collaboration [56], UK Panel [57], Health Council of the Netherlands [58] and US Preventive Services Task Force [53] have evaluated the evidence of randomized controlled trials and observational trials for benefits and harms of breast cancer screening. A significant breast cancer mortality reduction (about 20 %) could be shown in the age group 50–69 years. In 2015, the International Agency for Research on Cancer (IARC) published an independent evaluation of the mammography screening on the basis of RCTs and, in particular, observational studies [52], as some of the aforementioned RCTs are in the focus of criticism due to their age and further improvement in screening technique and quality. In summary, the IARC confirms the sufficient evidence that mammography screening for breast cancer has an impact on a reduction in breast cancer mortality with up to 40 % in women of the age group 50–69 years. Additionally, breast cancer mortality reduction was also reported for the age group 70–79 years; however, the effect of breast cancer mortality reduction in women 40–49 years is limited. In terms of absolute numbers, great differences in results on prevented breast cancer death by mammography screening occur in the literature depending on the follow-up time used [59]: 1–2 in 1000 women (10 years of follow-up) [60], 4 in 1000 women (25 years of follow-up) [57] and 7–9 in 1000 women (30 years of follow-up) [61].

Regarding possible harms of screening, the IARC also stated sufficient evidence of overdiagnoses, false-positive results and increased risk of radiation-induced breast cancer due to mammography screening with a wide range in results due to different study designs and statistical model. The IARC concluded that the significant net benefit of mammography screening for women in the age group 50–69 years (reduction of breast cancer mortality) outweighs possible harms and side effects [52]. This is in line with the prior recommendations of the UK Panel [57], Health Council of the Netherlands [58] and US Preventive Services Task Force [53].

Evidence for a reduction of breast cancer mortality due to other imaging techniques such as tomosynthesis, ultrasound or MRI additionally to mammography screening is still insufficient [52].

Counselling of women in the target group for screening should include a balanced discussion on the potential benefits and harms of mammography screening. For the future, the results of risk-adapted screening programs could help to improve the decision making for or against a screening participation.

7.4 Prognosis

In the recent decades, the survival rates of breast cancer have shown a significant increase worldwide. The age-standardized 5-year net survival[2] is 80 % or higher for women in 34 countries diagnosed with breast cancer in 2005–2009. In most developed countries, 5-year survival has improved. Survival is high in North America and Oceania (84–89 %), but generally low in Europe with bigger geographic differences. Low net survival is observed in South Africa (53 %), Mongolia (57 %), India (60 %) and Malaysia (68 %) [62].

As breast cancer is a complex and heterogeneous disease with a wide variety in morphology, molecular characteristics, clinical behaviour and response to therapy, prognostic factors such as tumour characteristics, demographic information and biomarkers are of great importance in the personalized oncologic patient care to predict outcomes as recurrence and overall survival [63].

[2] 5-year net survival is the cumulative probability that cancer patients would have survived 5 years or more after diagnosis when background mortality was eliminated and differences in population mortality is not entered in the comparisons.

In breast cancer, the most useful prognostic factors are mostly clinically based and include traditional factors such as tumour size, lymph node status, presence of metastasis, tumour histology, presence of peri-tumoural vascular invasion and expression of molecular markers such as oestrogen receptor (ER), progesterone receptor (PR) status and cell membrane-bound tyrosine kinase receptor (HER2) [64, 65]. Some of the prognostic factors are combined in prognostic indices such as the well-known TNM classification or other validated tools such as scoring systems that have been recently introduced to combine clinical parameters such as age, tumour stage, hormone receptor status and tumour grading to be used as prediction models for recurrence and death of breast cancer, e.g. the Nottingham Prognostic Index (NPI) and the Adjuvant Online (Adjuvant!). [66–68].

Tumour size and lymph node involvement (composed of the TNM classification together with the presence of the metastasis) are strong prognostic indicators for recurrence rate and survival in breast cancer patients. [68]. While 5-year relative survival of patients with localized breast cancer is very high (99 %), locally or regionally advanced cancers are associated with lower survival (80 %) and 5-year relative survival of women with metastasized breast cancer is even lower (23 %) [69]. Age-standardized 5-year net survival for node-negative breast cancer is 92–98 % in Europe and the USA, whereas large, node-negative tumours have lower survival (84–93 %) [70].

Even though limited by the high degree of interobserver variability, grading of the tumour is another recognized prognostic marker [71]. Independent from the TNM classification, histological grading is associated with disease-free and overall survival [72]. The mostly used grading system is the semiquantitative Elston and Ellis modification of the Scarff–Bloom–Richardson classification which ranges from well to poorly differentiated (Grade I–III) to score tubule formation, nuclear pleomorphism and mitotic rate of the tumour [65, 72, 73].

Invasive breast cancers presenting an ER-positive and PR-positive status have shown a better prognosis and longer disease-free survival than ER-/PR-negative tumours. ER is one of the most important molecular markers and is present in around 75–80 % of breast cancers [74]. Although the prognostic value of hormone receptors is only weak to moderate [71, 75, 76], it is a strong predictor of response to hormone therapy, especially in ER- and PR-positive tumours [65].

HER2 overexpression is present in approximately 20–30 % of breast cancer [74]. Even though the presence of HER2 is associated with an aggressive behaviour, high recurrence and increase of mortality rate [65, 77], it is a weak-to-moderate independent predictor of survival in patients, at least for node-negative involvement [78, 79].

In addition to the traditional clinic pathological prognostic factors in breast cancer patients, the use of intrinsic molecular subtypes provides an improvement in prognostication and treatment decisions in the heterogeneous character of breast cancer [71, 80]. Intrinsic subtypes combine routine histology and immunohistochemical evaluation and are grouped into four subtypes [64, 74, 81]:

- Luminal A: ER-positive, HER2-negative, Ki-67 low and PR high
- Luminal B:
  - (HER2-negative)—ER-positive, HER2-negative and either Ki-67 high or PR low
  - (HER2-positive)—ER-positive, HER2 overexpressed or amplified, any Ki-67 and any PR
- HER2-enriched: HER2 overexpressed or amplified, ER and PR absent
- Basal-like: ER and PR absent and HER2-negative

Luminal tumours show a wide range of behaviours with Luminal A tumours being described as less aggressive, but more chemoresistant and bearing a higher risk of late recurrence. In contrast, Luminal B tumours present with an increased level of aggressiveness, but a higher sensitivity to chemotherapy. HER2-enriched and basal-like tumours are most responsive to chemotherapy, but are representing the tumour group with the highest proliferation rates and most aggressive potential, leading to early recurrence of the disease (mostly < 5 years) [74].

References

1. World Health Organization, International Agency for Research on Cancer. GLOBOCAN 2012: Estimated Cancer Incidence, Mortality and Prevalence Worldwide in 2012. 2012 [December 9, 2012]; Available from: http://globocan.iarc.fr/.
2. Stewart EW, Wild CP. World cancer report 2014. Lyon: International Agency for Research on Cancer; 2014.
3. Howlader N, Noone AM, Krapcho M, Garshell J, Miller D, Altekruse SF, et al. SEER cancer statistics review 1975–2012 Bethesda, MD: National Cancer Institute; 2015 [updated based on November 2014 SEER data submission, posted to the SEER web site, April 2015, January 6, 2016]; Available from: http://seer.cancer.gov/csr/1975_2012/.
4. Youlden DR, Cramb SM, Yip CH, Baade PD. Incidence and mortality of female breast cancer in the Asia-Pacific region. Cancer biol Med. 2014;11(2):101–15 Epub 2014/07/11.
5. Song Q-K, Li J, Huang R, Fan J-H, Zheng R-S, Zhang B-N, et al. Age of diagnosis of breast cancer in China: almost 10 years earlier than in the United States and the European Union. Asian Pac J Cancer Prev. 2015;15(22):10021.
6. Fentiman IS, Fourquet A, Hortobagyi GN. Male breast cancer. Lancet. 2006;367(9510):595–604 Epub 2006/02/21.
7. Robert Koch-Institute. Cancer in Germany 2009/2010 [Krebs in Deutschland 2009/2010]. 9th ed. Berlin 2013.
8. Cancer Research UK 2014. Breast cancer in men. 2014 [updated July 30, 2014, December 16, 2015]; Available from: http://www.cancerresearchuk.org/about-cancer/type/rare-cancers/rare-cancers-name/breast-cancer-in-men.

9. Association of the Nordic Cancer Registries (NORDCAN). NORDCAN, Cancer stat fact sheets. 2015 [updated December 11, 2015, December 16, 2015]; Available from: http://www-dep.iarc.fr/NORDCAN/english/StatsFact.asp?cancer=200&country=0.
10. American Cancer Society. What are the key statistics about breast cancer? 2015 [updated October 6, 2015 December 16, 2015]; Available from: http://www.cancer.org/cancer/breastcancer/detailedguide/breast-cancer-key-statistics.
11. GEKID. [GEKID Atlas - Tabellenabfrage]. 2012 [January 05, 2016]; Available from: http://www.gekid.de/Atlas/Tabellen/Tabellen_D.php?Method=INCIDENCE_EU&ICD10=C50&Year_from=2012&Year_to=2012&Men=on&Women=on&Cases=on.
12. World, Health, Organization. Global Health Observatory, Visualizations, Causes of death - Ten leading causes of death. 2012 [December 10, 2015]; Available from: http://www.who.int/gho/mortality_burden_disease/causes_death/top_10/en/.
13. Cancer Research UK 2013. Cancer mortality by age. 2013 [updated December 4, 2013 January 6, 2016]; Available from: http://www.cancerresearchuk.org/content/cancer-mortality-by-age#heading-Two.
14. Singletary SE. Rating the risk factors for breast cancer. Ann Surg. 2003;237(4):474–82 Epub 2003/04/05.
15. Pharoah PD, Day NE, Duffy S, Easton DF, Ponder BA. Family history and the risk of breast cancer: a systematic review and meta-analysis. Int J Cancer J Int du Cancer. 1997;71(5):800–9 Epub 1997/05/29.
16. Collaborative Group on Hormonal Factors in Breast Cancer. Familial breast cancer: collaborative reanalysis of individual data from 52 epidemiological studies including 58,209 women with breast cancer and 101,986 women without the disease. Lancet. 2001;358(9291):1389–99 Epub 2001/11/14.
17. Slattery ML, Kerber RA. A comprehensive evaluation of family history and breast cancer risk. The Utah Population Database. JAMA. 1993;270(13):1563–8 Epub 1993/10/06.
18. Dossus L, Benusiglio PR. Lobular breast cancer: incidence and genetic and non-genetic risk factors. Breast Cancer Res: BCR. 2015;17:37 Epub 2015/04/08.
19. Lalloo F, Evans DG. Familial breast cancer. Clin Genet. 2012;82(2):105–14 Epub 2012/02/24.
20. Chompret A, Brugieres L, Ronsin M, Gardes M, Dessarps-Freichey F, Abel A, et al. P53 germline mutations in childhood cancers and cancer risk for carrier individuals. Br J Cancer. 2000;82(12):1932–7 Epub 2000/06/23.
21. Couch FJ, Nathanson KL, Offit K. Two decades after BRCA: setting paradigms in personalized cancer care and prevention. Science. 2014;343(6178):1466–70 Epub 2014/03/29.
22. Easton DF, Pooley KA, Dunning AM, Pharoah PD, Thompson D, Ballinger DG, et al. Genome-wide association study identifies novel breast cancer susceptibility loci. Nature. 2007;447(7148):1087–93 Epub 2007/05/29.
23. Stone J, Thompson DJ, Dos Santos Silva I, Scott C, Tamimi RM, Lindstrom S, et al. Novel associations between common breast cancer susceptibility variants and risk-predicting mammographic density measures. Cancer Res. 2015;75(12):2457–67 Epub 2015/04/12.
24. Zhang B, Shu XO, Delahanty RJ, Zeng C, Michailidou K, Bolla MK, et al. Height and breast cancer risk: evidence from prospective studies and mendelian randomization. J Natl Cancer Inst. 2015;107(11). Epub 2015/08/25.
25. van den Brandt PA, Spiegelman D, Yaun SS, Adami HO, Beeson L, Folsom AR, et al. Pooled analysis of prospective cohort studies on height, weight, and breast cancer risk. Am J Epidemiol. 2000;152(6):514–27 Epub 2000/09/21.
26. McTiernan A. Behavioral risk factors in breast cancer: can risk be modified? Oncologist. 2003;8(4):326–34 Epub 2003/08/05.
27. Collaborative Group on Hormonal Factors in Breast Cancer. Menarche, menopause, and breast cancer risk: individual participant meta-analysis, including 118 964 women with breast cancer from 117 epidemiological studies. Lancet Oncol. 2012;13(11):1141–51 Epub 2012/10/23.
28. National Breast and Ovarian Cancer Centre (NBOCC). Breast cancer risk factors: a review of the evidence. 2009.
29. Collaborative Group on Hormonal Factors in Breast Cancer. Breast cancer and breastfeeding: collaborative reanalysis of individual data from 47 epidemiological studies in 30 countries, including 50302 women with breast cancer and 96973 women without the disease. Lancet. 2002;360(9328):187–95 Epub 2002/07/23.
30. Renehan AG, Zwahlen M, Minder C, O'Dwyer ST, Shalet SM, Egger M. Insulin-like growth factor (IGF)-I, IGF binding protein-3, and cancer risk: systematic review and meta-regression analysis. Lancet. 2004;363(9418):1346–53 Epub 2004/04/28.
31. Gierisch JM, Coeytaux RR, Urrutia RP, Havrilesky LJ, Moorman PG, Lowery WJ, et al. Oral contraceptive use and risk of breast, cervical, colorectal, and endometrial cancers: a systematic review. Cancer Epidemiol Biomark Prev. 2013;22(11):1931–43 Epub 2013/09/10, A Publication of the American Association for Cancer Research, Cosponsored by the American Society of Preventive Oncology.
32. Narod SA. Hormone replacement therapy and the risk of breast cancer. Nat Rev Clin Oncol. 2011;8(11):669–76 Epub 2011/08/03.
33. Friis S, Kesminiene A, Espina C, Auvinen A, Straif K, Schuz J. European code against cancer 4th edition: medical exposures, including hormone therapy, and cancer. Cancer Epidemiol. 2015;39(Suppl 1):S107–19 Epub 2015/09/24.
34. McCormack VA, dos Santos Silva I. Breast density and parenchymal patterns as markers of breast cancer risk: a meta-analysis. Cancer Epidemiol Biomark Prev. 2006;15(6):1159–69 Epub 2006/06/16, A Publication of the American Association for Cancer Research, cosponsored by the American Society of Preventive Oncology.
35. Dyrstad SW, Yan Y, Fowler AM, Colditz GA. Breast cancer risk associated with benign breast disease: systematic review and meta-analysis. Breast Cancer Res Treat. 2015;149(3):569–75 Epub 2015/02/01.
36. Seitz HK, Pelucchi C, Bagnardi V, La Vecchia C. Epidemiology and pathophysiology of alcohol and breast cancer: Update 2012. Alcohol and alcoholism (Oxford, Oxfordshire). 2012;47(3):204–12. Epub 2012/03/31.
37. Aune D, Chan DS, Vieira AR, Rosenblatt DA, Vieira R, Greenwood DC, et al. Fruits, vegetables and breast cancer risk: a systematic review and meta-analysis of prospective studies. Breast Cancer Res Treat. 2012;134(2):479–93 Epub 2012/06/19.
38. Zheng JS, Hu XJ, Zhao YM, Yang J, Li D. Intake of fish and marine n-3 polyunsaturated fatty acids and risk of breast cancer: meta-analysis of data from 21 independent prospective cohort studies. BMJ. 2013;346:f3706 Epub 2013/07/03.
39. Hu F, Wang Yi B, Zhang W, Liang J, Lin C, Li D, et al. Carotenoids and breast cancer risk: a meta-analysis and meta-regression. Breast Cancer Res Treat. 2012;131(1):239–53 Epub 2011/09/09.
40. Zhang YF, Shi WW, Gao HF, Zhou L, Hou AJ, Zhou YH. Folate intake and the risk of breast cancer: a dose-response meta-analysis of prospective studies. PloS One. 2014;9(6):e100044. Epub 2014/06/17.
41. Monninkhof EM, Elias SG, Vlems FA, van der Tweel I, Schuit AJ, Voskuil DW, et al. Physical activity and breast cancer: a

systematic review. Epidemiology. 2007;18(1):137–57 Epub 2006/11/30.
42. Colditz GA, Bohlke K. Priorities for the primary prevention of breast cancer. CA Cancer J Clin. 2014;64(3):186–94 Epub 2014/03/22.
43. Hartmann LC, Schaid DJ, Woods JE, Crotty TP, Myers JL, Arnold PG, et al. Efficacy of bilateral prophylactic mastectomy in women with a family history of breast cancer. New Engl J Med. 1999;340(2):77–84 Epub 1999/01/14.
44. Howell A, Anderson AS, Clarke RB, Duffy SW, Evans DG, Garcia-Closas M, et al. Risk determination and prevention of breast cancer. Breast cancer research: BCR. 2014;16(5):446. Epub 2014/12/04.
45. Fisher B, Costantino JP, Wickerham DL, Redmond CK, Kavanah M, Cronin WM, et al. Tamoxifen for prevention of breast cancer: report of the national surgical adjuvant breast and bowel project P-1 study. J Natl Cancer Inst. 1998;90(18):1371–88 Epub 1998/09/25.
46. Visvanathan K, Hurley P, Bantug E, Brown P, Col NF, Cuzick J, et al. Use of pharmacologic interventions for breast cancer risk reduction: American Society of Clinical Oncology clinical practice guideline. J Clin Oncol. 2013;31(23):2942–62 Epub 2013/07/10, Official journal of the American Society of Clinical Oncology.
47. Domchek SM, Friebel TM, Singer CF, Evans DG, Lynch HT, Isaacs C, et al. Association of risk-reducing surgery in BRCA1 or BRCA2 mutation carriers with cancer risk and mortality. JAMA. 2010;304(9):967–75 Epub 2010/09/03.
48. Rebbeck TR, Friebel T, Lynch HT, Neuhausen SL, van 't Veer L, Garber JE, et al. Bilateral prophylactic mastectomy reduces breast cancer risk in BRCA1 and BRCA2 mutation carriers: the PROSE Study Group. J Clin Oncol. 2004;22(6):1055–62 Epub 2004/02/26, Official journal of the American Society of Clinical Oncology.
49. Claus EB, Risch N, Thompson WD. The calculation of breast cancer risk for women with a first degree family history of ovarian cancer. Breast Cancer Res Treat. 1993;28(2):115–20 Epub 1993/11/01.
50. Gail MH, Brinton LA, Byar DP, Corle DK, Green SB, Schairer C, et al. Projecting individualized probabilities of developing breast cancer for white females who are being examined annually. J Natl Cancer Inst. 1989;81(24):1879–86 Epub 1989/12/20.
51. Tyrer J, Duffy SW, Cuzick J. A breast cancer prediction model incorporating familial and personal risk factors. Stat Med. 2004;23 (7):1111–30 Epub 2004/04/02.
52. Lauby-Secretan B, Scoccianti C, Loomis D, Benbrahim-Tallaa L, Bouvard V, Bianchini F, et al. Breast-cancer screening–viewpoint of the IARC Working Group. New Engl J Med. 2015;372 (24):2353–8 Epub 2015/06/04.
53. U.S. Preventive Task Force. Screening for breast cancer: U.S. Preventive Services Task Force recommendation statement. Annals of internal medicine. 2009;151(10):716–26, W-236. Epub 2009/11/19.
54. Kosters JP, Gotzsche PC. Regular self-examination or clinical examination for early detection of breast cancer. The Cochrane database of systematic reviews. 2003(2):CD003373. Epub 2003/06/14.
55. Weiss NS. Breast cancer mortality in relation to clinical breast examination and breast self-examination. Breast J. 2003;9(Suppl 2):S86–9 Epub 2003/04/26.
56. Gotzsche PC, Jorgensen KJ. Screening for breast cancer with mammography. The Cochrane database of systematic reviews. 2013;6:CD001877. Epub 2013/06/06.
57. Independent UK. Panel on breast cancer screening. The benefits and harms of breast cancer screening: an independent review. Lancet. 2012;380(9855):1778–86 Epub 2012/11/03.
58. The Hague, Netherlands HCot. Health Council of the Netherlands. Population screening for breast cancer: expectations and developments. 2014;publication no. 2014/01.
59. Fügemann H, Kääb-Sanyal V. Mammographie-Screening: Nutzen-Schaden-Abwägung im internationalen Vergleich. Deutsches Ärzteblatt. 2016;113(3).
60. Gesundheitswesen IfQuWi. Einladungsschreiben und Merkblatt zum Mammographie-Screening. Rapid Report. IQWiG-Berichte – Nr. 288. 2015.
61. Paci E, Group EW. Summary of the evidence of breast cancer service screening outcomes in Europe and first estimate of the benefit and harm balance sheet. J Med Screen. 2012;19(Suppl 1):5–13 Epub 2012/11/08.
62. Allemani C, Weir HK, Carreira H, Harewood R, Spika D, Wang XS, et al. Global surveillance of cancer survival 1995-2009: analysis of individual data for 25,676,887 patients from 279 population-based registries in 67 countries (CONCORD-2). Lancet. 2015;385(9972):977–1010 Epub 2014/12/04.
63. Clark GM. Prognostic and Predictive Factors for Breast Cancer. Breast Cancer (Tokyo, Japan). 1995;2(2):79–89. Epub 1995/10/31.
64. Senkus E, Kyriakides S, Ohno S, Penault-Llorca F, Poortmans P, Rutgers E, et al. Primary breast cancer: ESMO clinical practice guidelines for diagnosis, treatment and follow-up. Ann Oncol. 2015;26(Suppl 5):v8–30 Epub 2015/09/01, Official journal of the European Society for Medical Oncology/ESMO.
65. Ly ALS, Dillon D. Prognostic factors for patients with breast cancer: traditional and new. Surg Pathol. 2012;5:775–85.
66. Blamey RW, Pinder SE, Ball GR, Ellis IO, Elston CW, Mitchell MJ, et al. Reading the prognosis of the individual with breast cancer. Eur J Cancer. 2007;43(10):1545–7 Epub 2007/02/27.
67. Ravdin PM, Siminoff LA, Davis GJ, Mercer MB, Hewlett J, Gerson N, et al. Computer program to assist in making decisions about adjuvant therapy for women with early breast cancer. J Clin Oncol. 2001;19(4):980–91 Epub 2001/02/22, Official Journal of the American Society of Clinical Oncology.
68. Soerjomataram I, Louwman MW, Ribot JG, Roukema JA, Coebergh JW. An overview of prognostic factors for long-term survivors of breast cancer. Breast Cancer Res Treat. 2008;107 (3):309–30 Epub 2007/03/23.
69. Holleczek B, Brenner H. Provision of breast cancer care and survival in Germany—results from a population-based high resolution study from Saarland. BMC Cancer. 2014;14:757 Epub 2014/10/12.
70. Allemani C, Sant M, Weir HK, Richardson LC, Baili P, Storm H, et al. Breast cancer survival in the US and Europe: a CONCORD high-resolution study. Int J Cancer J Int du Cancer. 2013;132 (5):1170–81 Epub 2012/07/21.
71. Subramaniam DS, Isaacs C. Utilizing prognostic and predictive factors in breast cancer. Curr Treat Options Oncol. 2005;6(2):147–59 Epub 2005/02/19.
72. Elston CW, Ellis IO. Pathological prognostic factors in breast cancer. I. The value of histological grade in breast cancer: experience from a large study with long-term follow-up. Histopathology. 1991;19(5):403–10 Epub 1991/11/01.
73. Bloom HJ, Richardson WW. Histological grading and prognosis in breast cancer; a study of 1409 cases of which 359 have been followed for 15 years. Br J Cancer. 1957;11(3):359–77 Epub 1957/09/01.
74. Kos Z, Dabbs DJ. Biomarker assessment and molecular testing for prognostication in breast cancer. Histopathology. 2016;68(1):70–85 Epub 2016/01/16.
75. Tinnemans JG, Beex LV, Wobbes T, Sluis RF, Raemaekers JM, Benraad T. Steroid-hormone receptors in nonpalpable and more advanced stages of breast cancer. A contribution to the biology and

natural history of carcinoma of the female breast. Cancer. 1990;66 (6):1165–7 Epub 1990/09/15.
76. Fisher B, Redmond C, Fisher ER, Caplan R. Relative worth of estrogen or progesterone receptor and pathologic characteristics of differentiation as indicators of prognosis in node negative breast cancer patients: findings from National Surgical Adjuvant Breast and Bowel Project Protocol B-06. J Clin Oncol. 1988;6(7):1076–87 Epub 1988/07/01, Official Journal of the American Society of Clinical Oncology.
77. Weigel MT, Dowsett M. Current and emerging biomarkers in breast cancer: prognosis and prediction. Endocr Relat Cancer. 2010;17(4):R245–62 Epub 2010/07/22.
78. Reed W, Hannisdal E, Boehler PJ, Gundersen S, Host H, Marthin J. The prognostic value of p53 and c-erb B-2 immunostaining is overrated for patients with lymph node negative breast carcinoma: a multivariate analysis of prognostic factors in 613 patients with a follow-up of 14–30 years. Cancer. 2000;88(4):804–13 Epub 2000/02/19.
79. Menard S, Balsari A, Casalini P, Tagliabue E, Campiglio M, Bufalino R, et al. HER-2-positive breast carcinomas as a particular subset with peculiar clinical behaviors. Clin Cancer Res. 2002;8 (2):520–5 Epub 2002/02/13, An official journal of the American Association for Cancer Research.
80. Toss A, Cristofanilli M. Molecular characterization and targeted therapeutic approaches in breast cancer. Breast Cancer Res: BCR. 2015;17:60 Epub 2015/04/24.
81. Coates AS, Winer EP, Goldhirsch A, Gelber RD, Gnant M, Piccart-Gebhart M, et al. Tailoring therapies-improving the management of early breast cancer: St Gallen International Expert Consensus on the Primary Therapy of Early Breast Cancer 2015. Ann Oncol. 2015;26(8):1533–46 Epub 2015/05/06, Official journal of the European Society for Medical Oncology/ESMO.
82. Hankinson S, Tamini R, Hunter D. Breast cancer. In: Adami HO, Hunter D, Trichopoulos D, editors. Textbook of cancer epidemiology. 2nd ed 2008.

Breast Cancer Screening

8

Ismail Jatoi

Breast cancer screening is a major public health issue. Although its potential impact on breast cancer mortality has received much attention, screening has also had a huge global impact on quality of life and healthcare expenditures. In this chapter, we will review the evidence with respect to breast cancer screening. Women who wish to consider breast cancer screening should be informed about not only its potential for benefit, but also its potential for harm.

Breast cancer screening has been one of the most controversial topics in modern medicine. For instance, there is considerable controversy as to what age breast cancer screening should begin (40 vs. 50 years of age), at what age it should stop, and even whether the overall benefits outweigh the risks. Although we generally associate breast cancer screening with mammography screening, there are several breast cancer screening methods available today, and it is important that we evaluate these critically and base screening recommendations on good evidence rather than assumptions. In our society, there is a deeply rooted belief that the early detection of cancer is invariably beneficial, and evidence to the contrary is often viewed with skepticism.

Over the years, a few investigators have steadfastly maintained that breast cancer is systemic at inception and that screening would have little impact on reducing mortality [1, 2]. Proponents of this paradigm argued that the early detection and timely extirpation of the primary breast tumor would not alter the natural history of the disease. Indeed, a prominent physician once argued that we were missing the forest (the systemic problem) because our efforts were primarily directed at the tree (the breast tumor) [3]. However, most clinicians never accepted this view. For many years, the prevailing view has been that breast cancer begins as a cell or clone of cells that multiply and grow in size [4]. At some point during the growth of this breast mass, metastasis occurs, and the resulting metastatic deposits lead to the death of the patient. This paradigm led to the belief that the early detection and treatment of breast cancer (before the onset of symptoms) could significantly reduce mortality. Therefore, considerable interest has focused on screening as a means of reducing breast cancer mortality.

Today, there are five breast cancer screening methods that are commonly utilized: mammography, clinical breast examination (CBE), breast self-examination (BSE), magnetic resonance imaging (MRI), and ultrasound [5]. Various studies have examined the efficacy of screening in reducing breast cancer mortality, and this chapter reviews these studies (Table 8.1). It is also important to note that breast screening programs target large, healthy (asymptomatic) populations, and very few women who undergo screening will actually be diagnosed with breast cancer. Thus, the potential risks of breast cancer screening must be weighed against its potential for benefit. The risks and benefits of breast cancer screening are emphasized in this chapter.

8.1 Cancer Screening Principles

Cancer therapy is generally directed toward patients who have symptoms. However, proponents of screening have long argued that the asymptomatic period in the natural history of cancer represents a "window of opportunity" for treatment [6]. The total preclinical phase (TPCP) refers to the period from the initiation of cancer to the onset of symptoms [7]. Generally, the beginning of the TPCP is not known. However, the detectable preclinical phase (DPCP) is a component of the TPCP and refers to the period when the cancer is detectable with a screening test. The starting point of the DPCP depends on the screening test used. A screening test that detects cancer very early in its natural history will be associated with a longer DPCP when compared with a test that detects it later. The sensitivity of a screening test refers to the proportion of patients with a disease who have a positive result (true positive rate); the

I. Jatoi (✉)
Division of Surgical Oncology and Endocrine Surgery, University of Texas Health Science Center, 7703 Floyd Curl Drive, Mail Code 7738, San Antonio, TX 78229, USA
e-mail: Jatoi@uthscsa.edu

I. Jatoi and A. Rody (eds.), *Management of Breast Diseases*, DOI 10.1007/978-3-319-46356-8_8

Table 8.1 Evidence of mortality benefit for the breast cancer screening modalities

Screening modality	Randomized controlled trials to assess mortality benefit		Significant reduction in breast cancer mortality
Mammography	HIP Malmo Two-country Stockholm	Gothenburg Edinburg CNBSS I CNBSS II UK age trial	25 % in women aged 50 and older (7–9 years of follow-up) 18 % in women aged 40–49 (>12 year of follow-up)
Breast self-examination (BSE)	St. Petersburg, Russia, Shanghai, China		No proven benefit
Clinical breast examination (CBE)	India		Results not yet available
Ultrasound	Japan		Results not yet available
Magnetic resonance imaging (MRI)			No randomized controlled trials to assess mortality benefit

HIP health insurance plan; *CNBSS* Canada national breast screening study

specificity of a test refers to the proportion of patients without the disease who have a negative result (true negative rate) [8]. A longer DPCP is associated with a more sensitive screening test. Prevalence refers to the total number of persons who have a disease at a particular time; incidence refers to the number of persons who develop a disease over a period [9]. In any screening program, the first screening round is referred to as the prevalent screen, and the cancers detected are known as the prevalent cancers. The number of cancers detected during the prevalent screen depends on the DPCP (i.e., a longer DPCP is associated with a greater number of prevalent cases). Following the prevalent screen, the subsequent screening rounds are known as the incident screens, and the cancers detected are referred to as the incident cancers. Cancers diagnosed between screening sessions generally present as symptomatic cases and are referred to as interval cancers [9]. Anderson et al. [9] showed that, as a group, the prevalent cancers generally have a more favorable tumor biology and better prognosis than cancers detected at the incident screens. The interval cancers generally have the worst prognosis [10].

Cole and Morrison argued that before the screening of any cancer was initiated, three conditions had to be met [7]. First, there must be effective treatment for the cancer, and the treatment must be more effective in screen-detected cases than in clinically detected cases. Obviously, if there is no available treatment for the cancer, then screening will provide no survival advantage. Additionally, if treatment is equally effective in screen-detected and clinically detected cases, then, again, screening will provide no survival advantage. Second, there should be a high prevalence among persons who undergo screening. A high prevalence is necessary to justify the expense of a screening program. Lastly, the cancer should have serious consequences (i.e., a high mortality rate or significant morbidity).

Many investigators believe that breast cancer meets the three conditions outlined by Cole and Morrison. Numerous studies have been undertaken to determine the efficacy of breast cancer screening in reducing mortality. However, before discussing these breast cancer screening studies, we must first consider the biases inherent in those studies. Three biases merit particular attention: lead time, length, and selection.

8.1.1 Lead-Time Bias

Screening detects cancers "early," but this alone cannot justify screening. Screening can only be justified if it prevents or delays the time of death from cancer. Survival refers to the period from diagnosis of cancer to death. "Lead-time bias" refers to the interval between the diagnosis of cancer by screening and by usual clinical detection [11]. As screening advances the time of breast cancer diagnosis, patients with screen-detected cancers will appear to have better survival rates than those with clinically detected cancers, even if screening does nothing to delay death. As a result of lead-time bias, screening may appear to prolong life, when it simply extends the period over which the cancer is observed. The effect of lead-time bias is illustrated in Fig. 8.1.

8.1.2 Length Bias

Slower growing cancers exist for a longer period in the preclinical phase and are more likely to be detected by screening. In contrast, faster growing tumors exist for a

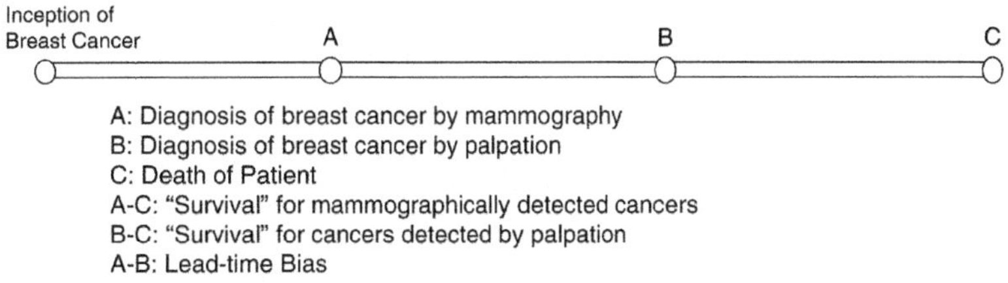

Fig. 8.1 Breast cancer timeline

shorter period in the preclinical phase and are more likely to be detected in the intervals between screening sessions. This phenomenon is termed length bias [12]. Indeed, we now know that there are differences in the biologic properties of the mammographically detected (screen-detected) breast cancers and those detected clinically. When histologic differentiation, tumor necrosis, mitotic counts, estrogen and progesterone receptors, histological type, DNA ploidy, and S-phase fraction are compared, the mammographically detected cancers are generally found to have a more favorable tumor biology [13].

8.1.3 Selection Bias

Women who are health conscious are more likely to volunteer for periodic breast cancer screening. In general, these women are more likely to eat nutritional foods, exercise regularly, and maintain a healthy lifestyle. As a result, volunteers have a lower mortality rate from all causes than women who do not volunteer for breast cancer screening. This is sometimes referred to as the healthy-screenee effect [14]. Thus, studies that compare volunteers for breast cancer screening with nonvolunteer controls are subject to a selection bias. The lower mortality of women who undergo screening might not necessarily be due to screening but due to other factors associated with healthy volunteers. The effect of selection bias was suggested in a case–control study from the UK. Moss et al. compared volunteers and nonvolunteers for breast cancer screening [15]. Women from two separate communities were compared. In one community, women had the opportunity to undergo periodic screening (screening district), whereas in the other community, no screening program was available (comparison district). These authors found that breast cancer mortality was higher among the nonvolunteers of the screening district compared with women in the comparison district. This difference in mortality was attributed to selection bias.

Various studies examined the efficacy of breast cancer screening: case–control, retrospective, and prospective; however, the best way to exclude the biases discussed here is to conduct randomized prospective clinical trials with all-cause mortality as the endpoint. Unfortunately, clinical trials that use all-cause mortality as the endpoint require huge numbers of subjects and are therefore not practical. Thus, the breast cancer screening trials have used cause-specific (breast cancer) mortality as a surrogate endpoint. These randomized prospective trials are discussed in the following sections.

8.2 Mammography Screening

The distinction between diagnostic mammography and screening mammography should be emphasized [16]. Diagnostic mammography is used to evaluate patients with breast symptoms (such as a breast lump). In contrast, mammography screening targets asymptomatic women. In this chapter, we consider the merits of mammography screening, and diagnostic mammography is discussed elsewhere in this book.

The concept of mammography screening for asymptomatic women has evolved over many years. Salomon, a surgeon, is credited with initiating mammography in 1913, using gross mastectomy specimens [17]. Subsequently, in 1930, Warren reported on the use of mammography in patients [18]. The concept of mammography screening for asymptomatic women was proposed by Gershon-Cohen et al. [19] in the 1950s. In the 1950s and 1960s, Gershon-Cohen et al. and Egan [20, 21] published reports indicating that mammography could detect impalpable cancers in asymptomatic women. Soon after, randomized prospective trials were initiated to determine the efficacy of mammography screening in reducing mortality from breast cancer.

Nine randomized prospective trials have examined the efficacy of mammography screening [22]. These are the health insurance plan (HIP) trial of New York, Swedish Two County, Gothenburg, Stockholm, Malmo, Edinburgh, Canadian National Breast Screening Study I (CNBSS I), CNBSS II, and the UK age trial. A total of about 661,000 women have been enrolled in these nine trials, and approximately 331,000 were below the age of 50 at the start of these trials.

There is considerable heterogeneity with respect to the design of these trials (Table 8.2). Some of the trials evaluated the efficacy of screening with mammography and CBE, whereas others evaluated the efficacy of screening with

Table 8.2 Characteristics of the randomized controlled trials of mammography screening

Trial	Entry years	Age at entry	Screening method	Randomization	Screening frequency	No. of women
HIP	1963–1969	40–64	2-view MM and PE	Individual	Annually, 4 rounds	60, 696
Malmo	1976–1986	45–69	1-or 2-view MM	Cluster: birth cohort	18–20 mo, 5 rounds	41, 478
Two-County	1977–1985	40–74	1-view MM	Cluster: geographic	24–33 mo, 4 rounds	133, 065
Stockholm	1981–1985	40–64	1-view MM	Cluster: birth cohort	28 mo, 2 rounds	59, 176
Gothenburg	1982–1988	40–59	2-view MM	Individual (age <50 year) Cluster (age >50 year)	18 mo, 4 rounds	49, 553
Edinburg	1978–1985	45–64	1-or 2-view MM and PE	Cluster: physician	24 mo, 4 rounds	54, 671
CNBSS I	1980–1987	40–49	2-view MM and PE	Individual: volunteer	Annually, 5 rounds	50, 430
CNBSS II	1980–1987	50–59	2-view MM and PE versus PE	Individual: volunteer	Annually 5 rounds	39, 405
UK age trial	1991–1997	40–41	2-view MM at first year; 1-view MM subsequently	Individual	Annually	160, 921

HIP health insurance plan; *CNBSS* Canada national breast screening study; *PE* physical exam; *MM* mammography

mammography alone. In some, mammography screening was undertaken with one view per breast, while other trials included two views per breast. The screening interval in these trials ranged from 12 to 33 months, and the ages of the women enrolled ranged from 39 to 74 years. Additionally, the randomization method varied (i.e., cluster or individual).

8.2.1 Health Insurance Plan Trial

The HIP trial was initiated in New York in 1963 and involved 60,696 women between the ages of 40 and 64 at entry [23]. Women were randomized either to undergo periodic screening or to receive usual medical care. Screening consisted of mammography and CBE. Analysis of the cancers detected by screening in the HIP trial revealed the following: 45 % were detected by CBE alone, 33 % by mammography alone, and 22 % by mammography and CBE. Thus, any reduction in breast cancer mortality in the screened group cannot be attributed to mammography alone. Indeed, any mortality reduction in the study group may also mean that CBE is an effective screening modality.

At 10-year follow-up, the HIP trial demonstrated a 29 % reduction in breast cancer mortality in the screened group [24]. This result also can be described in terms of a relative risk (RR) reduction (RR of 1.0 indicates no difference between the screened and control groups). Thus, after 10 years of follow-up, the RR of death from breast cancer in the study group was 0.71 (95 % confidence interval (CI), 0.55–0.93). The CI does not cross 1.0, indicating that the result is statistically significant.

There has been considerable interest in comparing the effect of screening in women who were below and above 50 years at the start of the trials [25]. If these two subsets are examined separately, differences emerge. In the HIP trial, at 10 years of follow-up, the RR of death from breast cancer for women below the age of 50 in the screened group was 0.77 (95 % CI, 0.50–1.16), whereas for those above age 50, it was 0.68 (95 % CI, 0.49–0.96). Thus, there was no significant benefit to screening women below age 50, but for those over age 50, periodic screening significantly reduced breast cancer mortality. With further follow-up to 18 years, however, the benefit of screening younger women in the HIP trial begins to approach statistical significance, with RR of death from breast cancer of 0.77 (95 % CI, 0.53–1.11) compared with controls. This trend is seen in other trials as well and is further discussed below.

8.2.2 Swedish Trials

Four randomized prospective trials on breast cancer screening were conducted in Sweden: the Two County (Kopparberg and Ostergotland), Malmo, Stockholm, and Gothenburg trials [26]. These trials were initiated between the years 1976 and 1982 and enrolled approximately 283,000 women between the ages of 40 and 74. In these trials, women were randomized either to undergo periodic screening with mammography alone or to receive usual care. CBE was used as a screening modality in the HIP, Edinburgh, and Canadian trials, but not in any of the Swedish trials.

In 1993, Nystrom et al. [26] published an overview of the four Swedish trials based on 5–13 years of follow-up. For women of all ages, a significant reduction in breast cancer mortality was seen in the screened group, with RR of 0.76 (95 % CI, 0.66–0.87). For women aged 40–49 at the start of the trials, however, there was an insignificant reduction in breast cancer mortality in the study group, with RR 0.87 (95 % CI, 0.63–1.20). In 1996, another overview was conducted, with an additional 4 years of follow-up [27]. In that overview, the benefit of screening for women aged 40–49 at the start of the Swedish trials approached statistical significance, with RR 0.77 (95 % CI, 0.59–1.01). A further follow-up overview of the Swedish trials was reported in 1997 by Hendrick et al. [28]. In that study, the RR of breast cancer death in the screened group was 0.71 (95 % CI, 0.57–0.89) for women aged 40–49 years at the start of the trials. Thus, with long-term follow-up, a statistically significant benefit to screening younger women finally emerges in the Swedish trials.

8.2.3 Edinburgh Trial

The Edinburgh randomized trial of breast cancer screening recruited 44,288 women between the ages of 45 and 64 from 1978 to 1981 [29, 30]. This initial recruitment included 11,391 women between the ages of 45 and 49 at entry (cohort one). Subsequently, an additional 10,383 women were recruited in two cohorts during the periods 1982–1983 (cohort two) and 1984–1985 (cohort three) [31]. Thus, the Edinburgh trial included a total of 54,671 women who were between the ages of 45 and 64 at the start of the study.

The design of the trial was similar to that of the HIP trial. Women were randomized either to undergo periodic screening with mammography and CBE or to receive usual care. For women of all ages, after 10 years of follow-up, the RR of death from breast cancer in the screened group was 0.82 (95 % CI, 0.61–1.11). For women below age 50 at entry, the RR was 0.78 (95 % CI, 0.46–1.31). Alexander et al. [31] reported the results of 14 years of follow-up for all women enrolled in the Edinburgh trial. The RR of death in the screened group, when compared with the control group, was 0.87 (95 % CI, 0.70–1.06). After adjusting for the socioeconomic status of the general medical practices from which the participants in the study were recruited, the rate ratio was 0.79 (95 % CI, 0.60–1.02).

8.2.4 Canadian Trials

The CNBSS consisted of two separate randomized prospective trials (CNBSS I and CNBSS II), both initiated in 1980 [32, 33]. The CNBSS I was specifically designed to assess the efficacy of screening women below age 50 and included 50,430 women between the ages of 40 and 49 at the start of this study. Women were randomized either to undergo periodic screening or to receive usual care. Screening consisted of annual mammography and CBE. After an average follow-up of 7 years, there was an insignificant excess in breast cancer mortality in the screened group, with RR 1.36 (95 % CI, 0.84–2.21). This insignificant excess in mortality persisted even after 10.5 years of follow-up, with RR 1.14 (95 % CI, 0.83–1.56).

The CNBSS II examined the efficacy of screening women who were between the ages of 50 and 59 at the start of the trial. The design of the CNBSS II study was different from that of the CNBSS I. Women were randomized to undergo either screening with annual mammography and CBE (study group) or CBE alone (control group). Surprisingly, after 7 years of follow-up, breast cancer mortality in the two groups was nearly identical, with the RR of death in the study group 0.97 (95 % CI, 0.62–1.52). Similar results were reported after 13 years of follow-up; the number of breast cancer deaths in the study and control groups was 107 and 105, respectively, and the cumulative rate ratio was 1.02 (95 % CI, 078–1.33) [34]. More recently, the twenty-five years of follow-up results of the Canadian National Breast Screening study were reported, and it was found that annual mammography screening did not reduce breast cancer mortality among women aged 40–59 [35]. These results might be interpreted to mean that mammography screening does nothing to reduce breast cancer mortality beyond that which can be achieved by screening with CBE alone when adjuvant therapy is freely available. The potential use of CBE as a screening method is discussed later in this chapter.

8.2.5 UK Age Trial

To further assess the efficacy of mammography screening for women aged 40–49, a randomized prospective trial was undertaken in the UK [36]. This trial involved 160,921 women, of whom, a third received annual screening invitations and two-thirds received usual care. Women were aged 40 or 41 at the start of the trial to ensure that all results were based solely on mammography screening in women before age 50. At 17 years of follow-up, there was no significant reduction in breast cancer mortality in the screened group, with the RR of death being 1.02 (95 % CI, 0.80–1.30) [37]. Thus, the results of this study are consistent with those of previous trials showing no significant benefit to mammography screening in younger women.

8.3 Overview (Meta-analyses) of the Mammographic Screening Trials

Several overviews (meta-analyses) of the mammography screening trials have been published. Many have focused on the results for women who were between the ages of 40 and 49 years at the start of the trials, but have not included the results of the recent UK age trial, which is unlikely to substantively change the conclusions of earlier meta-analyses. In 1995, Kerlikowske et al. [38] published a meta-analysis of the eight randomized controlled trials and four case–control studies on mammography screening that had been undertaken up to that point in time. This meta-analysis showed that, for women between the ages of 50 and 74 at the start of the studies, a significant reduction in breast cancer mortality was evident in the screened group after 7–9 years of follow-up, with RR 0.74 (95 % CI, 0.66–0.83). Longer follow-up did not alter the magnitude of this benefit. In contrast, for women between the ages of 40 and 49 at the start of these studies, the duration of follow-up did affect the risk of death from breast cancer. For these younger women, the RR of death from breast cancer in the screened group was 1.02 (95 % CI, 0.73–1.27) after 7–9 years of follow-up and 0.83 (95 % CI, 0.65–1.06) after 10–12 years of follow-up. That same year, Smart et al. reported a meta-analysis of all published and presented data on the eight mammographic screening trials [39]. For women in the screened group between the ages of 40 and 49 at the start of the trials, the RR of death from breast cancer was 0.84 (95 % CI, 0.69–1.02).

In 1996, an updated meta-analysis of the eight mammographic screening trials reported in Falun, Sweden [27]. In that study, the RR of death from breast cancer in the screened group for women aged 40–49 at entry was 0.85 (95 % CI, 0.71–1.01) compared with controls. The following year, Hendrick et al. [28] published a meta-analysis of the eight mammographic screening trials, with average follow-up time of 12.7 years. For women aged 40–49 at the start of the screening trials, a significant reduction in breast cancer mortality was seen in the screened group, the RR being 0.82 (95 % CI, 0.71–0.95). A subsequent meta-analysis demonstrated that screening mammography every 1–2 years in women 40–49 years of age results in a 15 % decrease in breast cancer mortality after 14 years of follow-up [RR, 0.85 (95 % CI, 0.73–0.99)] [40]. Thus, the various overviews indicate that a statistically significant benefit of screening younger women emerges with longer follow-up.

Clearly, these results indicate that the impact of mammography screening differs between younger and older women. For women who are over age 50 at the start of the screening trials, a significant reduction in breast cancer mortality is apparent after 7–9 years of follow-up, and longer follow-up does not change the magnitude of that benefit. In contrast, for women below age 50 at the start of the screening trials, the benefit of screening emerges gradually, with a significant reduction in breast cancer mortality appearing after 12 or more years of follow-up.

Gotzsche and Olsen scrutinized data from eight randomized controlled trials on mammography screening and argued that most of these trials were flawed (with the exception of the Canadian trials and the Malmo trial in Sweden) [41]. These authors reported discrepancies in the number of women randomized to the screened and control arms of the studies and also differences in the mean ages of women in the two arms of the studies. In their meta-analysis, the authors only included trials that they believed were adequately randomized, and concluded that mammography screening had no effect on breast cancer mortality (pooled RR 1.04, 95 % CI, 0.84–1.27). This review was widely criticized [42, 43]. In 2006, Gotzsche and Nielsen updated this controversial overview, and included six trials in their meta-analysis (two trials that they considered adequately randomized and four that were considered as having suboptimal randomization) [44]. In their updated overview, the authors concluded that mammography screening reduces breast cancer mortality by about 20 % (RR > 0.80, 95 % CI, 0.73–0.88). However, the authors pointed out that the risks of mammography screening were considerable. False-positive results were far more common than true positives, and many women who underwent mammography screening were likely "overdiagnosed" as having breast cancer ("overdiagnosis" is discussed later in this chapter).

A recent systematic review and meta-analysis of the US Preventive Services Task Force (USPSTF) reported RR of breast cancer mortality attributable to mammography screening of 0.92 for women aged 39–49 (95 % CI, 0.75–1.02), 0.86 for those aged 50–59 (CI, 0.68–0.97), 0.67 for those aged 60–69 (CI, 0.54–0.83), and 0.80 for those aged 70–74 (CI, 0.51–1.28) [45]. Thus, although mammography screening may reduce breast cancer mortality, the estimates are not statistically significant at all ages and the magnitudes of the effect are small.

8.4 Effect of Age on Mammographic Screening

The effectiveness of mammography screening for women aged 40–49 has been a topic of intense controversy for many years. Several medical organizations have further fueled this controversy by issuing guidelines on mammography screening that were at odds with one another [46]. Despite opposition from a few medical groups, mammography screening for younger women has been widely recommended in the USA. This is not necessarily the case in Europe, however. Indeed, for many years, the USA has stood alone among the major industrialized countries in encouraging mammography screening for women between the ages of 40 and 49. There are several possible reasons for the difference between the American and European positions on this issue [47]. For instance, the "fee for service" healthcare system in the USA may encourage the use of mammography screening for younger women. Additionally, the medico-legal climate in the USA may contribute to the greater willingness of American physicians to recommend mammography screening for women below age 50. Yet despite the widespread use of mammography screening for younger women in the USA, the US breast cancer mortality rates continue to mirror those of many industrialized countries that do not recommend screening for this age group [48].

Why does it take longer to see a benefit for women who are below age 50 at the start of the mammography screening trials? There are several possible explanations [49]. One possibility is that screening may detect very slow-growing (indolent) tumors in younger women. Thus, a reduction in breast cancer mortality may take longer to appear. Kerlikowske has argued, however, that if this is the case, then detecting these slow-growing tumors after age *50* perhaps could provide the same reduction in risk of breast cancer deaths [50]. Alternatively, screening might not be very effective in younger women. Indeed, the delayed benefit of screening younger women actually might be attributed to screening these women after the age of 50. This possibility was studied by de Koning et al. [51] using a computer simulation model known as MISCAN (microsimulation screening analysis). Their study suggested that most of the reduction in breast cancer mortality for women who were between the ages of 40 and 49 at the start of the screening trials was, in fact, the result of screening these women beyond the age of 50.

Another important question is why the effect of mammography screening is different for women below and above age 50. Some investigators have argued that there is no rational basis for the abrupt change in the effectiveness of mammographic screening at age 50 [52]. Yet age 50 corresponds approximately to the age of the menopause, and the biology and epidemiology of breast cancer differ in premenopausal and postmenopausal women [53]. There is a steep rise in breast cancer incidence until about age *50,* followed by a less rapid increase after that age [54]. We have pointed out that there are important qualitative age interactions with respect to the etiology, prognosis, and treatment of breast cancer, and these interactions may suggest that breast cancers in younger and older women are different diseases, derived from different pathways [55]. A qualitative age interaction is defined as the reversal of RRs or rates according to age at diagnosis. Once thought rare, qualitative age interactions are commonly reported in studies that examine the etiology, prognosis, and treatment of breast cancer [56]. For instance, nulliparity, obesity, and oral contraceptives decrease breast cancer risk in younger women but increase risk in older women [50]. Additionally, high-risk tumors are common in younger women, whereas low-risk tumors are more common in the elderly, with bimodal peak frequencies at ages 50 and 70, respectively. By this we mean that premenopausal women have a higher proportion of larger tumors (>2 cm), node-positive tumors, and estrogen receptor-negative tumors than do postmenopausal women [55, 57]. Therefore, the results of the mammography screening trials are consistent with the results of other studies showing differences in the biology and epidemiology of breast cancers in younger and older women. Baines has drawn attention to the "mortality paradox" associated with mammography screening in younger women [58]. Baines points out that, during the initial years of follow-up, many of the screening trials actually show an increased number of deaths associated with mammography screening in younger women, with a decrease in the number of deaths evident after longer follow-up. In contrast, mammography screening in older women is associated with an immediate reduction in mortality.

Why might mammography screening be less effective in premenopausal women than in postmenopausal women? This question cannot be answered with any degree of certainty at the present time, but several possibilities should be considered. As screening advances the time of breast cancer diagnosis and allows for the early initiation of therapy, one might speculate that postmenopausal women benefit more from early therapy than do premenopausal women. Another possibility is that the sensitivity of mammography might be lower in premenopausal women, making it less effective as a screening test. Finally, Tabar et al. [59] suggested that tumors of premenopausal women grow more rapidly than those of postmenopausal women. In fact, the incidence of interval cancers (diagnosed between screening sessions) appears to be greater in premenopausal than in postmenopausal women. Thus, Tabar et al. suggest that reducing the interval between screening sessions (from 2 to 1 year) may improve the efficacy of mammographic screening for younger women.

8.4.1 Mammography Screening in Elderly Women

Much interest centers on the optimal age for initiation of mammography screening (40 vs. 50), while the upper age limit for screening has received less attention. Although organizations in the USA may recommend mammography screening for women aged 70 and older, little data support these recommendations [60]. Analysis of data from the Swedish trials might be interpreted to mean that mammography screening for women over age 70 is not effective [61]; however, meaningful conclusions cannot be drawn because few women over age 70 were included in these trials. Because a woman's risk of developing breast cancer increases with age, the efficacy of mammography screening for older women remains an important issue. Using a mathematical model (the Markov model), Kerlikowske et al. [62] studied the effect of mammography screening in older women. Their analysis suggests that mammography screening after age 69 is moderately cost-effective and results in a small gain in life expectancy for women with high bone mineral density (BMD) but is more costly in those with low BMD. These investigators calculated that, to prevent one death, either 1064 women with high BMD or 7143 women with low BMI, would need to be screened routinely from ages 69 to 79. Clearly, the risks and benefits of mammography screening should be weighed carefully before recommending it for older women. The risks of screening are discussed later in this chapter.

Of the nine randomized trials that have examined the efficacy of mammography screening, only the Swedish Two County trial included women 70 years and older (women were aged 40–74 at entry), but participation in this age group was low and a subgroup analysis found no mortality benefit for those aged 70–74 at entry [26]. Indeed, it seems unlikely that older women would benefit significantly from mammography screening, and the harms (discussed later in this chapter) may outweigh any potential small benefits [63]. In particular, the risk of overdiagnosis (discussed later in this chapter) is quite substantial in older women, and this may increase the risk of mortality from unnecessary treatments [63]. Moreover, in the population, it takes approximately 10 years for the mortality benefit of mammography screening to emerge, and because older women have an increased risk of death from other causes, few would be expected to benefit from such a delayed effect of screening [64]. Also, the benefits of screening diminish as treatments improved (discussed later in this chapter), and in this era of modern effective adjuvant systemic therapy, mammography screening is unlikely to provide any added benefit in the elderly [65].

8.5 Screening Breast Ultrasound

Breast ultrasound (sonography) is primarily used to evaluate specific abnormalities discovered either on CBE or mammography. However, in recent years, there has been growing interest in the use of screening ultrasound as a supplement to mammography screening for women at increased risk for breast cancer and for those with dense breasts [66]. It has been suggested that ultrasound screening might be indicated for women with dense fibroglandular breast tissue, where the sensitivity of mammography is diminished. The American College of Radiology Imaging Network (ACRIN) conducted a large prospective evaluation of mammography screening and ultrasound in approximately 2809 women who were at increased risk for breast cancer and had heterogeneously dense or extremely dense breast parenchyma in at least one breast quadrant [67]. In this study, screening with mammography and ultrasound was associated with a 55 % increased breast cancer detection rate when compared to screening with mammography alone. However, the addition of screening ultrasound was associated with a substantial increase in the number of false-positive results. To date, the impact of screening ultrasound on breast cancer mortality is not known. A large-scale randomized controlled trial is now underway in Japan to assess the impact of screening with both mammography and ultrasound on breast cancer mortality [68]. In the Japan Strategic Anti-cancer Randomized Trial (J-START), 72,998 asymptomatic women aged 40–49 were randomly assigned to undergo screening mammography and ultrasonography (intervention group) versus screening mammography alone (control) twice in two years between 2007 and 2011 [69]. Recently reported results indicate that sensitivity was significantly higher in the intervention versus the control group, but specificity was lower [69]. Longer follow-up will be required to determine whether screening ultrasonography has any impact in reducing breast cancer-specific mortality.

8.6 Screening Breast MRI

Several nonrandomized prospective studies have evaluated annual MRI screening (in conjunction with mammography screening) for women at increased risk for developing breast cancer [70]. These studies have been undertaken in several countries throughout the world. Women who participated in these studies were BRCA 1 and BRCA 2 mutation carriers and others with a strong family history of breast cancer. In several of these studies, women were also sometimes screened with mammography, breast ultrasound, and/or CBE. These studies showed that the sensitivity of MRI ranged from 77 to 100 %, while the sensitivity of mammography or ultrasound ranged from 16 to 40 %. Although the sensitivity of MRI is greater than that of mammography, its specificity is lower. Kriege et al. [71] reported that the specificity of MRI was 88 % compared to 95 % for mammography. Furthermore, there are no data indicating whether or not the improved sensitivity of MRI screening translates to a greater reduction in breast cancer mortality. In April 2007, the American cancer society (ACS) issued guidelines for the use of MRI as an adjunct to mammography in breast cancer screening [72]. The ACS panel recommended breast MRI screening for BRCA mutation carriers, first-degree relatives of known BRCA mutation carriers who have not undergone genetic testing, women who have received radiation treatment to the chest, such as for Hodgkin's disease, and women with an approximately 20–25 % or greater lifetime risk of breast cancer.

8.7 Screening by Clinical Breast Examination

CBE can be used either for screening (detecting cancers in asymptomatic women) or for diagnosis (evaluating breast complaints). Screening by CBE differs from screening by BSE in that it requires the use of trained personnel. Since the advent of mammography screening, the role of CBE as a screening modality has diminished. Indeed, there is evidence to suggest that the increased use of mammography screening in the USA generally has been accompanied by a decline in the use of CBE as a screening modality [73]. Yet several influential medical organizations, such as the American College of Radiology, the ACS, and the American Medical Association, recommend screening with CBE in addition to mammography [74]. It is also important to note that about 5–10 % of all breast cancers are detectable by CBE but not by mammography [74]. Although the impact of screening by CBE on breast cancer mortality has not been fully elucidated, it seems premature to abandon screening by CBE. Furthermore, screening programs should train their personnel to perform proper CBE.

CBE readily detects cancers larger than 1 cm [75]. Additionally, in the US breast cancer detection and demonstration project (BCDDP), 39 % of mammographically detected cancers smaller than 1 cm also were detectable by CBE [76]. Mittra et al. [75] suggested that careful screening by CBE would fail to detect in situ cancers and 22 % of the mammographically detected invasive cancers smaller than 1 cm. They argued that this advantage of mammography over CBE is not likely to be clinically significant.

A large randomized prospective trial was initiated in the Philippines in the late 1990s to assess the impact of screening CBE on breast cancer mortality [77]. Women were randomized to receive either a combination of screening by CBE and instructions on the technique of breast self-examination or usual care. Women were aged 35–64 at entry, and a total of 404,947 women were randomized (216,884 of these to the intervention arm and 188,063 to the control arm). Five rounds of screening were planned at intervals of 1–2 years, and the primary endpoint of the study was mortality. However, the study was terminated in December 1997 (after the first screening round) because of poor compliance among the screen-positive women (many women with abnormalities detected on CBE declined further investigations or treatment).

It should be noted that four of the mammography screening trials have also included CBE as a screening modality: HIP, Edinburgh, and the Canadian NBSS I and II [25, 30, 33, 34]. The results of these four trials suggest that screening with CBE can effectively detect breast cancers. Barton et al. [78] calculated that screening by CBE has a sensitivity of approximately 54 % and a specificity of about 94 %.

In the HIP trial, women were randomized to screening with mammography and CBE or no screening [25]. This study was conducted during the early years of the development of mammography, and a disproportionately large number of cancers were detected by CBE. Overall, in the HIP trial, 67 % of the cancers in the screened population were detected by CBE. Of these, *45 %* were detected by CBE alone and 22 % by CBE and mammography. Only 33 % of the cancers were detected by mammography alone. In the HIP trial, age seemed to influence the effectiveness of CBE in detecting breast cancer. For women aged 50–59, 40 % of the cancers were detected by CBE alone and 42 % by mammography alone; however, for women aged 40–49, CBE was much more effective in detecting tumors than mammography, with 61 % of cancers detected by CBE alone and 19 % by mammography alone. Thus, CBE might have contributed much to the reduction in breast cancer mortality observed in the screened group of the HIP trial.

In the Edinburgh trial, women were randomized to screening with mammography and CBE or no screening [30]. In that study, 74 % of the cancers in the screened group were detected by CBE, with 3 % detected by CBE alone and 71 % by mammography and CBE. Mammography alone detected 26 % of the cancers in the screened population. Thus, the Edinburgh trial also suggests that screening by CBE is effective in detecting cancers.

In the CNBSS I, women aged 40–49 were randomized to either screening with mammography and CBE or no screening [33]. The results of the CNBSS I trial are consistent with those of other trials, showing no benefit to screening younger women during the first 7–9 years of follow-up. In the CNBSS II, women aged 50–59 at entry were randomized to either screening with CBE alone or CBE and mammography [34]. While other trials showed a benefit to mammography screening for this age group, the CNBSS II found that it provided no survival advantage. This result might be interpreted to mean that mammography screening contributes nothing to breast cancer mortality reduction beyond that achievable with screening with CBE alone when adjuvant systemic therapy is freely available. In the CNBSS, CBE detected *59 %* of the cancers in women aged 40–49. Of these, 32 % were detected by CBE alone and 27 % by CBE and mammography. For women aged 50–59, 44 % of the cancers were detected by CBE, with 18 % detected by CBE alone and 26 % detected by CBE and mammography. The results of the CNBSS are therefore consistent with those of the HIP trial, indicating that screening by CBE is more effective in detecting cancers of younger women.

Although screening by CBE is effective in detecting breast cancer, its impact on breast cancer mortality is not known. If screening by CBE could reduce breast cancer mortality, it might be particularly useful in developing countries, where mammography screening is not affordable and breast cancer mortality rates are rising. As mentioned previously, a large trial to assess the efficacy of screening CBE on breast cancer mortality was initiated in the Philippines in the late 1990s, but terminated because of poor compliance [77]. However, another large trial was initiated in India in 1998 under the direction of Dr. Indraneel Mittra [79]. In the Indian trial, 120,000 women between the ages of 30–60 were randomized to either an intervention arm (consisting of screening CBE, teaching of screening BSE, and visual inspection of the cervix by trained female health workers), or usual care. The women randomized to the intervention arm received screening every 18 months for 6 years, with total follow-up period of 10 years. Mittra et al. [80] have reported significant downstaging of tumors in the screening arm of the trial. A similar downstaging of breast cancers were reported in a cluster randomized controlled trial initiated in the Trivandrum district in Kerala, India, in 2006 [81]. This trial included 115, 652 women aged 30–69 randomized to screening CBE or no screening.

Mittra et al. [75] have argued that there is also a need for a clinical trial whereby women are randomized to either receive screening with mammography or CBE. They have argued that there is compelling evidence to indicate that screening with CBE is a potentially effective screening modality, and that a direct comparison with screening mammography is therefore warranted.

8.8 Screening by Breast Self-examination

Screening by BSE has been advocated since the early part of the twentieth century [82]. Today, it is widely promoted by various medical societies, breast cancer advocacy groups, and the media as an effective screening tool (generally in conjunction with mammography screening). Many hospitals and clinics throughout the USA sponsor classes where women are taught BSE techniques. BSE is a very appealing screening method because it is inexpensive, self-generated, and nonintrusive. Yet its efficacy in reducing breast cancer mortality has never been demonstrated.

Two randomized controlled trials have examined the efficacy of screening by BSE on breast cancer mortality. The first of these was the World Health Organization trial of BSE undertaken in St. Petersburg, Russia [83]. Women in this study were recruited from 1985 to 1989. There were 57,712 women from 14 randomly selected outpatient hospitals who were taught BSE. Another 64,759 women from another 14 outpatient hospitals served as controls. Semiglazov et al. [83] reported the preliminary results of this trial in 1992. The number of breast cancers detected in the two arms of the study was nearly identical (190 cases in the BSE group and 192 in the control group), and there was no significant difference in mortality between the two groups. Additionally, no significant differences were found between the two groups with respect to the size of the primary tumor or incidence of nodal metastasis. Of note, the BSE-trained group had a higher number of excisional biopsies for benign lesions, the RR being *1.5* in the BSE group compared with controls (95 % CI, 1.1–1.9). Semiglazov et al. [84] reported a further update of this study in 1999 and again found no significant difference in the death rates between the BSE and control groups.

Another BSE trial was initiated in Shanghai, China, between 1989 and 1991 [85]. In that trial, 267,040 women were randomly assigned on the basis of work sites (520 textile factories) to receive either intensive BSE instruction (study group) or sessions on the prevention of low back pain (control group). After *5* years of follow-up, the number of breast cancer cases and the rate of breast cancer mortality were nearly identical in the two groups. Yet there was more than a twofold increase in the number of breast biopsies in the BSE group compared with the control group.

A meta-analysis of the Russian and Shanghai trials was reported by Kosters and Gotzsche [79] from the Nordic Cochrane Center. There was no statistically significant difference in breast cancer mortality between the BSE screening and control groups, RR 1.05 (95 % CI, 0.90–1.24). However, almost twice as many breast biopsies with benign results were performed in the BSE groups when compared to the controls groups, RR 1.88 (95 % CI, 1.77–1.99). Thus, screening by BSE is not without risk. There is evidence that it can generate considerable anxiety among women. Furthermore, false-positive and false-negative results may incur considerable costs and risks.

8.9 The Impact of Advances in Therapy on the Efficacy of Screening

Improvements in breast cancer therapy might be diminishing the benefit of breast cancer screening [65]. The historical overview of the nine mammography screening trials seems to support this notion. The HIP trial of New York, initiated in 1963, showed that mammography screening reduced breast cancer mortality by about 30 %, but none of the subsequent mammography screening trials has matched those results, despite improvements in breast imaging technology [65]. The three most recent trials (Canadian National Breast Screening Studies I and II, and the UK age trial) found no benefit to mammography screening at all [35, 37]. Two factors likely account for the diminishing benefit of screening. First, there has been an increase in breast cancer awareness which, over time, has resulted in smaller tumors in the control arms of the screening trials. For example, it has been reported that the average tumor size in the control arm of the Swedish Two County trial was 2.8 cm, while it was only 1.9 cm in the more recent Canadian trials [65]. Secondly, and perhaps more importantly, it is likely that improvements in therapy have substantially reduced the benefit of screening. Breast cancer adjuvant systemic therapy was implemented in the 1980s and was freely available to patients enrolled in the Canadian National Breast Cancer Screening Study I and II and the UK Age trials, but not in the earlier mammography screening trials. The failure of mammography screening to show any benefit in these three more recent trials may at least partly be attributable to the availability of adjuvant systemic therapy for women enrolled in those trials.

The benefit of cancer screening is closely intertwined with the benefit of cancer therapy [65]. For screening to be effective, the benefit of screen-detected cancers must be more effective than that of clinically detected cancers. If breast cancer were curable at every clinical stage or, alternatively, if therapy were ineffective, then screening would offer no advantage. Moreover, as therapy improves, both the relative and absolute benefits of screening will decline. Thus, advances in breast cancer therapy would be expected to reduce the effectiveness of breast cancer screening. Consider, for example, a situation where mammography screening reduces the risk of breast cancer death from 40 to 30 % over a 20-year period (a relative benefit of 25 % and an absolute benefit of 10 %). Now let us also assume that an adjuvant therapy regimen with a relative benefit of 20 % becomes available. Patients who receive this therapy would lower their risk of breast cancer death from 40 to 32 % over a 20-year period. The effect of screening should now be considered in the context of a 32 % risk of death over a 20-year period, and screening (if we assume that its relative benefit remains constant at 25 %) would lower the risk of death from 32 to 24 %. Thus, prior to the advent of this particular adjuvant therapy regimen, the absolute benefit of screening would have been 10 %, but after its introduction, the absolute benefit of screening would decrease to 8 %.

However, the relative benefit of screening will also diminish with improvements in therapy. Consider three categories of breast cancer patients: those curable only with screening, those curable with clinical detection, and those who cannot be cured with either screening or clinical detection. Improvements in therapy will increase the number of patients curable following clinical detection, by decreasing the numbers curable only with screening or not curable at all. Thus, the relative benefit of screening will decrease.

8.10 Potential Hazards of Screening

The randomized controlled trials discussed in this chapter indicate that mammography screening can reduce breast cancer mortality by about 25 % in postmenopausal women. Additionally, screen-detected cancers are generally smaller than those detected clinically and are therefore more amenable to treatment with conservative surgery (i.e., lumpectomy, quadrantectomy, or segmental resection) than cancers detected clinically. Furthermore, breast MRI might be a particularly useful screening tool for women at high risk for breast cancer (such as mutation carriers), because its sensitivity is greater than that of mammography.

Yet there are certain hazards associated with breast cancer screening. Five potentially harmful consequences of screening merit consideration: lead time, false-positives, radiation exposure, overdiagnosis, and cost (Table 8.3).

Table 8.3 Potential hazards of screening

Lead time	Advanced notice of a cancer diagnosis without tangible gain
Radiation exposure (mammography)	Possible increased risk of breast cancer in patients susceptible to the effects of low-dose radiation
False-positives	Results in unnecessary breast biopsies
Overdiagnosis	Adverse financial/emotional consequences of being falsely labeled as a cancer patient
Cost	Costs of breast cancer screening may divert resources away from more mundane healthcare needs

8.10.1 Lead Time

Screening advances the time of breast cancer diagnosis, but this does not benefit all women. The randomized controlled trials indicate that mammography screening in postmenopausal women reduces breast cancer mortality by about 25 %. Thus, for most women, advancing the time of breast cancer diagnosis by mammography screening does not change the outcome. As a result of screening, many women are simply given advanced notice of a cancer diagnosis with no tangible gain. This "lead time" effect of screening (in the absence of any tangible benefit) may have an adverse impact on quality of life.

8.10.2 False-Positives

False-positives are cases that are reported as suspicious or malignant on screening that, on further evaluation (such as a breast biopsy), prove benign. False-positives have an adverse effect on quality of life and result in additional healthcare expenditures. For mammography screening, the false-positive rate is much greater in the USA than in Europe, perhaps because of the fear of litigation in the USA, resulting in a greater unwillingness of American radiologists to commit themselves to a benign diagnosis [86].

Elmore et al. [87] calculated that, after ten mammograms, a woman in the USA has about a 49 % cumulative risk of a false-positive result. Overall, approximately 10.7 % of all screening mammograms in the USA lead to a false-positive result. For women between the ages of 40–49, the cumulative risk is about 56 %, whereas for those aged 50–79, the cumulative risk of a false-positive result after ten mammograms is about 47 %. In contrast, the cumulative 10-year risk of a false-positive mammogram in the Norwegian Breast Cancer Screening program is about 21 % [88].

Evidence from the CNBSS II suggests that there are fewer false-positives associated with screening by CBE [76]. In that study, women aged 50–59 were randomized to either screening with CBE or screening with mammography and CBE. No significant difference was found in the mortality between the two arms of the study. The rate of biopsy of benign breast lumps was 3 times higher with combined screening, however, compared with screening with CBE alone.

One study found that women are generally aware that mammography screening can produce false-positive results [89]. The study also indicated that most women consider false-positives an acceptable consequence of mammography screening and are willing to tolerate such results. Indeed, the survey found that 63 % of all women thought that 500 or more false-positives per life saved were reasonable, and 37 % were willing to tolerate as many as 10,000 false-positives per life saved. Yet analyses of data from the US national health interview survey (NHIS) indicate that false-positive mammograms have an adverse effect on the quality of life [90]. In this random sampling of the US population, women who had previously experienced false-positive mammograms were more likely to report symptoms of anxiety and depression.

8.10.3 Radiation Exposure

Bailar was one of the first to suggest that low-dose radiation exposure from mammography screening might induce breast cancer [91]. Subsequently, Beemsterboer et al. [92] developed a computer simulation model to estimate breast cancer deaths caused from exposure to low-dose radiation and the number of lives saved as a result of mammography screening. These estimates were based on data from the Swedish mammography screening trials and the Netherlands breast cancer screening program. In their model, the ratio between the number of breast cancer deaths prevented with those induced as a result of mammography screening for women aged 50–69 was 242:1, assuming a 2-year screening interval and a mean glandular dose of 4 mGy to each breast from a two-view mammogram. When mammography screening was expanded to include women aged 40–49, the ratio was 97:1. Thus, according to this model, the potential hazards of low-dose radiation are greatly increased if mammography screening is initiated below age 50.

Swift et al. [93] called attention to the potential hazards of mammography screening in carriers of the gene for ataxia-telangiectasia (AT). These carriers are at increased risk for developing breast cancer after exposure to relatively low doses of radiation. Approximately 1.4 % of all individuals are heterozygote carriers of the gene for AT, so the population potentially at risk from the harmful effects of low-dose radiation is large. Identifying these persons before mammography screening would be a huge, expensive undertaking and is probably not feasible. The amount of radiation required to induce breast cancer in a heterozygote carrier of the gene for AT is not clear. Some investigators speculate that a total dose of 20 mGy would be required [94]. If so, a carrier of the AT gene who undergoes mammography screening every 2 years might accumulate a hazardous dose of ionizing radiation over a 10-year period, assuming a mean glandular dose of 4 mGy to each breast from a two-view mammogram.

Women who carry mutations in the *BRCA1* and *BRCA2* genes have an increased risk of developing breast cancer. Over the years, medical organizations have recommended that BRCA 1 and BRCA 2 mutation carriers begin annual mammography screening at the age of 25–30 [95]. These recommendations did not consider, however, the potential hazards of low-dose radiation associated with mammography screening. The *BRCA 1* and *BRCA2* genes are required for DNA repair, and it has been suggested that women who carry mutations in these genes might be very sensitive to the effects of low doses of radiation [96, 97]. The cumulative lifetime risk of radiation-induced breast cancer mortality is higher in younger women, and a study suggests that there is no net benefit for mammography screening in BRCA mutation carriers who are younger than age 35 [98]. These concerns make breast MRI a particularly attractive screening option for young women who carry the BRCA 1 or BRCA 2 mutation. In contrast to mammography, there is no radiation exposure associated with MRI screening.

8.10.4 Overdiagnosis

During the last 30 years, breast cancer incidence in the USA has increased dramatically, partly because of the impact of "overdiagnosis" attributable to mammography screening. Peeters and colleagues defined overdiagnosis as "a histologically established diagnosis of intraductal or invasive cancer that would never have developed into a clinically manifest tumor during the patient's normal life expectancy if no screening examination had been carried out" [99]. Long-term follow-up of the Malmo screening trial suggests that about a quarter of the breast cancers detected with mammography screening represent overdiagnosis [100]. A recent study suggests that, in the USA, nearly one-third of all breast cancers would never have been diagnosed in the absence of mammography screening [101]. This alarming rate of overdiagnosis may have an adverse effect on quality of life and it may even adversely impact mortality. Indeed, overdiagnosis of breast cancer with mammography screening exposes women to the risk of unnecessary treatments and this may produce a small excess in treatment-related mortality.

To understand how screening might result in the overdiagnosis of invasive breast cancer, consider the following hypothetical situation. A 65-year-old woman with severe coronary artery disease undergoes routine mammography screening. As a result of that screening, an occult (nonpalpable) invasive breast cancer is discovered. This cancer is treated with surgery, radiotherapy, and tamoxifen. One year later, this patient dies of a myocardial infarction (MI). As mammography screening advances the time of breast cancer diagnosis by about 2–4 years, this patient's breast cancer probably would not have been discovered without screening. She probably would have died of a MI, never knowing that she had breast cancer and would have been spared the treatments resulting from her cancer diagnosis. This example illustrates how screening might unmask invasive cancers that would not have become clinically symptomatic or pose a threat to a woman's normal life expectancy. Zahl et al. [102] suggested that some of the occult invasive breast cancers detected by mammography screening might ultimately have undergone spontaneous regression.

However, an even greater problem associated with mammography screening is the overdiagnosis of noninvasive (in situ) cancers [103]. Since the advent of mammography screening, the incidence of ductal carcinoma in situ (DCIS) has increased dramatically [104]. DCIS is rarely palpable and therefore seldom detected by clinical examination. Most cases of DCIS are diagnosed by mammography screening. Indeed, before the advent of mammography screening, DCIS accounted for only 1–2 % of all breast cancer cases in the USA [105]. In more recent years, DCIS has accounted for more than 12 % of all breast cancer cases and about 30 % of those discovered mammographically [106].

Many clinicians have long assumed that DCIS is a preinvasive cancer that, if left untreated, invariably progresses to invasive breast cancer. This assumption was based on two observations. First, after simple excision of DCIS, recurrences often occur, many of which are invasive breast cancers. Second, DCIS often is adjacent to invasive breast cancer, suggesting that DCIS was the precursor to the invasive tumor. Evidence now suggests, however, that most cases of DCIS would not progress to manifest breast cancers clinically during a woman's lifetime. Nielsen et al. [107] reported the results of 110 medico-legal autopsies performed at the Fredericksburg Hospital in Copenhagen, Denmark. These autopsies were performed on women who had died of accidents. DCIS was found incidentally in 15 % of these women, a prevalence of 4–5 times greater than the number of overt cancers expected to develop over a 20-year period. Additionally, in two separate studies, Rosen et al. [108] and Page et al. [109] retrospectively reviewed benign breast biopsies and found numerous instances where the initial pathologist overlooked DCIS. In both studies, only about 25 % developed clinically manifest invasive breast cancers after 15–18 years of follow-up. Finally, in women with a previous diagnosis of breast cancer, Alpers and Wellings found DCIS in about 48 % of contralateral breasts at autopsy, but only about 12.5 % of these women would be expected to develop contralateral breast cancer over a 20-year period [110]. Together, these studies suggest that perhaps only one of every four or five cases of DCIS detected mammographically would progress to a clinically manifest breast cancer during a woman's lifetime.

8.10.5 Cost

Healthcare resources are often limited, particularly in developing countries. Ideally, these resources should be distributed equitably across a wide range of healthcare programs to obtain the maximum benefit. Again, it is important to emphasize that women who are invited to participate in breast cancer screening programs are not "patients" and most do not become patients. Yet breast cancer screening programs often use expensive technology. Resources directed toward maintaining breast cancer screening programs could lower resources available for more pressing and mundane healthcare programs, adversely affecting the health of an entire community. To put this matter into perspective, Kattlove et al. [111] estimated, in 1995, the cost of potentially saving one life over a 10-year period with mammography screening. For women aged 40–49, the estimated cost of screening was considerably higher when compared to the cost of screening for women aged 50–59, which in turn was higher than the cost for women aged 60–69. If healthcare resources are limited, then age should be considered when deciding how best to appropriate scarce resources. Additionally, it is important to consider that the cost-effectiveness of CBE screening for breast cancer in developing countries such as India may compare favorably with that of mammography screening in the developed countries [112].

8.11 Conclusion

More is known about screening for breast cancer than for any other type of cancer. In this chapter, the commonly used breast cancer screening methods were discussed. These are mammography, CBE using trained personnel, BSE, ultrasound, and MRI. Randomized controlled trials indicate that mammography screening in postmenopausal women can reduce breast cancer mortality by about 25 %; however, its effect in premenopausal women is disputed. To date, no data are available from randomized prospective trials comparing the effect of screening by CBE with no screening on breast cancer mortality. However, several mammography screening trials incorporated CBE as a screening modality, and the results of these trials suggest that CBE might be an effective screening tool. A large, randomized, prospective study has been initiated in India to study this possibility further. Thus far, data from two large, randomized, prospective trials indicate that screening with BSE has no effect in reducing breast cancer mortality.

In the lay media, considerable emphasis is placed on the potential benefits of breast cancer screening, and little attention is paid to its potential risks. Women who volunteer for breast cancer screening are generally healthy, and the vast majority will derive no tangible gain from screening. Many women seem to be poorly informed about the impact of screening on their risk of dying of breast cancer. Black et al. [113] surveyed 200 women between the ages of 40 and 50 with no history of breast cancer and found that these women overestimated their probability of dying of breast cancer by more than 20-fold and the effectiveness of screening in reducing mortality by sixfold. Thus, a more balanced presentation about breast cancer risk and the effectiveness of screening is warranted. Not only should the potential for benefit be discussed with each woman prior to screening, but the potential risks outlined as well.

Yet it is also important to note that several recent studies have suggested that breast cancer screening has contributed to declines in population-based breast cancer mortality rates [114, 115]. Inequalities in the use of screening (as well as differences in the effectiveness of screening) might also partly account for the widening racial disparity in breast cancer mortality rates in the USA [116]. Clearly, a closer scrutiny of population-based statistics is needed to better discern the overall impact of breast cancer screening.

References

1. MacDonald I. Biological predeterminism in human cancer. Surg Gynecol Obstet. 1951;92:443–52.
2. Black MM, Speer FD. Biological variability of breast carcinoma in relation to diagnosis and therapy. NY State J Med. 1953;53:1560–3.
3. Devitt JE. Breast cancer: have we missed the forest because of the tree? Lancet. 1994;344:734–5.
4. Haagensen CD. Diseases of the breast. Philadelphia: WB Saunders; 1956.
5. Jatoi I. Breast cancer screening. Am J Surg. 1999;177:518–24.
6. Jatoi I. Breast cancer: a systemic or local disease? Am J Clin Oncol. 1997;20:536–9.
7. Cole P, Morrison AS. Basic issues in population screening for cancer. J Natl Cancer Inst. 1980;64:1263–72.
8. Nielsen C, Lang RS. Principles of screening. Med Clin North Am. 1999;83:1323–37.
9. Anderson TJ, Lamb J, Alexander F, et al. Comparative pathology of prevalent and incident cancers detected by breast cancer screening: Edinburgh breast screening project. Lancet. 1986;1:519–23.
10. Gilliland FD, Joste N, Stauber PM, et al. Biologic characteristics of interval and screen-detected breast cancer. J Natl Cancer Inst. 2000;92:743–9.
11. Xu IL, Prorok PC. Non-parametric estimation of the post-lead-time survival distribution of screen-detected cancer cases. Stat Med. 1995;14:2715–25.
12. Black WC, Welch HG. Advances in diagnostic imaging and overestimation of disease prevalence and the benefits of therapy. N Engl J Med. 1993;328:1237–43.
13. Kiemi PJ, Joensuu H, Toikkanen S, et al. Aggressiveness of breast cancers found with and without screening. Br Med J. 1992;304:467–9.
14. Schmidt JG. The epidemiology of mass breast cancer screening—a plea for a valid measure of benefit. J Clin Epidemiol. 1990;43:215–22.
15. Monsees BS, Destouet JM. A screening mammography program: staying alive and making it work. Radiol Clin North Am. 1992;30:211–9.
16. Hurley SF, Kaldor JM. The benefits and risks of mammographic screening for breast cancer. Epidemiol Rev. 1992;14:101–30.

17. Salomon A. Beitrage zur pathologie und klinik der maminacrcinome. Arch f klin Chir. 1913;101:573–668.
18. Warren SL. A roentgenologic study of the breast. Am J Roentgenol. 1930;24:113–24.
19. Gershon-Cohen I, Ingleby H, Moore L. Can mass X-ray surveys be used in detection of early cancer of the breast? JAMA. 1956;161:1069–71.
20. Gershon-Cohen I, Hermel MB, Berger SM. Detection of breast cancer by periodic X-ray examinations. JAMA. 1961;176: 1114–6.
21. Egan RL. Mammography, an aid to diagnosis of breast carcinoma. JAMA. 1962;182:839–43.
22. Fletcher SW, Black W, Harris R, et al. Report of the international workshop on screening for breast cancer. J Natl Cancer Inst. 1993;85:1644–56.
23. Shapiro S, Venet W, Strax P, et al. Ten-to fourteen-year effect of screening on breast cancer mortality. J Natl Cancer Inst. 1982;69:349–55.
24. Eddy DM, Hasselblad V, McGivney W, et al. The value of mammography screening in women under age 50 years. JAMA. 1988;259:1512–9.
25. Shapiro S, Venet W, Strax P, et al. Periodic screening for breast cancer: the health insurance plan project and its Sequelae, 1963–1986. Baltimore: Johns Hopkins University; 1988.
26. Nystrom L, Rutqvist LE, Wall S et al. Breast cancer screening with mammography: overview of Swedish randomized trials. Lancet. 1993;34(l):973–8.
27. Organizing Committee and Collaborators. Breast cancer screening with mammography in women aged 40–49 years: report of the Organizing Committee and Collaborators, Falun Meeting, Falun, Sweden (21 and 22 March 1996). Int J Cancer. 1996;68:693–9.
28. Hendrick RE, Smith RA, Rutlege JH, et al. Benefit of screening mammography in women aged 40–49: a new meta-analysis of randomized controlled trials. Monogr Natl Cancer Inst. 1997;22:87–92.
29. Alexander FE, Anderson TI, Brown H, et al. The Edinburgh randomised trial of breast cancer screening: results after 10 years of follow-up. Br J Cancer. 1994;70:542–8.
30. Alexander FE. The Edinburgh randomized trial of breast cancer screening. Monogr Natl Cancer Inst. 1997;22:31–5.
31. Alexander FE, Anderson TI, Brown HK, et al. 14 years of follow-up from the Edinburgh randamised trial of breast cancer screening. Lancet. 1999;353:1903–8.
32. Miller AB, Baines CI, To T, et al. Canadian national breast screening study I. Breast cancer detection and death rates among women aged 40 to 49 years. Can Med Assoc J. 1992;147:1459–76.
33. Miller AB, Baines CJ, To T, et al. Canadian national breast screening study II. Breast cancer detection and death rates among women aged 50 to 59 years. Can Med Assoc J. 1992;147:1477–88.
34. Miller AB, To T, Baines CI, Wall C. Canadian national breast screening study-2: 13-year results of a randomized trial in women aged 50–59 years. J Natl Cancer Inst. 2000;92:1490–9.
35. Miller AB, Wall C, Baines CJ, Sun P, To T, Narod SA. Twenty five year follow-up for breast cancer incidence and mortality of the Canadian National Breast Screening Study: randomised screening trial. Br Med J. 2014;348:g366.
36. Mosss SM, Cuckle H, Evans A, Johns L, Waller M, Bobrow L. Trial management group. Effect of mammographic screening from age 40 years on breast cancer mortality at 10 years' follow-up: a randomized controlled trial. Lancet. 2006;368 (9552):2053–60.
37. Moss SM, Wale C, Smith R, Evans A, Cuckle H, Duffy SW. Effect of mammographic screening from age 40 years on breast cancer mortality in the UK Age trial at 17 years' follow-u: a randomised controlled trial. Lancet Oncology. 2015;16:1123–32.
38. Kerlikowske K, Grady D, Rubin SM, et al. Efficacy of screening mammography. A meta-analysis. JAMA. 1995;273:149–54.
39. Smart CR, Hendrick RE, Rutledge JH III, et al. Benefit of mammography screening in women ages40 to 49 years: current evidence from randomized controlled trials. Cancer. 1995; 75:1619–25.
40. Humphrey LL, Helfand M, Chan BK, Woolf SH. Breast cancer screening: a summary of the evidence for the U.S. preventive services task force. Ann Intern Med. 2002;137:347–60.
41. Gotzsche PC, Olsen O. Is screening for breast cancer with mammography justifiable? Lancet. 2000;355:129–34.
42. Duffy SW, Tabar L. Screening mammography re-evaluated. Lancet. 2000;355:747–8.
43. Dean PB. Final comment. The articles by Gotzsche and Olsen are not Official Cochrane reviews and lack scientific merit. Lakartidningen. 2000;97:3106.
44. Gotzsche PC, Nielsen M. Screening for breast cancer with mammography. Cochrane Database Syst Rev. 2006;(4): CD001877.
45. Nelson HD, Fu R, Cantor A, Pappas M, Daeges M, Humphrey L. Effectiveness of breast cancer screening: systematic review and meta-analysis to update the 2009 U.S. preventive services task force recommendation. Ann Intern Med. 2016;164(4):1–12.
46. Jatoi I. The case against mammographic screening for women in their forties. In: Jatoi I, editor. Breast cancer screening. Austin: Landes Biosciences; 1997. p. 35–49.
47. Jatoi I, Baum M. American and European recommendations for screening mammography in younger women: a cultural divide? RMJ. 1993;307:1481–3.
48. Davis DL, Love SM. Mammographic screening. JAMA. 1994;271:152–3.
49. Fletcher SW. Breast cancer screening among women in their forties: an overview of the issues. Monogr Natl Cancer Inst. 1997;22:5–9.
50. Kerlikowske K. Efficacy of screening mammography among women aged 40 to 49 years and 40 to 69 years: comparison of relative and absolute benefit. Monogr Natl Cancer Inst. 1997;22:79–86.
51. de Koning HJ, Boer R, Warmerdam PG, et al. Quantitative interpretations of age-specific mortality reductions from the Swedish breast cancer screening trials. J Nati Cancer Inst. 1995;87:1217–23.
52. Kopans DB. The case in favor of mammographic screening for women in their forties. In: Jatoi I, editor. Breast cancer screening. Austin: Landes Biosciences; 1997. p. 9–34.
53. Elwood JM, Cox B, Richardson AK. The effectiveness of breast cancer screening by mammography in younger women. Online J Curr Clin Trials. 1993 (Doc No. 32).
54. Clemmensen J. Carcinoma of the breast: results from statistical research. Br J Radiol. 1948;21:583.
55. Jatoi I, Anderson WF, Rosenberg PS. Qualitative age-interactions in breast cancer: a tale of two diseases? Am J Clin Oncol. 2008;31:504–6.
56. Willett W. Nutritional epidemiology. New York: Oxford University; 1990.
57. Henderson IC. Biologic variations of tumors. Cancer. 1992;69:1888–95.
58. Baines CJ. Mammography screening: are women really giving informed consent? J Natl Cancer Inst. 2003;95(20):1512–3.
59. Tabar L, Fagerberg G, Day NE, et al. What is the optimum interval between mammographic screening examinations? An analysis based on the latest results of the Swedish two-county breast cancer screening trial. Br J Cancer. 1987;55:547–51.

60. Leitch AM, Dodd GD, Constanza M, et al. American cancer society guidelines for the early detection of breast cancer: update 1997. CA Cancer J Clin. 1997;47:150–3.
61. Larsson LG, Nystrom L, Wall S, et al. The Swedish randomized mammography screening trials. J Med Screen. 1996;3:129–32.
62. Kerlikowske K, Salzmann P, Phillips KA, et al. Continuing screening mammography in women aged 70 to 79 years: impact on life expectancy and cost-effectiveness. JAMA. 1999; 282:2156–63.
63. Jatoi I, Miller AB. Breast cancer screening in elderly women: primum non nocere. JAMA Surgery. 2015;150(12):1107–8.
64. Jatoi I, Miller AB. Why is breast cancer mortality declining? Lancet Oncology. 2003;4:251–4.
65. Jatoi I. The impact of advances in treatment on the efficacy of mammography screening. Prev Med. 2011;53:103–4.
66. Kuhl CK. The "coming of age" of nonmammographic screening for breast cancer. JAMA. 2008;299(18):2203–5.
67. Berg WA, Blume JD, Cormack JB. Combined screening with ultrasound and mammography vs mammography alone in women at elevated risk of breast cancer. JAMA. 2008;299(18): 2151–63.
68. Tohno E, Ueno E, Watanabe H. Ultrasound screening of breast cancer. Breast Cancer. 2009;16(1):18–22.
69. Ohuchi N, Suzuki A, Sobue T, et al. Sensitivity and specificity of mammography and adjunctive ultrasonography to screen for breast cancer in the Japan Strategic Anti-cancer Randomized Trial (J-START): a randomised controlled trial. Lancet. 2016;387:341–8.
70. Jatoi I, Anderson WF. Management of women who have a genetic predisposition for breast cancer. Surg Clin North Am. 2008;88(4):845–61.
71. Kriege M, Brekelmans CT, Boetes C, et al. Efficacy of MRI and mammography for breast cancer screening in women with a familial or genetic predisposition. N Engl J Med. 2004;351 (5):427–37.
72. Saslow D, Boetes C, Burke W, et al. American cancer society guidelines for breast screening with MRI as an adjunct to mammography. CA Cancer J Clin. 2007;57(2):75–89.
73. Bums RB, Freund KM, Ash AS, et al. As mammography use increases, are some providers omitting clinical breast examination? Arch Intern Med. 1996;156:741–4.
74. Saslow D, Hannan J, Osuch J, et al. Clinical breast examination: practical recommendations for optimizing performance and reporting. CA Cancer J Clin. 2004;54:327–44.
75. Mittra I, Baum M, Thornton H, et al. Is clinical breast examination an acceptable alternative to mammographic screening? BMJ. 2000;321:1071–3.
76. Report of the Working Group to review the National Cancer Institute-American Cancer Society breast cancer detection demonstration projects. J Nati Cancer Inst. 1979;62:639–709.
77. Pisani P, Parkin DM, Ngelangel C, Esteban D, et al. Outcome of screening by clinical examination of the breast in a trial in the Philippines. Int J Cancer. 2006;118(1):149–54.
78. Barton MB, Harris R, Fletcher SW. Does this patient have breast cancer? The screening clinical breast examination: should it be done? How? JAMA. 1999;282:1270–80.
79. Kosters JP, Gotzsche PC. Regular self-examination or clinical examination for early detection of breast cancer. Cochrane Database Syst Rev. 2003;2(CD003373). doi:10.1002/14651858. CD003373.
80. Mittra I, Mishra GA, Singh S, et al. A cluster randomized, controlled trial of breast and cervix cancer screening in Mumbai, India: methodology and interim results after three rounds of screening. Int J Cancer. 2010;126:976–84.
81. Sankaranarayanan R, Ramadas K, Thara S, et al. Clinical breast examination: preliminary results from a cluster randomized controlled trial in India. J Natl Cancer Inst. 2011;103:1–5.
82. Adair FE. Clinical manifestations of early cancer of the breast—with a discussion on the subject of biopsy. N Engl J Med. 1933;208:1250–5.
83. Semiglazov VF, Moiseyenko VM, Bavli JL, Migmanova N, et al. The role of breast self-examination in early breast cancer detection (results of the 5-year USSR/WHO randomized study in Leningrad). Eur J Epidemiol. 1992;8(4):498–502.
84. Semiglazov VF, Moiseyenko VM, Manikhas AG, Protsenko SA, Kharikova RS, Ivanow VG, et al. Role of breast self-examination in early detection of breast cancer: Russia/WHO prospective randomized trial in St. Petersburg. Cancer Strategy. 1999;1:145–51.
85. Thomas DB, Gao DL, Ray RM, Wang WW, Allison CJ, Chen FL, et al. Randomized trial of breast self-examination: final results. J Natl Cancer Inst. 2002;94(19):1445–57.
86. Fletcher SW, Elmore JG. False-positive mammograms—can the USA learn from Europe? Lancet. 2005;365:7–8.
87. Elmore JG, Barton MB, Moceri VM, et al. Ten-year risk of false-positive screening mammograms and clinical breast examinations. N Engl J Med. 1998;338:1089–96.
88. Hofvind S, Thorsen S, Tretli S. The cumulative risk of a false-positive recall in the Norwegian breast cancer screening program. Cancer. 2004;101:1501–7.
89. Schwartz LM, Woloshin S, Sox HC, et al. U.S. women's attitudes to false-positive mammography results and detection of ductal carcinoma in situ: cross sectional survey. BMJ. 2000;320:1635–40.
90. Jatoi I, Zhu K, Shah M, Lawrence W. Psychological distress in U. S. women who have experienced false-positive mammograms. Breast Cancer Res Treat. 2006;101:191–200.
91. Bailar JC. Mammography: a contrary view. Ann Intern Med. 1976;84:77–84.
92. Beemsterboer PM, Warmerdam PG, Boer R, et al. Radiation risk of mammography related to benefit in screening programmes: a favourable balance? J Med Screen. 1998;5:81–7.
93. Swift M, Morrell D, Massey RB, et al. Incidence of cancer in 161 families affected by ataxia-telangiectasia. N Engl J Med. 1991;325:1831–6.
94. Werneke U. Ataxia telangiectasia and risk of breast cancer. Lancet. 1997;350:739–40.
95. Robson M, Offit K. Clinical practice. Management of an inherited predisposition to breast cancer. N Engl J Med. 2007;357(2):154–62.
96. Vaidya JS, Baum M. Benefits and risks of screening mammography in women with BRCA1 and BRCA2 mutations. JAMA. 1997;278:290.
97. Pijpe A, Andrieu N, Easton DF, et al. Exposure to diagnostic radiation and risk of breast cancer among carriers of BRCA ½ mutations: retrospective cohort study (GENE-RAD-RISK). Br Med J. 2012;345:1–15.
98. de Gonzalez AM, Berg CD, Visvanathan K, Robson M. Estimated risk of radiation-induced breast cancer from mammographic screening for young BRCA mutation carriers. J Natl Cancer Inst. 2009;101:205–9.
99. Peeters PH, Verbeek AL, Straatman H, et al. Evaluation of over-diagnosis of breast cancer in screening with mammography: results of the Nijmegen programme. Int J Epidemiol. 1989;18:295–9.
100. Zackrisson S, Andersson I, Janzon L, Manjer J, Garne JP. Rate of over-diagnosis of breast cancer 15 years after end of Malmo mammographic screening trial: follow-up study. Br Med J. 2006;332(7543):689–92.

101. Bleyer A, Welch HG. Effect of three decades of screening mammography on breast cancer incidence. N Engl J Med. 2012;367:1998–2005.
102. Zahl P, Maehlen J, Welch HG. The natural history of invasive breast cancers detected by screening mammography. Arch Intern Med. 2008;168(21):2311–6.
103. Jatoi I, Baum M. Mammographically detected ductal carcinoma in situ: are we overdiagnosing breast cancer? Surgery. 1995;118:118–20.
104. Welch HG, Woloshin S, Schwartz LM. The sea of uncertainty surrounding ductal carcinoma in situ—the price of screening mammography. J Natl Cancer Inst. 2008;100(4):228–9.
105. Moore MM. Treatment of ductal carcinoma in situ of the breast. Semin Surg Oncol. 1991;7:267–70.
106. Emster VL, Barclay J, Kerlikowske K, et al. Incidence of and treatment for ductal carcinoma in situ of the breast. JAMA. 1996;275:913–8.
107. Nielsen M, Thomsen JL, Primdahl S, et al. Breast cancer and atypia among young and middle aged women: a study of 110 medicolegal autopsies. Br J Cancer. 1987;56:814–9.
108. Rosen PR, Braun DW Jr, Kinne DE. The clinical significance of pre-invasive breast carcinoma. Cancer. 1980;46:919–25.
109. Page DL, Dupont WD, Rogers LW, et al. Intraductal carcinoma of the breast: follow-up after biopsy only. Cancer. 1982;49:751–8.
110. Alpers CE, Wellings SR. The prevalence of carcinoma in situ in normal and cancer-associated breasts. Hum Pathol. 1985;16: 796–807.
111. Kattlove H, Liberati A, Keeler B, et al. Benefits and costs of screening and treatment for early breast cancer: development of a basic benefit package. JAMA. 1995;273:142–8.
112. Okonkwo QL, Draisma G, der Kinderen A, Brown ML, de Koning HJ. Breast cancer screening policies in developing countries: a cost-effectiveness analysis for India. J Natl Cancer Inst. 2008;100:1290–300.
113. Black WC, Nease RF, Tosteson AN. Perceptions of breast cancer risk and screening effectiveness in women younger than 50 years of age. J Natl Cancer Inst. 1995;87:720–31.
114. Berry DA, Cronin KA, Plevritis SK, et al. Effect of screening and adjuvant therapy on mortality from breast cancer. N Engl J Med. 2005;353(17):1784–92.
115. Jatoi I, Chen BE, Anderson WF, Rosenberg PS. Breast cancer mortality trends in the United States according to estrogen receptor status and age at diagnosis. J Clin Oncol. 2007;25 (13):1683–90.
116. Jatoi I, Anderson WF, Rao SR, Devesa SS. Breast cancer trends among black and white women in the United States. J Clin Oncol. 2006;23(31):7836–41.

Breast Imaging

9

Anne C. Hoyt and Irene Tsai

9.1 Introduction

Mammography can be divided into two basic types: *screening* and *diagnostic*. Screening mammography continues to be the primary imaging modality for breast cancer screening and diagnosis. Diagnostic mammography is indicated in the imaging evaluation of a patient with a breast symptom. The introduction of digital mammography and, more recently, digital breast tomosynthesis (DBT) ranks as the most important technologic improvements in breast imaging. 97 % of all certified mammography facilities in the USA utilize digital imaging, and 29 % offer DBT, according to certification statistics from the US Food and Drug Administration (FDA) as of July 1, 2016. Advances in the overall quality of mammography performance are related to the efforts of programs established by both professional societies and government agencies. Introduction of the American College of Radiology (ACR) Mammography Accreditation Program in 1987 [1] and the Mammography Quality Standards Act in 1994 [2] are among the most significant of these efforts. In addition, the ACR breast imaging reporting and data system (BI-RADS) continues to improve the communication of mammography results, monitoring and tracking of patients and quality assurance activities, such as the medical audit [3]. Owing to its importance and now widespread international use, the BI-RADS-standardized lexicon should be understood by referring physicians and will be used throughout this chapter. The latest 5th edition of BI-RADS includes breast ultrasound and magnetic resonance imaging (MRI) [3].

Ultrasonography is the most important adjunctive imaging modality for mammography. Like mammography, ultrasonography also has undergone significant technical improvements that have extended its contributions to breast imaging. Other imaging modalities include breast MRI and radionuclide imaging. Advances in imaging-guided breast biopsy techniques led to the widespread use of stereotactic- and ultrasound-guided breast core needle biopsy (CNB) as the primary methods for breast biopsy.

9.2 Mammography

9.2.1 Screening Mammography

Screening mammography is an examination of an asymptomatic woman to detect clinically occult breast cancer. The standard screening examination includes two views of the breast: a mediolateral oblique (MLO) and a craniocaudal (CC) (Fig. 9.1) [4]. Screening mammography is the most studied examination of all screening tests. The effectiveness of screening mammography for mortality reduction from breast cancer has been confirmed by evaluations of randomized clinical trials (RCTs) [5]. While there is a general agreement that screening mammography reduces mortality from breast cancer in women over 50 years of age, there has been considerable debate over the effectiveness of screening mammography for women aged 40–49 [6]. Despite the controversy, 1 in 6 breast cancers occur in women age 40–49, 18 % of all breast cancer deaths occur among women diagnosed in their 40s, 27 % of all *person-years of life lost* (PYLL) are among women diagnosed between ages 40 and 49, and 70 % of women who died from breast cancer in their 40s at major Harvard teaching hospitals were among the 20 % of women who were not screened [7, 8]. A comprehensive study of the effectiveness of population-based service screening of women aged 40–49 years found a 29 % mortality reduction for women who attended screening [9].

A.C. Hoyt (✉)
Department of Radiological Sciences, UCLA, 200 UCLA Medical Plaza, RM. 165-53, Los Angeles, CA 90095, USA
e-mail: hoyt@mednet.ucla.edu

I. Tsai
Department of Radiological Sciences, UCLA, 200 UCLA Medical Plaza, Suite 165-47, Box #956952, Los Angeles, CA 90095, USA
e-mail: itsai@mednet.ucla.edu

I. Jatoi and A. Rody (eds.), *Management of Breast Diseases*, DOI 10.1007/978-3-319-46356-8_9

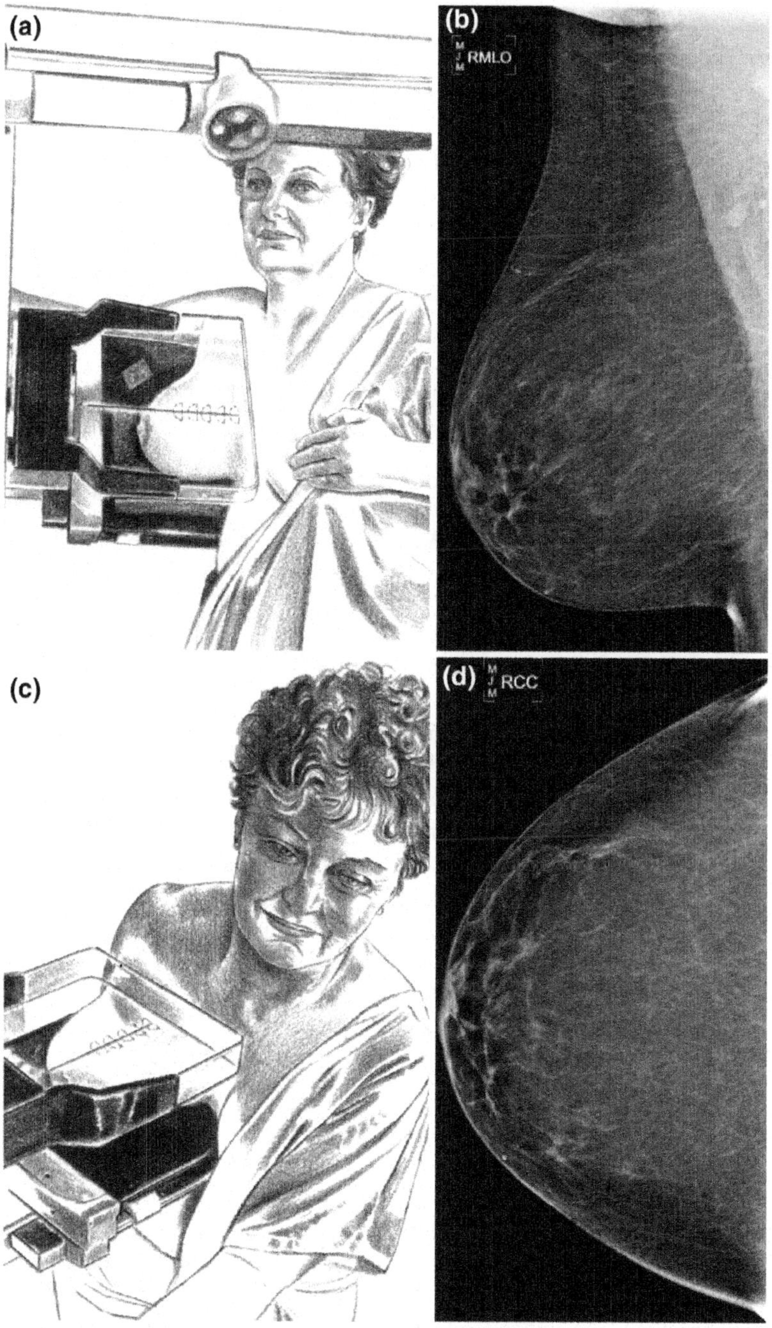

Fig. 9.1 Screening mammograms. **a** Positioning for the right mediolateral oblique (MLO) projection. **b** Right full-field digital mammography MLO image. **c** Positioning for the right craniocaudal (CC) view. **d** Right full-field digital mammography CC image

Organized service screening in 7 Swedish counties proved that the reductions in breast cancer mortality were principally due to mammography screening rather than advancements in treatment [10]. In this large trial that included approximately 33 % of the population of Sweden, outcomes were compared pre- and post-screening and then outcomes were compared among women exposed to screening and among women unexposed to screening. There was a significant reduction in mortality after the introduction of screening compared to the prescreening era. Mortality reduction was 40–45 % among women actually screened compared to 30 % in the *invited* population that includes women both exposed and unexposed to screening. The breast carcinomas cases were contemporaneously diagnosed and treated and were thus not affected by advancements in therapy over time. Therefore, most of the mortality reduction in screened counties after the introduction of screening could only be attributed to the availability of mammography screening.

Mammography screening has been shown to decrease breast cancer mortality across many study designs including randomized control trials, case–control studies, incidence-based mortality studies, and computer-based screening service models. When analyzing different study types, distinguishing between the relative mortality reduction between women *invited to screen* and women who actually underwent screening mammography is critical. **Randomized controlled studies** compare women invited to screening (not women actually screened) with those not invited. Thus, deaths from breast cancer in women invited to screening but not attending mammography count against the screened group (noncompliance). Similarly, women who are invited to screening but who choose to undergo mammography and avoid a breast cancer death due to earlier detection are counted in the unscreened group (contamination) [11, 12]. When compared to other study designs and actual clinical practice, RCTs underestimate the benefit of screening mammography due to noncompliance and contamination. Meta-analyses of RCTs show an 18–22 % mortality reduction in those *invited to screen* compared to the control group (*not invited to screen*) [13–17]. In contrast, **case–control studies** show mortality reductions of 31 % (invited to screen) [18] and 48–49 % (screened) [18, 19]. **Incidence-based mortality studies** show mortality reductions of 25 % (invited to screen) and 38 % (screened) [18]. Canadian and European **service screening studies** show a 38–40 % reduction in breast cancer mortality among women actually screened [18, 20]. **Computer-based studies** (CISNET) show mortality reduction of 40 % [21, 22].

Current screening guidelines for average-risk women vary among the major organizations (Table 9.1). All agree that screening mammography beginning at age 40 and performed annually saves the most lives. In addition, all organizations agree that benefits outweigh harms at all ages and informed decision making including and understanding of the benefits and limitations of screening is essential. However, the differences in recommendations reflect the different values that each group places on the relative importance of benefits and potential harms of screening mammography such as a false-positive mammogram (call-back), benign biopsy, potential overdiagnosis, and/or anxiety. The American College of Radiology (ACR), Society of Breast Imaging (SBI), National Comprehensive Cancer Network (NCCN), and American College of Obstetrics and Gynecology (ACOG) recommend annual mammography screening beginning at age 40. The American Cancer Society guidelines, updated in 2015, now recommend annual mammography for women of ages 45–54 with the opportunity to start annual screening between the ages 40–44, biennial or annual mammography for women 55 and older, and for screening to continue as long is the patient is able and life expectancy is more than 10 years. The age to begin screening was selected by the ACS based upon the 5-year absolute risk of breast cancer, which is similar in women aged 45–49 and women aged 50–54, but greater than the risk in women aged 40–44. The traditional comparison of 10-year age-groups (age 40–49 vs. age 50–59) obscured the change in disease burden that begins closer to age 45 rather than age 50 [23]. The United States Preventative Task Force (USPSTF) released new recommendations regarding breast cancer screening in 2016. The USPSTF recommends biennial screening for women aged 50–74. The decision to screen women aged 40–49 should be individualized. "For women in their 40s, the benefit still outweighs the harms, but to a smaller degree; this balance may therefore be more subject to individual values and preferences than it is in older women. Women who place a higher value on the potential benefit than the potential harms may choose to begin screening between the ages of 40 and 49" [24]. The USPSTF suggests screening continue until age 74. They

Table 9.1 2016 breast cancer screening guidelines

Organization	Age to begin	Screening interval	Stopping age
ACR, ACOG, NCCN, NCBC	40	Annual	ACR: Continue screening as long as health is good and life expectancy is at least 5–7 years, and there is willingness to undergo additional testing ACOG: Shared decisions 75 + NCCN: Consider comorbidity and therapeutic decisions
ACS, ASBS, ASCO	45, with option to begin at age 40	Annual 40–54; biennial 55+ with option to continue annually	Continue screening as long as health is good and life expectancy is at least 10 years
USTFPF, AAFP, ACP	50, the decision to begin screening between ages 40 and 49 should be individualized based on the risk and values	Biennial, 40+	74, insufficient evidence to recommend for or against screening

Source Modified from Smith RA. Guidelines for Breast Cancer Screening: A Rosetta Stone for Radiologists. Los Angeles Radiologic Society Summer Seminar in Breast Imaging; 2016 July 16

ACR American College of Radiology, *ACOG* American Congress of Obstetrics and Gynecology, *NCCN* National Comprehensive Cancer Network, *NCBC* National Consortium of Breast Centers, *ACS* American Cancer Society, *ASBS* American Society of Breast Surgeons, *ASCO* American Society of Surgical Oncology, *USPSTF* United States Preventative Services Task Force, *AAFP* American Academy of Family Physicians, ACP American College of Physicians cite a lack of sufficient evidence to recommend for or against screening mammography in women 75 and older.

The widespread use of mammography in the USA led to the detection of smaller, earlier stage tumors. This resulted in revision of the American Joint Committee on Cancer (AJCC) staging system for breast cancer [25]. Since most cancers were being detected at Stage 1 (invasive tumors ≤2 cm), the AJCC subdivided Stage 1 into these subcategories: (1) Tis: carcinoma in situ (preinvasive), (2) T1mic: microinvasion ≤1 mm, (3) T1a: >1–5 mm, (4) T1b: >5 mm–1 cm, and (5) T1c: >1–2 cm. The Chair of the Committee made this statement: "The need for substantial changes in the staging system for breast cancer stemmed from continuing developments in breast cancer diagnosis and management. First, with the widespread use of screening mammography, most breast tumors are now first detected when they are very small…"

9.2.2 Diagnostic Mammography

Diagnostic mammography, sometimes called problem-solving mammography, is indicated when there are clinical findings such as a palpable lump, localized pain, nipple discharge, or an abnormal screening mammogram that requires additional workup [26]. The diagnostic examination involves a complete workup tailored to a symptomatic patient or one with abnormal findings on a screening examination.

Diagnostic mammograms should always be performed when a biopsy is being considered for a palpable lump in a woman 30 years or older. The purpose of mammography prior to the biopsy is to better define the nature of the clinical abnormality and to find unexpected lesions, including multifocal carcinoma or intraductal component of an invasive carcinoma. The diagnostic mammogram could also reveal that the finding is benign and does not require a biopsy. An example of the latter would be a typical fibroadenoma or an area of fat necrosis due to the previous surgery. To correlate the clinical and imaging findings, a marker (e.g., radiopaque "BB" or other) is often placed over the area of clinical concern prior to performing the mammogram (Fig. 9.2a). The diagnostic workup may include additional views of the breast, spot compression and/or magnification techniques, tomosynthesis views, correlative clinical breast examination, and ultrasonography (Fig. 9.2b). With some exceptions, a radiologist should be on site to supervise the performance of a diagnostic examination and should discuss the results directly with the patient at the conclusion of the examination.

9.2.3 Digital Breast Tomosynthesis

DBT was approved for clinical use in conjunction with conventional digital mammography by the US Food and Drug Administration (FDA) in 2011. In DBT, the breast is positioned and compressed in the same manner as conventional digital mammography. However, instead of a single exposure, multiple very low-dose projection images are obtained while the X-ray tube moves through an arc of 10°–20°. The total dose of all of the projection images is essentially the same as a

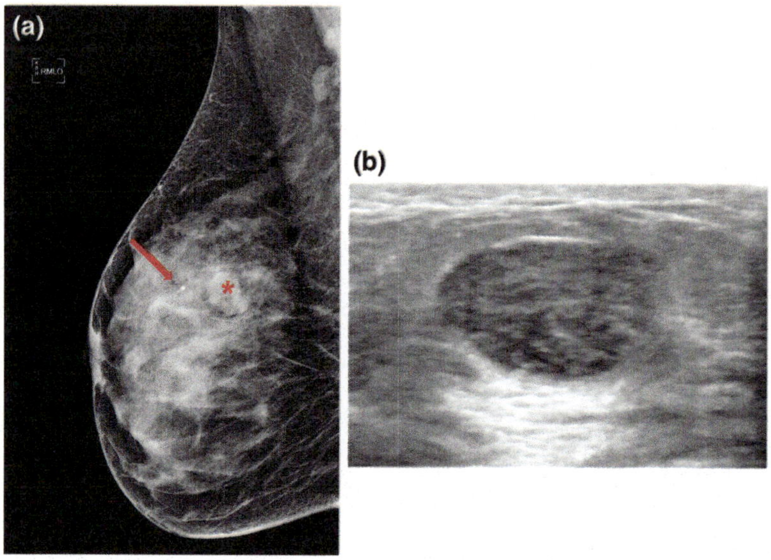

Fig. 9.2 Palpable mass. **a** Digital left MLO view. A metallic "BB" marker (*arrow*) was placed over the palpable mass prior to performing the image. An oval, partially circumscribed and partially obscured mass (*asterisk* *) is present and corresponds to the palpable abnormality. **b** Ultrasound over the palpable mass revealed an oval solid mass, parallel to the skin surface ("wider-than-tall"), with circumscribed margins, consistent with a fibroadenoma

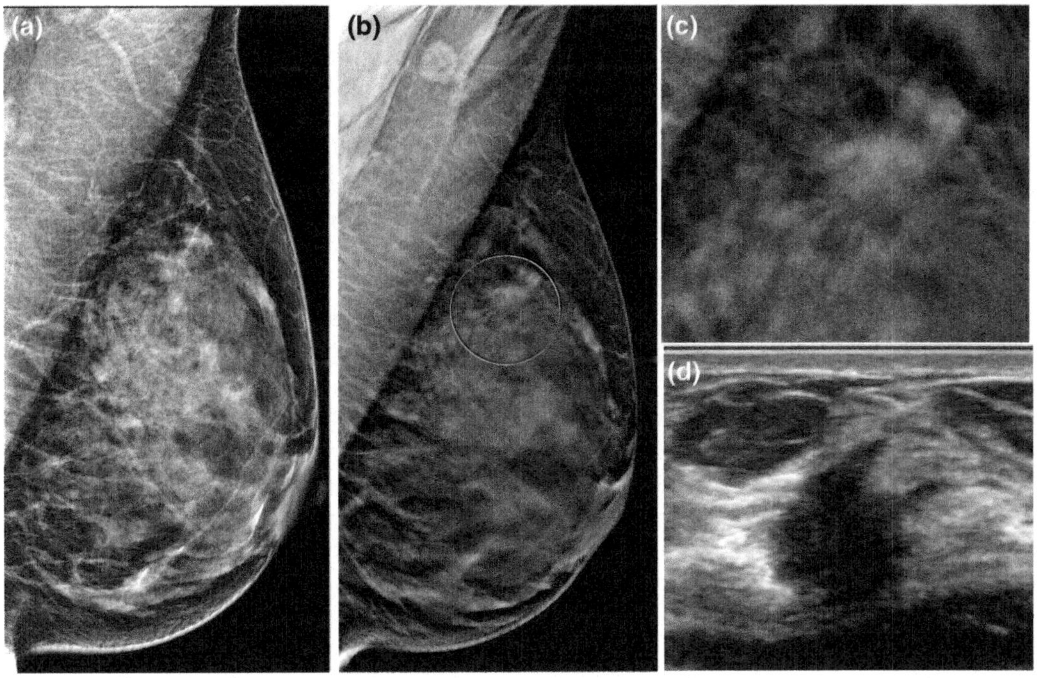

Fig. 9.3 Digital breast tomosynthesis allows identification of an otherwise mammographically occult breast cancer. **a** Conventional digital 2D mammogram shows no suspicious finding. **b** 1-mm-thick tomographic image shows an underlying highly suspicious spiculated mass in the upper breast that was obscured on the digital 2D mammogram by overlying breast tissue. **c** Photographic enlargement of the abnormal area shows the spiculated mass. **d** Corresponding ultrasound confirms the presence of an irregularly shaped solid mass with angular margins. Ultrasound-guided core needle biopsy shows invasive lobular carcinoma

single conventional digital mammographic exposure, the latter of which can be obtained during the same acquisition. The tomosynthesis projection images are then processed into a stack of 1-mm-thick tomographic images. The radiologist can then scroll through the 1-mm-thick tomographic images and examine the breast tissue layer-by-layer, removing the superimposed fibroglandular tissue. The process, which is akin to paging through a book, allows for the detection of breast tumors that otherwise may have been hidden by superimposed breast tissue (Fig. 9.3).

Multiple studies have shown that conventional digital mammography combined with DBT improves the detection of invasive breast cancers by approximately 40 % and decreases recall rates (fewer false positives) by approximately 15 % compared to conventional digital mammography alone. These findings apply to women of all breast densities in all age categories [27–32].

The limitations of DBT include higher costs, longer interpretation times, and when first FDA approved, a doubling of the radiation dose due to the requirement that DBT be performed in conjunction with conventional digital mammography. In 2013, software used to create a synthetic mammogram in place of a conventional digital mammogram received approval by the FDA, thus cutting the radiation dose in half with a dose essentially identical to a conventional digital mammogram. This synthetic view is a summation or composite view of the 1-mm tomographic images and effectively eliminates the need to obtain the conventional digital mammogram [33].

9.2.4 The Mammography Report

Prior to 1990, many radiologists and training programs had developed their own terminology and methods for reporting mammograms. Referring physicians often complained that the terminology was confusing, conclusions were equivocal, and recommendations were unclear. The American College of Radiology Breast Imaging and Reporting System (BI-RADS®) was a response to complaints from referring physicians about these problems [3]. The BI-RADS reporting system uses standardized descriptors and final assessment categories that are linked directly to recommended management protocols. In its development, there was input from the American College of Surgeons, College of American Pathologists, American Medical Association, National Cancer Institute, Centers for Disease Control and Prevention, FDA, and American Cancer Society. The BI-RADS standardized report includes six components: (1) the reason for the examination, (2) the overall breast tissue composition, (3) the description of the findings using standardized BI-RADS terminology, (4) comparison to prior examinations, if appropriate, (5) the final assessment category, and (6) management recommendations.

9.2.4.1 Reason for the Examination

Examples include "screening," "palpable mass," "additional workup of a screening detected abnormality," and "6-month follow-up of a probably benign finding."

9.2.4.2 Breast Tissue Composition

Since the sensitivity of mammography is directly related to the relative amounts of fat and fibroglandular tissue in the patient's breast, it is important for the referring physician to be aware of the overall breast tissue composition. The overall breast tissue composition can range from almost entirely fatty to extremely dense tissue. Breast cancers tend to be white (radiodense) on mammograms. Fatty tissue provides an excellent background (dark), in which to detect small breast cancers (white). On the other hand, dense tissue (white) can obscure or mask breast cancers (white). The four categories of breast tissue composition are as follows: (A) almost entirely fatty, (B) scattered areas of fibroglandular density, (C) heterogeneously dense which may obscure small masses, and (D) extremely dense which lowers the sensitivity of mammography (Fig. 9.4).

9.2.4.3 Description of Findings

Normal, benign, and suspicious findings are described using a standard lexicon. The descriptors reflect the probability of malignancy. Masses and calcifications are the most common abnormalities found on mammograms, and the BI-RADS descriptors of these abnormalities are found later in this chapter.

9.2.4.4 Comparison to Prior Examinations, if Appropriate

Sometimes, final assessments cannot be reached until comparison to prior examinations is performed to evaluate for change or stability of a finding. However, when a finding has either unequivocally benign characteristics, or unequivocally suspicious features, then comparison to prior studies may be irrelevant.

9.2.4.5 Assessment Categories and Management

The BI-RADS final *assessment* is currently placed into one of seven categories (categories 0–6) (Table 9.2). The mammography report ends with (1) a final assessment and (2) its associated management recommendation. If the report includes both a mammography examination and an ultrasound examination, there should be an overall *assessment* that summarizes the more actionable BI-RADS category for the two examinations. In other words, if the mammogram was "negative" (BI-RADS 1), but the ultrasound examination showed a "suspicious" mass, the overall *assessment* would be "category 4—suspicious."

BI-RADS Category 0—"*incomplete, need additional imaging evaluation and/or prior mammograms for comparison*"—is reserved for screening examinations that require additional workup before a final assessment can be made. Additional workup usually involves diagnostic mammography views and/or breast ultrasound. This category could also refer to the need for comparison to prior images, if available, to evaluate for interval change before a final assessment can be issued.

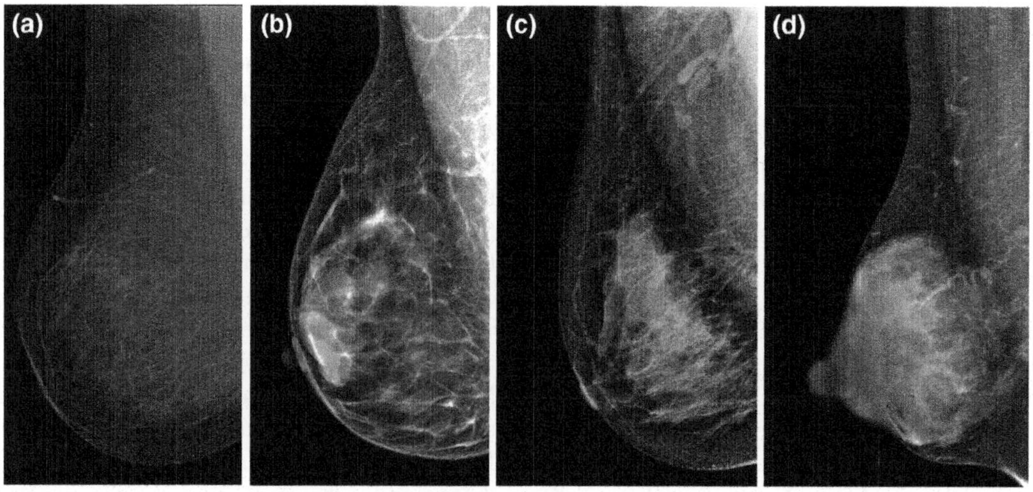

Fig. 9.4 Four BI-RADS descriptors for breast density (presented in right MLO digital mammograms). **a** Type A—almost entirely fatty. **b** Type B—scattered areas of fibroglandular density. **c** Type C—heterogeneously dense which may obscure small lesions. **d** Type D—extremely dense which lowers the sensitivity of mammography

Table 9.2 BI-RADS report final assessment categories

Category	Definition
0	Incomplete—need additional imaging evaluation and/or prior mammograms for comparison
1	Negative
2	Benign finding
3	Probably benign
4	Suspicious abnormality 4A: low suspicion for malignancy 4B: Moderate suspicion for malignancy 4C: High suspicion for malignancy
5	Highly suggestive of malignancy
6	Known biopsy-proven malignancy

BI-RADS Category 1—*Negative*: There is nothing to comment on.
BI-RADS Category 2—*Benign.* This means the examination is negative except for some typically benign finding(s).
BI-RADS Category 3—*Probably benign.* This is used for findings that have a high probability of being benign (≤2 % suspicion for malignancy).
BI-RADS Category 4—*Suspicious.* This includes abnormalities that do not have definite morphology of cancer but have enough concern to urge a biopsy. BI-RADS subdivides these into three subcategories: 4A (low suspicion: 2–10 % likelihood of malignancy), 4B (intermediate suspicion: 10–50 % likelihood of malignancy), and 4C (high suspicion: 50–94 % likelihood of malignancy) [3].
BI-RADS Category 5—*Highly suggestive of malignancy.* These cases show classic findings of breast cancer (≥95 % likelihood of malignancy).
BI-RADS Category 6—*Known Biopsy-Proven Malignancy.* These cases consist of biopsy-proven malignancies, in which no other actionable finding is identified, typically used to assess treatment response in patients with known malignancy.

Assigning a BI-RADS assessment category (0–6) to each mammography report provides a user-friendly mechanism for tracking and monitoring mammography patients, which does not require an understanding of medical terminology. Thus, office staff supervised by a healthcare provider can verify that the breast imaging recommendations are carried out.

The assignment of a final assessment to each examination also facilitates outcome analyses, such as the medical audit of a mammography practice or a community screening project. The medical audit is an MQSA-mandated annual quality assurance activity to determine the effectiveness of a mammography program. The audit compares the mammography interpretation to the outcome of a biopsy or 2-year follow-up [34]. For this purpose, the mammography examination must be categorized as *positive or negative* for cancer, and the outcome is based on the result of biopsies or clinical follow-up that verifies whether or not cancer was present.

If the final assessment for a screening mammogram is negative (category 1) or benign (category 2), the interpretation is categorized as *negative* for the medical audit. If the final assessment is probably benign (category 3), suspicious (category 4), or highly suggestive of malignancy (category 5), the interpretation is considered *positive* for the medical audit. A clinical follow-up or a biopsy will determine whether or not the imaging interpretation was correct.

9.2.5 Describing the Location of an Abnormality

When there is a palpable finding in the breast that is referred for imaging evaluation, it is very important that the referring healthcare provider provides the exact location of the palpable finding identified on the clinical examination (Fig. 9.5). Often, the patient does not know the location of the finding you are concerned about when she arrives for her imaging examination.

These are current recommendations for indicating the area of concern based on your clinical examination (your responsibility) and on the breast imaging reports (the radiologist's responsibility):

1. Right versus left breast.
2. Quadrant location: right upper outer (RUO), right upper inner (RUI), etc.
3. Clock-face location: RUO 10:00, LUO 2:00, etc.
4. In addition, it is really helpful if you provide the distance from the nipple (FN) of the area of concern. A palpable finding you are concerned about in the left upper outer breast at 2:00 could be anywhere from 1 to 10 cm from the nipple depending on the breast size.

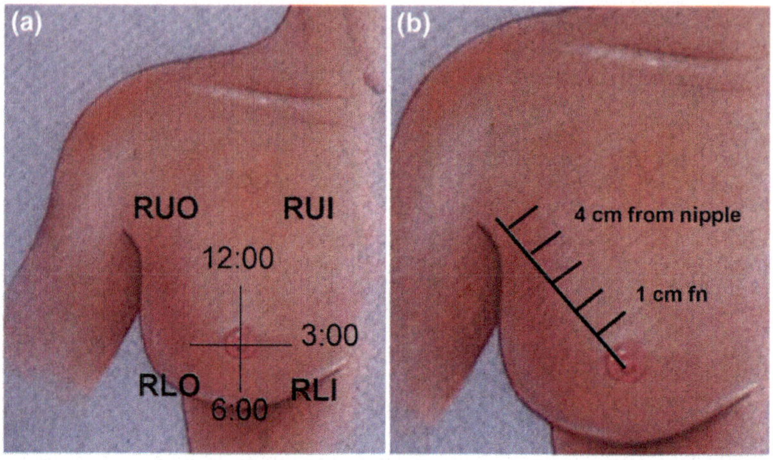

Fig. 9.5 Describing the exact location of a clinical or imaging finding. **a** Laterality, quadrant, and clock-face location. **b** Distance from the nipple

9.2.6 Masses

A *mass* is defined as a space-occupying lesion that is seen on at least two mammographic projections [3]. An "asymmetry" is an area of fibroglandular-density tissue that is seen only on one view. In BI-RADS, masses are described by their shape and margins (Fig. 9.6). The *shape* can be oval, round, or irregular. Oval and round masses are usually benign. An irregular shape suggests a greater likelihood of malignancy. The *margins* of masses are the most important indicator of the likelihood of malignancy [35]. The margins can be described as circumscribed, microlobulated, obscured (≥25 % of the margin is hidden by superimposed tissue), indistinct (ill-defined), or spiculated. *Circumscribed* margins favor a benign etiology, and the likelihood of malignancy for a circumscribed mass is very low, probably less than 2 % [36–38]. Additional workup may be necessary to verify that the margins are completely circumscribed. This workup usually involves additional projections of the mass and magnification spot compression views. Ultrasound is often necessary to determine whether a round or oval circumscribed mass is cystic or solid. If the mass is a simple cyst, no further workup is needed. If it is solid, the shape, the margins, and the clinical findings should be further evaluated. A solitary, nonpalpable, completely circumscribed solid mass is often managed with a 6-month follow-up to establish that it is stable (not growing). If available, the previous examinations should be compared. If stable, continued mammography surveillance is recommended for at least 2 years [39]. The presence of multiple circumscribed masses is even stronger evidence of benignity, indicating multiple cysts, fibroadenomas, or benign intramammary lymph nodes [40], and follow-up in 1 year is often sufficient. If one of the masses is "dominant," biopsy is indicated. Dominant masses would include those that are significantly larger, not circumscribed, growing or palpable. *Microlobulated* margins increase the likelihood of malignancy. If the mass is partially obscured by nearby fibroglandular tissue, additional imaging should be done to show the margins as completely as possible. The finding of an *indistinct* margin is suspicious for malignancy. A *spiculated* margin has lines radiating from its border, and this finding is highly suggestive of malignancy. An area of radiating spicules in the absence of a central mass is called an *architectural distortion*.

The *density* of a mass compared with normal fibroglandular tissue provides another clue as to its etiology. In general, benign masses tend to be lower in density than carcinomas; however, the density of a mass is not always a reliable sign for differentiating benign from malignant [41].

9.2.7 Calcifications

Calcifications are described on mammograms by their *morphology* and distribution (Fig. 9.7). Based on their *morphology*, calcifications can be divided into two groups: (1) *Typically benign* calcifications include skin, vascular, coarse, or "popcorn-like," large rod-like, round, rim, dystrophic, suture, and milk-of-calcium types; (2) *suspicious morphology* calcifications include amorphous, coarse heterogeneous, fine pleomorphic, and fine linear or fine-linear branching. The likelihood of malignancy for amorphous, coarse heterogeneous, and fine pleomorphic calcifications is 13–29 %; thus, they should be reported as a category 4B. While the likelihood of malignancy for fine linear or fine-linear branching calcifications is 70 %, a category 4C designation is appropriate.

Calcifications are also characterized by their *distribution* and include diffuse, regional, grouped, linear, and segmental descriptors. *Diffuse* calcifications are distributed randomly through both breasts and are almost always benign. *Regional* calcifications occupy a larger a volume of breast tissue and span 2 cm or greater, and are also likely benign. *Grouped*

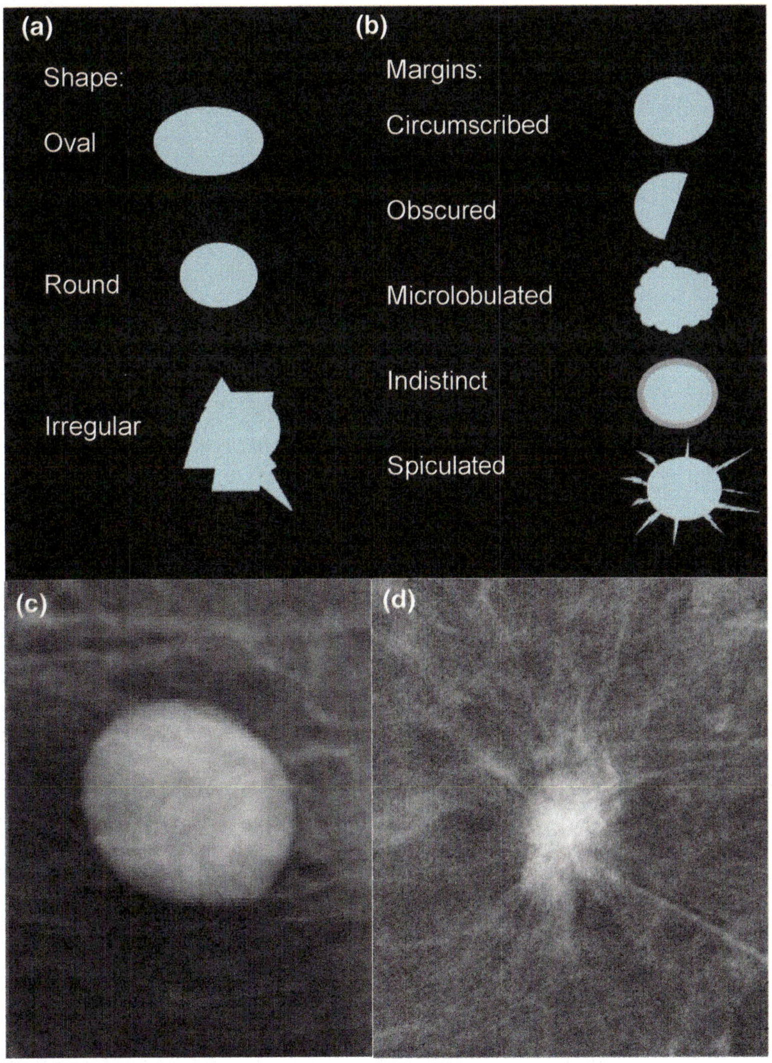

Fig. 9.6 BI-RADS standardized description of masses. **a** Shape varies from oval and round (most likely benign) to irregular (most likely malignant). **b** Margins vary from circumscribed (most likely benign) to spiculated (most likely malignant). **c** Round mass with circumscribed margins. **d** Irregular mass with spiculated margins. Biopsy revealed invasive ductal carcinoma

calcifications can be benign or malignant and range from as small as 5 calcifications within 1 cm of each other and as a large as >5 calcifications within 2 cm of each other [3, 42]. *Linear* calcifications are arranged in a line, and this distribution suggests an intraductal location, thus raising the suspicion of malignancy. *Segmental* calcifications are triangular in distribution with the apex toward the nipple. This distribution suggests deposits in a duct and its branches, further raising the possibility of malignancy, including multifocal carcinoma (Fig. 9.8).

9.2.8 Indirect and Secondary Signs of Malignancy

Other important findings that can be described in the BI-RADS report include indirect or subtle signs of malignancy, such as a new or developing asymmetry or an architectural distortion [43, 44]. Other secondary signs of malignancy include skin thickening, nipple retraction, and axillary node enlargement.

A new or developing asymmetry is identified by comparison with prior examinations and requires additional workup, which may include additional mammography views, ultrasound, and biopsy. Asymmetrically distributed fibroglandular tissue may be a normal variant, but could be subtle sign of underlying malignancy (Fig. 9.9).

An *architectural distortion* is described as radiating spicules without a central mass and may be difficult to perceive (Fig. 9.10). Both benign and malignant entities, including surgical scar, radial scar, and invasive carcinoma, may present as an architectural distortion on mammograms.

Skin thickening also can be seen with benign conditions, including postradiation change, mastitis, inflammatory breast carcinoma, lymphatic obstruction, and fluid-overload states, such as congestive heart failure and renal failure.

New skin or nipple retraction is often a sign of an underlying malignancy. In addition, unilateral axillary

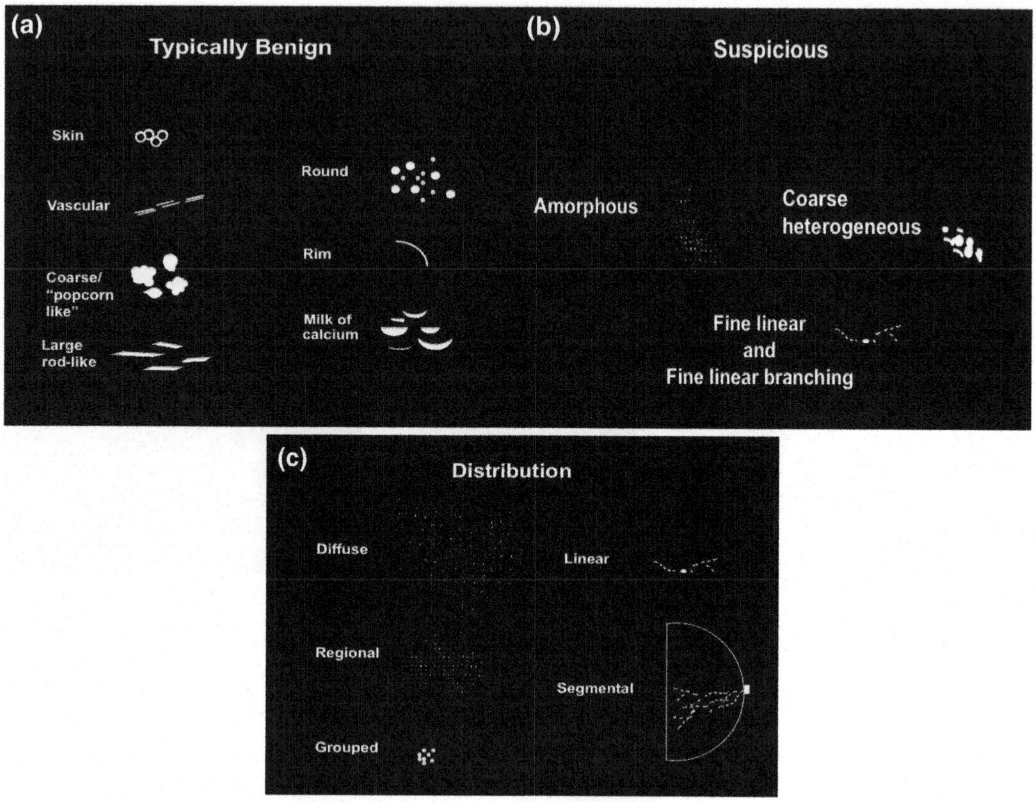

Fig. 9.7 BI-RADS standardized description of calcifications. Based on their morphology, calcifications are categorized as typically benign (**a**), including skin, vascular, coarse/popcorn-like, round, rim, and milk of calcium. Suspicious calcifications (**b**) include amorphous, coarse heterogeneous, or fine linear/fine-linear branching. Based on their distribution (**c**), calcifications are described as diffuse (not suspicious), regional (low suspicion), grouped (variable), linear (moderate to high suspicion), or segmental (high suspicion)

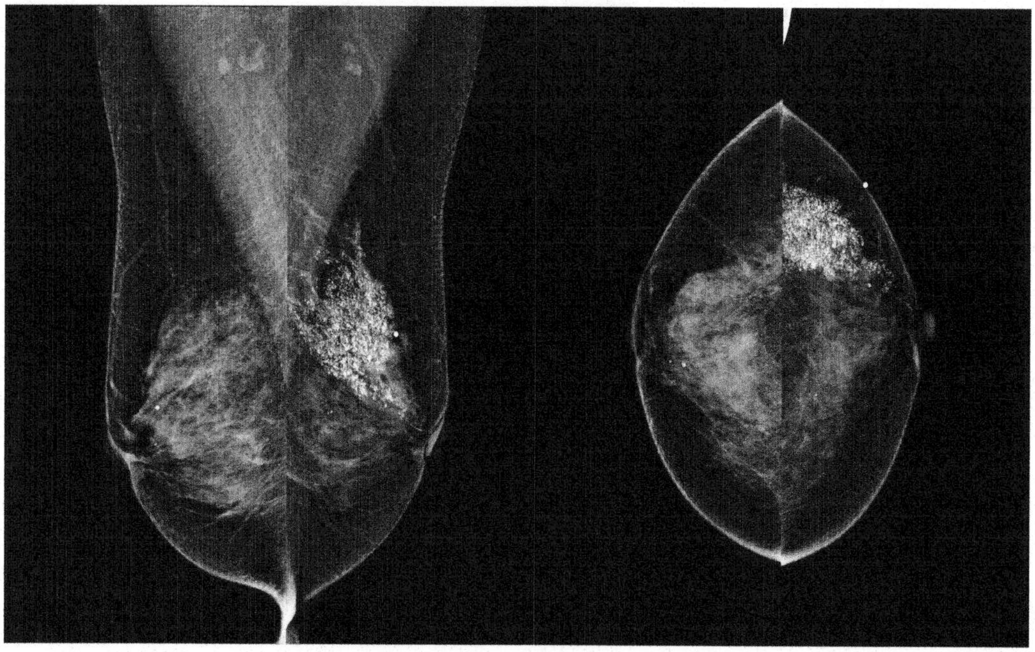

Fig. 9.8 Extensive fine-linear branching microcalcifications in a segmental distribution (**a–d**). Biopsy showed ductal carcinoma in situ (DCIS)

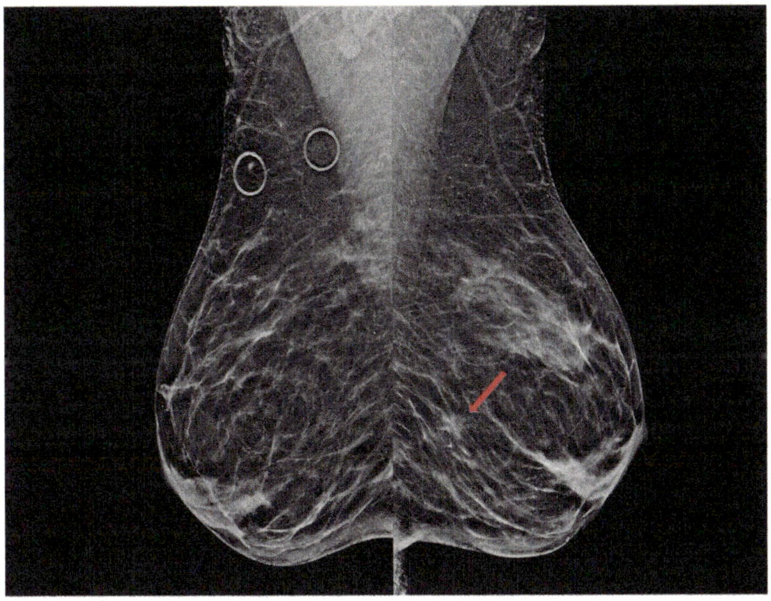

Fig. 9.9 **a** Right MLO and **b** left MLO synthetic mammograms show an asymmetry (*arrow*) in the left lower breast. Additional workup confirmed the asymmetry represented normal asymmetric breast tissue and had been stable for more than eight years

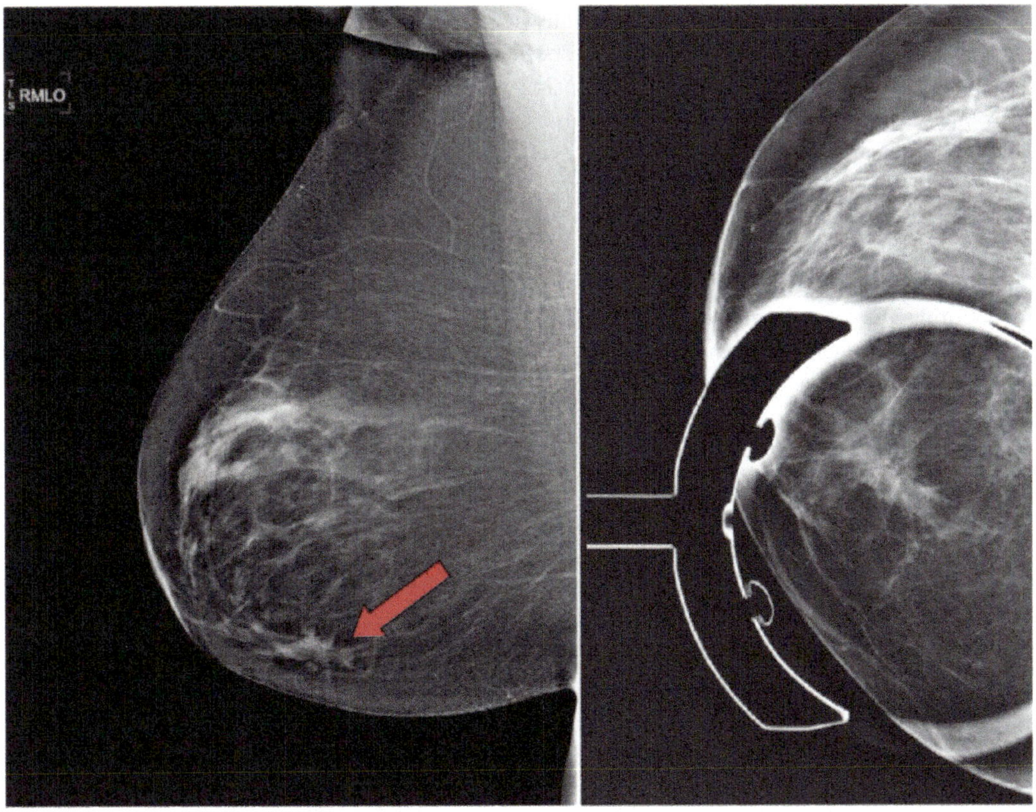

Fig. 9.10 Architectural distortion. **a** Right MLO digital mammogram shows an area of architectural distortion (*arrow*) in the inferior breast. **b** Spot compression views confirmed the persistence of the architectural distortion. Biopsy revealed invasive breast carcinoma

lymph node enlargement can result from a breast primary cancer, metastases from other cancers, or inflammatory conditions.

9.2.9 Potential Adverse Consequences of Screening

Referring healthcare providers should be aware of the possible adverse consequences of mammography screening, the likelihood of each and strategies to lower their likelihood. Potential adverse consequences of mammography include excessive biopsies, inadequate communication of results, anxiety associated with the need for additional views, pain and discomfort, false reassurance, and delay in diagnosis.

In the process of detecting as many early breast cancers as possible, a certain number of biopsies will be done for benign mammographic abnormalities. The positive predictive value of biopsies done for mammographic abnormalities (number of cancers detected/ number of biopsies) can vary significantly from one facility to another. The recommended positive biopsy rate for experienced interpreting physicians is 25–40 % [34]. The average in US facilities is close to 20 % [45]. Failing to communicate mammography results has been a relatively common problem in the past [46]. The failure to communicate results can lead to delay in diagnosis and treatment of breast cancer. The failure to communicate results in a *timely fashion* can lead to unnecessary anxiety in women. In addition to the formal report to the referring healthcare provider, women are notified of their results by the mammography facility. The Mammography Quality Standards Act requires that this notification is direct (no intermediary), in writing and in lay language for patients [2].

Substantial anxiety can be generated when a woman has to return for additional or repeat mammographic views. These extra views should be done as soon as feasible to reduce anxiety. Staff should be supportive and available to answer any questions.

When properly performed, mammography may be uncomfortable but rarely painful. If women have unnecessary pain and severe discomfort, they may not return for future screening examinations. Therefore, mammography should be performed using proper breast compression, so that women feel as little pain and discomfort as possible. Routine mammography should not be done when the breast is tender or in the week before menstruation for women who have breast pain associated with menses [47–49].

False reassurance occurs when a woman ignores a palpable abnormality because of a previous negative screening mammogram. Palpable abnormalities in women aged 30 or older should be evaluated with diagnostic mammography and breast ultrasound. Delay in diagnosis occurs when a clinical finding is not acted on because imaging studies turn out to be negative. Referring healthcare providers should inform women that a negative mammogram should not delay the evaluation of a clinically suspicious breast lump or other suspicious clinical finding. A lump or other abnormal clinical finding that develops after a negative screening examination should be evaluated as soon as possible and not delayed until the next screening examination.

9.2.10 False-Negative Mammograms

A false-negative mammogram is one that is interpreted as negative, but cancer is diagnosed within 1 year. Five medical specialties were named in 87 % of all breast cancer medical malpractice claims: radiology, obstetrics/gynecology (Ob/Gyn), internal medicine, and general surgery. In all cases that went to completion (closed claims), 43 % of those named in the claim were radiologists, with the most common causation being error in diagnosis. Ob/Gyn surgeons were associated with the second highest percentage of closed claims at 16 %. The average indemnity paid for claims involving radiologists and Ob/Gyn surgeons was $433,668 and $443,458 respectively [50].

Causes of false-negative mammograms include dense breast tissue, suboptimal technical quality, errors in interpretation, and failure of communication [51]. The most common cause of a false-negative mammogram is dense fibroglandular tissue [52]. The sensitivity of mammography decreases with increasing tissue density, though this effect may be partially mitigated by the use of DBT (Fig. 9.3).

The use of proper technical factors is particularly crucial in detecting breast cancer, especially in evaluating a woman with dense breast tissue. Suboptimal positioning and underexposure increase the risk of a false-negative mammogram. Using dedicated equipment, adequate compression and proper exposure can optimize the mammographic examination.

9.3 Breast Ultrasound

Breast ultrasound is an essential adjunct to mammography for the workup and diagnosis of palpable and mammographically detected abnormalities. Historically, breast ultrasound was used to differentiate solid and cystic masses. In the past decade and a half, advances in ultrasound technology have led to high-resolution ultrasound equipment and to the identification of sonographic features to help differentiate benign and malignant solid masses [53–55]. In addition to lesion characterization, breast ultrasound is used to guide interventional breast procedures, including cyst aspiration, CNB, fine needle aspiration, and preoperative needle localization.

9.3.1 Technical Advances

State-of-the-art breast ultrasound equipment systems utilize linear array, high-resolution transducers with advanced processing algorithms yielding superior image quality. Innovative techniques include shear-wave elastography (SWE), spatial compounding, and tissue harmonic imaging. Shear-wave elastography, which provides data on the stiffness of a lesion, in combination with other diagnostic ultrasound techniques, can be useful in differentiating benign from malignant lesions. Spatial compounding obtains multiple simultaneous images at different angles, which are then superimposed into a single compound image, resulting in reduced artifacts. Clinically, this translates into clearer visualization of cystic contents, improved contrast resolution and tissue differentiation, enhanced delineation of anatomic margins, and improved depiction of internal architecture of solid lesions [54, 55]. Tissue harmonic imaging minimizes artifacts leading to better lesion conspicuity and margin depiction when compared to conventional sonographic imaging [56, 57]. Power Doppler technology allows for visualization of vascular structures, including tiny, low-flow vessels, which may surround or penetrate breast tissue and masses. Knowledge of lesion vascularity is important in planning interventional procedures and is helpful in characterizing solid breast masses and certain breast conditions (e.g., mastitis and Mondor's disease).

9.3.2 Normal Anatomy

Breast ultrasound reveals the breast anatomic structures from the skin surface to the chest wall (Fig. 9.11). Normal skin measures less than 3 mm and is composed of two parallel echogenic (white) lines separated by a thin, hypoechoic (dark) band. Just deep to the skin lies the subcutaneous fat followed by the interwoven bands of fibroglandular tissue and breast fat. Both subcutaneous and breast fat are mildly hypoechoic (gray), whereas the fibroglandular tissue is hyperechoic (light gray to white). Deep to the fibroglandular tissue is the retroglandular fat, which lies against the chest wall. The chest wall is composed of the more superficial band of the pectoralis muscle, the ribs laying deep to the pectoralis muscle, and the parietal pleura. The pectoralis muscle, ribs, and pleura have characteristic sonographic features that are easily and reliably identified. The lung parenchyma is not sonographically visible as the ultrasound beam does not propagate well through air.

9.3.3 Cystic Masses

Breast ultrasound can reliably identify cystic masses. The BI-RADS descriptors for the three types of cystic masses are as follows: (1) *simple cyst,* (2) *complicated cyst, and* (3) *complex cystic and solid mass.*

The sonographic features of a *simple* cyst are a round or oval shaped, anechoic (black with no internal echoes) mass with circumscribed margins and increased posterior enhancement (Fig. 9.12). Increased posterior enhancement means it appears as if a flashlight is shining through the back of the cyst. Because cysts develop within the terminal duct lobular unit of the breast, it is not uncommon to see clusters of cysts or coalescing cysts. Simple cysts need no further workup unless a cyst aspiration is indicated. Indications for cyst aspiration include a painful cyst, a large cyst that

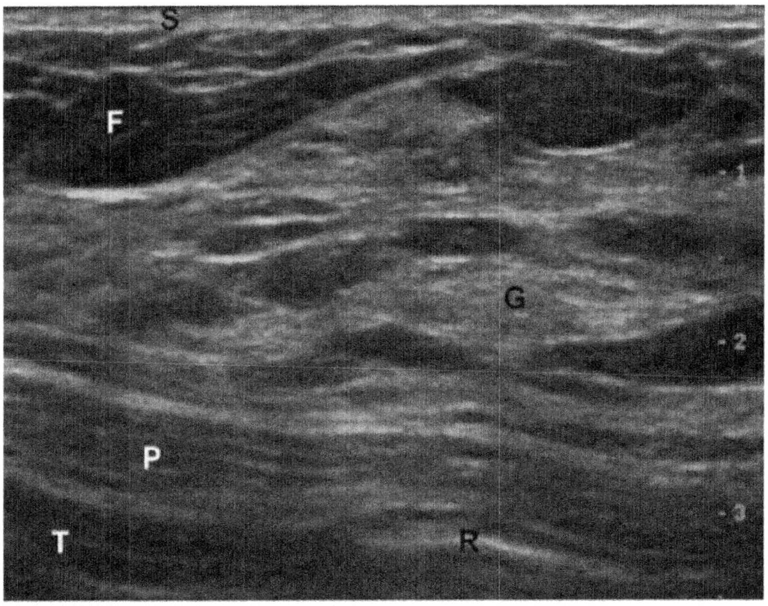

Fig. 9.11 Normal breast anatomy on ultrasound. The skin (*S*) is represented by horizontal echogenic lines. Below this, there is a layer of hypoechoic subcutaneous fat (*F*). This is followed by alternating bands of fibroglandular tissue (*G*). The retromammary fat lies on the chest wall. The pectoral muscle (*P*), ribs (*R*), and thoracic cavity (*T*) are deep to the retromammary fat

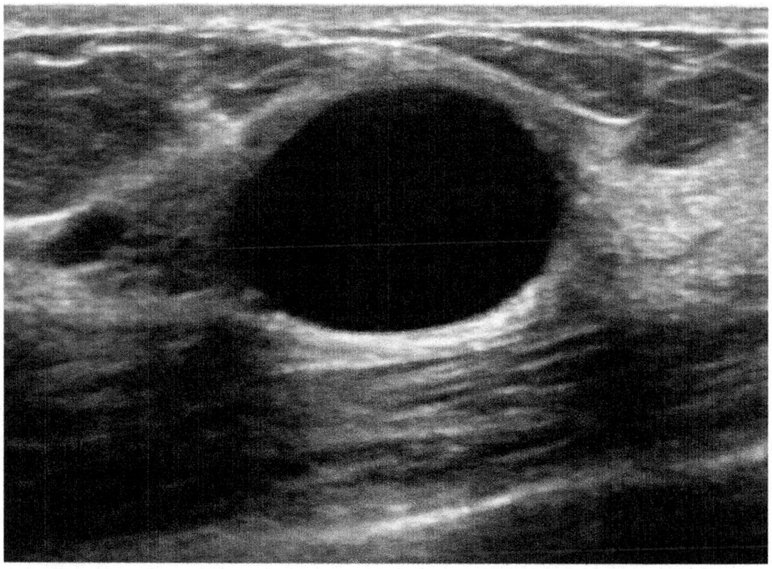

Fig. 9.12 Simple cyst. Ultrasound features are a round or oval, anechoic (*black* with no internal echoes) mass with circumscribed margins and increased posterior enhancement

compromises mammographic imaging, patient anxiety, or a debris-filled complicated cyst that needs to be aspirated to rule out a solid mass.

It is not uncommon to identify a "cyst" with fine internal echoes, such as a debris-filled cyst. These cystic masses do not fulfill the criteria for a simple cyst and are called *complicated* cysts. When a complicated cyst is suspected, further evaluation may be needed. Ultrasound-guided aspiration can be performed to verify its cystic nature, to exclude a solid mass, and to confirm complete resolution of the mass after aspiration.

A *complex* cystic and solid mass is defined as a mass with both cystic and solid components. Usually, the solid component is described as a mural nodule or an intracystic mass. A complex cystic and solid mass can also be composed of thick walls and anechoic center. A cyst with a solid component is suspicious for a malignancy, such as a papillary carcinoma or a necrotic infiltrating carcinoma. Benign papillomas can also present as a complex cystic and solid mass. The diagnostic evaluation of a complex cystic and solid mass is ultrasound-guided CNB of the solid component with micromarker placement or surgical excision.

9.3.4 Solid Masses

Criteria differentiating benign and malignant solid masses have evolved. Several studies have defined criteria to aid in the distinction of benign and malignant solid breast masses [53, 54]. Although no single or combination of sonographic features is 100 % diagnostic for a benign mass, careful use of established criteria can help differentiate benign and malignant solid masses and avoid biopsy of certain solid masses. Mass shape, margins, orientation relative to the skin surface, echogenicity, and posterior echoes are the minimum preliminary characteristics that should be assessed in solid masses.

Typically benign sonographic features of solid masses include an oval shape (which includes two or three undulations), orientation parallel to the skin surface, circumscribed margins, and *absence* of any malignant features (Fig. 9.13).

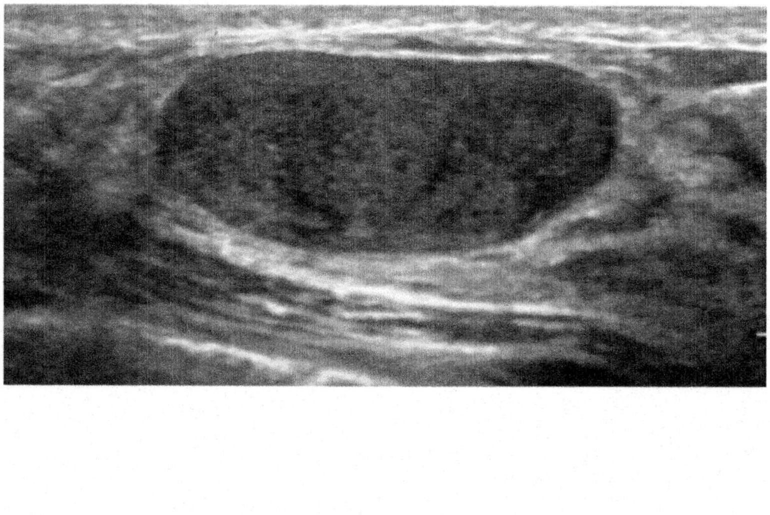

Fig. 9.13 Typical sonographic features of a benign solid mass. This mass is oval, oriented parallel to the skin, and has circumscribed margins. Findings are typical for a fibroadenoma

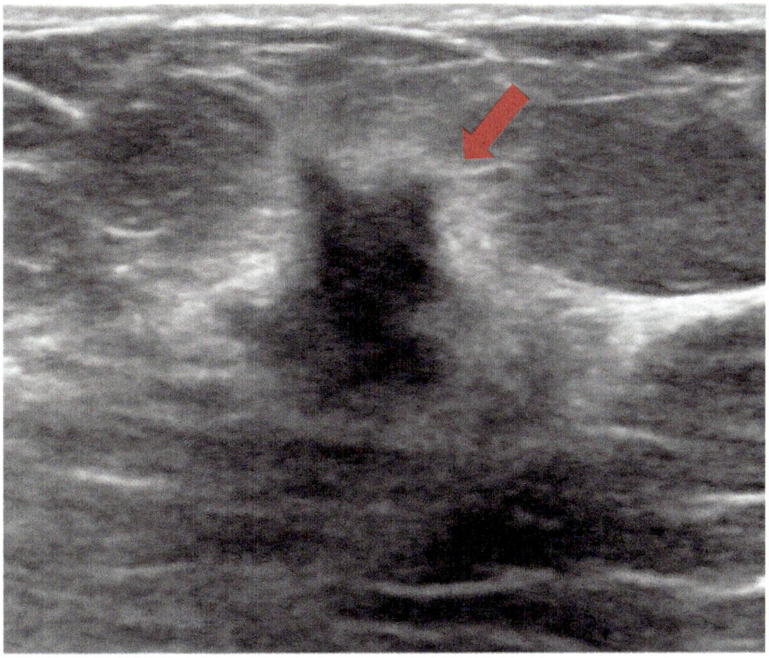

Fig. 9.14 Typical sonographic features of a malignant solid mass. This hypoechoic mass (*arrow*) manifests an irregular shape with angular and indistinct margins, and is orientated nonparallel to the skin. Biopsy revealed invasive ductal carcinoma

Malignant sonographic features of solid masses include an irregular shape, indistinct angular, microlobulated or spiculated margins; orientation not parallel to the skin surface; markedly hypoechoic (dark) echogenicity; posterior shadowing (black shadows posterior to the mass); and associated calcifications (Fig. 9.14).

In conclusion, the results of benign vs. malignant ultrasound features of solid masses are helpful. These features have potential for decreasing the number of biopsies performed for benign solid masses. Studies have also shown interobserver variability from one ultrasound interpreter to another in the evaluation for these features and in making a final diagnosis [58]. Furthermore, there appears to be overlap in these features, and some malignant masses may have features suggesting they are benign, which could lead to false-negative interpretations of malignant solid masses. Therefore, these sonographic diagnostic criteria should not be generally applied as the sole criteria in determining whether to perform a biopsy of a solid mass.

Solid masses with any suspicious mammographic or sonographic feature should undergo biopsy. Any palpable or growing benign-appearing solid mass warrants at least a needle biopsy. However, an incidentally identified, nonpalpable, solid mass that demonstrates benign mammographic and sonographic features may be managed with a 6-month follow-up examination.

9.3.5 Screening Ultrasound

Screening ultrasound is defined as bilateral whole breast ultrasound of an asymptomatic woman and always should be performed in combination with screening mammography. The sensitivity of screening mammography is decreased in women with dense breasts as the dense tissue may obscure underlying lesions. Several studies have shown that small, clinically and mammographically occult breast cancers may be detected with screening ultrasound in women with dense breast tissue [59–63]. This can be attributed to the ability of ultrasound to "look through" dense breast tissue and identify otherwise occult benign and malignant masses.

Despite the encouraging results from these studies, many potential drawbacks are associated with screening ultrasound. Of particular concern is the high number incidental benign masses encountered during screening ultrasound, for which either biopsy, aspiration, or short-interval follow-up ultrasound is recommended. Furthermore, there is lack of proven short-interval follow-up ultrasound criteria for probably benign, incidentally identified masses.

Several studies of screening ultrasound (37,085 total exams) detected 127 additional cancers, resulting in a prevalence of 0.34 % (3.4 additional cancers per 1000) [59–61, 63–65]. However, 2–6 % of women undergoing screening ultrasound will receive a recommendation for biopsy with an approximate positive predictive value of only 5–16 % [65] An additional 3–16 % of patients will receive a recommendation for short-interval follow-up ultrasound [59–65]. Additional problems include an extremely limited ability to detect ductal carcinoma in situ (DCIS), patient anxiety, and morbidity associated with additional biopsy procedures, added cost, lengthy examination times, and highly variable ultrasound performance skill levels among practicing technologists and radiologists.

The largest study of blinded screening breast ultrasound in high-risk women conducted by the American College of Radiology Imaging Network (ACRIN 6666) and the Avon Foundation was published in 2008, which was the first study to independently evaluate screening ultrasound compared to screening mammography [65, 66]. This study found that after one year of ultrasound and mammography screening in high-risk women, the supplemental yield of ultrasound screening was 4.2 per 1000. Furthermore, most ultrasound only detected tumors were invasive carcinomas, with a median size of 10 mm, and were lymph node-negative. However, it showed that screening ultrasound was associated with a higher risk of false positives (benign biopsy results and/or short-interval follow-up) and a low positive predictive value of 8.9 %, compared to mammography at 22.6 %. A 2015 study analyzing benefits, harms, and cost-effectiveness of screening ultrasound for women with dense breasts found supplemental ultrasonography screening would substantially increase costs while producing relatively small benefits [67].

9.4 Core Needle Biopsy

Several breast biopsy alternatives are available to the patient with a suspicious finding. Prior to 1990, the biopsy of imaging-detected breast lesions was limited to excisional biopsy. Introduced in 1990, CNB has become a desirable alternative to excisional biopsy because it is less costly, results in less morbidity, and leaves minimal to no scar. CNB of the breast overcomes the limitations of fine needle aspiration (FNA) because insufficient samples are less frequent, and the interpretation can be performed by a pathologist without special training in cytopathology. Furthermore, CNB can differentiate invasive from in situ breast cancer and provide adequate tissue to determine tumor biomarkers (estrogen receptor, progesterone receptor, HER2/neu) [68, 69].

CNBs are performed with a large-bore (7–14 gauge) needle in combination with imaging guidance to sample a clinical or imaging identified abnormality. Imaging guidance can be provided by ultrasound, mammography (conventional digital or DBT), or MRI. Stereotactic-guided CNB uses two mammographic views acquired at different angles to determine the location of a lesion in the breast. Choice of ultrasound versus stereotactic-guided CNB is based on which modality best demonstrates the abnormality and the location of the abnormality in the breast. However, ultrasound is usually preferred because it is faster and more comfortable for the patient (Fig. 9.15). MRI biopsy should only be performed when the suspicious imaging finding can only be confidently visualized on MRI.

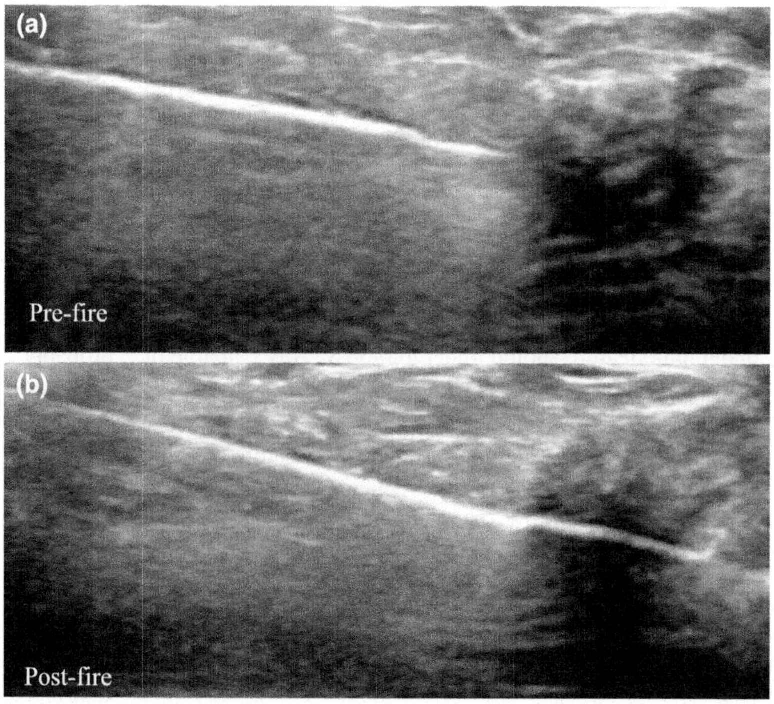

Fig. 9.15 Ultrasound-guided core needle biopsy. **a** Prefire image shows the biopsy needle tip at the edge of the mass undergoing biopsy. **b** Post-fire image confirms that the biopsy needle is within the mass

9.4.1 Indications, Relative Contraindications, and Complications

Imaging-guided CNB is indicated for most nonpalpable, mammographically suspicious abnormalities [70]. Abnormalities categorized as "probably benign" (BI-RADS 3), "suspicious" (BI-RADS 4), and "highly suggestive of malignancy" (BI-RADS 5) can undergo biopsy. Overuse of the technique for sampling of "probably benign" (BI-RADS 3) abnormalities that would otherwise be managed with a 6-month follow-up can increase the cost of screening with little to no benefit [71]. CNB of "highly suggestive of malignancy" (BI-RADS 5) lesions can expedite surgical planning by avoiding the need to perform intraoperative frozen-section analysis to verify malignancy prior to definitive surgical treatment.

Stereotactic CNB is contraindicated in patients who exceed the weight limit of the biopsy table or have extremely thin breasts that preclude safely firing the biopsy device. Abnormalities located just under the skin or areola, or deep against the chest wall may be inaccessible. Patients, who are unable to cooperate, lie prone, or still; who have bleeding disorders; or who are on anticoagulation therapy, may not be suitable candidates. The location of the abnormality in the breast of a woman with breast implants dictates whether biopsy is feasible.

CNB of the breast has proven to have few complications. Potential complications include neck, back, arm, and shoulder pain related to patient positioning, bleeding, infection, and vasovagal reactions. In patients with normal coagulation profiles and no predisposition to infection, the risk of serious bleeding or infection is minimal (less than 1 %).

9.4.2 Appropriate Post-core Needle Biopsy Follow-up

CNB is a sampling technique; hence, appropriate post-CNB follow-up to ensure lesion stability is critical in all patients with a benign biopsy result. The rate of false-negative CNB results is not known with certainty, but it is believed to be approximately 2 % [72]. This percentage is likely to be much lower at centers performing a large number of biopsies, and those that correlate their radiological and pathological results on a regular basis. Several steps can be followed to minimize false-negative biopsy results. An adequate number of core samples should be obtained at biopsy to avoid sampling error, and specimen radiography should be performed in all cases where calcifications are sampled to verify that an adequate sampling of the targeted calcifications is contained within the biopsy core samples. Once the biopsy result is reported, radiologic–pathologic concordance or discordance should be assessed. *Concordance* means that the pathological result adequately explains the imaging finding. *Discordance* means that the pathological result does not adequately explain the imaging. In our practice, any patient with radiologic–pathologic discordance undergoes excisional biopsy of the abnormality.

In addition, a number of CNB controversial histologic diagnoses may require excisional biopsy. There is consensus that a CNB diagnosis of atypical ductal hyperplasia mandates excisional biopsy. There is still controversy about the need for excisional biopsy after CNB diagnosis of radial scar, papilloma, lobular carcinoma in situ (LCIS), and atypical lobular hyperplasia (ALH) [73–78]. More recent studies of LCIS and ALH cases diagnosed at CNB have shown upgrade rates to malignancy at excisional biopsy to be approximately 17–19 %. This approaches the upgrade rate in patients with ADH [79, 80]. For this reason, in our practice, we recommend surgical excision when radial scar, papilloma, or LCIS/ALH is identified at CNB.

Patients with definitely benign CNB results can return to age appropriate follow-up. If there is any question that a benign pathology result is definitely benign, then 6-month short-interval imaging follow-up using the imaging modality that best demonstrated the finding is indicated. Any interval growth or suspicious change on imaging or clinical grounds warrants surgical excision. If discordance is suspected, then excisional biopsy should be performed following the CNB.

9.5 Magnetic Resonance Imaging of the Breast

The initial studies to determine the potential value of MRI for detecting breast cancer were performed in the 1980s. In these studies, MRI without contrast was not found to be reliable for the detection or diagnosis of breast cancer [81]. Later investigations using intravenous gadolinium-based MR contrast agents showed a high sensitivity for the detection of breast cancer [82–86]. However, specificity varies as both benign conditions and breast cancer can enhance (Fig. 9.16). Noncontrast MRI has been applied successfully for the evaluation of silicone breast implants for intracapsular and extracapsular rupture but, in the absence of contrast, does not assess for breast cancer [87].

There are now several established indications for contrast-enhanced breast MRI: (1) screening of high-risk women; (2) assessment of ipsilateral extent of disease and performance of contralateral screening in patients with newly diagnosed breast cancer; (3) identifying multifocal and multicentric lesions; (4) evaluating women presenting with metastatic axillary adenopathy and an occult primary breast malignancy (Fig. 9.17); (5) identifying recurrent

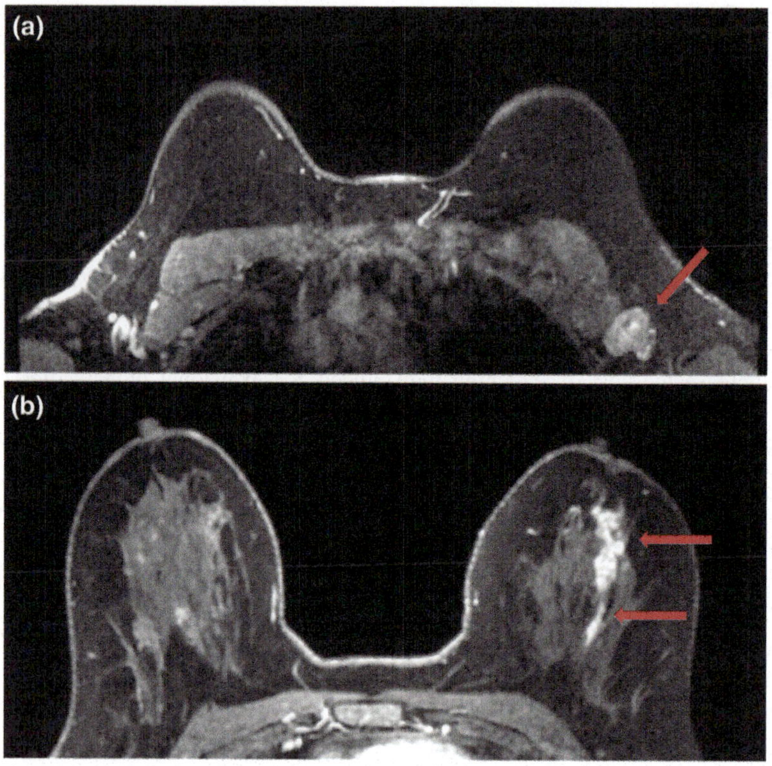

Fig. 9.16 A 35-year-old BRCA-2-positive woman referred for high-risk screening MRI. The contrast-enhanced MRI coronal (looking at the patient from the front, anterior to posterior) image shows contrast uptake in a lobular mass with dark internal septations (*arrow*) typical for fibroadenoma. A biopsy was performed as requested by the patient and confirmed a fibroadenoma

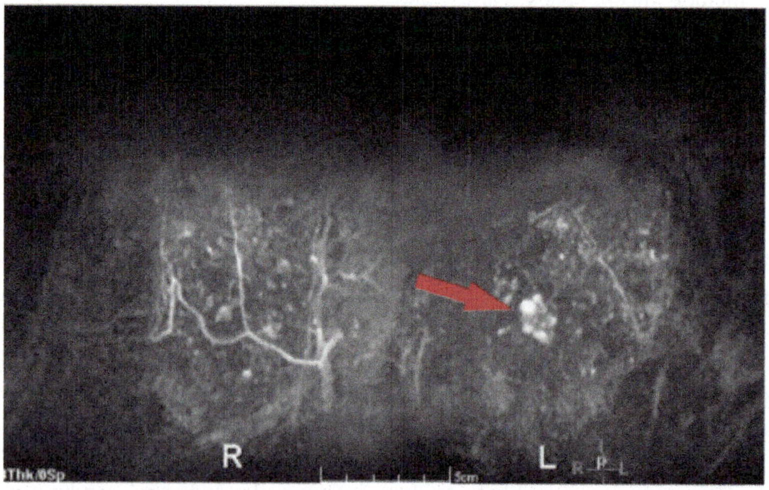

Fig. 9.17 A 51-year-old woman with an enlarged axillary lymph node that proved on core needle biopsy to be metastatic breast cancer. Mammograms and ultrasound were negative. **a** Axial contrast-enhanced breast MRI at the level of the axillae shows an enlarged 2.5-cm left axillary lymph node (*arrow*) with a replaced fatty hilum consistent with metastatic disease. **b** Axial contrast-enhanced MRI at the level of the central retroareolar breast shows segmental nonmass enhancement (*arrow*) which was occult on mammography and ultrasound. MRI-guided core needle biopsy revealed invasive mammary carcinoma with lobular features

carcinoma in the conservatively treated breast; (6) evaluating for response to neoadjuvant chemotherapy; and (7) guidance for CNB and preoperative wire localization of abnormalities only visualized on MRI.

9.5.1 Contrast-Enhanced Breast MRI for Screening in High-Risk Women

The use of MR in addition to mammography in screening women at high risk of breast cancer has become widely used in clinical practice. Multiple studies evaluating the performance of screening breast MRI in high-risk women show 77–100 % sensitivity and 81–99 % specificity with evidence that interpreting radiologist experience, high interpretation volume, and training are associated with improved efficacy [88–93]. One of these studies, a multi-institutional study conducted by Lehman et al. [88], concluded that women at high risk of breast cancer would benefit from screening MRI. In that study, high risk included women 25 years of age or older who were genetically at high risk, defined as BRCA-1/ BRCA-2 carriers or with at least a 20 % probability of carrying such a mutation. The study found that screening MRI imaging (1) had a higher biopsy rate with the PPV of biopsies performed as a result of MRI being 43 % and (2) helped detect more cancers than either mammography or ultrasound. The ACS recommends annual supplemental breast MRI (in conjunction with annual screening mammography) for women at high risk of breast cancer: BRCA-1/BRCA-2 mutation or first-degree relative with this mutation, a 20–25 % or greater lifetime risk of breast cancer, radiation to the chest wall between ages 10 and 30, history of Li-Fraumeni syndrome, Cowden syndrome, or Bannayan-Riley-Ruvalcaba syndrome, or first-degree relative with such syndromes [94].

Concerns about screening MRI cost, scan acquisition time, and interpretation time have led to investigation of abbreviated breast MRI screening protocols that are less costly and allows image acquisition in 3 min [95]. Expert radiologist interpretation time is rapid and yields a negative predictive value of 99.8 %, sensitivity of 100 %, and an additional cancer yield of 18.2 per 1000. Specificity (94.3 %) and PPV (24.4 %) are equivalent to more time-consuming full MRI protocols. Further experience with abbreviated protocols will ultimately determine whether this technique can replace current longer protocols.

9.6 Radionuclide Imaging

Another area of active investigation involves radionuclide scanning of the breast after the injection of the radionuclide-labeled substances that concentrate in breast tumors. Technetium^{99m} (Tc^{99m}) methoxyisobutyl isonitrile (MIBI) breast scintimammography has been under the investigation for several years now. Early reports indicated high sensitivity (>90 %) and specificity (slightly <90 %) [96]. Later reports, however, indicate a relatively low sensitivity for small cancers, those found only by mammography (56 %), and 1 cm or smaller (39 %) [97, 98].

Breast-specific gamma imaging (BSGI) utilizes the radionuclide Tc^{99m}-sestamibi, which has been used for cardiac studies, for the evaluation for breast cancer. BSGI has a relatively high sensitivity at 96.4 %, but a moderate sensitivity at 59.5 %. Additionally, the sensitivity of BSGI (and of all radionuclide imaging of the breast) is independent of breast density; however, the spatial resolution of BSGI limits its ability to reliably detect lesions less than 1 cm in size [99]. When BSGI is used as a supplemental screening tool in women with dense breasts and negative screening mammography, the cancer detection rate is 7.7 %, with a recall rate of 8.4 % [100]. One of the drawbacks to BSGI is its associated increased radiation dose that is approximately four times that of a conventional mammography with a total effective dose to the *body* of approximately 2.3 mSv [100]. Given the higher radiation dose to the body associated with Tc^{99m}-sestamibi imaging, additional research focused on lowering radiation dose may be indicated.

Positron emission tomography (PET) using fluorine-18 2-deoxy-2-fluoro-D-glucose (FDG) has also been used in the evaluation for breast cancer, as most breast cancers have been shown to demonstrate FDG uptake (Fig. 9.18) [101]. FDG also accumulates in axillary lymph nodes, providing information about nodal involvement. When combined with CT, PET-CT is a powerful tool to assess for metastatic disease and for staging.

Tc^{99m} sulfur colloid has been proven useful and is widely used for the identification of sentinel lymph nodes [102, 103]. Prior to surgery, the isotope is injected into the breast in the vicinity of a biopsy-proven breast cancer. The injected isotope drains through the lymphatic chain, identifying the initial, or sentinel lymph nodes. At surgery, the sentinel nodes are identified using a radioisotope probe and are then removed and evaluated histologically. If the sentinel nodes are negative for tumor, axillary node dissection and its associated complications can be avoided.

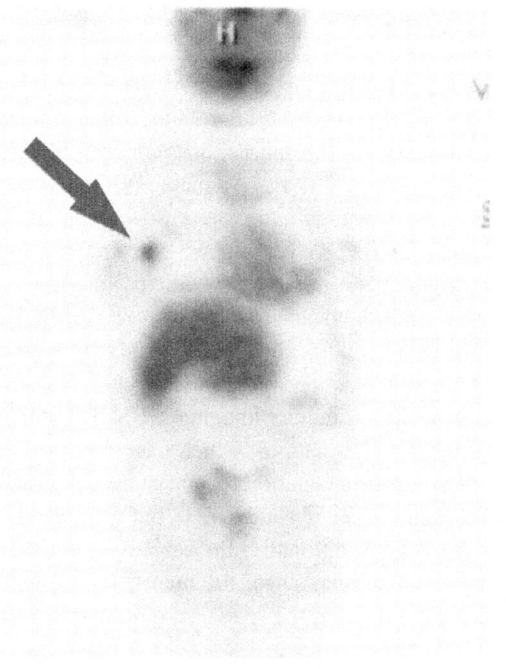

Fig. 9.18 Positron emission tomography (PET) image shows an area of radionuclide enhancement (*arrow*) at the site of an invasive cancer in the right breast

References

1. McLelland R, Hendrick RE, Zinninger MD, et al. The American college of radiology mammography accreditation program. Am J Roentgenol. 1991;157:497.
2. Mammography Quality Standards Act of 1992. Public Law 102539.
3. D'Orsi CJ, Sickles EA, Mendelson EB, Morris EA, et al. ACR BI-RADS Atlas, breast imaging reporting and data system. Reston, VA: American College of Radiology; 2013.
4. American College of Radiology. Standards for the performance of screening mammography. [Adopted by the ACR Council 1990, Revised 1994]. In: ACR digest of official actions. Reston, VA: ACR; 1994.
5. Tabar L, Fagerberg CJ, Gad A, et al. Reduction in mortality from breast cancer after mass screening with mammography: randomized trial from the breast cancer screening working group of the Swedish National Board of Health and Welfare. Lancet. 1985;1:829–32.
6. National Institutes of Health Consensus Development Panel. National Institutes of Health Consensus Development Panel: breast cancer screening for women 40–49. J Natl Cancer inst. 1997;39:1015–26.
7. Howlander N, Noone A, Krapcho M, et al. SEER cancer statistics review, 1975–2012. Bethesda, MD: National Cancer Institute; 2015.
8. Webb ML, Cady B, Michaelson JS, Bush DM, Calvillo KZ, Kopans DB, Smith BL. A failure analysis of invasive breast cancer: most deaths from disease occur in women not regularly screened. Cancer. 2014;120(18):2839–46. doi:10.1002/cncr.28199.
9. Hellquist BN, Duffy SW, Abdsaleh S, et al. Effectiveness of population-based service screening with mammography for women ages 40-49 years: evaluation of the Swedish mammography screening in young women (SCRY) cohort. Cancer. 2011;117(4):714–22. doi:10.1002/cncr.25650 (Epub 2010 Sep 29).
10. Duffy SW, Tabar L, Chen HH, et al. The impact of organized mammography service screening on breast carcinoma mortality in seven Swedish counties. Cancer. 2002;95:458–69.
11. Freer P, Moy L, Demartini WB. Breast cancer screening: understanding the randomized controlled trial. SBI News. 2015;3:25–7.
12. Joe B, Price E, Parkinson B. Screening in the 40–49 age group. SBI News. 2016;1:12–4.
13. Independent UK. Panel on breast cancer screening. The benefits and harms of breast cancer screening: an independent review. Lancet. 2012;380:1778–86.
14. Smith RA, Duffy SW, Gabe R, Tabar L, Yen AM, Chen TH. The randomized trials of breast cancer screening: what have we learned? Radiol Clin North Am. 2004;42:793–806.
15. Tabar L, Yen AM, Wu WY, et al. Insights from the breast cancer screening trials: how screening affects the natural history of breast cancer and implications for evaluating service screening programs. Breast J. 2015;21:13–20.
16. Duffy SW, Yen AMF, Chen THH, et al. Long-term benefits of breast screening. Breast Cancer Manage. 2012;1:31–8.
17. Gotzsche PC, Jorgensen KJ. Screening for breast cancer with mammography. Cochrane Database Syst Rev. 2013;6: CD001877.
18. Broeders M, Moss S, Nystrom L, et al. The impact of mammographic screening on breast cancer mortality in Europe: a review of observational studies. J Med Screen. 2012;19(suppl 1):14–25.
19. Nickson C, Mason KE, English DR, Kavanagh AM. Mammographic screening and breast cancer mortality: a case-control study and meta-analysis. Cancer Epidemiol Biomark Prev. 2012;21:1479–88.
20. Coldman A, Phillips N, Wilson C, et al. Pan-Canadian study of mammography screening and mortality from breast cancer. J Natl Cancer Inst. 2014;106(11):dju261.
21. Cancer Intervention and Surveillance Modeling Network. (CISNET) Collaborators. Effect of screening and adjuvant therapy on mortality from breast cancer. N Engl J Med. 2005;353:1784–92.
22. Hendrick RE, Helvie MA. Mammography screening: a new estimate of number needed to screen to prevent one breast cancer death. AJR Am J Roentgenol. 2012;198(3):723–8.
23. Oeffinger KC, Fontham ETH, Etzioni R. Breast cancer screening for women at average risk 2015 guideline update from the American Cancer Society. JAMA. 2015;314(15):1599–614.
24. Siu AL. Screening for breast cancer: U.S. preventive services task force recommendation statement. Ann Intern Med. 2016;164:279–96.
25. Singletary SE, Allred C, Ashley P, et al. Staging system for breast cancer: revisions for the 6th edition of the AJCC cancer staging manual. Surg Clin North Am. 2003;83(4):803–19.
26. American College of Radiology (ACR). Clinical Practice Guideline for the performance of diagnostic mammography and problem-solving breast evaluation [Adopted by the ACR Council 1994]. In: ACR digest of official actions. Reston, VA: ACR; 1994.
27. Destounis SV, Morgan R, Arieno A. Screening for dense breasts: digital breast tomosynthesis. AJR Am J Roentgenol. 2015;204:261–4.

28. McDonald ES, Oustimov A, Weinstein SP, et al. Effectiveness of digital breast tomosynthesis compared with digital mammogram: outcome analysis from 3 years of breast cancer screening. JAMA Oncol. 2016;6:737–43.
29. Rose SL, Tidwell AL, Gujnoch LJ, et al. Implementation of breast tomosynthesis in a routine screening practice: an observational study. AJR Am J Roentgenol. 2013;200(6):1401–8.
30. Skaane P, Bandos AI, Gullien R, et al. Comparison of digital mammography alone and digital mammography plus tomosynthesis in a population-based screening program. Radiology. 2013;267(1):47–56.
31. Friedewald SM, Rafferty EA, Rose SL, et al. Breast cancer screening using tomosynthesis in combination with digital mammography. JAMA. 2014;311(24):2499–507.
32. Ciatto S, Houssami N, Bernardi D, et al. Integration of 3D digital mammography with tomosynthesis for population breast-cancer screening (STORM): a prospective comparison study. Lancet Oncol. 2013;14(7):583–9.
33. Skaane P, Bandos AI, Eben EB, et al. Two-view digital breast tomosynthesis screening with synthetically reconstructed projection images: comparison with digital breast tomosynthesis with full-field digital mammographic images. Radiology. 2014;271 (3):655–63. doi:10.1148/radiol.13131391 (Epub 2014 Jan 24).
34. Linver MN, Osuch JR, Brenner RJ, et al. Mammography medical audit: primer for the mammography quality standards act (MQSA). AJR Am J Roentgenol. 1995;165:19–25.
35. Gold RH, Montgomery CK, Rambo ON. Significance of margination of benign and malignant infiltrative mammary lesions: roentgenologic-pathologic correlation. Am J Roentgenol. 1973;118:881–94.
36. Hall FM, Storella JM, Silverstone DZ, et al. Nonpalpable breast lesions: recommendations for biopsy based on suspicion of carcinoma at mammography. Radiology. 1988;167:353–8.
37. Moskowitz M. The predictive value of certain mammographic signs in screening for breast cancer. Cancer. 1983;51:1007–11.
38. Sickles EA. Nonpalpable, circumscribed, noncalcified solid breast masses: likelihood of malignancy based on lesion size and age of patient. Radiology. 1994;192:439–42.
39. Brenner RJ, Sickles EA. Acceptability of periodic follow-up as an alternative to biopsy for mammographically detected lesions interpreted as probably benign. Radiology. 1989;171:645–6.
40. Feig SA. Breast masses: mammographic and sonographic evaluation. Radiol Clin North Am. 1992;30:67–92.
41. Jackson VP, Dines KA, Bassett LW, et al. Diagnostic importance of radiographic density of noncalcified breast masses: analysis of 91 lesions. AJR Am J Roentgenol. 1991;157:25–8.
42. Bassett LW. Mammographic analysis of calcifications. Radiol Clin North Am. 1992;30:93–105.
43. Sickles EA. Mammographic features of 300 Consecutive nonpalpable breast cancers. Am J Roentgenol. 1986;146:661–3.
44. Sickles EA. Mammographic features of "early": breast cancer. Am J Roentgenol. 1984;143:461–4.
45. Brown ML, Houn F, Sickles EA, et al. Screening mammography in community practice: positive predictive value of abnormal finding and yield of follow-up diagnostic procedures. Am J Roentgenol. 1995;165:1373–7.
46. Robertson CL, Kopans DB. Communication problems after mammographic screening. Radiology. 1989;172:443–4.
47. Brew MD, Billings JD, Chisholm RJ. Mammography and breast pain. Australas Radiol. 1989;33:335–6.
48. Jackson VP, Loex AM, Smith DJ. Patient discomfort during screen-film mammography. Radiology. 1998;168:421–3.
49. Stomper PC, Kopans DB, Sadowsky NL, et al. Is mammography painful? A multicenter patient study. Arch Intern Med. 1988;148:521–4.
50. Physician Insurer's Association of America. PIAA breast cancer study, MPL cancer claims mini series: volume 1. Washington, DC: Physician Insurers Association of America; 2013.
51. Feig SA, Shaber GS, Patchefsky A, et al. Analysis of clinically occult and mammographically occult breast tumors. Am J Roentenol. 1977;128:403–8.
52. Mann BD, Giuliano AE, Bassett LW, et al. Delayed diagnosis of breast cancer as a result of normal mammograms. Arch Surg. 1983;118:23–4.
53. Fornage BD, Lorigan JG, Andry E. Fibroadenoma of the breast: sonographic appearance. Radiology. 1989;172:671–5.
54. Stavros AT, Thickman D, Rapp CL, et al. Solid breast nodules: use of sonography to distinguish between benign and malignant lesions. Radiology. 1995;196:123–34.
55. Entrekin R, Jackson P, Jago JR, Porter BA. Compound Imaging in breast ultrasound: technology and early clinical experience. Medicamundi. 1999;43(3):35–43.
56. Rosen EL, Soo MS. Tissue harmonic imaging sonography of breast lesions: improved margin analysis, conspicuity and image quality compared to conventional ultrasound. Clin Imaging. 2001;25(6):379–84.
57. Mesurolle B, Helou T, El-Khoury M, et al. Tissue harmonic imaging, frequency compound imaging and conventional imaging: use and benefit in breast sonography. J Ultrasound Med. 2007;26(8):1041–51.
58. Rahbar G, Sie AC, Hansen GC, et al. Benign versus malignant solid breast masses: US differentiation. Radiology. 1999;213:889–94.
59. Gordon PB, Goldenberg SL. Malignant breast masses detected only by ultrasound: a retrospective review. Cancer. 1995;76: 626–60.
60. Buchberger W, Niehoff A, Obrist P, et al. Clinically and mammographically occult breast lesions: detection and classification with high resolution sonography. Semin Ultrasound CT MR. 2002;21:325–36.
61. Kaplan SS. Clinical utility of bilateral whole-breast US in the evaluation of women with dense breast tissue. Radiology. 2001;221:641–9.
62. Crystal P, Strano SD, Shcharynski S, et al. Using sonography to screen women with mammographically dense breasts. Am J Roentgenol. 2003;181:177–82.
63. Kolb TM, Lichy J, Newhouse JH. Occult cancer in women with dense breasts: detection with screening US—diagnostic yield and tumor characteristics. Radiology. 1998;207:191–9.
64. Kolb TM, Lichy J, Newhouse JH. Comparison of the performance of screening mammography, physical examination, and breast US and evaluation of factors that influence them: an analysis of 27, 825 patient evaluations. Radiology. 2002;225:165–75.
65. Berg WA. Rationale for a trial of screening breast ultrasound: American college of radiology imaging network (ACRIN) 6666. Am J Roentgenol. 2003;180:1225–8.
66. Berg WA, Blume JD, Cormack JB et al. ACRIN 6666 Investigators. Combined screening with ultrasound and mammography vs mammography alone in women at elevated risk of breast cancer. JAMA. 2008;299(18):2151–63. doi:10.1001/jama. 299.18.2151.
67. Sprague BL, Stout NK, Schechter C, et al. Benefits, harms, and cost-effectiveness of supplemental ultrasonography screening for women with dense breasts. Ann Intern Med. 2015;162(3):157–66. doi:10.7326/M14-0692.
68. Parker SH, Lovin JD, Jobe WE, et al. Stereotactic breast biopsy with a biopsy gun. Radiology. 1990;176:741–7.
69. Jackson VP, Bassett LW. Stereotactic fine-needle aspiration biopsy for nonpalpable breast lesions. Am J Roentgenol. 1990;154:1196–7.

70. Bassett LW, Winchester DP, Caplan RB, et al. Stereotactic core-needle biopsy of the breast. CA Cancer J Clin. 1997;47:171–90.
71. Sickles EA, Parker SH. Appropriate role of core breast biopsy in the management of probably benign lesions. Radiology. 1993;199:315.
72. Lee CH, Philpotts LE, Horvath LJ, et al. Follow-up of breast lesions diagnosed as benign with stereotactic coreneedle biopsy: frequency of mammographic change and false negative rate. Radiology. 1999;212:189–94.
73. Brem RF, Behrndt VS, Sanow L, et al. Atypical ductal hyperplasia: histologic underestimation of carcinoma in tissue harvested from impalpable breast lesions using 11-G stereotactically guided directional vacuum-assisted biopsy. Am J Roentgenol. 1999;172:1405–7.
74. Jackman RJ, Nowels W, Rodriguez-Soto J, et al. Stereotactic, automated, large-core needle biopsy of nonpalpable breast lesions: false-negative rates and histologic underestimation rates after long-term follow-up. Radiology. 1999;210:799–805.
75. Liberman L, Bracero N, Vuolo MA, et al. Percutaneous large-core biopsy of papillary breast lesions. Am J Roentgenol. 1999;172:331–7.
76. Liberman L, Sama M, Susnik B, et al. Lobular carcinoma in situ at percutaneous breast biopsy: surgical biopsy findings. Am J Roentgenol. 1999;173:291–9.
77. Philpotts LE, Shaheen NA, Carter D, et al. Comparison of rebiopsy rates after stereotactic core-needle biopsy of the breast with 11-G vacuum suction probe vs. 14-G automatic gun. Am J Roentgenol. 1999;172:683–7.
78. Brenner RJ, Jackman RJ, Parker SH, et al. Percutaneous core needle biopsy of radial scars of the breast: when is excision necessary? Am J Roentgenol. 2002;179:1179–84.
79. Foster MC, Helvie MA, Gregory NE, et al. Lobular carcinoma in situ or atypical lobular hyperplasia at coreneedle biopsy: is excisional biopsy necessary? Radiology. 2004;231:813–9.
80. Mahoney MC, Robinson-Smith TM, Shaughnessy EA. Lobular neoplasia at 11-gauge vacuum-assisted stereotactic biopsy: correlation with surgical excisional biopsy and mammographic follow-up. Am J Roentgenol. 2006;187:949–54.
81. El Yousef SJ, O'Connell DM, Duchesneau RH, et al. Benign and malignant breast disease: magnetic resonance and radiofrequency pulse sequences. Am J Roentgenol. 1985;145:1–8.
82. Heywang SH, Hahn D, Schmidt H, et al. MR imaging of the breast using gadolinium-DTPA. J Comput Asst Tomogr. 1986;10:199–204.
83. Kaiser WA (1992) MRM promises earlier breast cancer diagnosis. Diagn Imaging Int. 11:44–50.
84. Heywang-Kobrunner SH. Contrast-enhanced MRI of the breast-overview after 1250 patient examinations. Electromedica. 1993;2:43–52.
85. Harms SE, Flamig DP, Hesley KL, et al. MRI of the breast with rotating delivery of excitation off resonance: clinical experience with pathologic correlation. Radiology. 1993;186:493.
86. Gilles R, Guinebretiere JM, Lucidarme O, et al. Nonpalpable breast tumors: diagnosis with contrast-enhanced subtraction dynamic MRI. Radiology. 1994;191:625–31.
87. Gorczyca DP, Sinha S, Ahn CY, et al. Silicone breast implants in vivo: MR imaging. Radiology. 1992;185:407–10.
88. Lehman CD, Blume JD, Weatherall P, et al. Screening women at high risk for breast cancer with mammography and magnetic resonance imaging. Cancer. 2005;103:1898–905.
89. Kriege M, Brekelmans CT, Boetes C, et al. Efficacy of MRI and mammography for breast-cancer screening in women with a familial or genetic predisposition. N Engl J Med. 2004;351:427–37.
90. Kuhl CK, Schrading S, Leutner CC, et al. Mammography, breast ultrasound, and magnetic resonance imaging for surveillance of women at high familial risk for breast cancer. J Clin Oncol. 2005;23:8469–76.
91. Leach MO, Boggis CR, Dixon AK, et al. Screening with magnetic resonance imaging and mammography of a UK population at high familial risk of breast cancer: a prospective multicentre cohort study (MARIBS). Lancet. 2005;365:1769–78.
92. Sardanelli F. Breast MRI imaging in women at high risk of breast cancer. Is something changing in early breast cancer detection? Eur Radiol. 2007;73: 873–87.
93. Warner E, Plewes DB, Hill KA, et al. Surveil-lance of *BRCA1* and *BRCA2* mutation carriers with magnetic resonance imaging, ultrasound, mammography, and clinical breast examination. JAMA. 2004;292:1317–25.
94. Saslow D, Boetes C, Burke W, et al. American cancer society guidelines for breast screening with MRI as an adjunct to mammography. CA Cancer J Clin. 2009;57:75–89. doi:10.3322/canjclin.57.2.75.
95. Kuhl CK, Schrading S, Strobel K, et al. Abbreviated breast magnetic resonance imaging (MRI): first postcontrast subtracted images and maximum-intensity projection-a novel approach to breast cancer screening with MRI. Clin Oncol. 2014;32(22):2304–10. doi:10.1200/JCO.2013.52.5386 (Epub 2014 Jun 23).
96. Khalkhali I, Mena I, Jouanne E, et al. Prone scintimammography in patients with suspicion of carcinoma of the breast. J Am Coll Surg. 1994;178:491–7.
97. Tolmos J, Cutrone JA, Wang B, et al. Scintimammographic analysis of non palpable breast lesions previously identified by conventional mammography. J Natl Cancer Inst. 1998;90:846–9.
98. Prats E, Carril J, Herranz R, et al. Spanish multicenter scintigraphic study of the breast using Tc99 m MIBI: report of results. Rev Esp Med Nucl. 1998;17:338–50.
99. Brem RF, Floerke AC, Rapelyea JA, et al. Breast-specific gamma imaging as an adjunct imaging modality for the diagnosis of breast cancer. Radiology. 2008;247(3):651–7.
100. Shermis RB, Wilson KD, Doyle MT, et al. Supplemental breast cancer screening with molecular breast imaging for women with dense breast tissue. AJR Am J Roentgenol. 2016;17:1–8.
101. Adler LP, Crowe JP, Al-Kasisi NK, et al. Evaluation of breast masses and axillary lymph nodes with (F-18) 2-Deoxy-2-fluro-D-glucose PET. Radiology. 1993;187:743–50.
102. Winchester DJ, Sener SF, Winchester DP, et al. Sentinel lymphadencotomy for breast cancer: experience what 180 consecutive patients: efficacy of filtered technetium 99 m sulphur colloid with overnight migration time. J Am Coll Surg. 1999;188:597–603.
103. Schwartz GF, Guiliano AE, Veronesi U. Consensus conference committee. Proceeding of the consensus conference of the role of sentinel lymph node biopsy in carcinoma or the breast scr; 2002.
104. Bassett LW, Hendrick RE, Bassford TL, et al. Quality determinants of mammography; clinical practice guideline. No 13. AHCPR Publication 95-0632. Rockville, MD: Agency for Health Care Policy and Research, Public Health Service, U.S. Department of Health and Human Services, October 1994.

10 Premalignant and Malignant Breast Pathology

Hans-Peter Sinn

10.1 Introduction

In recent years, many concepts on the pathology of premalignant and malignant breast disease have been greatly influenced by progress in the understanding of their molecular biology, and its impact on adjuvant and neoadjuvant therapy and risk estimation. However, molecular classification has not yet replaced the traditional, morphologically oriented tumor classification of breast cancer because the many facets of breast cancer can still being described most accurately in terms of classic histopathology. This also relates to the methodology of diagnosing breast cancer that is slowly, but steadily changing away from a descriptive morphological view of the disease towards a more quantitative and molecularly oriented estimation of the tumor tissue. Much of this has been driven by the need of oncologists for precise information on the tumor biology in order to more accurately guide adjuvant and neoadjuvant therapy. Therefore, breast pathology nowadays is both morphologically and molecularly oriented with the focus on a unifying view of these two aspects of breast cancer.

It is not possible to comprehensively cover all aspects of the pathology of premalignant and malignant breast disease in this chapter. Therefore, we will give an overview on the current and innovative aspects of breast pathology and growing points of translational research. For the precursor lesions, this mostly relates to the risk estimation and recommendation for the management of the lesions. For the invasive carcinomas, aspects of morphological classification, as well as the evaluation of operative and non-operative specimens are covered.

H.-P. Sinn (✉)
Department of Pathology, University of Heidelberg, Im Neuenheimer Feld 224, 69124 Heidelberg, Baden-Württemberg, Germany
e-mail: Peter.sinn@med.uni-heidelberg.de

10.2 Premalignant Lesions

In the following paragraphs, a short overview will be given to neoplastic, but preinvasive disease including ductal carcinoma in situ (DCIS). In the European guidelines for quality assurance in breast cancer screening and diagnosis [1], the category of *lesions of uncertain malignant potential* (B3 category) includes lesions with an increased risk of malignancy at open excision. These lesions are usually detected with breast ultrasound-guided or vacuum-assisted (stereotactic) core biopsy at breast cancer screening or at prophylactic mammography and may or may not require surgical excision after being diagnosed. The B3 category includes lesions which are benign but carry an increased risk of in situ or invasive malignant disease because of their frequent heterogeneity (such as papillomas or phyllodes tumor), but also low-grade neoplastic lesions, such as lobular neoplasia of flat epithelial atypia. This makes an important difference for the management of B3 lesions, because not all B3 lesions are neoplasia with low malignant potential. The risk potential of premalignant lesions in the B3 category generally is lower than risk of low-grade DCIS, which are categorized as B5a, together with other DCIS cases.

The recommendations for excision of precursor lesions are dependent upon the natural history, subtype, and extent of the lesion, as well on other patient and lesion-related parameters. Over the last years, the evidence base to guide management of the management of precursor lesions with low and uncertain malignant potential detected on screen mammography has grown, and this has led to a more conservative approach in general (Table 10.1) [2]. A cautious attitude towards the management of these lesions requires a close collaboration between the radiologist and the pathologist and should ideally be discussed at a screening or preoperative multidisciplinary conference. The pathologic diagnosis on a core biopsy per se is not sufficient for recommendation of further treatment, because it may or may not be representative of the radiological lesion, and even if it is representative, the most significant pathologic findings

I. Jatoi and A. Rody (eds.), *Management of Breast Diseases*, DOI 10.1007/978-3-319-46356-8_10

Table 10.1 Recommendations for treatment of precursor lesions after diagnosis on core biopsy

Atypical ductal hyperplasia (ADH) – All patients referred for surgical consultation and excision
Atypical lobular hyperplasia (ALH) – Patients with incidental ALH offered surveillance
Lobular carcinoma in situ (LCIS) – Patients with incidental classical LCIS may be offered surveillance; patients with non-classic variants should undergo excision

Source Data from Calhoun [2]

(such as LCIS) may not be the one that is visible radiologically and has led to the core biopsy. The published literature on preneoplastic precursor lesions (except DCIS) mostly consists of single-institution, non-randomized retrospective case series, often with the lack of careful pathological–radiological correlation, and concern about possible selection bias for open biopsy. This may explain for the variations in the published upgrade risks to invasive or noninvasive cancer on open biopsy and is part of the reason for the variability of the clinical management of precursor lesion in different institutions.

10.2.1 Ductal Carcinoma in Situ

10.2.1.1 Terminology

The term *carcinoma* in situ has been criticized in the last years, especially in the context of screening mammography where low-risk lesions with uncertain malignant potential are not infrequently detected. It has been argued that the patient with a lesion which is not capable of metastasis should not be confronted with the term "carcinoma" [3], and the term "overdiagnosis" has been used in this context [4, 5]. However, this is unfortunate, because "overdiagnosis" suggests "misdiagnosis." The discussion of the correct management of DCIS in breast cancer screening should therefore be focussed on the question of possible overtreatment rather than overdiagnosis [6]. Actually, preinvasive neoplasia of the breast (DCIS and lobular neoplasia) have all characteristic features of noninvasive carcinoma both histologically and molecularly, and therefore truly represent in situ malignancy.

10.2.1.2 Incidence and Clinical Presentation

Ductal carcinoma in situ (DCIS) is characterized as having an inherent, but not necessarily obligate tendency for progression to invasive breast cancer. Over the last decades, the incidence of DCIS has increased markedly. A systematic review gave an estimated incidence of DCIS of 1.87 per 100,000 in 1973–1975 and 32.5/100,000 in 2004 in USA [7]. The relative proportion of DCIS in the SEER breast cancer database in 1983 was 0.3 % compared to 12 % in 1992 [8], and 21 % in 2014 [9]. It is believed that the main reason for this rise in incidence is routine mammography in the asymptomatic patient and population-based screening programs. In mammography screening, the standardized detection rate of DCIS was estimated as 1.60/1000 women in the UK [10], and lower numbers were reported internationally [11]. Clinically, 80 % of DCIS are asymptomatic, and only 20 % present as symptomatic disease [7].

10.2.1.3 Natural History and Mortality of DCIS

Recently, there has been some debate on the value of early detection of DCIS and its treatment (Morrow JNCI 2015), because of the very low mortality of 3.3 % of pure DCIS in the SEER cancer registry (20-year breast cancer specific mortality rate). This is 1.8 times greater than the expected mortality of age-matched controls in the US population [12]. This study has been cited frequently to prove the low malignant potential of DCIS, and because of the low mortality associated with DCIS, and with low-grade DCIS in particular, the term DCIS itself was put into question and it was proposed to instead call it "borderline breast disease" [13]. However, since it must be assumed that the great majority of cases in the SEER registry were adequately treated by complete surgical excision with or without radiotherapy, and therefore the low mortality of documented cases of DCIS more likely represents the mortality which is caused by occult invasive disease. For this reason, it may not be appropriate to use this epidemiological data as a measure of the natural course of DCIS. Only the study of untreated patients with DCIS could give such evidence. In the Nurse's health study, 6 out of 13 patients with DCIS that had been misdiagnosed as having a benign disease, later developed invasive breast cancer in the same breast. Based on these cases, the odds ratio for development of invasive carcinoma with DCIS that has been overlooked and untreated was estimated as 13.5, and the mean time interval until invasive cancer occurred was 9.0 years [14]. It was concluded by the authors that patients with untreated DCIS are at high risk for progression to invasive breast carcinoma. Other studies indicate that over a period of 10 years, 14–53 % of women diagnosed with DCIS subsequently develop invasive ductal carcinoma (IDC) if the DCIS is left untreated or inadequately treated [15].

10.2.1.4 Grading and Risk Assessment of DCIS

Much of the uncertainty regarding clinical management of DCIS is due to the fact that DCIS is a heterogeneous disease with variable malignant potential, and that invasive disease can only be excluded when the lesion has been thoroughly examined pathologically. Therefore, the evaluation of pathological factors is an important cornerstone in determining the risk of progression and based on that, the management of DCIS. Pathologically, the variable malignant potential of DCIS is reflected by its histological grade, the architectural pattern, by the size of the disease, and (to some extent) its immunohistological phenotype. More recently, gene-expression analysis has also been proposed to more precisely evaluate the aggressiveness of DCIS. Among all these parameters, the architectural pattern is the weakest predictor of prognosis after the diagnosis of DCIS, and secondary to grade and the presence of necrosis of comedo type.

Grading is one of the most important risk factors for outcome in DCIS [16]. In the current WHO classification of breast cancer, grading of DCIS is based upon its nuclear features, and, in contrast to the preceding WHO classification, the diagnosis of DCIS of low nuclear grade is not precluded by the presence of focal punctate or comedo-type necrosis. This grading system has superseded previously reported grading systems, including the Silverstein classification of DCIS [17], and the 1997 consensus on classification of DCIS [18]. With high nuclear grade DCIS, comedo-type necrosis is commonly seen, but not obligatory. Cytonuclear grading was shown to be a strong risk factor for both ipsilateral invasive and noninvasive tumor recurrence, and especially for a subgroup with additional extensive confluent comedo-type necrosis in more than 50 % of ducts [19].

10.2.1.5 Molecular Pathology and Special Types of DCIS

One of the arguments for the role of DCIS as a non-obligate precursor of invasive breast cancer is that the molecular subtyping of DCIS similar to that of invasive breast cancer; however, DCIS differs with respect to the relative proportions of the subgroups (Fig. 10.1). About 76 % of DCIS fall into the luminal category, being positive for estrogen and/or progesterone receptors. 14 % of DCIS are characterized by HER2 overexpression with negative hormone receptors, and 13 % were HER2 and ER positive. This 27 % or HER2-positive DCIS cases is in contrast to only 12.7 % HER2-positive invasive carcinomas in the same case series [20]. Similar frequencies were reported in other cases series [21, 22]. The much higher prevalence of HER2-positive pure DCIS than in invasive carcinoma has been reported in the literature consistently, but the HER2 expression status in invasive carcinoma, and its intraductal component is concordant in >90 % of cases. Therefore, it has been concluded that HER2 plays no significant role in progression to invasive carcinoma [23]. Special DCIS subtypes include molecular-apocrine DCIS, hypersecretory DCIS, and basal-like DCIS. Basal-like DCIS are rare (<10 %), and this subtype of DCIS is believed to be a precursor lesion for invasive basal-like carcinoma [24]. The molecular mechanisms that cause DCIS to progress to invasive cells are still unknown and no clear correlation between molecular subtype of DCIS and recurrence has been established. Therefore, there is no practical relevance to the subtyping of DCIS yet.

10.2.1.6 Pathologic Working Up of DCIS Specimens

It should be emphasized that the methods used in the pathology laboratory for working up specimens containing DCIS are

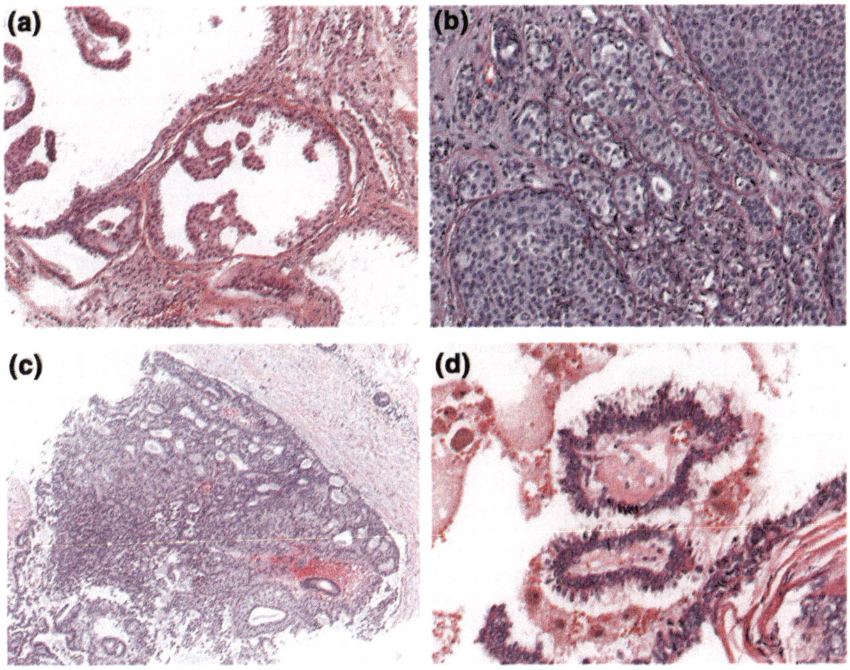

Fig. 10.1 Ductal carcinoma in situ (DCIS), some growth patterns: **a** DCIS G1, micropapillary type. **b** DCIS G2, solid type. **c** DCIS G1, encapsulated type. **d** DCIS G1, hypersecretory type

critical for the correct evaluation of the disease. This concerns the size of the lesion and the margin status, but most importantly the problem of detecting occult tumor invasion. To this end, it has been recommended that the entire region of the targeted lesion should be examined microscopically and, when practical, the entire specimen should be submitted in a sequential fashion for histologic examination [25, 26]. If the lesion is a nonpalpable imaging finding, a specimen radiography may be necessary to identify the lesion [25], and the most straightforward method to accomplish this is specimen radiography of the sliced breast conserving or mastectomy specimen. Actually, it can be recommended to process all excisional specimens in this way, and to perform specimen slice radiography in order to be able to submit appropriate tissue for histology [27]. This facilitates the identification of the lesions and of critical margins which can be adequately sampled according to the results of the radiography. The preferred method is serial sequential sampling. Without specimen radiography and systematic sampling, occult foci of invasion and invasion of margins may be easily missed, especially in large operative specimens, such as skin-sparing or nipple-sparing mastectomy.

Determination of the size of DCIS is not required for staging of the disease, but nevertheless important for pathological–radiological correlation and management of the patient [28]. The larger the DCIS, the more likely is the presence of residual disease, the involvement of margins, the likelihood of local recurrence, and the possibility of invasion [29–34]. The DCIS size frequently is underestimated based on mammographic assessment or specimen radiography, but also may be overestimated, in cases with well-differentiated DCIS and a background of proliferating breast disease. Usually, DCIS cannot be measured directly on the histology slide, unless it is <1 cm, but the size can be estimated by calculating the extent of DCIS on histology in a serially sampled specimen. It must be kept in mind that gaps in ductal involvement may be present, particularly in low-grade DCIS, and the pathology report it is recommended to calculate the total size including these gaps, not the size of each focus [26]. Also, in case that DCIS has been resected in multiple parts, it should be attempted by the pathologist to estimate the size of the DCIS by taking into account the topography of the individual specimens [25].

Microinvasion in DCIS is present when there are one or more invasive foci measuring ≤0.1 cm [35]. Care must be taken not to over diagnose microinvasion on core biopsy or on the excisional specimen, because the involvement of lobules or the involvement of sclerosing adenosis by DCIS may closely mimic microinvasion. Immunohistochemistry with basal markers (preferably p63) should be performed routinely in difficult cases in order to rule out or to confirm microinvasion [36, 37]. In a series of 21 cases with microinvasion, 15 had axillary staging, and in two of these cases, one positive lymph node was found [38]. In another case series axillary lymph node metastases were present in 9 out of 46 patients with DCIS and microinvasion [39]. This underlines the clinical significance of microinvasion in DCIS.

10.2.2 Atypical Ductal Hyperplasia (ADH)

10.2.2.1 Terminology

The term "atypical ductal hyperplasia" (ADH) has been defined to describe small atypical ductal lesions with insufficient criteria for a definite diagnosis of DCIS. The relative risk for breast cancer in women with ADH has been calculated as 4.5 in a recent update of the Nurses' Health Study, compared to 1.6 for women with nonproliferative breast disease [40]. There is no general agreement on the diagnostic criteria to distinguish ADH from a very small lesion of low-grade DCIS, and different definitions have been applied. Commonly, ADH is either defined as partial involvement of the terminal duct-lobular unit by monomorphic, low-grade atypical ductal epithelia with architectural disturbances, such as rigid bridges or micropapillae but not completely filling the duct [41], or as an unifocal or multifocal lesion that fulfils all criteria of low-grade DCIS except for a maximum size of 2 or 3 mm [42]. Uncommon variants of ADH include atypical apocrine hyperplasia and atypical ductal proliferations developing within a preexisting benign proliferative lesion such as sclerosing adenosis, usual-type ductal hyperplasia, or papilloma [43]. Atypical ductal hyperplasia may be distinguished pathologically from usual ductal hyperplasia by the use of basal cytokeratins, especially cytokeratin 5/6 [44].

There are two terminological problems with ADH: Firstly, ADH clearly is not a hyperplastic lesion but has all features of an early neoplastic process, and for this reason, ADH is also considered part of the classification system of ductal intraepithelial neoplasia [45]. Secondly, the term "atypical epithelial proliferation of ductal type" is preferred over the term ADH in the European Screening Mammography guidelines [1], because it has been argued that a lesion with criteria of ADH on core biopsy may prove to be part of a larger low-grade DCIS on excision specimen and a definitive diagnosis of ADH on needle core biopsies may not be possible. On the other hand the use of the term "atypical epithelial proliferation of ductal type" may create the false impression of the presence of a lesion with low risk and a non-neoplastic nature, which would be misleading. Therefore, we prefer to continue using the term ADH also in core biopsies, knowing that at the time of biopsy a substantial proportion will turn out to be low-grade DCIS.

10.2.2.2 Molecular Similarity of ADH and DCIS

The current concept of ADH being the immediate precursor of low-grade DCIS (lg-DCIS) is based not only on morphologic similarities between both lesions, but also on a high degree of genomic similarity with almost identical kinds of chromosomal imbalances [46–48]. A loss at chromosome 16q and 17p was concurrently observed when comparing ADH and DCIS lesions [46, 47], also in a study of nine ADHs, a total of 18 copy number changes were identified with recurrent losses of 16q and 17p and frequent gains on chromosome 1q [46], similar to observations in lg-DCIS. This genomic similarity of lg-DCIS and ADH may give rise to questioning the validity of making a difference between both lesions. However, because of the prognostic differences of ADH and lg-DCIS, it is fair to interpret the molecular data as supportive of the assumption that ADH is not just a small low-grade DCIS, but a closely related precursor lesion [49].

10.2.2.3 Significance of ADH in Core Biopsy

Atypical ductal hyperplasia (ADH) has a higher upgrade risk after diagnosis on core biopsy than other lesions of uncertain malignant potential for several reasons, one of them being that the criteria for diagnosis of ADH were established in open biopsies some 30 years ago and are now being applied to core biopsies and vacuum-assisted biopsies. Given the fact that the criteria for diagnosing ADH are, in part, quantitative, the upgrade risk for ADH mostly represents an underestimation of risk for ductal carcinoma in situ (DCIS). In one recent study, 82 % of the open biopsies upgraded after the diagnosis of ADH contained DCIS [50].

Clinically, an excisional biopsy is recommended when ADH is identified in core needle biopsy or in a vacuum-assisted biopsy specimen [1, 51, 52]. This is because of the relatively high probability of underestimating a DCIS or invasive cancer on needle biopsy. The question about the risk of upgrade of an ADH lesion found in needle biopsy has been addressed in several studies and has been reported to range between 22 and 56 %. The high variability of these upgrade rates has been attributed to different biopsy techniques (i.e., core biopsy versus vacuum-assisted biopsy), and to pathologic criteria used in these studies. Clearly, the diameter of the needle biopsy is one of the most important determinants of the probability of finding a higher grade lesion, but also the number of ADH foci in the needle biopsies. However, it has been concluded that, neither by using 11- or 9-gauge needles, nor by counting the ADH foci, a group of patients that does not require excisional biopsy can be delineated with sufficient accuracy [53].

10.2.3 Lobular Neoplasia and Its Variants

Lobular neoplasia (LN) or lobular intraepithelial neoplasia (LIN) is the preferred terms for noninvasive neoplasia with lobular phenotype, and they include the lesser developed atypical lobular hyperplasia (ALH) and several forms of lobular carcinoma in situ (LCIS) [54]. It is a spectrum of morphologically heterogeneous, but clinically and biologically related lesions (Table 10.2). It has been pointed out that, because of the large spectrum of LN, the term LN is not very useful in clinical diagnosis, and more specific terms such as ALH, LCIS, and its variants should be used [55]. All forms of LN are regarded as non-obligatory precursor lesions of invasive breast cancer, or, more specifically as preinvasive neoplasia, and at the same time LN is an indicator lesion for an increased ipsilateral and contralateral breast cancer risk of the patient. Rare pleomorphic or florid variants of LCIS should be distinguished from classical LCIS. Morphologic features of lobular neoplasia include variable distention of terminal ductulo-lobular units by discohesive, isomorphic-atypical epithelial cells.

Table 10.2 Classification of lobular neoplasia

(1) Atypical lobular hyperplasia
(2) Lobular carcinoma in situ (LCIS) (a) Usual variant (b) High-risk variants (i) Pleomorphic and pleomorphic-apocrine LCIS (ii) Florid LCIS (iii) Signet ring cell LCIS

10.2.3.1 Incidence and Clinical Presentation

The incidence of lobular neoplasia is relatively low, but an increasing incidence has been reported in the last decades with a rise of 39 % from 2000 until 2009 [56]. It is believed that this increased incidence is due to an increased detection rate by mammography screening and the use of large core biopsies for the assessment of occult mammographic lesions, but the increase may also be associated with an increasing use of hormone replacement therapy (HRT) [57]. No specific clinical or radiological abnormality is indicative of LN, and usually LN is seen in the assessment of microcalcifications that are found in screening mammography. In this context, LN frequently is associated with columnar changes, flat epithelial atypia, or sclerosing adenosis which may account for the microcalcifications, but LN itself is an incidental finding in this context. Rarely is comedo-type necrosis present in LN or LN presents as a mass lesion, and only in these situations, LN may explain the imaging findings [58]. When a diagnosis of LN is made on core biopsy, the risk for upgrade on open biopsy (to DCIS or invasive cancer) was estimated to be 13 % [59], but this figure is highly dependent on the clinical and radiological context. When histological and radiological findings are concordant, the risk for upgrade on resection is 3 % and, in the case of discordance, as high as 38 % [60]. This is consistent with upgrade rates

<10 % for occult lesions with LIN on core biopsy [61, 62]. Lobular neoplasia is classified as a lesion of unknown malignant potential (B3) [1], but pleomorphic LCIS or LCIS with mixed duct and lobular features is classified as B5a. The treatment in cases of LN should be based upon the individual situation, and various risk factors should be considered when making this decision.

10.2.3.2 Atypical Lobular Hyperplasia (ALH)

ALH is an incidental finding at core needle biopsy and usually occurs in association with benign microcalcifications. Histologically, it is distinguished from LCIS by distension and distortion of less than 50 % [63] or 75 % [55] of affected acinar units, but otherwise has similar histological characteristics. It is important to distinguish ALH from solid types of blunt duct adenosis or microglandular adenosis. ALH can be observed as a part of other lesions, such as papilloma, fibroadenoma, or radial scar, but when this occurs, ALH does not confer a malignant potential to these lesions, and no other treatment other than excisional biopsy is indicated. ALH mostly has characteristics of a risk lesion, not a precursor lesion, and Page et al. [64] found an increased relative risk for ALH of 5.8, which was similar to atypical ductal hyperplasia (RR 4,7) compared with women who had nonproliferative lesions.

10.2.3.3 Lobular Carcinoma In Situ (LCIS Classical Variant)

In contrast to ALH, the classical variant of LCIS is characterized by slightly to markedly distended terminal ductulo-lobular which are completely filled by isomorphic-atypical cells, replacing normal acinar cells. LCIS may extend into the ducts in a peculiar fashion called pagetoid spread, undermining and replacing ductal epithelial cells. But the term "pagetoid" is an unfortunate misnomer in this context, because LCIS is not related in any way to Paget's disease of the nipple, and there is no morphologic resemblance to it. Not infrequently LCIS may involve preexisting benign proliferative lesions, such as sclerosing adenosis, yielding a complex picture, and possibly creating the false impression of invasive carcinoma.

In a review of follow-up data from 252 women who had received breast biopsies with lobular neoplasia between 1950 and 1985, Page et al. [65] showed that invasive carcinoma was three times more likely in the same breast that had been diagnosed with lobular neoplasia than in the contralateral breast and that the tumor type was much more likely to be lobular than ductal. Additionally, molecular studies have revealed that the molecular profile of lobular neoplasia and synchronous invasive lobular carcinoma is similar [66, 67], suggesting that in these cases LN indeed is the precursor lesion. Even more convincing for LCIS as a preinvasive carcinoma is the fact that invasive lobular carcinoma indeed is clonally related to lobular neoplasia occurring years earlier [68]. With extensive follow-up, the risk of invasive carcinoma was calculated as 35 % in patients 35 years after initial biopsy of the lesion [69].

A subclassification of lobular neoplasia into different grades of severity (LIN1, LIN2, LIN3) has been proposed [70] but did not gain wide acceptance. This classification is based on the degree of acinar distension, necrosis, and nuclear pleomorphism (Fig. 10.2). Higher grades, especially LIN3, were more frequently associated with invasive carcinoma [70], but other outcome data which would confirm the clinical value of this classification, especially for the management of core needle biopsies, is lacking. Nevertheless, this LIN classification may be clinically useful, because more aggressive subtypes of LCIS, such as pleomorphic LCIS or florid LCIS fall into the LIN3 category, and therefore there is an overlap of this LIN grading system with LCIS subtyping. On the low-risk side, LIN1 indicates minimal involvement of acini, and this overlaps with the ALH.

10.2.3.4 High-Risk Variants of LCIS

Some histologic variants of LCIS which are associated with an increased risk have been described in the literature. This includes pleomorphic LCIS and florid LCIS. *Pleomorphic LCIS* and *pleomorphic-apocrine LCIS* are characterized by high-grade cellular atypia and can be associated with massive distension of the lobules and extension into the ducts with the formation of necrosis and calcifications [71]. When involvement of the ducts is a prominent feature, pleomorphic LCIS resembles DCIS histologically, but it can be distinguished by the loss of E-Cadherin expression [72]. In case of mixed e-Cadherin positivity, the term mixed ductulo-lobular carcinoma is used.

Another high-risk variant of LCIS is *florid LCIS* [73–75]. In contrast to pleomorphic LCIS, it is composed of cells typical for classical LCIS, but many adjacent ductal and lobular units are maximally distended, almost to the point of confluence. Comedo-type necroses are commonly seen with florid LCIS and on a molecular basis recurrent genomic alterations could be detected, including losses in the chromosomal regions 11q-, 17p-, and 8p- and gains in the region 11q13.3 [75]. Not infrequently, amplifications in the region 17q21 (concerning the HER2 gene) may occur, resulting in a HER2 overexpression on immunohistology. Clinically, florid LN also may be associated with extensive microcalcifications or forming a tumor mass (tumor-like LN) [76]. With florid LCIS, a complete excision of the lesion with clear margins is recommended, or a re-resection in case of close margins and massive acinar distension immediately adjacent to the resection margin [77, 78].

High-risk LCIS may contain clusters of signet ring cells [73, 79], but a pure signet ring cell variant of LCIS is quite rare, and usually associated with ILC with predominant

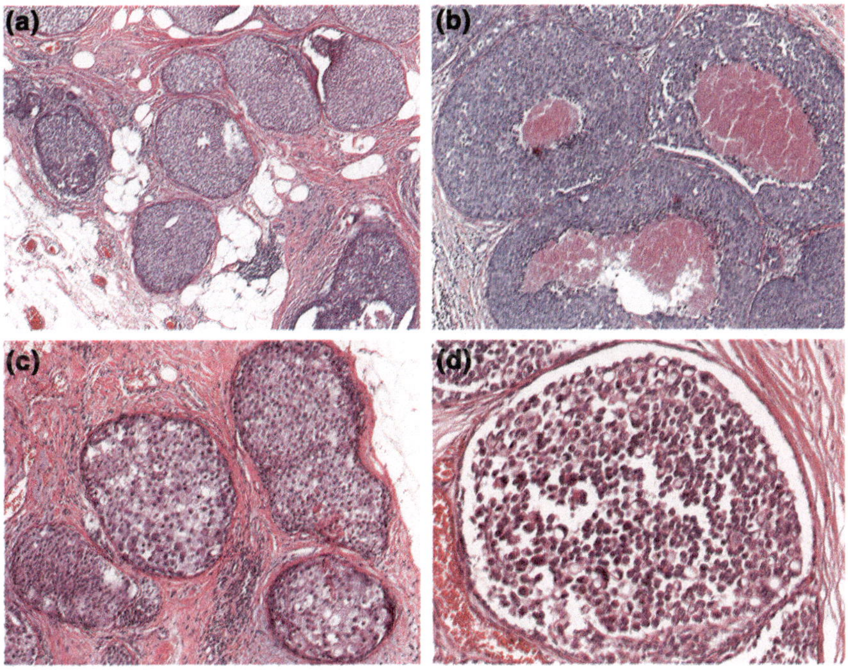

Fig. 10.2 Lobular carcinoma in situ (LCIS), high-grade variants: **a** Florid LCIS, classic variant, with foci of invasion. **b** LCIS, pleomorphic type with confluence and comedo-type necrosis. **c** Pleomorphic-apocrine LCIS. **d** High-grade LCIS, signet ring cell type

signet ring cell differentiation. Microinvasion can be detected in high-risk variants of LCIS not infrequently [80], and therefore special attention must be paid in the workup of high-risk LCIS to exclude microinvasion. As in pure DCIS, this includes complete embedding of the lesion and serial sectioning.

10.2.4 Immunohistology and Molecular Biology

Because of the different therapy implications for the diagnosis of LCIS versus DCIS, it is important to clearly distinguish both types of preinvasive disease with certainty from one another, or to diagnose mixed duct-lobular carcinoma in situ. If the histology on H&E is ambiguous, a E-Cadherin immunohistology will be helpful, possibly in conjunction with p120 Catenin or Beta-catenin [81]. Generally, LN is characterized by loss of E-Cadherin expression with simultaneous expression of p120 Catenin [81]. HER2 overexpression and gene amplification may be present in pleomorphic LCIS, especially in pleomorphic-apocrine LCIS, or in florid LCIS, and therefore is not an argument against the diagnosis of LN. With carcinoma in situ of mixed duct and lobular phenotype, the therapy should be performed like in pure DCIS. It should be noted that a loss in E-Cadherin expression is not a proof for the presence of lobular neoplasia, because triple-negative DCIS may show a reduced E-cadherin expression [81] also. Therefore, the diagnosis of lobular neoplasia always requires that conventional histologic criteria are present, and a routine E-cadherin stain is discouraged.

10.3 Invasive Carcinoma

10.3.1 Breast Cancer Classification and Grading

The current WHO classification of breast cancer [42] is based on the morphologic definition of tumor types. It includes more than 30 types of invasive carcinoma, and most of them are quite rare (Table 10.3). The most common tumor types are invasive carcinoma of no special type (NST), and invasive lobular carcinoma (ILC). These two tumor type account for about 80–90 % of all breast cancers, the other tumor types are much rarer. As a result, the molecular and clinical heterogeneity of breast cancer cannot be adequately reflected by the current, morphologically oriented tumor classification (Fig. 10.3). Except for the rarer special subtypes, the WHO classification is of limited clinical significance and must be complemented by tumor grading, immunohistological and molecular characterization of breast in order to be clinically useful [82].

Table 10.3 Breast cancer classification and ICD-0-3 codes

Invasive carcinoma of no special type (NST)	8500/3
– Pleomorphic carcinoma	8022/3
– Carcinoma with osteoclast-like stromal giant cells	8035/3
– Carcinoma with choriocarcinomatous features	
– Carcinoma with melanotic features	
Invasive lobular carcinoma	8520/3
– Classic lobular carcinoma	
– Solid lobular carcinoma	
– Alveolar lobular carcinoma	
– Pleomorphic lobular carcinoma	
– Tubulo-lobular carcinoma	
– Mixed lobular carcinoma	
Tubular carcinoma	8211/3
Cribriform carcinoma	8201/3
Mucinous carcinoma	8480/3
Carcinoma with medullary features	
– Medullary carcinoma	8510/3
– Atypical medullary carcinoma	8513/3
– Invasive carcinoma NST with medullary features	8500/3
Carcinoma with apocrine differentiation	
Carcinoma with signet ring cell differentiation	
Invasive micropapillary carcinoma	8507/3
Metaplastic carcinoma of no special type	8575/3
– Low-grade adenosquamous carcinoma	8570/3
– Fibromatosis-like metaplastic carcinoma	8572/3
– Squamous cell carcinoma	8070/3
– Spindle cell carcinoma	8032/3
– Metaplastic carcinoma with mesenchymal differentiation	
– Chondroid differentiation	8571/3
– Osseous differentiation	8571/3
– Other types of mesenchymal differentiation	8575/3
– Mixed metaplastic carcinoma	8575/3
– Myoepithelial carcinoma	8982/3
Epithelial–myoepithelial tumors	
Adenomyoepithelioma with carcinoma	8983/3
Adenoid cystic carcinoma	8200/3
Rare types	
Carcinoma with neuroendocrine features	
– Neuroendocrine tumor, well-differentiated	8246/3
– Neuroendocrine carcinoma poorly differentiated (small cell carcinoma)	8041/3
– Carcinoma with neuroendocrine differentiation	8574/3
Secretory carcinoma	8502/3
Invasive papillary carcinoma	8503/3

(continued)

Table 10.3 (continued)

Acinic cell carcinoma	8550/3
Mucoepidermoid carcinoma	8430/3
Polymorphous carcinoma	8525/3
Oncocytic carcinoma	8290/3
Lipid-rich carcinoma	8314/3
Glycogen-rich clear cell carcinoma	8315/3
Sebaceous carcinoma	8410/3

10.3.2 Invasive Carcinoma of No Special Type (NST)

This group of breast cancers comprises all tumors without special differentiating features and applies to more than 70 % of breast cancers. The diagnosis of a carcinoma of no special type (NST) is made by exclusion of recognized special types of breast cancers.

The terminology for this most common type of breast cancer has changed in the WHO classification from "invasive ductal carcinoma, not otherwise specified" (2003) [83] into "invasive carcinoma of no special type" (NST) (2012) [42]. The definition of invasive carcinomas of no special type is identical with the previous edition of the WHO classification of breast cancer; only the name "ductal" was omitted in the new terminology. The rationale for this is that there is no clear histogenetic difference between histologic tumor types and NST tumors that are not a uniform group of carcinomas. For these reasons, the term "ductal" does not represent a distinguishing pathological feature for breast cancers of special type or no special type. The terms "invasive ductal carcinoma" or "ductal NOS" are accepted as alternative terminology options, but the use of "carcinoma of no special type" is the preferred term. Rare morphological variants of invasive carcinoma NST include pleomorphic carcinoma, carcinoma with osteoclast-like stromal giant cells, carcinoma with choriocarcinomatous features, and carcinoma with melanotic features. Carcinomas of mixed type have a specialized pattern in at least 50 % of the tumor and a non-specialized pattern between 10 and 49 %. These tumors are designated as mixed invasive NST and special type or mixed invasive NST and lobular carcinoma.

The pathological and molecular evaluation of differentiating features in NST carcinomas is important for the proper surgical and adjuvant treatment. This includes tumor grading, and the recognition of special features, such as an extensive intraductal tumor component (EIC), the presence or absence of angioinvasion, and the presence of multifocality or multicentricity. With EIC and/or multifocal disease, a breast conserving approach is still possible [84], but the chances for the later occurrence of an in-breast recurrence

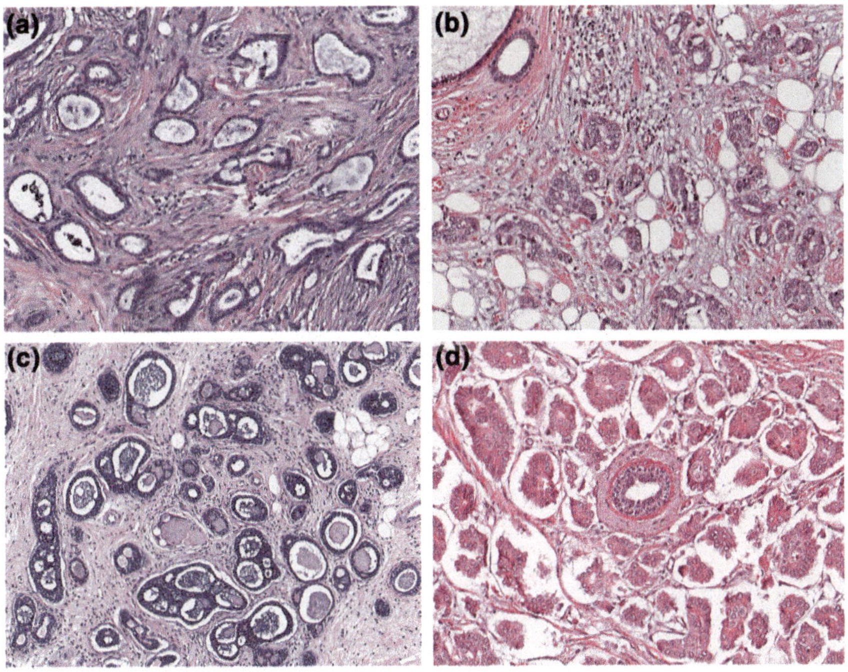

Fig. 10.3 Invasive carcinoma with low-grade nuclear morphology: **a** Invasive tubular carcinoma. **b** Invasive carcinoma, no special type (NST), grade 1. **c** Adenoid cystic carcinoma. **d** Invasive carcinoma, micropapillary type

are increased [85, 86]. In a similar way, lymphatic and blood vessel invasion is considered an adverse local factor and is associated with an increased frequency of lymph node metastasis [87].

10.3.3 Invasive Lobular Carcinoma

10.3.3.1 Clinical Presentation

Invasive lobular carcinoma (ILC) is the most common special tumor type and accounts for up to 15 % of invasive breast cancer [88, 89]. It has distinct biological, epidemiological, and clinical features [90–93]. The mean age of patients with ILC has been calculated to be 4 years higher than with invasive carcinoma of no special type (NST) [92, 93], and about 10 years higher that the age of patients with LCIS, who present at 52 years of age on average [94]. The majority of patients with ILC present with a palpable tumor [95] and, on mammography, an architectural disturbance abnormality is the most frequent finding. However, 6–16 % of patients present without a mammographic abnormality [96, 97]. Patients with hormone replacement therapy are at 2–3 times higher risk for ILC compared to NST [98].

Clinically, and radiologically, an increased tendency for multicentricity and bilaterality was described [99]. This, and the difficulty of exact determination of the size and the extent of ILC, has prompted the recommendation of routine mammography in ILC [100] but does not achieve survival benefits or reduction in re-resection rates [101, 102]. In about 25 % of ILC multifocal tumor extensions are detectable [103]. Multifocality and the underestimation of tumor size in ILC have to be considered in the operative therapy of ILC [104]. According to the SEER database, on average, ILC are larger, having a mean tumor diameter of 2.0 cm in comparison to invasive breast cancer NST with a tumor size of 1.6 cm [92].

10.3.3.2 Classical and Variant Forms of ILC

ILC in its classical form is characterized by a diffuse infiltrative growth of small epithelial tumor cells with a narrow cytoplasmic rim [42]. The nuclear grading and the Nottingham grading [105] usually is G2. Periductal and perilobular growth patterns are frequent, as is adjacent LCIS. ILC often has a relatively low cellularity, and desmoplastic stromal reaction may be missing. This can explain the clinically ill-defined tumor mass and the mammographic aspect. Histologic variants of ILC includes solid, pleomorphic, signet ring cells, and tubulo-lobular or alveolar growth patterns [106, 107], as well as mixed forms, often intermingling with classical differentiation. Among these variants, the pleomorphic and solid variants of ILC are associated with a higher risk of recurrence [108, 109], while the tubulo-lobular variant is associated with a better prognosis [110] (Fig. 10.4).

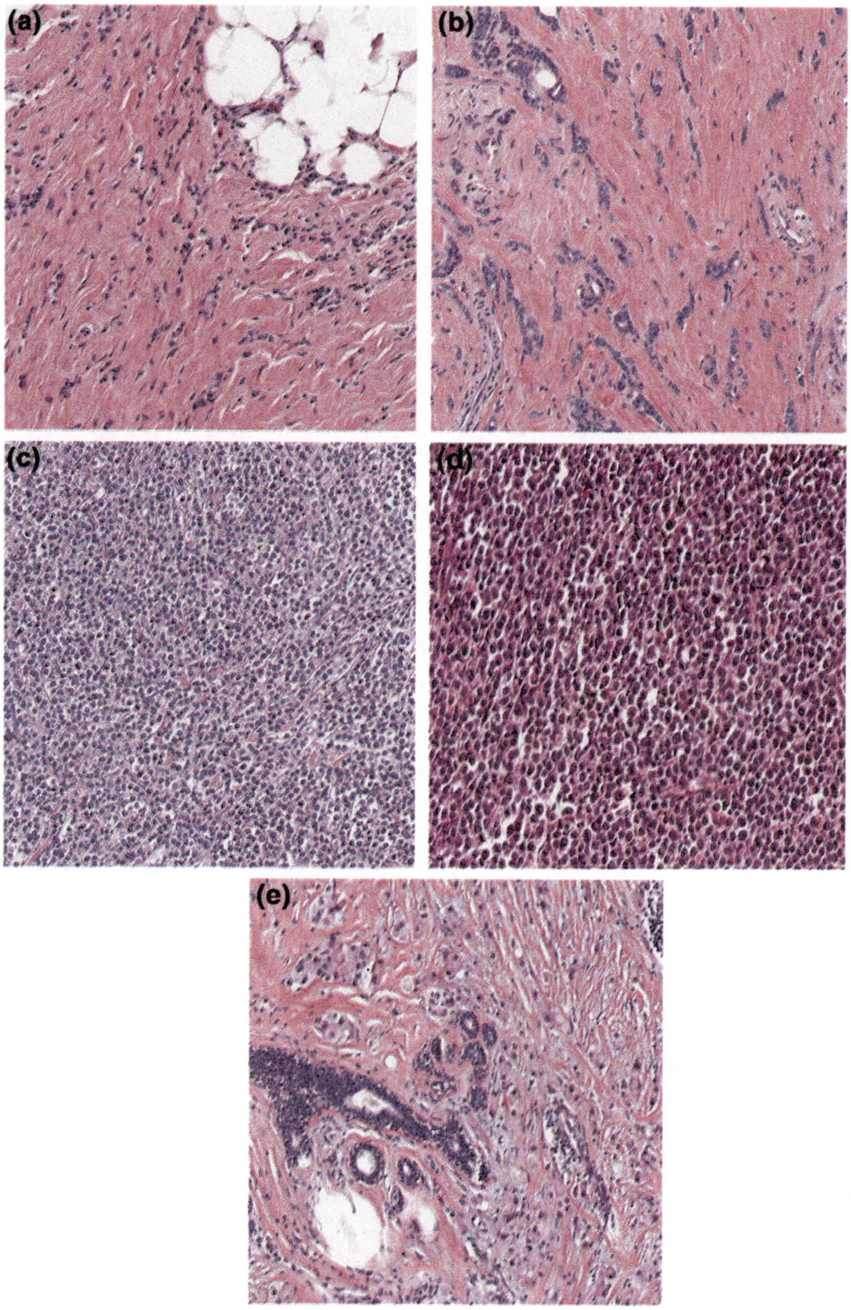

Fig. 10.4 Variant forms of invasive lobular carcinoma. **a** Classic variant (G2). **b** Tubulo-lobular variant (G1). **c** Solid variant (G2). **d** Pleomorphic variant (G3). **e** Histiocytic-apocrine variant (G3)

10.3.3.3 Prognostic Factors

ILC generally are associated with a better biologic phenotype, being more likely estrogen and progesterone receptor positive, HER2 negative, and diploid [111], but also more likely to occur in older patients and being larger in size. Nevertheless, long-term survival of ILC is similar to NST carcinomas [111–113], but, when matched for stage survival analysis, better survival rates were shown for ILC [114]. With regard to tumor grade, intermediate grade of differentiation is most frequently found in ILC and the relationship of G1:G2:G3 has been reported as 12 %:76 %:12 %, with the grade 3 tumors being mostly the pleomorphic variant [115]. In the great majority of cases, ILC present as luminal A and B subtypes, independent of classical or variant differentiation, and this molecular subtype was of higher prognostic significance than that of a ILC variant [110]. Hematogenous metastasis in ILC is more frequently observed in Bone, GI-Tract, uterus, meninges, ovary, and peritoneal serosa, but less frequently in lung, pleura, or the CNS [116–121].

10.3.4 Other Special Types of Breast Cancer

The main strength of morphologic classification of breast cancer is that the correct identification of rare tumor subtypes provides important prognostic and otherwise clinically useful information, such as the tendency for lymph node metastasis [82]. *Invasive tubular carcinoma* represents about 4 % of all newly diagnosed breast cancer, and its excellent prognosis is well-documented, being superior to the prognosis of invasive carcinoma NST, grade 1 [122]. In a large study of 7372 consecutive patients with invasive luminal type breast cancer, Colleoni et al. [123] identified only invasive *cribriform carcinoma* with similarly good prognosis as invasive tubular carcinoma. In the past, invasive *mucinous carcinoma* often had been included among the more favorable histologic subtypes, but Colleoni et al. [123, 124] and other studies showed similar prognostic significance as invasive breast cancer of no special type (NST). Invasive *medullary carcinoma* is a special type also often linked to a good outcome. However, the good prognosis in invasive medullary carcinoma is evident only when strict criteria are being applied to the histologic diagnosis [125]. This makes it a very rare subtype in its pure form and the WHO classification now recommends the use of the term *breast cancer with medullary features* in order to avoid confusion with medullary carcinoma in its strict sense [42]. Special subtypes with outcomes similar to or worse than invasive carcinoma NST include invasive *apocrine carcinoma* [126] and invasive *micropapillary carcinoma*. The latter subtype is characterized by its tendency to lymphangioinvasion and lymph node metastasis [127]. *Metaplastic carcinoma* is a mixed bag of invasive carcinomas with mostly basal phenotype [128] and they include tumors with metaplastic looking elements such as spindle cell carcinoma, chondroid or osseous differentiation, and squamous cell carcinoma of the breast [42]. With the exception to low-grade metaplastic spindle cell carcinoma and low-grade adenosquamous carcinoma, metaplastic carcinomas tend to follow an aggressive course and are mostly lymph node negative tumors [129].

10.3.5 Sarcoma and Malignant Pyhllodes Tumors

Angiosarcoma of the breast is the most frequent sarcoma of the breast. Three different forms of angiosarcoma must be distinguished: (1) Primary angiosarcoma, which occurs de novo in young patients, having a median age of onset between 30 and 50 years; (2) secondary angiosarcoma with patients that underwent radiotherapy for breast conserving surgery, and a median onset about 10 years after initial treatment; and (3) angiosarcoma developing in the upper extremity after mastectomy and radiotherapy and chronic lymphoedema (Stewart-Treves Syndrome) [130] which is rare nowadays. Angiosarcoma generally has a dismal prognosis and requires aggressive surgical therapy [131]. The role of adjuvant therapy in primary angiosarcoma has not been firmly established, but evidence is emerging for a beneficial role of paclitaxel [132] and adjuvant radiotherapy [133]. Other sarcomas of the breast are rarer and are not discussed here. Malignant phyllodes tumor is an infrequent form of phyllodes tumor in the breast with malignant, sarcomatous stroma. Its biology and clinical behavior has been reviewed recently [134]. A wide local excision has been recommended as the treatment of choice, which means mastectomy in the majority of cases because of the tumor size and the tendency of satellite nodules within the breast. Therefore, a wide surgical margin of 1 cm or more is required [135]. Adjuvant radiotherapy was shown to be beneficial [136], but there is no clear indication for adjuvant chemotherapy.

10.3.6 Tumor Grading

The Nottingham grading system (NGS), which was initially proposed by Elston and Ellis in 1992 [105], is a modification of the Scarff–Bloom–Richardson grading system [137] and is applicable to all types of invasive breast cancer, including special types. The NGS is the most widely used grading system and has been endorsed by the WHO [42], the UICC [138], the AJCC [35], and by the Royal College of Pathologists [139], among others. It is based on the evaluation of three morphological features: (a) degree of tubule or gland formation, (b) nuclear pleomorphism, and (c) mitotic count. Grading is the second strongest prognostic factor in breast cancer, next to lymph node status. 5-year survival rates for invasive carcinoma NST were 98.1, 94.4, and 84.3 % for G1, G2, and G3 tumors, respectively, in the SEER database [140], and the NGS was shown to be largely independent of tumor size and lymph node status [141]. These three morphologically defined prognostic parameters were combined to a widely used prognostic score, the Nottingham Prognostic Index (NPI) [142], and the NPI also is part of the Adjuvant Online prognostic tool [143].

When tumor grading is compared to molecular features of breast cancer, it becomes apparent that low-grade and high-grade breast cancers are different diseases at the genomic, gene-expression, and immunohistologic level, leading to the hypothesis of two different pathways of breast cancer evolution: low-grade and high-grade pathways [144]. This concept of a two-tier grading scheme is supported by studies that directly compared histologic grading with molecular features leading to the concept of molecular tumor grade [145, 146]. This genomic grade index not only has prognostic impact, but also is predictive of the outcome of neoadjuvant chemotherapy [147, 148], similar to conventional grading [149]. Not surprisingly, histologic grading also is strongly related to molecular prognostic scores, such as Oncotype DX [150–153].

There have been criticisms of tumor grading as a prognostic factor for being too subjective and lacking consistency and reproducibility [154], but several studies did in fact show acceptable inter- and intra-observer variability [155–157] and that inter-observer variability can be improved by training [158]. For an overview of inter- and intra-observer agreement of grading see [159]. The authors conclude that histologic grade is still relevant in the molecular area.

References

1. Perry N, Broeders M, Wolf C. European guidelines for quality assurance in breast cancer screening and diagnosis. Luxembourg: European Commission; 2006. 416 p.
2. Calhoun BC, Collins LC. Recommendations for excision following core needle biopsy of the breast: a contemporary evaluation of the literature. Histopathology. 2016;68(1):138–51.
3. Wells CJ, O'Donoghue C, Ojeda-Fournier H, Retallack HE, Esserman LJ. Evolving paradigm for imaging, diagnosis, and management of DCIS. J Am Coll Radiol. 2013;10(12):918–23.
4. Drukker CA, Schmidt MK, Rutgers EJ, Cardoso F, Kerlikowske K, Esserman LJ, et al. Mammographic screening detects low-risk tumor biology breast cancers. Breast Cancer Res Treat. 2014;144(1):103–11.
5. Esserman LJ, Thompson IM Jr, Reid B. Overdiagnosis and overtreatment in cancer: an opportunity for improvement. JAMA. 2013;310(8):797–8.
6. Morrow M, Katz SJ. Addressing overtreatment in DCIS: what should physicians do now? J Natl Cancer Inst. 2015;107(12): djv290.
7. Virnig BA, Tuttle TM, Shamliyan T, Kane RL. Ductal carcinoma in situ of the breast: a systematic review of incidence, treatment, and outcomes. J Natl Cancer Inst. 2010;102(3):170–8.
8. Ernster VL, Barclay J, Kerlikowske K, Grady D, Henderson C. Incidence of and treatment for ductal carcinoma in situ of the breast. JAMA. 1996;275(12):913–8.
9. Siegel R, Ma J, Zou Z, Jemal A. Cancer statistics, 2014. CA Cancer J Clin. 2014;64(1):9–29.
10. Duffy SW, Dibden A, Michalopoulos D, Offman J, Parmar D, Jenkins J, et al. Screen detection of ductal carcinoma in situ and subsequent incidence of invasive interval breast cancers: a retrospective population-based study. Lancet Oncol. 2016;17 (1):109–14.
11. Lynge E, Ponti A, James T, Majek O, von Euler-Chelpin M, Anttila A, et al. Variation in detection of ductal carcinoma in situ during screening mammography: a survey within the International Cancer Screening Network. Eur J Cancer. 2014;50(1):185–92.
12. Narod SA, Iqbal J, Giannakeas V, Sopik V, Sun P. Breast cancer mortality after a diagnosis of ductal carcinoma in situ. JAMA Oncol. 2015;1(7):888–96.
13. Masood S. New insights from breast pathology: should we consider low grade DCIS NOT a cancer? Eur J Radiol. 2012;81 (Suppl 1):S93–4.
14. Collins LC, Tamimi RM, Baer HJ, Connolly JL, Colditz GA, Schnitt SJ. Outcome of patients with ductal carcinoma in situ untreated after diagnostic biopsy—results from the nurses' health study. Cancer. 2005;103(9):1778–84.
15. Erbas B, Provenzano E, Armes J, Gertig D. The natural history of ductal carcinoma in situ of the breast: a review. Breast Cancer Res Treat. 2006;97(2):135–44.
16. Shamliyan T, Wang SY, Virnig BA, Tuttle TM, Kane RL. Association between patient and tumor characteristics with clinical outcomes in women with ductal carcinoma in situ. J Natl Cancer Inst Monogr. 2010;2010(41):121–9.
17. Silverstein MJ, Poller DN, Waisman JR, Colburn WJ, Barth A, Gierson ED, et al. Prognostic classification of breast ductal carcinoma-in-situ. Lancet. 1995;345(8958):1154–7.
18. Committee TC. Consensus conference on the classification of ductal carcinoma in situ. Hum Pathol. 1997;28(11):1221–5.
19. Pinder SE, Duggan C, Ellis IO, Cuzick J, Forbes JF, Bishop H, et al. A new pathological system for grading DCIS with improved prediction of local recurrence: results from the UKCCCR/ANZ DCIS trial. Br J Cancer. 2010;103(1):94–100.
20. Tamimi RM, Baer HJ, Marotti J, Galan M, Galaburda L, Fu Y, et al. Comparison of molecular phenotypes of ductal carcinoma in situ and invasive breast cancer. Breast Cancer Res. 2008;10(4):R67.
21. Livasy CA, Perou CM, Karaca G, Cowan DW, Maia D, Jackson S, et al. Identification of a basal-like subtype of breast ductal carcinoma in situ. Hum Pathol. 2007;38(2):197–204.
22. Clark SE, Warwick J, Carpenter R, Bowen RL, Duffy SW, Jones JL. Molecular subtyping of DCIS: heterogeneity of breast cancer reflected in pre-invasive disease. Br J Cancer. 2011;104 (1):120–7.
23. Park K, Han S, Kim HJ, Kim J, Shin E. HER2 status in pure ductal carcinoma in situ and in the intraductal and invasive components of invasive ductal carcinoma determined by fluorescence in situ hybridization and immunohistochemistry. Histopathology. 2006;48(6):702–7.
24. Bryan BB, Schnitt SJ, Collins LC. Ductal carcinoma in situ with basal-like phenotype: a possible precursor to invasive basal-like breast cancer. Mod Pathol. 2006;19(5):617–21.
25. Lester S, Bose S, Chen Y, Connolly J, de Baca M, Fitzgibbons P, et al. Protocol for the examination of specimens from patients with ductal carcinoma in situ of the breast. Arch Pathol Lab Med. 2009;133(1):15–25.
26. Pinder SE. Ductal carcinoma in situ (DCIS): pathological features, differential diagnosis, prognostic factors and specimen evaluation. Mod Pathol. 2010;23(Suppl 2):S8–13.
27. Kallen ME, Sim MS, Radosavcev BL, Humphries RM, Ward DC, Apple SK. A quality initiative of postoperative radiographic imaging performed on mastectomy specimens to reduce histology cost and pathology report turnaround time. Ann Diagn Pathol. 2015;19(5):353–8.
28. Silverstein MJ, Lagios MD, Recht A, Allred DC, Harms SE, Holland R, et al. Image-detected breast cancer: state of the art diagnosis and treatment. J Am Coll Surg. 2005;201(4):586–97.
29. Dillon MF, Mc Dermott EW, O'Doherty A, Quinn CM, Hill AD, O'Higgins N. Factors affecting successful breast conservation for ductal carcinoma in situ. Ann Surg Oncol. 2007;14(5):1618–28.
30. Maffuz A, Barroso-Bravo S, Najera I, Zarco G, Alvarado-Cabrero I, Rodriguez-Cuevas SA. Tumor size as predictor of microinvasion, invasion, and axillary metastasis in ductal carcinoma in situ. J Exp Clin Cancer Res. 2006;25(2):223–7.

31. Sigal-Zafrani B, Lewis JS, Clough KB, Vincent-Salomon A, Fourquet A, Meunier M, et al. Histological margin assessment for breast ductal carcinoma in situ: precision and implications. Mod Pathol. 2004;17(1):81–8.
32. Cheng L, Al-Kaisi NK, Gordon NH, Liu AY, Gebrail F, Shenk RR. Relationship between the size and margin status of ductal carcinoma in situ of the breast and residual disease. J Natl Cancer Inst. 1997;89(18):1356–60.
33. MacDonald HR, Silverstein MJ, Mabry H, Moorthy B, Ye W, Epstein MS, et al. Local control in ductal carcinoma in situ treated by excision alone: incremental benefit of larger margins. Am J Surg. 2005;190(4):521–5.
34. Asjoe FT, Altintas S, Huizing MT, Colpaert C, Marck EV, Vermorken JB, et al. The value of the Van Nuys Prognostic Index in ductal carcinoma in situ of the breast: a retrospective analysis. Breast J. 2007;13(4):359–67.
35. American-Joint-Committee-on-Cancer. AJCC cancer staging manual. 7th ed. New York; London: Springer; 2010. xiv, 648 p.
36. Bianchi S, Vezzosi V. Microinvasive carcinoma of the breast. Pathol Oncol Res. 2008;14(2):105–11.
37. Werling RW, Hwang H, Yaziji H, Gown AM. Immunohistochemical distinction of invasive from noninvasive breast lesions: a comparative study of p63 versus calponin and smooth muscle myosin heavy chain. Am J Surg Pathol. 2003;27(1):82–90.
38. Prasad ML, Osborne MP, Giri DD, Hoda SA. Microinvasive carcinoma (T1mic) of the breast: clinicopathologic profile of 21 cases. Am J Surg Pathol. 2000;24(3):422–8.
39. Lee SK, Cho EY, Kim WW, Kim SH, Hur SM, Kim S, et al. The prediction of lymph node metastasis in ductal carcinoma in situ with microinvasion by assessing lymphangiogenesis. J Surg Oncol. 2010;102(3):225–9.
40. Collins LC, Aroner SA, Connolly JL, Colditz GA, Schnitt SJ, Tamimi RM. Breast cancer risk by extent and type of atypical hyperplasia: An update from the nurses' health studies. Cancer. 2016;122(4):515–20.
41. Page D, Rogers L. Combined histologic and cytologic criteria for the diagnosis of mammary atypical ductal hyperplasia. Hum Pathol. 1992;23(10):1095–7.
42. Lakhani SR, Ellis I, Schnitt S, Tan PH, Vijver M. WHO classification of tumours of the breast. IARC, ed. Lyon: IARC Press; 2012. 240 p.
43. Böcker W. Preneoplasia of the breast. A new conceptual approach to proliferative breast disease. Munich: Saunders, Elsevier; 2006. XIX, 587 S p.
44. Nofech-Mozes S, Holloway C, Hanna W. The role of cytokeratin 5/6 as an adjunct diagnostic tool in breast core needle biopsies. Int J Surg Pathol. 2008;16(4):399–406.
45. Bratthauer GL, Tavassoli FA. Assessment of lesions coexisting with various grades of ductal intraepithelial neoplasia of the breast. Virchows Arch. 2004;444(4):340–4.
46. Gong G, DeVries S, Chew KL, Cha I, Ljung BM, Waldman FM. Genetic changes in paired atypical and usual ductal hyperplasia of the breast by comparative genomic hybridization. Clin Cancer Res. 2001;7(8):2410–4.
47. Amari M, Suzuki A, Moriya T, Yoshinaga K, Amano G, Sasano H, et al. LOH analyses of premalignant and malignant lesions of human breast: frequent LOH in 8p, 16q, and 17q in atypical ductal hyperplasia. Oncol Rep. 1999;6(6):1277–80.
48. Lakhani SR, Collins N, Stratton MR, Sloane JP. Atypical ductal hyperplasia of the breast: clonal proliferation with loss of heterozygosity on chromosomes 16q and 17p. J Clin Pathol. 1995;48(7):611–5.
49. Reis-Filho J, Lakhani S. The diagnosis and management of pre-invasive breast disease: genetic alterations in pre-invasive lesions. Breast Cancer Res. 2003;5(6):313–9.
50. Menes TS, Rosenberg R, Balch S, Jaffer S, Kerlikowske K, Miglioretti DL. Upgrade of high-risk breast lesions detected on mammography in the breast cancer surveillance consortium. Am J Surg. 2014;207(1):24–31.
51. Arpino G, Laucirica R, Elledge R. Premalignant and in situ breast disease: biology and clinical implications. Ann Intern Med. 2005;143(6):446–57.
52. Yeh IT, Dimitrov D, Otto P, Miller AR, Kahlenberg MS, Cruz A. Pathologic review of atypical hyperplasia identified by image-guided breast needle core biopsy. Correlation with excision specimen. Arch Pathol Lab Med. 2003;127(1):49–54.
53. Kohr JR, Eby PR, Allison KH, Demartini WB, Gutierrez RL, Peacock S et al. Risk of upgrade of atypical ductal hyperplasia after stereotactic breast biopsy: effects of number of foci and complete removal of calcifications. Radiology. 2010;255(3):723–30.
54. Jorns J, Sabel MS, Pang JC. Lobular neoplasia: morphology and management. Arch Pathol Lab Med. 2014;138(10):1344–9.
55. Hoda SA, Brogi E, Koerner FC, Rosen PP. Rosen's breast pathology, 4nd ed. Philadelphia: Lippincott Williams & Wilkins; 2014. 1399 p.
56. Portschy PR, Marmor S, Nzara R, Virnig BA, Tuttle TM. Trends in incidence and management of lobular carcinoma in situ: a population-based analysis. Ann Surg Oncol. 2013;20(10):3240–6.
57. Li CI, Malone KE, Porter PL, Lawton TJ, Voigt LF, Cushing-Haugen KL, et al. Relationship between menopausal hormone therapy and risk of ductal, lobular, and ductal-lobular breast carcinomas. Cancer Epidemiol Biomarkers Prev. 2008;17 (1):43–50.
58. Hussain M, Cunnick GH. Management of lobular carcinoma in-situ and atypical lobular hyperplasia of the breast—a review. Eur J Surg Oncol. 2011;37(4):279–89.
59. Lewis JL, Lee DY, Tartter PI. The significance of lobular carcinoma in situ and atypical lobular hyperplasia of the breast. Ann Surg Oncol. 2012;19(13):4124–8.
60. Murray MP, Luedtke C, Liberman L, Nehhozina T, Akram M, Brogi E. Classic lobular carcinoma in situ and atypical lobular hyperplasia at percutaneous breast core biopsy: outcomes of prospective excision. Cancer. 2013;119(5):1073–9.
61. Rendi MH, Dintzis SM, Lehman CD, Calhoun KE, Allison KH. Lobular in-situ neoplasia on breast core needle biopsy: imaging indication and pathologic extent can identify which patients require excisional biopsy. Ann Surg Oncol. 2012;19(3):914–21.
62. D'Alfonso TM, Wang K, Chiu YL, Shin SJ. Pathologic upgrade rates on subsequent excision when lobular carcinoma in situ is the primary diagnosis in the needle core biopsy with special attention to the radiographic target. Arch Pathol Lab Med. 2013;137 (7):927–35.
63. Page DL, Kidd TE Jr, Dupont WD, Simpson JF, Rogers LW. Lobular neoplasia of the breast: higher risk for subsequent invasive cancer predicted by more extensive disease. Hum Pathol. 1991;22(12):1232–9.
64. Page DL, Dupont WD, Rogers LW, Rados MS. Atypical hyperplastic lesions of the female breast. A long-term follow-up study. Cancer. 1985;55(11):2698–708.
65. Page DL, Schuyler PA, Dupont WD, Jensen RA, Plummer WD Jr, Simpson JF. Atypical lobular hyperplasia as a unilateral predictor of breast cancer risk: a retrospective cohort study. Lancet. 2003;361(9352):125–9.
66. Hwang E, Nyante S, Yi Chen Y, Moore D, DeVries S, Korkola J, et al. Clonality of lobular carcinoma in situ and synchronous invasive lobular carcinoma. Cancer. 2004;100(12):2562–72.
67. Vos CB, Cleton-Jansen AM, Berx G, de Leeuw WJ, ter Haar NT, van Roy F, et al. E-cadherin inactivation in lobular carcinoma

in situ of the breast: an early event in tumorigenesis. Br J Cancer. 1997;76(9):1131–3.
68. Aulmann S, Penzel R, Longerich T, Funke B, Schirmacher P, Sinn HP. Clonality of lobular carcinoma in situ (LCIS) and metachronous invasive breast cancer. Breast Cancer Res Treat. 2008;107(3):331–5.
69. Bodian CA, Perzin KH, Lattes R. Lobular neoplasia. Long term risk of breast cancer and relation to other factors. Cancer. 1996;78 (5):1024–34.
70. Bratthauer GL, Tavassoli FA. Lobular intraepithelial neoplasia: previously unexplored aspects assessed in 775 cases and their clinical implications. Virchows Arch. 2002;440(2):134–8.
71. Khoury T, Karabakhtsian RG, Mattson D, Yan L, Syriac S, Habib F, et al. Pleomorphic lobular carcinoma in situ of the breast: clinicopathological review of 47 cases. Histopathology. 2014;64(7):981–93.
72. Reis-Filho JS, Simpson PT, Jones C, Steele D, Mackay A, Iravani M, et al. Pleomorphic lobular carcinoma of the breast: role of comprehensive molecular pathology in characterization of an entity. J Pathol. 2005;207(1):1–13.
73. Alvarado-Cabrero I, Picon Coronel G, Valencia Cedillo R, Canedo N, Tavassoli FA. Florid lobular intraepithelial neoplasia with signet ring cells, central necrosis and calcifications: a clinicopathological and immunohistochemical analysis of ten cases associated with invasive lobular carcinoma. Arch Med Res. 2010;41(6):436–41.
74. Fadare O, Dadmanesh F, Alvarado-Cabrero I, Snyder R, Stephen Mitchell J, Tot T, et al. Lobular intraepithelial neoplasia [lobular carcinoma in situ] with comedo-type necrosis: a clinicopathologic study of 18 cases. Am J Surg Pathol. 2006;30(11):1445–53.
75. Shin SJ, Lal A, De Vries S, Suzuki J, Roy R, Hwang ES, et al. Florid lobular carcinoma in situ: molecular profiling and comparison to classic lobular carcinoma in situ and pleomorphic lobular carcinoma in situ. Hum Pathol. 2013;44(10):1998–2009.
76. Stein LF, Zisman G, Rapelyea JA, Schwartz AM, Abell B, Brem RF. Lobular carcinoma in situ of the breast presenting as a mass. AJR Am J Roentgenol. 2005;184(6):1799–801.
77. Masannat YA, Bains SK, Pinder SE, Purushotham AD. Challenges in the management of pleomorphic lobular carcinoma in situ of the breast. Breast. 2013;22(2):194–6.
78. Brogi E, Murray MP, Corben AD. Lobular carcinoma, not only a classic. Breast J. 2010;16(Suppl 1):S10–4.
79. Middleton LP, Palacios DM, Bryant BR, Krebs P, Otis CN, Merino MJ. Pleomorphic lobular carcinoma: morphology, immunohistochemistry, and molecular analysis. Am J Surg Pathol. 2000;24(12):1650–6.
80. Ross DS, Hoda SA. Microinvasive (T1mic) lobular carcinoma of the breast: clinicopathologic profile of 16 cases. Am J Surg Pathol. 2011;35(5):750–6.
81. Dabbs DJ, Schnitt SJ, Geyer FC, Weigelt B, Baehner FL, Decker T, et al. Lobular neoplasia of the breast revisited with emphasis on the role of E-cadherin immunohistochemistry. Am J Surg Pathol. 2013;37(7):e1–11.
82. Viale G. The current state of breast cancer classification. Ann Oncol. 2012;23(Suppl 10):x207–10.
83. Tavassoli FA, Devilee P. Tumours of the breast and female genital organs. Pathology and genetics. Iarc ed. Lyon: IARC Press; 2003. 432 p.
84. Eggemann H, Kalinski T, Ruhland AK, Ignatov T, Costa SD, Ignatov A. Clinical implications of growth pattern and extension of tumor-associated intraductal carcinoma of the breast. Clin Breast Cancer. 2015;15(3):227–33.
85. Sinn H, Anton H, Magener A, von Fournier D, Bastert G, Otto H. Extensive and predominant in situ component in breast carcinoma: their influence on treatment results after breast-conserving therapy. Eur J Cancer. 1998;34(5):646–53.
86. Tot T, Gere M, Pekar G, Tarjan M, Hofmeyer S, Hellberg D, et al. Breast cancer multifocality, disease extent, and survival. Hum Pathol. 2011;42(11):1761–9.
87. Gujam FJ, Going JJ, Edwards J, Mohammed ZM, McMillan DC. The role of lymphatic and blood vessel invasion in predicting survival and methods of detection in patients with primary operable breast cancer. Crit Rev Oncol Hematol. 2014;89 (2):231–41.
88. McCart Reed AE, Kutasovic JR, Lakhani SR, Simpson PT. Invasive lobular carcinoma of the breast: morphology, biomarkers and omics. Breast Cancer Res. 2015;17:12.
89. Ellis IO, Galea M, Broughton N, Locker A, Blamey RW, Elston CW. Pathological prognostic factors in breast cancer. II. Histological type. Relationship with survival in a large study with long-term follow-up. Histopathology. 1992;20(6):479–89.
90. Bertucci F, Orsetti B, Negre V, Finetti P, Rouge C, Ahomadegbe JC, et al. Lobular and ductal carcinomas of the breast have distinct genomic and expression profiles. Oncogene. 2008;27(40):5359–72.
91. Gruel N, Lucchesi C, Raynal V, Rodrigues MJ, Pierron G, Goudefroye R, et al. Lobular invasive carcinoma of the breast is a molecular entity distinct from luminal invasive ductal carcinoma. Eur J Cancer. 2010;46(13):2399–407.
92. Anderson WF, Pfeiffer RM, Dores GM, Sherman ME. Comparison of age distribution patterns for different histopathologic types of breast carcinoma. Cancer Epidemiol Biomarkers Prev. 2006;15(10):1899–905.
93. Li CI, Uribe DJ, Daling JR. Clinical characteristics of different histologic types of breast cancer. Br J Cancer. 2005;93(9):1046–52.
94. Claus EB, Stowe M, Carter D, Holford T. The risk of a contralateral breast cancer among women diagnosed with ductal and lobular breast carcinoma in situ: data from the connecticut tumor registry. Breast. 2003;12(6):451–6.
95. Winchester DJ, Chang HR, Graves TA, Menck HR, Bland KI, Winchester DP. A comparative analysis of lobular and ductal carcinoma of the breast: presentation, treatment, and outcomes. J Am Coll Surg. 1998;186(4):416–22.
96. Hilleren DJ, Andersson IT, Lindholm K, Linnell FS. Invasive lobular carcinoma: mammographic findings in a 10-year experience. Radiology. 1991;178(1):149–54.
97. Newstead GM, Baute PB, Toth HK. Invasive lobular and ductal carcinoma: mammographic findings and stage at diagnosis. Radiology. 1992;184(3):623–7.
98. Slanger TE, Chang-Claude JC, Obi N, Kropp S, Berger J, Vettorazzi E, et al. Menopausal hormone therapy and risk of clinical breast cancer subtypes. Cancer Epidemiol Biomarkers Prev. 2009;18(4):1188–96.
99. Weinstein SP, Orel SG, Heller R, Reynolds C, Czerniecki B, Solin LJ, et al. MR imaging of the breast in patients with invasive lobular carcinoma. AJR Am J Roentgenol. 2001;176(2):399–406.
100. Mann RM, Veltman J, Barentsz JO, Wobbes T, Blickman JG, Boetes C. The value of MRI compared to mammography in the assessment of tumour extent in invasive lobular carcinoma of the breast. Eur J Surg Oncol. 2008;34(2):135–42.
101. Houssami N, Turner R, Morrow M. Preoperative magnetic resonance imaging in breast cancer: meta-analysis of surgical outcomes. Ann Surg. 2013;257(2):249–55.
102. Turnbull L, Brown S, Harvey I, Olivier C, Drew P, Napp V, et al. Comparative effectiveness of MRI in breast cancer (COMICE) trial: a randomised controlled trial. Lancet. 2010;375(9714):563–71.

103. Mitze M, Meyer F, Goepel E, Kleinkauf-Houcken A, Jonat W. Besonderheiten in Klinik und Verlauf beim invasiven lobulären Mammakarzinom. Geburtshilfe Frauenheilkd. 1991;51(12):973–9.
104. Sakr RA, Poulet B, Kaufman GJ, Nos C, Clough KB. Clear margins for invasive lobular carcinoma: a surgical challenge. Eur J Surg Oncol. 2011;37(4):350–6.
105. Elston CW, Ellis IO. Pathological prognostic factors in breast cancer. I. The value of histological grade in breast cancer: experience from a large study with long-term follow-up. Histopathology. 1991;19(5):403–10.
106. Hanby A, Hughes T. In situ and invasive lobular neoplasia of the breast. Histopathology. 2008;52(1):58–66.
107. Orvieto E, Maiorano E, Bottiglieri L, Maisonneuve P, Rotmensz N, Galimberti V, et al. Clinicopathologic characteristics of invasive lobular carcinoma of the breast: results of an analysis of 530 cases from a single institution. Cancer. 2008;113(7):1511–20.
108. Talman ML, Jensen MB, Rank F. Invasive lobular breast cancer. Prognostic significance of histological malignancy grading. Acta Oncol. 2007;46(6):803–9.
109. Monhollen L, Morrison C, Ademuyiwa FO, Chandrasekhar R, Khoury T. Pleomorphic lobular carcinoma: a distinctive clinical and molecular breast cancer type. Histopathology. 2012;61 (3):365–77.
110. Iorfida M, Maiorano E, Orvieto E, Maisonneuve P, Bottiglieri L, Rotmensz N, et al. Invasive lobular breast cancer: subtypes and outcome. Breast Cancer Res Treat. 2012;133(2):713–23.
111. Arpino G, Bardou VJ, Clark GM, Elledge RM. Infiltrating lobular carcinoma of the breast: tumor characteristics and clinical outcome. Breast Cancer Res. 2004;6(3):R149–56.
112. Pestalozzi BC, Zahrieh D, Mallon E, Gusterson BA, Price KN, Gelber RD, et al. Distinct clinical and prognostic features of infiltrating lobular carcinoma of the breast: combined results of 15 international breast cancer study group clinical trials. J Clin Oncol. 2008;26(18):3006–14.
113. Rakha EA, El-Sayed ME, Powe DG, Green AR, Habashy H, Grainge MJ, et al. Invasive lobular carcinoma of the breast: response to hormonal therapy and outcomes. Eur J Cancer. 2008;44(1):73–83.
114. Wasif N, Maggard MA, Ko CY, Giuliano AE. Invasive lobular vs. ductal breast cancer: a stage-matched comparison of outcomes. Ann Surg Oncol. 2010;17(7):1862–9.
115. Rakha EA, El-Sayed ME, Menon S, Green AR, Lee AH, Ellis IO. Histologic grading is an independent prognostic factor in invasive lobular carcinoma of the breast. Breast Cancer Res Treat. 2008;111(1):121–7.
116. Borst MJ, Ingold JA. Metastatic patterns of invasive lobular versus invasive ductal carcinoma of the breast. Surgery. 1993;114 (4):637–41.
117. Harris M, Howell A, Chrissohou M, Swindell RI, Hudson M, Sellwood RA. A comparison of the metastatic pattern of infiltrating lobular carcinoma and infiltrating duct carcinoma of the breast. Br J Cancer. 1984;50(1):23–30.
118. Jain S, Fisher C, Smith P, Millis RR, Rubens RD. Patterns of metastatic breast cancer in relation to histological type. Eur J Cancer. 1993;29A(15):2155–7.
119. Sastre-Garau X, Jouve M, Asselain B, Vincent-Salomon A, Beuzeboc P, Dorval T, et al. Infiltrating lobular carcinoma of the breast. Clinicopathologic analysis of 975 cases with reference to data on conservative therapy and metastatic patterns. Cancer. 1996;77(1):113–20.
120. Silverstein MJ, Lewinsky BS, Waisman JR, Gierson ED, Colburn WJ, Senofsky GM, et al. Infiltrating lobular carcinoma. Is it different from infiltrating duct carcinoma? Cancer. 1994;73 (6):1673–7.
121. Toikkanen S, Pylkkanen L, Joensuu H. Invasive lobular carcinoma of the breast has better short- and long-term survival than invasive ductal carcinoma. Br J Cancer. 1997;76(9):1234–40.
122. Rakha EA, Lee AH, Evans AJ, Menon S, Assad NY, Hodi Z, et al. Tubular carcinoma of the breast: further evidence to support its excellent prognosis. J Clin Oncol. 2010;28(1):99–104.
123. Colleoni M, Rotmensz N, Maisonneuve P, Mastropasqua MG, Luini A, Veronesi P, et al. Outcome of special types of luminal breast cancer. Ann Oncol. 2012;23(6):1428–36.
124. Bae SY, Choi MY, Cho DH, Lee JE, Nam SJ, Yang JH. Mucinous carcinoma of the breast in comparison with invasive ductal carcinoma: clinicopathologic characteristics and prognosis. J Breast Cancer. 2011;14(4):308–13.
125. Jensen ML, Kiaer H, Andersen J, Jensen V, Melsen F. Prognostic comparison of three classifications for medullary carcinomas of the breast. Histopathology. 1997;30(6):523–32.
126. Dellapasqua S, Maisonneuve P, Viale G, Pruneri G, Mazzarol G, Ghisini R, et al. Immunohistochemically defined subtypes and outcome of apocrine breast cancer. Clin Breast Cancer. 2013;13 (2):95–102.
127. Chen L, Fan Y, Lang RG, Guo XJ, Sun YL, Cui LF, et al. Breast carcinoma with micropapillary features: clinicopathologic study and long-term follow-up of 100 cases. Int J Surg Pathol. 2008;16 (2):155–63.
128. Weigelt B, Kreike B, Reis-Filho JS. Metaplastic breast carcinomas are basal-like breast cancers: a genomic profiling analysis. Breast Cancer Res Treat. 2009;117(2):273–80.
129. Tse GM, Tan PH, Putti TC, Lui PC, Chaiwun B, Law BK. Metaplastic carcinoma of the breast: a clinicopathological review. J Clin Pathol. 2006;59(10):1079–83.
130. Hui A, Henderson M, Speakman D, Skandarajah A. Angiosarcoma of the breast: a difficult surgical challenge. Breast. 2012;21 (4):584–9.
131. Vorburger SA, Xing Y, Hunt KK, Lakin GE, Benjamin RS, Feig BW, et al. Angiosarcoma of the breast. Cancer. 2005;104 (12):2682–8.
132. Farid M, Ong WS, Lee MJ, Jeevan R, Ho ZC, Sairi AN, et al. Cutaneous versus non-cutaneous angiosarcoma: clinicopathologic features and treatment outcomes in 60 patients at a single Asian cancer centre. Oncology. 2013;85(3):182–90.
133. Penel N, Marreaud S, Robin YM, Hohenberger P. Angiosarcoma: state of the art and perspectives. Crit Rev Oncol Hematol. 2011;80(2):257–63.
134. Tan BY, Acs G, Apple SK, Badve S, Bleiweiss IJ, Brogi E, et al. Phyllodes tumours of the breast: a consensus review. Histopathology. 2016;68(1):5–21.
135. Mitus J, Reinfuss M, Mitus JW, Jakubowicz J, Blecharz P, Wysocki WM, et al. Malignant phyllodes tumor of the breast: treatment and prognosis. Breast J. 2014;20(6):639–44.
136. Gnerlich JL, Williams RT, Yao K, Jaskowiak N, Kulkarni SA. Utilization of radiotherapy for malignant phyllodes tumors: analysis of the National Cancer Data Base, 1998–2009. Ann Surg Oncol. 2014;21(4):1222–30.
137. Bloom HJ, Richardson WW. Histological grading and prognosis in breast cancer; a study of 1409 cases of which 359 have been followed for 15 years. Br J Cancer. 1957;11(3):359–77.
138. Sobin LH, Gospodarowicz MK, Wittekind C, International Union against Cancer. TNM classification of malignant tumours, 7th ed. Chichester, West Sussex, UK; Hoboken, NJ: Wiley; 2010, xx, 309 p.
139. NHS. Pathology reporting of breast disease 2005 [A joint document incorporating the third edition of the NHS breast screening programme's guidelines for pathology reporting in breast cancer screening and the second edition of the royal college of pathologists' minimum dataset for breast cancer

histopathology]. Available from: http://www.cancerscreening.nhs.uk/breastscreen/publications/nhsbsp58.html.
140. Wachtel MS, Halldorsson A, Dissanaike S. Nottingham grades of lobular carcinoma lack the prognostic implications they bear for ductal carcinoma. J Surg Res. 2011;166(1):19–27.
141. Schwartz AM, Henson DE, Chen D, Rajamarthandan S. Histologic grade remains a prognostic factor for breast cancer regardless of the number of positive lymph nodes and tumor size: a study of 161 708 cases of breast cancer from the SEER Program. Arch Pathol Lab Med. 2014;138(8):1048–52.
142. Galea MH, Blamey RW, Elston CE, Ellis IO. The nottingham prognostic index in primary breast cancer. Breast Cancer Res Treat. 1992;22(3):207–19.
143. Mook S, Schmidt MK, Rutgers EJ, van de Velde AO, Visser O, Rutgers SM, et al. Calibration and discriminatory accuracy of prognosis calculation for breast cancer with the online Adjuvant! program: a hospital-based retrospective cohort study. Lancet Oncol. 2009;10(11):1070–6.
144. Simpson PT, Reis-Filho JS, Gale T, Lakhani SR. Molecular evolution of breast cancer. J Pathol. 2005;205(2):248–54.
145. Sotiriou C, Wirapati P, Loi S, Harris A, Fox S, Smeds J, et al. Gene expression profiling in breast cancer: understanding the molecular basis of histologic grade to improve prognosis. J Natl Cancer Inst. 2006;98(4):262–72.
146. Loi S, Haibe-Kains B, Desmedt C, Lallemand F, Tutt AM, Gillet C, et al. Definition of clinically distinct molecular subtypes in estrogen receptor-positive breast carcinomas through genomic grade. J Clin Oncol. 2007;25(10):1239–46.
147. Liedtke C, Hatzis C, Symmans WF, Desmedt C, Haibe-Kains B, Valero V, et al. Genomic grade index is associated with response to chemotherapy in patients with breast cancer. J Clin Oncol. 2009;27(19):3185–91.
148. Metzger Filho O, Ignatiadis M, Sotiriou C. Genomic grade index: an important tool for assessing breast cancer tumor grade and prognosis. Crit Rev Oncol Hematol. 2011;77(1):20–9.
149. Schneeweiss A, Katretchko J, Sinn H, Unnebrink K, Rudlowski C, Geberth M, et al. Only grading has independent impact on breast cancer survival after adjustment for pathological response to preoperative chemotherapy. Anticancer Drugs. 2004;15(2):127–35.
150. Allison KH, Kandalaft PL, Sitlani CM, Dintzis SM, Gown AM. Routine pathologic parameters can predict Oncotype DX recurrence scores in subsets of ER positive patients: who does not always need testing? Breast Cancer Res Treat. 2012;131(2):413–24.
151. Mattes MD, Mann JM, Ashamalla H, Tejwani A. Routine histopathologic characteristics can predict oncotype DX(TM) recurrence score in subsets of breast cancer patients. Cancer Invest. 2013;31(9):604–6.
152. Auerbach J, Kim M, Fineberg S. Can features evaluated in the routine pathologic assessment of lymph node-negative estrogen receptor-positive stage I or II invasive breast cancer be used to predict the Oncotype DX recurrence score? Arch Pathol Lab Med. 2010;134(11):1697–701.
153. Klein ME, Dabbs DJ, Shuai Y, Brufsky AM, Jankowitz R, Puhalla SL, et al. Prediction of the Oncotype DX recurrence score: use of pathology-generated equations derived by linear regression analysis. Mod Pathol. 2013;26(5):658–64.
154. Gilchrist KW, Kalish L, Gould VE, Hirschl S, Imbriglia JE, Levy WM, et al. Interobserver reproducibility of histopathological features in stage II breast cancer. An ECOG study. Breast Cancer Res Treat. 1985;5(1):3–10.
155. Longacre TA, Ennis M, Quenneville LA, Bane AL, Bleiweiss IJ, Carter BA, et al. Interobserver agreement and reproducibility in classification of invasive breast carcinoma: an NCI breast cancer family registry study. Mod Pathol. 2006;19(2):195–207.
156. Fisher ER, Redmond C, Fisher B. Histologic grading of breast cancer. Pathol Annu. 1980;15(Pt 1):239–51.
157. Robbins P, Pinder S, de Klerk N, Dawkins H, Harvey J, Sterrett G, et al. Histological grading of breast carcinomas: a study of interobserver agreement. Hum Pathol. 1995;26(8):873–9.
158. Ellis IO, Coleman D, Wells C, Kodikara S, Paish EM, Moss S, et al. Impact of a national external quality assessment scheme for breast pathology in the UK. J Clin Pathol. 2006;59(2):138–45.
159. Rakha EA, Reis-Filho JS, Baehner F, Dabbs DJ, Decker T, Eusebi V, et al. Breast cancer prognostic classification in the molecular era: the role of histological grade. Breast Cancer Res. 2010;12(4):207.

Breast Cancer Molecular Testing for Prognosis and Prediction

11

Nadia Harbeck

11.1 Biomarkers

Biomarkers in oncology are properties of the tumor or the host that can be measured in tissue or blood and that can aid in therapy decision-making.

11.1.1 Prognostic Markers

Prognostic markers are associated with clinical outcome either in the absence of therapy, thereby reflecting the natural course of the disease, or in a population of homogenously treated patients. Their clinical use is mostly to identify a patient population that has such a good outcome that additional therapy may not be necessary or that has such a poor outcome that additional therapy may be warranted. In breast cancer, prognostic markers are mostly needed in early breast cancer to identify those luminal breast cancers that are so aggressive that adjuvant chemotherapy is needed in addition to endocrine therapy.

11.1.2 Predictive Markers

Predictive markers are biomarkers that are associated with the benefit or lack of a particular therapy. Predictive biomarkers guide physicians in therapy selection, i.e., in choosing one therapy over another one. In certain cases, the biomarker itself constitutes a therapeutic target.

So far, the most important biomarkers in breast cancer are estrogen and progesterone receptor (ER, PgR) as well as HER2. In clinical routine, these markers are determined by immunohistochemistry. These markers are somewhat prognostic but more importantly, they are therapeutic targets and thus predictive for therapy response to the respective targeted agents.

Before routine use of new biomarkers in clinical practice, the markers need to be validated analytically as well as clinically, and clinical utility needs to be demonstrated [1]. The highest level of evidence (LOE IA) is ideally obtained by a prospective trial designed to validate the biomarker or by a meta- or pooled analysis [2]. As prospective trials may require several years before results are available, a revised level of evidence for biomarkers was subsequently proposed that enabled prospectively planned retrospective validation in formalin-fixed paraffin-embedded (FFPE) tissue specimens from well-controlled clinical trials or well-characterized tumor banks. In this classification, level I evidence can also be obtained by several prospectively planned analyses of archival specimens [3].

11.2 Molecular Subtypes in Breast Cancer and Therapy Concepts

The current understanding of breast cancer as a heterogenous disease consisting of several molecular subtypes is based on the seminal work of Perou and Sørlie in the early years of this millennium. They showed that there were at least four clinically relevant subtypes: luminal A and B, HER2-enriched, and basal-like [4, 5]. As molecular subtyping is not readily available in most centers, these subtypes are usually reconstructed using immunohistochemical markers for clinical routine [6]: Hormone receptor-positive tumors (ER- and/or PgR-positive) are considered luminal. ER- and/or PgR-positive tumors with low proliferation are classified as luminal A and those with high proliferation as luminal B. Proliferation is usually assessed by immunohistochemically determined Ki67. So far, there is no prospectively validated internationally standardized cutoff for low versus high Ki67 to be used for clinical decision-making. Immunohistochemical staining or in situ hybridization is used for the assessment of HER2 status. Last but not least, there is a

N. Harbeck (✉)
Breast Center, University of Munich, Marchioninistrasse 15, 81377 Munich, Germany
e-mail: nadia.harbeck@med.uni-muenchen.de

I. Jatoi and A. Rody (eds.), *Management of Breast Diseases*, DOI 10.1007/978-3-319-46356-8_11

substantial overlap between the basal subtype and triple-negative tumors which are characterized by the absence of ER and PR and HER2 [7].

For the 2016 ASCO recommendations for biomarkers suitable for guiding therapy decisions in early breast cancer (EBC), an extensive literature search was performed. Next to established markers ER, PgR, and HER2, only four multigene assays (Oncotype DX, EndoPredict, PAM50, and Breast Cancer Index) and one protein-based test (uPA/PAI-1) were found to have sufficient clinical utility [8]. Most of these recommended newly developed assays have only prognostic utility; only few have additional predictive potential for response to adjuvant chemotherapy. Yet, none of these new markers is predictive for a particular drug or regimen.

11.3 Multigene Assays in Early Breast Cancer

In EBC, systemic therapy recommendations are based on tumor subtype [6]. Whereas well-defined systemic therapy standards exist for HER2-positive (chemotherapy + anti-HER2 therapy) and triple-negative disease (chemotherapy), the key clinical question in luminal disease is whether to also indicate adjuvant chemotherapy prior to the guideline recommended endocrine therapy. For this question, established clinical–pathological factors are not sufficient for adequate risk assessment and thus additional biomarkers are needed (see Fig. 11.1).

For risk assessment in EBC, several multigene assays have been developed over the last decade. They all consist of a specific prognostic signature, i.e., some cases combined with clinical criteria for enhanced prognostic information. In some cases, data also exist for a predictive impact regarding response to adjuvant chemotherapy. Whereas most signatures have been thoroughly validated in archival cohorts, only two signatures have been validated by prospective clinical trials specifically designed to validate the signature as a primary or secondary end point. So far, some of these results are still pending.

In the 2016, ASCO recommended only four multigene assays (Oncotype DX, EndoPredict, PAM50, and Breast Cancer Index) for routine use in EBC because of their validated clinical utility [8]. In addition, a fifth multigene assay, MammaPrint, is also discussed in this chapter as it is recommended by the AGO (Working Group for Gynecological Oncology Breast Commission) guidelines [9]. Data from a prospective clinical trial for MammaPrint were presented at AACR 2016, i.e., after the publication of the ASCO recommendations.

Tests differ in patient collectives used for clinical validation and quality and quantity of available evidence (see Table 11.1).

11.3.1 21-Gene Signature (Oncotype DX, Recurrence Score)

The 21 Gene Assay (Oncotype DX™ Breast Cancer Assay (Genomic Health Inc., Redwood City, USA) quantifies gene expression for 21 genes by qRT-PCR. This test for FFPE tissue is performed on a single central analytic platform, where qRT-PCR conditions are validated and reproducible with certified quality assurance [10]. The assay consists of 15 genes that mainly represent proliferation, estrogen receptor (ER) regulation, HER2 pathway, and invasion, and are analyzed together with five control genes. Test result is a numerical score (recurrence score, RS) between 0 and 100. Tumors are classified into three risk categories based on their recurrence score (RS): low (RS < 18), intermediate (RS 18–30), or high risk (RS ≥ 31). Initial test development was done in archival tissue from tamoxifen-treated node-negative patients from the NSABP B14 trial [11]. In an additional

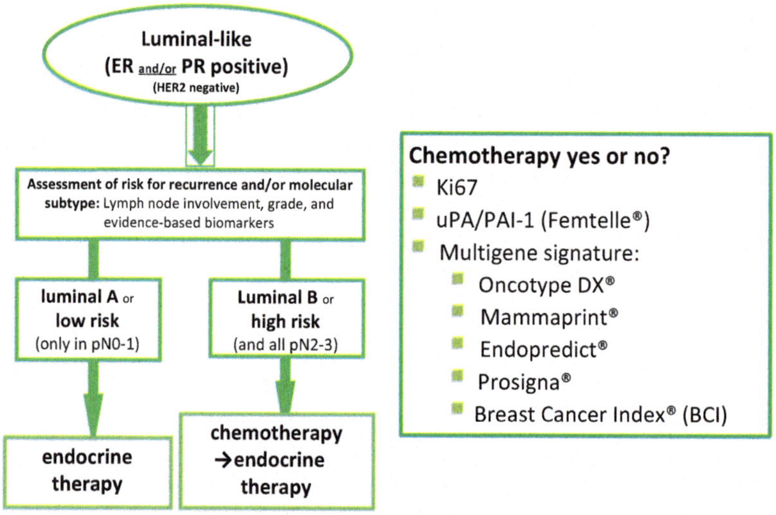

Fig. 11.1 Therapy concepts in luminal early breast cancer

Table 11.1 Multigene Assays in early breast cancer as recommended by ASCO 2016 [8] and AGO 2016 [9]

Multigene assay	Oncotype DX	MammaPrint	EndoPredict	Prosigna (PAM50)	Breast cancer index (BCI)
Manufacturer	Genomic health	Agendia	Sividon	Nanostring	bioTheranostics
Assay	21 gene recurrence score (RS)	70 gene assay	11 gene assay	50 gene assay (PAM50, ROR score)	HoxB13/IL17BR (H/I) Molecular grade index (MGI)
Testing	Central laboratory (USA)	Central laboratory (Netherlands, USA)	Decentral	Decentral	Central laboratory (USA)
Accreditation	CLIA, CAP	FDA (IVDMIA)	CE mark	FDA (510k), CE mark	n.a.
Molecular subtype	No	Yes (Blueprint)	No	Yes (not reported in USA)	No
Prognostic information	Yes	Yes	Yes	Yes	Yes
Predictive information	Yes (chemotherapy)	Yes (chemotherapy)	No data so far	No data so far	Yes (extended endocrine therapy)
Retrospective validation	NSABP B14 & B20 TransATAC ECOG 9127 SWOG 8814	Multicenter	ABCSG 6 & 8 TransATAC GEICAM 9906	ABCSG 8 TransATAC NCIC CTG MA.21	Stockholm trial NCIC CTG MA.14 multicenter
Prospective clinical validation trials	WSG-Plan B WSG ADAPT TAILORx RxPONDER	MINDACT	None	None	None

All tests are suitable for FFPE tissue specimens

analysis using archival tissues from the NSABP B20 trial, it was shown that benefit from adjuvant chemotherapy (CMF) is greatest in patients with high-risk recurrence score, whereas patients with low RS do not derive any benefit and benefit in intermediate RS patients is uncertain [12]. Subsequently, prognostic and predictive impacts of RS were retrospectively validated also for node-positive patients in archival tissue from the SWOG 8814 trial. RS was prognostic in the tamoxifen-alone cohort. While there was no benefit from CAF chemotherapy in low RS patients, patients in the chemotherapy group with high-risk RS did have an improved disease-free survival (DFS) [13]. TransATAC showed that RS was provided similar prognostic information in node-negative and node-positive postmenopausal patients treated by adjuvant tamoxifen or aromatase inhibitor [14]. Most importantly, this retrospective analysis showed that while RS is prognostic in node-positive patients independent of number of involved nodes, baseline risk in patients with 4 and more involved lymph nodes even with low RS is too high to consider omitting adjuvant chemotherapy. Yet, in patients up to three lymph nodes, an RS up to 11 is associated with a 9-year risk of distant recurrence of about 10 %. As this percentage is within the rate where absolute benefit from chemotherapy may not exceed potentially severe-side effects, sparing patients the additional toxicity of adjuvant chemotherapy can be considered. These data form the basis for the prospective clinical trials with Oncotype DX that used RS 11 as a cutoff for low versus intermediate-risk groups instead of the commercial cutoff of 18.

Large population-based registries studies such as the Kaiser Permanente case–control study (n = 790) [15], the SEER database (n = 38,568) [16], or the Israeli Clalit registry (n = 1594) [17] have further validated the clinical utility of the Oncotype DX test.

In addition, there are three prospective international clinical trials using prospective Oncotype DX results for patient stratification or randomization: TAILORx (pN0), RxPONDER (pN1), and WSG-Plan B (pN0-1). In TAILORx and RxPONDER, intermediate-risk patients (RS 11–25) are randomized between chemoendocrine therapy and endocrine therapy alone. While RyPONDER is still ongoing, the low-risk arm of TAILORx has already been reported: Low (0–10) RS patients treated by endocrine therapy alone had a 5-year invasive DFS of 93.8 % and OS of 98 % [18]. The WSG-Plan B study confirmed the excellent outcome of low-risk (0–11) RS patients treated by endocrine therapy alone even with up to three involved lymph nodes with a 3-year DFS of 98 % compared to 98 % in intermediate RS (12–25) and 92 % (RS > 25) patients treated by adjuvant chemotherapy [19] (see Fig. 11.2). Five-year results for low

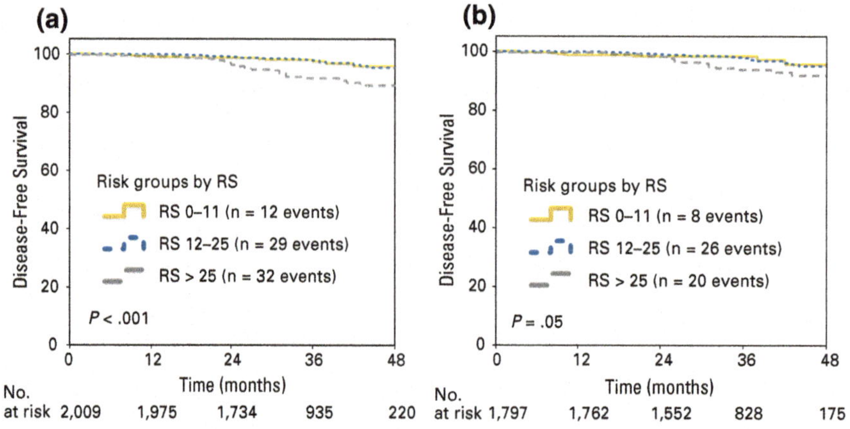

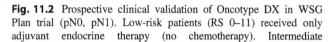

Fig. 11.2 Prospective clinical validation of Oncotype DX in WSG Plan trial (pN0, pN1). Low-risk patients (RS 0–11) received only adjuvant endocrine therapy (no chemotherapy). Intermediate (RS 12–25) and high-risk (>25) patients received adjuvant chemotherapy prior to adjuvant endocrine therapy. Reprinted with permission © 2016 American Society of Clinical Oncology. Gluz et al. [19]

RS patients were 94 % for DFS and 99 % for OS and did not differ substantially between pN0 and pN1 patients [20].

11.3.2 70-Gene Signature (MammaPrint)

The 70 Gene Assay (MammaPrint™; Agendia, Amsterdam, the Netherlands) is based on DNA microarray technology. It was developed using archival frozen tissue and a case–control design [21] and subsequently validated in a larger cohort of young (<53 years), node-negative, and node-positive EBC patients from the Netherlands Cancer Institute [22]. The test gives a dichotomized test result, distinguishing a genomically low-risk from a high-risk group. To facilitate its use in a diagnostic setting, the 70-gene prognosis profile was translated into a customized microarray (MammaPrint) which received approval as an in vitro diagnostic multivariate index assay (IVDMIA) by the US Food and Drug Administration in February 2007 [23]. Subsequently, the platform was adjusted to enable the analysis of FFPE tissue samples from clinical routine with an overall equivalence of 91.5 % between fresh frozen and FFPE and highly reproducible results in FFPE analysis of >97 % precision and repeatability [24]. An 80-gene signature now also enables molecular subtyping of FFPE breast cancer specimens [25].

Clinical validation was achieved by several retrospective studies such as TransBIG [26] or the prospective community-based RASTER study [27]. In a pooled case series (n = 541), a predictive impact regarding response to adjuvant chemotherapy was shown [28]. While in MammaPrint low-risk patients, 5-year breast cancer specific survival (BCSS) was similar with or without adjuvant chemotherapy, and 5-year BCSS was significantly higher in patients who received adjuvant chemotherapy prior to endocrine therapy.

The MINDACT (Microarray in Node-Negative Disease May Avoid Chemotherapy) Trial (EORTC, Breast International Group BIG) was designed to prospectively validate the MammaPrint test in >6000 EBC patients and to evaluate the role of adjuvant chemotherapy in patients who have discordant results between clinical–pathological and genomic risk assessment [29]. MINDACT (n = 6693) reached its primary end point by demonstrating a 94.7 % (95 % CI 92.5–96.4 %) 5-year OS in EBC patients at clinical high-risk whose tumors tested low-risk by MammaPrint and who did not receive any adjuvant chemotherapy after randomization [30].

11.3.3 Endopredict

Endopredict (Endopredict®; Sividon Diagnostics GmbH, Cologne, Germany; distributed by Myriad) is based on quantification of mRNA levels of 8 selected genes by qRT-PCR, with 3 additional control genes. The test renders a numerical value (Endopredict® score) and a dichotomized result (low vs. high risk); together with two clinical risk factors (nodal status and tumor size), it results in a comprehensive risk score, EPclin [31]. The test was developed and validated in archival specimens from the two ABCSG (Austrian Breast and Colorectal Cancer Study Group) studies 6 and 8 in postmenopausal patients with ER-positive, HER2-negative EBC receiving adjuvant endocrine therapy [32]. Endopredict does not just provide information on the first 5 years but also on late recurrences which may be used in order to indicate extended adjuvant therapy [33]. A retrospective analysis from the GEICAM 9906 trial validated EndoPredict also in node-positive patients who received adjuvant chemotherapy. Moreover, it showed that the test has a prognostic impact in pre- and postmenopausal patients [34].

In an additional GEICAM 9906 substudy comparing EP and ROR, no significant difference between the tests was found. Both signatures provided prognostic information beyond clinical factors and reliably predicted risk of distant metastasis in node-positive ER+ HER2− EBC patients treated by chemo- and endocrine therapy. Addition of clinical parameters to the risk scores improved their prognostic impact [35].

In a small study in seven different international laboratories with 10 different tumors, decentral testing resulted in excellent 100 % concordance [36]. There is also excellent concordance between core biopsy and matching surgical specimens with a 95 % overall agreement in risk classification [37].

11.3.4 Prosigna (PAM50)

Prosigna™ (PAM50; Breast Cancer Prognostic Gene Signature Assay: Nanostring Technologies, Seattle, USA) received European Union regulatory clearance (CE mark) in September 2012 and 510(k) clearance from the US Food and Drug Administration (FDA) in 2013. This assay is based on the original molecular intrinsic breast cancer subtypes and allows their determination using a minimal gene set (PAM50) in FFPE tissue. The test renders a numerical ROR score (low/intermediate/high) and the molecular subtype (which is not reported in the US) [38]. The ROR score reported for clinical routine incorporates clinical information from tumor size and nodal status. Prosigna has been validated for decentralized testing using the Nanostring nCounter technology [39].

In ABCSG 8, patients who were all treated by adjuvant endocrine therapy alone, PAM50 ROR score was clinically validated ($n = 1478$) regarding its prognostic impact. ROR score provided relevant prognostic information beyond clinical risk factors and luminal A tumors were associated with a significantly lower risk of recurrence at 10 years than luminal B tumors [40]. In addition, PAM50 and ROR score provide significant prognostic information in addition to clinical factors also for late recurrences between years 5 and 15 [41]. In the TransATAC cohort, PAM50 ROR provided significant prognostic information over a clinical treatment score (CTS). When compared to recurrence score, its intermediate-risk group was smaller, and the gain of prognostic information versus the CTS seemed greater [42]. Combined analysis from TransATAC and ABCSG 8 ($n = 2137$) validated the prognostic impact of PAM50 ROR as being superior to that provided by clinical information for late relapses [43]. It also substantiated its prognostic impact for node-positive patients [44].

In a retrospective analysis of NCIC CTG MA.21 ($n = 1094$), high ROR was associated with poor and luminal A subtype with favorable relapse-free survival in node-positive or high-risk node-negative patients (<60 years) who received AC-paclitaxel (AC-T), dose-dense CEF, or dose-dense, dose-intense EC-paclitaxel (EC-T). While intrinsic subtypes were not predictive of treatment benefit (AC-T vs. dose-dense chemotherapy), subgroup analysis indicated that subtype (non-luminal vs. luminal) was predictive of taxane benefit [45].

11.4 Breast Cancer Index (BCI)

The Breast Cancer Index™ (BCI) (bioTheranostics Inc, San Diego, CA, USA) is a gene expression-based algorithm incorporating two gene signatures, the HOXB13:IL17BR ratio (H/I) and the Molecular Grade Index (MGI). BCI is a real-time RT-PCR assay that measures the expression of H/I, MGI, and four normalization genes. The *BCI Prognostic* score is calculated as a value from 0 to 10 and categorized into risk levels for late (high vs. low) and overall (high, intermediate, low) distant recurrence. Moreover, *BCI Predictive* provides the likelihood of benefit from extended adjuvant endocrine therapy beyond 5 years. The test was validated in the archival tumor samples from the Stockholm study (node-negative, post-menopausal, $n = 317$ tamoxifen-treated, $n = 283$ untreated) as well as from a multiinstitutional cohort which included also larger tumors, premenopausal patients, and patients treated by adjuvant chemotherapy [46]. In both cohorts, continuous BCI was the most significant prognostic factor beyond clinicopathological factors for early (up to 5 years) and late relapses (beyond 5 years). In the TransATAC study, BCI provided prognostic information beyond the CTS and beyond recurrence score. BCI enabled restratification of the low and intermediate RS risk groups into subgroups with significantly different distant recurrence rates. In contrast, RS did not achieve a clinically meaningful restratification of BCI risk groups [47]. BCI but not RS predicted early and relapses in the TransATAC cohort [48]. In a case–control series in ER+ node-negative EBC without adjuvant chemotherapy, BCI was significantly associated with 10-year OS [49]. In a NCIC CTG MA.14 substudy, BCI provided prognostic information for node-negative and node-positive patients [50].

11.5 Clinical Use of Multigene Assays for Decision-Making in Early Breast Cancer

Several assays have been compared retrospectively in archival tissue samples from prospective trials regarding their prognostic impact such as in TransATAC or prospectively regarding their impact on clinical decision-making. The English OPTIMA program suggests that current multigene assays tend to provide similar risk information in

ER-positive EBC but that risk assessment and molecular subtype results may differ for an individual patient [51]. When comparing several tests in archival cohorts, risk group classifications may need to be mathematically modeled and thus not reflect actual risk group stratification as used in the clinic (e.g., tertiles or quartiles instead of dichotomization). Moreover, patient collectives from those archival cohorts may not necessarily always reflect prospective testing in patients who usually have a clinically high enough risk to warrant consideration of adjuvant chemotherapy (pN0-1). Thus, results from those retrospective test comparisons do not necessarily adequately reflect the clinical utility of each individual test.

In summary, several multigene assays are available for risk assessment in EBC. They are best suited for HER2-negative luminal EBC with up to 3 involved axillary lymph nodes. In these patients, accurate risk assessment based on multigene assays may prevent over—but also undertreatment by adjuvant chemotherapy. Prospective clinical trials have now validated the retrospective evidence for two tests (Oncotype DX and MammaPrint) with regard to risk group assessment: Patients with up to three lymph nodes and low-risk test result have an excellent 5-year outcome with adjuvant endocrine therapy alone and thus can safely be spared adjuvant chemotherapy. The prospective results regarding the benefit from adjuvant chemotherapy in intermediate-risk patients are still missing.

In clinical practice, a test for the individual patient will to be chosen based on the available evidence, also for particular subgroups such as node-positive patients or pre-menopausal patients. Moreover, provision of molecular subtype information, test logistics, costs, reimbursement policies, and local and/or national guidelines play an important role. Given the observed discordant results for individual patients, use of multiple tests in a single patient is strongly discouraged. In particular, patients definitely need to be counseled about adjuvant chemotherapy if one evidence-based test renders a high-risk result.

11.6 Molecular Testing for Therapy Prediction

So far, next to ER, PR, and HER2, no molecular factors have validated clinical utility for the prediction of therapy response or resistance to a specific drug or therapy regimen. Multiple molecular markers for prediction of therapy response or resistance have been proposed over the last decade. Yet, none of them has demonstrated clinical utility so far.

Hepatic cytochrome P450 2D2 (**CYP 2D6**) is essential for metabolism of tamoxifen into the active metabolite endoxifen. Several publications have linked CYP 2D6 polymorphisms to reduced efficacy of adjuvant tamoxifen. However, a metaanalysis covering 25 studies (n = 13629) concluded that there is insufficient evidence to recommend CYP 2D6 genotyping to guide tamoxifen treatment [52].

Topoisomerase II alpha has been suggested as a marker for anthracycline response in breast cancer as it is one of the intracellular anthracycline targets. The gene (TOP2A) is located on chromosome 17q12-21. While individual studies suggested an association between TOP2A amplification and response to anthracyclines, a meta-analysis of 5 prospective randomized trials was not able to validate these observations [53].

PIK3CA mutations are the most frequent mutations in breast cancer. They have been implicated with resistance to anti-HER2 therapy in the neoadjuvant setting. In a meta-analysis of five clinical trials (n = 967) in which patients received either trastuzumab or lapatinib or a combination thereof together with taxane chemotherapy, pCR rates were significantly lower in PIK3CA mutant versus PIK3CA wild-type tumors (16.2 % vs. 29.6 %; $P < 0.001$). The effect was most pronounced in luminal HER2-positive tumors. Definite conclusions regarding survival can not be drawn so far [54]. Recent data from MBC suggest that patients with alterations of the PI3K pathway may derive benefit from the addition of everolimus to trastuzumab therapy [55]. Circulating free DNA has been suggested as a clinically useful alternative to tissue analysis. High diagnostic accuracy has already been demonstrated [56].

These examples show that despite of a convincing pre-clinical rationale, clinical utility could not be demonstrated for of several interesting biomarkers. Particularly in MBC, it has not bene established which tissue is most suited for molecular marker analysis. Circulating tumor DNA is readily available and can also be used for repeated analyses over time. Thus, ctDNA may be a promising source for novel molecular markers in the future.

11.7 Conclusions

So far, next to ER, PgR, and HER2, few novel biomarkers have been introduced into clinical management in breast cancer. Considering the advent of several highly effective targeted agents over the recent years, new molecular biomarkers, in particular for prediction of therapy response, are urgently needed for individualization of treatment concepts. Molecular analysis methods and modern high-throughput techniques provide great promise for identification of new biomarkers. Circulating tumor DNA (ctDNA) holds great promise as a new tissue source for future validation of molecular markers. Yet, a bad biomarker can potentially be as dangerous for patients as a bad drug. Technical feasibility alone is thus not sufficient for adoption of a marker into clinical management. Thorough technical and clinical validations together with undisputed clinical utility are thus perquisites for introducing new markers into the clinic.

References

1. Hayes DF. Considerations for implementation of cancer molecular diagnostics into clinical care. Am Soc Clin Oncol Educ Book. 2016;35:292–6.
2. Hayes DF, Bast RC, Desch CE, et al. Tumor marker utility grading system: a framework to evaluate clinical utility of tumor markers. J Natl Cancer Inst. 1996;88(20):1456–66.
3. Simon RM, Paik S, Hayes DF. Use of archived specimens in evaluation of prognostic and predictive biomarkers. J Natl Cancer Inst. 2009;101(21):1446–52.
4. Perou CM, Sørlie T, Eisen MB, et al. Molecular portraits of human breast tumours. Nature. 2000;406(6797):747–52.
5. Sørlie T, Perou CM, Tibshirani R, et al. Gene expression patterns of breast carcinomas distinguish tumor subclasses with clinical implications. Proc Natl Acad Sci USA. 2001;98(19):10869–74.
6. Coates AS, Winer EP, Goldhirsch A, et al. Tailoring therapies–improving the management of early breast cancer: St Gallen International Expert Consensus on the primary therapy of early breast cancer 2015. Ann Oncol. 2015;26(8):1533–46.
7. Anders CK, Abramson V, Tan T, Dent R. The evolution of triple-negative breast cancer: from biology to novel therapeutics. Am Soc Clin Oncol Educ Book. 2016;35:34–42.
8. Harris LN, Ismaila N, McShane LM, et al. Use of biomarkers to guide decisions on adjuvant systemic therapy for women with early-stage invasive breast cancer: American Society of Clinical Oncology clinical practice guideline. J Clin Oncol. 2016;34 (10):1134–50.
9. AGO recommendations 2016 for diagnosis and treatment of early and advanced breast cancer. Available from: www.ago-online.de.
10. Cronin M, Sangli C, Liu ML, et al. Analytical validation of the Oncotype DX genomic diagnostic test for recurrence prognosis and therapeutic response prediction in node-negative, estrogen receptor-positive breast cancer. Clin Chem. 2007;53(6):1084–91.
11. Paik S, Shak S, Tang G, et al. A multigene assay to predict recurrence of tamoxifen-treated, node-negative breast cancer. N Engl J Med. 2004;351(27):2817–26.
12. Paik S, Tang G, Shak S, et al. Gene expression and benefit of chemotherapy in women with node-negative, estrogen receptor-positive breast cancer. J Clin Oncol. 2006;24(23):3726–34.
13. Albain KS, Barlow WE, Shak S, et al. Breast Cancer Intergroup of North America. Prognostic and predictive value of the 21-gene recurrence score assay in postmenopausal women with node-positive, oestrogen-receptor-positive breast cancer on chemotherapy: a retrospective analysis of a randomised trial. Lancet Oncol. 2010;11(1):55–65.
14. Dowsett M, Cuzick J, Wale C, et al. Prediction of risk of distant recurrence using the 21-gene recurrence score in node-negative and node-positive postmenopausal patients with breast cancer treated with anastrozole or tamoxifen: a TransATAC study. J Clin Oncol. 2010;28(11):1829–34.
15. Habel LA, Shak S, Jacobs MK, et al. A population-based study of tumor gene expression and risk of breast cancer death among lymph node-negative patients. Breast Cancer Res. 2006;8(3):R25.
16. Shak S, Petkov VI, Miller DP, et al. Breast cancer specific survival in 38,568 patients with node negative hormone receptor positive invasive breast cancer and oncotype DX recurrence score results in the SEER database. SABCS 2015: P5-15-01.
17. Stemmer SM, Steiner M, Rizel S, et al. Real-life analysis evaluating 1594 N0/Nmic breast cancer patients for whom treatment decisions incorporated the 21-gene recurrence score result: 5-year KM estimate for breast cancer specific survival with recurrence score results ≤30 is >98 %. SABCS 2015: P5-08-02.
18. Sparano JA, Gray RJ, Makower DF, et al. Prospective validation of a 21-gene expression assay in breast cancer. N Engl J Med. 2015;373(21):2005–14.
19. Gluz O, Nitz U, Christgen M, et al. The WSG phase III PlanB trial: first prospective outcome data for the 21-gene recurrence score assay and concordance of prognostic markers by central and local pathology assessment. J Clin Oncol. 2016;34(20):2341–9.
20. Gluz O, Nitz U, Christgen M, et al. Prognostic impact of 21 gene recurrence score, IHC4, and central grade in high-risk HR+/HER2− early breast cancer (EBC): 5-year results of the prospective Phase III WSG PlanB trial. J Clin Oncol. 2016;34:(suppl; abstr 556).
21. van 't Veer LJ1, Dai H, van de Vijver MJ, et al. Gene expression profiling predicts clinical outcome of breast cancer. Nature. 2002;415(6871):530–6.
22. van de Vijver MJ, He YD, van't Veer LJ, et al. A gene-expression signature as a predictor of survival in breast cancer. N Engl J Med. 2002;347(25):1999–2009.
23. Glas AM, Floore A, Delahaye LJ, et al. Converting a breast cancer microarray signature into a high-throughput diagnostic test. BMC Genom. 2006;30(7):278.
24. Sapino A, Roepman P, Linn SC, et al. MammaPrint molecular diagnostics on formalin-fixed, paraffin-embedded tissue. J Mol Diagn. 2014;16(2):190–7.
25. Krijgsman O, Roepman P, Zwart W, et al. A diagnostic gene profile for molecular subtyping of breast cancer associated with treatment response. Breast Cancer Res Treat. 2012;133(1):37–47.
26. Buyse M, Loi S, van't Veer L, et al. TRANSBIG consortium. Validation and clinical utility of a 70-gene prognostic signature for women with node-negative breast cancer. J Natl Cancer Inst. 2006;98(17):1183–92.
27. Bueno-de-Mesquita JM, van Harten WH, Retel VP, et al. Use of 70-gene signature to predict prognosis of patients with node-negative breast cancer: a prospective community-based feasibility study (RASTER). Lancet Oncol. 2007;8(12):1079–87.
28. Knauer M, Mook S, Rutgers EJ, et al. The predictive value of the 70-gene signature for adjuvant chemotherapy in early breast cancer. Breast Cancer Res Treat. 2010;120(3):655–61.
29. Cardoso F, Van't Veer L, Rutgers E, et al. Clinical application of the 70-gene profile: the MINDACT trial. J Clin Oncol. 2008;26 (5):729–35.
30. Piccart M, Rutgers E, van't Veer L, et al. On behalf of TRANSBIG consortium and MINDACT investigators. Primary analysis of the EORTC 10041/ BIG 3-04 MINDACT study: a prospective, randomized study evaluating the clinical utility of the 70-gene signature (MammaPrint) combined with common clinical-pathological criteria for selection of patients for adjuvant chemotherapy in breast cancer with 0–3 positive nodes. AACR 2016: CT039.
31. Dubsky P, Filipits M, Jakesz R, et al. Austrian Breast and Colorectal Cancer Study Group (ABCSG). EndoPredict improves the prognostic classification derived from common clinical guidelines in ER-positive, HER2-negative early breast cancer. Ann Oncol. 2013;24(3):640–7.
32. Filipits M, Rudas M, Jakesz R, et al. EP Investigators. A new molecular predictor of distant recurrence in ER-positive, HER2-negative breast cancer adds independent information to conventional clinical risk factors. Clin Cancer Res. 2011;17 (18):6012–20.
33. Dubsky P, Brase JC, Jakesz R, et al. Austrian Breast and Colorectal Cancer Study Group (ABCSG). The EndoPredict score

provides prognostic information on late distant metastases in ER+/HER2− breast cancer patients. Br J Cancer. 2013;109(12): 2959–64.
34. Martin M, Brase JC, Calvo L, et al. Clinical validation of the EndoPredict test in node-positive, chemotherapy-treated ER +/HER2- breast cancer patients: results from the GEICAM 9906 trial. Breast Cancer Res. 2014;16(2):R38.
35. Martin M, Brase JC, Ruiz A, et al. Prognostic ability of EndoPredict compared to research-based versions of the PAM50 risk of recurrence (ROR) scores in node-positive, estrogen receptor-positive, and HER2-negative breast cancer. A GEICAM/9906 sub-study. Breast Cancer Res Treat. 2016;156 (1):81–9.
36. Denkert C, Kronenwett R, Schlake W, et al. Decentral gene expression analysis for ER+/Her2− breast cancer: results of a proficiency testing program for the EndoPredict assay. Virchows Arch. 2012;460(3):251–9.
37. Müller BM, Brase JC, Haufe F, et al. Comparison of the RNA-based EndoPredict multigene test between core biopsies and corresponding surgical breast cancer sections. J Clin Pathol. 2012;65(7):660–2.
38. Wallden B, Storhoff J, Nielsen T, et al. Development and verification of the PAM50-based Prosigna breast cancer gene signature assay. BMC Med Genomics. 2015;22(8):54.
39. Nielsen T, Wallden B, Schaper C, et al. Analytical validation of the PAM50-based Prosigna Breast Cancer Prognostic Gene Signature Assay and nCounter Analysis System using formalin-fixed paraffin-embedded breast tumor specimens. BMC Cancer. 2014;13(14):177.
40. Gnant M, Filipits M, Greil R, et al. Austrian Breast and Colorectal Cancer Study Group. Predicting distant recurrence in receptor-positive breast cancer patients with limited clinicopathological risk: using the PAM50 Risk of Recurrence score in 1478 postmenopausal patients of the ABCSG-8 trial treated with adjuvant endocrine therapy alone. Ann Oncol. 2014;25(2):339–45.
41. Filipits M, Nielsen TO, Rudas M, et al. Austrian Breast and Colorectal Cancer Study Group. The PAM50 risk-of-recurrence score predicts risk for late distant recurrence after endocrine therapy in postmenopausal women with endocrine-responsive early breast cancer. Clin Cancer Res. 2014;20(5):1298–305.
42. Dowsett M, Sestak I, Lopez-Knowles E, Sidhu K, Dunbier AK, Cowens JW, Ferree S, Storhoff J, Schaper C, Cuzick J. Comparison of PAM50 risk of recurrence score with oncotype DX and IHC4 for predicting risk of distant recurrence after endocrine therapy. J Clin Oncol. 2013;31(22):2783–90.
43. Sestak I, Cuzick J, Dowsett M, et al. Prediction of late distant recurrence after 5 years of endocrine treatment: a combined analysis of patients from the Austrian breast and colorectal cancer study group 8 and arimidex, tamoxifen alone or in combination randomized trials using the PAM50 risk of recurrence score. J Clin Oncol. 2015;33(8):916–22.
44. Gnant M, Sestak I, Filipits M, et al. Identifying clinically relevant prognostic subgroups of postmenopausal women with node-positive hormone receptor-positive early-stage breast cancer treated with endocrine therapy: a combined analysis of ABCSG-8 and ATAC using the PAM50 risk of recurrence score and intrinsic subtype. Ann Oncol. 2015;26(8):1685–91.
45. Liu S, Chapman JA, Burnell MJ, et al. Prognostic and predictive investigation of PAM50 intrinsic subtypes in the NCIC CTG MA.21 phase III chemotherapy trial. Breast Cancer Res Treat. 2015;149(2):439–48.
46. Zhang Y, Schnabel CA, Schroeder BE, et al. Breast cancer index identifies early-stage estrogen receptor-positive breast cancer patients at risk for early- and late-distant recurrence. Clin Cancer Res. 2013;19(15):4196–205.
47. Sestak I, Zhang Y, Schroeder BE, et al. Cross stratification and differential risk by breast cancer index and recurrence score in women with hormone receptor positive lymph-node negative early stage breast cancer. Clin Cancer Res. 2016.
48. Sgroi DC, Sestak I, Cuzick J, et al. Prediction of late distant recurrence in patients with oestrogen-receptor-positive breast cancer: a prospective comparison of the breast-cancer index (BCI) assay, 21-gene recurrence score, and IHC4 in the TransATAC study population. Lancet Oncol. 2013;14(11): 1067–76.
49. Habel LA, Sakoda LC, Achacoso N, Ma XJ, Erlander MG, Sgroi DC, Fehrenbacher L, Greenberg D, Quesenberry CP Jr. HOXB13:IL17BR and molecular grade index and risk of breast cancer death among patients with lymph node-negative invasive disease. Breast Cancer Res. 2013;15(2):R24.
50. Sgroi DC, Chapman JA, Badovinac-Crnjevic T, et al. Assessment of the prognostic and predictive utility of the Breast Cancer Index (BCI): an NCIC CTG MA.14 study. Breast Cancer Res. 2016; 18(1):1.
51. Bartlett JM, Bayani J, Marshall A, et al. OPTIMA TMG. Comparing breast cancer multiparameter tests in the OPTIMA prelim trial: no test is more equal than the others. J Natl Cancer Inst. 2016;108(9).
52. Lum DW, Perel P, Hingorani AD, Holmes MV. CYP2D6 genotype and tamoxifen response for breast cancer: a systematic review and meta-analysis. PLoS ONE. 2013;8(10):e76648.
53. Di Leo A, Desmedt C, Bartlett JM, et al. HER2/TOP2A Meta-analysis Study Group. HER2 and TOP2A as predictive markers for anthracycline-containing chemotherapy regimens as adjuvant treatment of breast cancer: a meta-analysis of individual patient data. Lancet Oncol. 2011;12(12):1134–42.
54. Loibl S, Majewski I, Guarneri V, et al. PIK3CA mutations are associated with reduced pathological complete response rates in primary HER2-positive breast cancer: pooled analysis of 967 patients from five prospective trials investigating lapatinib and trastuzumab. Ann Oncol. 2016.
55. André F, Hurvitz S, Fasolo A, et al. Molecular alterations and everolimus efficacy in human epidermal growth Factor receptor 2-overexpressing metastatic breast cancers: combined exploratory biomarker analysis from BOLERO-1 and BOLERO-3. J Clin Oncol. 2016;34(18):2115–24.
56. Zhou Y, Wang C, Zhu H, et al. Diagnostic Accuracy of PIK3CA mutation detection by circulating free DNA in breast cancer: a meta-analysis of diagnostic test accuracy. PLoS ONE. 2016;11(6): e0158143.

Molecular Classification of Breast Cancer

12

Maria Vidal, Laia Paré, and Aleix Prat

Abbreviations

ER	Estrogen receptor
PR	Progesterone receptor
HER2	Human epidermal growth factor 2
IHC	Immunohistochemistry
5NP	5 Negative Profile
TN	Triple-negative
pCR	Pathologic complete response
qRT-PCR	Quantitative reverse transcriptase polymerase chain reaction
CNAs	Copy number aberrations
CDH1	E-cadherin

12.1 Introduction

Breast cancer remains the most common cancer diagnosed in women in Europe and the USA. Screening programs, education, and improved adjuvant treatment have decreased the mortality rates from this disease. However, more than 450,000 estimated deaths due to breast cancer are expected annually worldwide [1]. The most plausible explanation for this scenario is that we lack a complete picture of the biologic heterogeneity of breast cancers. Importantly, this complexity is not fully reflected by the main clinical parameters (such as tumor size, lymph node involvement, histological grade, age) and pathological markers (estrogen receptor [ER], progesterone receptor [PR], and human epidermal growth factor 2 [HER2]), all of which are routinely used in the clinic to stratify patients for prognostic predictions, to select treatments and to include patients in clinical trials.

Gene expression profiling has had a considerable impact on our understanding of breast cancer biology allowing researchers to carry out simultaneous expression of thousands of genes in a single experiment in order to create molecular profiles. During the last 15 years, we and others have identified and extensively characterized 5 intrinsic molecular subtypes of breast cancer (Luminal A, Luminal B, HER2-enriched, basal-like, and claudin-low) and a normal breast-like group [2–6]. In 2000, Perou and colleagues published the first article classifying breast cancer into intrinsic subtypes based on gene expression profiling [2]. Using DNA microarrays from 38 breast cancer cases, 4 molecular subtypes were identified: Luminal, HER2, basal-like, and normal breast. The subsequent expansion of this work in a larger cohort of patients showed that the

M. Vidal · A. Prat (✉)
Medical Oncology, Hospital Clinic of Barcelona, St. Villaroel, 170, Gate stair 2-5 Floor, 08036 Barcelona, Spain
e-mail: aprat@vhio.net; alprat@clinic.ub.es

M. Vidal
e-mail: mjvidal@clinic.cat

L. Paré
Translational Genomics and Targeted Therapeutics in Solid Tumors Lab, August Pi I Sunyer Biomedical Research Institute (IDIBAPS), Rosselló, 149, 1 Floor, Barcelon, Spain
e-mail: lpare@clinic.cat

I. Jatoi and A. Rody (eds.), *Management of Breast Diseases*, DOI 10.1007/978-3-319-46356-8_12

Luminal subgroup could be divided into at least two groups (Luminal A and B) [7].

In 2009, Parker et al. [8] published a clinically applicable gene expression-based predictor, known as PAM50, which was developed using microarray and quantitative reverse transcriptase polymerase chain reaction (qRT-PCR) data from 189 prototypic samples which fell into one of the 4 main intrinsic subtypes: Luminal A, Luminal B, HER2-enriched, basal-like, and normal-like. By comparing global gene expression data from microarray and qRT-PCR, a minimized set of 50 genes was identified that could reliably classify each tumor into one of the intrinsic subtypes with 93 % accuracy. Over the past 7 years, the PAM50 intrinsic subtypes have shown to provide significant prognostic and predictive information beyond standard parameters [9–12]. The PAM50 assay is now clinically implemented worldwide using the nCounter platform [13–19].

A particular result that highlights the importance of intrinsic subtyping in breast cancer comes from one of the most complete molecular characterization studies that has ever been performed in breast cancer. In this study, led by The Cancer Genome Atlas Project (TCGA), more than 500 primary breast cancers were extensively profiled at the DNA (i.e., methylation, chromosomal copy number changes, and somatic and germ line mutations), RNA (i.e., miRNA and mRNA expressions), and protein (i.e., protein and phosphor-protein expression) levels using the most recent technologies [6]. In a particular analysis of over 300 primary tumors [6], 5 different data types (i.e., all except DNA mutations) were combined together in a cluster of clusters in order to identify how many biological homogenous groups of tumors one can identify in breast cancer. The consensus clustering results showed the presence of 4 main entities of breast cancer but, more importantly, these 4 entities were found to be recapitulated very well by the 4 main intrinsic subtypes (Luminal A, Luminal B, HER2-enriched, and basal-like) as defined by mRNA expression only [8]. Overall, these results suggest that intrinsic subtyping captures a great amount of biological diversity that occurs in breast cancer.

12.2 Intrinsic Subtyping Based on Gene Expression Versus Histopathology

To date, numerous studies have evaluated and compared the classification of tumors based on the PAM50 gene expression predictor with the pathology-based surrogate definitions [6, 11, 20–34]. To better understand the concordance between the 2 classification methods, we have combined the data from all of these studies for a total of 5994 independent samples (Fig. 12.1). The vast majority of these studies performed central determination of pathology-based biomarkers, so this needs to be taken into account, since this is not what is currently being done in the clinical setting where each hospital determines these biomarkers. Of note, large discrepancies (~20 %) between local and central determination of ER, PR, Ki67, and HER2 are expected [35–39].

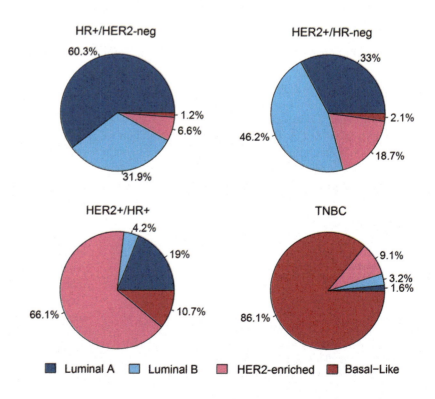

In this combined analysis, the discordance rate between both classifications was found to be present in almost 30.72 % across all patients. Across the IHC-based subtypes,

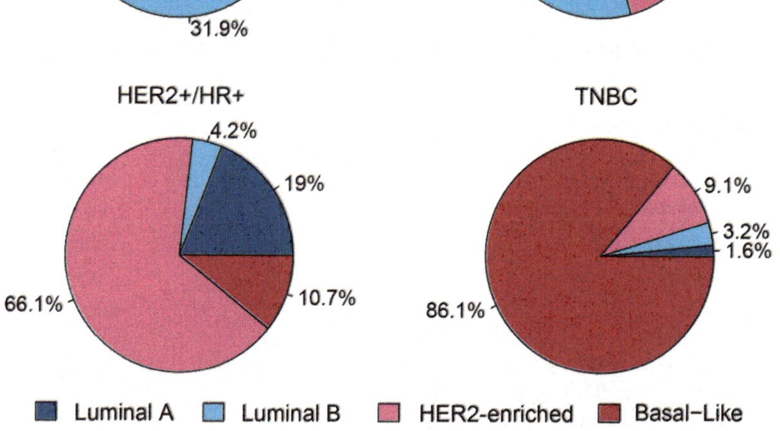

Fig. 12.1 Distribution of the PAM50 intrinsic subtypes within each pathology-based group. The data have been obtained from the different publications. Several studies have performed a standardized version of the PAM50 assay (RT-qPCR-based or nCounter-based) from formalin-fixed paraffin-embedded tumor tissues [11, 22, 25, 27–30], while others have performed the microarray-based version of the PAM50 assay [6, 24, 26, 31–34]

the discordance rate was 37.8, 48.9, 53.8, 33.9, and 13.9 % for the IHC-Luminal A, IHC-Luminal B, IHC-Luminal B/HER2+ (to identify PAM50 Luminal B), HR-/HER2+ (to identify PAM50 HER2-enriched), and triple-negative (to identify PAM50 basal-like) subtypes, respectively. The most likely explanation for these results is that 3 or 4 biomarkers do not fully recapitulate the intrinsic subtypes of breast cancer. In fact, during the development of the clinically applicable PAM50 intrinsic subtype predictor, 50 genes were found to be the minimum number of genes needed to robustly identify the 4 main intrinsic subtypes without compromising its accuracy [4].

The protein expression of Ki-67 has been studied as a potential IHC marker that could distinguish Luminal B from Luminal A subtypes in HR+ breast tumors. In the article published by Cheang et al. [40], 357 breast tumors were profiled and tumor subtypes were assigned using the 50-gene qRT-PCR 'PAM50' subtype predictor. By linking the available immunohistochemical data with the expression profile assignments, the authors identified 84 and 60 H+/HER2− tumors as Luminal A and B, respectively. Thus, the Luminal A subtype was defined as being HR+/HER2− and low for Ki-67, and the Luminal B subtype as being HR+/HER2− and high for Ki-67 or HR+/HER2+. Further validation of this surrogate IHC panel in an independent population-based cohort of 4046 tumors demonstrated the prognostic value of this Luminal B IHC definition within homogeneously treated patient subsets. However, we must keep in mind that although the HR+/HER2 −/Ki67-high/low IHC panel will distinguish the majority of Luminal B from A tumors, this definition does not identify all the tumors within the Luminal B expression-defined subtype since up to 20 and 7 % of Luminal B tumors are clinically ER +/HER2+ and ER−/HER2−, respectively.

12.3 Main Molecular Features of the Intrinsic Subtypes

12.3.1 Luminal Disease

At the RNA and protein level, Luminal A and B subtypes are largely distinguished by the expression of two main biological processes: proliferation/cell cycle-related pathways and luminal/hormone-regulated pathways (Fig. 12.2).

The Luminal A breast cancer is the most common subtype, representing 50–60 % of the total. It is characterized by the expression of genes activated by the ER transcription factor that are typically expressed in the luminal epithelium lining the mammary ducts. It also presents a low expression of genes related to cell proliferation [41]. The Luminal A immunohistochemistry (IHC) profile is characterized by the expression of ER, PGR, Bcl-2, and cytokeratin CK8/18, an absence of HER2 expression, a low rate of proliferation measured by Ki67, and a low histological grade. Moreover, the GATA3 marker expresses its highest level in the Luminal A subgroup.

Compared to Luminal A tumors, Luminal B tumors have higher expression of proliferation/cell cycle-related genes or proteins (e.g., MKI67 and AURKA) and lower expression of several luminal-related genes or proteins such as the PR [42] and FOXA1, but not the ER [30], which is found similarly expressed between the two luminal subtypes and can only help distinguish luminal from non-luminal disease. At the DNA level, Luminal A tumors show a lower number of somatic mutations across the genome, lower number of chromosomal copy number changes (e.g., lower rates of CCND1 amplification), less TP53 mutations (12 % vs. 29 %), similar GATA3 mutations (14 % vs. 15 %), and more PIK3CA (45 % vs. 29 %) and MAP3K1 mutations (13 % vs. 5 %) compared to Luminal B tumors [6] (Table 12.1). Interestingly, a subgroup of Luminal B tumors is found hypermethylated, and a subgroup of Luminal A (6.3–7.8 %) and Luminal B (16.4–20.8 %) tumors show HER2-amplification/overexpression.

Within HR+/HER2-negative breast cancer, 90–95 % of tumors fall into the Luminal A and B subtypes. In early breast cancer, Luminal B disease has worse baseline distant recurrence-free survival at 5 and 10 years regardless of adjuvant systemic therapy compared to Luminal A disease (Fig. 12.3). Regarding prognosis, the Luminal A subtype has shown repeatedly to have a better outcome than the rest of subtypes across many datasets of patients with early breast cancer, including 6 phase III clinical trials (i.e., CALGB9741 [43], GEICAM9906 [44], TransATAC [11], ABCSG08, MA.5 [45], and MA.12 [25] trials) coming from different countries and populations and with different adjuvant systemic therapies (i.e., endocrine-only, chemotherapy-only, and both).

Of note, the vast majority of these studies with long-term follow-up show that the survival curves of Luminal B tumors cross the survival curves of basal-like disease at around ~10 years of follow-up. Thus, although at 5 years of follow-up, basal-like disease had a worse outcome than Luminal B tumors, and this is not the case at 10 years. This result suggests that we should focus on finding additional therapies for Luminal B disease since this tumor subtype is very frequent (i.e., represent ~30–40 % of all breast cancer diagnoses), and chemotherapy and endocrine therapies are not enough for the majority of these patients.

Apart from predicting baseline prognosis, the Luminal A vs B classification, together with tumor size and nodal status, predicts the residual risk of recurring at a distant site within the 5–10 years of follow-up (the so-called late recurrence)

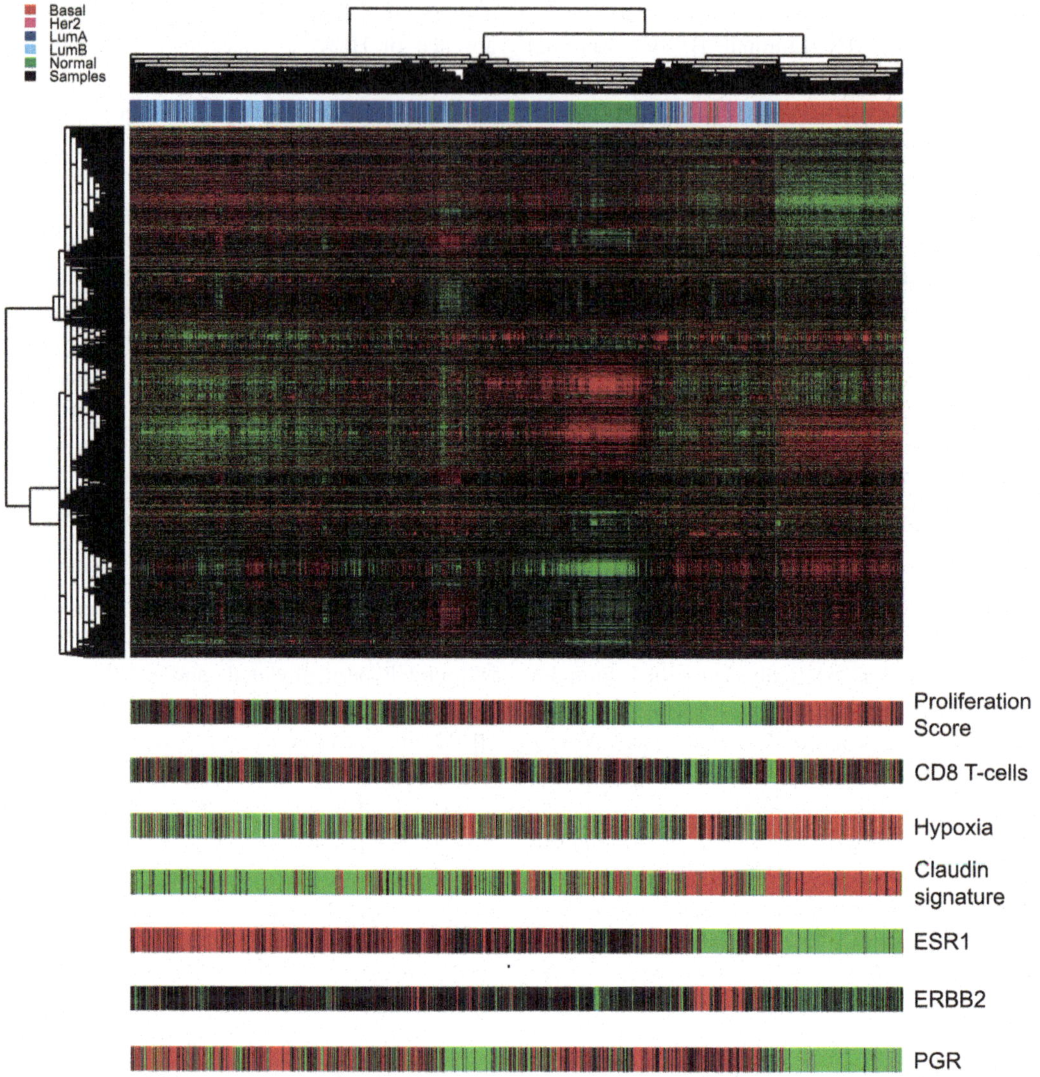

Fig. 12.2 Intrinsic subtype identification using the PAM50 subtype predictor. PAM50 unsupervised gene expression heatmap of 1197 breast cancer samples profiled at the TCGA download portal. The subtype calls of each sample are shown below the array tree. Each *square* represents the relative transcript abundance

Table 12.1 More frequently mutated genes in 3303 primary breast cancers

Gene	Frequency
PIK3CA	32.4
TP53	30.5
CDH1	11.2
GATA3	9.9
MAP3KI	7.1
KMT2C	7
MUC12	5.5
MUC4	5.4
FLG	4.6
SYNE1	4.4

Source Data from TCGA, [110–112]

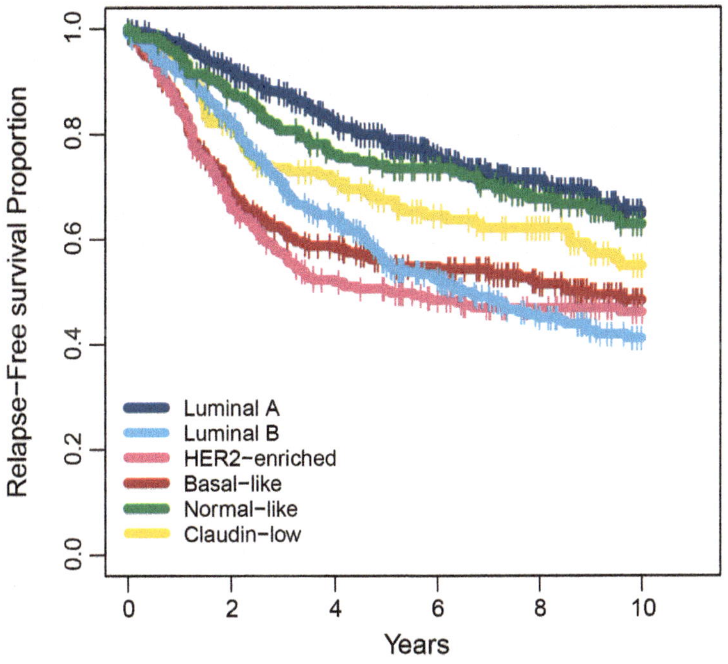

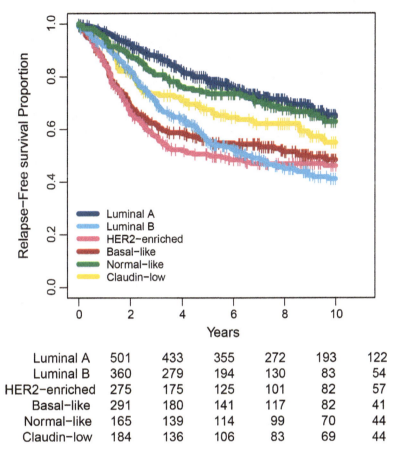

Luminal A	501	433	355	272	193	122
Luminal B	360	279	194	130	83	54
HER2–enriched	275	175	125	101	82	57
Basal–like	291	180	141	117	82	41
Normal–like	165	139	114	99	70	44
Claudin–low	184	136	106	83	69	44

Fig. 12.3 Kaplan–Meier curves of relapse-free survival based on intrinsic subtype in 2629 patients from a combined cohort (GSE12276 [113], GSE18229 [5], GSE18864 [114], GSE2034 [115, 116], GSE22219 [117], GSE25066 [118, 119], GSE2603 [120], GSE2990 [121], GSE4922 [122, 123], GSE7390 [124], and GSE7849 [125]) of breast cancer patients. *Dark blue*, Luminal A; *light blue*, Luminal B; *red*, basal-like; *pink*, HER2-enriched; *yellow*, claudin-low

[46–48], suggesting that intrinsic subtype has the ability to inform decisions concerning the length of endocrine therapy (i.e., 5 vs. 10 years), being the low-risk Luminal A tumors with low tumor burden (e.g., tumor size 1 cm and node-negative) the group were 5 years of endocrine therapy might be sufficient.

Most of the direct evidence of general chemosensitivity of the Luminal A and B subtypes comes from the neoadjuvant setting. For example, in a cohort of 208 patients with luminal disease treated with anthracycline/taxane-based chemotherapy and with pathologic complete response (pCR) data, the pCR rates in patients with the Luminal A and B subtypes were 3 and 16 % (odds ratio = 6.01, p-value = 0.003), respectively [4, 49–52]. Overall, these data suggest that among the 2 luminal subtypes, the Luminal A tumors are less chemosensitive than Luminal B tumors. This hypothesis is further sustained by the fact that pCR is not predictive of survival outcome in IHC-Luminal A tumors [51] and in patients with HR+/HER2−/low-grade [53], but it is predictive of outcome in IHC-Luminal B/HER2-negative [51] and in HR+/HER2−/high-grade [53]. Further studies are needed to determine whether Luminal A tumors benefit from chemotherapy or specific chemotherapeutic agents/regimens or even CDK4/6 inhibitors. This answer would be especially relevant in the clinic for those patients with Luminal A tumors with high tumor burden (intermediate or high risk).

Regarding the benefit from endocrine therapy, both tumor subtypes have shown to derive a similar relative benefit by looking at the proportional fall in the proliferation marker Ki67 upon treatment with an aromatase inhibitor in the neoadjuvant setting [24]. However, since Luminal A tumors have a lower baseline proliferation status than Luminal B tumors, a larger proportion can achieve low post-treatment values.

12.3.2 HER2-Enriched

The HER2-enriched subtype is characterized at the RNA and protein level by the high expression of HER2-related and proliferation-related genes and proteins (e.g., ERBB2/HER2 and GRB7), intermediate expression of luminal-related genes and proteins (e.g., ESR1 and PGR), and low expression of basal-related genes and proteins (e.g., keratin 5 and FOXC1). At the DNA level, these tumors show the highest number of mutations across the genome, and 72 and 39 % of HER2-enriched tumors are TP53- and PIK3CA-mutated, respectively (Table 12.2). Although the majority (68 %) of HER2-enriched tumors have ERBB2/HER2 overexpression/amplification, we should expect to identify the HER2-enriched subtype within HER2-negative disease. Interestingly, the HER2-enriched subtype has been found uniquely enriched for tumors with high frequency of APOBEC3B-associated mutations [54]. APOBEC3B is subclass of APOBEC cytidine deaminases, which convert cytosine to uracil and has been implicated as a source of mutations in many cancer types [55].

Similar to the other pathology-based groups, all the intrinsic molecular subtypes can be identified within clinically HER2-positive disease albeit with different proportions. In our combined analysis of 831 HER2+ tumors (Fig. 12.1), 44.6, 26.8, 17.6, and 11.0 % were identified as HER2-enriched, Luminal B, Luminal A, and basal-like.

From a biological perspective, a particular unanswered question was how different is an intrinsic subtype based on HER2 status. For example, how different is HER2+/Luminal A disease from a classical HER2-negative/Luminal A disease? We recently approached this question by interrogating The Cancer Genome Atlas (n = 495) and Molecular Taxonomy of Breast Cancer International Consortium (METABRIC) datasets (n = 1730) of primary breast cancers for molecular data derived from DNA, RNA, and protein, and determined intrinsic subtype. Within each subtype, only 0.3–3.9 % of genes were found differentially expressed between HER2+ and HER2-negative tumors. As expected, the vast majority of differentially expressed genes originated in the 17q12 DNA amplicon where the ERBB2 gene is located. Within HER2+ tumors, HER2 gene and protein expression were statistically significantly higher in the HER2-enriched subtype than either luminal subtype. Thus, this result suggests that intrinsic subtype dominates the biological phenotype within HER2+ and HER2-negative disease.

Two large studies have evaluated the prognostic value of HR status (i.e., a surrogate manner of looking at luminal vs

Table 12.2 Highlights of genomic, clinical, and proteomic features of the intrinsic subtypes

Subtype	Luminal A	Luminal B	Basal-like	HER2E
$ER^+/HER2^-$ (%)	87	82	10	20
$HER2^+$ (%)	7	15	2	68
TNBCs (%)	2	1	80	9
TP53 pathway	*TP53* mut (12 %); gain of *MDM2* (14 %)	*TP53* mut (32 %); gain of *MDM2* (31 %)	*TP53* mut (84 %); gain of *MDM2* (14 %)	*TP53* mut (75 %); gain of *MDM2* (30 %)
PIK3CA/PTEN pathway	*PIK3CA* mut (49 %); *PTEN* mut/loss (13 %); *INPP4B* loss (9 %)	PIK3CA mut (32 %) PTEN mut/loss (24 %) INPP4B loss (16 %)	PIK3CA mut (7 %); PTEN mut/loss (35 %); INPP4B loss (30 %)	PIK3CA mut (42 %); PTEN mut/loss (19 %); INPP4B loss (30 %)
RB1 pathway	Cyclin D1 amp (29 %); *CDK4* gain (14 %); low expression of *CDKN2C*; high expression of *RB1*	Cyclin D1 amp (58 %); *CDK4* gain (25 %)	*RB1* mut/loss (20 %); cyclin E1 amp (9 %); high expression of *CDKN2A*; low expression of *RB1*	Cyclin D1 amp (38 %); *CDK4* gain (24 %)
mRNA expression	High ER cluster; low proliferation	Lower ER cluster; high proliferation	Basal signature; high proliferation	HER2 amplicon signature; high proliferation
Copy number	Most diploid; many with quiet genomes; 1q, 8q, 8p11 gain; 8p, 16q loss; 11q13.3 amp (24 %)	Most aneuploid; many with focal amp; 1q, 8q, 8p11 gain; 8p, 16q loss; 11q13.3 amp (51 %); 8p11.23 amp (28 %)	Most aneuploid; high genomic instability; 1q, 10p gain; 8p, 5q loss; *MYC* focal gain (40 %)	Most aneuploid; high genomic instability; 1q, 8q gain; 8p loss; 17q12 focal *ERRB2* amp (71 %)
DNA mutations	*PIK3CA* (49 %); *TP53* (12 %); *GATA3* (14 %); *MAP3K1* (14 %)	*TP53* (32 %); *PIK3CA* (32 %); *MAP3K1* (5 %)	*TP53* (84 %); *PIK3CA* (7 %)	*TP53* (75 %); *PIK3CA* (42 %); *PIK3R1* (8 %)
DNA methylation	–	Hypermethylated phenotype for subset	Hypomethylated	–
Protein expression	High estrogen signaling; high MYB; RPPA reactive subtypes	Less estrogen signaling; high FOXM1 and MYC; RPPA reactive subtypes	High expression of DNA repair proteins, PTEN and INPP4B loss signature (pAKT)	High protein and phospho-protein expression of EGFR and HER2

Source Reprinted by permission from Macmillan Publishers Ltd: Nature [93], copyright 2012
Percentages are based on 466 tumor overlap list. *Amp* Amplification; *mut* Mutation

non-luminal disease) within HER2+ breast cancer [56, 57]. In the 4 year follow-up of the N9831 and National Surgical Adjuvant Breast and Bowel Project B-31 adjuvant trials of trastuzumab in HER2 + disease (n = 4045), HR-positive disease was found statistically significantly associated with approximately 40 % increased disease-free survival and overall survival, compared to hormone receptor-negative disease [38]. This association of hormone receptor status with survival was found to be independent of the main clinical–pathological variables, including trastuzumab administration. Similar results were observed in a prospective cohort study of 3394 patients with stage I to III HER2+ breast cancer from National Comprehensive Cancer Network centers [57]. In both studies, HR-negative disease experienced more cancer relapse in the first 5 years than HR-positive [57]. Interestingly, patients with HR-negative tumors were less likely to experience first recurrence in bone and more likely to recur in brain, compared to patients with hormone receptor-positive tumors [57]. Better outcomes independently of treatment in the HR-positive group compared to the HR-negative have also been observed in the NeoALTTO [58] and ALTTO [59] clinical trials.

Regarding intrinsic subtyping, we have recently evaluated the prognostic value of these entities in a large retrospective cohort of 1730 patients from the UK and Canada with and without HER2+ disease treated in the adjuvant setting with different treatments except trastuzumab [32]. The results revealed that intrinsic subtypes are an independent prognostic variable beyond tumor size and nodal status, and HER2+/Luminal A tumors showed a similar outcome compared to HER2-negative/Luminal A tumors [31]. Overall, these data suggest that Luminal A disease could be used, in the future, together with tumor size and nodal status, to help better identify those patients with a low risk of relapsing and thus safely treated with less intense chemotherapy such as the adjuvant regimen paclitaxel and trastuzumab recently proposed for "small" (i.e., <3.0 cm) and node-negative HER2+ breast cancer [60].

The intrinsic subtypes might be to help identify those patients with HER2+ early breast cancer that might be successfully treated with dual HER2 blockade (+/− endocrine therapy) but without chemotherapy since their tumors are exquisitely sensitive to anti-HER2 therapy. Interestingly, in a recently reported neoadjuvant study, the TBCRC023, comparing 12-week versus 24-week lapatinib + trastuzumab treatment (and endocrine therapy if HR+), the pCR rate in the HR+ tumors was 33.2 %, suggesting that longer treatment in HR+ tumors might reach similar pCR rates as chemotherapy plus two anti-HER2 agents [61]. However, no data on intrinsic subtype are available to date from these studies. Based on the prior knowledge, one can speculate that regardless of HR status, the HER2-enriched subtype enriches for the identification of patients that are more likely to achieve a pCR with dual HER2 blockade without chemotherapy. We are currently testing this hypothesis in a prospective neoadjuvant clinical trial called PAMELA (NCT01973660), which is similar to TBCRC006 and TBCRC023 trials, but the treatment lasts for 18 weeks.

12.3.3 Basal-Like

The basal-like subtype is characterized at the RNA and protein level by the high expression of proliferation-related genes (e.g., MKI67) and keratins typically expressed by the basal layer of the skin (e.g., keratins 5, 14, and 17), intermediate expression of HER2-related genes, and very low expression of luminal-related genes. At the DNA level, these tumors show the second highest number of mutations across the genome, mostly hypomethylated, and 80 and 9 % of basal-like tumors are TP53- and PIK3CA-mutated, respectively. BRCA1-mutated breast cancer is associated with basal-like disease [62, 63]. Finally, ERBB2/HER2 overexpression/amplification is found in 2.1–17.4 % of tumors with a basal-like profile.

Previous studies (including our own) have tried to define basal-like carcinomas based on immunohistochemical (IHC) surrogate profiles. For example, EGFR and keratins 5/6 (CK5/6) have been proposed as positive IHC markers on top of the ER-PR-HER2-definition (the "five-marker method," also known as the Core Basal group). This definition has previously been shown to identify basal-like tumors versus microarray-based classifications with 76 % sensitivity and 100 % specificity [29]. Furthermore, in a series of 4046 breast tumors [64], 17 % (639 of 3744) were defined as the triple-negative (TN), whereas 9.0 % were basal-like by the five-marker core basal definition. Interestingly, when the triple-negative group was segregated into core basal and the "5 Negative Profile" (5NP), the Core Basal group showed a significantly worse outcome compared to the 5NP group.

12.3.3.1 Basal-Like Classification: Biological and Epidemiological Implications

The TCGA comprehensive molecular characterization of breast cancer confirmed that among all the intrinsic subtypes, the basal-like is the most distinct [6]. This observation fits with previous molecular studies and with clinical data that show that triple-negative breast cancer tends to affect young women, is associated with BRCA1 mutations, and is a highly aggressive disease [65]. However, how different is basal-like disease from the rest of breast cancer subtypes?

Two recent studies have addressed this question from a biological perspective [66, 67]. In the first one, we evaluated global microarray-based gene expression profiles of a combined dataset composed of 6 different cancer types obtained from the TCGA project and that included 542 primary breast cancers [66]. The unsupervised results revealed that a subgroup of breast cancers, virtually all basal-like by PAM50, should be considered a molecular entity by itself just like ovarian or colorectal cancer, and that >70 % of basal-like breast cancers were more similar to squamous cell lung cancer than to Luminal A or B disease [66]. In the second study, the panCancer TCGA study group combined all the available molecular data (except mutations) across 12 cancer types, including 845 primary breast cancers [67]. Unsupervised classification using all data types revealed a similar finding as the previous study, namely that basal-like breast cancer is a unique entity and much different from the rest of breast tumors. Interestingly, the other cancer type that showed such a large biological heterogeneity was bladder cancer which could be reclassified into 3 distinct molecular entities, one being similar to the basal-like breast cancer subtype [67].

Despite in vivo preclinical data suggesting that breast cancer disease arises from the transformation of a common luminal progenitor [68–70], this biological result with human tumors strongly suggest that 2 very different cell types of origin exist in the mammary gland; one whose transformation gives rise to basal-like disease and another one whose transformation gives rise to non-basal-like disease.

An example is work by Millikan et al. [71] looking at risk factors of breast cancer in a population-based, case–control study of African-American, and white women. The results revealed that Luminal A disease exhibits risk factors typically reported as protective for the development of breast cancer, including increased parity and younger age at first full-term pregnancy; on the other hand, basal-like cases exhibits several associations that were opposite to those observed for Luminal A, including increased risk for parity and younger age at first term full-term pregnancy [71]. Moreover, longer duration breastfeeding, increasing number of children breastfed, and increasing number of months breastfeeding per child were each associated with reduced risk of basal-like breast cancer, but not Luminal A [71]. Overall, these data suggest that we should clearly separate these two entities when we talk about breast cancer.

Within HR+/HER2-negative early disease, it is expected to identify a subpopulation of non-luminal subtypes (i.e., HER2-enriched and basal-like) by gene expression (Fig. 12.1). Basal-like tumors represent around ~ 1 %. Based on the molecular features of these two non-luminal subtypes, one would expect to identify these tumors in patients with tumors that express low ER. In fact, a study performed intrinsic subtyping in 25 tumor samples with 1–9 % ER-positive tumor cells and found that 80 % were non-luminal (48 % basal-like and 32 % HER2-enriched) [72]. On the other hand, a combined analysis of 48 borderline cases (1–10 % ER+ tumor cells) from the MA.5, MA.12, and GEICAM9906 revealed that 46.0 % were non-luminal (29 % HER2-enriched and 17 % basal-like) [73]. Moreover, HER2-enriched and basal-like tumors can still be identified in tumors that have very high expression of ER as exemplified by the 6 non-luminal tumors (representing 2.9 % of the entire cohort) identified in the Z1031 trial where patients' tumors were all Allred ER score of 6–8.

In terms of survival outcome, we evaluated the prognostic value of the intrinsic subtypes in a cohort of 1380 patients with ER+/HER2-unknown early breast cancer treated with 5 years of adjuvant tamoxifen-only across several retrospective studies [74]. Non-luminal subtypes represented 9 % (7 % HER2-enriched and 2 % basal-like) of the samples, and each non-luminal subtype showed a significant worse outcome compared to Luminal A subtype in both node-negative and node-positive disease.

In the past, we have used the word TN and basal-like interchangeably. However, within TN disease, all the intrinsic molecular subtypes can be identified, although the vast majority fall into the basal-like subtype (86 %; range 56–95 %, depending on the study). In our combined analysis of 868 TN tumors, 86.1, 9.1, 3.2, and 1.6 % were identified as basal-like, HER2-enriched, Luminal B, and Luminal A, respectively. Although the correlation between pathological and gene expression profiling is moderate, this pathology-based subset is the one with the greatest consistency between both classifications. Of note, we did not evaluate the presence of the claudin-low subtype [5].

At the same time, other gene expression-based classifications of TN disease have emerged over the years. For example, Lehmann and colleagues described 6 molecular subtypes of TN breast cancer: two basal-like (BL1 and BL2), an immunomodulatory (IM), a mesenchymal (M), a mesenchymal stem-like (MSL), and a luminal androgen receptor subtype (LAR) [75, 76]. As expected, Lehmann's classification identified most TN tumors as basal-like (80.6 %) [76] and, with the exception of LAR group, all other subtypes were mostly identified as basal-like by PAM50 (BL1 99 %, BL2 95 %, IM 84 %, M 97 %, MSL 50 %). Interestingly, the LAR subtype was predominantly identified as either HER2-enriched (74 %) or Luminal B (14 %). In another recent study, Burstein et al. [77] classified TN disease into 4 main groups: LAR, mesenchymal (MES), basal-like immune-suppressed (BLIS), and basal-like immune-activated (BLIA). Again, most PAM50 non-basal-like tumors were identified as LAR by this classification, and most PAM50 basal-like were BLIS and BLIA. Thus, we can conclude that TN disease is biologically heterogeneous and that although basal-like disease predominates (+/− immune activation and/or infiltration), there is a small group of non-basal-like tumors (mostly LARs, or HER2-enriched) [23, 78]. These TN tumors with a non-basal-like or LAR profile might benefit from androgen receptor inhibition.

No data are available regarding the prognostic impact of the intrinsic molecular subtypes defined by PAM50 within TN disease. Regarding the Lehmann's classification, the 7 subtypes have been evaluated retrospectively in several publicly available cohorts of TN disease treated with different adjuvant therapies [75, 76, 78]. Although no clear results were obtained, several tendencies were observed in both studies. For example, the M group showed the worse outcome and the IM group showed a relatively better outcome. Regarding the LAR group, one study showed a worse outcome and another one a tendency for the best outcome. In Burstein et al. [77], the only group that showed a different outcome from the rest was the BLIA, which is consistent with the known prognostic impact of immune infiltration in TN disease [79–81]. However, the BLIA group, or the basal-like with immune infiltration, has a high risk of relapsing (~20 %). Thus, these data suggest that subtyping within TN will not have a clinical impact based on prognosis-only since no group has such an outstanding.

12.3.4 Claudin-Low

In 2007, Herschkowitz et al. [82] analyzed 232 human breast samples by semi-unsupervised hierarchical clustering and compared their gene expression profiles versus 108 mammary tumors from multiple genetically engineered mouse models. In this report, a potential new intrinsic subtype, apparent in both mouse and human datasets, was identified; this 'claudin-low' subtype was characterized by the low expression of genes involved in tight junctions and cell–cell adhesion. Interestingly, most of the defining characteristics of the claudin-low human tumors were conserved in several mouse models including 3 models with engineered BRCA1 and/or p53 deficiencies.

After, we have reported a more comprehensive characterization of this rare intrinsic subtype [5]. Hierarchical clustering analysis of 320 human breast tumors and 17 normal breast samples using a 1900 gene intrinsic list [8] places the claudin-low group next to the basal-like subtype, indicating that both tumor types share some gene expression features. These shared features include low expression of the HER2 and the luminal gene clusters, as well as the genes HER2, ESR1, GATA3, and the luminal keratins 8 and 18. However, two intrinsic gene clusters are uniquely expressed (or not expressed) in the claudin-low subtype. One of these clusters is enriched with cell–cell adhesion proteins and is found to show low expression within claudin-low tumors. Among the 20 genes that compose this cluster are claudin 3, 4, 7, cingulin, and occludin that are involved in tight junctions, and E-cadherin that is a calcium-dependent cell adhesion protein. Conversely, the other cluster, which is composed of 40 genes, is highly enriched with immune system response genes and is highly expressed in claudin-low samples. Many of these genes are known to be expressed by T- and B-lymphoid cells (i.e., CD4 and CD79a), indicating high immune cell infiltration in this tumor subtype. However, the origin of other immune-related genes highly expressed in claudin-low tumors, such as interleukin 6 or CXCL2 might be produced by the actual tumor cells, or immune cells, or both.

Clinically, the majority of claudin-low tumors are poor prognosis ER-negative (ER−), PR-negative (PR−), and HER2-negative (HER2−) (i.e., triple-negative) invasive ductal carcinomas with a high frequency of metaplastic and medullary differentiation. Preliminary data show that they have a response rate to standard neoadjuvant chemotherapy that is intermediate between basal-like and luminal tumors [5]. Furthermore, claudin-low tumors are enriched with unique biologic properties linked to mammary stem cells (MaSCs) [83], a Core EMT signature [84], and show features of tumor-initiating cells (TICs, also known as cancer stem cells [CSCs]) [85, 86], the study of which is leading to the formulation of new hypothesis regarding the "cell of origin" of the different subtypes of breast cancers.

No differences in survival were observed between claudin-low tumors and other poor prognosis subtypes (Luminal B, HER2-enriched, and basal-like), or even between claudin-low tumors versus all other tumors combined.

Metaplastic and medullary carcinomas have also been linked with the claudin-low profile [3, 86]. These two special histological types represent less than 5–7 % of all breast cancer diagnoses and generally are poorly differentiated triple-negative tumors. However, while metaplastic carcinomas are associated with poor prognosis and treatment resistance [87], medullary carcinomas tend to show good outcomes despite their aggressive pathological features [88].

In a combined dataset of 400 tumors/patients (UNC337 [5] and MDACC133 [89], 49 % of TN tumors were basal-like, 30 % claudin-low, 9 % HER2-enriched, 6 % Luminal B, 5 % Luminal A, and 1 % normal breast-like; if the claudin-low classification is ignored, then 72 % of triple-negative tumors are basal-like. Conversely, 6–29 % [7, 90] and 9–13 % of basal-like tumors are ER+ or HER2+, respectively. Thus, the triple-negative surrogate for basal-like makes both kinds of mistakes in that it includes samples that are not basal-like and it fails to identify a significant number of basal-like tumors.

Overall, claudin-low tumors are the least frequent subtype (prevalence 12–14 %) and are mostly high-grade and ER−/PR−/HER2− (i.e., triple-negative) tumors similar to the basal-like subtype, which is concordant with the low expression of the luminal and HER2 intrinsic gene clusters observed in both tumor types. However, it is important to note that 15–25 % of claudin-low tumors are hormonal receptor-positive (HR+) and 10 % of basal-like tumors are also HR+.

12.4 Novel Subgroups of Breast Cancer

In 2012, Curtis et al [91.] proposed a new molecular classification of breast cancer based on the combination of two different genomic views derived from primary fresh-frozen tissue from 2000 women with breast cancer from the METABRIC cohort. The authors presented an integrated analysis of copy number changes and gene expression in a discovery and validation set of 997 and 995 primary breast tumors, respectively, with long-term clinical follow-up. The results revealed a total of 10 different subtypes [92]:

Integrative cluster (IntClust) 1 is constituted by ER-positive tumors, predominantly classified into the Luminal B intrinsic subtype. The subgroup typically has an intermediate prognosis, similar to that of IntClust 6 and 9. All encompass a high proportion of higher proliferation ER+/Luminal B tumors and are characterized by relatively high levels of genomic instability. The defining molecular feature of IntClust 1 is amplification of the 17q23 locus. IntClust 1 also has the highest prevalence of *GATA3* mutations across all of the 10 clusters.

Integrative cluster 2 is comprised of ER-positive tumors and includes both Luminal A and Luminal B tumors. Remarkably, this subgroup is associated with the worst prognosis of all ER-positive tumors with a 10-year disease-specific survival rate of only around 50 %. The defining molecular feature of this subtype is amplification of 11q13/14.

Integrative cluster 3 is composed primarily of Luminal A cases and is enriched for histopathological subtypes that have a good prognosis such as invasive lobular and tubular carcinomas. At the molecular level, the subtype is characterized by low genomic instability, a very low prevalence of *TP53* mutations, and a paucity of copy number and *cis*-acting alterations. However, of note, tumors within this subtype have the highest frequency of *PIK3CA*, *CDH1*, and *RUNX1* mutations. Importantly, the subgroup is associated with the best prognosis of all the 10 integrative clusters with a 10-year disease-specific survival of around 90 %.

Integrative cluster 4 is a unique cluster incorporating both ER-positive (n = 238/343) and ER-negative (n = 105/343) cases, including 26 % of all triple-negative tumors, and a mixture of intrinsic subtypes including basal-like cases. Importantly, the subtype is associated with favorable outcome and a 10-year disease-specific survival of around 80 %. Similarly to IntClust 3, IntClust4, the largest subtype of breast cancer (up to 17 % of cases), is characterized molecularly by low levels of genomic instability and a "CNA-devoid" flat copy number landscape. Many of the tumors within this subgroup show evidence of extensive lymphocytic infiltration, and the observed deletions are the consequences of the somatic TCR rearrangement present in the infiltrating T cells.

Integrative cluster 5 encompasses the ERBB2-amplified cancers composed of both HER2-enriched ER-negative (58 %) and luminal ER-positive cases (42 %). Women in the METABRIC study were enrolled before the general availability of trastuzumab, and as expected, this group demonstrated the worst disease-specific survival at 10 years of around 45 %. In addition to specific ERBB2 amplification at 17q12, these tumors demonstrate intermediate levels of genomic instability and a high proportion of *TP53* mutations (in >60 % cases).

Integrative cluster 6 represents a distinct subgroup of ER-positive tumors, comprising both Luminal A and Luminal B cases. Clinically, this cluster shows an intermediate prognosis and a 10-year disease-specific survival of around 60 %. Molecularly, this subtype is characterized by specific amplification of the 8p12 locus and high levels of genomic instability. Notably, tumors within this cluster demonstrate the lowest levels of *PIK3CA* mutations across all of the ER-positive cancers.

Integrative cluster 7 is comprised predominately of ER-positive Luminal A tumors and identifies a good prognostic subgroup with 10-year disease-specific survival rates of around 80 %. It is characterized by intermediate levels of genomic instability, specific 16p gain, and 16q loss, as well as a higher frequency of 8q amplification.

Integrative cluster 8 shares similarities with IntClust7 and encompasses ER-positive tumors predominately of the Luminal A intrinsic subtype with a good prognosis. This subgroup, however, is characterized molecularly by the classical 1q gain/16q loss event. Furthermore, tumors within IntClust 8 demonstrate high levels of *PIK3CA*, *GATA3*, and *MAP2K4* mutations.

Integrative cluster 9 is comprised of a mixture of intrinsic subtypes but includes a large number of ER-positive cases of the Luminal B subgroup. IntClust 9 shows an intermediate prognosis with a 10-year disease-specific survival of around 60 %. This cluster is characterized by high levels of genomic instability and the highest level of *TP53* mutations among the ER-positive subtypes.

Integrative cluster 10 incorporates mostly triple-negative tumors (n = 190/320 classify into this cluster) from the core basal-like intrinsic subtype. Although the subtype represents a high-risk group in the first 5 years after diagnosis, beyond 5 years the prognosis for this subgroup is relatively good. These breast cancers have the highest rates of *TP53* mutations despite displaying only intermediate levels of genomic instability.

12.5 Intrinsic Subtypes in the Metastatic Setting

A better understanding of the biological changes occurring during metastatic progression of breast cancer is needed to identify new biomarkers, targets, and novel treatment strategies. Although the TCGA results provide a valuable landmark of genomic/genetic information, a critical point is that the TCGA analyses were performed in non-treated primary breast tumors and not in post-treated, resistant, or metastatic tumors. This is important as recent studies that are starting to characterize resistant or metastatic tumors are identifying frequent genomic alterations that were found to be rare in the TCGA dataset [93].

One example is the molecular alterations in the ER gene [94] (i.e., somatic mutations, gene amplifications, or gene fusions), which are found in ~20 % of metastatic luminal tumors, and which we (in collaboration with Washington Univ. St. Louis, USA) and others have shown that they might play an important role in the development of endocrine resistance [95, 96]. Recent studies have identified mutations in *ESR1* affecting the ligand-binding domain (LBD) of the ER-α protein [97]. In preclinical models, mutant receptors drive ER-dependent transcription and proliferation in the absence of estrogen and reduce the efficacy of ER antagonists, suggesting that LBD-mutant forms of the ER are involved in mediating clinical resistance to endocrine therapy and that more potent ER antagonists may be of substantial therapeutic benefit.

Regarding the intrinsic changes from primary to metastatic tumors, our data obtained after comparing expression changes of a set of 105 genes between 30 paired luminal primary and metastatic tumors in the CONVERTHER trial [98] suggest that a potential driver of treatment resistance and aggressiveness in luminal disease (i.e., high proliferation) is the fibroblast growth factor receptor 4 (FGFR4), a tyrosine kinase cell surface receptor, which we have found to be highly upregulated in metastatic tumor samples. Interestingly, upregulation of this gene is a main feature of the HER2-enriched subtype [99], a subtype known to have high RAS-/MAPK-pathway signaling and be endocrine-resistant [26]. Interestingly, many Luminal A and B metastatic samples have a FGFR4 expression above the mean expression of this gene in primary HER2-enriched tumors. In contrast, ERBB2 expression was not found upregulated in metastatic luminal disease. Our results showed that intrinsic subtype is mostly maintained during metastatic progression, except primary Luminal A disease which becomes non-Luminal A in the majority of the cases.

Recently, we published [100] an unplanned retrospective analysis of 821 tumor samples (85.7 % primary and 14.3 % metastatic) from the EFG30008 phase III trial[101] in which postmenopausal women with HR-positive invasive breast cancer and no prior therapy for advanced or metastatic disease were randomized to letrozole with or without lapatinib. In this retrospective study, we showed that intrinsic subtype is the strongest prognostic factor independently associated with progression-free survival and overall survival in all patients, being the first study to reveal an association between intrinsic subtype and outcome in first-line HR-positive metastatic breast cancer. The clinical value of intrinsic subtyping in HR-positive metastatic breast cancer warrants further investigation.

12.6 Frequently Mutated Genes in Breast Cancer

In estrogen receptor-positive (ER+) breast cancer, mutations in PIK3CA represent the most common genetic events, occurring at a frequency of 30–50 %. As we can see in Table 12.1, there are other frequently mutated genes in breast cancer. Less commonly observed are mutations in PTEN (2–4 %), AKT1 (2–3 %), and phosphatidylinositol-3-kinase regulatory subunit alpha (PIK3R1: 1–2 %). Similar findings were observed in HER2-positive breast cancer. In contrast, triple-negative breast cancer (TNBC) is associated with a lower incidence of PIK3CA mutations (<10 %).

The frequent occurrence of PI3K pathway activation makes it an attractive therapeutic target in breast (Table 12.1). The recognition of its importance in tumorigenesis and cancer progression has led to the development of a number of agents that target various components of this pathway as cancer therapeutics. Promising results with these agents have been observed in the treatment of advanced estrogen receptor-positive (ER+) breast cancer. However, the therapeutic efficacy of single-agent PI3K pathway inhibitors is likely limited by feedback regulations among its pathway components and cross talk with other signaling pathways. Strategies that combine PI3K pathway inhibitors with inhibitors against RTKs, or inhibitors against MEK, MYC, PARP, or STAT3 pathways, or agents that activate autophagy and apoptosis machineries, are being explored. In addition, there is continued effort to identify resistance mechanisms and predictors of therapeutic response.

Germ line mutations in p53 occur in a high proportion of individuals with the Li-Fraumeni cancer susceptibility syndrome, which confers an increased risk of breast cancer [102]. This implies an important role for p53 inactivation in mammary carcinogenesis, and the structure and expression of p53 have been widely studied in breast cancer. Loss of heterozygosity (LOH) in the p53 gene was shown to be a common event in primary breast carcinomas [103], and this is accompanied by mutation of the residual allele in some cases. Although the overall frequency of p53 mutation in breast cancer is approximately 20 %, certain types of the disease are associated with higher frequencies. For example, a number of studies have identified an increased rate of p53 mutations in cancers arising in carriers of germ line BRCA1 and BRCA2 mutations. Moreover, a distinct spectrum of p53 mutations occurs in such carcinomas. Strikingly, in typical medullary breast carcinomas, p53 mutation occurs in 100 % of cases. This is of particular interest, since it is now well recognized that medullary breast cancers share clinico-pathological similarities with BRCA1-associated cases. Indeed, methylation-dependent silencing of BRCA1 expression occurs commonly in medullary breast cancers. Molecular pathological analysis of specific components of the p53 pathway is likely to have diagnostic and prognostic utility in breast cancer. Moreover, a number of innovative strategies have been proposed to restore p53 function to tumors. It will be of great interest to observe how these and other novel therapeutic approaches targeted to the p53 pathway impact on clinical outcome in breast cancer [104].

HER2 somatic mutations have been described in the last years, with an overall HER2 mutation rate of approximately 1.6 % of breast cancers. Some of them are activating mutations, including G309A, D769H, D769Y, V777L, P780ins, V842I, and R896C that are likely driver events in their cancer [105]. It is important to note that recurrence did not predict the phenotype of the mutation (activating, drug resistant, or neomorphic). Therefore, the presence of recurrence in these HER2 mutations tends to predict a functional effect, but lack of recurrence cannot be used to rule out an effect by the mutation. Several HER2-targeted drugs were tested on these mutations, and it has been observed that neratinib was a very potent inhibitor for all of the HER2 mutations. Lobular breast cancer may have an increased frequency of HER2 somatic mutations, but the number of cases sequenced to date is small (3 patients with lobular breast cancer with HER2 somatic mutation among 39 lobular breast cases in the TCGA study and 3 patients with HER2 mutations among 113 lobular cases in Shah et al. [106]. The HER2 mutation frequency in relapsed or metastatic breast cancer patients is currently unknown and potentially could be higher than 1.6 %. Because of the low mutation rate, prospective clinical trials using HER2 gene-sequencing results will need to screen a large number of patients, and the cooperation of many academic institutions and treatment centers is essential.

12.6.1 Lobular Breast Cancer

Invasive lobular carcinoma (ILC) is the second most prevalent histologic subtype of invasive breast cancer, constituting ~10–15 % of all cases. The classical form [107] is characterized by small discohesive neoplastic cells invading the stroma in a single-file pattern. The discohesive phenotype is due to dysregulation of cell–cell adhesion, primarily driven by lack of protein expression observed in ~90 % of ILCs. This feature is the ILC hallmark, and immunohistochemistry (IHC) scoring for CDH1 expression is often used to discriminate between lesions with borderline ductal versus lobular histological features. ILC variants have also been described, yet all display loss of E-cadherin expression [108].

The first TCGA breast cancer study reported on 466 breast tumors assayed on six different technology platforms. ILC was represented by only 36 samples, and no lobular-specific features were noted besides mutations and decreased mRNA and protein expression of CDH1. In 2012, Ciriello et al. [109.] profiled 817 breast tumors, including 127 ILC, 490 ductal (IDC), and 88 mixed IDC/ILC. As expected, they could identify CDH1 loss at the DNA, mRNA, and protein level in almost all ILC cases. Moreover, 12/27 *CDH1* mutations in non-ILC cases occurred in *mixed* tumors strongly resembling ILC at the molecular level. Surprisingly, they did not identify DNA hypermethylation of the CDH1 promoter in any breast tumor, suggesting that E-cadherin loss is not epigenetically driven. Besides E-cadherin loss, they identified mutations targeting PTEN, TBX3, and FOXA1 as ILC-enriched features. PTEN loss associated with increased AKT phosphorylation was highest in ILC among all breast cancer subtypes. Spatially clustered FOXA1 mutations correlated with increased FOXA1 expression and activity. Conversely, GATA3 mutations and high expression characterized Luminal A IDC, suggesting differential modulation of ER activity in ILC and IDC. Proliferation and immune-related signatures determined three ILC transcriptional subtypes associated with survival differences. Mixed IDC/ILC cases were molecularly classified as ILC-like and IDC-like, revealing no true hybrid features. This multidimensional molecular atlas sheds new light on the genetic bases of ILC and provides potential clinical options.

12.7 Conclusions

Breast cancer is a clinically and biologically heterogeneous disease. However, the vast majority of the biological diversity coming from the DNA, mRNA, miRNA, and protein is captured by the 4 main intrinsic subtypes defined by gene expression only. At the same time, and contrary to popular belief, intrinsic biology is not sufficiently captured by standard clinical–pathological variables. In this chapter, we have argued how intrinsic biology identified by gene expression analyses provides today, and especially in the future, clinically relevant information beyond the current pathology-based classification. In the upcoming years, we should expect more wealth of data regarding the clinical utility of intrinsic subtyping in a variety of clinical scenarios, and in combination with other biomarkers such as somatic mutations will allow the development of new targeted therapeutics now being tested in ongoing clinical trials.

These findings have led us to understand that this is not just one disease, but many, and that each patient entails a particular case where personalized medicine could play a crucial role. The last decade has changed the way researchers understand, classify, and study breast cancer, and it has reshaped the way doctors diagnose and treat this disease. In addition, it has undoubtedly changed the search for alternative therapies by integrating molecular studies and the selection of study populations based on their molecular markers into clinical trials. The therapeutic advances made to date have been achieved by performing large randomized clinical trials. The problem is that these trials were designed to determine the best therapeutic approach for the median population, not for a specific individual. Furthermore, we have learned through trial and error that new targeted therapies have to be developed in targeted populations, selected on the basis of a given biomarker. The good news is that the molecular studies that have been developed over the past decade have opened a broad field in cancer research that allows basic and translational researchers to look for new potential therapeutic targets and to test them in the clinic.

References

1. La Vecchia C, Bosetti C, Lucchini F, Bertuccio P, Negri E, Boyle P, et al. Cancer mortality in Europe, 2000–2004, and an overview of trends since 1975. Ann Oncol. 2010;21(6):1323–60.
2. Perou CM, Sorlie T, Eisen MB, van de Rijn M, Jeffrey SS, Rees CA, et al. Molecular portraits of human breast tumours. Nature. 2000;406(6797):747–52.
3. Prat A, Perou CM. Deconstructing the molecular portraits of breast cancer. Mol Oncol. 2011;5(1):5–23.
4. Prat A, Parker JS, Fan C, Perou CM. PAM50 assay and the three-gene model for identifying the major and clinically relevant molecular subtypes of breast cancer. Breast Cancer Res Treat. 2012;135(1):301–6.
5. Prat A, Parker JS, Karginova O, Fan C, Livasy C, Herschkowitz JI, et al. Phenotypic and molecular characterization of the claudin-low intrinsic subtype of breast cancer. Breast Cancer Res. 2010;12(5):R68.
6. Cancer Genome Atlas. N. Comprehensive molecular portraits of human breast tumours. Nature. 2012;490(7418):61–70.
7. Sorlie T, Perou CM, Tibshirani R, Aas T, Geisler S, Johnsen H, et al. Gene expression patterns of breast carcinomas distinguish tumor subclasses with clinical implications. Proc Natl Acad Sci USA. 2001;98(19):10869–74.
8. Parker JS, Mullins M, Cheang MC, Leung S, Voduc D, Vickery T, et al. Supervised risk predictor of breast cancer based on intrinsic subtypes. J Clin Oncol. 2009;27(8):1160–7.
9. Liu S, Chapman JA, Burnell MJ, Levine MN, Pritchard KI, Whelan TJ, et al. Prognostic and predictive investigation of PAM50 intrinsic subtypes in the NCIC CTG MA.21 phase III chemotherapy trial. Breast Cancer Res Treat. 2015;149(2):439–48.
10. Gnant M, Filipits M, Greil R, Stoeger H, Rudas M, Bago-Horvath Z, et al. Predicting distant recurrence in receptor-positive breast cancer patients with limited clinicopathological risk: using the PAM50 risk of recurrence score in 1478 postmenopausal patients of the ABCSG-8 trial treated with adjuvant endocrine therapy alone. Ann Oncol. 2014;25(2):339–45.
11. Dowsett M, Sestak I, Lopez-Knowles E, Sidhu K, Dunbier AK, Cowens JW, et al. Comparison of PAM50 risk of recurrence score with oncotype DX and IHC4 for predicting risk of distant recurrence after endocrine therapy. J Clin Oncol. 2013;31 (22):2783–90.
12. Caan BJ, Sweeney C, Habel LA, Kwan ML, Kroenke CH, Weltzien EK, et al. Intrinsic subtypes from the PAM50 gene expression assay in a population-based breast cancer survivor cohort: prognostication of short- and long-term outcomes. Cancer Epidemiol Biomarkers Prev. 2014;23(5):725–34.
13. Sestak I, Cuzick J, Dowsett M, Lopez-Knowles E, Filipits M, Dubsky P, et al. Prediction of late distant recurrence after 5 years of endocrine treatment: a combined analysis of patients from the Austrian breast and colorectal cancer study group 8 and arimidex, tamoxifen alone or in combination randomized trials using the PAM50 risk of recurrence score. J Clin Oncol. 2015;33(8): 916–22.
14. Prat A, Galván P, Jimenez B, Buckingham W, Jeiranian HA, Schaper C, et al. Prediction of response to neoadjuvant chemotherapy using core needle biopsy samples with the Prosigna assay. Clin Cancer Res. 2016;22(3):560–6.
15. Martin M, Prat A, Rodriguez-Lescure A, Caballero R, Ebbert MT, Munarriz B, et al. PAM50 proliferation score as a predictor of weekly paclitaxel benefit in breast cancer. Breast Cancer Res Treat. 2013;138(2):457–66.
16. Martín M, González-Rivera M, Morales S, de la Haba-Rodriguez J, González-Cortijo L, Manso L, et al. Prospective study of the impact of the Prosigna assay on adjuvant clinical decision-making in unselected patients with estrogen receptor positive, human epidermal growth factor receptor negative, node negative early-stage breast cancer. Curr Med Res Opin. 2015;31(6):1129–37.
17. Jorgensen CL, Nielsen TO, Bjerre KD, Liu S, Wallden B, Balslev E, et al. PAM50 breast cancer intrinsic subtypes and effect of gemcitabine in advanced breast cancer patients. Acta Oncol. 2014;53(6):776–87.
18. Filipits M, Nielsen TO, Rudas M, Greil R, Stoger H, Jakesz R, et al. The PAM50 risk-of-recurrence score predicts risk for late distant recurrence after endocrine therapy in postmenopausal women with endocrine-responsive early breast cancer. Clin Cancer Res. 2014;20(5):1298–305.
19. Boccia RV. Translating Research into Practice: the Prosigna® (PAM50) Gene Signature Assay. Clin Adv Hematol Oncol. 2015;13(6 Suppl 6):3–13.
20. Prat A, Lluch A, Albanell J, Barry WT, Fan C, Chacon JI, et al. Predicting response and survival in chemotherapy-treated triple-negative breast cancer. Br J Cancer. 2014;111(8):1532–41.
21. Sikov W, Barry W, Hoadley K, Pitcher B, Singh B, Tolaney S, et al. Impact of intrinsic subtype by PAM50 and other gene signatures on pathologic complete response (pCR) rates in triple-negative breast cancer (TNBC) after neoadjuvant chemotherapy (NACT) +/− carboplatin (Cb) or bevacizumab (Bev): CALGB 40603/150709 (Alliance). San Antonio Breast Cancer Symp. 2014;2012:S4–05.
22. Bastien RR, Rodriguez-Lescure A, Ebbert MT, Prat A, Munarriz B, Rowe L, et al. PAM50 breast cancer subtyping by RT-qPCR and concordance with standard clinical molecular markers. BMC Med Genomics. 2012;5(1):44.
23. Prat A, Adamo B, Cheang MC, Anders CK, Carey LA, Perou CM. Molecular characterization of basal-like and non-basal-like triple-negative breast cancer. Oncologist. 2013;18(2):123–33.

24. Dunbier AK, Anderson H, Ghazoui Z, Salter J, Parker JS, Perou CM, et al. Association between breast cancer subtypes and response to neoadjuvant anastrozole. Steroids. 2011;76(8):736–40.
25. Chia SK, Bramwell VH, Tu D, Shepherd LE, Jiang S, Vickery T, et al. A 50-Gene intrinsic subtype classifier for prognosis and prediction of benefit from adjuvant tamoxifen. Clin Cancer Res. 2012;18(16):4465–72.
26. Ellis MJ, Suman VJ, Hoog J, Lin L, Snider J, Prat A, et al. Randomized Phase II neoadjuvant comparison between letrozole, anastrozole, and exemestane for postmenopausal women with estrogen receptor-rich stage 2 to 3 breast cancer: clinical and biomarker outcomes and predictive value of the baseline PAM50-based intrinsic subtype—ACOSOG Z1031. J Clin Oncol. 2011;29(17):2342–9.
27. Gnant M, Filipits M, Greil R, Stoeger H, Rudas M, Bago-Horvath Z, et al. Predicting distant recurrence in receptor-positive breast cancer patients with limited clinicopathological risk: using the PAM50 risk of recurrence score in 1478 postmenopausal patients of the ABCSG-8 trial treated with adjuvant endocrine therapy alone. Ann Oncol. 2014;25(2):339–45.
28. Martín M, González-Rivera M, Morales S, de la Haba J, González-Cortijo L, Manso L, et al. Prospective study of the impact of the Prosigna™ assay on adjuvant clinical decision-making in women with estrogen receptor-positive, HER2-negative, node-negative breast cancer: a GEICAM study. In: San Antonio Breast Cancer Symposium 2012; P6-08-10, 2014.
29. Nielsen TO, Parker JS, Leung S, Voduc D, Ebbert M, Vickery T, et al. A comparison of PAM50 intrinsic subtyping with immunohistochemistry and clinical prognostic factors in tamoxifen-treated estrogen receptor-positive breast cancer. Clin Cancer Res. 2010;16(21):5222–32.
30. Prat A, Cheang MC, Martin M, Parker JS, Carrasco E, Caballero R, et al. Prognostic significance of progesterone receptor-positive tumor cells within immunohistochemically defined luminal A breast cancer. J Clin Oncol. 2013;31(2):203–9.
31. Prat A, Carey LA, Adamo B, Vidal M, Tabernero J, Cortés J, et al. Molecular features and survival outcomes of the intrinsic subtypes within HER2-positive breast cancer. J Natl Cancer Inst. 2014;106(8).
32. Curtis C, Shah SP, Chin S-F, Turashvili G, Rueda OM, Dunning MJ, et al. The genomic and transcriptomic architecture of 2,000 breast tumours reveals novel subgroups. Nature. 2012;486(7403):346–52.
33. Prat A, Bianchini G, Thomas M, Belousov A, Cheang MC, Koehler A, et al. Research-based PAM50 subtype predictor identifies higher responses and improved survival outcomes in HER2-positive breast cancer in the NOAH study. Clin Cancer Res. 2014;20(2):511–21.
34. Carey L, Berry D, Ollila D, Harris L, Krop I, Weckstein D, et al. Clinical and translational results of CALGB 40601: a neoadjuvant phase III trial of weekly paclitaxel and trastuzumab with or without lapatinib for HER2-positive breast cancer. Proc Am Soc Clin Oncol: a500. 2013.
35. Prat A, Ellis MJ, Perou CM. Practical implications of gene-expression-based assays for breast oncologists. Nat Rev Clin Oncol. 2012;9(1):48–57.
36. Dowsett M, Nielsen TO, A'Hern R, Bartlett J, Coombes RC, Cuzick J, et al. Assessment of Ki67 in breast cancer: recommendations from the international Ki67 in Breast Cancer Working Group. J Natl Cancer Inst. 2011.
37. Hammond MEH, Hayes DF, Dowsett M, Allred DC, Hagerty KL, Badve S, et al. American society of clinical oncology/college of american pathologists guideline recommendations for immunohistochemical testing of estrogen and progesterone receptors in breast cancer. J Clin Oncol. 2010;28(16):2784–95.
38. Wolff AC, Hammond MEH, Hicks DG, Dowsett M, McShane LM, Allison KH, et al. Recommendations for human epidermal growth factor receptor 2 testing in breast cancer: American Society of Clinical Oncology/College of American Pathologists Clinical practice guideline update. J Clin Oncol. 2013;31(31):3997–4013.
39. McCullough A, Dell'Orto P, Reinholz M, Gelber R, Dueck A, Russo L, et al. Central pathology laboratory review of HER2 and ER in early breast cancer: an ALTTO trial [BIG 2-06/NCCTG N063D (Alliance)] ring study. Breast Cancer Res Treat. 2014;143(3):485–92.
40. Cheang MC, Chia SK, Voduc D, Gao D, Leung S, Snider J, et al. Ki67 index, HER2 status, and prognosis of patients with luminal B breast cancer. J Natl Cancer Inst. 2009;101(10):736–50.
41. Eroles P, Bosch A, Perez-Fidalgo JA, Lluch A. Molecular biology in breast cancer: intrinsic subtypes and signaling pathways. Cancer Treat Rev. 2012;38(6):698–707.
42. Prat A, Cheang MCU, Martín M, Parker JS, Carrasco E, Caballero R, et al. Prognostic significance of progesterone receptor-positive tumor cells within immunohistochemically defined luminal A breast cancer. J Clin Oncol. 2013;31(2):203–9.
43. Liu M, Pitcher B, Mardis E, Davies S, Snider J, Vickery T, et al. PAM50 gene signature is prognostic for breast cancer patients treated with adjuvant anthracycline and taxane based chemotherapy. In: San Antonio Breast Cancer Symposium 2012; P2-10-01.
44. Martín M, Prat A, Rodríguez-Lescure Á, Caballero R, Ebbert MW, Munárriz B, et al. PAM50 proliferation score as a predictor of weekly paclitaxel benefit in breast cancer. Breast Cancer Res Treat. 2013;138(2):457–66.
45. Cheang MC, Voduc KD, Tu D, Jiang S, Leung S, Chia SK, et al. Responsiveness of intrinsic subtypes to adjuvant anthracycline substitution in the NCIC.CTG MA.5 randomized trial. Clinical Cancer Res (an official journal of the American Association for Cancer Research). 2012;18(8):2402–12.
46. Filipits M, Nielsen TO, Rudas M, Greil R, Stöger H, Jakesz R, et al. The PAM50 Risk-of-recurrence score predicts risk for late distant recurrence after endocrine therapy in postmenopausal women with endocrine-responsive early breast cancer. Clinical Cancer Res. 2014.
47. Sestak I, Cuzick J, Dowsett M, Lopez-Knowles E, Filipits M, Dubsky P, et al. Prediction of late distant recurrence after 5 years of endocrine treatment: a combined analysis of patients from the austrian breast and colorectal cancer study group 8 and arimidex, tamoxifen alone or in combination randomized trials using the PAM50 risk of recurrence score. J Clin Oncol. 2015;33(8):916–22.
48. Sestak I, Dowsett M, Zabaglo L, Lopez-Knowles E, Ferree S, Cowens JW, et al. Factors predicting late recurrence for estrogen receptor–positive breast cancer. J Natl Cancer Inst. 2013.
49. Usary J, Zhao W, Darr D, Roberts PJ, Liu M, Balletta L, et al. Predicting drug responsiveness in human cancers using genetically engineered mice. Clin Cancer Res. 2013;19(17):4889–99.
50. von Minckwitz G, Blohmer JU, Costa SD, Denkert C, Eidtmann H, Eiermann W, et al. Response-guided neoadjuvant chemotherapy for breast cancer. J Clinl Oncol. 2013.
51. von Minckwitz G, Untch M, Blohmer J-U, Costa SD, Eidtmann H, Fasching PA, et al. Definition and impact of pathologic complete response on prognosis after neoadjuvant chemotherapy in various intrinsic breast cancer subtypes. J Clin Oncol. 2012;30(15):1796–804.
52. Carey LA, Dees EC, Sawyer L, Gatti L, Moore DT, Collichio F, et al. The triple negative paradox: primary tumor chemosensitivity of breast cancer subtypes. Clin Cancer Res. 2007;13(8):2329–34.

53. Cortazar P, Zhang L, Untch M, Mehta K, Costantino JP, Wolmark N, et al. Pathological complete response and long-term clinical benefit in breast cancer: the CTNeoBC pooled analysis. Lancet 384. 2014;(9938):164–72.
54. Roberts SA, Lawrence MS, Klimczak LJ, Grimm SA, Fargo D, Stojanov P, et al. An APOBEC cytidine deaminase mutagenesis pattern is widespread in human cancers. Nat Genet. 2013;45 (9):970–6.
55. Kuong KJ, Loeb LA. APOBEC3B mutagenesis in cancer. Nat Genet. 2013;45(9):964–5.
56. Vaz-Luis I, Ottesen R, Hughes M, Marcom PK, Moy B, Rugo H, et al. Impact of hormone receptor status on patterns of recurrence and clinical outcomes among patients with human epidermal growth factor-2-positive breast cancer in the National Comprehensive Cancer Network: a prospective cohort study. Breast Cancer Res. 2012;14(5):R129.
57. Perez EA, Romond EH, Suman VJ, Jeong J-H, Davidson NE, Geyer CE, et al. Four-year follow-up of trastuzumab plus adjuvant chemotherapy for operable human epidermal growth factor receptor 2–positive breast cancer: joint analysis of data from NCCTG N9831 and NSABP B-31. J Clin Oncol. 2011;29 (25):3366–73.
58. de Azambuja E, Holmes AP, Piccart-Gebhart M, Holmes E, Di Cosimo S, Swaby RF, et al. Lapatinib with trastuzumab for HER2-positive early breast cancer (NeoALTTO): survival outcomes of a randomised, open-label, multicentre, phase 3 trial and their association with pathological complete response. Lancet Oncol. 2014;15(10):1137–46.
59. Piccart-Gebhart M, Holmes A, Baselga J, De Azambuja D, Dueck A, Viale G, et al. First results from the phase III ALTTO trial (BIG 2-06; NCCTG [Alliance] N063D) comparing one year of anti-HER2 therapy with lapatinib alone (L), trastuzumab alone (T), their sequence (T → L), or their combination (T + L) in the adjuvant treatment of HER2-positive early breast cancer (EBC). Proc Am Soc Clin Oncol: LBA4. 2014.
60. Tolaney SM, Barry WT, Dang CT, Yardley DA, Moy B, Marcom PK, et al. Adjuvant paclitaxel and trastuzumab for node-negative, HER2-positive breast cancer. N Engl J Med. 2015;372(2):134–41.
61. Rimawi M, Niravath P, Wang T, Rexer B, Forero A, Wolff A, et al. TBCRC023: A randomized multicenter phase II neoadjuvant trial of lapatinib plus trastuzumab, with endcorine therapy and without chemotherapy, for 12 vs. 24 weeks in patients with HER2 overexpressing breast cancer. In: San Antonio Breast Cancer Symposium 2012;S6-02, 2014.
62. Prat A, Cruz C, Hoadley K, Díez O, Perou C, Balmaña J. Molecular features of the basal-like breast cancer subtype based on BRCA1 mutation status. Breast Cancer Res Treat. 2014;147(1):185–91.
63. Foulkes WD, Stefansson IM, Chappuis PO, Bégin LR, Goffin JR, Wong N, et al. Germline BRCA1 mutations and a basal epithelial phenotype in breast cancer. J Natl Cancer Inst. 2003;95 (19):1482–5.
64. Cheang MC, Voduc D, Bajdik C, Leung S, McKinney S, Chia SK, et al. Basal-like breast cancer defined by five biomarkers has superior prognostic value than triple-negative phenotype. Clin Cancer Res. 2008;14(5):1368–76.
65. Schneider BP, Winer EP, Foulkes WD, Garber J, Perou CM, Richardson A, et al. Triple-negative breast cancer: risk factors to potential targets. Clin Cancer Res. 2008;14(24):8010–8.
66. Prat A, Adamo B, Fan C, Peg V, Vidal M, Galvan P, et al. Genomic analyses across six cancer types identify basal-like breast cancer as a unique molecular entity. Sci Rep. 2013;3:3544.
67. Hoadley KA, Yau C, Wolf DM, Cherniack AD, Tamborero D, Ng S, et al. Multiplatform analysis of 12 cancer types reveals molecular classification within and across tissues of origin. Cell. 2014;158(4):929–44.
68. Lim E, Vaillant F, Wu D, Forrest NC, Pal B, Hart AH, et al. Aberrant luminal progenitors as the candidate target population for basal tumor development in BRCA1 mutation carriers. Nat Med. 2009;15(8):907–13.
69. Molyneux G, Geyer FC, Magnay F-A, McCarthy A, Kendrick H, Natrajan R, et al. BRCA1 basal-like breast cancers originate from luminal epithelial progenitors and not from basal stem cells. Cell Stem Cell. 2010;7(3):403–17.
70. Keller PJ, Arendt LM, Skibinski A, Logvinenko T, Klebba I, Dong S, et al. Defining the cellular precursors to human breast cancer. Proc Natl Acad Sci. 2012;109(8):2772–7.
71. Millikan R, Newman B, Tse C-K, Moorman P, Conway K, Smith L, et al. Epidemiology of basal-like breast cancer. Breast Cancer Res Treat. 2008;109(1):123–39.
72. Iwamoto T, Booser D, Valero V, Murray JL, Koenig K, Esteva FJ, et al. Estrogen receptor (ER) mRNA and ER-related gene expression in breast cancers that Are 1 % to 10 % ER-positive by immunohistochemistry. J Clin Oncol. 2012;30 (7):729–34.
73. Cheang M, Martin M, Nielsen T, Prat A, Rodriguez-Lescure A, Ruiz A, et al. Quantitative hormone receptors, triple-negative breast cancer (TNBC), and molecular subtypes: a collaborative effort of the BIG-NCI NABCG. Proc Am Soc Clin Oncol: a1008. 2012.
74. Prat A, Parker JS, Fan C, Cheang MCU, Miller LD, Bergh J, et al. Concordance among gene expression-based predictors for ER-positive breast cancer treated with adjuvant tamoxifen. Ann Oncol. 2012;23(11):2866–73.
75. Lehmann BD, Bauer JA, Chen X, Sanders ME, Chakravarthy AB, Shyr Y, et al. Identification of human triple-negative breast cancer subtypes and preclinical models for selection of targeted therapies. J Clin Invest. 2011;121 (7):2750–67.
76. Lehmann BD, Pietenpol JA. Identification and use of biomarkers in treatment strategies for triple-negative breast cancer subtypes. J Pathol. 2014;232(2):142–50.
77. Burstein MD, Tsimelzon A, Poage GM, Covington KR, Contreras A, Fuqua S, et al. Comprehensive genomic analysis identifies novel subtypes and targets of triple-negative breast cancer. Clinical Cancer Res. 2014.
78. Masuda H, Baggerly KA, Wang Y, Zhang Y, Gonzalez-Angulo AM, Meric-Bernstam F, et al. Differential response to neoadjuvant chemotherapy among 7 triple-negative breast cancer molecular subtypes. Clinical Cancer Res (An Official Journal of the American Association for Cancer Research). 2013;19(19): 5533–40.
79. Loi S, Michiels S, Salgado R, Sirtaine N, Jose V, Fumagalli D, et al. Tumor infiltrating lymphocytes are prognostic in triple negative breast cancer and predictive for trastuzumab benefit in early breast cancer: results from the FinHER trial. Ann Oncol. 2014;25(8):1544–50.
80. Ali HR, Provenzano E, Dawson S-J, Blows FM, Liu B, Shah M, et al. Association between CD8+ T-cell infiltration and breast cancer survival in 12 439 patients. Ann Oncol. 2014;25(8): 1536–43.
81. Rody A, Karn T, Liedtke C, Pusztai L, Ruckhaeberle E, Hanker L, et al. A clinically relevant gene signature in triple negative and basal-like breast cancer. Breast Cancer Res. 2011; 13(5):R97.
82. Herschkowitz JI, Simin K, Weigman VJ, Mikaelian I, Usary J, Hu Z, et al. Identification of conserved gene expression features between murine mammary carcinoma models and human breast tumors. Genome Biol. 2007;8(5):R76.

83. Lim E, Vaillant F, Wu D, Forrest NC, Pal B, Hart AH, et al. Aberrant luminal progenitors as the candidate target population for basal tumor development in BRCA1 mutation carriers. Nat Med. 2009;15(8):907–13.
84. Taube JH, Herschkowitz JI, Komurov K, Zhou AY, Gupta S, Yang J, et al. Core epithelial-to-mesenchymal transition interactome gene-expression signature is associated with claudin-low and metaplastic breast cancer subtypes. Proc Natl Acad Sci USA. 2010;107(35):15449–54.
85. Phillips JE, Petrie TA, Creighton FP, Garcia AJ. Human mesenchymal stem cell differentiation on self-assembled monolayers presenting different surface chemistries. Acta Biomater. 2010;6(1):12–20.
86. Hennessy BT, Gonzalez-Angulo AM, Stemke-Hale K, Gilcrease MZ, Krishnamurthy S, Lee JS, et al. Characterization of a naturally occurring breast cancer subset enriched in epithelial-to-mesenchymal transition and stem cell characteristics. Cancer Res. 2009;69(10):4116–24.
87. Hennessy BT, Krishnamurthy S, Giordano S, Buchholz TA, Kau SW, Duan Z, et al. Squamous cell carcinoma of the breast. J Clin Oncol. 2005;23(31):7827–35.
88. Vu-Nishino H, Tavassoli FA, Ahrens WA, Haffty BG. Clinicopathologic features and long-term outcome of patients with medullary breast carcinoma managed with breast-conserving therapy (BCT). Int J Radiat Oncol Biol Phys. 2005;62(4):1040–7.
89. Hess KR, Anderson K, Symmans WF, Valero V, Ibrahim N, Mejia JA, et al. Pharmacogenomic predictor of sensitivity to preoperative chemotherapy with paclitaxel and fluorouracil, doxorubicin, and cyclophosphamide in breast cancer. J Clin Oncol. 2006;24(26):4236–44.
90. Nielsen TO, Hsu FD, Jensen K, Cheang M, Karaca G, Hu Z, et al. Immunohistochemical and clinical characterization of the basal-like subtype of invasive breast carcinoma. Clin Cancer Res. 2004;10(16):5367–74.
91. Curtis C, Shah SP, Chin SF, Turashvili G, Rueda OM, Dunning MJ, et al. The genomic and transcriptomic architecture of 2,000 breast tumours reveals novel subgroups. Nature. 2012;486(7403):346–52.
92. Dawson SJ, Rueda OM, Aparicio S, Caldas C. A new genome-driven integrated classification of breast cancer and its implications. EMBO J. 2013;32(5):617–28.
93. Comprehensive molecular portraits of human breast tumours. Nature. 2012;490(7418):61–70.
94. Robinson DR, Wu Y-M, Vats P, Su F, Lonigro RJ, Cao X, et al. Activating ESR1 mutations in hormone-resistant metastatic breast cancer. Nat Genet. 2013;45(12):1446–51.
95. Liu Y, Colditz GA, Gehlert S, Goodman M. Racial disparities in risk of second breast tumors after ductal carcinoma in situ. Breast Cancer Res Treat. 2014;148(1):163–73.
96. Jeselsohn R, Yelensky R, Buchwalter G, Frampton G, Meric-Bernstam F, Gonzalez-Angulo AM, et al. Emergence of constitutively active estrogen receptor-α mutations in pretreated advanced estrogen receptor-positive breast cancer. Clin Cancer Res. 2014;20(7):1757–67.
97. Segal CV, Dowsett M. Estrogen receptor mutations in breast cancer–new focus on an old target. Clin Cancer Res. 2014;20(7):1724–6.
98. de Dueñas E, Hernández A, Zotano Á, Carrión R, López-Muñiz J, Novoa S, et al. Prospective evaluation of the conversion rate in the receptor status between primary breast cancer and metastasis: results from the GEICAM 2009-03 ConvertHER study. Breast Cancer Res Treat. 2014;143(3):507–15.
99. Parker JS, Mullins M, Cheang MCU, Leung S, Voduc D, Vickery T, et al. Supervised risk predictor of breast cancer based on intrinsic subtypes. J Clin Oncol. 2009;27(8):1160–7.
100. Prat A, Maggie C, Galván P, Nuciforo P, Paré L, Adamo B, Muñoz M, Viladot M, Press F, Gagnon R, Ellis C, Johnston S. Intrinsic subtype, prognosis, and benefit of lapatinib therapy in first line hormone-receptor positive metastatic breast cancer treated with letrozole. JAMA Oncol. 2016;2(10).
101. Johnston S, Pippen J, Pivot X, Lichinitser M, Sadeghi S, Dieras V, et al. Lapatinib combined with letrozole versus letrozole and placebo as first-line therapy for postmenopausal hormone receptor-positive metastatic breast cancer. J Clin Oncol. 2009;27(33):5538–46.
102. Malkin D, Li FP, Strong LC, Fraumeni JF Jr, Nelson CE, Kim DH, et al. Germ line p53 mutations in a familial syndrome of breast cancer, sarcomas, and other neoplasms. Science. 1990;250(4985):1233–8.
103. Davidoff AM, Kerns BJ, Pence JC, Marks JR, Iglehart JD. p53 alterations in all stages of breast cancer. J Surg Oncol. 1991;48(4):260–7.
104. Gasco M, Shami S, Crook T. The p53 pathway in breast cancer. Breast Cancer Res. 2002;4(2):70–6.
105. Bose R. A neu view of invasive lobular breast cancer. Clin Cancer Res. 2013;19(13):3331–3.
106. Shah SP, Morin RD, Khattra J, Prentice L, Pugh T, Burleigh A, et al. Mutational evolution in a lobular breast tumour profiled at single nucleotide resolution. Nature. 2009;461(7265):809–13.
107. Foote FW Jr, Stewart FW. A histologic classification of carcinoma of the breast. Surgery. 1946;19:74–99.
108. Dabbs DJ, Schnitt SJ, Geyer FC, Weigelt B, Baehner FL, Decker T, et al. Lobular neoplasia of the breast revisited with emphasis on the role of E-cadherin immunohistochemistry. Am J Surg Pathol. 2013;37(7):e1–11.
109. Ciriello G, Gatza ML, Beck AH, Wilkerson MD, Rhie SK, Pastore A, et al. Comprehensive molecular portraits of invasive lobular breast cancer. Cell. 2015;163(2):506–19.
110. cBioportal for Cancer Genomics.
111. Cerami E, Gao J, Dogrusoz U, Gross BE, Sumer SO, Aksoy BA, et al. The cBio cancer genomics portal: an open platform for exploring multidimensional cancer genomics data. Cancer Discov. 2012;2(5):401–4.
112. Gao J, Aksoy BA, Dogrusoz U, Dresdner G, Gross B, Sumer SO, et al. Integrative analysis of complex cancer genomics and clinical profiles using the cBioPortal. Sci Signal. 2013;6(269):pl1.
113. Bos PD, Zhang XH, Nadal C, Shu W, Gomis RR, Nguyen DX, et al. Genes that mediate breast cancer metastasis to the brain. Nature. 2009;459(7249):1005–9.
114. Silver DP, Richardson AL, Eklund AC, Wang ZC, Szallasi Z, Li Q, et al. Efficacy of neoadjuvant Cisplatin in triple-negative breast cancer. J Clin Oncol. 2010;28(7):1145–53.
115. Li Y, Zou L, Li Q, Haibe-Kains B, Tian R, Li Y, et al. Amplification of LAPTM4B and YWHAZ contributes to chemotherapy resistance and recurrence of breast cancer. Nat Med. 2010;16(2):214–8.
116. Juul N, Szallasi Z, Eklund AC, Li Q, Burrell RA, Gerlinger M, et al. Assessment of an RNA interference screen-derived mitotic and ceramide pathway metagene as a predictor of response to neoadjuvant paclitaxel for primary triple-negative breast cancer: a retrospective analysis of five clinical trials. Lancet Oncol. 2010;11(4):358–65.
117. Buffa FM, Camps C, Winchester L, Snell CE, Gee HE, Sheldon H, et al. microRNA-associated progression pathways

and potential therapeutic targets identified by integrated mRNA and microRNA expression profiling in breast cancer. Cancer Res. 2011;71(17):5635–45.

118. Hatzis C, Pusztai L, Valero V, Booser DJ, Esserman L, Lluch A, et al. A genomic predictor of response and survival following taxane-anthracycline chemotherapy for invasive breast cancer. JAMA. 2011;305(18):1873–81.
119. Itoh M, Iwamoto T, Matsuoka J, Nogami T, Motoki T, Shien T, et al. Estrogen receptor (ER) mRNA expression and molecular subtype distribution in ER-negative/progesterone receptor-positive breast cancers. Breast Cancer Res Treat. 2014;143(2):403–9.
120. Minn AJ, Gupta GP, Siegel PM, Bos PD, Shu W, Giri DD, et al. Genes that mediate breast cancer metastasis to lung. Nature. 2005;436(7050):518–24.
121. Sotiriou C, Wirapati P, Loi S, Harris A, Fox S, Smeds J, et al. Gene expression profiling in breast cancer: understanding the molecular basis of histologic grade to improve prognosis. J Natl Cancer Inst. 2006;98(4):262–72.
122. Ivshina AV, George J, Senko O, Mow B, Putti TC, Smeds J, et al. Genetic reclassification of histologic grade delineates new clinical subtypes of breast cancer. Cancer Res. 2006;66(21):10292–301.
123. Desmedt C, Piette F, Loi S, Wang Y, Lallemand F, Haibe-Kains B, et al. Strong time dependence of the 76-gene prognostic signature for node-negative breast cancer patients in the TRANSBIG multicenter independent validation series. Clin Cancer Res. 2007;13(11):3207–14.
124. Patil G, Valliyodan B, Deshmukh R, Prince S, Nicander B, Zhao M, et al. Soybean (Glycine max) SWEET gene family: insights through comparative genomics, transcriptome profiling and whole genome re-sequence analysis. BMC Genom. 2015;16:520.
125. Anders CK, Acharya CR, Hsu DS, Broadwater G, Garman K, Foekens JA, et al. Age-specific differences in oncogenic pathway deregulation seen in human breast tumors. PLoS ONE. 2008;3(1):e1373.

Ductal Carcinoma In Situ

13

Ian H. Kunkler

13.1 Introduction

Ductal carcinoma in situ may be defined as a disorder of the breast resulting from the accumulation of malignant epithelial cells within the terminal ductal lobular network. It forms part of a spectrum of preinvasive lesions arising within normal breast tissue with histological progression from atypical hyperplasia to invasive breast cancer [1]. It is the direct but non-obligate and non-life-threatening precursor of invasive breast cancer. Women with biopsy confirmed DCIS has in excess of a 10-fold increased risk of developing invasive breast cancer compared to those without DCIS [2]. However, irrespective of treatment the 10-year risk of death as a result of invasive cancer is 1.1–2.6 % [3–6]. DCIS is heterogeneous in terms of genetic and molecular changes, cytological features and architecture. While there is no universally accepted classification of DCIS, categorisation based on nuclear grade alone into low, intermediate and high grade in combination with comedo necrosis is widely accepted.

The clinical importance of DCIS is rising with advances in imaging and the arrival of drugs licensed for reducing breast cancer risk [7]. Before the advent of breast screening, DCIS commonly presented as a lump. However, the development of screening programmes has increased the diagnosis of DCIS, frequently on the basis of mammographic calcifications. Management remains controversial and practice varies substantially. Local treatment options include conservative surgery with or without postoperative radiotherapy, unilateral or bilateral mastectomy. Adjuvant endocrine therapy with tamoxifen is also an option for hormone receptor positive patients. There is no role for chemotherapy in DCIS. All patients should have access to a multidisciplinary opinion on their management. Adequate time must be allowed for patients to consider the various options offered by the surgeon and to make an informed decision. Patients should be reassured that taking 1–2 weeks to come to a considered decision on treatment is not going to compromise their outcome.

Approximately 13–35 % of DCIS will recur within 10 years of conservative surgery [8]. Half of the recurrences after excision of DCIS are invasive [9, 10]. While postoperative and adjuvant endocrine therapy can reduce the risks of recurrent DCIS and invasive cancer, there is no current reliable clinico-pathological or molecular factor which predicts which DCIS lesions will progress to invasive cancer or which ones will recur after primary therapy. The consequence may be overtreatment or undertreatment. Practice varies widely [1, 11–16]. Little is known about the natural history of DCIS since surgical excision precludes studying their evolution [7]. There is a small longitudinal study of 28 women with small, non-comedo DCIS on follow-up for in excess of 30 years after biopsy alone. The risk of transformation to invasive cancer was about 40 %. Five patients developed metastatic disease [17].

13.2 Biology

Chromosomal loss or gain at multiple loci occurs as hyperplastic lesions progress to DCIS and invasive cancer. Loss of heterozygosity is observed in 70 % of high-grade DCIS compared to 35–40 % of atypical hyperplasia and 0 % of normal breast tissue [18–20]. HER2 is overexpressed in excess of half of DCIS. ER is expressed in over 70 % of DCIS. p53 is mutated about a quarter of DCIS and rarely in normal breast tissue or benign proliferative lesions. The majority, if not all, of clinically relevant factors (ER status, oncogene expression and histological grade) are probably determined by the time DCIS has evolved [21–24]. This is the probable explanation for the heterogeneous nature of breast cancer mirroring that of DCIS.

I.H. Kunkler (✉)
Institute of Genetics and Molecular Medicine (IGMM), University of Edinburgh, Crewe Road, Edinburgh, Scotland, EH4 2XU, UK
e-mail: i.kunkler@ed.ac.uk

I. Jatoi and A. Rody (eds.), *Management of Breast Diseases*, DOI 10.1007/978-3-319-46356-8_13

The histological progression through atypical hyperplasia, ductal carcinoma in situ, and mutational profiling suggests that the acquisition of invasive potential is a relatively late event [25]. It is unclear what factors contribute to the development and progression of DCIS. If these could be identified, then it might be possible to inhibit them. Analysis of genomic data implies that tumour cell gene expression changes happen at the transition from normal tissue to DCIS with relatively few changes at the transition from DCIS to invasive breast cancer [26, 27]. Non-epithelial cells are implicated in the progression to invasive disease [28, 29]. In the normal breast, a layer of contractile myoepithelial cells surrounds the epithelial ductal and alveolar structures. These myoepithelial cells are required for the expulsion of milk as well as for normal mammary gland development as they exert influence on ductal branching, polarity in addition to milk production [30]. One of the features of progression from DCIS to invasive breast cancer is breaching of the myoepithelial cell layer and basement membrane. It is thought [25] that the myoepithelial cells have an active role in tumour suppression by downregulating metalloproteinases [31, 32], secreting protease inhibitors and synthesising tumour-suppressive proteins such as maspin [33]. Russell et al. [25] have described a preclinical model studying myoepithelial integrity. p63 loss was an early indicator, calponin loss intermediate and alpha smooth muscle actin a more delayed measure of compromised myoepithelium.

It is possible that the hypoxic intraduct microenvironment leads to the survival and adaptation of premalignant cells which might lead to genetic instability and selection of malignant cells with invasive potential [34]. Autophagy is the pathway which is activated to promote survival in the presence of hypoxic and nutrient stress. Autophagy is known to occur at the same sites as areas of hypoxic stress in models of epithelial tumours [35]. It may be that autophagy is a major survival mechanism employed by DCIS cells to survive and proliferate in the stressful intraductal space. It is postulated that autophagy might aid cell migration through regions of degraded matrix by processing matrix breakdown products that undergo phagocytosis by the migrating cells.

13.3 Presentation

In excess of 90 % of DCIS are found at breast screening. Approximately 6 % of patients with symptomatic breast cancer are preinvasive [36]. Presentations include Paget's disease of the nipple, nipple discharge or a palpable mass. DCIS which presents with clinical signs is more likely to be extensive and has an invasive component [37]. Men may present with a bloodstained nipple discharge or a retroareolar mass.

13.4 Diagnosis

Microcalcifications on screening mammography are the commonest abnormality. Architectural distortion, masses, nodules and ductal asymmetry are also seen. Image-guided biopsy or vacuum-assisted biopsy is recommended. A meta-analysis has shown that a 14-gauge core biopsy halves the risk of missing a coexisting invasive cancer by half ($p = -0.006$) [38]. Magnetic resonance imaging (MRI) has an increasing role in assessing the extent of DCIS [39]. MRI may detect occult multifocal or contralateral disease.

13.5 Surgery

Some form of surgery whether microdochectomy, breast conserving or mastectomy is recommended for all patients, since a biopsy diagnosis of DCIS cannot exclude the presence of invasive cancer. For this reason, observation is not an advised option. Many DCIS lesions are diagnosed on mammography which prove to be microscopically more extensive than the radiological appearance and cannot be excised locally with clear margins. Approximately 35 % of patients in the UK with DCIS undergo mastectomy and 72 % breast-conserving surgery [36]. For some patients, prophylactic contralateral mastectomy is performed. Sentinel node biopsy is not recommended unless the patient is at high risk of invasive disease [40]. There is no role for axillary dissection since the rates of axillary involvement are extremely low [41]. The choice between mastectomy and breast-conserving surgery is determined by the extent of DCIS and preference of the patient. After wide local excision, the specimen is X-rayed to verify that all microcalcifications have been removed. However, many DCIS lesions cannot be managed by breast-conserving surgery while achieving satisfactory cosmesis. After mastectomy, imaging of the specimen slices aids the pathologist in determining the extent of the disease [37]. Patients with extensive DCIS may be candidates for immediate breast reconstruction.

Surgical margins for DCIS remain a subject for debate. They are an important prognostic factor for recurrence. The adequacy of the margin relates to local control but is not precisely assessed by margin status alone [42]. The NSABP B-17 trial which showed that adjuvant whole breast irradiation was effective in reducing local recurrence was criticised for its lack of definition of an adequate margin. Around a quarter of cases had positive or unknown margins. Practice varies. Some clinicians are content with tumour at the inked margins as long as all the microcalcifications have been removed and the patients are treated by adjuvant radiotherapy. In general, a margin of 2–3 mm is considered acceptable as long as postoperative RT is given [43] or narrower (1–2 mm) [42] or at least 1 mm for circumferential margins [37]. The pathologist has a key role in determining the adequacy of the margin. If the margins are <1 mm, a reexcision should be undertaken to clear the margins.

13.6 Adjuvant Radiotherapy

There are four randomised trials (Table 13.1) which have assessed the role of postoperative whole breast irradiation and breast-conserving surgery NSABP-B17 [9], EORTC 108 [44, 45, 53], UK/ANZ [46, 47] and SweDCIS [48]. All these five trials show that adjuvant whole breast irradiation significantly reduces the risk of local recurrence. The first was the NSABP B-17 which randomised 818 patients to wide excision alone or wide excision plus whole breast irradiation. At a mean follow-up of 90 months, there was a statistically significant reduction in local recurrence of DCIS from 13.4 % with surgery alone compared to 8.2 % with combined treatment ($p = 0.007$). For invasive disease, the reduction was even greater from 13.4 to 3.9 % ($p < 0.0001$). Benefit from radiation was seen in all patients and pathological subgroups with the largest gain in patients with necrosis [5]. There have been some criticisms of the NSABP B-17 trial. These include lack of rigorous mammographic and pathological quality assurance, variation between institutions in the definition of tumour-free margins and lack of examination of pathological subtypes [49, 50].

In the EORTC 10853 trial, 1002 patients were randomised to wide excision with or without whole breast irradiation. In the initial report [44] with a median follow-up of 4.25 years, the 4-year relapse-free survival was 84 % in the group treated by wide excision and 91 % in the group treated by wide excision plus radiation (p-0.005). There were similar reductions of DCIS 35 % ($p = 0.06$) and invasive disease 40 % ($p = 0.04$). In an update of the trial [45] at a median follow-up of 10.5 years, radiotherapy reduced the recurrence of DCIS and invasive recurrence by 48 % ($p = 0.001$) and 42 %, respectively. The magnitude of benefit from RT was slightly greater than in the original report (HR at 4.25 years: 0.62 and at 10.5 years: 0.53). On multivariate analysis, factors associated with an increased risk of local recurrence were young age (=/<40 years), symptomatic presentation, intermediate- or high-grade disease, cribriform or solid growth pattern, doubtful margins and treatment by wide local excision alone. The effect of radiotherapy was homogeneous across all the risk factors assessed. All the subgroups examined had a risk of recurrence of more than 10 % when treated by wide excision alone with the exception of patients with a clinging or micropapillary architecture. Well-differentiated DCIS had a lower risk of recurrent DCIS but not of invasive cancer. The absolute benefit of radiotherapy in low-grade DCIS was smaller than in intermediate and high grade. Both the NSABP B-17 and the EORTC 10853 trials showed a relatively high local recurrence rate at 10 years of 15 % after RT. Neither trial was a boost to the site of the excision used. In invasive cancer, it has been shown that a boost of 16 Gy in 8 fractions after

Table 13.1 Outcomes of treatment for DCIS with breast-conserving surgery and radiotherapy

Study	Period	No. of patients	% of screen detected	% of negative margins	Median follow-up (months)	Local recurrence rate (%)	% of local recurrences being invasive
Bijker et al. [45] EORTC	1986–96	507	71	84	126	15	53
Cuzick et al. [47] UK/ANZ DCIS	1990–98	267	>90	100	152	9	42
Holmberg et al. [54] SweDCIS	1987–99	526	79	80	101	12	59
Wapnir et al. [10] NSABP B-17 and B-24	1985–90	410	80	87	207	20	54
Solin et al. [56] J of Clin Onc	1998–2006	636	NS	100	85	0.9	42

Source Data from Boxer et al. [57]

whole breast irradiation of 50 in 25 daily fractions to the site of excision further reduced the risk of recurrence with a HR of 0.59 [51]. At a median follow-up of 17.2 years, ipsilateral breast tumour recurrence was 13 % in the 'no boost' group versus 9 % in the 'boost' group, HR 0.65 (99 % CI 0.52–0.81, $p < 0.0001$) [52]. The role of a breast boost in 'non-low-risk' DCIS is being investigated in the TransTasman Radiation Oncology Group BIG 3-07 boost trial. This is a 2 × 2 phase III trial studying the role of a tumour bed boost (16 Gy in 8 fractions). There are 4 arms: (1) whole breast RT alone using shorter fractionation (42.6 Gy in 16 fractions); (2) whole breast irradiation alone with standard fractionation (50 Gy in 25 fractions); (3) whole breast irradiation with shorter fractionation followed by tumour bed boost; and (4) whole breast irradiation with standard fractionation followed by tumour bed boost. The primary endpoint is local recurrence. Its target accrual of 1600 patients internationally has been reached. It is now in follow-up phase. A French phase III trial, BONBIS, is currently recruiting evaluating the role of a boost after conventional fractionation for DCIS following breast-conserving surgery and whole breast irradiation. The primary endpoint is local recurrence. Target accrual is 1950 patients.

There was no evidence that high-grade DCIS seemed to progress more rapidly to invasive cancer than low-grade DCIS. However, a higher number of women ($n = 12$) died as a result of invasive cancer compared to 2 women with well-grade DCIS and 3 with intermediate-grade DCIS. There was no survival difference between irradiated and non-irradiated groups. The death rate due to metastatic breast cancer was 2 % in both groups and is similar to death rates following mastectomy [4].

In the UK UK/ANZ boost trial [47], 1701 patients were randomised to radiotherapy and tamoxifen, radiotherapy alone or tamoxifen alone or to no further therapy after breast-conserving surgery. Radiotherapy reduced the incidence of ipsilateral recurrence of DCIS ($p < 0.0001$) and invasive disease ($p < 0.0001$). Tamoxifen reduced all new breast cancer events including contralateral breast cancer but did not reduce ipsilateral invasive disease. The tamoxifen effect appeared only to occur in patients who did not receive radiotherapy. Nonetheless, only 523 of the patients treated with radiotherapy were in the tamoxifen group. A test for interaction between treatments was not significant. An effect of tamoxifen in irradiated patients was, however, observed in the NSABP B-24 trial [53]. The effect of radiotherapy was slightly greater (HR 0.32) than in the original report of the trial (HR 0.38) [46]. The impact of radiotherapy was the same irrespective of whether patients received tamoxifen or not.

In the Swedish DCIS trial [49], 1046 patients were randomised after sector resection to radiotherapy or no further adjuvant treatment. The primary endpoint was local recurrence. Microscopic radical removal was not required. It was at the discretion of the surgeon based on operative findings, specimen radiography and pathology report whether a further excision was attempted or not. Microscopically clear margins were not a prerequisite. Whole breast irradiation (50 Gy in 25 fractions) or 54 Gy in two series with a two-week gap was given without a boost to the tumour bed. The 5-year cumulative incidence of local recurrence was 7 % in the RT group (95 % CI 5–10 %) and 22 % in the non-irradiated group (95 % CI 18–26 %). There was no evidence of a difference in the impact of radiotherapy on DCIS and invasive recurrence. In a subsequent report of the trial [54] at a median follow-up of 8.4 years, there was a 16 % risk reduction in ipsilateral breast events from RT at 10 years (95 % CI 10.3–21.6 %). Invasive recurrences occurred in 59.4 % of the irradiated group and 45.4 % of the control group. The impact of radiotherapy increased with age. The cumulative incidence of recurrence in the RT group was 20 % in the youngest group, falling to 8 % in women aged 65 or older. The authors could not identify a low-risk group among non-irradiated patients with less than 1 % local recurrence risk per year.

The Oxford overview of trials of adjuvant radiotherapy in DCIS brought together data on 3729 women [8]. The absolute 10-year risk of recurrence was reduced by 15.2 % (SE 1.6 %, 12.9 % vs. 28.1 %, 2P < 0.00001). The rate of ipsilateral breast events is roughly halved into all four trials studied (Fig. 13.1). Radiotherapy reduced local recurrence irrespective of age, type of surgery (local or sector excision) and whether tamoxifen was given or not. The proportional effect of radiotherapy was higher in older women.

The authors noted that breast screening has become more common since the periods of recruitment of the four trials with the result that DCIS lesions are smaller. In addition, there is a greater attention now in achieving clear margins. There was no difference in the risk of death between irradiated and non-irradiated patients.

Is there a subgroup of patients from postoperative radiotherapy can be safely omitted?

Given that DCIS carries virtually no mortality and there are risks of acute and late toxicity from radiotherapy, identifying patients with DCIS at low enough for radiotherapy to be omitted has been an important objective. In the ECOG-ACRIN E5194 study [55], patients were enrolled into two cohorts. In the first cohort, 1 561 women with grade 1 or 2 DCIS <2.5 cm treated by breast-conserving surgery with margins =/>1 mm (or no residual disease on reexcision). Cohort 2 is comprised of high-grade DCIS =/<1 cm (104 patients). No tamoxifen was allowed. In the initial report [55] at a median follow of 3.3 years, the number of local recurrences reached the threshold defined by the study stopping rules. The 5-year local recurrence rate was 12 %. The study was stopped. In a recently published follow-up of

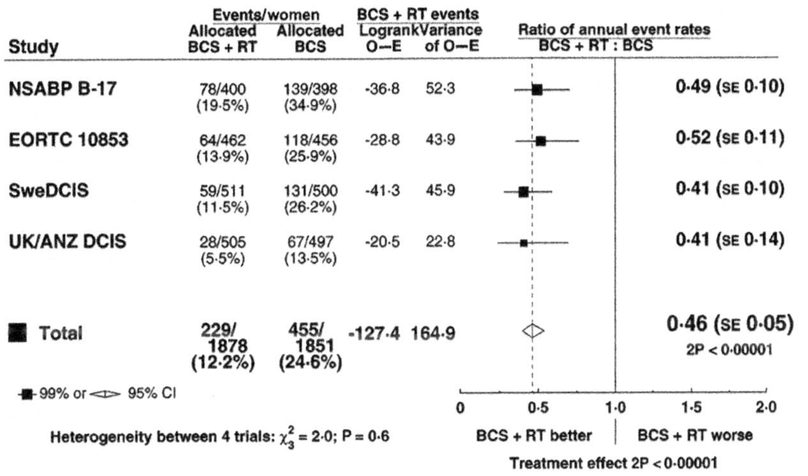

Figure 2. Effect of radiotherapy (RT) after breast-conserving surgery (BCS): ratio of annual event rates of any ipsilateral breast event by trial. SE = standard error; CI = confidence interval.

Fig. 13.1 Overview of the randomised trials of radiotherapy in ductal carcinoma in situ of the breast. (Reprinted from Abe et al. [64], with the permission of Oxford University Press)

the trial [56] at a median follow-up of 12.3 years, there had been 99 ipsilateral breast events of which 51 (52 %) were invasive. The ipsilateral breast rates were 14.4 % for cohort 1 and 24.6 % for cohort 2. The 12-year rates for an invasive recurrence for the two cohorts were 7.5 and 13.4 %, respectively. Over the 12-year period, the risks of invasive recurrence increased without any plateau. The ipsilateral breast event rate was 1.2 % for cohort 1 and 0.6 % for invasive recurrence. As Boxer et al., (2013) point out in their review [57], the median size of DCIS in the low- and intermediate-grade groups in the E5194 study was 6 mm while in the high-grade group it was 5 mm. They caution the extrapolating the results to the general patient population since the patients in E5194 were highly selected.

The Oxford overview [8] identified 291 women with small (1–20 mm) with low nuclear grade and clear margins. Their risk of local recurrence at 5 and 10 years after breast-conserving surgery alone was 20.6 and 30.1 %, respectively.

Results are awaited from the radiation therapy (RTOG) 9804 RCT comparing postoperative radiotherapy after breast-conserving surgery to control in 'low-risk' DCIS. Eligible patients were mammographically detected, <2.5 cm in size with low- or intermediate-grade DCIS with clear margins of at least 3 mm. Adjuvant tamoxifen was permissible but not a prerequisite.

Overall there remains considerable uncertainty in identifying a 'true low'-risk group from whom postoperative radiotherapy may be safely omitted. This uncertainty is largely due to inconsistencies in prospective and observational studies in relation to the predictive value of clinico-pathological risk factors [58].

13.7 Partial Breast Irradiation

There is no established role for partial breast irradiation in DCIS and very limited level 1 evidence. A non-randomised prospective study of partial breast irradiation using high dose rate brachytherapy (34 Gy over 5 days) by Mammosite balloon catheter [59] in 41 patients treated by breast-conserving surgery showed a worryingly high local recurrence rate of 9.8 % at a median follow-up of 5.3 years. A recently published multicentre phase III non-inferiority trial [60] from the GEC-ESTRO compared postoperative whole breast irradiation versus multicatheter brachytherapy after breast-conserving surgery in 1134 patients with low-risk invasive and ductal carcinoma. Adjuvant accelerated partial breast irradiation (ABPI) was shown to be non-inferior to whole breast irradiation. However. only 36 (6 %) of patients with DCIS were enrolled in the ABPI arm and 24 (4 %) in the whole breast arm. The numbers of patients with DCIS are too small to draw any firm conclusions on the safety of ABPI in this setting. Partial breast irradiation in DCIS should be regarded as investigational.

13.8 Adjuvant Hormonal Therapy

In contrast to postoperative whole breast irradiation, the role of adjuvant tamoxifen is less well established in DCIS. No survival advantage has been shown for adjuvant tamoxifen in this setting so its use is optional but not mandatory [7]. Most DCIS lesions are ER positive. In the NSABP B-24 trial, ER positivity was observed in 72 % of cases in a subset analysis [61].

In the NSABP B24 trial, adjuvant tamoxifen (20 mg) after breast-conserving surgery and postoperative whole breast irradiation resulted in a 37 % reduction in all breast events, although ER status was unknown at median follow-up of 6.2 years. In a retrospective subset analysis of the 40 % of patients with tissue available for assessment of ER status, and long-term follow-up of 14.5 years, tamoxifen reduced the risk of breast cancer events (ipsilateral DCIS and invasive recurrence and contralateral disease from 31 to 20.5 % (HR 0.38, $p = 0.0015$)). ER negative patients derived no benefit from tamoxifen. These findings were consistent with the results of the UK/ANZ DCIS trial [47] as discussed earlier. A meta-analysis of both trials [62] showed no reduction in mortality from tamoxifen +/− radiotherapy. Tamoxifen reduced all breast cancer events by 33 % (absolute reduction 5 %). The principal benefit of tamoxifen was in reducing contralateral non-invasive disease (RR 0.41, 95 % CI 0.20–0.82). Contralateral invasive disease was not reduced. Tamoxifen reduced invasive recurrence by 1 % but had no impact on recurrent DCIS. Both trials are based on 5 years of adjuvant tamoxifen. Consideration also has to be given to the risks of thrombo-embolism of tamoxifen, particularly in women over the age of 50. Whether there is an advantage of longer term tamoxifen (which has been shown in invasive cancer [63]) is uncertain.

References

1. Burstein HJ, Polyak K, Wong JS, Lister SC, Kaelin CM. Ductal carcinoma of the breast. N Eng J Med. 2004;350:1430–41.
2. Page DL, Dupont WD, Rogers LW, Jenson RA, Schuyler PA. Continued local recurrence of carcinoma 15–25 years after a diagnosis of low grade ductal carcinoma in situ of the breast treated only by biopsy. Cancer. 1995;76:1197–200.
3. Kerlikowske K. Epidemiology of ductal carcinoma in situ. J Natl Cancer Inst Monogr. 2010;41:139–41.
4. Ernster VL, Barclay J, Kerlikowske K, Wilkie H, Ballard-Barbash R. Mortality among women with ductal carcinoma in situ of the breast in the population based surveillance epidemiology and end results program. Arch Intern Med. 2000;160:953–8.
5. Fisher B, Dignam J, Wolmark N, Mamounas E, Costantino J, Poller W. Lumpectomy and radiation therapy for the treatment of intraductal breast cancer: finding from national surgical adjuvant breast and bowel project. B-17. J Clin Oncol. 1998;16:441–52.
6. Kerlikowske K, Molinero A, Cha I, Ljung BM, Ernster VL, Stewart K. Characteristics associated with recurrence among women with ductal carcinoma In situ treated by lumpectomy. J Natl Cancer Inst. 2003;95:1692–702.
7. Morrow M, Schnitt S, Norton L. Current management of lesions associated with an increased risk of breast cancer. Nat Rev Clin Oncol. 2015;12:227–38.
8. Early Breast Cancer Trialists Collaborative Group (EBCTCG), Correa C, McGale P, Taylor C, Wang Y, Clarke M et al. Overview of the randomised trials of radiotherapy in ductal carcinoma in situ of the breast. J Nat Inst Monogr. 2010;41:162–7.
9. Fisher ER, Dignam J, Tan-Chiu E, Costantino J, Fisher B, Paik S, et al. Pathologic findings from the National Surgical Adjuvant Breast Project (NSABP): eight year update of Protocol B-1.7. Cancer. 1999;86:429–38.
10. Wapnir I, Dignam J, Fisher B, Mamounas E, Anderson S, Julian T, et al. Long term outcomes of invasive ipsilateral breast tumor recurrence after lumpectomy in NSABP B-7 and B-24 randomised clinical trials for DCIS. J Nati Cancer Inst. 2011;103:478–88.
11. Allegra CJ, Aberle DR, Ganschow P, Hahn SM, Lee CN, Millon-Underwood S et al. National Institutes of Health State-of the-Science conference statement: diagnosis and management of ductal carcinoma in situ. September 22–24 2009. J Inst Natl Caner Inst. 2010;102:161–9.
12. Schwartz GF, Solin LJ, Olivotto IA, Ernster V, Pressman PI. The Consensus Conference Committee. Consensus conference on the treatment of in situ ductal carcinoma in situ of the breast. April 22–25, 1999. Cancer 2000;88:946–54.
13. Zujewskin JA, Harlan LC, Morrell DM, Stevens JL. Ductal carcinoma in situ: trends in treatment over time in the US. Breast Cancer Res Treat. 2011;127:251–7.
14. Dodwell D, Clements K, Lawrence G, Kearins O, Thomson CS, Dewar J, et al. Radiotherapy following breast-conserving surgery for screen-detected ductal carcinoma in situ: indications and utilization in the UK—interim findings from the Sloane Project. Br J Cancer. 2007;97:725–9.
15. Baxter NN, Virnig BA, Durham SB, Tuttle TM. Trends in the treatment of ductal carcinoma in situ of the breast. J Natl Cancer Inst. 2004;96:228–443.
16. Smith GL, Smith BD, Haffty BG. Rationalization and regionalization of treatment for ductal carcinoma of the breast. Int J Rad Oncol Biol Phys. 2006;65:1397–403.
17. Sanders MD, Schuyter PA, Dupont WD, Page DL. The natural history of low-grade ductal carcinoma in situ of the breast in women treated by biopsy only revealed over 30 years of long-term follow-up. Cancer. 2005;103:2481–4.
18. O'Connell P, Pekkel V, Fuqua SA, Osborne CK, Clark GM, Allred RC. Analysis of loss of heterozygosity in 300 premalignant breast lesions at 15 genetic loci. J Natl Cancer Inst. 1998;90:697–703.
19. Aubele MM, Cummings MC, Mattis AE, Zitzelsberger HF, Walch AK, Kremer M, et al. Accumulation of chromosomal imbalances from intraductal proliferative lesions to adjacent in situ and invasive ductal breast cancer. Diagn Mo Pathol. 2000;9:14–9.
20. Farabegoli F, Champene M, Bieche I, Santini D, Ceccarelli C, Derenzini M, et al. Genetic pathways in the evolution of breast ductal carcinoma in situ. J Pathol. 2002;196:280–6.
21. Lampejo OT, Barnes DM, Smith P, Millis RR. Evaluation of infiltrating ductal carcinoma with a DCIS component: correlation with the histological type of the in situ component with grade of the infiltrating component. Semin Diag Pathol. 1994;11:15–22.
22. Gupta AK, Douglas-Jones AG, Fenn N, Morgan JM, Mansel RE. The clinical behaviour of breast carcinoma is probably determined at the preinvasive stage (ductal carcinoma in situ). Cancer. 1997;85:869–74.
23. Warnberg F, Norgren H, Bergkvist L, Holmberg L. Tumour markers in breast carcinoma correlate with grade rather than with invasiveness. Br J Cancer. 2001;869–74.
24. Buerger H, Otterbach F, Simon R, Schafer KL, Poremba C, Diallo R et al. Different genetic pathways in the evolution of invasive breast cancer are associated with distinct morphological subtypes. J Pathol. 199;189:521–6.
25. Russell TD, Sonali J, Agunbiade S, Gao D, Troxell M, Borges VF et al. Myoepithelial cell differentiation markers in ductal carcinoma

in situ progression. Am J Pathol. 2015; pii: S0002–9440(15) 00430-7. doi:10.1016/j.ajpath.2015.07.004. [Epub ahead of print].
26. Ma XL, Salunga R, Tuggle JT, Gaudet J, Enright E, McQuary P et al. Gene expression profiles of human breast cancer progression. Proc Nat Sci USA. 2003;100:5974–9.
27. Lee S, Stewart S, Nagtegaal I, Luo J, Wu Y, Colditz G, et al. Differentially expressed genes regulating the progression of ductal carcinoma in situ to invasive breast cancer. Cancer Res. 2012;72:4574–86.
28. Allincn M, Beroukhim R, Cai L, Brennan C, Lahti-Domenici J, Huang H, et al. Molecular characterization of the tumor microenvironment in breast cancer. Cancer Cell. 2004;6:17–32.
29. Bombonati A, Sgroi DC. The molecular pathology of breast cancer progression. J Pathol. 2011;223:307–17.
30. Moumen M, Chiche A, Cagnet S, Petit V, Raymond K, Faraldo MM, et al. The mammary myoepethial cell. Int J Dev Biol. 2011;55:763–71.
31. Barsky SH, Karlin NH. Myoepithelial cells: autocrine and paracrine suppressors of breast cancer progression. J Mammary Gland Biol Neoplasia. 2005;10:249–60.
32. Hu M, Yao J, Carroll DK, Weremowicz S, Chen H, Carrasco D, et al. Regulation of in situ to invasive breast carcinoma transition. Cancer Cell. 2008;13:394–406.
33. Zou Z, Anisowicz A, Hendrix MJ, Thor A, Neven M, Sheng S. Maspin. A serpin with tumor-suppressing activity in human mammary epithelial cells. Science. 1994;263:526–9.
34. Espina V, Liotta L. What is the malignant nature of human carcinoma in situ? Nat Rev Cancer. 2011;11:68–75.
35. Matthew R, Karantza-Wordsworth B, White E. Assessing metabolic stress and autophagy: status in epithelial tumours. Meth Enzymol. 2009;453:53–81.
36. NHS cancer screening programmes. All breast cancer report. An analysis of all symptomatic patients and screen detected breast cancers diagnosed in 2006. NHS Breast Screening Programme Oct 2009.
37. Barnes NP, Ooi L, Yarnold J, Bundred NJ. Ductal carcinoma in situ of the breast. BMJ. 2012;344:e797.
38. Brennan ML, Turner RM, Ciatto S, Marinovich ML, French JR, Macaskill P, et al. Ductal carcinoma in situ at core-needle biopsy meta-analysis of underestimation and predictors of invasive breast cancer. Radiology. 2011;260:119–28.
39. Lehman CD. Magnetic resonance imaging in the evaluation of ductal carcinoma in situ. J Natl Cancer Monogr. 2010;2010:150–1.
40. Francis AM, Haugen CE, Grimes LM, Crow JR, Yi M, Mittendorf EA et al. is sentinel lymph node dissection warranted for patients with a diagnosis of ductal carcinoma in situ. Ann Surg Oncol. 2015. [Epub ahead of print].
41. Silverstein MJ, Rosser RJ, Gierson ED, Waisman JR, Gamagami P, Hoffman RS, et al. Axillary lymph node dissection for intraductal breast carcinoma—is it indicated. Cancer. 1987;69:1819–24.
42. Vaidya Y, Vaidya P, Vaidya T. Ductal carcinoma in situ of the breast. Indian J Surg. 2015;77:141–6.
43. Boughey JC, Gonzalez RJ, Bonner E, Kuere HM. Current treatment and clinical trial development for ductal carcinoma of the breast. Oncologist. 2007;11:1276–87.
44. Julien J-P, Bijker N, Fentiman IS, Peterse JL, Delledonne V, Rouanet P, et al. Radiotherapy in breast-conserving treatment for ductal carcinoma in situ: first results of the EORTC randomised phase III trial 10853. EORTC Breast Cancer Cooperative Group and EORTC Radiotherapy Group. Lancet. 2000;355:528–33.
45. Bijker N, Maijnon P, Peterse JL, Bogaerts J, Van Hoorebeek I, Julien P, et al. Breast conserving treatment with or without radiotherapy in ductal carcinoma in situ. Ten year results of European Organisation for Research and Treatment of Cancer Randomised phase 111 trial 10852—Study by the EORTC breast cancer cooperative group and EORTC Radiotherapy Group. J Clin Oncol. 2006;24:3381–7.
46. Houghton J, George WD, Cuzick J, Duggan C, Fentiman IS, Spittle M, et al. Radiotherapy and tamoxifen in women with completely excised ductal carcinoma in situ of the breast in UK, Australia and New Zealand. Lancet. 2003;362:95–102.
47. Cuzick J, Sestak I, Pinder SE, Ellis IO, Forsyth S, Bundred NJ, et al. Effect of tamoxifen and radiotherapy in women with locally excised ductal carcinoma in situ: long-term results from the UK/ANZ DCIS trial. Lancet Oncol. 2011;12:21–9.
48. Emdin SO, Bengt G, Ringberg A, Sandelin K, Arnession L-G, Nordgren J, et al. SweDCIS: Radiotherapy after sector resection for ductal carcinoma in situ of the breast. Results of a randomised trial in a population offered mammography screening. Acta Oncol. 2006;45:536–43.
49. Page DL, Lagios MD. Pathologic analysis of the National Surgical Adjuvant Breast Project (NSABP) B-17 trial Unanswered questions remaining unanswered considering current concepts of ductal carcinoma in situ. Cancer. 1995;75:1219–22.
50. Morrow M. Understanding carcinoma in situ: a step in the right direction. Cancer. 1999;86:375–7.
51. Bartelink H, Horiot JC, Poortmans P, Struikmans H, Van de Bogaert W, Barillot I, et al. Recurrence rates after treatment of breast cancer with standard radiotherapy with or without an additional radiation. N Eng J Med. 2001;345:1378–87.
52. Bartelink H, Maingnon P, Poortmans P, Weitens C, Fourquet A, Jager J, et al. Whole breast irradiation with or without a boost for patients treated with breast-conserving surgery for early breast cancer. 20-year follow-up of a randomised phase 3 trial. Lancet Oncol. 2015;16:47–56.
53. Fisher B, Land S, Mamounas E, Dignam J, Fisher ER, Wolmark N. Prevention of invasive breast cancer in women with ductal carcinoma in situ: an update of the National Surgical Adjuvant Breast and Bowel Project experience. Semin Oncol. 2001;28: 400–18.
54. Holmberg L, Garmo H, Granstrand B, Ringberg A, Arnesson L-G, Sandelin PK, et al. Absolute risk reductions for local recurrence after postoperative radiotherapy after sector resection for ductal carcinoma in situ. J Clin Oncol. 2008;8:1247–52.
55. Wong JS, Kaelin CM, Troyan SL, Gadd MA, Gelman R, Lester SC et al. Prospective study of wide excision alone for ductal carcinoma in situ. J Clin Oncol. 2006;24:1031–6.
56. Solin LJ, Gray R, Hughes LL, Wood WC, Lowen MA, Badwe SS et al. Surgical excision without radiation for ductal carcinoma in situ of the breast: 12 year results from the ECOG-ACRIN E5194 study. J Clin Oncol. published ahead of print on Sept 14, 2015 as 10.1200/JCO.2015.60.8588.
57. Boxer MM, Delaney GP, Chua BH. A review of the management of ductal carcinoma in situ following breast conserving surgery. Breast. 2013;22:1019–25.
58. Cutuli B, Bernier J, Poortmans P. Radiotherapy for DCIS: an underestimated benefit? Radiother Oncol. 2014;112:1–8.
59. Abbott AM, Portschy PR, Lee C, Le Chap T, Han LK, Washington T, et al. Prospective multicentre trial evaluating balloon catheter partial breast irradiation for ductal carcinoma in situ. Int J Rad Oncol. 2013;87:494–8.
60. Strnad V, Ott OJ, Hildebrandt G, Kauer-Dorner D, Knauerhase H, Major T. 5-year results of accelerated partial breast irradiation using sole interstitial multicatheter brachytherapy versus whole-breast irradiation with boost after breast-conserving surgery for low-risk invasive and in-situ carcinoma of the female breast: a randomised, phase 3, non-inferiority trial. Lancet. 2016;387:229–38.
61. Allred DC, Anderson SJ, Paik S, Wickerham DL, Naqtegaal ID, Swain SM, et al. Adjuvant tamoxifen reduces subsequent breast cancer in women with oestrogen receptor positive ductal

carcinoma in situ: a study based on NSABP protocol B-24. J Clin Oncol. 2012;30:1268–73.
62. Petrelli F, Barni S. Tamoxifen added to radiotherapy and surgery for the treatment of ductal carcinoma in situ of the breast: a meta-analysis of 2 randomized trials. Radiother Oncol. 2011;10:195–9.
63. Davies C, Pan H, Godwin J, Gray R, Arriagada R, Raina V, et al. Adjuvant Tamoxifen: Longer against Shorter. (ATLAS) Collaborative Group. Longterm effects of continuing adjuvant tamoxifen to 10 years versus stopping at 5 years after diagnosis of oestrogen receptor positive breast cancer. ATLAS, a randomised trial. Lancet. 2013;381:805–16.
64. Abe O, et al. Overview of the randomized trials of radiotherapy in ductal carcinoma in situ of the breast. JNCI Monogr. 2010;41: 162–77.

Surgical Considerations in the Management of Primary Invasive Breast Cancer

14

Carissia Calvo and Ismail Jatoi

14.1 Introduction

Surgical considerations and standards of care in the management of breast cancer have transformed since the early nineteenth century as advances in the knowledge and treatment of breast cancer have emerged. Although significant progress has been made in the modern treatment of primary breast cancer owing to the integration of breast-conserving surgery, radiation, and systemic treatments, surgery remains a principal cornerstone in overall breast cancer management. The primary aim of this chapter was to highlight the historical background, modern recommendations, and continuing developments in the surgical treatment of primary breast cancer.

14.2 Historical Background

In the nineteenth century, German pathologist Rudolf Virchow (Fig. 14.1) studied the morbid anatomy of breast cancer. He undertook a series of postmortem dissections and postulated that breast cancer spreads along fascial planes and lymphatic channels [1]. Little importance was given to the hematogenous spread of cancer. Virchow's hypothesis influenced the work of the American surgeon, William Halsted (Fig. 14.2). In the late nineteenth century, Halsted described radical mastectomy (MT), which is performed for the treatment of breast cancer [2]. This operation removed the breast, the underlying pectoralis muscles, and the ipsilateral axillary lymph nodes. Thus, in keeping with the postulates of Virchow' s hypothesis, the lymphatic channels connecting the breast and axillary lymph nodes were extirpated *en bloc.* Halsted argued that resection of a node-negative breast cancer was curative, believing that such tumors were extirpated before they spread through the lymphatics. Halsted also maintained that the extent of both the MT and axillary dissection were important determinants of outcome. Therefore, breast cancer recurrence and distant metastases were often attributed to inadequate surgery.

By the early twentieth century, the radical MT had become widely accepted as the standard treatment for breast cancer. The risk of local recurrence was far less with the radical MT than with other contemporary procedures. The radical MT was also credited with improving survival from breast cancer during the early years of the twentieth century [3]. This improvement in survival was probably largely attributable to the effect of lead time bias, rather than to any advancement in surgical technique. Indeed, by the turn of the century, patients were seeking medical attention sooner (with smaller tumors).

One important observation was inconsistent with the Halsted paradigm. About 30 % of node-negative breast cancer patients die of metastatic disease within 10 years after surgery [4]. This finding suggested that the lymphatics are not the only source for the distant spread of cancer. Yet, most surgeons in the early twentieth century were not willing to discard the Halstedian concept that the distant spread of breast cancer occurs solely through the lymphatics. Some proposed that metastatic spread through the internal mammary and supraclavicular lymph node chains might account for distant relapse in women whose axilla were free of nodal involvement [5, 6]. Extirpation of these additional nodal chains failed to improve outcome however, and these more extensive lymphadenectomies were soon abandoned [7, 8].

The radical MT remained the cornerstone for the treatment of breast cancer for about the first three quarters of the twentieth century. Thereafter, the operation lost favor. By the latter half of the twentieth century, many surgeons regarded the radical MT as too debilitating, and several centers reported good outcome with less extensive surgery

C. Calvo
Department of Surgery, University of Texas Health Science Center, 7703 Floyd Curl Drive, San Antonio, TX 7738, USA
e-mail: calvoc@uthscsa.edu

I. Jatoi (✉)
Division of Surgical Oncology and Endocrine Surgery, University of Texas Health Science Center, 7703 Floyd Curl Drive, Mail Code 7738, San Antonio, TX 78229, USA
e-mail: Jatoi@uthscsa.edu

I. Jatoi and A. Rody (eds.), *Management of Breast Diseases*, DOI 10.1007/978-3-319-46356-8_14

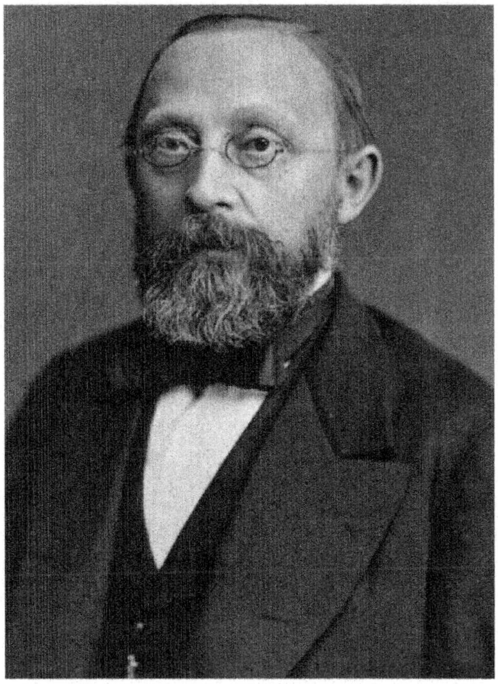

Fig. 14.1 Dr. Rudolph Virchow (courtesy of the national library of medicine archives)

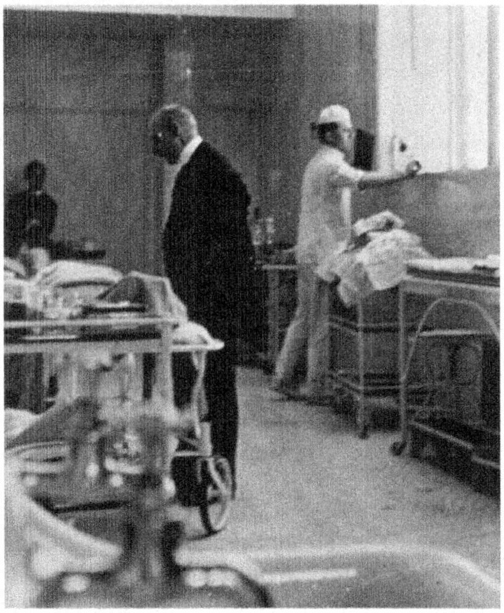

Fig. 14.2 Dr. William Halsted (courtesy of the national library of medicine archives)

[9, 10]. These lesser procedures included the modified radical MT (which spares the pectoralis muscles) and simple excision of the primary breast tumor. The trend toward less radical surgery was attributable to two important factors [11]. Firstly, surgeons during the latter half of the twentieth century were seeing patients with smaller tumors, and these were often amenable to local excision. Secondly, there were improvements in radiotherapy (RT) techniques, enabling tumoricidal doses to be delivered effectively without significant damage to surrounding tissues. Thus, many surgeons developed an interest in breast-conserving surgery (BCS), undertaken in conjunction with breast RT.

Skepticism concerning the merits of the Halsted radical MT surfaced in 1962, when Bloom et al. reported about the survival of 250 patients with primary breast cancer who received no treatment [12]. These patients were diagnosed clinically between the years 1805 and 1933 at the Middlesex Hospital in London, England, and the tissue diagnosis was established at autopsy. The survival rate of these untreated patients was almost identical to Halsted's patients who were treated with the radical MT. This seemed to suggest that surgery contributes little to reducing the risk of death from breast cancer but the impact of surgery 100 years ago might have been quite different from what it is today. Patients in the late nineteenth century generally presented with cancers at an advanced stage. In many instances, distant metastases were perhaps already present, and therefore, surgery might have had little impact on the natural history of the disease. In contrast, patients seen today generally present with early disease. Thus, in the absence of metastases, local therapy alone could cure some patients.

During the last 25 years, the tenets of the Halsted paradigm were put to test in several large, randomized prospective trials. These trials examined the effect of various surgical options in the treatment of breast cancer. None of these trials compared surgical treatment with any treatment, and so the true effect of surgery on breast cancer mortality was never established. The results of these trials suggested, however, that breast-conserving therapy (BCT) (partial removal of the breast in conjunction with RT) was a viable option for most women with breast cancer.

The National Surgical Adjuvant Breast Project-04 (NSABP-04) and King's/Cambridge trials randomized patients with clinically node-negative breast cancer to either early or delayed treatment of the axilla [13, 14]. In the NSABP-04 trial, 1665 clinically node-negative women received either no initial treatment to the axilla or initial treatment with either axillary lymph node dissection (ALND) or RT [13]. About 18 % of patients who received no initial axillary treatment developed axillary adenopathy and subsequently were treated with ALND. Yet, there was no significant difference in breast cancer mortality between patients in the three arms of the trial. In the King's/Cambridge trial, 2243 women with clinically node-negative breast cancer were randomly assigned to either total MT and immediate RT to the axilla or total MT and careful observation of the axilla [14]. In the group assigned to observation, RT was delayed until there was progression or recurrence of the disease in the axilla. No significant difference in breast cancer mortality was found between the two groups, however. The NSABP-04 and King's/Cambridge trials indicated that the

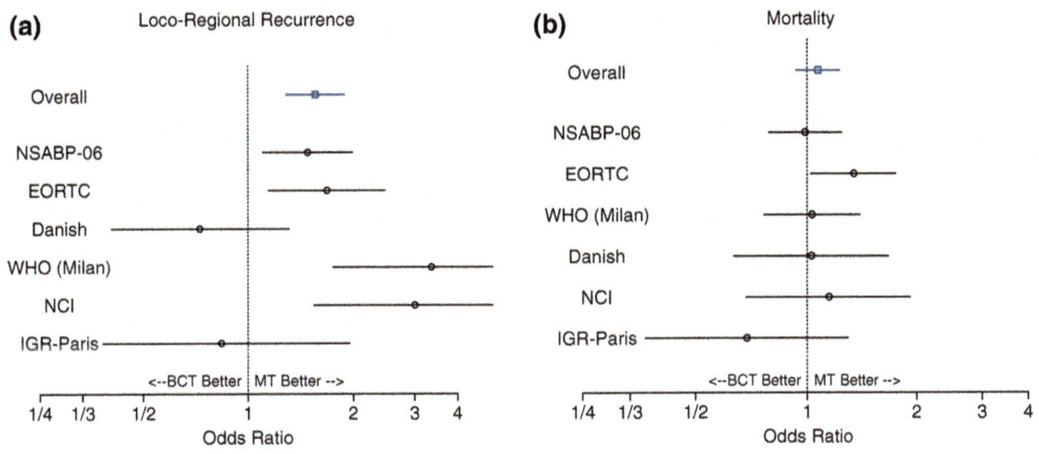

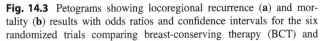

Fig. 14.3 Petograms showing locoregional recurrence (**a**) and mortality (**b**) results with odds ratios and confidence intervals for the six randomized trials comparing breast-conserving therapy (BCT) and mastectomy (MT) for early breast cancer. Reprinted with the permission from Jatoi and Proschan [28]

delayed treatment of the axilla does not adversely affect breast cancer mortality. This finding suggests that the axillary lymph nodes are not a nidus for the further spread of cancer, a finding that is inconsistent with the Halsted hypothesis.

Halsted also proposed that breast cancer is a locally progressive disease. He argued that metastases occurred by the contiguous and centrifugal spread of cancer from the primary tumor in the breast. If this were true, then the extent of the MT should influence survival. During the last 30 years, this hypothesis was tested in six large, randomized prospective trials. These were the Milan I, Institute of Gustave-Roussy (GR), NSABP-06, US National Cancer Institute, European Organization for the Research and Treatment of Cancer (EORTC), and Danish Group trials [15–20] (Fig. 14.3a, b). These trials compared either the radical MT or the modified radical MT with less extensive procedures (variously labeled as segmentectomy, lumpectomy, tylectomy, quadrantectomy, or wide local excision), undertaken in conjunction with an ALND. All these trials showed that the extent of the MT has no impact on breast cancer mortality.

The NSABP-06 was the largest of these six trials [17]. There were 1843 patients randomized to one of three groups: total MT and axillary dissection (modified radical MT), lumpectomy and axillary dissection, or lumpectomy and axillary dissection followed by breast RT. The NSABP-06 found no difference in survival between patients in the three arms of the study; however, the incidence of local breast tumor recurrence in the lumpectomy plus breast radiation group was significantly lower than in the lumpectomy group who received no radiation. Thus, RT is generally used today in conjunction with BCS in the treatment of primary breast cancer.

14.3 Local Recurrences

Local recurrences following total MT may occur on the chest wall; the skin overlying the chest wall; or the axillary, internal mammary, supraclavicular, and infraclavicular lymph nodes [21]. However, women treated with BCS are also at risk for recurrences in the ipsilateral breast [22]. Thus, breast cancer patients treated with BCS have, overall, a greater risk of local recurrence than those treated with total MT. For many years, Fisher argued that ipsilateral breast tumor recurrences following BCS are indicators of distant disease that is already present [23]. He argued that such recurrences were markers for poor prognosis but not the cause of the poor prognosis. Studies have shown that, following BCS, women who develop ipsilateral breast tumor recurrences have greater than a threefold increased risk of developing distant metastases when compared to those who do not develop such recurrences [24]. Also, patients who develop recurrences in the ipsilateral breast within 3–5 years following BCS seem to have a worse prognosis than those who develop such recurrences later [25].

Radiation therapy can reduce the risk of ipsilateral breast tumor recurrences. In the NSABP-06 study, the risk of ipsilateral breast tumor recurrences was about 40 % following lumpectomy and about 10 % following lumpectomy and RT [17]. For patients treated with total MT, the risk of ipsilateral breast tumor recurrences was essentially nil. Ipsilateral breast tumor recurrences are generally treated with salvage MT (total MT), and the 10-year actuarial survival for these patients is about 58 % [21]. In contrast, local recurrences in the chest wall, ipsilateral axilla, or supraclavicular and infraclavicular fossa carry a worse prognosis. More than 90 % of these patients will develop distant metastases, and most will die of their disease within 10 years after recurrence [26].

What factors influence the risk of ipsilateral breast tumor recurrence following BCS? Several investigators have addressed this question. Borger et al. studied 1026 patients treated at the Netherlands Cancer Institute with BCS and RT [27]. Univariate analysis showed that seven factors were associated with an increased risk of ipsilateral breast tumor recurrence: age, residual tumor at re-excision, histologic tumor type, presence of any components of carcinoma in situ component, vascular invasion, microscopic margin involvement, and whole-breast radiation dose. Only two factors remained independently significant after proportional hazard regression analysis: age and the presence of vascular invasion. Thus, ipsilateral breast tumor recurrence rates were 6 % for patients less than 40 years of age and 8 % for patients with tumors showing vascular invasion at 5 years. In the absence of these factors, the risk of ipsilateral breast tumor recurrence after BCS was only about 1 % at 5 years.

An overview of the six major randomized trials comparing MT versus BCT (BCS + RT) confirmed that there was a substantial increase in the risk of locoregional recurrence associated with BCT, pooled odds ratio 1.561, 95 % CI, 1.289–1.890; $p < 0.001$ [28] (Fig. 14.3a). Yet, in this analysis, there was no significant difference in mortality between the two groups, odds ratio 1.070, 95 % CI, 0.935–1.224; $p > 0.33$ (Fig. 14.3b). However, this meta-analysis may have lacked the statistical power to discern a small but significant effect of local recurrence on breast cancer mortality. Alternatively, competing causes of mortality (heart disease, stroke, etc.) may have obscured a potentially small effect of local recurrence on mortality in this meta-analysis. It should be noted that, in these trials, women were followed closely, and those who developed ipsilateral breast tumor recurrences following BCT were immediately treated with MT (salvage MT).

In recent years, there has been mounting evidence to indicate that local recurrences are indeed associated with an increase in breast cancer mortality. A pooled analysis of 15 trials comparing RT versus no RT after BCS showed that the omission of RT was associated with a threefold increase in ipsilateral breast tumor recurrences and a small (8.6 %) but statistically significant increase in mortality [29]. Also, the Early Breast Cancer Trialists' Collaborative Group (EBCTCG) reported the results of a collaborative meta-analysis of randomized trials of RT and various types of surgery for early breast cancer [30]. Comparisons were made between RT versus no RT, more surgery versus less surgery (with or without RT), and more surgery without RT versus less surgery with RT, etc. These investigators found that the avoidance of local recurrence, either in the conserved breast or elsewhere (chest wall, regional lymph nodes, etc.), was important in reducing breast cancer mortality. Over a 15-year period, one breast cancer death could be prevented for every four local recurrences avoided.

Turner et al. reported that women who carry a *BRCA* mutation (*BRCA1* or *BRCA2*) are more likely to develop ipsilateral breast tumor recurrences following BCS and RT [31]. However, the median time to ipsilateral breast tumor recurrence was 7.8 years for patients with *BRCA1* or *BRCA2* mutations, compared with 4.7 years for patients without such mutations. The longer time to recurrence in the carriers of these mutations suggests that these were second de novo primary tumors. The *BRCA* genes play an important role in DNA repair, and some studies seem to suggest that persons who carry mutations in these genes are extremely sensitive to the effects of RT [32]. Thus, one might speculate that RT administered following BCS may play a role in the development of de novo ipsilateral breast cancers in the carriers of *BRCA* mutations. Pierce and colleagues followed 160 BRCA carriers and 445 matched controls who underwent BCS following a diagnosis of breast cancer. These authors reported that mutation carriers who had not undergone oophorectomy were at increased risk for ipsilateral breast tumor recurrences, while those who had undergone oophorectomy were not [33]. Yet, BRCA mutation carriers also face a high risk of developing breast cancer in the contralateral breast, and many are now opting for contralateral prophylactic MT at the time of initial breast cancer diagnosis. A recent study found that BRCA mutation carriers in North America were more willing to accept contralateral prophylactic mastectomy following a breast cancer diagnosis than were their counterparts in Europe [34]. Large variations in the acceptance of contralateral prophylactic MT were reported, ranging from 0 % in Norway to 49.3 % in the USA.

14.4 Surgical Options

Today, a patient with primary breast cancer might consider three surgical options: modified radical MT, modified radical MT with contralateral prophylactic MT or BCS (Table 14.1). A modified radical MT refers to the removal of the breast and the ipsilateral lymph nodes (the sentinel lymph node is first removed, and if metastatic cancer is evident, then the patient generally undergoes an ALND). If the patient chooses this option, she can often avoid RT (although post-mastectomy RT is recommended for patients with large tumors (>5 cm) and/or extensive lymph node involvement [35]). Patients treated with the modified radical MT should generally be offered breast reconstructive surgery, which is discussed later. Also, some women with unilateral breast cancer might opt for a modified radical MT and a contralateral prophylactic MT (i.e., bilateral MT), particularly if they carry the BRCA 1 or BRCA 2 gene mutations or have anxiety over the possibility of developing a new cancer in the opposite breast.

Table 14.1 Surgical options for primary invasive breast cancer

Modified radical MT	Resection of entire breast
	Sentinel lymph node biopsy (SLNB)/axillary dissection
	Breast reconstruction
	Radiotherapy (RT) sometimes required
Modified radical MT and contralateral prophylactic MT	Resection of both breasts
	SLNB/axillary dissection on side containing the cancer
	Bilateral breast reconstruction
	RT sometimes required
Breast-conserving surgery	Resection of tumor and margin of normal tissue
	SLNB/axillary dissection
	RT generally required

Finally, a patient with unilateral breast cancer may choose to undergo a breast-conserving procedure along with removal of axillary lymph nodes. This is often the preferred option because it results in the best cosmetic and tactile outcome. If a patient elects this option, she will generally require RT to reduce the risk of ipsilateral breast tumor recurrence. However, lumpectomy plus adjuvant endocrine therapy alone (without RT) might be a suitable option for women 70 years of age or older with early estrogen-receptor-positive breast cancer [36].

Various terms are used to describe breast-conserving procedures, including segmental MT, lumpectomy, tylectomy, wide local excision, and quadrantectomy. Essentially, these terms refer to the extirpation of the breast tumor with various margins of normal breast tissue. The terms *segmental MT* and *lumpectomy are* used interchangeably. These terms refer to the resection of the breast tumor with enough surrounding normal tissue to result in microscopically tumor-free surgical margins. By definition, tumor cells may approach to within one cell's breadth of the surgical margin. The term *extended tylectomy* was used at the Guy's Hospital in London to describe resection of the breast tumor plus surrounding breast tissue within 3 cm of the tumor mass [37]. The microscopic status of the surgical margins was not defined. In the *quadrantectomy,* described by Veronesi et al. at the Tumor Institute of Milan, Italy, the entire quadrant of the breast containing the tumor is removed [15]. In the six randomized trials comparing BCT and MT, there was considerable heterogeneity with respect to the risk of ipsilateral breast tumor recurrence, and this was most likely attributable to variations in surgical procedures [28]. For example, in the Milan trial, patients treated with BCT underwent quadrantectomy (excision of the tumor with 2–3-cm margin of normal tissue around it), whereas in the Danish and US National Cancer Institute trials, a simple excision of the tumor (with no gross involvement of the margins) was performed.

After any breast-conserving procedure, RT is generally administered to eliminate occult tumor foci remaining in the ipsilateral breast. RT to the breast can be initiated 10–14 days after surgery. If chemotherapy is also planned, RT is postponed until one or more doses of chemotherapy are administered. RT is discussed in a separate chapter in this book.

Most patients with primary breast cancer are suitable candidates for BCS, but there are a few contraindications [31] (Table 14.2). These are only relative contraindications however, and each patient's circumstances should be examined closely [38]. For example, pregnant patients are generally advised not to undergo BCS because RT carries substantial risk to the fetus. Yet, it is important to remember that several months of chemotherapy are generally given before RT. Thus, if RT is to be administered after delivery, BCS is an acceptable option. Patients who have had previous RT to the breasts are also often advised not to undergo BCS. However, radiation oncologists may wish to consider the previous dose of radiation administered, and some of these patients might be successfully treated with BCS and RT. Additionally, certain coexisting medical problems, such as collagen vascular diseases, may adversely affect the cosmetic results after RT and thereby increase the risk of complications. Collagen vascular disease is an issue only when there is active disease.

Patients with large tumors often are advised to undergo a modified radical MT rather than a breast-conserving procedure [39]. The appropriate tumor size for BCS is poorly defined, however. The various clinical trials used different criteria to recruit patients for BCS. In the Milan trial, BCS was an option only for patients with tumors smaller than 2.5 cm, and those patients underwent excision of the entire quadrant of the breast (quadrantectomy) containing the tumor [15]. In the NSABP-06 trial, patients with tumors smaller than 4 cm were eligible for BCS (lumpectomy), whereas the subsequent NSABP trials accepted patients with

Table 14.2 Factors that may influence surgical option for primary breast cancer (breast-conserving surgery (BCS) vs. MT)

Patient preference	Multi-centricity
Pregnancy	Mutation carriers
Previous RT	
Active collagen vascular disease	
Tumor size in relation to breast size	
Multicentric disease	

tumors as large as 5 cm [17]. An important consideration is the size of the tumor in relation to the size of the breast. Today, in some centers, preoperative chemotherapy is used to decrease the size of large tumors, making BCS feasible for more women [40]. Thus, a patient with a large tumor and a small breast might be a suitable candidate for BCS if she is prepared to receive preoperative chemotherapy.

Some surgeons argue that BCS should be contraindicated if the tumor is close to or involves the nipple–areola complex. Yet, the nipple–areola complex can be easily excised along with the tumor. Although sacrifice of the nipple–areola complex may result in a cosmetic deformity, many women prefer this to losing the entire breast. Thus, the patient's wishes should be considered.

A patient with multicentric cancer (involving more than one quadrant of the breast) is generally not a suitable candidate for BCS. Careful physical examination of the breasts and a preoperative mammogram are helpful in determining the presence of multicentric disease. A patient with a suspicious breast mass should have a mammogram prior to any diagnostic biopsy. Mammograms obtained immediately after a breast biopsy are often difficult to interpret due to post-biopsy changes. Thus, if cancer is confirmed with a biopsy, a post-biopsy mammogram might make it difficult to determine whether a patient is a suitable candidate for a breast-conserving operation.

In recent years, breast magnetic resonance imaging (MRI) has been widely utilized in women with newly diagnosed breast cancers to help determine eligibility for BCT. MRI will occasionally identify additional cancer foci in either the ipsilateral or contralateral breast that are not evident on either clinical examination or mammography [41]. On the basis of MRI findings, MT (and even bilateral MT) might be recommended for patients who otherwise might have been considered suitable candidates for BCT. The use of breast MRI in the initial evaluation of women with primary breast cancer has therefore generated considerable controversy. Many investigators argue that the additional cancer foci detected on MRI might be adequately treated with RT and systemic therapy, and that the use of breast MRI needlessly increases MT rates. A retrospective study from the University of Pennsylvania compared women with early-stage breast cancer who underwent preoperative evaluation with or without breast MRI [42]. In this study, all women underwent BCT, but in some cases the eligibility for BCT was determined by MRI and conventional mammography, while in others it was determined by conventional mammography alone. The authors found that breast MRI at the time of initial diagnosis was not associated with improvements in outcome.

BCS is a more complex treatment than the modified radical MT. The procedure generally requires two separate incisions, one to remove the primary breast tumor and the other to remove the axillary lymph nodes. In addition, patients treated with BCS require postoperative RT. Nattinger et al. analyzed the US National Surveillance, Epidemiology, and End-Results Tumor Registry and found that, with the increased use of BCS, a greater number of patients were receiving inappropriate surgical treatment for primary breast cancer [43]. *Appropriate* surgical therapy was defined as either total MT with ALND (modified radical MT) or BCS with ALND and RT. During the period from 1983 through 1995, the proportion of women undergoing an inappropriate form of modified radical MT remained stable at 2.7 %. During this period, however, the proportion receiving an inappropriate form of BCS (omission of RT or ALND or both) increased from 10 % in 1989 to 19 % at the end of 1995.

Since publication of the results of the NSABP-06 trial, there has been a gradual increase in the use of BCS in the USA. There has also been considerable geographic variation in the acceptance of this procedure, however. Several years ago, Nattinger et al. reported that the frequency of BCS in the various states ranged from 3.5 to 21.2 % [44]. The highest frequency was reported in the mid-Atlantic (20 %) and New England states (17 %), and the lowest in the eastern (5.9 %) and western South-Central states (73 %). A similar geographic variation in the use of BCS was reported in an analysis of patients treated within the US Department of Defense (DoD) Healthcare System [45]. In the DoD system, physicians rotate through various hospitals in the USA and abroad. Yet, geographic variation in the use of BCS persists. Thus, patient preferences in various parts of the USA might differ, resulting in variation in the acceptance of one procedure over another.

In the USA, the use of unilateral MT for women with primary breast cancer declined from about 76.5 % in 1988 to 38 % in 2004, while use of BCS dramatically increased during this same period [46]. But this study also found that radiation is frequently omitted after BCS, particularly among racial/ethnic minorities and younger and older women. Paradoxically, in the USA, the use of bilateral mastectomies for early-stage unilateral breast cancer has more than doubled between the years 1998 and 2004 [47].

By 1990, 18 states had passed legislation requiring physicians to disclose options for the treatment of breast cancer. Nattinger et al. studied the effect of this legislation on the use of BCS [48]. They found that such legislation has only a small, transient effect on the rate of use of BCS. Dolan et al. reported that medically indigent women treated in public hospitals are less likely to receive BCS when compared with more affluent patients treated in private hospitals [49]. A recent study suggests that when fully informed of the two available options for the treatment of primary breast cancer (BCS or MT), many women will choose MT [50]. Women may choose MT for peace of mind or to avoid RT. Thus, several complex factors, and not insurance coverage alone, appear to be influencing trends in the surgical treatment of primary breast cancer.

14.4.1 Contralateral Prophylactic Mastectomy

Contralateral prophylactic mastectomy (CPM) refers to the surgical removal of the opposite, uninvolved breast in women diagnosed with unilateral breast cancer. A surprising trend toward the increased utilization of CPM began in the USA in the late 1990s (first reported in 2007) and is dramatically increasing worldwide. This trend is paradoxical as it exists in spite of an overall decrease in the risk of contralateral breast cancer development, which can be attributed to the widespread use of adjuvant systemic therapy for early-stage breast cancer. Thus, in recent years, the surgical treatment of breast cancer in the USA seems to be polarizing, with more and more women opting for either BCS or more aggressive surgery (bilateral MT), while use of unilateral MT diminishes.

There are several factors that may be attributed to the increased utilization of CPM. Firstly, there has been wider use of genetic testing for mutations such as BRCA1/BRCA2 that greatly increases the risk for contralateral breast cancer [51]. CPM is often recommended for women who harbor these mutations given the three- to fourfold increased risk for contralateral breast cancer development compared to the average risk patient. Secondly, wider use of preoperative breast MRI has improved the sensitivity of detection of potentially suspicious lesions in the contralateral breast and may thus prompt the decision toward CPM [52]. Recent evidence has supported that women who obtain a preoperative breast MRI are twice as likely to opt for CPM [53]. Additionally, increased use of CPM may be partially attributable to improvements in breast reconstruction techniques with some women opting for bilateral mastectomy with reconstruction over unilateral mastectomy with reconstruction on the premise of achieving better cosmetic symmetry [54]. Lastly, overestimation of the risk of development of contralateral breast cancer by patients themselves may potentially contribute to the recent trend toward CPM, despite the overall decreased rate of contralateral breast cancer development since the implementation of adjuvant systemic therapy (annual risk 0.1 % per year).

The impact of CPM on breast cancer mortality has never been studied in a randomized prospective trial. However, a large number of observational studies have suggested that CPM is associated with reductions in breast cancer specific and all-cause mortality (e.g., death from any cause) in women who are at an increased risk for developing contralateral breast cancer (BRCA1/BRCA2 mutation carriers as well as ER-negative tumors) as well as those with an average risk for the development of contralateral breast cancer (annual risk 0.1 % per year). It is important to note that datasets which form the basis for observational studies often omit important covariates, such as overall health and socioeconomic status/backgrounds, and these studies can therefore produce biased estimates of treatment effects. Close examination of the association between CPM and noncancer mortality, utilizing the 1998-2010 Surveillance, Epidemiology, and End-Results (SEER) dataset [55], confirmed that an association between CPM and reductions in breast cancer specific and all-cause mortality exists but, more importantly, demonstrated an even-stronger association between CPM and reduced noncancer mortality (e.g., death from a cause other than cancer) [56]. The overall stronger association between CPM and noncancer mortality is suggestive of the presence of selection bias in that unmeasured confounders may have contributed to the previously identified associations between CPM and lower breast cancer specific as well as all-cause mortality. Potential confounders that may influence preferential selection for CPM include generally healthier women (better able to tolerate a longer surgical procedure) or women from higher socioeconomic backgrounds.

Thus, the increased utilization of CPM (bilateral mastectomy for the treatment of unilateral breast cancer) is difficult to justify in most cases. CPM might be justifiable in women who harbor mutations (such as the BRCA 1 or BRCA 2) or in women who have previously received mantle radiation, where risk of developing contralateral breast cancer is high, but otherwise CPM should generally be discouraged.

14.4.2 Breast Reconstructive Surgery

For some patients with primary breast cancer, BCS is not a suitable option. As mentioned previously, for some pregnant patients, those with large or multicentric cancers, patients who have been previously treated with RT to the breast, and those with active collagen vascular disease, BCS might not be suitable. These patients are often advised to undergo modified radical MT (total breast removal and ALND). Most of these patients are good candidates for breast reconstructive surgery, which may be performed either at the time of surgery for primary breast cancer (immediate reconstruction) or later (delayed reconstruction). For several years, there were concerns that immediate reconstructive surgery might mask locoregional recurrences and thereby contribute to a worse outcome [57]. Thus, many investigators recommended delayed reconstruction; however, studies suggest that immediate reconstruction does not adversely affect outcome [58, 59]. Furthermore, immediate reconstruction allows two procedures (the cancer operation and reconstruction) to be performed with the use of one anesthetic and might even be associated with less psychosocial morbidity [60].

Several options are available for breast reconstruction, including the placement of implants or the creation of latissimus dorsi myocutaneous, transverse rectus abdominis myocutaneous (TRAM) and free flaps. Additionally, the deep inferior epigastric artery perforator (DIEP) flap has been gaining popularity in recent years [61]. A detailed review of breast reconstruction is found in a separate chapter in this text and in surgical atlases [62].

Reconstruction with breast implants is used widely [63]. Several methods are now available, including permanent implants, permanent expandable implants, and serial expansion of tissue with an expandable implant followed by implant exchange. Tissue expanders are placed beneath the pectoral muscles and then gradually inflated over several weeks by injecting saline through a subcutaneous port. Once a skin mound is produced that is slightly larger than required, a permanent implant is inserted. Tissue expanders are feasible only for women with small- or medium-sized breasts who have not had prior skin radiation. Both silicone gel and saline implants have been used. There have been concerns that silicone gel implants may result in an increased risk of connective tissue disorders. Indeed, this concern has resulted in considerable litigation and debate [64]. Several studies, however, failed to demonstrate any association between silicone implants and connective tissue disorders [65, 66].

A breast mound can be refashioned using a myocutaneous flap, where skin and muscle from one anatomic region are transferred to the chest wall, with the vascular pedicle remaining attached. The latissimus dorsi myocutaneous flap is quite popular and is suitable for patients with large breasts or who have been previously treated with RT [67]. Thus, it is often used in women who have had RT as part of BCS and who subsequently develop a recurrence requiring salvage MT. Unfortunately, it does not contain sufficient tissue bulk, and so an implant is generally required beneath the flap.

The TRAM has a greater risk of potential complications than does the latissimus dorsi flap [62]. It has several advantages as well however, and is now the most commonly used flap in the USA. The TRAM flap provides sufficient bulk of tissue so that an implant beneath the flap is not necessary. The TRAM flap is useful for patients with a moderate or excessive amount of lower abdominal fat who require additional soft tissue on the chest wall. Thus, it not only provides sufficient tissue for breast reconstruction, but also results in an abdominoplasty.

Finally, a breast mound can be refashioned using free flaps; the free TRAM flap is the most popular [68]. In a free flap, the skin and underlying muscle are detached from their vascular pedicle, and microvascular techniques are used to reestablish the blood supply once the flap is placed on the chest wall. The free TRAM flap has several advantages over the standard TRAM flap. Less rectus abdominis muscle is required, and the medial contour of the breast generally looks better because a tunnel for the vascular pedicle is not required. Surgeons must have special expertise in performing microvascular procedures.

Among women treated with MT, less than 20 % will undergo breast reconstruction [69]. In 1999, the Women's Health and Cancer Rights Act (WHCRA) was implemented, mandating insurance coverage for breast reconstruction after MT, and additional legislation was passed in 2001, imposing penalties on noncompliant insurers [70]. However, this legislation has not significantly increased the overall use of breast reconstruction in the USA or reduced variations across geographic regions and patient subgroups.

14.5 Management of the Axilla

Since the late nineteenth century, breast cancer surgery has been closely linked to surgery of the axilla. Today, axillary surgery remains an integral part of BCS and the modified radical MT. Nonetheless, surgical management of the axilla is a topic of intense controversy. Axillary lymph node metastases are no longer considered a prerequisite for distant metastases. Thus, the impact of axillary surgery on survival, local control, and staging is frequently debated.

ALND refers to the extirpation of lymph nodes in the axilla. The lymph nodes in the axilla are divided into three compartments based on their anatomic relationship to the pectoralis minor muscle [71]. Lymph nodes lateral to the pectoralis minor muscle are classified as level I nodes, those posterior to its lateral and medial borders are classified as level II nodes, and those medial to the muscle are classified as level III nodes. A *complete* ALND refers to the extirpation of lymph nodes from all three compartments. In contrast, a *partial* ALND refers to the extirpation of lymph nodes only from levels I and II, and axillary sampling indicates only resection of the level I nodes.

Metastases to the axillary lymph nodes generally occur in an orderly fashion. Thus, lymph nodes in level I are generally involved first, followed by involvement of nodes in level II and then level III. *Skip metastases* indicate the involvement of lymph nodes at level II or level III but not level I; these occur rarely. Veronesi et al. studied the distribution of nodal metastases in 539 patients who underwent complete ALND [72]. Level I nodes were involved in 58 % of patients, levels I and II in 22 %, and all three levels in 16 %. In their series, skip metastases were present in only 4 % of cases. Today, most authorities recommend extirpation of lymph nodes from levels I and II (a partial ALND); ten or more nodes are usually removed [73]. A partial ALND correctly stages 96 % of patients with primary breast cancer as either node-positive or node-negative and rarely gives rise to significant lymphedema of the upper extremity. The 4 % false-negative rate associated with a partial ALND is attributable to skip metastases. This false-negative rate can be further reduced with resection of nodes from levels I–III (complete ALND), but this may increase the risk of upper-extremity lymphedema.

The technique of partial ALND is discussed in surgical atlases [62]. Essentially, the procedure involves resection of lymph nodes superiorly to the level of the axillary vein, laterally to the latissimus dorsi muscle and medially to the medial border of the pectoralis minor muscle. Particular attention should be paid to identifying the long thoracic and thoracodorsal nerves. The long thoracic nerve (nerve of Bell) runs along the lateral aspect of the chest wall and supplies the serratus anterior muscle. Injury to this nerve results in a *winged scapula.* The thoracodorsal nerve accompanies the subscapular artery along the posterior aspect of the axilla and supplies the latissimus dorsi muscle.

What impact does ALND have on survival, local control, and staging in patients with primary breast cancer? In recent years, several clinical trials have shed some light on this question. The impact of ALND on the management of patients with primary breast cancer remains a contentious issue.

14.5.1 Survival

For many years, the ALND was considered an important determinant of survival for patients with primary breast cancer. Halsted and his disciples fostered this notion more than 100 years ago, arguing that breast cancer spreads first to the regional lymph nodes and then to distant sites. Subsequently, some investigators provided retrospective data suggesting that the extent of the ALND does influence survival for patients with primary breast cancer. Such data are misleading, because there is no accounting for a *stage migration effect.* Consider, as an example, a patient with a 1.5-cm tumor and one metastatic lymph node to the axilla. Surgeon A may perform an extensive lymph node dissection and remove that node. On the other hand, surgeon B may perform a less extensive lymph node dissection and fail to uncover the metastatic node. Thus, if treated by surgeon A, this patient would be diagnosed as having stage II breast cancer. If treated by surgeon B, the same patient would be diagnosed as having stage I disease. When survival rates are compared for any given stage, it may seem that patients treated by surgeon A do better, but this may be attributable to the stage migration effect rather than any therapeutic benefit of the more extensive lymph node dissection.

The best way to determine whether the ALND has any effect on mortality is to compare treatment with ALND and without ALND in a randomized prospective trial. Such a study has never been conducted, although the results of the NSABP-04 and the King's/Cambridge trials, discussed already, indicate that the delayed treatment of the axilla has no effect on breast cancer mortality [13, 14]. The results of these trials might be interpreted to mean that the axillary lymph nodes are not a nidus for the further spread of cancer. Nonetheless, some investigators argue that the NSABP04 and King's/Cambridge trials did not include sufficient numbers of patients to detect small differences in survival between those randomized to either early or delayed treatment of the axilla [74]. Additionally, meta-analyses of randomized trials seem to suggest that there is a survival benefit associated with ALND, but this benefit might diminish in women who receive adjuvant systemic therapy [30, 75].

14.5.2 Axillary Relapse

Axillary lymph node metastasis is found in 35–40 % of patients with palpable breast cancers [76]. In many instances, nodal involvement is not clinically evident when the patient first presents with primary breast cancer. Indeed, up to 30 % of clinically node-negative patients are shown to have nodal involvement following ALND [77]. In the absence of ALND, many of these patients eventually would develop clinical evidence of nodal involvement. The NSABP-04 and King's/Cambridge trials provide important information on the effect of axillary treatment in clinically node-negative patients. These trials indicate that RT and ALND are equally effective in achieving local control of the axilla. In the NSABP-04 trial, clinically node-negative patients with primary breast cancer received either no treatment to the axilla or treatment with ALND or RT [13]. About 18 % of the patients who received no initial axillary treatment went on to develop axillary adenopathy within 5 years. In contrast, axillary adenopathy developed in only 2 % of patients whose axilla had been treated. Similar results were reported in the King's/Cambridge trial, where clinically node-negative patients were randomized to receive total MT, and RT to the axilla or total MT and observation of the axilla [14]. Taken together, these studies suggest that treatment of the axilla (with either ALND or RT) will reduce the 5-year risk of axillary relapse by about 90 %.

The importance of axillary treatment on local control is also reported in retrospective studies. Baxter et al. reviewed the records of 112 breast cancer patients who underwent lumpectomy without ALND [78]. When these patients first presented with breast cancer, they had no evidence of axillary lymph node involvement on clinical examination. During the subsequent 10-year period, about 28 % of these patients developed axillary adenopathy. Axillary adenopathy developed in 10 % of patients who presented with tumors 1 cm or less in diameter, in 26 % of those who presented with tumors 1.1–2.0 cm, and in 33 % of those with primary tumors greater than 2.1 cm in diameter.

The extent of the ALND seems to influence the risk of axillary relapse. Graverson et al. reviewed the records of 3128 patients with primary breast cancer who were clinically node-negative at initial presentation [79]. The 5-year risk of axillary relapse ranged from 19 % when no nodes were removed to 3 % when more than five nodes were removed. In the NSABP-04 study, no patient who had more than six nodes removed developed a relapse in the axilla. Thus, an adequate ALND is essential in reducing the risk of relapse in the axilla.

Axillary relapse is generally considered a marker of tumor biology, indicating an increased risk of distant metastasis and death. These relapses are not considered the cause of poor prognosis. Yet, many women are emotionally devastated following axillary relapse. Additionally, axillary relapses can cause significant morbidity. Major vessels and nerves of the axilla sometimes are invaded by the tumor, causing lymphedema or pain. In such instances, the axilla is difficult to manage. Surgical clearance of such axilla often is associated with increased morbidity. Thus, adequate treatment of the axilla at the time of initial diagnosis of primary breast cancer is important.

14.5.3 Staging

For patients with primary breast cancer, clinical assessment of the axilla is notoriously inaccurate. About 30 % of patients with palpable axillary nodes prove to be node-negative following ALND, and about 30 % of clinically node-negative patients prove to have nodal involvement [77]. Thus, the ALND traditionally played a vital role in staging patients with primary breast cancer (as either node-negative or node-positive).

The prognostic significance of nodal metastasis is poorly understood. For many years, physicians assumed that nodal status was simply a chronological variable. Thus, it was argued that node-positive patients fare worse than node-negative patients because their cancers are discovered later in their natural history. However, a study using the San Antonio Tumor registry seemed to suggest that nodal status is also a marker of tumor biology, because nodal status at initial diagnosis was found to also predict outcome after relapse [80]. In that study, patients with four or more involved nodes at initial diagnosis were found to have a significantly worse outcome after relapse compared with node-negative cases. Additionally, node-positive, high-risk tumors (>2 cm, ER-negative, high grade, and node-positive) are more common in younger patients (with a peak age of onset at 50 years), while node-negative, low-risk tumors (<2 cm, ER-positive, low grade, and node-negative) tend to occur later in life (with a peak age of onset at 70 years) [81]. This observation is also consistent with the notion that nodal status is a predictor of tumor biology and not simply tumor chronology.

The importance of ALND as a staging procedure was underscored in a study from the Institute Curie in Paris, France [82]. In that study, 658 breast cancer patients treated with lumpectomy and breast RT were randomly assigned to either ALND or axillary RT. Adjuvant chemotherapy was administered to a few of these patients, and the decision to administer adjuvant therapy was based on nodal status. However, nodal status was not assessed in patients whose axillae were treated with RT, and so none of those patients received adjuvant chemotherapy. There was a small but significantly greater overall 5-year survival rate ($p > 0.014$) in the group treated with ALND (96.6 %) compared with the group treated with axillary RT (92.6 %). Many investigators attribute this small benefit to adjuvant chemotherapy. Therefore, if nodal status will influence the decision to administer adjuvant systemic therapy, the axilla should be managed with ALND and not with RT.

Node-positive patients have a worse prognosis than node-negative patients. Nodal status, however, does not predict response to therapy. Indeed, for both node-negative and node-positive patients, adjuvant systemic therapy reduces the annual odds of relapse and death by approximately 30 and 25 %, respectively [83], although the absolute benefit of adjuvant systemic therapy is greater in node-positive patients because their risk of relapse and death is greater. As an example, consider two groups of breast cancer patients: a node-positive group with a 60 % risk of death from breast cancer over the next 10 years and a node-negative group with a 20 % risk of death. For both groups, the appropriate systemic therapy would reduce the risk of death from breast cancer by about 25 %. For this node-positive group, however, the absolute benefit would be 15 % (25 % of 60 % is 15 %), whereas for this node-negative group, the absolute benefit would be only 5 % (25 % of 20 % is 5 %). Thus, nodal status provides important information not only about prognosis, but also about the impact of adjuvant systemic therapy. An older woman with a good prognosis, node-negative tumor might be less willing to accept the toxicity of systemic therapy compared with a younger woman with a poor prognosis, node-positive tumor. However, in more recent years, the adjuvant treatment of breast cancer has been increasingly based on tumor predictive factors (ER status and HER2 status), which determine the responsiveness of a particular tumor to a specific treatment [84]. Thus, endocrine therapy (either tamoxifen or aromatase inhibitors) is administered to patients with ER-positive tumors, and Herceptin is administered to patients with HER2-positive tumors.

14.6 Sentinel Lymph Node Biopsy

The ALND is not without risks. The procedure is associated with wound infections and morbidity of the upper extremity. Wound infection rates between 8 and 19 % have been reported, but the reasons for this are poorly understood [85–87]. Some investigators speculate that the high rate of axillary wound infection might be due to the dead space beneath devascularized skin flaps or to an altered local immune response from disruption of local lymphatics. The ALND is also associated with significant morbidity of the upper extremity. In one series, the following upper-extremity complications were reported: paresthesia in 70 % of patients, pain in 33 %, weakness in 25 %, arm lymphedema in 10 %, and stiffness in 10 % [88]. Today, more than half of the patients with primary breast cancer are node-negative. If identified appropriately, these patients could be spared the potential morbidity associated with ALND. In recent years, attention has turned to sentinel lymph node biopsy (SLNB) as a means of achieving this goal.

The sentinel lymph node is the first node to receive lymphatic drainage from a tumor. For any nodal basin, one might assume that if the sentinel lymph node is free of metastatic tumor, then all other nodes in the basin should be free of tumor as well. Alternatively, involvement of the sentinel lymph node may mean that other nodes in the basin are involved. Thus, the SLNB is a diagnostic test that is useful in determining the status of the regional lymph nodes. This technique allows the surgeon to determine the status of the regional lymph nodes and avoid the morbidity associated with a more extensive lymph node dissection. For patients with primary breast cancer, the contraindications to SLNB include the presence of palpable axillary lymph node metastasis and prior breast or axillary surgery that might interfere with lymphatic drainage [89].

The SLNB technique was first described by Cabanas in 1977 as a means of assessing patients with penile carcinoma who might benefit from inguinofemoroiliac dissection [90]. Subsequently, Morton et al. demonstrated the feasibility and accuracy of SLNB for nodal staging in melanoma. [91]. More recently, SLNB has been widely used to stage patients with primary breast cancer, with the goal of reducing the morbidity of ALND [92]. Once identified, the sentinel node is excised and sent for histopathologic evaluation. Several studies have shown that the SLNB is quite accurate in predicting the status of the axillary lymph nodes [93, 94]. Surgeons can identify the first draining (sentinel) lymph node by injecting blue dye or radioactive colloid intradermally around the primary tumor. Subareolar injection appears to be as accurate as peri-tumoral injection [95]. In fact, for nonpalpable, mammographically detected cancers, subareolar injection might be preferable. There has also been debate as to whether injection with radioactive colloid and blue dye is more accurate than injection with blue dye alone as a means of identifying the sentinel node. Morrow et al. compared the two methods in a randomized trial and found that they were equally effective [96]. Thus, the preferences of the surgeon determine which method is used.

Giuliano et al. compared 134 patients with primary breast cancer who received standard ALND with 164 patients who underwent SLNB followed by completion ALND [97]. The reported incidences of nodal metastasis were 29 and 42 %. Thus, the reported incidence of node-positive cases is greater with SLNB than with standard ALND. Following ALND, one or two sections of each nonsentinel lymph node are generally examined with routine hematoxylin and eosin (H and E) staining; however, pathologists pay more attention to the sentinel lymph node. These nodes often are evaluated with multiple sectioning, H and E staining and immunohistochemical staining for cytokeratin. Thus, the SLNB results in a focused histopathologic evaluation of a single lymph node, and the probability of identifying micrometastases is thereby increased.

The false-negative rate of SLNB might be as high as 10 %, compared with 4 % following a level I and II ALND [98]. The false-negative rate refers to the percentage of patients with nodal metastases who are incorrectly designated as node-negative. False-negatives may lead to incorrect decisions concerning adjuvant therapy, thereby affecting outcome. These and other concerns about SLNB will be addressed in ongoing trials comparing long-term outcome following SLNB or ALND. However, randomized trials have now shown that SLNB can significantly reduce the morbidity associated with ALND [99–101]. SLNB has therefore been widely accepted now in the management of early breast cancer.

14.6.1 Sentinel Lymph Node Biopsy Versus Axillary Lymph Node Dissection

SLNB has now become an integral part of the conservative treatment of early breast cancer. Multiple published single institutional, multi-institutional, and prospective randomized controlled studies have exhibited the safety of omitting ALND in women who are identified to have a negative SLNB (free of metastatic disease). The gold standard for achievement of locoregional control in those patients who are identified to have metastatic disease on SLNB has, until recently, been completion ALND. However, in approximately 40–60 % of patients with clinically node-negative disease, the sentinel node is identified as the only involved node [102]. Consequently, ALND may be viewed as overtreatment in a large majority of clinically node-negative patients, particularly when taking into account potential long-term complications of lymphedema, pain, and reduced upper-extremity mobility.

The American College of Surgeons Oncology Group (ACOSOG) Z0011 trial examined the effect on local–regional control in patients with early-stage breast cancer and positive SLNB who received completion ALND versus no further axillary treatment [103]. In the study, 856 patients with T1 or T2 N0 M0 disease treated with SLNB and lumpectomy were randomized to undergo completion ALND or no further axillary surgery after identification of sentinel node-positive metastatic disease. Women with clinically positive nodal disease (palpable lymphadenopathy), matted notes, or gross extranodal disease were excluded from the study as were patients identified to have a high tumor burden (3 or more positive sentinel nodes) on SLNB. Only 1.8 % of the patients who received SLNB alone (no further axillary surgery) were identified to have local recurrence at a medial follow-up of 6.3 years, compared with 3.6 % on the group that received standard completion ALND ($P = 0.11$). Regional recurrences were further noted to be similar between the two groups with 0.9 % in the group that underwent SLNB with no further axillary surgery and 0.5 % in the ALND group ($P = 0.45$). No significant difference in the locoregional recurrence free survival rate was noted between the two groups. The ACOSOG Z0011 study thus showed that SLNB without completion ALND in patients with early-stage breast cancer treated with breast-conserving therapy, whole-breast irradiation, as well as adjuvant systemic therapy can offer excellent locoregional control.

With the development of sentinel lymph node biopsy came more comprehensive methods of evaluating the sentinel lymph node for disease. Tumor-involved sentinel nodes can now be further classified into those with macrometastasis (>2 mm in diameter), micrometastasis (≥0.2–2 mm in diameter), and isolated tumor cells (ITCs) (<0.2 mm in diameter) [104]. Although the overall prognostic/clinical significance of micrometastasis and ITCs remains uncertain, completion ALND for patients with such low sentinel node tumor burdens is a controversial topic. Wherein the ACOSOG Z0011 trial evaluated SLNB in patients with macrometastasis, the International Breast Cancer Study Group (IBCSG) Trial 23-01 sought to compare outcomes in randomized patients with sentinel node micrometastasis and ITCs who received standard completion ALND versus no further treatment [105]. The study evaluated 931 clinically node-negative women with a primary breast tumor of <5 cm in maximum diameter who were found to have one or more micrometastatic (≥0.2–2 mm) foci in the sentinel node, without macrometastatic disease. The 5-year disease-free survival rate was noted to be 84.4 % (95 % CI, 80.7–88.1 %) for those patients who underwent ALND and 87.8 % (95 % CI, 84.4–91.2 %) for those who had no further axillary treatment. Additionally, the reported 5-year overall survival rate was 97.6 % (95 % CI, 96.0–99.2 %) for the ALND group and 97.5 % (95 % CI, 95.8–99.1 %) for the SLNB only (no further axillary treatment) group. No significant difference in either disease-free survival or overall survival was noted between the two groups. The study further demonstrated a low <1 % rate of regional recurrence in the group randomized to receive no further axillary treatment.

The AATRM trial additionally evaluated the notion that SLNB and close clinical follow-up alone can be safely utilized in women with early-stage breast cancer identified to have sentinel micrometastasis, specifically [106]. The prospective clinical trial randomized 233 women with newly diagnosed early-stage breast cancer (primary tumor <3.5 cm, N0, M0) who were identified to have micrometastic foci on SLNB to receive standard completion ALND versus clinical follow-up (no further axillary treatment). A total of four patients were identified to have disease recurrence over a 5-year period: 1 of 108 (1 %) women randomized to the ALND group and 3 of 119 women in the group that received SLNB and no further axillary treatment. In accordance with the results of the IBCSG 23-01 trial, no significant difference in disease-free survival was identified between the two groups ($P = 0.325$).

Conclusively, the IBCSG 23-01 and AATRM trials provided further evidence to support the recent ACOGSOG Z0011 findings that SLNB alone is safe in clinically node-negative patients with early-stage breast cancer and a low burden of positive sentinel node metastasis, provided they receive traditional whole-breast irradiation and systemic adjuvant treatment. Collectively, the ACOSOG Z0011, IBCSG 23-01, AATRM, and AMAROS (discussed below) trials have lead to a change in the clinical management of early-stage breast cancer patients with positive SNLB.

While the American Society of Clinical Oncology has recommended that ALND can be safely avoided in patients with 1–2 sentinel node macrometastases provided they undergo conventional whole-breast irradiation following breast-conserving surgery, based on the results of the Z0011 trial, other professional societies have criticized the study secondary to its lack of generalizability and lack of radiation therapy quality assurance. Specifically, the results of the Z0011 study are not applicable to mastectomy patients. An ongoing randomized, multi-center, noninferiority trial known as the UK–Austria New Zealand (UK-ANZ) "POsitive Sentinel NOde: Adjuvant therapy alone versus adjuvant therapy plus Clearance or axillary radiotherapy" trial (POSNOC) seeks to specifically address the limitations of the Z0011 study by evaluating patients undergoing both breast-conserving surgery and mastectomy [107]. One thousand nine hundred participants with uni-focal or multi-focal invasive breast cancer (primary lesion ≤5 cm) identified to have 1–2 positive sentinel nodes with macrometastases will be randomized to receive either adjuvant systemic therapy alone (chemotherapy and/or endocrine therapy; no further axillary specific treatment) versus adjuvant therapy plus ALND or axillary radiotherapy. The POSNOC trial will additionally include a radiotherapy quality assurance program. The primary designated end-point of the study is axillary recurrence at 5 years with secondary end-points including arm morbidity, quality of life, locoregional recurrence, and survival/economic evaluation. The results of the study will hopefully provide further evidence to clarify the safety and generalizability of the Z0011 study results.

14.6.2 Radiotherapy of the Axilla

Evidence from the NSABP-04 trial revealed that radiotherapy of the axilla has an equivalent rate (4 %) of axillary recurrence in comparison with ALND; however, this primary aim of this study, as previously discussed, was to evaluate early versus delayed treatment of the axilla. The multicenter, phase 3 noninferiority EORTC 10981-22023 AMAROS (After Mapping of the Axilla Radiotherapy or Surgery) trial sought to further evaluate the efficacy of axillary radiotherapy in comparison with ALND in achieving regional control by randomizing clinically node-negative patients with T1-2 breast cancer and a positive SNLB to either axillary lymph node dissection or axillary radiotherapy [108]. The results of study revealed a noninferior five-year axillary recurrence rate in the axillary RT group (1.19 %; 95 % CI, 0.31–2.08 %) in comparison with that in the ALND group (0.43 %; 95 % CI, 0.00–0.92 %). No significant difference in disease-free survival and overall survival between the two treatment groups was noted. The study thus demonstrated that for women with early-stage breast cancer and a clinically node-negative axilla who are recommended to undergo further axillary treatment (based on tumor size, grade, vascular invasion, and/or extra-capsular extension of tumor cells), axillary RT can be offered over ALND as it provides comparable regional control with considerably less morbidity secondary to development of lymphedema (Table 14.3).

14.6.3 Axillary Surgery in the Neo-Adjuvant Chemotherapy Setting

Neo-adjuvant chemotherapy is increasingly utilized for the treatment of early-stage breast cancer as it often allows for downstaging of the primary tumor and thus increases the likelihood of breast-conserving surgery. Among patients who present with clinical node-positive disease and receive neo-adjuvant chemotherapy, only 50–60 % are found to have residual axillary nodal disease. While sentinel lymph node biopsy has been established as a reliable means for staging the axilla while offering considerably less morbidity than axillary lymph node dissection, ideal timing for performance of SLNB for patients treated with neo-adjuvant chemotherapy is controversial. The prospective, multicenter cohort

Table 14.3 Studies evaluating sentinel lymph node biopsy

Trial	Number of patients	Design	Sentinel node metastases evaluated
ACOSOG Z0011	856	Sentinel node-positive: randomized to ALND versus not	Micrometastasis, macrometastasis
AMAROS	1425	Sentinel node-positive: randomized to ALND versus axillary radiotherapy	Micrometastasis, macrometastasis
AATRM	233	Sentinel node-positive: randomized to ALND versus not	Micrometastasis
IBCSG 23-01	931	Sentinel node-positive: randomized to ALND versus not	Micrometastasis, ITCs
POSNOC	1900 planned	Sentinel node-positive: randomized to adjuvant systemic therapy alone versus adjuvant systemic therapy + axillary treatment (either ALND or radiotherapy)	Macrometastasis

"SENTinel Neo-Adjuvant" (SENTINA) study sought to evaluate the false-negative rate of SLNB after administration of neo-adjuvant chemotherapy in clinically node-positive women as well as clinically node-negative women with positive sentinel nodes [109]. The study allocated patients into four treatment arms: Arm A consisted of patients with clinically node-negative disease who were found to have a negative SLNB prior to neo-adjuvant chemotherapy and received no further axillary treatment; arm B consisted of clinically node-negative patients identified to have a positive sentinel node before administration of neo-adjuvant chemotherapy who subsequently underwent a second SLNB after completing neo-adjuvant chemotherapy; arm C consisted of clinically node-positive (N1 or N2) patients who converted to a clinically negative axilla after neo-adjuvant chemotherapy and underwent both a SLNB and an ALND; and arm D consisted of node-positive patients who remained node-positive after neo-adjuvant chemotherapy and thus underwent gold-standard completion ALND. The sentinel lymph node detection rate was noted to be 99.1 % (95 % CI, 98.3–99.6 %) in clinically node-negative women who underwent SLNB before neo-adjuvant chemotherapy (arms A and B), whereas the detection rate was significantly lower at 80.1 % (95 % CI, 76.6–83.2 %) in patients who underwent SLNB after neo-adjuvant chemotherapy. Additionally, no more than two-thirds of sentinel nodes [detection rate 60.8 % (95 % CI, 55.6–65.9 %; 219 of 360)] were successfully detected in patients who underwent a second SLNB after neo-adjuvant chemotherapy (arm B). The false-negative rate was noted to be 14.2 % (95 % CI, 9.9–19.4 %) for patients who converted from a clinically node-positive to a clinically node-negative axilla after neo-adjuvant chemotherapy (arm C).

The ACOSOG Z1071 (Alliance) trial further sought to evaluate whether SLNB could be utilized for axillary staging following neo-adjuvant chemotherapy in women with initial node-positive cancer by determining its false-negative rate (FNR) [110]. The acceptable FNR has consistently been accepted as ≤10 %, based on the established rate for women with clinically node-negative disease undergoing SLNB. Seven hundred and one women with N1 or N2 disease were enrolled in the study and underwent both SLNB and ALND after completion of neo-adjuvant chemotherapy. A complete nodal pathologic complete response (pCR) rate of 41 % (95 % CI, 36.7–45.3 %) was identified. In concordance with findings from the SENTINA trial, the phase two clinical study demonstrated a FNR of 12.6 % (90 % Bayesian credible interval, 9.85–16.05 %) in women with cN1 disease who had at least 2 or more sentinel nodes examined, suggesting that SLNB cannot reliably detect the presence of all axillary lymph node metastasis following chemotherapy administration. One might speculate that the decreased accuracy of SLNB after chemotherapy may be attributed to increased fibrosis, which in turn disrupts lymphatic drainage and makes radiotracer update/surgical dissection more difficult. Alternatively, one might speculate that tumor cells in the sentinel nodes are preferentially ablated following neo-adjuvant chemotherapy, leaving disease in other nodes intact. Notably, the ACOSOG study additionally identified that the FNR was significantly lower when three or more sentinel nodes were evaluated (FNR 9.1 % (95 % CI, 5.6–13.7 %) for ≥3 SLNs versus 21.1 % (95 %, 13.2–31.0 %) for 2 SNLs) and when a combination of blue dye and radiolabeled colloid was utilized (FNR 10.8 %; 95 % CI, 7.2–15.3 %) with combination agents versus 20.3 % (95 % CI, 11.0–32.8 %; $P = 0.05$) with a single agent).

The prospective, multi-centric "Sentinel Node Biopsy Following Neo-adjuvant Chemotherapy" (SN FNAC) study also evaluated the accuracy of SLNB after chemotherapy in patients who presented with biopsy-proven node-positive breast cancer [111]. In this particular study, sentinel nodes were evaluated with standard hematoxylin and eosin staining, and if determined to be negative, further evaluation using immunohistochemistry was mandatory. In comparison with the ACOSOG Z1071 study wherein only sentinel nodes with metastasis >0.2 mm were considered positive, sentinel node metastases of any size were considered positive in the SN FNAC study. By mandating more sensitive pathologic analysis via immunohistochemistry and by including metastases of any size, the study reported an acceptable FNR of 8.4 % (95 % CI, 2.4–14.4 %) for SNLB after neo-adjuvant chemotherapy. A notable limitation of the study, however, is the relatively small sample size (153 patients).

The SENTINA, ACOSOG Z1071, and SN FNAC studies collectively suggest that for clinically node-positive patients undergoing neo-adjuvant chemotherapy greater sensitivity in patient selection and sentinel node evaluation may lower the FNR. An acceptable FNR ≤ 10 % would ultimately be necessary to support use of SLNB as an alternative to ALND in patients with early stage, clinically node-positive breast cancer who receive neo-adjuvant chemotherapy.

14.7 Conclusion

The modern surgical treatment of primary breast cancer dates back to the late nineteenth century, with Halsted's description of the radical MT. However, the radical MT is now rarely utilized in breast cancer management. Today, BCS with RT is the preferred option for most women with primary breast cancer. For those who are not suitable candidates for BCS, the modified radical MT is an acceptable alternative, and in recent years, greater numbers of women have been opting for modified radical MT and a contralateral prophylactic MT (i.e., bilateral MT). However, there is very little justification for use of bilateral mastectomy for the treatment of unilateral breast cancer, unless the patient is a mutation carrier or has a history of mantle irradiation, and in both these situations, the risk of contralateral breast cancer is dramatically increased. Patients treated with the modified radical MT or bilateral MT will generally seek breast reconstructive surgery. It should also be noted that it now appears that local recurrences may increase the risk of death from breast cancer, with four local recurrences resulting in one additional breast cancer death over a 15-year period. Thus, RT should be considered for most women who opt for BCS. Over the years, the management of the axilla has been a topic of considerable interest. Today, SLNB is considered the preferred alternative to the standard ALND. Several recently published randomized studies have provided additional evidence that SLNB alone is a safe alternative to completion ALND in women with early-stage breast cancer who have a low burden of axillary disease, particularly if these patients will be receiving adjuvant radiotherapy and adjuvant systemic therapy.

References

1. Virchow R. Cellular pathology. Philadelphia: JB Lippincott; 1863.
2. Halsted WS. The results of operations for the cure of cancer of the breast performed at the Johns Hopkins hospital from June 1889 to January 1894. Ann Surg. 1894;20:55–497.
3. Margoles RG. Surgical considerations for invasive breast cancer. Surg Clin North Am. 1999;79:1031–46.
4. Bonnadonna G, Valagussa P. The contribution of medicine to the primary treatment of breast cancer. Cancer Res. 1988;48:2314–24.
5. Urban JA, Marjoni MA. Significance of internal mammary lymph node metastases in breast cancer. AJR Am J Roentgenol. 1971;111:130–6.
6. Wagensteen OH. Another look at supraradical operation for breast cancer. Surgery. 1957;41:857–61.
7. Andreassen M, Dahl-Iversen E, Sorensen B. Extended exeresis of regional lymph nodes at operation for carcinoma of breast and the result of a 5-year follow-up of the first 98 cases with removal of the axillary as well as the supraclavicular glands. Acta Chir Scan. 1954;107:206–13.
8. Lacour J, Bucalossi P, Cacers E, et al. Radical mastectomy versus radical mastectomy plus internal mammary dissection. Cancer. 1976;37:206–14.
9. McWhirter R. Simple mastectomy and radiotherapy in treatment of breast cancer. Br J Radiol. 1955;28:128–39.
10. Mustakalio S. Conservative treatment of breast carcinoma—review of 25-year follow-up. Clin Radiol. 1972;23:110–6.
11. Margolese R. Surgical considerations in selecting local therapy. J Natl Cancer Inst Monogr. 1992;11:41–8.
12. Bloom HJG, Richardson WW, Harries EJ. Natural history of untreated breast cancer (1805–1933). BMJ. 1962;2:213–21.
13. Fisher B, Redmond C, Fisher ER, et al. Ten-year results of a randomized clinical trial comparing radical mastectomy and total mastectomy with or without radiation. N Eng J Med. 1985;312:674–81.
14. Cancer Research Campaign Working Party. Cancer research campaign (King's/Cambridge) trial for early breast cancer. Lancet. 1980;2:55–60.
15. Veronesi U, Cascinelli N, Mariani L, et al. Twentyyear follow-up of a randomized study comparing breastconserving surgery with radical mastectomy for early breast cancer. N Engl J Med. 2002;347:1227–32.
16. Arriagada R, Le MG, Rochard F, et al. Conservative treatment versus mastectomy in early breast cancer: patterns of failure with 15 years of follow-up data. J Clin Oncol. 1996;14:1558–64.
17. Fisher B, Anderson S, Bryant J, et al. Twenty-year follow-up of a randomized trial comparing total mastectomy, lumpectomy, and lumpectomy plus irradiation for the treatment of invasive breast cancer. N Engl J Med. 2002;347:1233–41.
18. Poggi MM, Danforth DN, Sciuto LC, et al. Eighteen-year results in the treatment of early breast carcinoma with mastectomy versus breast-conservation therapy. Cancer. 2003;98:696–702.
19. van Dongen JA, Voogd AC, Fentiman IS, et al. Longterm results of a randomized trial comparing breastconserving therapy with mastectomy: European organization for research and treatment of cancer 10801 trial. J Natl Cancer Inst. 2000;92:1143–50.
20. Bilchert-Toft M, Rose C, Anderson JA, et al. Danish randomized trial comparing breast-conservation therapy with mastectomy. J Natl Cancer Inst Monogr. 1992;11:19–25.
21. Lonning PE. Treatment of early breast cancer with conservation of the breast: a review. Acta Oncol. 1991;30:779–92.
22. Fowble B. Ipsilateral breast tumor recurrence following breast-conserving surgery for early stage invasive breast cancer. Acta Oncol. 1999;13(Suppl):9–17.
23. Fisher B. Personal contributions to progress in breast cancer research and treatment. Semin Oncol. 1996;23:414–27.
24. Fisher B, Anderson S, Fisher ER, et al. Significance of ipsilateral breast tumor recurrence after lumpectomy. Lancet. 1991;338: 327–31.
25. Kurtz JM, Spitalier JM, Amalric R, et al. The prognostic significance of late local recurrence after breastconserving therapy. Int J Radiat Oncol Biol Phys. 1990;18:87–93.
26. Donegan WL, Perez-Mesa CM, Watson FR. A biostatistical study of locally recurrent breast carcinoma. Surg Gynecol Obstet. 1966;122:529–40.
27. Borger J, Kemperman H, Hart A, et al. Risk factors in breast-conservation therapy. J Clin Oncol. 1994;12:653–60.
28. Jatoi I, Proschan MA. Randomized trials of breastconserving therapy versus mastectomy for primary breast cancer: a pooled analysis of updated results. Am J Clin Oncol. 2005;28(3): 289–94.
29. Ving-Hung V, Verschraegen C. Breast-conserving surgery with or without radiotherapy: pooled analysis for risks of ipsilateral breast tumor recurrence and mortality. J Natl Cancer Inst. 2004;96:114–21.
30. Early Breast Cancer Trialists' Collaborative Group. Effects of radiotherapy and of differences in the extent of surgery for early breast cancer on local recurrence and 15-year survival: an overview of the randomized trials. Lancet. 2005;366:2087–106.
31. Turner BC, Harrold E, Matloff E, et al. BRCA1/BRCA2 germline mutations in locally recurrent breast cancer patients after lumpectomy and radiation therapy: implications for breast-conserving management in patients with BRCA1/BRCA2 mutations. J Clin Oncol. 1999;17:3017–24.
32. Kinzler KW, Vogelstein B. Gatekeepers and caretakers. Nature. 1997;386:761–3.
33. Pierce LJ, Strawderman M, Narod SA, et al. Effect of radiotherapy after breast-conservig treatment in women with breast cancer and germline BRCA ½ mutations. J Clin Oncol. 2000;18(19):3360–9.

34. Metcalfe KA, Lubinski J, Ghadirian P, et al. Prediction of contralateral prophylactic mastectomy in women with a BRCA 1 or BRCA 2 mutation: the hereditary breast cancer clinical study group. J Clin Oncol. 2008;26(7):1093–7.
35. Benson J, Jatoi I. Management options breast cancer: case histories, best practice, and clinical decision-making. London: Informa Healthcare; 2009.
36. Hughes KS, Schnaper LA, Berry D, et al. Lumpectomy plus tamoxifen with or without irradiation in women 70 years of age or older with early breast cancer. N Engl J Med. 2004;351(10):971–7.
37. Atkins H, Hayward JL, Klugman OJ, et al. Treatment of early breast cancer: a report after ten years of a clinical trial. BMJ. 1972;2(5811):423–9.
38. Winchester O, Cox J. Standards for breast-conservation treatment. CA Cancer J Clin. 1992;42:134–62.
39. Foster RS, Wood WC. Alternative strategies in the management of primary breast cancer. Arch Surg. 1998;133:1182–6.
40. Veronesi D, Bonadonna G, Zurrida S, et al. Conservation surgery after primary chemotherapy in large carcinomas of the breast. Ann Surg. 1995;222:609–11.
41. Lehman CD, Gatsonis C, Kuhl CK, et al. MRI evaluation of the contralateral breast in women with recently diagnosed breast cancer. N Engl J Med. 2007;356:1295–303.
42. Solin LJ, Orel SG, Hwang SG, et al. Relationship of breast magnetic resonance imaging to outcome after breastconservation treatment with radiation for women with early stage invasive breast carcinoma or ductal carcinoma in situ. J Clin Oncol. 2008;26:386–91.
43. Nattinger AB, Hoffmann RG, Kneusel RT, et al. Relation between appropriateness of primary therapy for early stage breast carcinoma and increased use of breast conserving surgery. Lancet. 2000;356:1148–53.
44. Nattinger AB, Gottlieb MS, Veum J, et al. Geographic variation in the use of breast-conserving treatment for breast cancer. N Engl J Med. 1992;326:1147–9.
45. Kelemen JJ, Poulton T, Swartz MT, et al. Surgical treatment of early stage breast cancer in the department of defense healthcare system. J Am Coll Surg. 2001;192:293–7.
46. Freedman RA, He Y, Winer EP, Keating NL. Trends in racial and age disparities in definitive local therapy of early stage breast cancer. J Clin Oncol. 2009;27(5):713–9.
47. Tuttle TM, Haberman EB, Grund EH, et al. Increasing use of contralateral prophylactic mastectomy for breast cancer patients: a trend toward more aggressive surgical treatment. J Clin Oncol. 2007;25(33):5203–309.
48. Nattinger AB, Hoffmann RG, Shapiro R, et al. The effect of legislative requirements on the use of breastconserving surgery. N Engl J Med. 1996;335:1035–40.
49. Dolan J, Granchi TS, Miller CC, et al. Low use of breast-conservation surgery in medically indigent populations. Am J Surg. 1999;178:470–4.
50. Collins ED, Moore CP, Clay KF, et al. Can women with early stage breast cancer make an informed decision for mastectomy? J Clin Oncol. 2009;27(4):519–25.
51. Jatoi I, Benson JR, Liau SS, Chen Y, Cisco RM, Norton JA, et al. The role of surgery in cancer prevention. Curr Probl Surg. 2010;47(10):750–830.
52. Jatoi I, Benson JR. The case against routine preoperative breast MRI. Future Oncol. 2013;9(3):347–53.
53. Sorbero ME, Dick AW, Beckjord EB, Ahrendt G. Diagnostic breast magnetic resonance imaging and contralateral prophylactic mastectomy. Ann Surg Oncol. 2009;16(6):1597–605.
54. Murphy JA, Milner TD, O'Donoghue JM. Contralateral risk-reducing mastectomy in sporadic breast cancer. Lancet Oncol. 2013;14(7):e262–9.
55. Institute nc. surveillance epidemiology and end results program (2014) Available from: http://seer.cancer.gov.
56. Jatoi I, Parsons HM. Contralateral prophylactic mastectomy and its association with reduced mortality: evidence for selection bias. Breast Cancer Res Treat. 2014;148(2):389–96.
57. Dowden RV, Rosato FE, McGraw JB. Reconstruction of the breast after mastectomy for cancer. Surg Gynecol Obstet. 1979;149:109–15.
58. Johnson CH, van Heerden JA, Donohue JH, et al. Oncological aspects of immediate breast reconstruction following mastectomy for malignancy. Arch Surg. 1989;124:819–23.
59. Vinton AL, Traverso W, Zehring RD. Immediate breast reconstruction following mastectomy is as safe as mastectomy alone. Arch Surg. 1990;125:1303–8.
60. Dean C, Chetty D, Forrest APM. Effects of immediate breast reconstruction on psychosocial morbidity after mastectomy. Lancet. 1983;1:459–62.
61. Damen TH, Mureau MA, Timman R, et al. The pleasing end result after DIEP flap breast reconstruction: a review of additional operations. J Plast Reconstr Aesthet Surg. 2009;62(1):71–6.
62. Jatoi I, Kaufmann M, Petit JY. Atlas of breast surgery. Heidelberg: Springer; 2006.
63. Corral CJ, Mustoe TA. Special problems in breast cancer therapy: controversy in breast reconstruction. Surg Clin North Am. 1996;76:309–26.
64. Hulka BS, Kerkvliet NL, Tugwell P. Experience of a scientific panel formed to advise the federal judiciary on silicone breast implants. N Engl J Med. 2000;342:812–5.
65. Nyren O, Yin L, Josefsson S, et al. Risk of connective tissue disease and related disorders among women with breast implants: a nation-wide retrospective cohort study in Sweden. BMJ. 1998;316:417–22.
66. Janowsky EC, Kupper LL, Hulka BS. Meta-analyses of the relation between silicone breast implants and the risk of connective tissue diseases. N Engl J Med. 2000;342:781–90.
67. Schneider WJ, Hill HL Jr, Brown RG. Latissimus dorsi myocutaneous flap for breast reconstruction. Br J Plast Surg. 1977;30:277–81.
68. Amez Z, Smith R, Eder R. Breast reconstruction by the free lower transverse rectus abdominis muscular cutaneous flap. Br J Plast Surg. 1988;41:500–7.
69. Alderman AK, McMahon L, Wilkins EG. The national utilization of immediate and early delayed breast reconstruction and the impact of sociodemographic factors. Plast Reconstr Surg. 2003;111:695–703.
70. Alderman AK, Wei Y, Birkmeyer JD. Use of breast reconstruction after mastectomy following the Women's Health and Cancer Rights Act. JAMA. 2006;295(4):387–8.
71. Jatoi I. Management of the axilla in primary breast cancer. Surg Clin North Am. 1999;79:1061–73.
72. Veronesi U, Rilke R, Luini A, et al. Distribution of axillary node metastases by level of invasion. Cancer. 1987;59:682–7.
73. Morrow M. Axillary dissection: when and how radical? Semin Surg Oncol. 1996;12:321–7.
74. Harris JR, Osteen RT. Patients with early breast cancer benefit from effective axillary treatment. Breast Cancer Res Treat. 1985;5:17–21.
75. Samphao S, Eremin JM, El-Sheemy M, Eremin O. Management of the axilla in women with breast cancer: current clinical practice and a new selective targeted approach. Ann Surg Oncol. 2009;15 (5):1282–96.
76. Epstein RI. Routine or delayed axillary dissection for primary breast cancer? Eur J Cancer. 1995;31A:1570–3.
77. Sacks NPM, Baum M. Primary management of carcinoma of the breast. Lancet. 1993;342:1402–8.

78. Baxter N, McCready DR, Chapman JA, et al. Clinical behavior of untreated axillary nodes after local treatment for primary breast cancer. Ann Surg Oncol. 1996;3:235–40.
79. Graverson HP, Bilchert-Toft M, Andersen J, et al. Danish breast cancer cooperative group. Breast cancer: risk of axillary recurrence in node-negative patients following partial dissection of the axilla. Eur J Surg Oncol. 1988;14:407–12.
80. Jatoi I, Hilsenbeck SG, Clark GM, et al. The significance of axillary lymph node metastasis in primary breast cancer. J Clin Oncol. 1999;17:2334–40.
81. Jatoi I, Anderson WF, Rosenberg PS. Qualitative age interactions in breast cancer: a tale of two diseases? Am J Clin Oncol. 2008;31:504–6.
82. Cabanes PA, Salmon RI, Vilcoq JP, et al. Value of axillary dissection in addition to lumpectomy and radiotherapy in early breast cancer. Lancet. 1992;339:1245–8.
83. Gelber RD, Goldhirsch A, Coates AS. Adjuvant therapy for breast cancer: understanding the overview. J Clin Oncol. 1993;11:580–5.
84. Lonning PE. Breast cancer prognostication and prediction: are we making progress? Ann Oncol. 2007;18(Suppl 8):viii 3–7.
85. Bold RI, Mansfield PF, Berger DH, et al. Prospective, randomized, double-blind study of prophylactic antibiotics in axillary lymph node dissection. Am J Surg. 1998;176:239–43.
86. Coit DG, Peters M, Brennan MF. A prospective randomized trial of perioperative cefazolin treatment in axillary and groin dissection. Arch Surg. 1991;126:1366–72.
87. Rotstein C, Ferguson R, Cummings KM, et al. Determinants of clean surgical wound infections for breast procedures at an oncology center. Infect Control Hosp Epidemiol. 1992;13:207–14.
88. Ivens D, Hoe AL, Podd TJ, et al. Assessment of morbidity from complete axillary dissection. Br J Cancer. 1992;66:136–8.
89. Lyman GH, Giuliano AE, Somerfield MR, et al. American society of clinical oncology guideline recommendations for sentinel lymph node biopsy in early stage breast cancer. J Clin Oncol. 2005;23:7703–20.
90. Cabanas RM. An approach for the treatment of penile carcinoma. Cancer. 1977;39:456–66.
91. Morton DL, Wen DR, Wong JR, et al. Technical details of intraoperative lymphatic mapping for early stage melanoma. Arch Surg. 1992;127:392–9.
92. Chen AY, Halpern MT, Schrag MM, et al. Disparities and trends in sentinel lymph node biopsy among early stage breast cancer patients (1998–2005). J Natl Cancer Inst. 2008;100(7):462–74.
93. Giuliano AE, Jones RC, Brennan M. Sentinel lymphadenectomy in breast cancer. J Clin Oncol. 1997;15:2345–50.
94. Veronesi D, Paganelli G, Galimberti V. Sentinel node biopsy to avoid dissection in breast cancer with clinically negative lymph nodes. Lancet. 1997;349:1864–7.
95. Smith LF, Cross MJ, Klimberg VS. Subareolar injection is a better technique for sentinel node biopsy. Am J Surg. 2000;180:434–7.
96. Morrow M, Rademaker AW, Bethke KP, et al. Learning sentinel node biopsy: results of a prospective trial of two techniques. Surgery. 1999;126:714–20.
97. Giuliano AE, Dale PS, Turner RR, et al. Improved axillary staging of breast cancer with sentinel node lymphadectomy. Ann Surg. 1995;222:394–9.
98. McMasters KM, Giuliano AE, Ross MI, et al. Sentinel lymph node biopsy for breast cancer—not yet standard of care. N Engl J Med. 1998;339:990–5.
99. Veronesi U, Paganelli G, Viale G, et al. A randomized comparison of sentinel node biopsy with routine axillary dissection in breast cancer. N Engl J Med. 2003;349(6):546–53.
100. Lucci A, McCall LM, Beitsch PD, et al. Surgical complications associated with sentinel lymph node dissection (SLND) plus axillary lymph node dissection compared with SLND alone in the American College of Surgeons Oncology group trial Z0011. J Clin Oncol. 2007;25:3657–63.
101. Mansel RE, Fallowfield L, Kissin M, et al. Randomized multicenter trial of sentinel node biopsy versus standard axillary treatment in operable breast cancer: the ALMANAC trial. J Natl Cancer Inst. 2006;98(9):599–609.
102. Albertini JJ, Lyman GH, Cox C, et al. Lymphatic mapping and sentinel node biopsy in the patient with breast cancer. JAMA. 1996;276:1818–22.
103. Giuliano AE, McCall L, Beitsch P, et al. Locoregional recurrence after sentinel lymph node dissection with or without axillary dissection in patients with sentinel lymph node metastases: the American College of Surgeons Oncology Group Z0011 randomized trial. Ann Surg. 2010;252:426–32.
104. American Joint Committee on Cancer Breast Cancer Staging 7th edition. Available from: https://cancerstaging.org/. Accessed 28 May 2016.
105. Galimberti VV. Axillary dissection versus no axillary dissection in patients with sentinel-node micrometastases (IBCSG 23-01): a phase 3 randomised controlled trial. Lancet Oncol. 2013;14:297.
106. Solá MM. Complete axillary lymph node dissection versus clinical follow-up in breast cancer patients with sentinel node micrometastasis: final results from the multicenter clinical trial AATRM 048/13/2000. Ann Surg Oncol. 2013;20:120.
107. Goyal AA, Dodwell D. POSNOC: a randomised trial looking at axillary treatment in women with one or two sentinel nodes with macrometastases. J Clin Oncol (Royal College of Radiologists (Great Britain)). 2015;27:692.
108. Donker MM. Radiotherapy or surgery of the axilla after a positive sentinel node in breast cancer (EORTC 10981-22023 AMAROS): a randomised, multicentre, open-label, phase 3 non-inferiority trial. Lancet Oncol. 2014;15:1303.
109. Kuehn TT. Sentinel-lymph-node biopsy in patients with breast cancer before and after neoadjuvant chemotherapy (SENTINA): a prospective, multicentre cohort study. Lancet Oncol. 2013;14:609.
110. Boughey JCJ. Sentinel lymph node surgery after neoadjuvant chemotherapy in patients with node-positive breast cancer: the ACOSOG Z1071 (Alliance) clinical trial. JAMA. 2013;310: 1455.
111. Boileau JJ. Sentinel node biopsy after neoadjuvant chemotherapy in biopsy-proven node-positive breast cancer: the SN FNAC study. J Clin Oncol. 2015;33:258.

15 Management of the Axilla

John R. Benson and Vassilis Pitsinis

15.1 Introduction

Some form of axillary surgery is an integral component in the loco-regional management of early breast cancer. Surgical techniques have become progressively less extensive over the past 30 years in terms of both parenchymal and nodal resection of breast and axillary tissues, respectively. Despite the widespread introduction of breast conservation surgery (BCS), a formal axillary lymph node dissection (ALND) was, until recently, the standard procedure of choice for management of the axilla in the majority of patients irrespective of primary tumour characteristics. Breast screening programmes and heightened public awareness have led to smaller tumour size at presentation and a lower proportion of patients with nodal involvement. Approximately 25–30 % of patients now have nodal disease at the time of diagnosis compared with 50 % two decades ago [1]. For those patients with positive nodes, removal of axillary nodes containing tumour foci minimizes the chance of loco-regional relapse and can provide crucial information for guiding systemic adjuvant treatments. Moreover, axillary nodal status remains the single most important prognostic factor in breast cancer and has yet to be superseded by newer molecular indices [1, 2]. Nonetheless, for node-negative patients with favourable primary tumour parameters, ALND represents over-treatment and can be associated with significant morbidity [3, 4]. Increased rates of node negativity have spurred the investigation of non-invasive methods for imaging the axillary nodes. However, these alone are questionable as a staging modality due to limitations of resolution at the microscopic tumour level. Routine pre-operative axillary ultrasound in combination with percutaneous node biopsy for tissue acquisition provides crucial staging information on regional nodes [5]. The optimum method for managing the axilla in breast cancer patients remains controversial, but there is compulsion to apply surgical methods for purposes of staging in all patients with invasive cancer. The aforementioned stage shift coupled with failure of ALND dissection to confer any clear survival benefit [6, 7] has prompted exploration of less intrusive methods for surgical staging of the axilla. These alternative methods involve either a blind or targeted form of sampling in which a variable, though restricted number of nodes are removed (usually < 4–5 nodes). Non-targetted sampling of the axillary nodes has been championed by a surgical minority for several years, but this technique has now evolved into a targeted form of sampling using blue dye alone, the so-called blue dye-assisted node sampling (BDANS) [8]. Sentinel lymph node biopsy (SLNB) has been embraced around the world as a standard of care for breast cancer patients and ideally incorporates dual localization techniques using both blue dye and radioisotopic localization. Nonetheless, despite SLNB being the dominant method for staging the axilla in clinically node-negative patients, technical aspects await standardization and variations in details of practice persist. Breast cancer is a heterogeneous disease in terms of its pathobiology and this renders any blanket approach to management of the axilla inappropriate. A selective policy based on thresholds of probability for nodal involvement could include not only ALND, but also SLNB, BDANS and observation alone. It should be noted that it is not the absolute incidence of nodal involvement per se which is important, but rather the proportion of these metastases which develop into clinically relevant disease which is determined not only by surgical extirpation but also adjuvant therapies. The latter might be manifest either as loco-regional relapse or as distant metastases which have

J.R. Benson (✉)
Cambridge Breast Unit, Addenbrooke's Hospital, Cambridge University Hospitals NHS Trust, Cambridge, CB2 0QQ, UK
e-mail: john.benson@addenbrookes.nhs.uk

V. Pitsinis
Breast Unit, Ninewells Hospital and Medical School, NHS Tayside, Dundee, DD21UB, UK
e-mail: vpitsinis@nhs.net

I. Jatoi and A. Rody (eds.), *Management of Breast Diseases*, DOI 10.1007/978-3-319-46356-8_15

arisen from axillary deposits acting as a source for tertiary spread.

This chapter will address nodal anatomy and patterns of lymphatic dissemination in breast cancer together with underlying biological paradigms. Some basic clinical issues will be discussed including the indications for ALND and optimum axillary management in patients who do not require ALND either as a primary or delayed procedure.

15.2 Anatomy of the Axillary Lymph Nodes

An understanding of nodal anatomy is important in the surgical management of breast cancer. There is often confusion in designation of nodal groupings with classification based on clinical, anatomical or surgical criteria.

1. CLINICAL GROUPINGS—medial, lateral, anterior, posterior, apical
2. ANATOMICAL GROUPINGS—lateral, anterior (pectoral), posterior (subscapular), central, subclavicular, interpectoral (Rotter's)
3. SURGICAL—the axillary lymph nodes can be divided into 3 compartments which are defined in terms of their relationship to the pectoralis minor muscle [9].

LEVEL I—nodes below and lateral to the pectoralis minor muscle

LEVEL II—nodes deep to the muscle and lying posterior to the medial and lateral borders of the pectoralis minor muscle

LEVEL III—nodes above and medial to pectoralis minor

A complete ALND refers to removal of axillary nodes at levels I, II and III, whilst a partial ALND implies a more limited clearance of nodes at levels I and II only. The term sampling describes a blind or targeted resection of a variable number of nodes, usually at level I; the number of nodes removed is generally inversely related to the degree of targeting (Fig. 15.1).

15.3 Lymphatic System of the Breast

Metastases to regional lymph nodes is a common pattern of dissemination for solid epithelial tumours which commonly invade local structures and spread in a progressive and sequential manner from a primary tumour focus. The loco-regional pathways of spread lie in anatomical continuity with lymphatic vessels which act as a link between the index tumour and regional nodes. Metastatic dissemination of breast cancer occurs predominantly via the lymphatic system in accordance with the Halstedian paradigm, though it is acknowledged that a significant proportion of breast cancers are systemic at the outset as a result of tumour cells entering the bloodstream at an early stage of neoplastic development. Furthermore, such haematogenous dissemination is not conditional upon nodal involvement and access to the circulation can occur through both lymphatico-venous communications in regional nodes and the 'leaky' endothelium of the tumour neovasculature.

The lymphatics of the breast form an extensive and complex network of periductal and perilobular vessels which drain principally to the axillary nodes. The mammary gland is derived from ectoderm and develops from anterior thoracic wall structures. As noted by Haagensen [10], the lymphatics of the breast skin and parenchymal tissue are interconnected, and this accounts for preferential drainage of cutaneous malignancies to axillary nodes. Moreover, current practices in SLNB whereby tracer agents are injected intra-dermally are dependent upon the lymphatic system of the breast functioning as a single biological unit. Flow within this network of valveless vessels is passive and this results in a degree of plasticity which is relevant to malignant infiltration; the unidirectional flow of lymph may be diverted due to blockage at proximal sites by tumour emboli. The subepithelial lymphatics of the skin of the breast represent part of the superficial system of the neck, thorax and abdomen. These vessels are confluent over the surface of the body and the subepithelial plexus of lymphatics communicates directly with subdermal vessels to form a cutaneous plexus. Within the region of the nipple-areolar complex, this cutaneous plexus is linked to the Sappey subareolar plexus which receives lymphatics from the glandular tissue of the breast and has a key role in accommodating the dramatic surges of lymph flow occurring during lactation [11, 12]. From this subareolar and a related circumareolar plexus, lymph flows principally to the axillary nodes via a lateral lymphatic trunk. This together with minor inferior and medial lymphatic trunks drains along the surface of the breast to penetrate the cribriform fascia and reach the various groups of axillary nodes (Fig. 15.1).

Although the internal mammary nodes were recognized by Handley as a primary route for lymphatic drainage from medial and central zones of the breast [13], the majority of breast cancers metastasize to the axillary nodes irrespective of the index quadrant [14]. Fewer than 10 % of node-positive tumours exclusively affect the internal mammary nodes, and clinical manifestations of such metastases are rare. Furthermore, the biological significance of internal mammary node involvement is uncertain [15] and substantial morbidity can ensue from surgical extirpation of these nodes with no gains in overall survival from these more aggressive resections [16]. Veronesi examined the impact of extended radical mastectomy in which nodes along the internal mammary chain were excised. Amongst a group of 737 patients, 53.2 % were axillary node positive and an

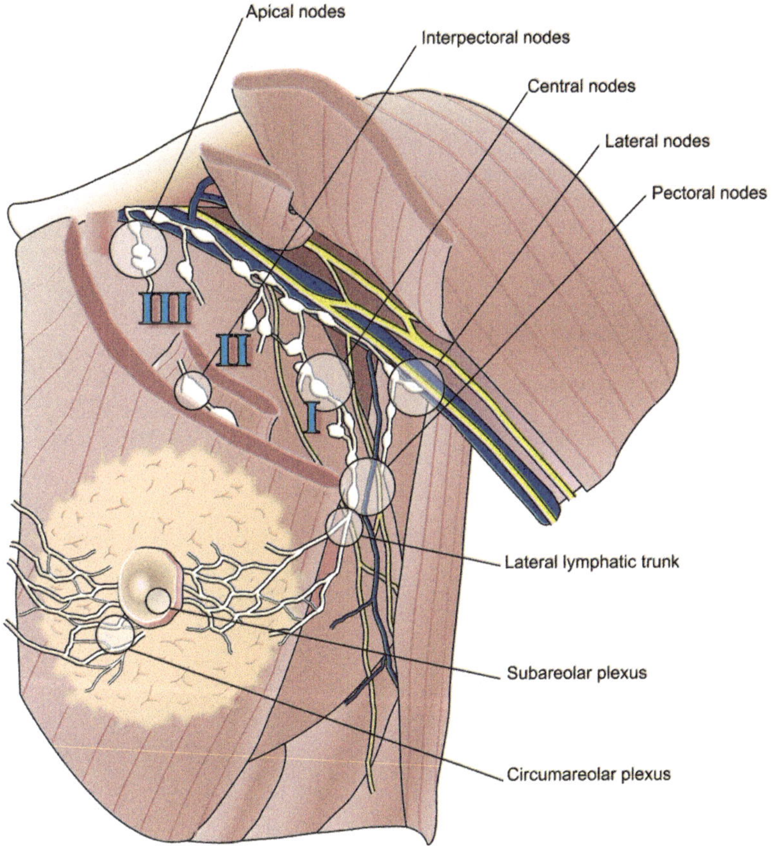

Fig. 15.1 The axillary lymph nodes are located at levels I, II and III; this is a surgical classification and indicating nodes which lie below/lateral, deep/posterior and above/medial to the pectoralis minor muscle, respectively. The lymphatic system of the breast is a complex network of arborizing vessels. A cutaneous plexus is linked to a subareolar plexus which receives lymphatics from the glandular tissue of the breast. From this subareolar and a related circumareolar plexus, lymph flows principally to the axillary nodes via a lateral lymphatic trunk

estimated 20.5 % had positive internal mammary nodes. The comparison group were radical mastectomy patients operated on in the 1960s who received no adjuvant treatment (radiotherapy, chemotherapy or endocrine therapy). No survival benefit was apparent from internal mammary node dissection within this study which was published at the turn of the millennium [17].

The internal mammary chain (IMC) represents one of the accessory drainage pathways of the breast and is considered to receive up to one-quarter of lymphatic flow. However, former estimates based on post-partum injection of colloidal gold suggested that as little as 3 % of the breast lymph flows to the IMC. The IMC is identified on routine lymphoscintigraphy during sentinel node localization in about 15 % of cases [14]. Accessory pathways of lymphatic drainage assume greater importance in more advanced states of disease when the main axillary drainage route has become obstructed [14, 18]. In addition to the IMC, these accessory pathways include the following routes:

1. substernal, crossover (contralateral IMC) [12, 19],
2. pre-sternal crossover (contralateral breast) [20],
3. mediastinal [20],
4. rectus abdominus muscle sheath to subdiaphragmatic and subperitoneal plexus (liver/peritoneal nodes).

Interestingly, with the advent of lymphoscintigraphy as part of sentinel lymph node mapping, drainage to the IMC is more likely when isotope is injected deep within the breast (close to the pectoral fascia) and uncommon when peri-areolar injections are employed [21].

The original definition of the sentinel lymph node was '*the first draining lymph node on the direct pathway from the primary tumour site*' [22]. In its purist form, this definition implied that there was a single node to which cancer cells drain first before proceeding on to higher echelon nodes. The sentinel node hypothesis is 'Halstedian' and presupposes a sequential and orderly spread of cancer cells from the primary tumour to the first draining or sentinel node (usually level I), from whence passage to level II and in turn level III nodes occurs. This hypothesis has proved to be slightly imperfect and does not accord with current understanding of lymphatic drainage patterns from anatomical studies nor the pathophysiology of disordered lymphatic flow [23]. The networks of lymphatic vessels arborize extensively in multiple directions [24] and converge towards a group of 3–5 lymph nodes at level I of the axilla [25] (Fig. 15.2). Detailed anatomical studies undertaken in the 1950s revealed no evidence of a single first or 'sentinel' lymph node at the 'gates of the axilla' towards which all lymphatic channels converge before passing to more distal nodes. As experience with SLNB has

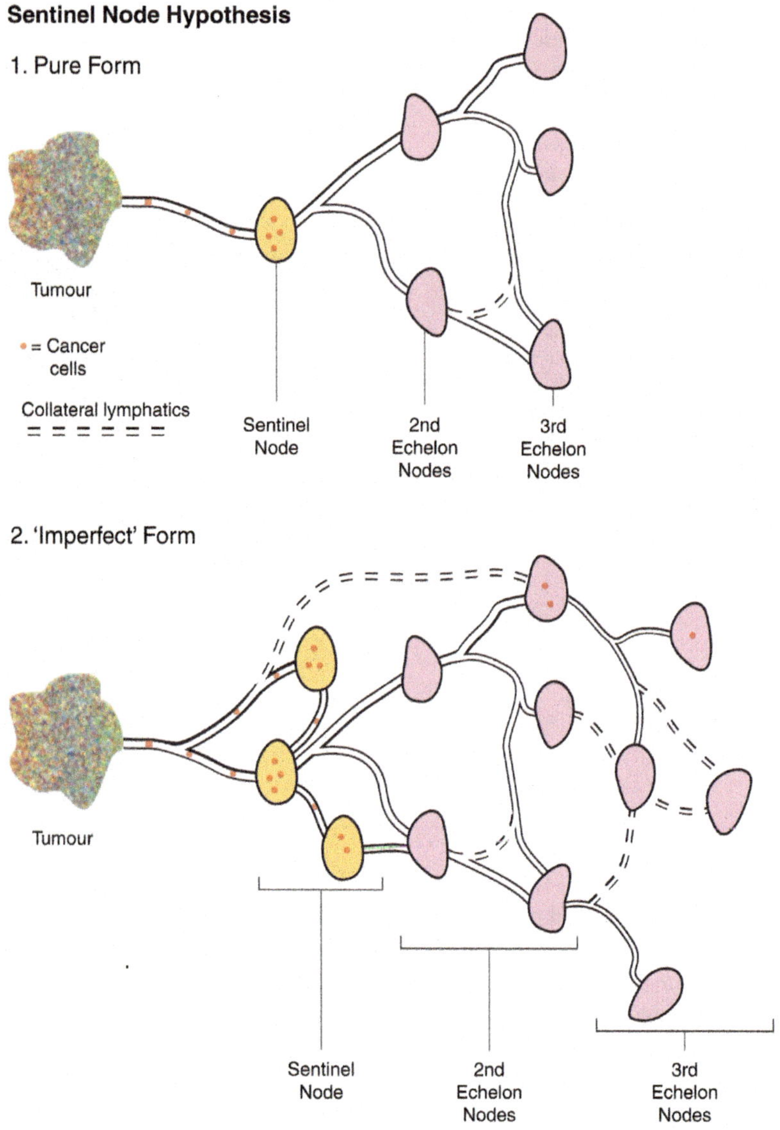

Fig. 15.2 (1) According to the sentinel node hypothesis in its 'pure' form, cancer cells pass from a primary tumour focus to a first draining or sentinel node from where sequential passage to second and third echelon nodes occurs. (2) In reality, cancer cells drain initially to a group of three to five nodes which are all 'sentinel' nodes if they are blue, hot, blue and hot or palpably suspicious. The plasticity of the lymphatic system permits cancer cells to travel via collaterals to non-sentinel nodes. This account for the finite false-negative rate of sentinel node biopsy

accrued using several different methodologies, the average number of nodes removed is between 2 and 3 with false-negative rates being minimized when multiple sentinel nodes are harvested [26]. Indeed, when palpably suspicious nodes are also removed at operation and classified as 'sentinel', many studies report an average of almost 4 nodes [23, 27]. This group of sentinel nodes may therefore correspond to the group of 3–5 nodes at level I from which there is a predictable passage of lymph towards level II and level III nodes. The 'plasticity' of the lymphatic system potentially allows skip metastases to occur in which nodes at levels II and III become involved in the absence of disease affecting level I nodes. In a study of the distribution of nodal metastases in more than 500 patients, Veronesi and colleagues reported skip metastases in only 4 % of cases [28]. In this study, level I nodes alone were found to be involved in 58 %, levels I and II nodes in 22 % and all 3 levels in 16 % of patients. Despite the occurrence of skip lesions, there is generally an orderly passage of lymph from nodes at level I through levels II and III. When nodes at levels I and II are tumour free, the chance of skip metastases at level III is only 2–3 %. For this reason, a standard ALND involves clearance of nodes at levels I and II (partial ALND) only. When at least 10 nodes have been removed during a partial ALND, the axilla should be correctly staged in 96 % of patients with primary breast cancer. When fewer than 10 negative nodes are resected, there is less confidence that the axillary basin is truly negative and involved nodes may have been left behind in a non-targetted dissection. Conversely, when overtly malignant nodes are present at levels I and II, it is customary to undertake a complete ALND which includes level III nodes. The ipsilateral supraclavicular nodes can subsequently be irradiated when extensive nodal involvement is confirmed histologically. More radical resection of axillary nodes is associated with greater upper limb morbidity including lymphoedema, shoulder stiffness, pain and paraesthesia [3, 4]. The benefits of ALND in terms of regional disease control, staging information and prognostication must be balanced against these potential sequelae of which lymphoedema is the most serious concern. The overall incidence of lymphoedema is cited between 10 and 30 % [4, 29–31]. Rates are generally lower for a level II ALND (10–15 %) compared with a level III ALND (25 %). The combination of a complete ALND with irradiation of the axilla can lead to rates of lymphoedema as high as 40 %. There is rarely any justification for combined axillary dissection and irradiation nowadays. Furthermore, surgeons often loosely refer to level II/III ALND in the literature and this confounds interpretation of data on rates of lymphoedema formation. It has been commented that removal of an additional 3–4 nodes maximum at level III is unlikely to significantly impact on documented rates of lymphoedema [32]. The latter remains a common complication which can lead to major physical and psychological morbidity [33] and in the longer term to the rare complication of lymphangiosarcoma (Stewart-Treves Syndrome) [34]. Though it is often the non-dominant upper limb which is affected (more breast cancers occur on the left side), lymphoedema causes symptoms of heaviness and discomfort with associated functional impairment and an unsightly appearance. The accumulation of protein-rich fluid within the extracellular compartment renders the limb prone to recurrent superficial infection which contributes to more chronic inflammatory changes with fibrosis. Disruption and blockage of the lymphatics raises hydrostatic pressure within other parts of the lymphatic system and promotes further tissue oedema by hampering absorption of excess fluid back into the lymphatic vessels. The precise aetiology of lymphoedema remains unclear, but it is related to the extent of extirpation of axillary nodes. The latter disrupts lymphatic drainage pathways and thus compromised function is more likely when surgical dissection is more extensive [33].

15.4 Axillary Lymph Node Dissection

15.4.1 Surgical Aspects

The axilla is a pyramidal space with an apex directed into the route of the neck and a base bounded infront by the anterior axillary fold (lower border of pectoralis major), behind by the posterior axillary fold (tendons of latissimus dorsi and teres major muscles) and medially by the chest wall [18]. The axillary tissue is composed of adipose and nodal elements. A partial (level II) ALND involves resection of all tissue inferior to the level of the axillary vein with no attempt to skeletonize the latter. All nodal/fatty tissue is cleared from the lateral edge of the latissimus dorsi muscle and to the medial border of pectoralis minor muscle. Wrapping of the arm during surgery permits flexion and adduction of the upper arm with relaxation of the pectoralis major muscle which facilitates dissection towards the apex of the axilla. The pectoralis minor muscle was previously either removed or divided to gain access to higher echelon nodes (namely at level III). The nerves to serratus anterior (long thoracic) and latissimus dorsi (thoracodorsal nerve) muscles are closely applied to the medial and posterior walls of the axilla, respectively. These are important motor nerves and should be preserved during axillary surgery unless encased by tumour. Damage to the long thoracic nerve results in a winged scapula and care should be taken not to inadvertently draw this structure laterally away from the chest wall during dissection of the axillary contents as it lies outside the fascia of serratus anterior. By contrast, the intercostobrachial nerve (ICBN) is purely sensory and crosses the axilla towards its base. It tends to be embedded in fatty/nodal tissue and its anatomical course renders it vulnerable during extirpative surgery. The ICBN has historically been considered a minor sensory nerve whose sacrifice during axillary surgery results in transient sensory loss and paraesthesia with minimal symptoms. In recent years, increasing attention has focused on chronic residual morbidity consequent to nerve division and pathophysiology of the ICBN. Provided the nerve is not encased by infiltrative tissue, oncological clearance is adequate and some surgeons advocate preservation of the ICBN, particularly when there is no macroscopic evidence of nodal involvement. Temple and colleagues found that more than one-third of patients in whom the ICBN was sacrificed reported symptoms of dysaesthesia/paraesthesia and concluded that nerve preservation reduces long-term morbidity [35]. However, the main nerve trunk often divides distally into smaller branches which can preclude preservation. Inadvertent division is not uncommon and the potential benefits of nerve preservation are dubious and poorly documented; nerve preservation does not eliminate potential sensory disturbances. Furthermore, randomized trials investigating preservation of the ICBN reveal no significant reduction in incidence of pain and paraesthesia with longer term follow-up. Nerve division can be associated with relatively normal sensation due to neural anastomoses in the vicinity of the shoulder and upper arm. Conversely, the majority of pain symptoms associated with nerve section are controlled with simple analgesia and resolve after a few months [36, 37]. It has been suggested that maintenance of an intact nerve can increase the chance of subsequent entrapment by scar tissue which can lead to troublesome and persistent symptoms.

A formal ALND is indicated for all patients with early-stage breast cancer who are clinically node positive (i.e. considered to have clinically malignant nodes). In addition, those patients with inflammatory cancers and some with clinically node-negative tumours measuring >5 cm in maximum diameter should undergo ALND considered at the outset. The chance of nodal involvement is related to tumour size and it is difficult to justify SLNB for larger tumours when there is a high probability of node positivity. Furthermore, there is no clinical trial data on the efficacy of SLNB as a staging procedure for tumours exceeding 5 cm for which false-negative rates are likely to be unacceptably high. Clinical examination of the axilla is notoriously inaccurate with a 30 % error rate either way; that is, 30 % of clinically node-negative patients will prove to have pathological nodal involvement whilst 30 % of clinically node-positive patients will have no evidence of axillary metastases. Pre-operative axillary ultrasound and percutaneous node biopsy is increasingly being used to identify node-positive patients who can then proceed to ALND as either primary surgical treatment or following induction chemotherapy. Percutaneous needle biopsy of lymph nodes will confirm positivity in more than 90 % of women with ≥4 positive nodes and select 40–50 % of node-positive cases overall [5, 38]. Those patients with non-inflammatory tumours ≤5 cm in size are eligible for some form of node sampling as a staging procedure (SLNB, BDANS or blind sampling) [39]. Notwithstanding previous comments, it remains unclear whether all patients with a negative axillary ultrasound and core biopsy are candidates for SLNB when tumour size exceeds 5 cm.

15.4.2 Overall Survival

Axillary metastases are viewed as indicators of risk for distant relapse and do not determine clinical outcome [40]. The majority of studies have not demonstrated any gains in survival from ALND, though the NSABP-B04 trial was confounded by salvage dissection for local recurrence and not powered to detect any benefit smaller in magnitude than 7 % [41]. Others have suggested that some benefit may be derived from more thorough node dissection [42–44]. A large meta-analysis of 3000 cases has claimed a survival benefit of 5.4 % from ALND [45]. Nonetheless, though meta-analyses can partly overcome the problem of under-powering, they cannot readily distinguish between the effects of removing nodal tissue per se and the effect of adjuvant systemic treatments on overall survival.

The issue of whether loco-regional treatment can directly impact on long-term survival was clarified by a milestone publication by the Early Breast Cancer Trialists Collaborative Group (EBCTCG) in 2005 [46]. This showed an overall survival benefit at 15 years from local radiation to either the breast following BCS or the chest wall after mastectomy. For those treatment comparisons where the difference in local recurrence at 5 years was less than 10 %, survival was unaffected. Where differences in local relapse were substantial (>10 %), there were moderate reductions in breast cancer specific and overall mortality. The absolute reductions were 19 % for local recurrence at 5 years and 5 % for breast cancer mortality at 15 years. This represents 1 life saved for every 4 loco-regional recurrences prevented by radiotherapy at 5 years. It is unclear precisely what the proportional contribution of local versus regional reductions in relapse was as absolute nodal recurrence rates were very low [46].

If ALND conferred a clear survival advantage, then this should be the standard of care for all patients with breast cancer. These data from the EBCTCG on longer term follow-up suggest that loco-regional recurrence may act as a determinant of distant disease in a subgroup of women. Loco-regional treatments are potentially curative in the absence of micrometastases when disease is confined to the breast and lymph nodes. Under these circumstances, when loco-regional management is incomplete, cancer cells or even 'oligometastases' may persist within the regional nodes and develop into distant metastases at a later date. For the majority of patients with adequate loco-regional therapy, local recurrence reflects the innate biological features of a tumour and is a marker of risk for distant relapse [47].

15.4.3 Axillary Relapse

Local control of disease is therefore important and can impact on longer term survival of breast cancer patients. The role of ALND in achieving loco-regional control is well established. The NSABP B-04 and King's/Cambridge trials provide key observations on the effect of axillary treatment in clinically node-negative patients and reveal that rates of recurrence are up to 6 fold higher for untreated axillae [41, 48]. In the NSABP B-04 study, rates of axillary recurrence at 10 years follow-up were 17.8 % for patients without axillary treatment (i.e. simple mastectomy only) versus less than 5 % for patients who underwent dissection (1.4 %) or irradiation of the axilla (3.1 %) [41]. Similar results were reported by the Kings/Cambridge trial in which clinically node-negative patients were randomized to the following treatment arms (a) total mastectomy and radiotherapy to the axilla or (b) total mastectomy and observation of the axilla [48]. Thus, treatment of the axilla with either surgery or irradiation will reduce the 5 year risk of relapse by almost 90 %. However, it is the avoidance of uncontrolled axillary relapse which is pertinent; this can cause significant morbidity with invasion of major nerves and blood vessels causing pain and lymphoedema. In the pre-screening era of radical and modified radical mastectomy, axillary recurrence often reflected intrinsically aggressive disease with chest wall infiltration which precluded satisfactory attempts at surgical or radioablation [49]. Most cases of axillary relapse after BCS for smaller tumours have a more 'benign' phenotype and are salvageable with either surgery or radiotherapy in 70–90 % of cases [50]. Though adequate management of the axilla at the time of initial diagnosis of breast cancer is essential, partial or complete ALND nowadays represents over-treatment for most patients in terms of loco-regional control (including some SLNB-positive patients). The axilla can be accurately staged with more restrictive methods of targeted sampling which identify pathologically node-negative patients who can safely avoid formal ALND. Overall rates of local recurrence following ALND typically vary from 0.8 to 2.5 % at 10 years. The median interval to regional recurrence after ALND is 19 months, and the chance of axillary recurrence is related to number of nodes removed [51].

It is essential that rates of axillary relapse after sampling techniques which deselect patients for ALND remain below those for this 'gold standard' procedure [52–57]. Though previous studies showed that the risk of axillary relapse was inversely related to the extent of ALND and the number of nodes removed [51], targeted approaches to node sampling should minimize false-negative rates and ensure that any residual disease within axillary nodes is low volume. Rates of axillary recurrence for SLNB remain low and range from 0 to 1.4 % with short-term follow-up of <5 years [52–57]. A systematic review of almost 15,000 patients reported an average rate of 0.3 % at a median follow-up of 34 months with most axillary recurrences occurring within 20 months of surgery [58]. Long-term follow-up of a single patient cohort involving more than 1500 patients revealed an axillary recurrence rate of 0.26 % with more than half of recurrences observed beyond 5 years [59] (Table 15.1 [52–59]).

15.5 Methods for Axillary Node Sampling

The recognition that axillary dissection was principally a staging procedure with concomitant morbidity led to investigation of alternative methods for surgical staging of the axilla. These included axillary sampling and more recently SLNB. Both of these methods aim to remove between 3 and 5 biologically relevant nodes compared with 10–20 nodes for a partial ALND [38]. SLNB is a sophisticated form of targeted axillary node sampling, and methods of blind axillary sampling have evolved into BDANS. There is generally an inverse relationship between the average number of nodes sampled and the degree of targeting, i.e. blue dye alone, isotope alone or a combined method. Accurate targeting of nodes reduces the chance of a false-negative result.

15.5.1 Four-Node Axillary Sampling

All methods of sampling are reliant on the sequential involvement of axillary node metastases from level I to level III with a low incidence of skip metastases [27]. Rosen noted that more than 50 % of node-positive T1 tumours involve only 1 or 2 nodes and these are usually within level I territory [60]. Axillary sampling was introduced more than 2 decades ago by Sir Patrick Forrest in Edinburgh and has been widely practiced 'north of the border' but more selectively elsewhere [61]. Initial studies showed that the original technique of a blind 4-node sample from level I could stage the axilla with an estimated accuracy of 97 % [62]. Four-node sampling has been compared with axillary clearance in randomized studies [63, 64] and harvesting of further nodes as part of a completion axillary dissection does not increase rates of node positivity [63]. Blind 4-node sampling is not associated with impaired loco-regional control [62], and there is no evidence to date of any detriment in overall survival [65]. For those patients found to be positive on node sampling, the axilla can either be irradiated (1–2 nodes positive) or surgically cleared (3–4 nodes positive) [62]. Rates of local control are excellent for both approaches and regional recurrence rates are 5 % at 10 years for patients with negative nodes who have been sampled only [62].

15.5.2 Blue Dye-Assisted Node Sampling (BDANS)

A potential problem with standard, or blind forms of sampling is lack of certainty that 4 nodes have been retrieved. It can be difficult to identify nodes amongst the fibro-fatty

Table 15.1 Rates of axillary recurrence following a negative sentinel node biopsy

Author	No. patients	Median follow-up	Axillary recurrences (%)
Chung et al. [54]	206	26 months	3 (1.4 %)
Blanchard et al. [55]	685	29 months	1 (0.1 %)
Naik et al. [53]	2340	31 months	3 (0.13 %)
Veronesi et al. [56]	953	38 months	3 (0.31 %)
Bergkvist et al. [57]	2246	37 months	27 (1.20 %)
Kiluk et al. [59]	1530	59 months	4 (0.26 %)

tissue of the axilla (even when the axillary tail has been mobilized). Blind sampling of axillary nodes requires skill and has been criticized for being too random and unreliable [66]. Standard 4-node axillary sampling has evolved into a blue dye-assisted variant which permits a more targeted sampling and better standardization of technique [8, 38]. A survey undertaken in 1999 revealed that 47 % of British surgeons used axillary sampling (either blind or dye-guided) and this figure increased to 64 % in 2001 [67]. In the absence of nuclear medicine facilities, the standard 4-node sample has been adapted as a 'blue dye-assisted node sample' (BDANS). This is a practical option for identification of 3–4 relevant nodes and avoids use of isotope which may present financial and logistical problems for some breast units. Some surgeons have opted to use BDANS despite availability of radioisotope and with increasing experience of SLNB, removal of 3–4 nodes seems optimal after all! Bleiweiss refers to a 'sentinel node plus' technique in which surgeons remove a similar number of nodes during an otherwise conventional SLNB as for a BDANS [23].

15.6 Sentinel Lymph Node Biopsy

The essence of the sentinel node hypothesis has been discussed above and presupposes a sequential spread of cancer cells to the 'sentinel node' from whence passage to higher echelon nodes occurs. If the sentinel node does not contain metastases, then the remaining non-sentinel lymph nodes (NSLN) are likewise presumed to be tumour free. Conversely, if tumour deposits are found in the sentinel node, then it is implicit that there is a finite probability of NSLN involvement and completion ALND is indicated. A crucial parameter is the false-negative rate which is the proportion of patients incorrectly diagnosed as node negative. The denominator for this calculation should be the number of node-positive patients and not the total number of patients which has been erroneously used in some reports. False-negative rates for SLNB are between 5 and 10 % which are slightly higher than for ALND and considered acceptable.

In practice, it appears that the axilla can be adequately staged by removal of 3–4 relevant nodes—as in sampling. McCarter found that 15 % of patients had 4 or more nodes removed at the time of SLNB and claimed that at least 3 nodes were required to identify 99 % of node-positive patients. False-negative rates are significantly higher when only one SLN is removed (16.5 %), but much lower when multiple nodes are harvested or 'sampled' [68]. Goyal and colleagues reported that amongst node-positive tumours, 99.6 % of metastases were contained within the first 4 nodes, suggesting that removal of more than 4 nodes is unnecessary [26]. It therefore appears that between 2 and 4 nodes should be removed for optimum staging. The sentinel lymph node is subjected to more detailed pathological scrutiny with multiple step-sections and immunohistochemical staining than is the case for routine nodal tissue. This more intense pathological examination of the sentinel lymph node potentially upstages disease and increases rates of node positivity to levels above those expected for standard ALND. Perhaps of more concern is the finding of macrometastases in NSLN when only micrometastases are present in the sentinel lymph node. This suggests that the latter has lower biological priority and that patterns of lymphatic flow exist which preferentially direct tumour cells to these non-sentinel nodes [69]. It has been suggested that when more than 3 'sentinel' nodes are removed, routine pathological processing may be sufficient and compatible with low false-negative rates [70]. Much published data on SLNB comes from validation studies in which clinically node-negative patients have undergone SLNB followed by immediate completion ALND. These studies have provided important information on the success rate and accuracy of SLNB, but have not yielded any comparative data for SLNB alone without concomitant ALND. Furthermore, these single and multi-institutional validation studies have involved relatively small numbers of patients. The NSABP B-32 trial recruited over 5000 women from 80 centres in the USA and Canada and is the largest of 5 randomized controlled trials comparing SLNB to conventional ALND in clinically node-negative patients [71]. Patients were randomized to either SLNB followed by ALND or SLNB alone. Both surgeons and pathologists followed specific protocols and performance audits were periodically done for purposes of quality control and consensual practice. Analysis of secondary endpoints pertaining to accuracy and technical aspects within the context of this trial confirmed SLNB to be a safe and accurate method for staging the axilla with an acceptable false-negative rate (9.8 %) and high negative predictive value. Omission of routine immunohistochemistry (IHC) helped avoid potential upstaging which would remove a subgroup of SLNB-negative patients who might otherwise lead to a decrement in overall survival. It is of crucial importance to ascertain whether the finite proportion of patients with residual disease in non-sentinel nodes suffer impaired overall survival. The NSABP B-32 trial was designed to detect a modest 2 % survival difference at 5 years, thereby acknowledging that any reduction in morbidity must not occur at the expense of impaired survival. At an average follow-up of 96 months, there were no significant differences in the primary endpoints of overall survival, disease-free survival and regional control. Interestingly there was a trend for improved survival in the ALND group with an unadjusted hazard ratio of 1.2 ($p = 0.12$) and an adjusted ratio of 1.19 ($p = 0.13$) which may be attributable to random events favouring the ALND group and positive non-sentinel lymph node prompting appropriate adjuvant systemic therapy (the unknown non-sentinel node-positive patients in group 2 would be treated as SLNB negative). The conclusions of this trial in terms of the appropriateness, safety and effectiveness of SLNB were justified for this population but may not necessarily apply to patients with larger T2 (2–5 cm) or multifocal tumours who commonly undergo SLNB. Nonetheless, results of NSABP B32 vindicate contemporary SLNB practice and supports a reduction in extent of axillary surgery for the majority of breast cancer patients [71, 72].

15.6.1 Technical Aspects

The technique of SLNB was initially assessed in peer-reviewed pilot studies using blue dye only (patent blue, isosulphan blue and methylene blue). These early studies identified the sentinel node in only two-thirds of cases and a learning curve for the technique was evident as further experience was accrued. Krag and colleagues introduced radioactive tracers (Technetium-99 m colloid) as an alternative method for identification of the sentinel lymph node [73], whilst others have used a dual localization method with detection of 'blue' and 'hot' nodes. Morrow and colleagues randomized patients to SLNB using either blue dye alone or blue dye combined with isotope and showed these to be of similar performance [74]. There is international consensus that dual localization methods are preferable and associated with a short learning curve and optimal performance indicators such as rates of identification and false negativity. In a review by the American Society of Clinical Oncology Expert Panel (ASCO), the overall false-negative rate for the SLNB technique was 8.4 % with a range of 0–29 % [75]. This analysis involved more than 10,000 patients who underwent SLNB followed by completion ALND for validation. Patients were distributed between 69 single and multi-institutional studies and yielded sensitivity rates varying from 71–100 %. The average false-negative rate in these non-randomized studies was comparable to that reported for the NSABP B-32 study (9.8 %) [71, 76]. The NSABP B32 [71], SNAC [77] and European Institute of Oncology (EIO) [78] trials compared SLNB alone with SLNB followed by ALND (A versus A + B), whilst the UK ALMANAC study randomized patients to SLNB versus ALND or node sampling (A versus B) [79] (Table 15.2). Within all trials, SLNB-positive patients underwent completion ALND. Therefore, dual localization with dye and isotope maximizes identification rates (>90 %) and is associated with high negative predictive values (>95 %) [80]. Furthermore, this method is recommended for 'beginners' and use of lymphoscintigraphy has also been advocated as an adjunct during the learning phase, particularly when isotope only is used for localization [81, 82]. However, lymphoscintigraphy does not generally yield additional staging information which influences management and ablative therapy is not routinely directed at extra-axillary nodal sites at the present time. A positive lymphoscintigram can be helpful, especially in the context of an IMC sentinel lymph node [83]. However, a negative lymphoscintigram does not preclude identification of axillary sentinel lymph nodes with standard intra-operative methods. There is probably no advantage in use of lymphoscintigraphy for most patients with tumours in the outer quadrants of the breast and a low likelihood of extra-axillary node involvement [84, 85].

Though intra-tumoral injection of dye/isotope is no longer used, peritumoral, subcutaneous, intra-dermal and subareolar sites are practiced (Fig. 15.3). Based on the evidence that the skin envelop shares a common pattern of lymphatic drainage with the parenchyma of the breast and these converge upon the same sentinel node (s)[10], there is a trend towards subareolar injection which gives less 'shine through' but requires more prolonged massage. The latter may encourage migration of tumour cells to the sentinel node (so-called traumatic metastases or 'traumets') [86]. Benign epithelial cells may be similarly displaced and be interpreted as a false-positive result on immunohistochemistry [87]. A randomized study comparing subareolar with peritumoral injection of blue dye alone for sentinel lymph node identification found a higher nodal yield for the peritumoral compared with the subareolar route (2.33+/−0.7 versus 1.64+/−0.6; $p < 0.001$ [88]. Peri-areolar injections give poorer visualization of the IMC, and when lymphoscintigraphy is employed, it is advisable to inject isotope deeper within the breast parenchyma (closer to the deep fascia). Technetium [99]-labelled nanocolloid or an equivalent radioisotope (20 MBq) is injected at least 2 h before surgery but can be administered on the preceding day if more convenient. It is sensible to use a slightly larger carrier molecule (e.g. sulphur colloid) in these circumstances in order to ensure retention within the lymphatic system up until the time of surgery. A special licence and training is required for handling of radioisotope and injection is best undertaken by nuclear medicine personnel. The dye of choice is injected by the surgeon at the time of surgery, and the breast is massaged for between 2 and 5 min. Some surgeons use 1–2 mls of undiluted dye, whilst others dilute 2 mls of dye with saline up to a final volume of 5 mls. However, larger volumes of injectate cause troublesome staining both of the breast tissues intra-operatively and of the skin post-operatively. Reduced volumes of dye may be appropriate in smaller breasted women and avoids more prolonged staining of the breast skin (of up to 12 months).

There is general consensus that SLNB should aim to remove all nodes which are blue, hot, blue and hot or

Table 15.2 Randomized trials of sentinel lymph node biopsy

Trial	Study population	Study groups
ALMANAC (UK) [79]	Any invasive tumour, Clinical No; (n = 1260)	ALND or ANS vs SLNB (if positive SLN, proceeded to ALND or RT to axilla; if negative SLN, observed)
NSABP-B32 (USA) [71]	Clinical T1–3, N0; (n = 4000)	SLNB + ALND vs SLNB (if positive SLN, proceeded to ALND; if negative SLN, observed)
SNAC (Australia/New Zealand) [77]	≤30 mm invasive tumour Clinical N0; (n = 1060)	SLNB + ALND vs SLNB (if positive SLN, proceeded to ALND; if negative SLN, observed)
European Institute of Oncology (Milan) [78]	T1, N0; (n = 516)	SLNB + ALND vs SLNB (if positive SLN, proceeded to ALND; if negative SLN, observed)
Cambridge [80]	≤30 mm invasive tumour Clinical N0; (n = 1060)	ALND vs SLNB (if positive, proceeded to ALND; if negative SLN, observed)

ANS Axillary node sampling, *RT* radiotherapy, *ALMANAC* Axillary lymphatic mapping against nodal axillary clearance, *SNAC* Sentinel node versus axillary clearance

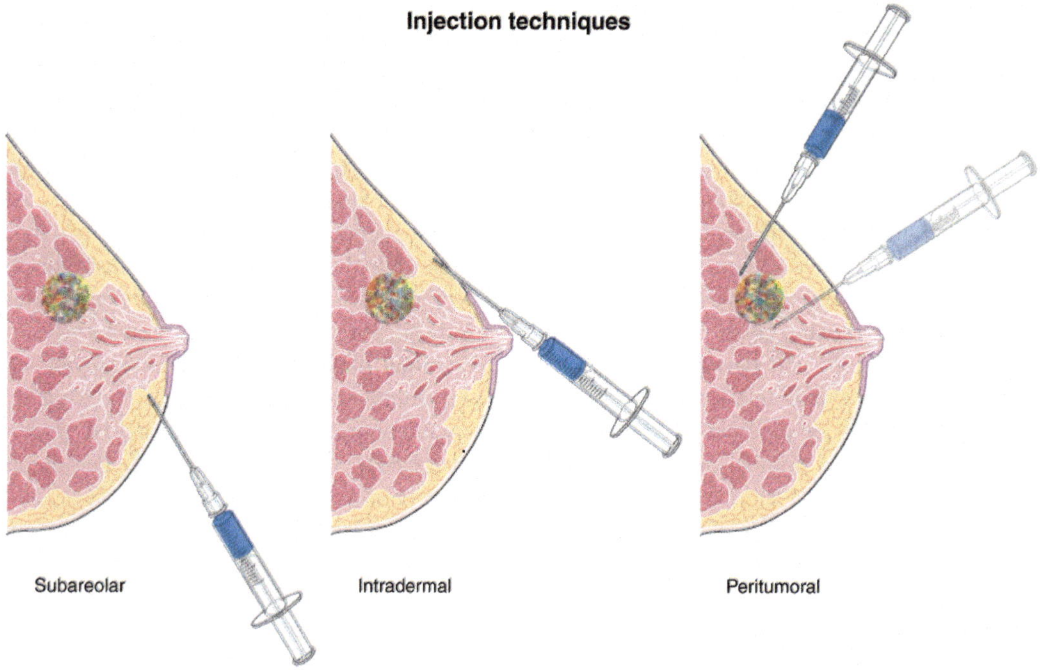

Fig. 15.3 Sites of injection of tracer agents (*blue dye*, *radiocolloid* or *indocyanine green*)

palpably suspicious. Some nodes are blue, but not hot and others are non-blue and hot. Sometimes it can be helpful to trace a blue lymphatic towards a node which may not necessarily be blue (but may be hot and should be removed). The decision when to stop sampling during surgery can be difficult; some surgeons consider any radioactive node to be hot, but use of count ratios can limit the number of nodes excised when activity levels are diffuse and high amongst three or more nodes. It is conventional to designate a node as being hot in terms of either the sentinel node:background count (3:1) or the ex vivo: background count (10:1). In the NSABP B32 trial, all nodes were removed containing at least 10 % of the activity of the hottest node [71]. Potential adverse effects of blue dye include allergic reactions and staining of cutaneous/surgical breast tissue (the latter can be a particular problem during skin-sparing mastectomy with concomitant SLNB). The Medicines and Healthcare Regulatory Authority (MHRA) issued a drug safety update in February 2012 emphasizing that occurrence of allergic reactions to blue dye was not uncommon and estimated to have an incidence of 0.1 % in the ALMANAC trial [79, 89]. Between 1975 and the beginning of 2012, a total of 70 cases of allergic reactions to blue dye had been reported to the MHRA. Of note, 58 of these cases had occurred since 2007 and included 26 serious allergic reactions. These reports of potentially serious allergic reactions have led many surgeons to dispense with routine use of blue dye when there is a strong radioactive signal in the axilla.

Evidence continues to emerge for the efficacy and safety of fluorescence mapping with the fluorochrome indocyanine green (ICG) as an alternative tracer agent for SLNB [90]. This technology relies on generation of molecular fluorescence by contact of ICG with plasma proteins in the lymphovascular system. This fluorochrome absorbs light at a wavelength of approximately 800 nm with the emission of a fluorescent signal when subatomic particles return from an excited to ground state. The illuminated subcutaneous lymphatic channels can be seen on a photodynamic eye (PDE) camera display and ICG tracked as it passes towards the axilla. The fluorescence is scattered by superficial tissues and cannot be detected at a depth of more than 1 cm with current equipment. The visual dimension of fluorescence with high optical sensitivity is a great advantage to radioisotope alone and could be complementary to radioisotope in the absence of blue dye.

Both blue dye and radioisotope have potential drawbacks including allergic reactions, staining of cutaneous and surgical breast tissue, radiation exposure and mandatory licencing. Therefore, problems exist with both tracer agents and exploration of alternative agents is warranted [91]. Identification rates approaching 100% have consistently been reported using ICG in combination with standard tracer agents (either blue dye or radioisotope) [92–95]. There has been a trend away from the use of blue dye for SLNB recently and ICG as a tracer agent may serve as an adjunct to radioisotope in the first instance. There are high levels of concordance (93.5 %) between ICG and radioisotope for sentinel lymph node identification [96] with recent evidence that ICG can outperform both blue dye and radioisotope in terms of detection of positive nodes [97]. Fluorescence imaging provides at least equivalent detection rates but offers an additional dimension of visual guidance and is safe with allergic reactions a rarity. Concerns about excessive nodal yields are not substantiated with average nodal yields of 1.5–3.7 and several recent reports citing nodal counts less than 2 [94, 95, 98]. A combination of radioisotope and ICG could represent a transition phase with ICG eventually becoming a sole tracer at a future stage when more clinical experience with its usage has accrued. It combines many of the advantages of blue dye and radioisotope without the disadvantages—in particular allergic reactions. Use of radioisotope alone can be challenging for less experienced surgeons, and in the longer term, there is a need to explore novel tracer agents such as ICG and magnetic particles [99] (Fig. 15.4).

No formal health economic evaluation of SLNB has yet been undertaken and it may prove to be cost neutral compared with ALND due to the additional costs of equipment, isotope, personnel, etc. Moreover, in some units, patients are now discharged early with drains in situ following ALND and this will reduce the relative cost of the latter procedure [100]. Methods for intra-operative assessment of sentinel lymph nodes obviate the need for delayed ALND in some patients, but reported rates of sensitivity and specificity remain problematic with no single method perceived as having any overall advantage in terms of performance, patient care, logistics and cost [101, 102]. Newer reverse transcriptase polymerase chain reaction (RT-PCR)-based techniques can potentially overcome difficulties of limited pathological sampling of nodes and operating parameters set at a threshold for detection of metastases >2 mm in size (i.e. macro- but not micrometastases nor isolated tumour cells (≤0.2 mm) [103]. Real-time PCR may permit quantitation of tumour load and more accurate differentiation between macro- and micrometastases. It should be appreciated that the definition of nodal micrometastases (>0.2 mm; ≤2 mm) is arbitrary and there is no sudden transition from low risk to high risk. The term staging implies a discontinuous concept, yet in reality there is a continuum in the extent of nodal involvement. Nodal status is the single most important prognostic factor in breast cancer and determines the propensity to form distant metastases. Nonetheless, for women with node-positive disease, a single node is affected in up to 60 % of cases amongst whom up to half contain micrometastases only. These observations are related to the more intensive pathological examination of the sentinel lymph node and were NSLNs to be assessed as thoroughly, some would probably be deemed positive which would otherwise be negative on routine pathological processing without step-sectioning nor immunohistochemistry. A further analysis of patients initially classified as node negative on the basis of H&E staining has confirmed that isolated tumour cells and micrometastases detected with immunohistochemistry only do not impact on survival outcomes. This substudy from the NSABP B32 study has provided further information on the prognostic significance of sentinel lymph node micrometastases detected by immunohistochemistry only [104]. Those patients who were node negative (without isolated tumour cells) had identical disease-free survival to those with micrometastases whereas patients with macrometastatic disease had poorer overall survival compared with node-negative patients or those with micrometastases.

15.6.2 Completion Axillary Lymph Node Dissection

This relatively high incidence of isolated sentinel node positivity with low-volume disease has created management dilemmas in terms of both further (completion) axillary surgery and systemic treatment. The chance of NSLN involvement is related to the volume of disease in the sentinel node. Cserni found on meta-analysis that when macrometastases (>2 mm) were present in the sentinel node, the incidence of

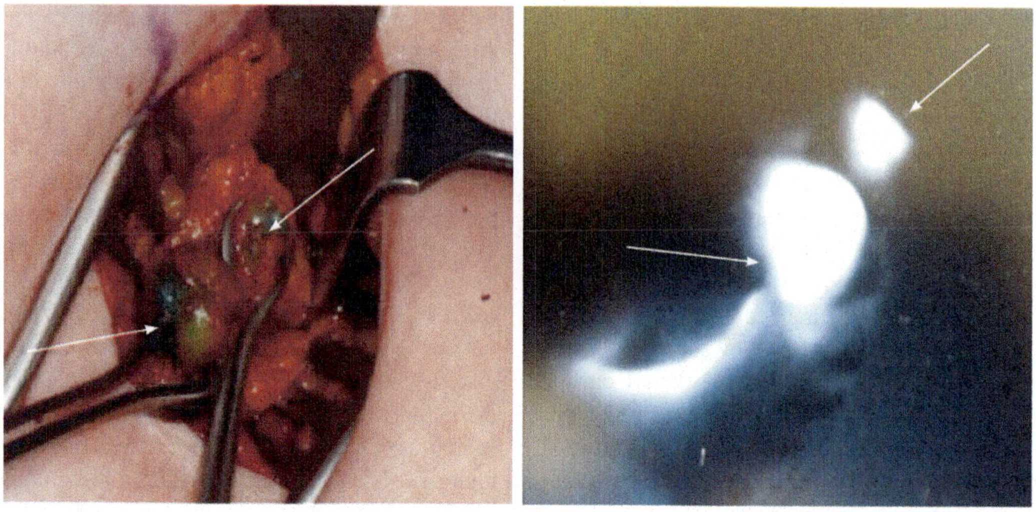

Fig. 15.4 Sentinel lymph nodes (1 and 2) observed in situ with fluorescence imaging using indocyanine green (combined with *blue dye*). An afferent lymphatic can be seen coursing towards the larger lymph node. (Reprinted from European Journal of Surgical Oncology, Volume 38, Wishart GC, Loh S-W, Jones L, Benson JR. A feasibility study (ICG-10) of indocyanine green (ICG) fluorescence mapping for sentinel lymph node detection in early breast cancer. Pages 651–656. Copyright 2012 with permission from Elsevier)

NSLN involvement was 50 %, but only 15 % for micrometastases (>0.2 mm ≤2 mm) and 9 % for isolated tumour cells (≤2 mm) [105]. However, there is much heterogeneity in terminology and definition of isolated tumour cells and micrometastases with lack of reproducibility between categories. The risk of residual NSLN disease for an individual patient can be estimated from a multivariate nomogram which incorporates several factors such as primary tumour size and grade [106]. However, nomograms devised locally for estimation of NSLN involvement may not be transferable to data sets generated from other institutions. Until recently, US guidelines recommend completion ALND for all patients with macro- or micrometastatic deposits in the sentinel lymph node, but not for isolated tumour cells. This includes micrometastases detected either by routine H&E staining or immunohistochemistry alone [75].

There is emerging evidence that selected groups of SLNB-positive patients can safely avoid completion ALND when omitted on a discretionary basis [107, 108]. Axillary ultrasound with core biopsy of nodes according to pre-defined criteria can potentially deselect a subgroup of patients for SLNB who have a positive nodal core biopsy (or fine needle aspirate) or suspicious nodes with a negative needle biopsy. This reduces the axillary tumour burden and the chance of non-sentinel lymph node positivity. Removal of axillary nodes containing foci of tumour provides regional control of disease and may remove a potential source of distant metastases but adjuvant therapies including radiotherapy and systemic treatments are also effective at eliminating residual tumour burden within axillary nodes [109, 110]. Nomograms devised for estimation of non-sentinel lymph node positivity from primary tumour and sentinel node parameters have been difficult to reliably apply in practice and are less accurate when the predicted incidence of non-sentinel lymph node involvement is low [111, 112]. The American College of Surgeons Oncology Group Z0011 trial potentially allows relaxation of informal policies and broadens the scope for omission of completion ALND in sentinel lymph node-positive patients [113]. This phase III non-inferiority trial examined disease-free and overall survival in a group of almost 900 patients undergoing breast conservation surgery for relatively good prognosis T1 and T2 tumours with macro- and micrometastases in 1 or 2 sentinel lymph nodes. Patients were randomized to completion ALND or observation only and all received tangential field whole breast irradiation and systemic therapy (chemotherapy/hormonal therapy). At a median follow-up of 6.3 years, there was no difference in either 5-year rates of loco-regional recurrence [SLNB alone = 1.6 % (95 % CI 0.7–3.3 %) versus ALND group = 3.1 % (95 % CI 1.7–5.2 %); $p = 0.11$] or overall survival [SLNB alone = 92.5 % (95 % CI 90.0–95.1 %) versus ALND group = 91.8 % (95 % CI 89.1–94.5 %)] between the two arms. The unadjusted hazard rate for treatment-related overall survival was 0.79 (90 % CI 0.56–1.11) and when adjusted for age and adjuvant therapy was closer to unity at 0.87 (90% CI 0.62–1.23). Both these values were less than a threshold hazard rate of 1.3 leading the authors to conclude that SLNB alone was *not* inferior to SLNB combined with completion ALND [113]. There have been concerns that this trial failed to accrue its target goal of 1900 patients and was underpowered. However, a lower rate of deaths than expected forced an early closure of the trial. It should be noted that the stage distribution and treatment context for this Z0011 trial are very different to those of NSAPB B-04 following which ALND prevailed despite equivalence of overall survival for patients with and without axillary treatment [6]. Due to limited follow-up, some breast cancer surgeons consider it premature to assume that results from Z0011 will change routine surgical practice. Nonetheless, more prolonged follow-up is unlikely to witness additional local recurrence which would translate into any meaningful survival decrement and overturn current trial conclusions [113].

The International Breast Cancer Study Group (IBCSG) 23-01 trial specifically aimed to determine whether ALND is necessary in patients with minimal SLN involvement [114]. Patients with micrometastases in ≥1 SLN were randomized to completion ALND or observation only. About 10 % of patients underwent mastectomy and in this respect the trial differed from Z0011 where all patients had breast conserving surgery with breast irradiation. More than 934 patients were randomized and there was also failure to meet the accrual target of 1960 patients, and the trial was likewise closed early due to a low event rate. As for Z0011, the majority of patients received some form of systemic treatment be this hormonal therapy alone, chemotherapy or chemohormonal therapy. At a median follow-up of 5.4 years, a total of 124 disease-free events were reported with no significant difference in the primary endpoint of disease-free survival, thereby satisfying the criteria for non-inferiority. Furthermore, overall survival was almost identical for the observation and completion ALND arms (97.5 and 97.6 %, respectively) and rates of axillary recurrence were very low. These results are potentially practice changing when taken together with those of Z0011.

A delayed ALND can be technically challenging, especially in the context of immediate breast reconstruction, although there is no evidence for increased morbidity with higher rates of lymphoedema for delayed ALND following a positive SLNB compared with a primary procedure [115]. Within the ALMANAC study, there was evidence of clinically significant morbidity from SLNB when analysed on an intention-to-treat basis [79]. This morbidity most likely relates to delayed ALND in sentinel lymph node-positive patients. For some patients, the risk: benefit ratio for detection of non-sentinel lymph node-positive cases may not justify completion ALND. The decision for further axillary surgery should be guided by variables such as primary tumour characteristics and nodal metastatic load together with patient preference. The proportion of retrieved nodes which contain metastases may be a critical factor in determining non-sentinel lymph node involvement [27].

There are several options for immediate change of practice in the aftermath of results from Z0011 and 23-01 trials which suggest that systemic therapies may effectively abort the process whereby circulating tumour cells from loco-regional disease undergo both arrest and proliferation to form viable metastatic foci. For patients with micrometastases (in any number of nodes), it is reasonable to consider omission of completion ALND irrespective of the type of breast surgery (mastectomy or lumpectomy) as there is a low statistical probability of non-sentinel lymph node tumour foci which are dependent on adjuvant treatments for elimination. Omission of completion ALND in the majority of patients who fulfil the criteria for Z0011 would represent a paradigm shift in surgical practice and undoubtedly leave some patients with persistent axillary disease post-operatively. More stringent inclusion criteria could reduce the chance of non-sentinel lymph node involvement even further and allay potential fears about inadequate treatment of residual tumour. This could, for example, take account of the sentinel lymph node metastatic ratio and might stipulate an upper size limit of 3 cm and exclude grade III tumours.

Whatever policy is adopted, it will be mandatory to audit patients carefully and consider establishment of a formal registration system (under the auspices of a formal authority). Furthermore, fully informed consent is essential in view of the above criticisms of the Z0011 trial in terms of accrual, power and limited follow-up. POSNOC (**PO**sitive **S**entinel Lymph **N**ode: **O**bservation vs **C**learance) is a non-inferiority trial which aims to accrue 1900 patients from 50 centres in the UK over a 2.5-year period with primary outcome results at 5.5 years and final trial results at 7.5 years. Pre-operative axillary ultrasound (+/− nodal needle biopsy) is mandatory, and unlike Z0011, this trial will include mastectomy patients and exclude those with sentinel node micrometastases (no further axillary surgery). Patients with 1 or 2 macrometastases in sentinel nodes will be randomized with the primary outcome measure being axillary recurrence [116].

15.7 Intra-operative Node Assessment

The main purpose for intra-operative nodal assessment is avoidance of completion ALND undertaken as a delayed, secondary procedure. Axillary reoperation can be technically challenging due to adhesions and fibrosis, but there is no objective evidence for increased morbidity when ALND follows SLN biopsy and median hospital stay is similar for delayed and primary ALND [115]. When completion ALND is performed as an *isolated* procedure, there are potential benefits from intra-operative assessment in terms of cost savings, patient convenience and avoidance of further general anaesthesia. When completion ALND rather than radiotherapy is recommended for patients with a positive SLN (tumour deposits >2 mm in size), this is sometimes combined with a breast surgical procedure—hence abrogating some disadvantages relating to cost and inconvenience [102]. For those patients who require a cavity re-excision or completion mastectomy for positive margins following wide excision, further axillary surgery can be done at the same time. The benefits of any intra-operative nodal assessment would be diminished for these patients in whom primary tumour characteristics mandate further surgery. There also exist subgroups of older patients and those with comorbidities for whom a single-stage axillary operation should be recommended at the outset. Similarly, selected women might safely avoid completion ALND with minimal chance of regional relapse or impact on longer term survival. In the 'post-Z0011' era, any decision for selective omission of completion ALND should be based on full histopathological parameters relating to both axillary nodes and primary tumour; ironically some patients may be committed to completion ALND when intra-operative node assessment is available and confirms positivity. Recently published results from the AMAROS trial suggest that axillary radiotherapy can substitute for completion ALND in some patients with low-volume nodal disease for whom intra-operative assessment would not apply [117].

It is appropriate to ask whether intra-operative nodal assessment can be justified for all patients having SLNB as a component of primary surgery in view of the inconsistent and variable sensitivity of both frozen section and touch imprint cytology (TIMC) which have not yet been surpassed by molecular assays based on quantitative reverse transcription polymerase chain reaction (RT-PCR). Both frozen section and TIMC employ rapid H&E staining methods but, like formalin-fixed tissue sections, examine less than 5 % of the node and have other limitations. Interpretation is subjective, and when only clusters of cells are examined, the distinction between micro- and macrometastases may be unclear. This might lead to ALND in some patients with micrometastases only ('false positive'). The reported patient-based sensitivities for both FS and TIMC are highly variable at 36–96 % and specificity of 95–100 % [118–121]. Frozen section examination has a false-negative rate of about 25 % and although TIMC is reported to be more accurate when immunohistochemical staining is used, a 'blinded' trial of a single-section approach using facing halves of a bivalved sentinel lymph node revealed equivalence of accuracy [122]. A meta-analysis reported a sensitivity of 75 % (95 % CI 65–84) and 63 % (95 % CI 57–69) for FS and TIMC, respectively, with TIMC having significantly lower pooled sensitivity for micrometastases (22 %) compared to macrometastases (81 %) [123].

Molecular-based technologies for intra-operative nodal assessment objectively measure expression of genes normally expressed in breast tissue but not lymph nodes such as the cytoskeleton protein CK19 which is expressed in most breast cancer cells [124]. Operating parameters are set such that quantitative RT-PCR detects macrometastases but not micrometastases nor isolated tumour cells. Validation studies suggest these molecular technologies are almost as accurate as conventional histological evaluation but examination of different nodal slabs ultimately prevents complete concordance [125]. Overall concordance levels between RT-PCR scores and permanent H&E sections were 93.7 % for the now extinct GeneSearch Breast lymph node assay (Veridex) and 98.2 % for the one-step nucleic acid assay (OSNA) which typically analyse 50 % of fresh nodal tissue [126]. The remaining commercially available molecular assay (OSNA) takes approximately 30 min to process one node (5 min per additional node) with a mean time saving of 18 min compared to TIMC or frozen section [127]. Though breast resection (wide local excision/mastectomy) is undertaken during this period, in reality intra-operative assessment incurs additional operating time of up to 30 min per case with cumulative delays and cost implications. SLNB-positive patients will subsequently require node clearance which consumes further operating time.

Intra-operative node examination may be more difficult to justify for all patients in the context of contemporary practice which either deselects patients for SLNB or dictates that completion ALND is performed alongside definitive or additional breast surgery. Formal cost analysis is warranted to compare intra-operative node assessment for all cases of SLNB in relation to the small number of cases of isolated completion ALND. Development of non-commercial open access molecular assays ('home recipes') as alternatives may significantly influence cost: benefit analyses of molecular methods for intra-operative assessment compared with TIMC or FS.

15.8 Indications for Sentinel Lymph Node Biopsy

Most of the validatory studies on SLNB were confined to tumours measuring 2 cm or less. With increasing tumour size, there is a greater probability of nodal involvement and gross metastatic disease within a lymph node may prevent uptake of dye and isotope. Lymph flow is passive and will be readily diverted to 'non-sentinel' nodes yielding a false-negative result [23]. A heavily infiltrated node which is non-blue and cold may once have constituted the 'true' sentinel node but subsequently been 'demoted' due to diversion of lymph flow within a complex lymphatic network. Patients with clinically positive nodes are more likely to have extensive pathological involvement and should not be offered SLNB. Some of these clinically node-positive patients will be found to have innocent nodes on axillary ultrasound and core biopsy/FNAC of a node may be negative. Provided the primary tumour is neither inflammatory nor locally advanced, these patients could be considered for SLNB. Although SLNB is usually contraindicated for tumours over 5 cm in size, Guiliano's group have reported the successful application of SLNB to tumours in excess of 5 cm [128]. Nonetheless, false-negative rates are higher when there is a greater chance of node positivity and current trials are evaluating the accuracy of SLNB for tumours measuring between 3 and 5 cm [77]. The Australian SNAC II trial examined SLNB in tumours exceeding 3 cm in size and includes both multifocal and multicentric tumours. Amongst a group of 100 patients from the SNAC trial database with tumours ≥3 cm (mean size—3.91 cm) almost two-thirds had axillary node metastases. The sentinel node(s) was successfully identified in 93/100 cases with an average yield of 1.75 nodes per case. More than 60 % of patients were SLNB-positive and over 40 % had positive non-sentinel nodes. Notably, the false-negative rate was 5 % which is comparable to outcomes for smaller tumours. However, the high positivity rate for both sentinel and non-sentinel nodes questions the rationale for SLNB in larger tumours—the latter may be more appropriately managed with primary axillary lymph node dissection [129].

15.8.1 Ductal Carcinoma in Situ

The indications for SLNB have broadened in recent years to include patients with widespread ductal carcinoma in situ (DCIS) undergoing mastectomy and even some localized forms of DCIS associated with a clinical or radiological mass lesion [130–132]. Despite earlier arguments against routine SLNB for patients with DCIS [133], there is now consensus that extensive high nuclear-grade (HNG) or intermediate nuclear-grade (ING) DCIS on imaging which mandates mastectomy or DCIS presenting as a palpable lesion are indications for SLNB. Typical cases of screen-detected localized areas of DCIS which represent up to 80 % of cases in a screening programme do not qualify for routine SLNB. An incidental invasive component is found in up to 20 % of cases of DCIS in which mastectomy is the choice of operation and extensive DCIS is a risk factor for invasive malignancy from historical studies [134]. The presence of HNG DCIS, comedo necrosis and mammographic size in excess of 4 cm are independent risk factors for invasion [135, 136]. A significant proportion of those patients with microinvasion (≤1 mm) diagnosed on core biopsy will have further invasive foci on definitive histology. SLNB is advisable for all patients with microinvasion, up to 10 % of whom will be sentinel lymph node positive [130]. Nonetheless, despite reports of node positivity rates approaching 15 % in higher risk DCIS and DCIS with microinvasion [137], many cases involve isolated tumour cells or micrometastases only which are of questionable biological significance and unlikely to be clinically relevant [131]. When the target of biopsy is not microcalcification, there is a greater chance patients will have further invasive foci on definitive histology which mandates some form of axillary staging. Moreover, between 10 and 15 % of lesions diagnosed as DCIS using large bore vacuum devices will show invasion on complete excision [138]. The risk of nodal involvement which is acceptable if left untreated is a subjective judgement and those with very low risk should be spared the minimal but finite morbidity of SLNB with concomitant cost savings.

15.8.2 Multifocal and Multicentric Tumours

Multifocal and multicentric tumours were initially found to be associated with high false-negative rates and were considered a contraindication to SLNB [139]. This was consonant with the misguided assumption that tumours located in different quadrants of the breast drain through mutually exclusive lymphatic pathways, and therefore, SLNB would lead to inaccurate axillary lymph node staging [140]. Subsequent publications have refuted this viewpoint and SLNB is no longer precluded by the presence of multiple tumour foci either within the same (multifocality) or different (multicentricity) quadrants of the ipsilateral breast [140–142]. Furthermore, evidence from lymphoscintigraphy supports the notion that the various quadrants of the breast share common lymphatic drainage channels which converge upon the subareolar region [143]. A meta-analysis evaluated almost one thousand patients with multifocal and multicentric tumours who underwent SLNB followed by ALND. Identification rates exceeded 95 % and the average false-negative rate was 6.3 % when those patients with relative contraindications (e.g. post-chemotherapy or tumours >5 cm) to SLNB were excluded from analysis. Nonetheless, the overall false-negative rate remained less than 10 % when all patients were included but caution is needed when recommending SLNB for multicentric and multifocal tumours where the largest tumour focus is >5 cm or SLNB follows neoadjuvant chemotherapy for such tumours [144]. A recent prospective validation study involving 30 patients with multicentric cancer confirms that SLNB is associated with high rates of identification (100 %) and low false-negative rates when dual localization techniques with blue dye and radioisotope are employed [145]. However, rates of node positivity were relatively high with 66.7 % of patients having axillary nodal metastases (albeit with immediate completion ALND for validation purposes).

15.8.3 Pregnancy

The development of breast cancer during pregnancy presents unique management challenges with a prominent emotional dimension. Though termination may be advocated in the first trimester, surgical treatments can be safely undertaken in any trimester of pregnancy [146]. Adjuvant therapies including radiotherapy and chemohormonal therapies are usually deferred until after delivery though chemotherapy (but *not* tamoxifen) can be safely administered in the second trimester when organogenesis is complete and teratogenic effects are minimal [147, 148]. Radiotherapy is absolutely contraindicated in the gravid state but interestingly the dose of radiation from exposure to technetium radiocolloid in SLNB is only 20 MBq. This is well below the safe upper limit for pregnant women, and therefore, SLNB using isotopic localization only could be employed; note that blue dye can stain placental and foetal tissue and should be avoided. If there are concerns about use of radioisotope during pregnancy, then axillary staging could be carried out as a delayed procedure (if ALND at the outset is deemed inappropriate) or blind sampling undertaken.

15.8.4 Elderly Patients

SLNB should be employed in most elderly patients with clinically node-negative breast cancer, but might be avoided in some older patients who have a low probability of nodal involvement. Perhaps a more pertinent issue is whether completion ALND should be undertaken for a positive sentinel lymph node in older patients. Even before publication of the ACOSOG Z0011 trial, completion ALND was selectively omitted in certain older patients, particularly those with only micrometastases in the sentinel lymph node. A publication from the Memorial Sloan-Kettering Cancer Centre reported that rates of axillary relapse in patients with a positive sentinel lymph node who for various reasons had no further axillary surgery are very low (2 % at 3 years) [149]. Some elderly patients will decline completion ALND when fully informed of risks and benefits of this procedure; this group of patients are very unlikely to have residual disease which would develop into any troublesome regional recurrence or compromise longer term survival in the setting of competing mortality risks.

15.8.5 Repeat Sentinel Lymph Node Biopsy

A particular challenge in contemporary breast cancer surgery is optimal management of the axilla in patients who develop IBTR following previous breast conservation therapy with a negative SLNB. Until recently, ALND was the default option for most SLNB-negative patients with local recurrence after BCS [150]. However, early reports suggested that SLNB was feasible in patients who had undergone axillary surgery for non-malignant conditions [151]. Several studies including a meta-analysis have now confirmed that repeat SLNB for this category of patients is associated with acceptable rates of identification and an inverse relationship is discernible between rates of successful repeat SLNB and the number of nodes previously removed at first surgery [152–154]. Hence, patients who had undergone ALND initially had failure rates exceeding 50 % which were more than twice those for patients having undergone prior SLNB only. An important concept when considering repeat SLNB is restoration of the lymphatic network following disruption from previous SLNB surgery. Although fibrosis occurs in this setting, there is collateralization of lymphatic vessels and connections are re-established between an area of breast tissue which harbours recurrent tumour and a 'new' sentinel lymph node within the territory of the operated axilla. Hence, rather than the adage 'one sentinel node forever' there is now recognition of 'always a new sentinel node' [152, 153]. Intra and colleagues reported their experience of repeat SLNB in patients with IBTR after BCS and a prior negative SLNB. They successfully performed SLNB in 196 out of 207 patients, all of whom had undergone lymphoscintigraphy prior to surgery (with identification of at least one node in 206 patients). Only 9 patients were node positive with micrometastases in 8 and isolated tumour cells in 1 patient. These and other authors have recommended repeat SLNB in selected patients based on results of lymphoscintigraphy; where facilities for the latter are not available, patients should undergo ALND rather than attempts at repeat SLNB which has a higher failure rate when not directed by pre-operative visualization of sentinel nodes on lymphoscintigraphy [155].

15.9 Neoadjuvant Chemotherapy

A dichotomy of practice has emerged in efforts to define how SLNB should be optimally incorporated into the neoadjuvant setting. Some breast units have opted for SLNB in conjunction with completion ALND *after* chemotherapy. This was practiced in prospective trials to assess the safety and accuracy of SLNB following a period of induction chemotherapy which might potentially alter patterns of lymphatic drainage in the axilla and increase false-negative rates. These latter concerns led others to recommend upfront SLNB performed *prior to* initiation of chemotherapy. The intrinsic accuracy of this technique in terms of parameters such as sentinel lymph node identification rates and false-negative rates would be no different to patients having primary surgical treatment.

15.9.1 Sentinel Lymph Node Biopsy Prior to Neoadjuvant Chemotherapy

Advantages—there will be minimal risk of an unacceptably high false-negative result and information derived from SLNB allows more accurate initial staging of patients when SLNB is undertaken prior to neoadjuvant chemotherapy [156, 157]. Identification rates for upfront SLNB are high and range from 98 to 100 % which is consistent with more extensive surgical experience of routine SLNB pre-treatment. It should be noted that nodal positivity rates are variable (29–67 %) within this patient population and reflect the heterogeneous nature of primary tumours within and between studies which nonetheless confirm that SLN biopsy has satisfactory performance characteristics for larger tumours [129]. A positive SLNB result would prompt a subsequent ALND following neoadjuvant chemotherapy, but otherwise no further axillary surgery is indicated and completion ALND can be safely avoided at time of definitive surgery, be this wide local excision, simple mastectomy or mastectomy with immediate breast reconstruction [70]. Upfront SLNB provides important information on prognostication and can guide treatment decisions for adjuvant radiotherapy, systemic therapy and axillary surgery. Although knowledge of the sentinel lymph node status at presentation may influence decisions on irradiation of regional nodes, precise nodal quantification of axillary metastatic load with an upfront approach is limited; for example, a single positive node only may be retrieved at the time of SLNB, but multiple nodes may be positive despite an innocent ultrasound examination of the axilla. In addition to established clinicopathological factors, molecular tests such as Oncotype DX (Genomic Health, Redwood, California) can assess estimated risk of recurrence in patients with early-stage breast cancer. Patients with larger tumours and a confirmed negative SLNB but low score on Oncotype DX could be treated with neoadjuvant hormonal therapy rather than chemotherapy. However, although prognostic tests provide information about risk of recurrence and death, predictive markers are needed to select optimum therapy for individual patients.

Disadvantages—upfront SLNB requires an additional operation for all neoadjuvant chemotherapy patients, irrespective of final nodal status. Nonetheless, selected node-positive patients will need additional surgery when SLNB follows chemotherapy and facilities for intra-operative node assessment are not available. Concerns have been expressed about possible delays in commencement of chemotherapy treatment when an upfront SLNB policy is employed, with delays consequent to either scheduling issues or wound complications such as seromas and infection. It may be prudent to wait at least 7 days from the time of SLNB before starting chemotherapy to minimize potential wound problems and consider surgical antibiotic prophylaxis in this group of patients.

A negative SLNB result prior to neoadjuvant therapy can be helpful as no further axillary treatment is necessary, and such information can reinforce any decision to withhold subsequent supraclavicular irradiation. However, patients selected for neoadjuvant chemotherapy have a higher chance of nodal involvement and, in the event of a positive SLNB, are then committed to completion ALND with no opportunity for nodal downstaging. An upfront SLNB can be useful in patients who do not require chemotherapy if SLN biopsy negative, but often age, primary tumour size, and information from core needle biopsy are sufficient to justify a recommendation for neoadjuvant chemotherapy.

15.9.2 Sentinel Lymph Node Biopsy After Neoadjuvant Chemotherapy

Advantages—when SLNB is undertaken after primary chemotherapy, it is possible to take advantage of potential nodal downstaging and avoidance of ALND [158]. A 'single' operation has the additional appeal of patient convenience and reduced costs when facilities for intra-operative node assessment are available. Rates of complete pathological nodal response vary from 20 to 36 % in patients with needle biopsy-confirmed positive-node pre-chemotherapy [159]. Most metastases diagnosed on needle biopsy are macrometastases (>2 mm), and it is conceivable that complete pathological response might be higher for nodes containing micrometastases only, though there is no current evidence to support this. There is a suggestion that knowledge of nodal response to chemotherapy is more relevant in terms of prognostication and decision-making for chest wall/supraclavicular radiotherapy than initial nodal status. In particular, those patients with a complete pathological response in both the breast and axilla appear to have a much better prognosis [160].

Disadvantages—primary chemotherapy may modify lymphatic drainage patterns within the axilla where there is a degree of plasticity within the lymphatic network of vessels [161]. Distortion of lymphatics may occur secondary to tumour shrinkage with creation of aberrant lymphatic drainage patterns which together with plugging of lymphatics by tumour emboli could increase false-negative rates. Notwithstanding these theoretical considerations, there is no conclusive evidence that such phenomena occur to any significant extent in neoadjuvant therapy patients and this may have encouraged a recent trend away from upfront SLNB in neoadjuvant chemotherapy patients [162]. Interestingly, chemotherapy is more likely to eradicate tumour within non-sentinel lymph nodes than the sentinel lymph

Table 15.3 Accuracy of sentinel lymph node biopsy after neoadjuvant chemotherapy

Study/author	Identification rate (%)	False-negative rate
NSAPB B-27 [169] (428 patients)	85	11 % (8 % [dye + RI]; 14 % [dye alone])
GANEA (French) [166] (195 patients)	90	11 % (9.4 % [node −ve]; 11.6 % [node +ve])
MD Anderson [164] (575 patients)	97.4	5.9 % (4.1 % [pre-chemotherapy]; p = 0.39)

node in which the tumour cell burden is likely to be greater. Thus although cancer cells spread first to the sentinel lymph node and thereafter to the non-sentinel nodes, the inverse sequence applies to chemotherapy effect and some have referred to a 'front to back, back to front' phenomenon in which chemotherapy is more likely to eradicate tumour within NSLN then the SLN in which the tumour cell burden is usually greater. Thus although cancer cells spread first to the sentinel node and thereafter to NSLNs, the inverse sequence applies to chemotherapy [163]. This would increase the negative predictive value of a negative SLNB after chemotherapy. However, if tumour deposits responded earlier in the sentinel than non-sentinel nodes, then a false-negative result would ensue.

An analysis by Hunt and colleagues revealed a false-negative rate of 5.9 % when SLNB followed neoadjuvant chemotherapy and 4.1 % for upfront SLNB [164]. Recent reports have shown false-negative rates in the region of 8–11 %; a meta-analysis of 21 single-institution studies involving more than 1200 patients undergoing post-chemotherapy SLNB with completion ALND reported a pooled false-negative estimate of 12 % when SLNB followed chemotherapy in clinically node-negative patients (Table 15.3) [165]. These figures are similar to false-negative rates for primary surgery, but it should be noted that these two clinical scenarios may not be strictly comparable as only a subset of patients in these neoadjuvant studies had SLNB post-chemotherapy with patient selection and surgeon experience introducing an element of bias [163]. There have been mixed reports on false-negative rates when there is needle biopsy (cytology or core biopsy)-proven positive nodes pre-chemotherapy with a limited number of published studies relating specifically to this group of patients (Table 15.4) [167–169]. Mamounas cited an overall false-negative rate of 11.1 % for SLNB post-neoadjuvant chemotherapy when there is confirmed nodal involvement at presentation [170]. These updated figures are reassuring but a note of caution has been sounded by Alvarado and colleagues who express concerns that false-negative rates can be unacceptably high when SLNB follows neoadjuvant chemotherapy in patients presenting with node-positive disease [171]. They reported an overall false-negative rate of 20.8 % although normalization of nodes on ultrasound post-chemotherapy reduced this rate to 16.1 % (compared with 27.8 % for those with abnormal node morphology including size and cortical thickness).

There is a paucity of data on omission of completion ALND in needle biopsy-proven node-positive patients with a subsequent negative SLNB after neoadjuvant chemotherapy. In particular, it is unclear from some reports whether cited rates relate to patients with positive or negative initial nodal status and there is confounding of studies due to some patients proceeding to ALND. Further information is needed on rates of regional recurrence specifically in those patients with a negative sentinel lymph node who did not have ALND. It is conceivable that axillary recurrence is higher when there is residual non-sentinel nodal disease after a false-negative SLNB post-chemotherapy (no further chemotherapy routinely given) [172].

Boughy and colleagues have provided important information from the American College of Surgeons Oncology Group (ACOSOG) Z1071 trial which examined false-negative rates for patients with core biopsy-proven node-positive breast cancer who underwent SLNB and concomitant ALND after primary chemotherapy [173]. The primary endpoint for this study was the false-negative rate for clinically node-positive patients who have at least 3 sentinel lymph nodes removed for pathological examination. Rates of identification were 92.5 % overall with an accuracy of 84 % for assignment of correct nodal status. Forty percentage of patients had a complete pathological nodal response with no

Table 15.4 False-negative rates for cytologically/core biopsy-proven positive nodes pre-chemotherapy

Author	No. patients	False-negative rate (%)
Shen et al. [167]	69	25
Lee et al. [168][a]	238	5.6
Newman et al. [169]	54	10.7
Alvarado et al. [171]	150	16.1
Boughy et al. [173]	649	12.6

[a]In this study, some patients were classified as node positive on the basis of suspicious nodes on ultrasound/PET scan

evidence of any residual tumour on routine H&E staining (metastases >0.2 mm). The false-negative rate was almost 20 % when only a single tracer agent was employed compared with 10.2 % for dual tracer localization and harvesting of a minimum of 2 nodes. It was recommended that at least 3 nodes be removed in this setting of SLNB post-chemotherapy. On the basis of these Z1071 results, SLNB after neoadjuvant chemotherapy for biopsy-proven nodal involvement at presentation can only be reliably used when dual localization methods have been employed and at least 2 nodes have been removed and examined.

The German SENTINA trial addressed the role of repeat SLNB in patients who had previously undergone the procedure prior to neoadjuvant chemotherapy [174]. Patients were allocated to one of four arms; initially clinically node-negative patients treated with upfront SLNB were designated arms A and B; if the sentinel lymph node was negative (arm A—662 patients), then no further axillary surgery was undertaken. If the sentinel lymph node was positive before chemotherapy, then repeat SLNB with ALND was performed after chemotherapy (arm B—360 patients). Patients who were initially clinically node positive were designated arms C and D; those who converted to clinically node-negative status after chemotherapy underwent SLNB with ALND (arm C—592 patients) whilst those who remained clinically node positive had a standard ALND (arm D—123 patients). The false-negative rate for repeat SLNB patients (arm B) exceeded 50 % (51.6 %; 95 % CI 38.7–64.2 %) and sometimes only a single node was removed. It was concluded that SLNB is unacceptable as a repeat procedure following neoadjuvant chemotherapy. The false-negative rate was also noted to be relatively high for those patients in arm C who converted from clinically node positive to negative after chemotherapy (14.2, 95 % CI 9.9–19.4 %).

There is increasing evidence that decisions for radiotherapy (chest wall/supraclavicular) should be based on tumour response to chemotherapy rather than the status of the regional nodes per se at presentation. Knowledge of sentinel lymph node negativity from downstaging after neoadjuvant chemotherapy (when there were biopsy confirmed nodal metastases at presentation) is very helpful when estimating benefit from radiotherapy. For clinically node-positive patients who become negative after neoadjuvant chemotherapy, there appears to be little benefit from radiotherapy. Hence, SLNB after neoadjuvant chemotherapy allows assessment of specific response within the regional nodes to chemotherapy whereas positive nodes might otherwise be removed with SLNB and preclude any comment on nodal response following formal ALND after neoadjuvant chemotherapy [158, 170].

A large randomized phase III trial (NSABP-51/RTOG-1304 trial) will evaluate post-mastectomy chest wall and regional nodal radiotherapy and post-lumpectomy regional nodal radiotherapy in patients with positive axillary nodes before neoadjuvant chemotherapy who convert to pathologically negative axillary nodes after neoadjuvant chemotherapy [175]. Thus amongst node-positive patients who convert to node-negative status, this trial will determine whether or not decisions concerning adjuvant radiotherapy should be based on nodal status at the time of initial presentation. Ultimately, the results of this trial will be an important consideration in the decision-making process for recommending SLNB either before or after administration of neoadjuvant chemotherapy.

There is now greater confidence in declaration of a 'negative' SLNB after primary chemotherapy for node-positive disease and withholding routine ALND in selected cases. Nonetheless, the significance of micrometastases and isolated tumour cells in this setting is uncertain and these may be of different biological consequence if they represent downstaged macrometastases. Any evidence of sentinel node tumour deposits on H&E staining (including isolated tumour cells) should be followed by completion ALND irrespective of the type of breast surgery.

15.10 Internal Mammary Node Biopsy

Substantial surgical morbidity can result from removal of internal mammary nodes with no demonstration of any gains in overall survival [16, 17]. It is uncommon for the internal mammary nodes to be involved in the absence of metastases in the axillary nodes, which undermines its value as additional staging information. The biological significance of internal mammary chain disease remains uncertain, and the use of adjuvant therapies is often prompted by concomitant axillary nodal disease. Thus, the necessity for internal mammary node biopsy is controversial; it is acknowledged that microscopic involvement of the internal mammary nodes may be significant for medially placed tumours with positive axillary nodes. It should be noted that trials of post-mastectomy radiotherapy which have shown an improvement of about 10 % in overall survival included irradiation of the internal mammary chain [176, 177]. The EORTC trial recruited axillary node-positive and node-negative patients with medial/central tumours. A total of 50 Gy was delivered in 25 fractions with a mixed technique of 6MV photons (26 Gy in 13 fractions) and 12 meV electrons (24 Gy in 12 fractions) [178]. A small improvement in overall survival at 5 years was noted which just reached statistical significance (HR 0.87; 95 % CI 0.76–1.00; $p = 0.056$). A meta-analysis of all three trials investigating irradiation of the internal mammary nodes (French, MA-20 and EORTC) reveals a benefit for overall and metastases-free survival (HR 0.88; 95 % CI 0.8–0.97; $p = 0.012$). Nonetheless, clinical manifestation of internal mammary node recurrence is rare. The indications for irradiation of the internal mammary nodes is unclear at the present time, but CT-based simulation with new planning techniques may minimize the volume of the heart and lungs exposed to radiation and hence related morbidities such as pericarditis and coronary artery disease. Internal mammary nodal irradiation is associated with low lung toxicity and a slight excess of cardiac deaths was noted in the French study, but numbers were small and not statistically significant. There is a delicate balance between cardiac versus breast cancer deaths, particularly for right-sided tumours. Patient selection is a major challenge and only a minority of stage 2 patients will have malignant involvement of internal mammary nodes. The odds of internal mammary nodal involvement increases from 2 to 20 % when lymphovascular invasion is present but nodes are negative. What are the implications of these findings for SLNB and how should sentinel node-positive patients be treated in the meantime? Some would argue that the main criterion for administration of internal mammary node irradiation should be a positive internal mammary node biopsy, although PET imaging may offer an alternative basis for declaring internal mammary node positivity. By implication, internal mammary node biopsy as a standard of care warrants consideration. There is likely to be a statistically significant benefit in overall survival from internal mammary node irradiation for internal mammary node-positive patients and high risk pN0 patients. Nonetheless, the role of internal mammary node irradiation in the era of SLNB remains unclear—especially bearing in mind that axillary lymph node dissection does not confer a survival advantage—so why should treatment of the internal mammary nodes be associated with any survival gain?

15.11 Conclusion

Approaches to management of the axilla have become more complex and present clinical decision-making challenges in terms of indications for SLNB and extent of surgery for SLNB-positive patients with limited axillary tumour burden. Axillary surgery encompasses both staging and therapeutic procedures, and it is important to select patients appropriately to avoid under- and over-treatment of patients, respectively. SLNB is now the dominant and preferred method for staging the axilla, but several questions remain unanswered. These relate to methodology, interpretation and the clinical significance of nodal metastases when SLNB is undertaken as a primary surgical procedure or following neoadjuvant chemotherapy. There has been a trend towards abandonment of blue dye for routine SLNB in recent years, but false-negative rates are minimized when dual localization techniques are used post-chemotherapy for needle biopsy-proven node-positive disease. For some patients, completion ALND may not be justified whilst for others any form of surgical axillary staging might be safely omitted. Collective results from the Z0011 and IBCSG 23-01 trials are considered practice changing in the USA, although a more cautious approach has been adopted in many European countries with a related POSNOC trial currently recruiting patients in the UK. Data from local audits suggest that results of Z0011 may not be applicable to practices in other units worldwide and pertain to a minority of SLNB-positive patients. Ironically, most patients with needle biopsy-proven nodal metastases at presentation are committed to an ALND, but some of these patients might be adequately treated with a SLNB which removes any positive nodes. Nonetheless, node-positive patients with larger, locally advanced or inflammatory cancers should undergo primary ALND. Individualized recommendations based on the risk of relapse in conjunction with benefits and cost of treatment is the ideal approach to management of the axilla. This strategy should incorporate a spectrum of options including ALND, targeted sampling and observation alone.

References

1. Carter CL, Allen C, Henderson DE. Relation of tumour size, lymph node status and survival in 24, 740 breast cancer cases. Cancer. 1989;73:505–8.
2. Rosen PP, Groshen S, Saigo PE, et al. Pathologic prognostic factors in stage I (T1N0M0) and stage II (T1N1M0) breast carcinoma: a study of 644 patients with median follow up of 18 years. J Clin Oncol. 1989;7:1239–125.
3. Kissin MW, Querci della Rovere G, Easton D, et al. Risk of lymphoedema following the treatment of breast cancer. Br J Surg. 1986;73:580–4.
4. Ivens D, Hoe AL, Podd TJ, et al. Assessment of morbidity from complete axillary dissection. Br J Cancer. 1992;66:136–8.
5. Britton PD, Goud A, Godward S, et al. Use of ultrasound-guided axillary node core biopsy in staging of early breast cancer. Eur Radiol 2008. doi:10.1007/s00330-008-1177-5.
6. Fisher B, Montague F, Redmond C, et al. Ten-year results of a randomized trial comparing radical mastectomy and total mastectomy with or without radiation. N Engl J Med. 1985;312:674–81.
7. Baum M, Coyle PJ. Simple mastectomy for early breast cancer and the behaviour of the untreated nodes. Bull Cancer. 1977;64:603–10.
8. Purushotham AD, MacMillan RD, Wishart G. Advances in axillary surgery for breast cancer—time for a tailored approach. Eu J Surg Oncol. 2005;31:929–31.
9. Jatoi I. Management of the axilla in primary breast cancer. Surg Clin North Am. 1999;79:1061–73.
10. Haagensen CD. Anatomy of the mammary glands. In Haagensen CD (ed): *Diseases of the breast* 3rd Edition, Philadelphia, 1986 WB Saunders.
11. Sappey M. Traite d'Anatomie Descriptive. 2nd Edition. Paris, 1888.
12. Rouviere H. Anatomie des lymphatiques de l'homme. Paris: Masson; 1932.
13. Handley RS, Thackray AC. The internal mammary lymph chain in carcinoma of the breast. Lancet. 1949;2:276.

14. Borgstein PJ, Meijer S, Pijpers RJ, et al. Functional lymphatic anatomy for sentinel node biopsy in breast cancer: echoes from the past and the periareolar blue dye method. Ann Surg. 2000;232:81–9.
15. Mansel RE, Goyal A, Newcombe RG. Internal mammary node drainage and its role in sentinel node biopsy: the initial ALMANAC experience. Clin Breast Cancer. 2004;5:279–84.
16. Veronesi U, Cascinella N, Greco M, et al. Prognosis of breast cancer patients after mastectomy and dissection of internal mammary nodes. Ann Surg. 1985;202:702–7.
17. Veronesi U, Marubini E, Mariou L, et al. The dissection of internal mammary nodes does not improve the survival of breast cancer patients. 30-year results of a randomized trial. Eur J Cancer. 1999;35:1320–5.
18. McMinn RMH. Last's Anatomy (Regional and Applied). 18th Edition Churchill Livingstone 1990.
19. Osborne MP, Jeyasingh K, Jewkes RF, et al. The pre-operative detection of internal mammary node metastases in breast cancer. Br J Surg. 1979;66:813.
20. Thomas JM, Redding WH, Sloane JP. The spread of breast cancer: importance of the intrathoracic lymphatic route and its relevance to treatment. Br J Cancer. 1979;40:540.
21. Tanis PJ, Neiweg OE, Valdes Olmos RA, et al. Anatomy and physiology of lymphatic drainage of the breast from the perspective of sentinel node biopsy. J Am Coll Surg. 2001;192:399–409.
22. Morton DL, Wen DR, Wong JH, et al. Technical details of intra-operative lymphatic mapping for early stage melanoma. Arch Surg. 1992;127:392–9.
23. Bleiweiss I. Sentinel lymph nodes in breast cancer after 10 years: rethinking basic principles. Lancet Oncol. 2006;7:686–92.
24. Romrell LJ, Bland KI. Anatomy of the breast, axilla, chest wall and related metastatic sites. Chapter 2. In: The Breast (Bland KI and Copeland EM Eds) Vol I 3rd Edition Saunders 2004. ISBN 0-7216-9490-X.
25. Turner-Warwick RT. The lymphatics of the breast. Br J Surg. 1959;46:574–82.
26. Goyal A, Newcombe RG, Mansell RE. Clinical relevance of multiple sentinel nodes in patients with breast cancer. Br J Surg. 2005;92:438–42.
27. Rescigno J, Taylor LA, Aziz MS, et al. Predicting negative axillary lymph node dissection in patients with positive sentinel lymph node biopsy: can a subset of patients be spared axillary dissection? Breast Cancer Res Treat. 2005;94:S35.
28. Veronesi U, Rilke R, Luini A, et al. Distribution of axillary node metastases by level of invasion. Cancer. 1987;59:682–7.
29. Jacobsson S. Studies of the blood circulation in lymphoedematous limbs. Scan J Plast Recon Surg. 1967;3:1–81.
30. Schuneman J, Willich N. Lympheodema of the arm after primary treatment of breast cancer. Anticancer Res. 1998;18:2235–6.
31. Mortimer PS, Bates DO, Brassington HD, et al. The prevalence of arm oedema following treatment for breast cancer. Q J Med. 1996;89:377–80.
32. Morrow M. Miami breast cancer conference. Florida, USA: Orlando; 2008.
33. Pain SJ, Purushotham AD. Lymphoedema following surgery for breast cancer. Br J Surg. 2000;87:1128–41.
34. Stewart FW, Treves N. Lymphangiosarcoma in post-mastectomy oedema. Cancer. 1948;1:64–81.
35. Temple WJ, Ketcham AS. Preservation of the intercostobrachial nerve during axillary dissection for breast cancer. Am J Surg. 1985;150:406–13.
36. Abdullah TI, Iddon J, Barr L, Baildam AD, Bundred NJ. Prospective randomized controlled trial of preservation of the intercostobrachial nerve. Br J Surg. 1998;85:1443–5.
37. Salmon RJ, Ansquer Y, Asselain B. Preservation versus section of the intercostobrachial nerve (ICBN) in axillary dissection for breast cancer—a prospective randomized trial. Eur J Surg Oncol. 1998;24:158–61.
38. MacMillan RD, Blamey RW. The case for axillary sampling. Advances in Breast Cancer. 2004;1:9–10.
39. Benson JR. Querci della Rovere G (and the Axilla Management Consensus Group). Management of the axilla in women with breast cancer. Lancet Oncology. 2007;8:331–48.
40. Fisher B. The evolution of paradigms for the management of breast cancer: a personal perspective. Cancer Res. 1992;52:2371–83.
41. Fisher B, Montague F, Redmond C, et al. Ten-year results of a randomized trial comparing radical mastectomy and total mastectomy with or without radiation. N Engl J Med. 1985;312: 674–81.
42. Harris JR, Osteen RT. Patients with early breast cancer benefit form effective axillary treatment. Breast Cancer Res Treat. 1985;5:17–21.
43. Gardner B, Feldman J. Are positive axillary nodes in breast cancer markers for incurable disease? Ann Surg. 1993;218:270–8.
44. Moffat FL, Sewofsky GM, Davis K, et al. Axillary node dissection for early breast cancer: some is good but all is better. J Surg Oncol. 1992;51:8.
45. Orr RK. The impact of prophylactic axillary node dissection on breast cancer survival: a Bayesian meta-analysis. Ann Surg Oncol. 1999;6:109–16.
46. Early Breast Cancer Trialists Collaborative Group. Effects of radiotherapy and of differences in the extent of surgery for early breast cancer on local recurrence and 15 year survival: an overview of the randomized trials. Lancet. 2005;366:2087–106.
47. Benson JR, Querci della Rovere G. The biological significance of ipsilateral local recurrence of breast cancer: determinant or indicator of poor prognosis. Lancet Oncol. 2002;3:45–9.
48. Cancer Research Campaign Working Party. Cancer research campaign (King's/Cambridge) trial for early breast cancer. Lancet. 1980;2:55–60.
49. Epstein RJ. Routine or delayed axillary dissection for primary breast cancer? Eu J Cancer. 1995;31A:1570–3.
50. Fowble B, Solin L, Schultz D, Goodman R. Frequency, sites of relapse and outcome of regional node failures following conservative surgery and radiation for early breast cancer. Int J Oncol Biol Phys. 1989;17:703–10.
51. Graverson HP, Blichert-Toft M, Andersen J, et al. for the Danish Breast Cancer Cooperative Group. Breast cancer: risk of axillary recurrence in node negative patients following partial dissection of the axilla. Eur J Surg Oncol 1988;14:407–412.
52. Veronesi U, Paganelli G, Viale G, et al. Sentinel lymph node biopsy as a staging procedure in breast cancer: update of a randomized controlled study. Lancet Oncol. 2006;7:983–90.
53. Naik AM, Fey J, Gemignani M, Heerdt A, et al. The risk of axillary relapse after sentinel lymph node biopsy for breast cancer is comparable with that of axillary lymph node dissection. Ann Surg. 2004;240:462–71.
54. Chung MA, Steinhoff MM, Cady B. Clinical axillary recurrence in breast cancer patients after a negative sentinel node biopsy. Am J Surg. 2002;184:310–4.
55. Blanchard DK, Donohue JH, Reynolds C. Relapse and morbidity in patients undergoing sentinel lymph node biopsy alone or with axillary dissection for breast cancer. Arch Surg. 2003;138:482–8.
56. Veronesi U, et al. Sentinel node biopsy in breast cancer: early results in 953 patients with negative sentinel lymph node and no axillary lymph node dissection. Eur J Cancer. 2005;41(2):231–7.
57. Bergkvist L, et al. Axillary recurrence rate after negative sentinel node biopsy in breast cancer: three-year follow up of the Swedish Multicentre Cohort Study. Ann Surg. 2008;247(1):150–6.

58. van der Ploeg IMC, Nieweg OE, van Rijk MC, et al. Axillary recurrence after a tumour negative sentinel lymph node biopsy in breast cancer patients: a systematic review and meta-analysis of the literature. Eur J Surg Oncol. 2008;34:1277–84.
59. Kiluk JV, Ly QP, Meade T, et al. Axillary recurrence rate following negative sentinel lymph node biopsy for invasive breast cancer: Long term follow-up. Ann Surg Oncol. 2011;18: S339–42.
60. Rosen PP, Siago PE, Braun DW, et al. Axillary micro- and macrometastases in breast cancer: prognostic significance of tumour size. Ann Surg. 1993;194:585–91.
61. Forrest APM, Everington D, McDonald C, Steele RJC, Chetty U, Stewart HJ. The Edinburgh randomized trial of axillary sampling or clearance after mastectomy. Br J Surg. 1995;82:1504–8.
62. Lambah A, Dixon JM, Prescott RJ, Jack W, Forrest APM, Rodger A. et al. Randomised study of axillary clearance versus four node sampling. Eur J Cancer. 2001; 37: (Suppl 5): 2.
63. Steel RJ, Forrest APM, Chetty U. The efficacy of lower axillary sampling in obtaining lymph node status in breast cancer: a controlled randomized trial. Br J Surg. 1985;72:368–9.
64. Chetty U. Axillary node sampling to evaluate the axilla. World J Surg. 2001;25:773–9.
65. Rampaul RS, Pinder SE, Morgan DAL, et al. Long term regional recurrence and survival after axillary node sampling for breast cancer. *Eur J Cancer* 2003; 39: (Suppl 1): 23.
66. Kissin M. Debate entitled *Management of the axilla in women with breast cancer*: Which is the best way of staging the axilla?. London: The Royal Society of Medicine; 2005.
67. Gaston MS, Dixon JM. A survey of surgical management of the axilla in UK breast cancer patients. Eur J Cancer. 2004;40:1738–42.
68. McCarter MD, Yeung H, Fey J, et al. The breast cancer patients with multiple sentinel nodes: when to stop? J Am Coll Surg. 2001;192:692–7.
69. Cserni G. Evaluation of sentinel nodes in breast cancer. Histopathology. 2005;46:697–702.
70. Dabbs DJ, Johnson R. The optimal number of sentinel lymph nodes for focused pathological examination. Breast J. 2004;10:101–5.
71. Krag D, Anderson SJ, Julian TB, et al. Sentinel lymph node resection compared with conventional axillary lymph node dissection in clinically node negative patients with breast cancer: overall survival findings from the NSABP B-32 randomised phase 3 trial. Lancet Oncol. 2010;11:927–33.
72. Benson JR. An alternative to axillary lymph node dissection. Lancet Oncol. 2010;11:908–9.
73. Krag D, Weaver D, Ashikaga T, et al. The sentinel node in breast cancer. A multicentre validation study. N Eng J Med. 1998;339:941–946.
74. Morrow M, Rademaker AW, Bethke KP, et al. Learning sentinel node biopsy: results of a prospective randomized trial of two techniques. Surgery. 1999;126:714–22.
75. Lyman GH, Guiliano AE, Somerfield MR, et al. The American society of clinical oncology guideline recommendations for sentinel lymph node biopsy in early stage breast cancer. J Clin Oncol. 2005;23:7703–20.
76. Krag DN, Anderson SJ, Julian TB, et al. Technical outcomes of sentinel-lymph node resection and conventional axillary lymph node dissection in patients with clinically node negative breast cancer: results from the NSABP B-32 randomised phase III trial. Lancet Oncol. 2007;8:881–8.
77. Gill PG. Sentinel lymph node biopsy versus axillary clearance in operable breast cancer. The RACS SNAC trial, A Multicenter randomised trial of the Royal Australian College of Surgeons (RACS) Section of Breast Surgery, in collaboration with the National Health and Medical Research Council Clinical Trials Center. Ann Surg Oncol. 2004;11:216S–21S.
78. Veronesi U, Paganelli G, Viale G, et al. A randomized comparison of sentinel node biopsy with routine axillary dissection in breast cancer. NEJM. 2003;349:546–53.
79. Mansel RE, Goyal A, Fallowfield L, et al. Sentinel node biopsy versus standard axillary treatment: results of the randomized multicentre UK ALMANAC trial. J Natl Cancer Inst. 2006;98:599–609.
80. Benson JR, Querci della Rovere G. Management of the axilla in women with breast cancer. Lancet Oncol. 2007;8:331–48.
81. Veronesi U. Sentinel node biopsy in breast cancer. Lancet. 1997;350:809.
82. O'Hea BJ, Hill ADK, El-Shirbiny AM, et al. Sentinel lymph node biopsy in breast cancer: initial experience at Memorial Sloan-Kettering Cancer Center. J Am Coll Surg. 1998;186:423–7.
83. Benamor M, Nos C, Freneaux P, Clough K. Impact of internal mammary sentinel node imaging in breast cancer. Clin Nucl Med. 2003;28:375–8.
84. McMasters KM, Wong SL, Tuttle TM, et al. Preoperative lymphoscintigraphy for breast cancer does not improve the ability to identify axillary sentinel nodes. Ann Surg. 2000;231:724–31.
85. Upponi SS, McIntosh SA, Wishart GC, et al. Sentinel lymph node biopsy in breast cancer—is lymphoscintigraphy really necessary. Eur J Surg Oncol. 2002;28(5):479–80.
86. Rosser RJ. Safety of sentinel lymph node dissection and significance of cytokeratin micrometastases. J Clin Oncol. 2001;19:1882–3.
87. Bleiweiss IJ, Legmann MD, Nagi CS, Jaffer S. Sentinel lymph nodes can be falsely positive due to iatrogenic displacement and transport of benign epithelial cells. J Clin Oncol. 2006;24:2013–8.
88. Kaklamanos IG, Birbas K, Syrigos K, et al. Prospective comparison of peritumoral and subareolar injection of blue dye alone for identification of sentinel lymph nodes in patients with early stage breast cancer. J Surg Oncol. 2011;104:37–40.
89. www.mhra.gov/Safetyinformation/DrugSafetyUpdate/.
90. Ahmed M, Purushotham A, Douek M. Novel techniques for sentinel lymph node biopsy in breast cancer: a systematic review. Lancet Oncol. 2014;15:351–62.
91. Benson JR. Evaluation of the clinical utility of the ICG fluorescence method in comparison to the radioisotope method for sentinel lymph node biopsy in breast cancer (commentary). Ann Surg Oncol. 2016;23:6–8.
92. Nimura H, Narimiya N, Mitsumori N, et al. Laparoscopic sentinel node navigation achieved by infra-red ray electronic endoscopy system in patients with gastric cancer. Br J Surg. 2004;91:575–9.
93. Kitai T, Inomoto T, Miwa M, Shikayama T. Fluorescence navigation with indocyanine green for detecting sentinel lymph nodes in breast cancer. Breast Cancer. 2005;12:2111–215.
94. Sugie T, Sawada T, Tagaya N, et al. Comparison of the Indocyanine green fluorescence and blue dye methods in detection of sentinel lymph nodes in early stage breast cancer. Ann Surg Oncol. 2012;. doi:10.1245/s10434-013-2890-0).
95. Wishart GC, Jones LC, Loh S-W, Benson JR. Fluorescence mapping with indocyanine green (ICG) for sentinel lymph node detection in early breast cancer—results of the ICG-10 study. Eur J Surg Oncol. 2012;38:651–6.
96. Ballardini B, Santoro L, Sangalli C, et al. The indocyanine green method is equivalent to the Tc-labelled radiotracer method for identifying the sentinel lymph node in breast cancer: a concordance and validation study. Eur J Surg Oncol. 2013;39:1332–6.
97. Verbeek FP, Troyan SL, Mieog JS, et al. Near-infrared fluorescence sentinel lymph node mapping in breast: a multicentre experience. Breast Cancer Res Treat. 2014;143:333–42.

98. Schaafsma BE, Verbeek FP, Riebergen DD, et al. Clinical trial of combined radio- and fluorescence-guided sentinel lymph node biopsy in breast cancer. B J Surg. 2013;100:1037–44.
99. Douek M, Monneypenny I, Kothari, et al. on behalf of the SentiMAG Trialists Group. Sentinel node biopsy using a magnetic tracer versus standard technique: the SentiMAG multicentre trial. Ann Surg Oncol 2013: published online Dec10. doi:10.1245/s10434-013-3379-6.
100. Chapman D, Purushotham A. Acceptability of early discharge with drains in situ after breast surgery. Br J Nursing. 2001;10:1447–50.
101. Salem AA, Douglas-Jones AG, Sweetland HM, Mansel RE. Intra-operative evaluation of axillary sentinel lymph nodes using touch imprint cytology and immunohistochemistry. Eur J Surg Oncol. 2006;32:484–7.
102. Benson JR, Wishart GC. In intraoperative node assessment essential in a modern breast practice? Eur J Surg Oncol. 2010;36:1162–4.
103. Julian TB, Blumencranz P, Deck K, et al. Novel intraoperative molecular test for sentinel lymph node metastasesin patients with early stage breast cancer. J Clin Oncol. 2008;26:3338–45.
104. Julian TB, Anderson SJ, Krag DN, et al. 10 Year follow up of NSABP B-32 randomised phase III clinical trial to compare sentinel node resection to conventional axillary dissection in clinically node negative patients. J Clin Onco. 2013;31:(Suppl abstr 100).
105. Cserni G, Gregori D, Merletti F, et al. Non-sentinel node metastases associated with micrometastatic sentinel nodes in breast cancer: metaanalysis of 25 studies. Br J Surg. 2004;91:1245–52.
106. Van Zee KJ, Manasseh DM, Bevilacqua JL, et al. A nomogram for predicting the likelihood of additional nodal metastases in breast cancer patients with a positive sentinel node biopsy. Ann Surg Oncol. 2002;10:1140–51.
107. Pal A, Provenzano E, Duffy SW, et al. A model for predicting non-sentinel lymph node metastatic disease when the sentinel lymph node is positive. Br J Surg. 2008;95:302–9.
108. Greco M, Agresti R, Cascinella N, Casalini P. et al. Breast cancer patients treated without axillary surgery. Ann Surg 2000;232(1):1–7.
109. Cserni G, Gregori D, Merletti F, et al. Non-sentinel node metastases associated with micrometastatic sentinel nodes in breast cancer: metaanalysis of 25 studies. Br J Surg. 2004;91:1245–52.
110. Fisher B, Joeng J-H, Anderson S, et al. Twenty-five year follow up of a randomized trial comparing radical mastectomy, total mastectomy and total mastectomy followed by irradiation. N Eng J Med. 2002;347:567–75.
111. Hellman S. Stopping metastases at their source. N Eng J Med. 1997;337:996–7.
112. Van Zee KJ, Manasseh DM, Bevilacqua JL, et al. A nomogram for predicting the likelihood of additional nodal metastases in breast cancer patients with a positive sentinel node biopsy. Ann Surg Oncol. 2002;10:1140–51.
113. Giuliano AE, Hunt K, Ballman K, et al. Axillary dissection vs no axillary dissection in women with invasive breast cancer and sentinel node metastases: a randomized clinical trial. JAMA. 2011;305:569.
114. Galimberti V, Cole BF, Zurrida S, et al. Update of International Breast Cancer Study Group Trial 23-01 to compare axillary dissection versus no axillary dissection in patients with clinically node negative breast cancer and micrometastases in the sentinel node. Cancer Res. 2011;71:102s.
115. Goyal A, Newcombe RG, Chhabra A, Mansel RE. Morbidity in breast cancer patients with sentinel node metastases undergoing delayed axillary lymph node dissection (ALND) compared with immediate ALND. Ann Surg Oncol. 2008;15(1):262–7.
116. Goyal A, Coleman RE, Dodwell D, et al. POSNOC: Positive sentinel node—adjuvant therapy alone versus adjuvant therapy plus clearance or axillary radiotherapy. A randomized trial looking at axillary treatment in early breast cancer (ISRCTN547652244). J Clin Oncol 2015; (Suppl; abstr TPS 1103).
117. Donker M, van Tienhoven G, Straver ME, et al. Radiotherapy or surgery of the axilla after a positive sentinel node in breast cancer (EORTC 10981-22033 AMAROS): a randomized multicenter, open-labelled, phase 3 non-inferiority trial. Lancet Oncol. 2014;15(1):1303–10.
118. Dixon JM, Mammam U, Thomas J. Accuracy of intraoperative frozen-section analysis of axillary nodes. Edinburgh breast unit team. Br J Surg. 1999;86:392–5.
119. Brogi E, Torres-Matundan E, Tan LK, Cody HS. The results of frozen section, touch preparation and cytological smear are comparable for intraoperative examination of sentinel lymph nodes: a study in 133 breast cancer patients. Ann Surg Oncol. 2005;12:173–8.
120. Dowlatshahi K, Fan M, Anderson JM, Bloom KJ. Occult metastases in sentinel nodes of 200 patients with operable breast cancer. Ann Surg Oncol. 2001;8:675–81.
121. Lambah PA, McIntyre MA, Chetty U, Dixon JM. Imprint cytology of axillary lymph nodes as an intraoperative diagnostic tool. Eur J Surg Oncol. 2003;29:224–8.
122. Vanderveen KA, Ramsamooj R, Bold RJ. A prospective, blinded trial of touch prep analysis versus frozen section for intraoperative evaluation of sentinel lymph nodes in breast cancer. Ann Surg Oncol. 2008;15:2006–11.
123. Tew K, Irwig L, Matthews A, et al. Meta-analysis of sentinel node imprint cytology in breast cancer. Br J Surg. 2005;92:1068–80.
124. Notomi T, Okayama H, Masubuchi H, et al. Loop-mediated isothermal amplication of DNA. Nucleic Acids Res. 2000;28: E63.
125. Mansel RE, Goyal A, Douglas-Jones A, et al. Detection of breast cancer metastasis in sentinel lymph nodes using intra-operative real time GeneSearch BLN Assay in the operating room: results of the Cardiff study. Breast Cancer Res Treat. 2009;115:595–600.
126. Tsujimoto M, Nakabayashi K, Yoshidome K, et al. One-step nucleic acid amplification for intra-operative detection of lymph node metastases in breast cancer patients. Clin Cancer Res. 2007;13:4807–16.
127. Bernet L, Martinez-Benaclocha M, Cano-Munoz R, et al. One-step nucleic acid amplification (OSNA) for sentinel node intra-operative diagnosis: advantages from the classical procedures. 7th European Breast Cancer Conference, Barcelona, 2010 [abstract 337].
128. Chung MH, Ye W, Guiliano AE. Role for sentinel lymph node dissection in the management of large (≥5 cm) invasive breast cancer. Ann Surg Oncol. 2001;8(9):668–92.
129. Beumer JD, Gill G, Campbell I, et al. Sentinel node biopsy and large (≥3 cm) breast cancer. ANZ J Surg. 2014;84:117–20.
130. Intra M, Zurrida S, Maffini F, et al. Sentinel lymph node metastasis in microinvasive breast cancer. Ann Surg Oncol. 2003;10:1160–5.
131. Klauber-DeMore N, Tan LK, Liberman L, et al. Sentinel lymph node biopsy: is it indicated in patients with high-risk ductal carcinoma in situ and ductal carcinoma in situ with microinvasion? Ann Surg Oncol. 2000;7:636–42.
132. Benson JR, Wishart GC, Forouhi P, Hill-Cawthorne G, Pinder SE. The role of sentinel node biopsy in patients with a pre-operative diagnosis of carcinoma in situ. Eur J Cancer. 2007;6(7):131.

133. Lagios MG, Silverstein MJ. Sentinel node biopsy for patients with DCIS: a dangerous and unwarranted direction. Ann Surg Oncol. 2001;8:275–7.
134. Meyer JE, Smith DN, Lester SC, et al. Large-core needle biopsy of non-palpable breast lesions. JAMA. 1999;281:1683–41.
135. Yen TWF, Hunt KK, Ross MI, et al. Predictors of invasive breast cancer in patients with an initial diagnosis of ductal carcinoma in situ: a guide to selective use of sentinel lymph node biopsy in management of ductal carcinoma in situ. J Am Coll Surg. 2005;200:516–26.
136. Tann JCC, McCready DR, Easson AM, Leong WL. Role of sentinel lymph node biopsy in ductal carcinoma in situ treated by mastectomy. Ann Surg Oncol. 2007;14:638–45.
137. Zavotsky J, Hansen N, Brennan MB, et al. Lymph node metastasis from ductal carcinoma in situ with micro-invasion. Cancer. 1999;85:2439–43.
138. Jackman RJ, Nowels KW, Rodriguez-Soto J, et al. Stereotactic, automated, large core needle biopsy of non-palpable breast lesions: false-negative and histologic underestimation rates after long-term follow up. Radiology. 1999;210:799–805.
139. Veronesi U, Paganelli G, Galimberti V, et al. Sentinel node biopsy to avoid axillary dissection in breast cancer with clinically negative nodes. Lancet. 1997;349:1864–7.
140. Goyal A, Newcombe RG, Mansell RE, et al. ALMANAC Trialist Group. Sentinel lymph node biopsy in patients with multifocal breast cancer. Eur J Surg Oncol. 2004;30:475–9.
141. Toumisis E, Zee KJV, Fey JV, et al. The accuracy of sentinel lymph node biopsy in multicentric and multifocal invasive breast cancers. J Am Coll Surg. 2003;197:529–34.
142. Holwitt DM, Gillanders WE, Aft RL, et al. Sentinel lymph node biopsy in patients with multicentric/multifocal breast cancer: low false-negative rate and lack of axillary recurrence. Am J Surg 2008; [Epub ahead of print].
143. Gentilini O, Trifiro G, Soleldo J, et al. Sentinel lymph node biopsy in patients with multicentric breast cancer. The experience of the European Institute of Oncology. Eur J Surg Oncol. 2006;32:507–10.
144. Moody LC, Wen X, McKnight T, Chao C. Indications for sentinel lymph node biopsy in multifocal and multicentric breast cancer. Surgery. 2012;152(3):389–96.
145. van la Parra RF, de Roos WK, Contant CM, et al. A prospective validation study of sentinel lymph node biopsy in multicentric breast cancer: SMMaC trial. *Eur J Surg Oncol* 2014;40 (10):1250–1255.
146. Theriault RL. Breast cancer during pregnancy. In: Singletary SE, Robb GL (Eds). Advanced therapy of breast disease. BC Decker Inc. Ontario 2000 Chapter 18, pp. 167–173.
147. Berry DL, Theriault RL, Holmes FA, et al. Management of breast cancer during pregnancy using a standardized protocol. J Clin Oncol. 1999;17:855–61.
148. Doll DC, Ringenberg QS, Yarbro JW. Antineoplastic agents and pregnancy. Semin Oncol. 1989;16:337–46.
149. Naik AM, Fey J, Gemignani M, et al. The risk of axillary relapse after sentinel lymph node biopsy for breast cancer is comparable with that of axillary lymph node dissection: a follow up study of 4008 procedures. Ann Surg. 2004;240:462–8.
150. Burger AE, Pain SJ, Peley G. Treatment of recurrent breast cancer following breast conserving surgery. Breast J. 2013;19:310–8.
151. Lyman GH, Temin S, Edge SB, et al. Sentinel lymph node biopsy for patients with early stage breast cancer: American society of clinical oncology clinical practice guideline update. J Clin Oncol. 2014;32:1365–83.
152. Port ER, Garcia-Etienne CA, Park J, et al. Re-operative sentinel lymph node biopsy: a new frontier in the management of ipsilateral breast tumour recurrence. Ann Surg Oncol. 2007;14:2209–14.
153. Taback B, Nguyen P, Hansen N, et al. Sentinel lymph node biopsy for local recurrence of breast cancer after breast conserving surgery. Ann Surg Oncol. 2006;13:1099–104.
154. Maaskant-Braat AJ, Roumen RM, Voogd AC, et al. Repeat sentinel node biopsy in patients with locally recurrent breast cancer: a systematic review and meta-analysis of the literature. Breast Cancer Res Treat. 2013;138:13–20.
155. Intra M, Viale G, Vila J, et al. Second axillary sentinel lymph node biopsy for breast tumour recurrence: Experience of the European Institute of Oncology. Ann Surg Oncol. 2015;22:2372–7.
156. Menard J-P, Extra J-M, Jacquemier J, et al. Sentinel lymphadenectomy for the staging of clinical axillary node negative breast cancer before neoadjuvant chemotherapy. Eur J Surg Oncol. 2009;35:916–20.
157. Straver ME, Rutgers EJT, Russel NS, et al. Towards rational axillary treatment in relation to neoadjuvant therapy in breast cancer. Eur J Cancer. 2009;45:2284–92.
158. Fisher B, Brown A, Mamounas E, et al. Effect of preoperative chemotherapy on local-regional disease in women with operable breast cancer: findings from national surgical adjuvant breast and bowel project B18. J Clin Oncol. 1997;15:2483–93.
159. Hennessy BT, Hortobagyi GN, Rouzier R, et al. Outcome after pathologic complete eradication of cytologically proven breast cancer axillary node metastases following primary chemotherapy. J Clin Oncol. 2005;23:9304–11.
160. Klaube-Demore N, Ollia DW, Moore DT, et al. Size of residual lymph node metastasis after neoadjuvant chemotherapy in locally advanced breast cancer patients is prognostic. Ann Surg Oncol. 2006;13:685–91.
161. Bleiweiss I. Sentinel lymph nodes in breast cancer after 10 years: rethinking basic principles. Lancet Oncol. 2007;7:686–92.
162. Sabel M. Sentinel lymph node biopsy before or after neoadjuvant chemotherapy: Pros and Cons. Surg Oncol Clin N Am. 2010;19:519–38.
163. Torisu-Itakura H, Lee JH, Scheri RP, et al. Molecular characteristization of inflammatory genes in sentinel and non-sentinel nodes in melanoma. Clin Cancer Res. 2007;13:3125–32.
164. Hunt KK, Yi M, Mittendorf EA, et al. Sentinel lymph node surgery after neoadjuvant chemotherapy is accurate and reduces the need for axillary dissection in breast cancer patients. Ann Surg. 2009;250:558–66.
165. van Deurzen CH, Vriens BE, Tjan-Heijnen VC, et al. Accuracy of sentinel lymph node biopsy after neoadjuvant chemotherapy in breast cancer patients: a systematic review. Eur J Cancer. 2009;45:3124–30.
166. Classe J-M, Bordes V, Campion L, et al. Sentinel lymph node biopsy after neoadjuvant chemotherapy for advanced breast cancer: results of Ganglion Sentinelle et Chimiotherapie Neoadjuvante, a French prospective multicentric study. J Clin Oncol. 2009;27:726–32.
167. Shen J, Gilcrease MZ, Babiera GV, et al. Feasibility and accuracy of sentinel lymph node biopsy after preoperative chemotherapy in breast cancer patients with documented axillary metastases. Cancer. 2007;109:1255–63.
168. Lee S, Kim EY, Kang SH, et al. Sentinel node identification rate, but not accuracy, is significantly decreased after pre-operative chemotherapy in axillary node positive breast cancer patients. Breast Cancer Res Treat. 2007;102:283–8.

169. Newman EA, Sabel MS, Nees AV, et al. Sentinel lymph node biopsy performed after neoadjuvant chemotherapy is accurate in patients with documented node positive breast cancer at presentation. Ann Surg Oncol. 2007;14:2946–52.
170. Mamounas EP, Brown A, Anderson S, et al. Sentinel node biopsy after neoadjuvant chemotherapy in breast cancer: results from national surgical adjuvant breast and bowel project protocol B-27. J Clin Oncol. 2005;23:2694–702.
171. Alvarado R, Yi M, Le-Petross H, et al. The role for sentinel lymph node dissection after neoadjuvant chemotherapy in patients who present with node positive breast cancer. Ann Surg Oncol. 2012;19:3177–84.
172. Sabel MS. Locoregional therapy of breast cancer: maximizing control, minimizing morbidity. Expert Rev Anticancer Ther. 2007;6:1261–79.
173. Boughy JC, Sumen VJ, Mittendorf EA, et al. Sentinel lymph node surgery after neoadjuvant chemotherapy in patients with node positive breast cancer: the ACOSOG Z1071 (ALLIANCE) clinical trial. JAMA. 2013;310(14):1455–61.
174. Kuehn T, Bauerfeind IGP, Fehm T, et al. Sentinel lymph node biopsy in patients with breast cancer before or after neoadjuvant chemotherapy (SENTINA): a prospective multicenter cohort study. Lancet Oncol. 2013;14(7):609–18.
175. NSABP Clinical Trials Overview [Internet]. Pittsburgh: National Surgical Adjuvant Breast and Bowel Project at the University of Pittsburgh [cited 2015 November 13]. Available from: www.nsabp.pitt.edu/B-51.asp.
176. Overgaard M, Hansen PS, Overgaard J, et al. Post-operative radiotherapy in high risk pre-menopausal women with breast cancer who receive adjuvant chemotherapy. N Eng J Med. 1997;337:949–55.
177. Ragaz J, Jackson SM, Le N, et al. Adjuvant radiotherapy and chemotherapy in node positive pre-menopausal women with breast cancer. N Eng J Med. 1997;337:956–62.
178. Poortmans P, Kouloulias VE, Venselaar JL, et al. Quality assurance of EORTC trial 22922/10925 investigating the role of internal mammary-medial supraclavicular irradiationnnnn in stage 1–111 breast cancer: the individual case review. Eur J Cancer. 2003;39(14):2035–42.

Breast Reconstructive Surgery

16

Yash J. Avashia, Amir Tahernia, Detlev Erdmann, and Michael R. Zenn

16.1 Introduction

Breast reconstruction following mastectomy can be achieved by a variety of techniques using alloplastic implants, autogenous tissues, or both. The established paradigm for breast reconstruction is to rebuild an identical and possibly symmetrical breast mound after mastectomy. In the last 30 years, breast reconstruction has progressed from a rarely requested procedure to one that has become an integral part of patient management. The modern era of breast reconstruction began in 1963 with the introduction of the silicone gel prosthesis. In 1972, Radovon described the use of tissue expansion for breast reconstruction [1]. The early introduction of free tissue transfer by Daniel and Taylor in 1973 broadened the scope of autologous breast reconstruction [2]. This technique allowed patients with more significant skin deficits to benefit from reconstruction. In the early 1980s, the use of autologous tissue for breast reconstruction was revolutionized by Hartrampf with the introduction of the transverse rectus abdominis muscle (TRAM) flap [3]. Later advances in microsurgical free tissue transfer reopened the door to a new range of options for autologous breast reconstruction. The advent of perforator flaps has now further refined microsurgical techniques, Donor site morbidity is minimized by perforator flaps by not requiring the violation or harvesting of abdominal musculature. Case example: DIEP vs Free TRAM Flap. The perforator flap allows us to harvest the skin/subcutaneous tissues with the vascular pedicle dissected through the fascia and muscle. The abdominal wall integrity is preserved compared to the TRAM flap. Furthermore, we can increase the number of donor sites based on perforators since there are a larger number of perforators throughout the body. With these developments, patients have benefited from improvements in cosmetic outcome, operative recovery, operative morbidity, and the overall expected outcomes.

Experience over time has also shown breast reconstruction to be an oncologically safe component of the overall treatment plan. Perhaps most importantly, breast reconstruction yields psychological benefits for women, offering a sense of normalcy, a "return to wholeness," and a way to leave the cancer experience behind them. Women gain the freedom to wear a variety of clothing, without the need for external prosthesis, which may be cumbersome and embarrassing.

Historically, almost all breast reconstructions were delayed for months or years after mastectomy. It was feared that immediate breast reconstruction would compromise adjuvant treatments and that it would increase postoperative complications. There were concerns of masking locoregional recurrences and rendering treatment of such disease as difficult. Today, studies not only have shown no increased risk for complications or oncologic risk but also have shown a psychological benefit and cost-effectiveness. In the right clinical scenario, patients can undergo immediate breast reconstruction with a minimum compromise to their overall cancer management and a maximum benefit.

Breast reconstruction has become an integral part of the multidisciplinary approach to breast cancer. In order to optimize results, patient selection is critical. Factors that need consideration prior to embarking upon a reconstruction include stage of the cancer, patient comorbidities, possible adjuvant radiotherapy, availability of autologous tissue, and, most importantly, the patient's own desires [4]. A certain group of women with early disease have the option of breast conservation therapy (BCT) instead of undergoing mastectomy. Prior studies have demonstrated an equivalent survival when comparing BCT with radiation to mastectomy. While the ultimate decision remains with the patient, both the oncologic surgeon and plastic surgeon should have a chance to counsel the patient.

Y.J. Avashia (✉) · D. Erdmann · M.R. Zenn
Surgery, Duke University Medical Center, 40 Duke Medical Circle, Durham, 27710, NC, USA
e-mail: yja@duke.edu

A. Tahernia
Plastic and Reconstructive Surgery, 9735 Wilshire Blvd, Suite 421, Beverly Hills, 90212, CA, USA

I. Jatoi and A. Rody (eds.), *Management of Breast Diseases*, DOI 10.1007/978-3-319-46356-8_16

In this chapter, we will review the indications, timing, principles, and techniques of breast reconstruction following mastectomy. We will also review the role of radiation and chemotherapy in breast reconstruction and how it impacts surgical decision-making.

16.2 Indications for Reconstruction

Patients who are candidates for breast reconstruction are those who have undergone mastectomy for cancer extirpation. However, with advances in the understanding of the genetic basis of breast cancer and identification of BRCA1 and BRCA2 genes, more patients with familial history of breast cancer are undergoing prophylactic mastectomies. Therefore, breast reconstruction is not only limited to patients with a diagnosis of breast cancer. Regarding indications for prophylactic mastectomy, the Society of Surgical Oncology updated their statement in 2007 with the following guidelines (Fig. 16.1).

Patients with metastatic disease are not candidates for reconstruction, and in those who have significant medical comorbidities, mastectomy may be the only reasonable surgical intervention, as the stress of reconstructive surgery may be prohibitive. Furthermore, there is no advantage to immediate reconstruction in the setting of mastectomy for inflammatory breast cancer (IBC) due to the high risk of recurrence, aggressive nature of the disease, and need to proceed expeditiously to adjuvant radiotherapy.

16.3 Skin-Sparing Mastectomy

The technique of skin-sparing mastectomy has greatly improved the esthetic outcomes of autologous breast reconstruction. It is an oncologically safe procedure in patients with stage I and II cancers. It allows the mastectomy to be performed with preservation of most of the natural breast skin envelope and inframammary fold.

The skin-sparing mastectomy technique involves a periareolar incision with or without some type of lateral extension for exposure and removal of breast tissue (Fig. 16.2). With the goal to minimize separate scars on the breast mound (for aesthetic purposes), designing the mastectomy scar to incorporate prior scars on the breast mound is done. This is with the understanding that the mastectomy is taking place after a prior breast biopsy which is the normal scenario here in the US. Although more time-consuming than traditional cancer ablation methods, this technique permits maximal preservation of skin and provides excellent cosmetic results. Several studies have validated its oncologic safety, and no studies have shown any statistically increased risk of tumor recurrence or compromised local control of the disease following skin-sparing mastectomies [5].

The use of complete skin-sparing mastectomy successfully reduces scar burden and skin color discrepancies, allows for optimal preservation of the preoperative breast shape, and may minimize the need for a contralateral procedure to achieve breast symmetry. The success of this procedure is dependent upon proper patient selection and ability of the oncologic surgeon to safely perform extensive skin flap mobilization in a precise plane through limited exposure and adequately remove all breast parenchyma. Patients with previous radiation, cup size larger than C, or surgeons unfamiliar with the technique should not have skin-sparing mastectomy [6].

The reconstruction of lumpectomy defects remains controversial. These patients have often received irradiation, which complicates revisional surgery. In most cases, if cosmesis is unacceptable, patients require completion mastectomy and reconstruction from scratch, removing the problematic irradiated tissues.

Suggested Indications for Prophylactic Mastectomy by the Society of Surgical Oncology

Women with no prior history of breast cancer
- Atypical hyperplasia
- Family history of premenopausal bilateral breast cancer
- Dense breats associated with atypical hyperplasia or family history of premenopausal bilateral breast cancer or both

Women with unilateral breast cancer
- Diffuse microcalcifications
- Labular carcinoma in situ
- Large breast,difficult to evaluate
- History of lobular carcinoma in situ followed by unilateral breast cancer
- History of atypical hyperplasia,primary family history, age at diagnosis < 40 y

Fig. 16.1 Table indications for prophylactic mastectomy

16.4 Nipple-Sparing Mastectomy

Nipple-sparing mastectomy (NSM) preserves the entire skin envelope of the breast, including the nipple–areola complex (NAC). This often includes intraoperative pathological assessment of the nipple. While neoplasia of the nipple is most often from Paget's disease of the breast, nipple involvement may also occur with ductal carcinoma in situ (DCIS) or invasive breast cancer. With earlier detection of disease and less tumor burden and with the increased popularity of prophylactic mastectomy, NSM is becoming the gold standard in properly selected patients.

Indications for NSM include prophylactic mastectomy and NSM in the treatment of breast cancer [7]. Optimal candidates for NSM are those with tumors 4 cm in diameter or less, 2 cm away from the nipple, clinically negative axilla

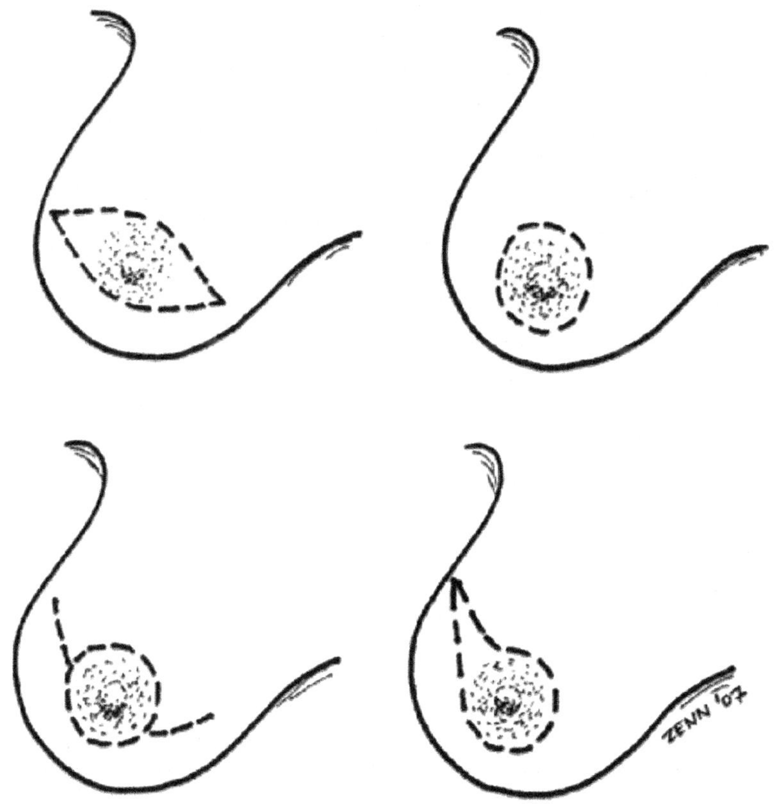

Fig. 16.2 Skin-sparing mastectomy incisions: varying incisions used in skin-sparing mastectomy. The incision is in part determined by the areas of previous biopsy. The goal is to minimize the area of scar on the skin envelope by incorporating biopsy incisions

or sentinel node negative, no skin involvement, and no inflammatory breast cancer [8]. The final decision to spare the nipple in cases of active disease must await frozen and then definitive pathologic section. With the caveat of an accepted false-negative rate for frozen section, the permanent pathology results will later provide definitive information to dictate management.

A plastic surgeon should screen possible candidates for NSM to make certain that it is technically realistic. Patients with larger or more ptotic breasts will be more likely to encounter nipple and/or flap necrosis. In cases where the skin flaps would be too long, such as cup size larger than C cup or ptosis greater than grade 2 (inferior displacement of the nipple–areola complex below the IMF), the nipple should not be saved and a SSM approach should be used. Regarding technique, reports have suggested that the best incisions are lateral, radial, lateral mammary fold (LMF), and inframammary fold (IMF). The IMF incision provides the best cosmesis but may be difficult for some oncologic surgeons to reach the upper portion of the breast safely [9]. Reconstructive options remain the same in these patients, but may be technically more challenging due to smaller incisions limiting exposure.

16.5 Timing of Breast Reconstruction

While most patients are candidates for "delayed reconstruction" following the completion of their breast cancer treatment, many patients are eligible for "immediate reconstruction" during which they undergo breast reconstruction at the time of their mastectomy. Factors influencing this decision include the patient, disease, and treatment-related factors. In the past, combining a reconstructive procedure with the mastectomy presented several concerns with the possibility of increased complications and possible delays in postoperative delivery of adjuvant treatment. These concerns, however, have been shown to be unwarranted. In some cases, the reconstruction may be performed a few weeks after the mastectomy to allow pathologic examination of the specimen and surgical "delay" of ischemic skin flaps to strengthen them. This technique has been termed "staged-immediate" [10].

Immediate reconstruction is usually reserved for stage I and some stage II breast cancer patients [11]. Immediate reconstruction is more convenient for patients as it limits the number of exposures to anesthesia and has psychological benefits. With immediate reconstruction, esthetics is improved, since incisions tend to be shorter and there is less skin removal. Immediate reconstruction is not an alternative for the patient not psychologically prepared for a reconstructive procedure. Some patients are simply overwhelmed by their new diagnosis and cannot make decisions beyond cancer treatment.

Immediate reconstruction is contraindicated in a patient with skin ulceration or inflammatory breast cancer. Furthermore, if the patient is planned to receive postmastectomy radiation therapy (PMRT), immediate reconstruction with autologous tissue should be avoided due to the negative effects of radiation on the reconstruction. Radiation therapy to an implant or expander causes problematic sequelae of capsular contracture and may lead to breakdown of the incision site overtime with prosthesis exposure. As references, a common technique used to avoid increased insult to the mastectomy flap is to deflate the expander prior to radiation. This will release any pressure on the skin flap during radiation therapy. By leaving the expander in place, it still preserves the pocket for resuming expansions after radiation therapy [12].

Delayed reconstruction may be the only option in some patients for various reasons. Some may not have access to a reconstructive surgeon at the time of the mastectomy. Others may feel that they need to deal individually with each step of the cancer treatment protocol. This will allow them to weigh all their options with regard to type of reconstructive method and selection of a reconstructive surgeon. As mentioned previously, delayed reconstruction is recommended for patients with advanced disease who will require PMRT. Some of the problems radiotherapy may produce include fat necrosis, shrinkage of autogenous tissue flaps, thinning of overlying chest skin, and periprosthetic capsular contracture. These patients should be reassured that a delayed reconstruction is in their best long-term interest and that esthetic results can be equal to immediate reconstruction. Most delayed reconstructions can be initiated 4 months after the completion of chemotherapy and 6 months after radiation therapy [13].

16.6 Alloplastic Versus Autogenous Reconstruction

16.6.1 Alloplastic Reconstruction

Today, most mastectomy patients are candidates for tissue expander/implant reconstruction. In general, the best results are seen in patients with moderate breast size and minimal ptosis (inferior displacement of the nipple–areola complex). The best candidate for implant-based breast reconstruction is one who is not obese, with moderate-sized breasts, and with mild or no breast ptosis [14]. These patients may also be considering contralateral augmentation or mastopexy as part of their reconstruction.

Morbid obesity is considered a relative contraindication for breast reconstruction with tissue expanders and implants. In these patients, the breast "footprint" is wide and there will be significant volume below the projected surface of the chest wall making even the largest implant reconstruction suboptimal. The delivery of radiotherapy before breast reconstruction with prosthetic devices is also a relative contraindication as the skin will simply not stretch due to radiation changes. While occasionally successful, attempts to perform prosthetic reconstruction after PMRT result in an unacceptable rate of severe complications with implant extrusion, capsular contracture, or implant displacement [15].

All breast reconstructions require more than one operation, and the process may extend over many months. Alloplastic reconstruction with the use of tissue expanders/implants is the simplest technique and the one chosen by over 75 % of patients who undergo breast reconstruction. Potential advantages of expander/implant reconstruction over other techniques include the following: (1) relative simplicity of the surgical procedure, (2) the use of adjacent tissue of similar color, texture, and sensation, (3) elimination of distant donor site morbidity, (4) minimal incisional scarring, and (5) reduced operative time and postoperative recovery compared to tissue reconstruction. Many women may choose prosthetic breast reconstruction so that they may resume physical activities quicker or with little disruption. In addition, these patients will continue to remain candidates for autologous reconstruction in the event of prosthetic failure or personal preference.

While implant reconstruction yields the best results in patients with moderate breast volumes (500 g or less), reconstruction of the large breast can be accomplished. In patients with large or markedly ptotic breasts, matching surgery on the contralateral breast may be necessary in order to achieve symmetry. This would be accomplished with breast reshaping, either by a breast reduction or by a breast lift (mastopexy). In some cases, a "Wise pattern" mastectomy may allow for single-stage reconstructions with symmetrical inverted-T scars with the contralateral breast reduction.

Prosthetic reconstruction can be performed in many ways, but the most common include (1) single-stage reconstruction with the use of primary implants, (2) two-staged reconstruction with the use of initial tissue expanders followed by the exchange for permanent implants, and (3) implants combined with tissue procedures [16]. Before looking at each of these modalities, a brief review of the technique of implant placement will allow for a better understanding of the anatomic considerations which are essential to optimal outcomes. Breast implants or tissue expanders traditionally are placed in the submuscular position (Fig. 16.3). This is due to the fact that after a mastectomy, no gland remains and so healthy vascularized soft tissue coverage is lacking. All implants induce a foreign body reaction and formation of a discrete fibrous shell or capsule. Under the influence of a variety of factors, this capsule may undergo the process of capsular contracture which can distort breast shape. Submuscular placement helps cover the implant with healthy tissue which hides capsular distortion and may help prevent it. Many variables can influence the development of capsular contracture and they include type of implant surface, implant placement, infection, and the use of radiation. We will revisit the issue of capsular contracture later in the Complications of Implant Reconstruction section. The key landmark for any breast reconstruction is the inframammary fold (IMF). Every effort is made to recreate a natural fold that matches the contralateral fold in position and symmetry. The critical measurement to consider when selecting an implant is the base diameter of the breast. Other factors to be considered are the height and projection of the breast. These factors are all accounted for preoperatively with the appropriate marks made on the patient's chest before the creation of the submuscular pocket. After the completion of the mastectomy, the viability of the mastectomy flaps is assessed. Poorly perfused tissue is excised, and if there is any doubt as to the adequacy of soft tissue coverage, the reconstruction should be delayed. If all looks well, an area under the pectoralis muscle is dissected forming a submuscular pocket for the implant. This dissection involves identification and elevation of the lateral border of the pectoralis major muscle and release of the muscles from its origin on the 5th rib. Dissection can sometimes be carried laterally, elevating the serratus anterior muscle. The location of the pocket will ultimately determine the level of the IMF.

16.6.2 Implant Types

The silicone gel-filled breast implant was first developed in 1963 for women with small breasts who desired augmentation. This was later applied to breast reconstruction to restore shape and contour in women following mastectomies. The implants that are currently available vary in shape, surface texture, size, and filler material. All implants, regardless of whether they are saline- or silicone gel-filled, have a silicone outer shell. The most commonly available shapes are round and anatomic or teardrop-shaped implants. Both shapes are commonly used and achieve excellent results. Choice is largely physician-driven. Placement and fixation of an anatomic implant is critical as it forms the entire mound and can be noticeable if mispositioned. Round implants are more forgiving as they can look the same even when rotated. This is not true with anatomic implants which need to stay in the position originally placed without rotation. Textured surface implants generally have more tissue ingrowth and tend to hold their position better. They have been shown to be less associated with capsular contracture, theoretically due to disorganized scarring around the implant that the textured

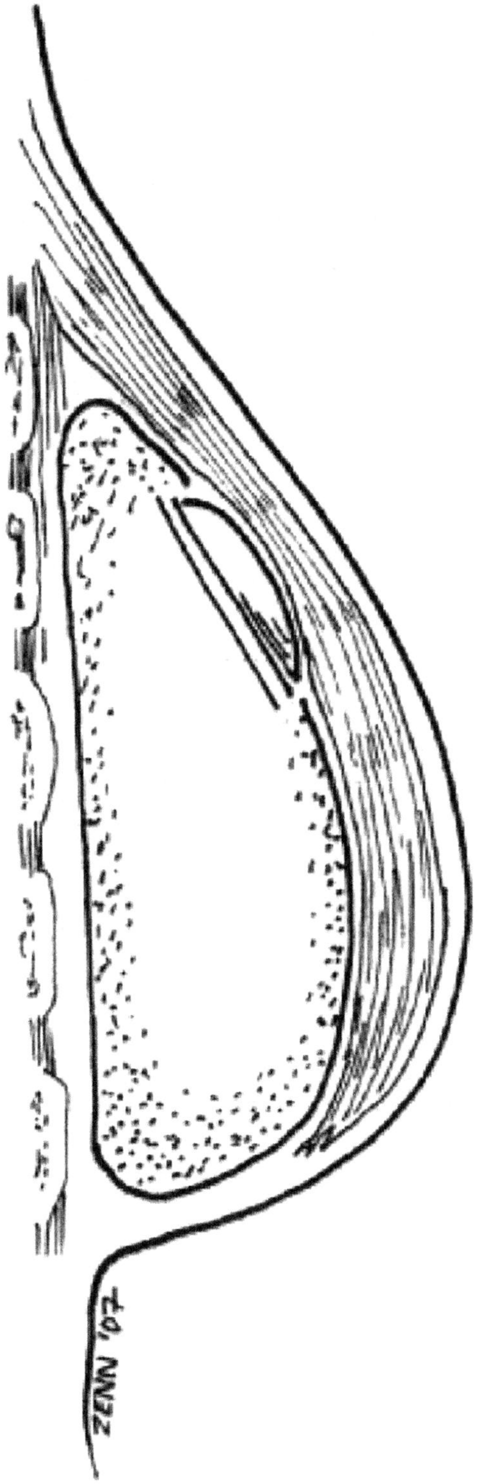

Fig. 16.3 Implant/expander placement: Tissue expanders can be placed in a subpectoral or submuscular position. This figure demonstrates a subpectoral prosthesis with most of the implant covered with pectoralis major muscle. In a true submuscular position, the rectus abdominis and serratus anterior muscles would be covering the inferomedial and inferolateral aspects of the prosthesis, respectively

surface induces. All shapes and textures are used regularly with excellent results. In 1992, the US Food and Drug Administration established a moratorium on the use of silicone gel-filled implants until 2005 in the USA. These implants were only available under the protocol for reconstructive purposes. The concern with the silicone implants was presumed to be in association with connective tissue disorders as well as metachronous development of breast cancer. Multiple retrospective studies over the past 20 years have shown this to be invalid, and as such, these implants were reapproved for use in the USA by the FDA in 2005.

Following the 1992 FDA moratorium on silicone gel implants, there was an expected surge in the use of saline-filled implants. An advantage with these implants is that a desired volume can be achieved with intraoperative instillation of saline into an empty implant. The advantages of saline implants include smaller scars for placement, customization of fill volume, and lack of silicone exposure if the implant ruptures. Several problems have been associated with saline implant use such as firmness, wrinkling of the implant, and complete deflation of the mound upon rupture. In comparison, newer silicone implants are softer, have a more natural appearance, and are filled with cohesive gel which maintains its shape upon outer shell failure [17].

16.6.3 Two-Stage Expander/Implant Reconstruction

Two-stage reconstruction using an initial expander followed by secondary permanent implant placement is the gold standard for implant reconstruction. It is especially desirable when there is insufficient tissue after mastectomy or when the desired size and shape of the breast cannot be safely and consistently achieved with a single-stage procedure [18]. The two-stage approach allows adjustments to the implant pocket at the time of the second procedure, allowing a more consistent reconstruction of the moderately sized breast with mild ptosis. Prosthetic reconstruction in patients with large breasts and significant ptosis requires a contralateral reduction or mastopexy to achieve symmetry, a symmetry that will only occur in clothes.

The procedure for expander placement creates a submuscular pocket of pectoralis and sometimes serratus muscles. Expander selection is based on the height and width of the desired breast. Most plastic surgeons favor textured expanders with integrated valves. They allow direct instillation of fluid through insensate mastectomy skin, which is not painful to the patient. Following skin closure, a magnet is used to identify the port and an initial volume of saline is instilled, from zero to 300 mL or more. Additional expansion continues postoperatively 2 weeks after expander placement. The patient is seen in clinic, and 50–100 cc is instilled every 2–3 weeks. Usually, this is carried out over a 2-month period until the desired amount of expansion has occurred. Most surgeons overexpand by 10 % as there is some retraction of the soft tissue once the expander is replaced with the permanent implant. If the patient is receiving chemotherapy, the exchange procedure is delayed up to 4 weeks after the completion of treatment to avoid issues with wound healing that may result. Following the completion of expansion, the exchange of the expander for a permanent implant involves reopening of the access incision, removal of the expander, adjustments of the pocket and IMF, and permanent implant placement (Fig. 16.4). Suction drains are placed, and patient is placed in support bra for 10–14 days to keep the implant properly oriented. If postoperative radiation therapy is planned, the expander is irradiated at final volume and exchange is delayed from 4 to 6 months, depending on radiation-induced edema and induration. Some radiation oncologists require deflation of the expander for optimal chest wall irradiation, and after the 5-week therapy, the expander is reinflated quickly over 2 weeks and then exchanged at 9 months.

16.6.4 Single-Stage Reconstruction with Implants

When nipple-sparing mastectomy is selected, immediate breast reconstruction may take place by replacing the excised mammary parenchyma with a similarly sized permanent implant. Depending on the nipple viability, either a final implant or tissue expander is placed. ICG laser angiography (SPY) can be useful in helping the surgeon evaluate viability [19]. For high-risk patients (i.e., previous surgery or radiation), delayed nipple-sparing mastectomies have been described that have shown to improve nipple vascularity at the time of the second-stage NSM.

With skin-sparing mastectomy of a small breast, placement of an implant can be done immediately. The goal is to maintain the breast envelope and fill it with volume. Since the skin after mastectomy is thin and relatively ischemic, healthy vascularized muscle is required to ensure implant longevity. In the one-stage approach, tissue expansion of the pectoralis does not occur and so effective muscle coverage must be obtained in another way. This is accomplished with either latissimus dorsi muscle transfer or an ADM sling (acellular dermal matrix). Currently, most surgeons will use ADM rather than sacrifice muscle. That said, at the time of mastectomy, the latissimus can be harvested via an open or endoscopic approach and rotated to the anterior chest where it drapes over the final breast implant. Immediate single-stage reconstruction is best suited for patients with small, round breasts with a resection weight of about 300 g. The implant is traditionally placed in a subpectoral pocket.

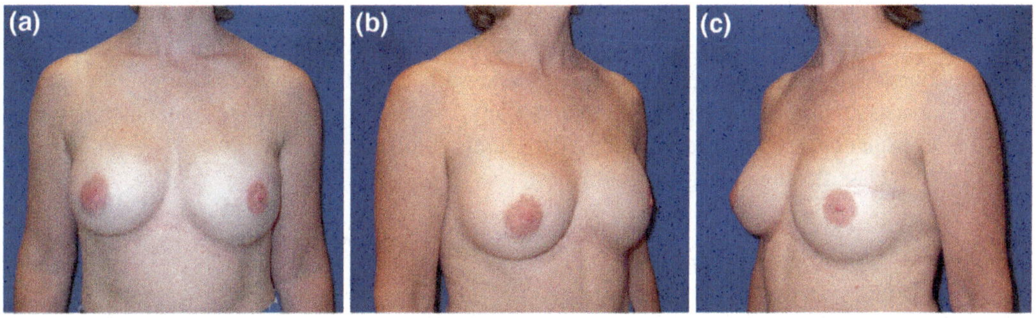

Fig. 16.4 Tissue expansion/exchange: This is a 45-year-old patient who underwent immediate placement of a tissue expander on the left, subsequent expansion, and exchange for an implant. At the implant exchange, she had a contralateral breast augmentation for better symmetry. These photographs represent her 9-month postoperative visit

Newer techniques not involving muscle are currently being tried (see "pre-pectoral" below).

16.6.5 Permanent Tissue Expander/Implant Reconstruction

One-stage breast reconstruction with permanent expander implants was introduced in 1984 with expandable double-lumen silicone gel/saline-filled prosthesis. This technique is largely of historical interest only. The implant can be partially filled at the time of reconstruction and gradually inflated postoperatively over a 3–6-month period, until symmetry is achieved. The device is placed in a similar manner as previously described. The major drawback of breast reconstruction with anatomic expander implants is that it is hard to get the skin to expand in a breast shape. This is the advantage of having a second stage—better shape. Disadvantages of this approach include superficial infection and discomfort often associated with the port. In addition, a second procedure is needed to remove the port.

16.6.6 Prosthetic Reconstruction with Acellular Dermal Matrix

Achieving the total muscle coverage of the implant and natural ptosis is a key technical challenge. In the past decade, the use of acellular dermal matrices has been adopted to supplement the pectoralis major muscle at the lower and lateral aspects for implant coverage. The reported benefits of ADM compared to total muscle coverage techniques include improved lower pole expansion, increased intraoperative fill volume for tissue expanders, and reduced number of expansions. Throughout its use, concerns with the use of ADM have been raised. Despite variability in study design and sample size, numerous studies have sought to evaluate the observed incidence and complication profile (infection and seroma rate) of ADM-assisted techniques. Both direct-to-implant and two-stage ADM-assisted immediate breast reconstruction have been described and are commonly used today in practice. "Pre-pectoral ADM-assisted breast reconstruction" where no muscle is used and full coverage of the implant is achieved with ADM only is coming into vogue. The obvious advantages include no muscle dysfunction, less postoperative pain, and no "animation" deformities when the pectoralis muscles are flexed.

16.6.7 Complications of Implant Reconstruction

As would be expected with any foreign body, there are certain risks associated with the use of implants. Infection, extrusion, malposition, and capsular contracture are among the most common. The incidence of infection of breast implants is generally around 2 %, but studies have shown an increased risk in the setting of chemotherapy, radiation, and previous axillary node dissection [20]. As a result, the incidence implant infection in the setting of breast reconstruction is higher, with some studies reporting infection in up to 10 % of patients. Treatment of implant infection or extrusion requires removal of the implant followed by antibiotic therapy. A period of 4–6 months should pass before embarking on a secondary reconstruction. Extrusion of implants can be secondary to infection or poor soft tissue coverage. For this reason, many surgeons prefer "total muscle" coverage of the implant at the time of surgery. It is thought that covering the entire implant with muscle will still protect the implant in the setting of a skin dehiscence, which would otherwise potentially expose an implant that has less soft tissue coverage. Poor tissue coverage will sometimes necessitate tissue flap coverage.

All implants induce a foreign body reaction and formation of a discrete fibrous shell or "capsule." Deformity can occur when the capsule thickens and contracts, leaving the implant space smaller and creating visible ripples in the reconstruction. Many variables influence the occurrence of significant capsular contracture, such as implant type, textured surface, filler substance, submuscular placement, and subclinical infection. Capsular contracture is classified based on severity. The Baker classification categorizes this as follows:

Grade 1: The breast is soft and natural appearing.
Grade 2: The breast is less soft with palpable distortion but still appears natural.
Grade 3: The breast is firm with visible distortion.
Grade 4: The breast is firm, painful, and visibly distorted.

Using this classification as a guide and evaluating each patient individually, severe cases of contracture (grades 3 and 4) may require surgery for removal of the capsule and replacement of the prosthesis (Fig. 16.5). Factors that have been shown to reduce the incidence of this complication include submuscular placement of the implant and use of a textured surface implant.

A less common but worrisome complication of implant use is anaplastic large cell lymphoma (ALCL). In January 2011, the FDA announced a safety communication, pointing out a possible association between breast implants and ALCL [21]. Breast implant ALCL (BI-ALCL) is distinct from primary breast lymphoma, which is a disease of the breast parenchyma and predominantly B cell in origin. BI-ALCL is a T cell lymphoma arising from an effusion or scar capsule surrounding the breast implant. Since the first report of BI-ALCL in 1997, greater than 90 cases have been published. Knowledge about BI-ALCL has evolved over the past 2 decades with a better understanding and recognition of this disease process. Patients with concerning findings should have tissue and fluid specimens sent for pathology review. Operative management includes removal of the implant and entire capsule with lymph node dissection. Adjunctive treatment modalities have been described and are now under further investigation. These include chemotherapy, radiation therapy, immunotherapy, and stem cell transplantation.

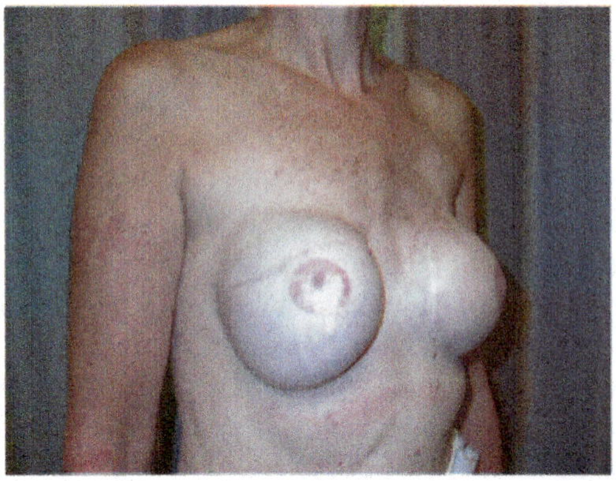

Fig. 16.5 Capsular contracture: This is a 57-year-old patient 5 years after right implant reconstruction and left implant reconstruction with a latissimus flap due to radiation. Note the distorted shapes of the breasts and thinning skin envelope

16.7 Autogenous Reconstruction

Advances in breast reconstruction during the past 30 years offer women the option of undergoing breast reconstruction with their own tissue and without the need for breast implants or expanders. The first application of autogenous transfer for breast reconstruction occurred in 1977 with the use of the latissimus dorsi muscle flap [22]. Myocutaneous flaps permit the movement of additional skin, underlying fat, and muscle for reconstruction of the breast. The most common donor sites for autogenous tissue are the lower abdomen, back, thighs, and gluteal regions. These areas are considered to have tissue excess and can be contoured to produce a more esthetic appearance. Flap reconstructions are particularly useful when there is a significant skin deficiency following mastectomy. With immediate breast reconstruction, the use of a flap can permit the creation of a breast that is relatively symmetrical with the contralateral breast with similar tissue characteristics.

The transfer of myocutaneous flaps is possible due to the blood supply to the overlying skin and subcutaneous tissue from the underlying muscle via musculocutaneous perforators. The transfer of myocutaneous flaps can be accomplished as pedicled flaps or free flaps. Pedicled flaps refer to tissue blocks that are transferred from the lower abdomen or back to the mastectomy site following elevation of the myocutaneous unit from its bed. The pedicle, consisting of an artery and a vein(s), may be skeletonized, but is left intact and serves as the axis of rotation of the flap. Free tissue transfer relies on the technique of microsurgery and in breast reconstruction applies to the transfer of tissue from remote regions of the body to the chest wall. This involves elevating the tissue needed, identifying its major vascular pedicle and dividing it. This is followed by the relocation of the tissue to the chest along with microvascular anastomosis of the donor vessels to the recipient vessels. In breast reconstruction, the most common recipient vessels are the internal mammary vessels and the thoracodorsal vessels.

Autogenous reconstruction can be performed in both the immediate and delayed settings. Today, when patients are felt to be at very high risk for radiotherapy, autogenous reconstruction is performed in a delayed fashion. Immediate reconstruction should occur when the risk of postoperative radiation is low, such as when sentinel node sampling reveals no evidence of lymph node metastasis or tumor size is small. Overall, autogenous breast reconstruction yields the most durable and natural appearing results with the greatest applicability. It has several advantages over implant reconstruction:

1. A large volume of the patient's tissue is available.
2. Prosthesis is not required, obviating problems such as implant infection, prosthesis, contracture, and extrusion.
3. It offers versatility in shaping the new breast with the creation of natural ptosis and fill of the infraclavicular hollow and anterior axillary fold.
4. It can withstand postoperative radiotherapy much better than implant reconstruction.
5. The excellent vascularity of the tissues allows for improved wound healing, especially in an irradiated chest wall.

The autogenous tissues available in decreasing order of frequency of use are the abdomen (pedicled TRAM flap, free TRAM flap, DIEP, SIEA), latissimus dorsi flap, superior and inferior gluteal flaps, upper thigh flaps (TUG, PAP), lateral transverse thigh flap, and deep circumflex iliac artery (DCIA) flap. Each of these flaps can be raised as a myocutaneous flap or a perforator flap, which spares the accompanying muscle and only lives off the perforating blood vessels in the flap. These flaps require microsurgical expertise. We will review these flaps and adjunctive methods available for optimal reconstructive outcomes.

16.7.1 Pedicled TRAM Flap/Unipedicled Flap

The pedicled TRAM flap was first described in 1982 by Hartrampf. Since then, the procedure has gained popularity and it remains the most commonly performed method of autologous breast reconstruction [23]. A lower abdominal transverse skin island is designed overlying the rectus abdominis muscles. This is the same tissue removed during an abdominoplasty, hence its appeal. The overlying skin and subcutaneous tissue receive their blood supply from perforating vessels from the underlying rectus muscle.

The rectus abdominis muscle receives a dual blood supply from the superior and inferior epigastric vessels. The pedicled flap is based on the superior epigastric vessels due to a better point of rotation to reach the chest. The vessels are the continuation of the internal mammary vessels and are distant from the lower abdomen. This means the degree of perfusion of the overlying skin and fat is limited and care must be exercised in deciding how much tissue to carry. It does not require microsurgical skills and is therefore more applicable to most plastic surgeons. The muscle with its overlying adipose tissue and skin is simply tunneled through the upper abdomen to the chest wall into the contralateral or ipsilateral mastectomy defect (Fig. 16.6).

The concept of perfusion becomes relevant when looking at flap survival and partial flap loss called "fat necrosis." Fat necrosis manifests as a subcutaneous or deep firmness, which often compromises the esthetic outcomes of the reconstruction. In addition, it causes anxiety in patients and surgeons in view of its differential diagnosis as a cancer recurrence. A simple way of thinking about this is that the risk of fat necrosis increases as the distance from the muscle perforators increases. The concept of angiosomes was first introduced by Taylor over 30 years ago [24]. An angiosome represents a three-dimensional tissue unit supplied by a source artery. Each source artery directly supplies perforators to the muscle and skin of a discrete area called the primary angiosome. A neighboring area may still be supplied by this source artery through secondary, less reliable "choke vessels," and these areas are secondary angiosomes. The primary blood supply territory of the superior epigastric artery is the upper abdomen. The lower abdomen is supplied in a pedicled TRAM flap by connections between the superior epigastric system (secondary) and the inferior epigastric system (primary to the lower abdomen) (Fig. 16.7). Intuitively, the best supplied tissues are present over the rectus muscles in direct continuity with the muscular

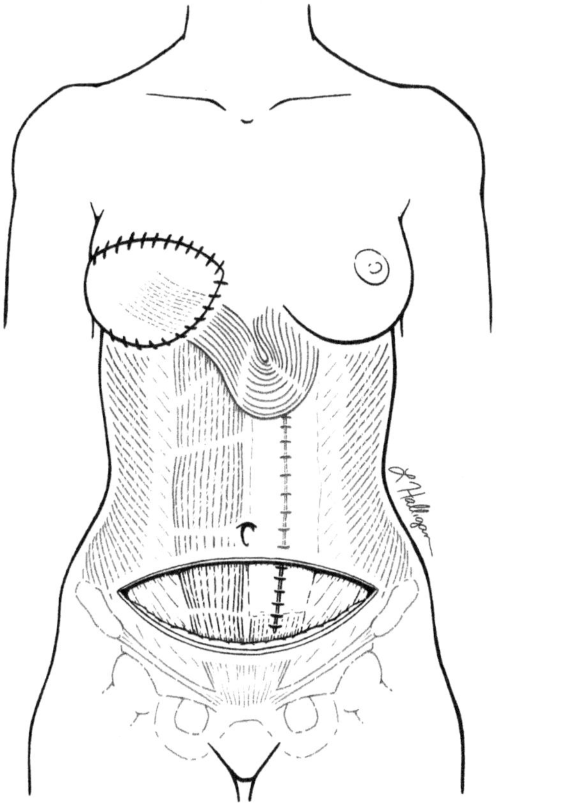

Fig. 16.6 Unipedicled TRAM flap: This picture demonstrates the unipedicled TRAM flap. This flap has been transposed to the contralateral chest. The pedicled TRAM flap can also be transferred onto the ipsilateral chest (Duke University Department of Surgery)

perforators. This is referred to as Zone 1 of the TRAM flap (Fig. 16.8). As shown in the figure, there are a total of 4 zones of a TRAM flap. Zone 2 represents the area medial to the elevated rectus across the midline, and Zone 3 represents the area lateral to elevated rectus. Zone 4 is the furthest from the elevated rectus, representing the area with the most tenuous blood supply present in the TRAM flap. The risk of fat necrosis is higher in patients with the history of COPD, diabetes mellitus, hypertension, obesity, and smoking history. In these patients, the pedicled TRAM may not be the best choice for reconstruction. Free TRAM transfer, bipedicled TRAM, and pedicled TRAM after delay may be more appropriate in these settings.

Following harvest and transposition of the flap to the mastectomy defect, the TRAM flap is inset or positioned in place. Attention is turned to recreating a symmetrical breast, with IMF at the same level and breast volume and projections also being similar. Often the volume of TRAM is in excess of what is needed, and in this setting, the zones furthest from the pedicle, demonstrating the poorest perfusion, can be partially resected down to the volume desired. The skin of the flap can also be de-epithelialized to leave behind enough epidermis to only bridge the mastectomy skin defect.

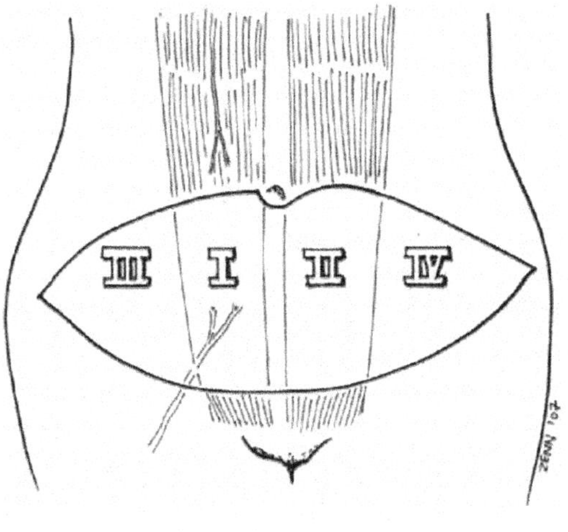

Fig. 16.8 TRAM vascular zones: The lower abdominal tissue that is transferred in a TRAM flap is divided into 4 zones based on the degree of perfusion. Zone 1 has the best perfusion as it is the area directly over the deep inferior epigastric artery. Zone 2 is the area directly medial and has the second best perfusion. Zone 3 is the area lateral to Zone 1 with a less robust blood supply than Zone 2. Zone 4 is the area farthest from the pedicle and thus has the most tenuous blood supply. Because of its relatively poor perfusion, Zone 4 is the first area discarded in flap transfer if debulking of the tissue block is necessary prior to inset

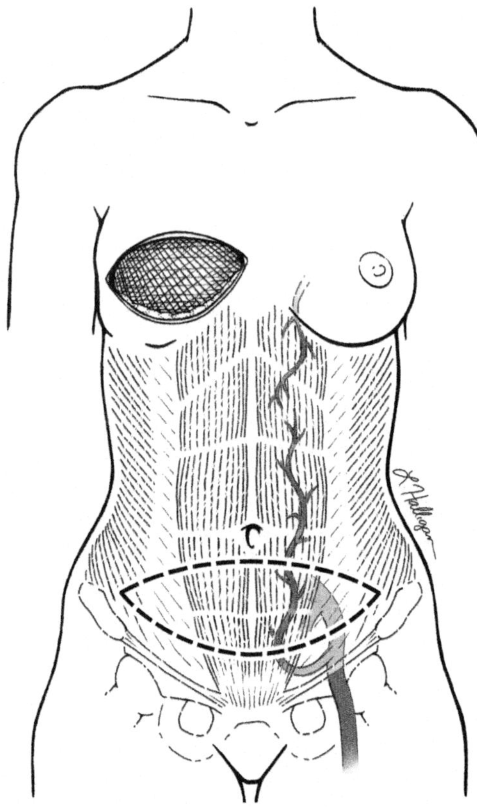

Fig. 16.7 Unipedicled TRAM flap: This picture demonstrates the vascular supply (superior epigastric artery) that runs superficial to the rectus fascia (Duke University Department of Surgery)

The donor site also needs careful attention to avoid hernias and bulges. With the rectus muscle harvested on one side, the chance of hernia is about 5 %. For this reason, mesh reconstruction of the muscle defect should be considered when primary closure is not possible or is tenuous. Despite these adjunctive procedures, up to 30 % of patients still experience a bulge or hernia in the lower abdomen with full muscle harvest. The clinical significance of this is debated.

16.7.2 Bipedicled TRAM Flap

The use of the two rectus muscle pedicles increases the blood flow to the overlying skin and fat, thereby increasing the reliability and size of the flap. However, indications are limited because of the morbidity associated with abdominal wall damage from the loss of both rectus muscles. It is used primarily to augment circulation in obese patients, smokers, and diabetes. It is also used in patients with limited abdominal tissue; hence, all zones are required for reconstruction and in patients who are unwilling to undergo reduction of the contralateral breast. It has been shown that patients who undergo unipedicled reconstruction have a 40 % decrease in abdominal muscle strength compared to a 64 % decrease in bipedicled flaps. With previous abdominal midline scars, some surgeons have reported acceptable results in these patients using the bipedicled TRAM. In larger centers, free flap reconstruction has largely supplanted the use of the bipedicled TRAM.

16.7.3 Midabdominal TRAM Flap

In the morbidly obese patients who would be considered high risk for the standard lower abdominal TRAM flap, the midabdominal TRAM represents an acceptable alternative. In this variant, the horizontal location of the abdominal ellipse is moved upward toward the midabdomen in order to increase the blood flow to the overlying skin and fat. The supplying superior epigastric vessels are not so distant, and perfusion of the tissue, now a primary angiosome, is improved. It is ironic that the obese patient with a significant abdominal pannus is a poor candidate for a standard TRAM. This is because the tissues, though significant, are poorly vascularized and edematous. The use of the ample mid- or upper abdomen avoids the use of these poorer tissues in the reconstruction, avoiding complications. Abdominal closure is facilitated by the large pannus. The main disadvantage, the highly visible scar in the mid- or upper abdominal area, is less of a concern for the morbidly obese patients, who benefit somewhat from the reduction of abdominal redundancy.

16.7.4 Free TRAM Flaps

The free TRAM flap utilizes the primary blood supply of the lower abdomen, the deep inferior epigastric vessels. It thus has better vascularity and less risk of ischemia in the peripheral zones (abdominal zones 2, 3, and 4). Because of this improved tissue perfusion, there is a lower incidence of fat necrosis when compared to the pedicled TRAM flap. Additionally, this flap reliably carries a larger amount of skin and adipose tissue than the pedicled TRAM. Since it is not possible to pedicle a flap based on the inferior epigastrics to the chest, these vessels must be divided and microscopically reconnected.

These vessels are connected with either the thoracodorsal or the internal mammary vessels (Fig. 16.9). In immediate breast reconstruction, the thoracodorsal vessels are usually targeted since they are usually fully exposed by the oncologic surgeon during axillary node dissection. In the delayed setting, the internal mammary vessels are more often chosen for the microvascular anastomosis. This recipient site has the advantage of being free of previous scarring around vessels, being centrally located facilitating microsurgery, and allowing a more medial positioning of the flap.

Studies from numerous cancer centers show distinct advantages of the free TRAM over its pedicled counterpart. There is a less than 10 % chance of fat necrosis with free flap reconstruction compared to 30 % with the pedicled TRAM [25]. As in the pedicled TRAM, the free TRAM flap is also associated with abdominal wall bulges and hernias, but less so. One study quoted the incidence of hernia to be

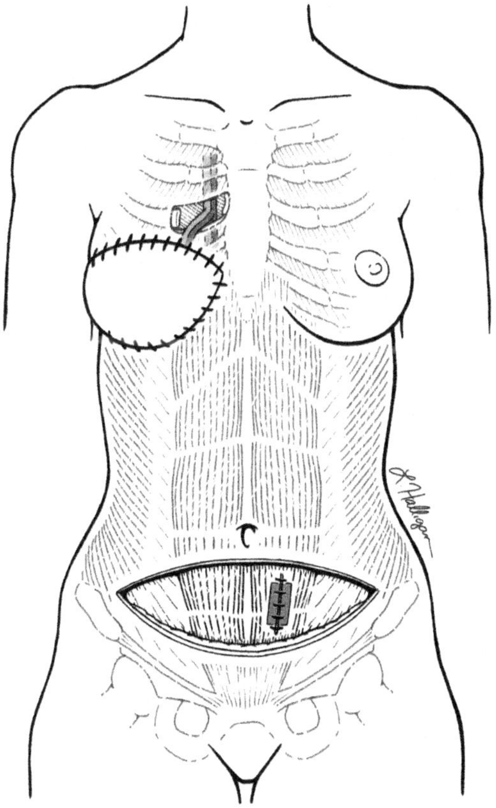

Fig. 16.9 Free TRAM flap: This figure demonstrates a muscle-sparing free TRAM flap where only a small portion of the rectus muscle and fascia surrounding the deep inferior epigastric pedicle is included. The pedicle can be co-apted to either the thoracodorsal or internal mammary system. Here, the anastomosis is to the internal mammary vessels that is often exposed by removing a portion of the 3rd rib cartilage (Duke University Department of Surgery)

12 % in the pedicled TRAM and 3–6 % in the free TRAM flap [26]. The free TRAM also avoids the bulge in the epigastrium and the disruption of the IMF that is required by the tunneling of the pedicled flap from the lower abdomen. Free flaps do not require tunnel formation, and a sharply demarcated IMF is possible during the first operation.

For the free TRAM flap, muscle-sparing variations have been described. In the muscle-sparing TRAM variant (Fig. 16.10), only the central portion of muscle surrounding the deep inferior epigastric pedicle is taken with the flap leading to less disruption of the rectus fibers as compared to the conventional free TRAM, where the complete transverse width of the muscle is removed. Comparing the degrees of muscle spared, the rate of fat necrosis gradually increases from complete transection of the rectus muscle in a free TRAM to a perforator-based abdominal flap which theoretically spares the entire muscle. This is related to the number of perforators used with each technique. Muscle sparing uses all perforators present, while a perforator flap isolates just a few. In the muscle-sparing TRAM, muscle continuity is maintained as is a significant portion of the muscle innervation, so the rates of hernia and bulge are less. In contradistinction, pedicled flap reconstruction mandates elevation of the entire rectus muscle leaving behind a large area of the lower abdomen often requiring mesh reinforcement. Although sacrificing the rectus muscle will not leave a patient completely disabled, patients may notice a considerable difference in flexion strength and abdominal contour when the rectus muscles are sacrificed. Objective measures of abdominal wall strength after pedicled or free TRAM reconstruction have consistently shown a deficit in strength which may persist long term. Several comparative studies have not shown a significant difference in long-term abdominal wall function between these two techniques.

16.7.5 Abdominal Perforator Flaps

Perforator flaps represent the newest generation of free flap reconstruction. The concept of a perforator flap emphasizes the blood vessels, not the muscles. The skin island and accompanying fat are isolated on perforating vessels that come through muscle from the source artery, leaving intact innervated muscle. In breast reconstruction, the dominant perforator flap used is the deep inferior epigastric perforator (DIEP) flap. The superficial inferior epigastric artery (SIEA) perforator flap has also been used; however, it is less available due to the anatomic variability seen in patients [27].

The DIEP flap preserves the whole rectus muscle and its sheath (Fig. 16.11). It can be based on a single large perforator or as many as 4 or 5 perforators (Fig. 16.12). When skeletonizing the perforators, the rectus sheath above and below the perforator is incised for a short distance to identify the vessel connection with the deep inferior epigastric system. The advantages of the DIEP flap include avoidance of muscle sacrifice and decreased abdominal wall morbidity, decreased postoperative pain, and decreased hospital stay. It usually also avoids the problems of a tight fascial closure and can preclude the need for synthetic mesh. Although the DIEP, based on a few perforators, has less perfusion than a free TRAM flap which is based on all perforators, the incidence of fat necrosis is similar and perfusion is still superior to a pedicled TRAM. One of the disadvantages of the DIEP flap is the technically more challenging dissection.

The free SIEA flap provides the same abdominal skin and fat for reconstruction as the DIEP flap. The SIEA flap is not a true "perforator" flap as the vessel is a primary branch of the femoral system [28]. Of the two flaps, the SIEA causes less donor site morbidity. Since the superficial epigastric vessels are superficial to rectus fascia, no incision must be made in the abdominal fascia and no vessel dissection is performed through the rectus abdominis muscle. The flap, however, is limited by the variability in its vascular anatomy.

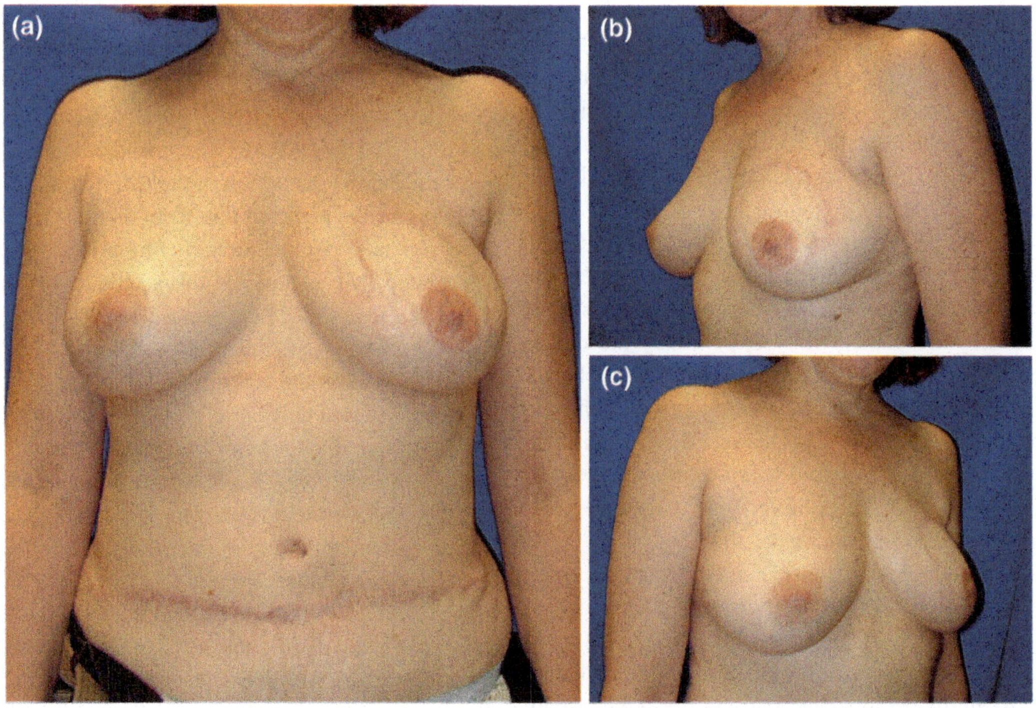

Fig. 16.10 Pedicled TRAM: This is a 43-year-old patient who underwent immediate breast reconstruction with a pedicled TRAM. These are 1-year postoperative photographs. The areola was reconstructed with tattoos and the nipple by nipple sharing from the contralateral nipple

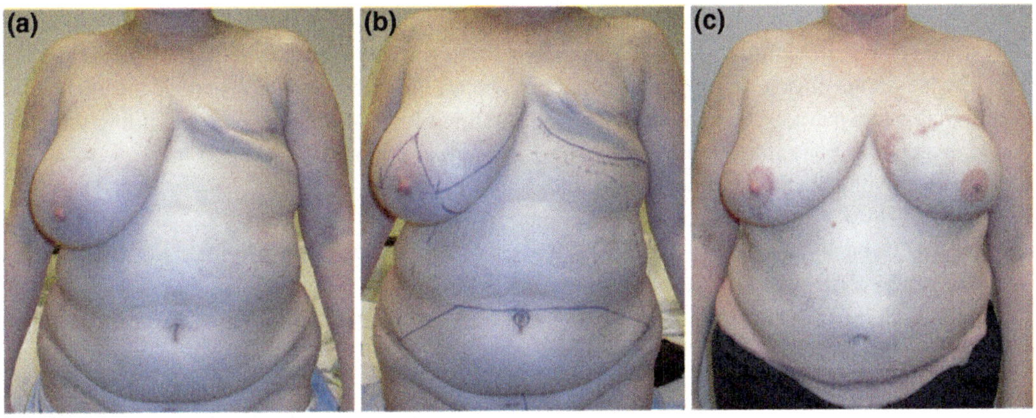

Fig. 16.11 Breast reduction with free TRAM: This is a 40-year-old patient who underwent delayed reconstruction. (**a**, **b**) Preoperative defect and markings. Her right breast was too large to match, so she had a reduction *on the right* and a muscle-sparing free TRAM flap *on the left* (**c**, **d**). These photographs are at 1-year follow-up

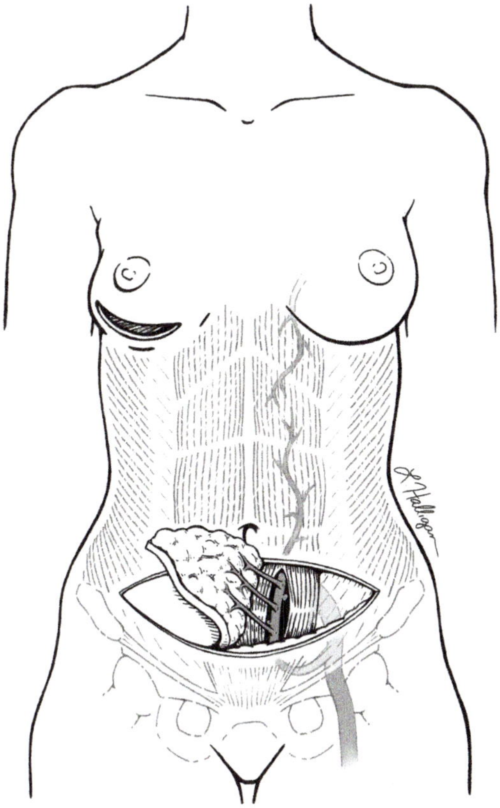

Fig. 16.12 DIEP flap: This figure demonstrates the split rectus abdominis muscle from which emanates the deep inferior epigastric artery perforator supplying vasculature to the abdominal adipocutaneous flap. The recipient site in this figure is the left breast as demonstrated by a nipple-sparing mastectomy incision (Duke University Department of Surgery)

The SIEA and vein are only inconsistently present in sufficient caliber to reliably support sufficient tissue for breast reconstruction. Disadvantages of the SIEA flap are a smaller pedicle diameter and shorter pedicle length than TRAM or DIEP flaps. The SIEA pedicle can be a valuable source of blood supply when the proposed flap requires a bipedicle approach (blood supply from both sides of the abdomen for a single flap). When performed successfully, esthetic results of SIEA flap breast reconstruction are indistinguishable from a TRAM or DIEP flap [29].

16.7.6 Latissimus Dorsi Musculocutaneous Flap

As previously alluded to, the latissimus dorsi muscle can be used for autogenous breast reconstruction. It is often combined with implant reconstruction in patients with moderate-sized breasts, and in those with smaller breasts, it can be used alone. With this operation, skin and muscle from the back are transferred to the mastectomy defect. It is safe with a reliable blood supply. The blood supply to the pedicled latissimus flap is the thoracodorsal vessels. In the event that these vessels are injured during surgery, the latissimus can still be raised based on the serratus branch of the thoracodorsal vessel. In this situation, retrograde flow from the intercostal system through the serratus branch maintains tissue perfusion.

The indications for use of the latissimus dorsi muscle in breast reconstruction include (1) primary reconstruction with or without implant/tissue expander; (2) patients with inadequate abdominal tissue, or patients who are unwilling to have an abdominal scar; (3) secondary reconstruction with implant after radiation therapy; and (4) as a salvage procedure for implant or tissue reconstruction when failure of reconstruction has occurred.

The skin paddle on the back over the muscle is quite healthy and is well perfused when placed directly over the latissimus muscle (primary angiosome). A patient who has undergone a skin-sparing mastectomy may require mainly muscle and only a small circle of skin to replace the nipple–areola complex. The latissimus muscle flap is usually used in combination with implant/expanders to achieve a desired breast volume to match the contralateral breast. In some patients who need added volume but do not want implants, the extended latissimus dorsi flap can be used. With this method, a more aggressive fat and skin harvest increases the bulk of flap and forms a larger breast. Disadvantages of this technique include the high incidence of seroma at the donor site and a large scar deformity on the back.

16.7.7 Gluteal Musculocutaneous and Perforator Flaps

Gluteal tissues are a distant second or third choice for total autogenous breast reconstruction. They are a distant choice due to the popularity of the abdominal tissue donor site and the difficulty of the gluteal vessel dissection. The gluteus maximus myocutaneous free flap was first described in 1983. Muscle is no longer harvested with these flaps as they are raised as perforator flaps. The superior gluteal free flap is based on the superior gluteal vessels (S-GAPs), and the inferior gluteal flap is based on the inferior gluteal vessels (I-GAPs) [30]. This has the added benefit of a longer vascular pedicle for ease of flap inset and microanastomosis. For any flap, the width of the skin island may be up to 13 cm and allow a primary donor closure, while the length varies from 10 to 30 cm. While there is ample adipose tissue to allow for reconstruction in the gluteal region, gluteal fat is more fibrous than abdominal wall fat. This can make shaping of the tissue more difficult during insetting of the flap and limit the final appearance of the reconstruction. Important anatomic differences exist between the superior and inferior gluteal flaps (Fig. 16.13). The superior gluteal artery is shorter and must be connected to the internal mammary system for the tissues to be placed properly on the chest. The inferior gluteal artery is longer and can reach the thoracodorsal vessels if needed. Dissection of the inferior gluteal artery can put the inferior gluteal and posterior femoral cutaneous nerves at risk, not an issue with the superior gluteal artery dissection. While harvest of the gluteal tissue can leave a deformity of the buttock, the superior flap mimics more a buttock "lift" and is better tolerated. Ultimately, the choice of superior versus inferior will depend on the distribution of the gluteal fat. For both gluteal flaps, dissection of the pedicles is more tedious when compared to the dissection of vessels in a free TRAM flap and often requires position changes for harvest and/or inset.

Newer perforator flaps are beginning to become more popular as our understanding of the anatomy improves and more surgeons become comfortable with microsurgery. These flaps (i.e., profunda artery perforator or PAP) and new flaps yet discovered will have in common the harvest of excess tissues in another part of the body based on perforating blood vessels for use in building a breast mound with minimal donor site morbidity [31].

16.8 Secondary Breast Reconstruction

16.8.1 Nipple–Areola Reconstruction

Creating a nipple–areola complex is an integral part of the breast reconstruction. It enhances the final cosmetic result and creates a more natural-looking reconstructed breast. It is typically performed 3 months after the mound reconstruction. It is delayed in the setting of a reconstruction that is to be radiated. It is the last step in the process of postmastectomy surgical rehabilitation [32].

The nipple can be reconstructed with local tissue of the reconstructed breast or as a nipple graft from the contralateral breast. When utilizing local tissue, flaps can be designed to wrap skin and fat into conical shapes to recreate a projecting nipple. Examples of such flaps include the skate, C-V, bell, and tab flaps, among others. All local flaps suffer from shrinkage during the healing phase and may not match the contralateral nipple [33]. Large nipples can best be matched with "nipple sharing" when the contralateral nipple is bisected, half used as a free nipple graft for reconstruction.

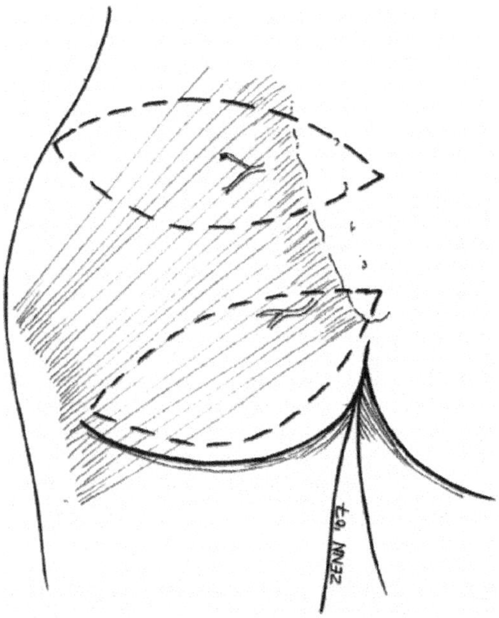

Fig. 16.13 Gluteal artery flaps: This figure demonstrates the zones of the superior and inferior gluteal artery flaps. These flaps can be harvested as musculocutaneous or perforator flaps

This reduces the large nipple and creates an opposite twin from like tissue.

The areola is reconstructed so that it is symmetrical and similar in color and diameter to the areola of the opposite breast. Methods used for reconstruction include skin grafts, areolar sharing from the other breast, and tattooing. Tattooing is the most common method as it is simple and avoids the need for a skin graft. If skin grafting is performed, further intradermal tattooing may be required to achieve symmetry to the opposite nipple–areola complex.

16.8.2 Autologous Fat Grafting

In pursuit of improving reconstructive shape, contour, and symmetry of the breast, autologous fat grafting has been adopted as the most common secondary reconstructive procedure performed for revision over the course of the past decade. This growth in popularity stems from it, being a reliable technique with low morbidity and improved esthetic results. Indications for fat grafting in breast reconstruction as a secondary procedure are expanding but involve improving contour, shape, and volume [34]. The harvesting and injection technique includes low-pressure syringe liposuction with small aliquot injections at the necessary sites. Implant-based reconstructions can benefit from upper pole injection to aid the transition from implant to upper chest wall and for implant rippling often associated with implants. In addition, abdomen-based flaps may benefit from contour irregularities and volume deficiencies. As with all autologous fat grafting, there is a certain amount of resorption that is encountered. Reported volume loss has been between 40 and 60 % within the first 4 to 6 months. Due to its low morbidity, fat grafting may be repeated as necessary to maximally improve final results.

16.8.3 Contralateral Breast

While breast reconstruction can nicely replace a breast lost to mastectomy, it rarely produces a breast that is symmetrical with the unaffected contralateral breast. As a result, the patient with a unilateral reconstruction may require alteration of the opposite breast to achieve symmetry. The options available for the contralateral breast include mastopexy, breast reduction, implant augmentation, and prophylactic mastectomy with reconstruction [35].

Mastopexy, or a breast lift procedure, is performed to correct a ptotic breast. The procedure involves lifting of the nipple–areola complex and reshaping of the breast cone to match the reconstructed breast in size and position. Breast reduction can effect similar changes but also reduces the volume of the contralateral breast (Fig. 16.10). In patients who have a reconstructed breast that is larger than their native breast and the patient prefers this size, augmentation mammoplasty of the opposite breast can be performed. Lastly, patients who request contralateral mastectomy must understand that a reconstruction can achieve a reasonable breast form but is not an equal substitute for a natural breast.

16.9 Radiation and Breast Reconstruction

Irradiation is known to cause permanent damage to cells involved in wound healing and as such can negatively impact healing of a flap or graft. Following the milestone publications in 1997 in the *New England Journal of Medicine* of randomized clinical trials performed in Denmark and British Columbia which demonstrated a survival benefit in patients with postmastectomy radiation (PMRT), the use of radiotherapy in the appropriate setting has become standard of care. Current indications for PMRT include (1) tumors with positive margins, (2) tumors that are T3 or greater (>5 cm), and (3) the presence of 4 or more positive axillary nodes. Although the role of PMRT in breast cancer patients has been well defined, its reported effects on breast reconstruction are variable. Radiation therapy subjects the skin surface to progressive change through a chronic inflammatory process. Early effects occur within 90 days and include skin dryness, epilation, pigmentation changes, and erythema. Late effects manifest with a progressive induration and thinning of the skin, fibrosis, and edema. Microscopic examination of radiated tissues demonstrate signs of vascular obliteration and chronic ischemia. A number of studies have looked at the long-term outcomes of radiation therapy on both implant and autologous reconstruction.

A review by Spear et al. of 40 patients who underwent implant reconstruction followed by PMRT showed that over 45 % of patients required revisional surgery with either implant replacement or autogenous tissue as compared to 10 % in patients who did not receive radiation [16]. They showed a 33 % rate of capsular contracture in the irradiated group compared to 0 % in the control group. Cosmetic outcomes are also considered inferior in the irradiated reconstructed breast. The risk of implant exposure and infection is higher following PMRT. Autogenous reconstruction is also negatively impacted by irradiation. A study by MD Anderson compared irradiation of immediate TRAM flaps to irradiation of delayed TRAM flaps. The study demonstrated a similar incidence of early complications. These included vessel thrombosis, partial flap loss, and mastectomy flap necrosis. However, the immediate TRAM flap group had a higher incidence of late complications (fat necrosis, volume loss, and contracture) with 28 % of patients requiring revisional surgery. Recent studies of postmastectomy irradiation of free TRAM and DIEP flaps showed a higher rate of fat necrosis with DIEP flaps, possibly reflecting their relative vascularity [36]. With PMRT in the setting of implant reconstruction, another consideration is the delivery of the radiation. The implant/expander can cause technical problems with the design of the radiation fields, particularly as it pertains to the internal mammary nodes. Therefore, the presence of an implant may result in the exclusion of the internal mammary chain with increasing doses delivered to the lung and heart.

Due to the high incidence of complications, most reconstructive surgeons will not pursue implant reconstruction in the patient who will need radiation. Most will perform a delayed reconstruction after completion of radiation. It is, however, often difficult to predict preoperatively who will be a candidate for immediate breast reconstruction and who will need radiation. In patients who are undergoing prophylactic mastectomies, immediate reconstruction can be pursued. In breast cancer patients, if the tumor is greater than 5 cm, then the patient will need PMRT and immediate reconstruction should be avoided. In patients without clear indications for PMRT, the ultimate need for radiation is unknown. In this situation, when immediate reconstruction is required, a separate sentinel lymph node sampling procedure can be performed. If the sentinel lymph node is negative, most reconstructive surgeons will pursue immediate reconstruction, assuming that it is the wish of the patient. As described previously, patients with plans for PMRT with sufficient skin envelope after skin-sparing mastectomy may have the option for immediate reconstruction using a tissue expander, with the understanding that this expander may need to be deflated prior to radiation.

As indications for postmastectomy radiation and other treatment modalities continue to change, the approach to breast reconstruction needs to adapt to maintain an appropriate balance between minimizing the risk of recurrence and providing the most durable and best esthetic reconstructive outcome. Delayed reconstruction is typically performed 6 months after the cessation of PMRT to allow full healing of the chest to limit healing difficulties [37].

16.10 Chemotherapy

As part of the postmastectomy regimen, patients with breast cancer may need chemotherapy. It is well known that certain chemotherapeutic agents can hinder wound healing and this can impact the breast reconstruction in the immediate postoperative period. Once the wound is healed (typically 3–4 weeks), chemotherapy can be initiated. In the long term, the effect of chemotherapy on breast reconstruction is negligible, and a history of previous chemotherapy has virtually no adverse effects. However, development of a chronic, non-healing wound after an immediate reconstruction can delay the administration of chemotherapy until the wound has healed. For this reason, in patients undergoing breast reconstruction who are scheduled to undergo chemotherapy, secondary procedures such as exchange of tissue expanders for implants or tissue flap revision are delayed 2–3 months after the cessation of adjuvant chemotherapy.

16.11 Conclusion

Modern breast reconstruction techniques provide a reliable source of rehabilitation and return to normalcy for patients following treatment for breast cancer. It has become an integral aspect of breast cancer management. As a member of the multidisciplinary breast cancer team, the reconstructive surgeon provides valuable input on the appropriate timing and techniques for reconstruction. Breast reconstruction can be done safely and effectively at the time of mastectomy or as a delayed procedure.

Irrespective of the timing of reconstruction, a spectrum of techniques is available from which the patient and surgeon can choose. These can involve breast implants, autologous tissue, or both. Implant reconstruction is a relatively simple and effective method of breast reconstruction, but may not be suitable for all patients, particularly those who need or have had radiation therapy. Autologous methods in contrast are more surgically demanding, but they consistently yield better esthetic results than implant reconstruction, particularly when combined with skin-sparing mastectomy.

The goal of breast reconstruction is to restore the size, shape, and appearance of the breast as closely as possible after mastectomy. This aids in the restoration of body image and makes it possible for patients to wear virtually all types of clothing with confidence. As we see further refinements in microsurgical techniques, it becomes possible to reconstruct a breast with a minimum morbidity and a lifetime benefit.

References

1. Radovan C. Breast reconstruction after mastectomy using the temporary expander. Plast Reconstr Surg. 1982;69(2):195–208.
2. Taylor GI, Daniel RK. The free flap: composite tissue transfer by vascular anastomosis. Aust N Z J Surg. 1973;43(1):1–3.
3. Elliott LF, Hartrampf CR Jr. Breast reconstruction: progress in the past decade. World J Surg. 1990;14(6):763–775 (Review).
4. Bostwick J. Breast reconstruction following mastectomy. CA Cancer J Clin. 1995;45:289–304.
5. Hidalgo D, Borgen P, Petrek J, Cody H, Disa J. Immediate reconstruction after complete skin-sparing mastectomy with autologous tissue. J Am Coll Sur. 1998;187(1):17–21.
6. Chiu E, Ahn C. Breast reconstruction. In: McCarthy J, editor. Current therapy in plastic surgery. Philadelphia: Saunders; 2006. p. 352–61.

7. Spear SL, Hannan CM, Willey SC, Cocilovo C. Nipple-sparing mastectomy. Plast Reconstr Surg. 2009;123(6):1665–73.
8. Tokin C, Weiss A, Wang-Rodriguez J, Blair SL. Oncologic safety of skin-sparing and nipple-sparing mastectomy: a discussion and review of the literature. Int J Surg Oncol. 2012;2012:921821.
9. Rawlani V, Fiuk J, Johnson SA, Buck DW 2nd, Hirsch E, Hansen N, Khan S, Fine NA, Kim JY. The effect of incision choice on outcomes of nipple-sparing mastectomy reconstruction. Can J Plast Surg. 2011;19(4):129–33.
10. Zenn MR. Staged immediate breast reconstruction. Plast Reconstr Surg. 2015;135(4):976–9.
11. Malata C, Mc Intosh A, Purushotham A. Immediate breast reconstruction after mastectomy for cancer. Br J Surg. 2000;87:1455–72.
12. Pomahac B, May J, Slavin S. New trends in breast cancer management: is the era of immediate breast reconstruction changing? Ann Surg. 2006;244(2):282–8.
13. Kronowitz S, Kuerer H. Advances and surgical decision-making for breast reconstruction. Cancer. 2006;107(5):893–907.
14. Agha-Mohammadi S, De La Cruz C, Hurwitz D. Breast reconstruction with alloplastic implants. J Surg Oncol. 2006;94:471–8.
15. Ascherman J, Hanasono M, Hughes D. Implant reconstruction in breast cancer patients treated with radiation therapy. Plastic Reconstr Surg. 2006;117(2):358–65.
16. Spear S, Spittlet C. Breast reconstruction with implants and expanders. Plastic Reconstr Surg. 2001;107(1):177–87.
17. Nahabedian MY, Mesbahi AN. Breast Reconstruction with Tissue Expanders and Implants. In Nahabedian MY, ed. Elsevier, 2009. 1:1–19.
18. Nava MB, Expander-implants breast reconstructions. In Neligan PC, eds. Plastic Surgery. Elsevier, 2013. 13:336–369.
19. Gurtner GC, Jones GE, Neligan PC, Newman MI, Phillips BT, Sacks JM, Zenn MR. Intraoperative laser angiography using the SPY system: review of the literature and recommendations for use. Ann Surg Innov Res. 2013;7(1):1.
20. Alderman A, Wilkins E, Kim H, Lowery J. Complications in postmastectomy breast reconstruction: two-year results of the michigan breast reconstruction outcome study. Plastic Reconstr Surg. 2002;109(7):2266–75.
21. Aladily TN, Medeiros LJ, Amin MB, Haideri N, Ye D, Azevedo SJ, Jorgensen JL, de Peralta-Venturina M, Mustafa EB, Young KH, You MJ, Fayad LE, Blenc AM, Miranda RN. Anaplastic large cell lymphoma associated with breast implants: a report of 13 cases. Am J Surg Pathol. 2012;36(7):1000–8.
22. Shons A, Mosiello G. Postmastectomy breast reconstruction: current techniques. Cancer Control. 2001;8(5):419–4226.
23. Neligan PC, Buck DW. Autologous breast reconstruction using abdominal flaps. In: Neligan PC, Buck DW, editors. Elsevier; 2014. 18:278–308.
24. Taylor GI, Palmer JH. The vascular territories (angiosomes) of the body: experimental study and clinical applications. Br J Plast Surg. 1987;40(2):113–41.
25. Chevray P. Breast reconstruction with superficial inferior epigastric artery flaps: a prospective comparison with TRAM and DIEP flaps. Plastic Reconstr Surg. 2004;114(5):1077–83.
26. Wang H, Olbrich K, Erdmann D, Georgiade G. Delay of TRAM flap reconstruction improves flap reliability in the obese patient. Plastic Reconstr Surg. 2005;116(2):613–8.
27. Granzow J, Levine J, Chiu E, LoTempio M, Allen R. Breast reconstruction with perforator flaps. Plastic Reconstr Surg. 2007;120(1):1–12.
28. Elliot F. Breast reconstruction- free flap techniques. In: Thorne C, editor. Grabb & Smith Plastic Surgery. Philadelphia: Lippincott Williams & Wilkins; 2006. p. 648–56.
29. Zenn MR. Insetting of the superficial inferior epigastric artery flap in breast reconstruction. Plastic Reconstr Surg. 2006;117(5):1407–11.
30. Zenn MR, Millard JA. Free inferior gluteal harvest with sparing of the posterior femoral cutaneous nerve. J Reconstr Microsurg. 2006;22(7):509–12.
31. Allen RJ, Haddock NT, Ahn CY, Sadeghi A. Breast reconstruction with the profunda artery perforator flap. Plast Reconstr Surg. 2012;129(1):16e–23.
32. Jabor M, Shayani P, Collins D, Karas T, Cohen B. Nippleareola reconstruction: satisfaction and clinical determinants. Plastic Reconstr Surg. 2002;110(2):458–64.
33. Zenn M, Garofalo J. Unilateral nipple reconstruction with nipple sharing: time for a second look. Plastic Reconstr Surg. 2009;123 (6):1640–53.
34. Losken A, Pinell XA, Sikoro K, Yezhelyev MV, Anderson E, Carlson GW. Autologous fat grafting in secondary breast reconstruction. Ann Plast Surg. 2011;66(5):518–22.
35. Hsieh F, Kumiponjera D, Malata CM. An algorithmic approach to abdominal flap breast reconstruction in patients with pre-existing scars—results from a single surgeon's experience. J Plast Reconstr Aesthet Surg. 2009;62(12):1650–60.
36. Rogers NE, Allen RJ. Radiation effects on breast reconstruction with the deep inferior epigastric perforator flap. Plast Reconstr Surg. 2002;109(6):1919–24.
37. Kronowitz S, Robb G. Breast reconstruction with postmastectomy radiation therapy: current issues. Plastic Reconstr Surg. 2004;114 (4):950–60.

The Role of Radiotherapy in Breast Cancer Management

17

Mutlay Sayan and Ruth Heimann

Abbreviations

CHF	Congestive heart failure
CT	Computed tomography
DCIS	Ductal carcinoma in situ
DIBH	Deep inspiration breath-hold
EORTC	European Organization for Research and Treatment of Cancer
IMNs	Internal mammary nodes
IMRT	Intensity-modulated radiation therapy
LINAC	Linear accelerator
MLC	Multileaf collimator
MRI	Magnetic resonance imaging
NIH	National Institutes of Health
NSABP	National Surgical Adjuvant Breast and Bowel Project
PET	Positron-emission tomography
US	Ultrasound

17.1 Introduction to Radiation Oncology

At the end of the nineteenth century (1895), Wilhelm Roentgen announced the discovery of "a new kind of ray" that allows the "photography of the invisible." The biologic and therapeutic effects of the newly discovered X-rays were soon recognized, particularly because of the dermatitis and epilation they caused. In the early 1896, a few weeks after the public announcement of Roentgen's discovery, among the first therapeutic uses, Emil Grubbe in Chicago irradiated a patient with recurrent carcinoma of the breast and Herman Gocht in Hamburg Germany, irradiated a patient with locally advanced inoperable breast cancer and another patient with recurrent breast cancer in the axilla [1]. Despite the technical limitations of the early equipment, tumor shrinkage and at times complete elimination of the tumor were noticed. However, the full potential of radiation therapy could not be achieved in those early days because of the limited knowledge regarding fractionation, treatment techniques and uncertainties in how to calculate the tissue dose so as to deliver safe and effective doses of radiation.

M. Sayan · R. Heimann (✉)
Department of Radiation Oncology,
University of Vermont Medical Center,
111 Colchester Avenue, Burlington, VT 05401, USA
e-mail: Ruth.Heimann@uvmhealth.org

M. Sayan
e-mail: Mutlay.Sayan@med.uvm.edu

17.1.1 Physics of Radiation Therapy

The X-rays and gamma rays are part of the spectrum of electromagnetic radiation that also includes radio waves, infrared, visible, and ultra violet light. They are thought of as small packets of energy called photons. The X-rays reaching

I. Jatoi and A. Rody (eds.), *Management of Breast Diseases*, DOI 10.1007/978-3-319-46356-8_17

the tissue deposit their energy and because the energy is quite high, it causes ejection of orbital electrons from the atoms, resulting in ionization, hence the term ionizing radiation. Once the energy is deposited, many interactions occur, resulting in the generation of more free electrons and free radicals. Because the human body is made mostly of water, the energy absorption leads to a chain reaction, resulting in the formation of multiple, reactive free radical intermediates. Any of the cell constituents such as proteins, lipids, RNA, and DNA can be damaged. Apoptosis, signal transduction, and lipid peroxidation are all altered as a result of direct or indirect effects of radiation; however, DNA double-strand breaks seem to be the most critical damage that if unrepaired or incorrectly repaired will result in cell death.

The radiation dose is measured in terms of the amount of energy absorbed per unit mass. Presently, the measurement unit is gray (1 Gy is equal to 1 J/kg). The past measurement unit was the Rad, and 100 Rads = 1 Gy. The beam energy determines its medical usefulness. The clinically useful energy ranges of the electromagnetic radiation are superficial radiation 10–125 keV, orthovoltage 125–400 keV, and supervoltage, over 1000 keV (>1 meV). As the beam energy increases, it can penetrate deeper and more uniformly into tissue, and the skin sparing increases. The reason for skin sparing is that the electrons that are created from the interaction between photons and the tissue travel some time before they interact with tissue molecule and deposit the maximum dose. In the superficial and orthovoltage ranges, because of the lower energies, most of the dose is deposited at or very close to the skin (i.e., with significant skin dose), a significant dose is absorbed in bones, and useful beam energy cannot reach tissues at more than a couple of centimeters deep, resulting in marked dose inhomogeneity in the tissue. The great advantage of the supervoltage/megavoltage photons is that as the energy increases, the penetration of the X-ray increases, absorption into bone is not higher than the surrounding tissue and skin sparing increases. Therefore, maximum dose does not occur on the skin but at depth in the tissue, and more homogeneity can be achieved in the targeted volume.

The era of modern radiation therapy started approximately 50–60 years ago when supervoltage machines became widely available because of advances in technology resulting from atomic energy research, the development of the radar, and advances in computing. The availability of high-energy beam revolutionized the field of radiation oncology. Initially, the cobalt machine, a by-product of atomic research, and subsequently the linear accelerator (LINAC) generating beams with the energy ranging from 4 to 24 meV became available; currently, LINACs are mostly in use. A photograph of a LINAC is shown in Fig. 17.1. In the LINAC, electrons are accelerated to very high speeds. The high-speed electrons are guided to strike a tungsten target to produce the X-rays.

For certain clinical circumstances, the electron beam is preferred. Electrons differ in the way they deposit energy in the tissue. With electrons, the maximum dose is reached close to the skin surface with minimum skin sparing; however, there is a marked fall in radiation dose at certain depth in the tissue. This depth can be carefully chosen depending on the energy of the electron beam. Electron beams are mostly used for therapy of superficial tumors or to supplement (boost) photon therapy.

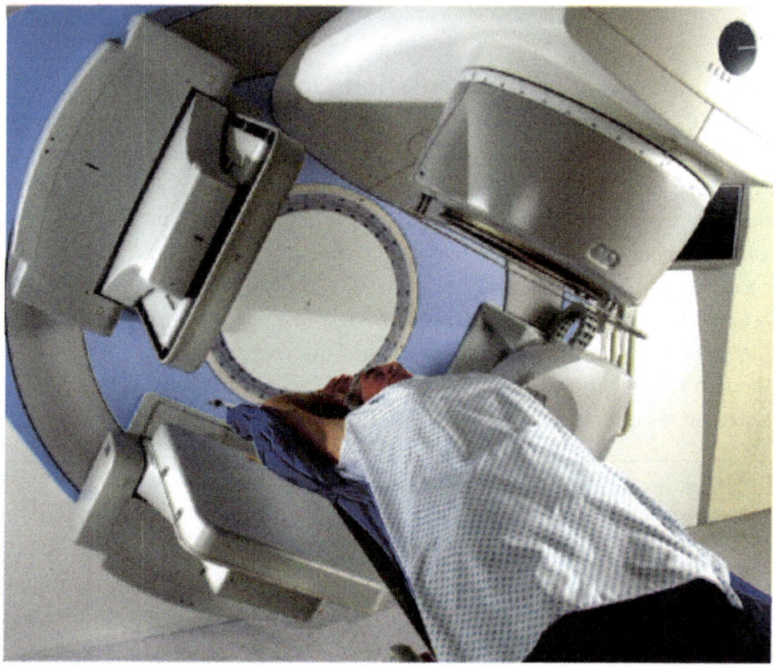

Fig. 17.1 A linear accelerator (LINAC) used for radiation therapy treatments (*photograph* courtesy of Elekta)

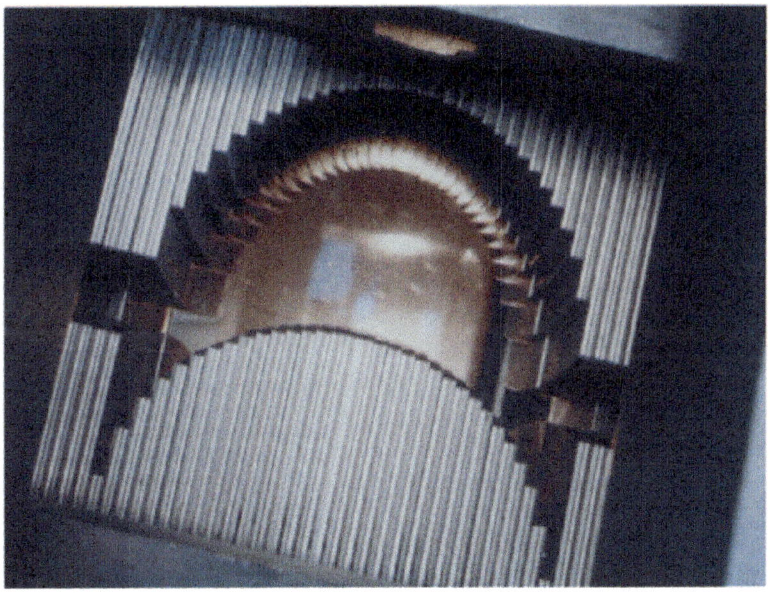

Fig. 17.2 The multileaf collimator (MLC) used to shape the treatment beam (*photograph* courtesy of Elekta)

Protons are heavy-charged particles generated in cyclotrons. Due to relatively large mass and charge protons have a limited range, little lateral scatter and small exit dose. Protons are well suited for pediatric brain tumors and tumors in close proximity to the spinal cord. There is no established use for protons in breast cancer.

To conform to the tumor shape and anatomy, the radiotherapy beam is tailored to each individual patient by using beam modifiers placed in the path of the beam. They may include such devices as collimators, tissue compensators, individually constructed blocks, or, more recently, the multileaf collimator (MLC). An image of a MLC is shown in Fig. 17.2. From the early days of manual computing when dose was calculated in a single point in the treated volume, recent computing advances led us to calculate dose in 3D in the tumor and surrounding tissue and account for differences in tissue density (i.e., lung, bone) as well as modify the dose inside the target area by "dose painting" or intensity-modulated radiation therapy (IMRT). We are now able to deliver more accurate radiation treatments and tailor treatments to individual patient anatomy with increased efficacy and less morbidity. When dose can be delivered more accurately to the tumor and more normal surrounding tissue can be spared, dose intensification can be attempted to achieve higher cure rates without increased complications. Uniform dose distribution and reduced dose in the surrounding tissue result in decreased acute and long-term side effects. Exclusion of as much normal tissue as possible from the path of the radiation beam is always of great importance, since many patients are also receiving chemotherapy that may result in higher probability of late complications.

17.1.2 Radiation, Surgery, and Chemotherapy

Radiation therapy is a local-regional curative modality that can be used either alone or in combination with surgery and chemotherapy. The rationale for combining surgery and radiation is because their patterns of failure are different. Radiation is less effective and failures occur more at the center of the tumor where there is the largest volume of tumor cells, some necrotic and in hypoxic conditions. Radiation is most effective at the margins where the tissue is well vascularized and the volume of tumor cells is the lowest. The extent of the surgery on the other hand is usually limited by the normal structures in the proximity of the tumor. The bulk of the tumor can be usually excised, but to remove all microscopic disease, at times, the surgery may need to be too extensive. Hence, the failures of surgery are usually at the margins of excision and that is where radiation is the most effective. To increase its therapeutic effectiveness, the radiation can also be combined with chemotherapeutic and biologic agents. Because these modalities have different mechanisms of cell kill and can interfere with different phases of the cell cycle, the combined effects may be additive, synergistic, or the systemic agents may act as sensitizer to the effects of radiation; however, it also increases the probability of side effects.

17.1.3 Technical Aspects of Radiation Planning and Delivery

Radiation therapy is an integral part of the management of all stages of breast cancer. Prior to embarking on radiation treatments, careful treatment planning is necessary. This includes decisions regarding patient positioning and immobilization. Both are essential for accuracy of therapy to ensure day to day reproducibility, and patient comfort. The treatment planning is done with the aid of a simulator, which is a machine with identical geometrical characteristics as the treatment machine; however, instead of high-energy treatment rays it generates diagnostic X-rays to image the target (i.e., the irradiated volume). More recently, computed tomography (CT), ultrasound (US), magnetic resonance imaging (MRI), and positron-emission tomography (PET) have been incorporated into the simulator, allowing even more accurate target identification in the actual treatment position. After the target and normal structures have been delineated in 3D, alternative treatment plans are generated and optimized. The plan that gives the best coverage of the target with minimal dose to the surrounding tissue and minimal inhomogeneities is chosen. The dose and homogeneity in the target are of great importance. Cold and hot spots have to be minimized because cold spots in the target will leave cancer undertreated, thus a source of disease recurrence, while hot spots may increase the risk of complications. The treatment planning is a team effort between the physician, physicist, dosimetrist, and technologist. It is an interactive process that usually goes through multiple iterations until the optimal plan is reached.

In the treatment of nonmetastatic breast cancer, the radiation is aimed at the breast/chest wall, and depending on the clinical situation, also at the regional lymphatics such as the supraclavicular, axillary, and internal mammary lymph nodes. The treatment goal is eradication of tumor with minimal side effects. The CT scanner can be used to delineate the targeted area and the critical structures to which dose should be limited. The beam arrangement that traverses the least amount of normal critical organs is chosen. In the treatment of the intact breast or chest wall, medial and lateral tangential beams are used (Fig. 17.3). Tangential beams allow the encompassing of the breast tissue while including limited amounts of lung or heart. Using 3D or IMRT treatment planning software, the dose distribution is calculated for the entire breast volume. Beam modifiers are incorporated to minimize the volume of tissue receiving higher or lower than the prescribed dose and minimize the dose to the

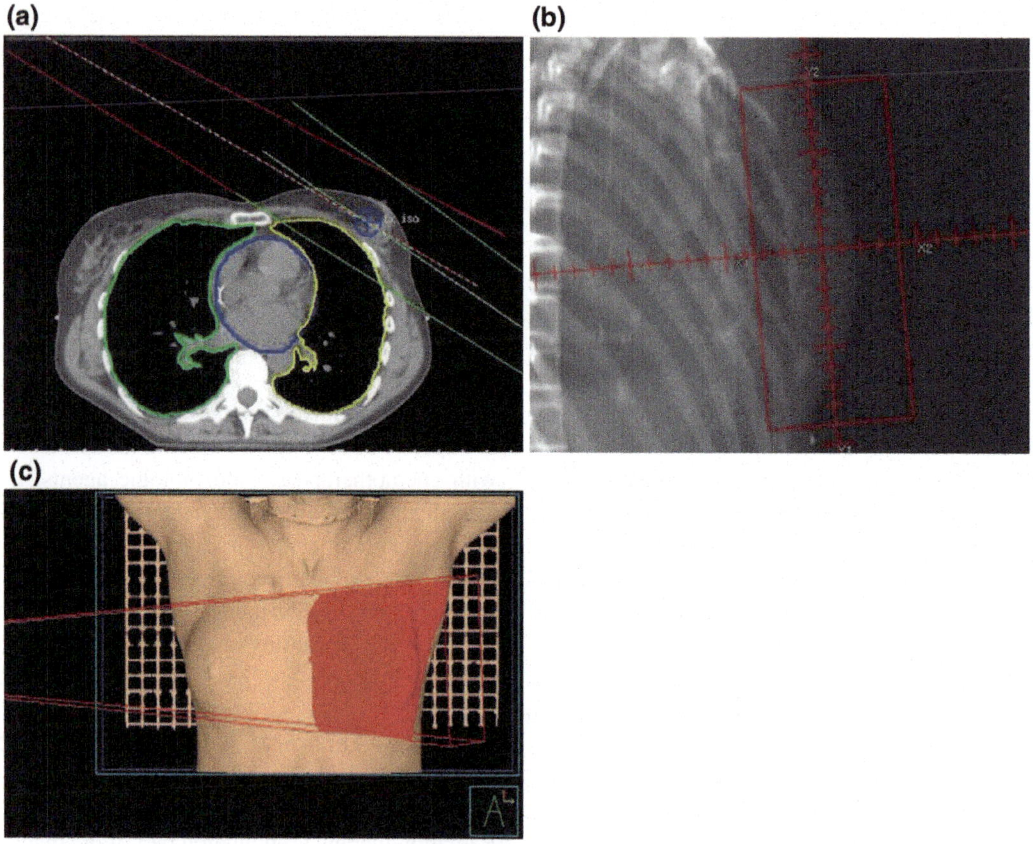

Fig. 17.3 Tangential beam arrangement for the treatment of the intact breast or chest wall. **a** An axial view showing the medial and lateral tangential beams covering the breast tissue. **b** The view from the beam direction, "beams eye view." Note the small amount of lung or heart in the treated volume. **c** The projection of the tangential beams on the patient's skin. These views were obtained from computer tomography (CT)-based simulation workstation

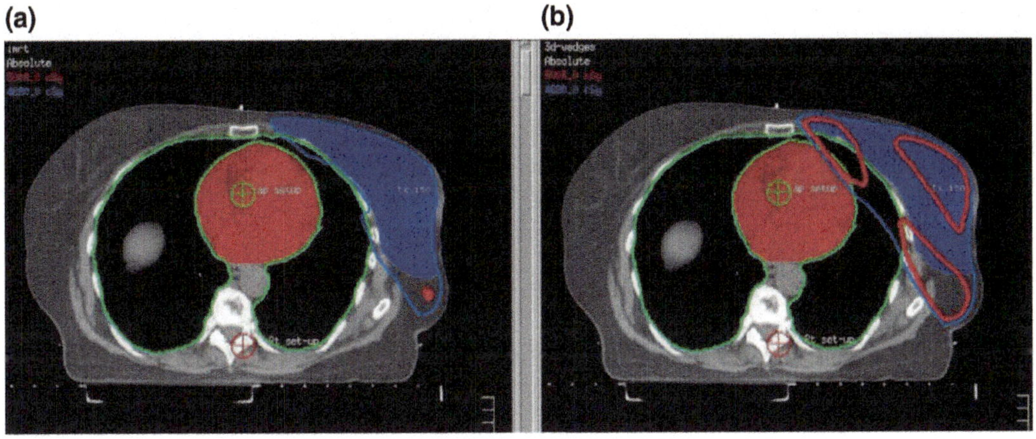

Fig. 17.4 Dose distribution in the breast using intensity-modulated radiation therapy (IMRT) planning (**a**) and 3D treatment planning (**b**). Note the elimination of "hot spots" in the IMRT plan

skin surface while ensuring that the glandular tissue several millimeters under the skin is not undertreated. IMRT allows the generation of a more homogenous plan, thus resulting in less acute side effects such as moist desquamation, pain, and breast lymphedema [2, 3]. Figure 17.4 demonstrates the more homogeneous dose achieved with IMRT, eliminating the "hot spots."

In many situations, IMRT also affords better conforming of the dose around the breast tissue, thus decreasing the dose to heart, lung, contralateral breast, and axilla, as well as less scatter dose [4]. More recently, development of the deep inspiration breath-hold (DIBH) technique has been shown to reduce incidental cardiac irradiation. Deep inspiration enables anatomical displacement of the heart medially, inferiorly, and posteriorly (i.e., away from the chest wall) resulting in decreased incidental cardiac irradiation. To treat the supraclavicular or axillary nodes and limit the dose to the spinal cord, a field shown in Fig. 17.5 is used. This field is usually an anterior/posterior field slightly angled to exclude the upper thoracic and lower cervical spinal cord. Various techniques are used to perfectly match all the fields so as to prevent an overlap or a gap between them. Depending on the clinical situation, radiation treatments are given daily for 5 1/2–6 1/2 weeks. In standard fractionation schedule, 1.8 or 2.0 Gy fractions are being used. Fractionation is necessary to keep the normal tissue complications to a minimum while achieving maximum tumor control. Several hypofractionated schedules using 15 fractions of 2.66–3.20 Gy in 3–5 weeks have been tested in randomized trials [5, 6]. In the selected patients, results show equivalence for local control and cosmesis to the schedule of 2.0 Gy in 5 weeks.

Proton therapy is currently being studied as an alternative potential strategy to achieve an optimized dose distribution [7]. At present time, protons are not being generally used in the treatment of breast cancer.

17.1.4 Adverse Effects of Radiation to the Breast

Treatments are usually well tolerated. Acute side effects may include fatigue, breast edema, skin erythema, hyperpigmentation, and at times desquamation mostly limited to the inframammary fold and axilla. Acute skin changes usually should resolve 1–2 weeks posttreatment. Higher treatment fraction sizes may result in more breast edema and fibrosis, thus jeopardizing the cosmetic outcome. The cosmesis posttreatment is usually good to excellent in a large majority of patients. However, there are no good objective quantitative criteria to evaluate the cosmetic outcome. Posttherapy, there is a gradual improvement in the appearance of the breast, hyperpigmentation resolves, skin color returns to normal, and breast edema resolves. The return to normal color and texture happens in a large majority of patients [8], but in some, it may take 2 or even up to 3 years.

With modern megavoltage therapy and treatment planning, the long-term side effects are limited. They depend on the radiation dose, fraction size, the energy of the beam, and the volume of radiated tissue. Most of the side effects can be limited with appropriate treatment planning.

Symptomatic pneumonitis is exceedingly rare, occurring in less than 1 % of patients, particularly in those treated only with tangential fields and not receiving chemotherapy. The risk is 3–5 % if chemotherapy is given and if the supraclavicular nodes need to be treated. It has been noted that if chemotherapy and radiation are given sequentially instead of concomitantly, the risk is lower. A study by Lingos et al. showed that the risk of radiation pneumonitis was 1 % if chemotherapy and radiation were given sequentially and could be as high as 9 % if the treatments were concurrent [9]. The risk also depends on the type, dose, and scheduling of the chemotherapeutic agents. The risk is further reduced by using 3D or IMRT treatment planning techniques. Those

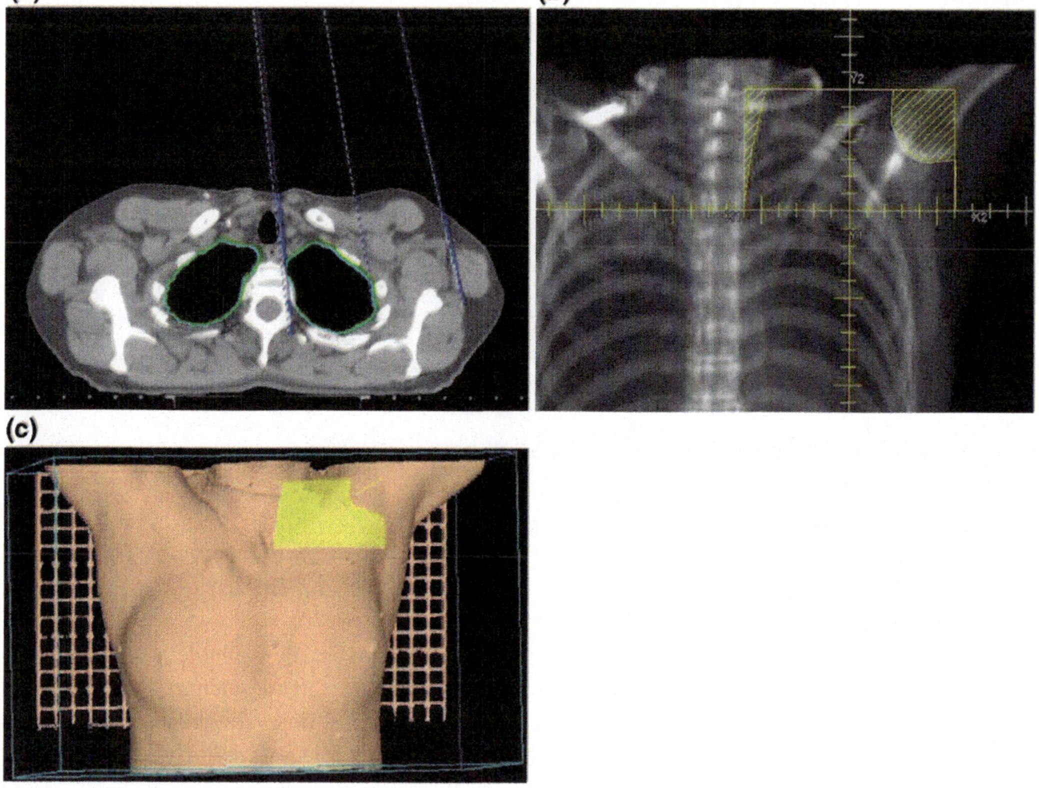

Fig. 17.5 The beam arrangement for the supraclavicular and axillary apex area. **a** An axial view. Note how the beam is directed to avoid the spinal cord. **b** The view from the beam angle also showing the blocking of the spinal cord and humeral head. **c** The beam as it projects on the patient skin

patients in whom symptomatic pneumonitis develops, it is usually mild and reversible either spontaneously or after a short course of steroids. Damage to the brachial plexus may develop in less than 1 % of the women treated with the currently used doses and fraction sizes. Larger fraction size may result in an increased risk of brachial plexopathy. There is a small risk of rib fractures, and soft tissue necrosis is exceedingly rare. In more than 2000 patients treated at the University of Chicago Center [8], no rib fractures or soft tissue necrosis were noted. Radiation may cause damage to the heart. The effects are dependent on the radiation technique used. The early trials of postmastectomy radiation have shown an increase in cardiac deaths in the long-term survivors [10]. However, in those days, an anteroposterior photon beam was used to treat the internal mammary nodes (IMNs), resulting in full-dose radiation to a large segment of the heart [11]. More recent reports show less risk of cardiac disease [12, 13]. The effects on the heart may include pericarditis [14], acceleration of coronary artery disease, cardiomyopathy, congestive heart failure (CHF), valvular heart disease, pericardial disease, and conduction block [15–19]. Although subclinical abnormalities may occur soon after irradiation such as microvascular injury and accelerated atherosclerosis, the resulting symptoms may not be apparent until decades later. With the currently used CT-based 3D and IMRT treatment planning techniques, excessive dose to a large part of the heart can be avoided. Moreover, utilizing the DIBH technique can further reduce incidental cardiac irradiation [20–22]. Many of the active and currently used chemotherapeutic agents (Adriamycin, Taxol) may also have deleterious effects on the heart. Except in rare occasions, the radiation and these chemotherapeutic agents are not given concurrently. No significantly increased risk of heart-related complication has been noted using sequential chemotherapy and radiation treatments. However, the long-term combined effects of cardiotoxic chemotherapeutic agents and radiation are not yet completely known because the newer drugs have not been used that long. Cardiac disease may become evident 10 to even 20 years posttherapy. Thus, longer follow-up will be needed before firm conclusions are reached. There has been substantial increase in the use of trastuzumab in the treatment of breast cancer. There are no data showing increased cardiac toxicity when combining radiation and trastuzumab, but longer follow-up will be necessary for more definitive data. In the interim, particular attention should be given to the treatment planning of left-sided breast cancer after cardiotoxic chemotherapy, even more so if the IMNs need to be treated.

Lymphedema may develop following axillary dissection and can be exacerbated with radiation. Although not life-threatening, it can significantly impact on quality of life. The risk of lymphedema depends on the extent of axillary node dissection and the extent of the radiation to the axilla. With a complete axillary dissection, including all three levels of axillary nodes and radiation therapy, the risk of lymphedema may be more than 40 %. However, if the surgery is only limited to level I and II dissections and the axilla is not radiated, some lymphedema may develop in up to 30 % of women, but the risk of significant lymphedema is only 3–5 %. The lymphedema is significantly less if surgery to the axial is limited to a sentinel node biopsy [23]. When compared to axillary lymph node dissection, axillary radiation following a positive sentinel lymph node biopsy results in reduced risk of lymphedema (11 % vs. 23 % at 5 years) [24]. The risk can be reduced by preventing trauma or infections to the arm on the dissected side. The condition can be chronic. It can be stabilized with physical therapy and manual lymphatic decompression but at times is difficult to eliminate. Early physical therapy and manual lymphatic decompression are very important and may reverse early stages of lymphedema.

There is a small risk of second malignancies in the long-term breast cancer survivors treated with radiation [25]. In general, for a woman with breast cancer, the risk of contralateral breast cancer is approximately 0.5–1 % per year, of which 3 % or less could be attributed to previous radiation [26, 27]. In the study by Boice et al., most of the risk was seen among women radiated before age 45. After age 45, there was little, if any, risk of radiation-induced secondary breast cancers. This has been further confirmed in a case control study in a cohort of more than 56,000 mostly perimenopausal and postmenopausal women. The dose to the contralateral breast was calculated to be 2.51 Gy, and the overall risk of contralateral breast cancer was not increased in patients receiving radiation therapy. The secondary tumors were evenly distributed in various quadrants of the breast, also arguing against radiation-related contralateral breast cancer [28]. In patients, treated at the University of Chicago, with mastectomy between 1927 and 1987, there was no increase in contralateral breast cancer in women who also received chest wall radiation [29].

Other treatment-related malignancies include lung cancer, sarcoma, and leukemia. The risk of treatment-related lung cancer is small. Studies from the Connecticut Tumor registry of patients treated between 1945 and 1981 show that in 10-year survivors, approximately nine cases of radiotherapy-induced lung cancer per year would be expected to occur among 10,000 treated women [30]. The risk is significantly increased with smoking [31]. The reported cumulative risk of sarcoma in the radiation field is 0.2 % at 10 years [32]. The risk of leukemia is minimal with radiation only; however, in combination with alkylating agents, the risk may be higher [33]. There are conflicting reports regarding the risk of esophageal cancer [34, 35]. Possibly, the increased risk in some studies is related to radiation techniques that used an anterior/posterior field to treat the IMN. In general, in most contemporary plans, the esophagus is excluded from the path of the beam. Many published studies tend to report the risk of second malignancies as the relative risks. It is important to realize when reading and evaluating the clinical literature that from the patients' and physicians' perspective, the concept of relative risk is not very informative because the relative risk of an event with radiation may be very high compared to no radiation, but if the absolute risk is very low, it has no management or practical clinical value. Thus, absolute numbers or percentages of the risk are much more relevant and informative.

17.2 Radiation Therapy in the Early-Stage Breast Cancer

17.2.1 Ductal Carcinoma in Situ

Ductal carcinoma in situ (DCIS), noninvasive ductal carcinoma, or intraductal carcinoma refers to proliferation of malignant cells confined within the basement membrane. DCIS, a premalignant condition, if untreated, is likely to progress to invasive breast cancer [36, 37]. Management of DCIS remains one the most controversial aspects of breast cancer treatment. It is a disease of the mammographic era with a significant increase in the incidence rate in the last decade. The nonpalpable DCIS, which comprises the majority of currently diagnosed disease, was almost unknown 25–30 years ago. In 2015, more than 60,000 women were diagnosed with DCIS [38]. The natural history is long, and although the incidence has been increasing in recent years, there are few studies of the alternative treatment options that have sufficient power and length of follow-up to have definite answers. The treatment options include simple mastectomy, or local excision, with or without radiation. Several factors are important in the management decision of a patient with DCIS. Any evidence that the disease is or could be extensive such as diffuse, suspicious, or indeterminate microcalcifications or multicentricity, as well as a mammogram, which is difficult to follow, or if there is uncertainty that the patient can comply with a program of routine mammograms for follow-up are contraindications for breast-conserving surgery. Status of the margin following local excision and the histologic subtype are important when making treatment decisions, and as always, patient wishes and comorbidities need be considered. If negative margins of excision cannot be obtained, breast conservation attempts have to be abandoned. Among histologic subtypes, high-grade nuclei and comedo necrosis appear to be more aggressive variants and seem to have a higher risk of recurrence or progression to invasive breast cancer. However, it is not clear if the risk of recurrence is higher with comedo DCIS, or just that the recurrences appear sooner and if the follow-up were long enough, the recurrence rate would be the same in patients with comedo or noncomedo histology.

Mastectomy was traditionally the standard of therapy for DCIS. The recurrence rates following mastectomy were 1 % or less and the cancer-related mortality 2 % [39]. However, after the documented success with breast-conserving therapy in infiltrating ductal carcinoma, it became increasingly difficult in the daily practice to recommend mastectomy to women with DCIS. Paradoxically, women who were adhering to a strict regimen of screening and were detected as having DCIS could be "rewarded" with mastectomy, while if they just would have waited a few years for the disease to progress to invasion, they could have breast-sparing surgery. There are no randomized trials that compare mastectomy to breast-conserving therapy; however, a decision analysis of trade-offs shows that there may only be a 1–2 % difference in the actuarial survival rates at 10 and 20 years if the initial therapy is breast-conserving surgery and radiation compared to mastectomy [40]. The small difference is most likely because at least half of the recurrences after breast conservation are DCIS and among the other half that are invasive, most are detected at an early stage. As in many other clinical dilemmas in breast cancer management, the National Surgical Adjuvant Breast and Bowel Project (NSABP) investigators significantly contributed to the changes in practice and redefined the standard of care in DCIS. NSABP-17 is a large, prospective randomized trial of 818 women that shows, with a median follow-up of 8 years, that radiation therapy following breast-conserving surgery reduces both the invasive and noninvasive ipsilateral breast cancer recurrences and the particular impact was on the reduction of invasive breast cancer recurrences. The incidence of noninvasive cancer was reduced from 13 to 9 %, and invasive breast cancer from 13 to 4 % [41]. All patients benefited from radiation irrespective of tumor size or pathologic characteristics. No features could be identified that would allow selection of patients in whom radiation could be eliminated [42, 43]. With a longer follow-up time, the combined data from NSABP-17 and NSABP-24 confirm the significant decrease in invasive breast cancer recurrence and improved survival [44]. A separate analysis of the effects of radiation on DCIS in the earlier NSABP-06 trial also showed a reduction in local failure with radiation [45]. A randomized trial performed by the European Organization for Research and Treatment of Cancer (EORTC) breast cancer cooperative group confirmed the NSABP-17 finding [46]. With radiation, the local recurrences at 10 years decreased from 26 to 15 %. In multivariate analysis, the addition of radiation, the architecture, grade of DCIS and margins status were independent predictors of recurrence. It is clear that negative margins are important for local control; however, controversy exists regarding the definition of adequate negative margins. Both the width of margins and the radiation dose influence local control. Boost radiotherapy has been shown to significantly decrease the risk of relapse in young women [47]. Excellent local control was also achieved when boost was given even when margins were defined as DCIS not touching the ink [48]. Although with longer follow-up and more information from the combined prospective and retrospective studies, the data may change, with the current information available in patients who are candidates for breast conservation, the local recurrence after excision alone is 20–30 %, and this can be reduced with radiation to approximately 10–15 %. To further improve the outcome, NSABP performed a study in which all patients who were candidates for breast conservation were treated with local excision followed by radiation and randomized to tamoxifen or placebo. This study, NSABP-24, enrolled more than 1800 women [49]. Tamoxifen therapy resulted in 32 % decrease in recurrences compared to radiation only without tamoxifen.

In several retrospective studies, attempts were also made to determine the patients in whom radiation can be eliminated. Silverstein et al. devised a scoring system combining the size of the DCIS, margins, grade, and necrosis [50]. This scoring was subsequently modified showing that margins alone are predictive of local recurrence [51]. Using the information regarding pathologic margins, the authors attempted to develop criteria when DCIS can be satisfactorily treated by local excision, when radiation therapy should be added, and when mastectomy is required. However, because the number of events in relation to the number of patients was low, the differences were not statistically significant and firm conclusions could not be reached [52]. They showed that in the low-risk patients when margins of excision are more than 1 cm, the 12-year local recurrence rate is 13.9 % compared to 2.5 % if postexcision radiation is given [53]. The widths of the margins can significantly compromise cosmesis. In breast conservation surgery, the surgical margins' width is in close inverse correlation with cosmesis. When performing the surgical excision, the surgeon is carefully balancing an oncologic surgery to achieve adequate margins and cosmesis because wide margins and removal of large amount of tissue may significantly impact on cosmesis. It is also important to recognize that because of the pathologic characteristics of DCIS, it is frequently difficult to determine the exact size of the DCIS and many pathologists are reluctant to do so. Thus, since many times the pathologic size is unavailable or cannot be accurately ascertained, some studies report DCIS size in millimeters, others in number of slides with DCIS, while others by using its mammographic size. This heterogeneity makes the comparison of local recurrence rates between studies difficult. A prospective study reported by Wong et al. attempted to select patients with DCIS in whom radiation following conservative surgery can be eliminated [54]. They included grade 1 and 2 DCIS, ≤2.5 cm, excised with more than 1-cm margins. The rate of local recurrence was 2.4 % per year, corresponding to a 5-year recurrence rate of 12 %. The study closed early because the number of recurrences met the predetermined stopping rules. This study demonstrated that it is very difficult to select patients in whom radiation can be omitted. RTOG 9804 demonstrated that even in good-risk DCIS where the local recurrence rate is low addition of RT further decreases the risk of recurrence [55]. Some small, incidental DCIS and small, low-grade DCIS excised with wide margins (>1 cm) can be followed after the local excision without radiation [56]. DCIS size, margins, histology, mammographic presentation, age, comorbidities, life expectancy, and patient preference are all factors in decision making regarding the optimal management of each individual patient.

17.2.2 Invasive Breast Cancer

17.2.2.1 Breast Conservation

In 1990, the National Institutes of Health (NIH) convened a Consensus Conference to address the issue of breast-conserving therapy in stage I and II breast cancer [57]. The participants concluded that breast-conserving therapy is equivalent and possibly better than mastectomy. The summary statement is presented in Fig. 17.6. The conclusions were based on six randomized trials that all showed equal survival in patients treated with breast-conserving therapy compared to those undergoing mastectomies. With additional follow-up and update, the results have been further

NIH Consensus Conference (1990)
Early-Stage Breast Cancer (38)

Breast conservation therapy is an appropriate method of primary therapy for the majority of women with stage I and II breast cancer and is <u>*preferable*</u> because it provides <u>*survival equivalent*</u> to the total mastectomy and axillary dissection while preserving the breast.

Fig. 17.6 The National Institutes of Health (NIH) consensus conference statement

confirmed and they are holding [58–63] (Table 17.1). Breast-conserving therapy with radiation may be even associated with better survival than mastectomy [64]. Breast-conserving therapy means local excision of the bulk of the tumor followed by moderate doses of radiation to eradicate residual foci of tumor cells in the remaining breast. Despite the NIH Consensus Conference conclusions, it seems that the acceptance of breast-conserving therapy is far from uniform and greatly varies by geographical areas [65, 66]. Overall, breast conservation rates vary from 60 to 70 %. There are significant barriers for utilization of breast-conserving therapy [67–70]. Medical contraindications and patient choice do not seem to be the major factors in the under utilization of breast-conserving surgery [71]. More than 80 % of the women, independent of age or race, if given the option, will opt for breast conservation.

The role of the radiation is to decrease the risk of local failure in the breast, but it also contributes to survival [34, 72–75]. It accomplishes what mastectomy would have done, i.e., treatment to the entire breast. Treatments are usually delivered to the whole breast and are followed with an additional radiation, "boost" to the lumpectomy site. Careful pathologic studies of mastectomy specimens have shown that microscopic residual disease is present away from the primary (index) tumor; however, the highest burden is in the same quadrant less than 4 cm from the primary tumor [76]. Extrapolation from early radiation therapy studies established the appropriate dose to eradicate microscopic foci of disease in the range of 45–50 Gy. This is the dose usually given to the entire breast. The higher burden of microscopic disease around the primary site is encompassed in the "boost" volume. Reported local control rates in the randomized trials and retrospective studies vary from 70 to 97 % [8, 61, 77]. Many factors have been suggested as having an impact on local control rates. Some have been confirmed in multiple studies while some were shown not to be of importance when longer follow-up and more data became available. Higher radiation doses to the lumpectomy site that are achieved by using a "boost" have been shown to improve the local control rates [78]. Most local recurrences following mastectomy occur in the first 3–5 years post-surgery; however, postbreast-conserving therapy recurrences have been documented to occur up to 20 years. Up to 5–8 years from diagnosis, most of the recurrences are in the same quadrant as the primary. Subsequently, the proportion changes in favor of tumor "elsewhere" in the breast [79]. These are most likely second primaries.

The determination whether a patient is candidate for breast-conserving surgery and radiation is a multidisciplinary effort in which close communication between the surgeon, the mammographer, the pathologist, the medical oncologist, and the radiation oncologist is necessary. Contraindications for breast-conserving surgery [80, 81] include:

Table 17.1 Overall survival (%) in six randomized trials of breast-conserving treatment compared to mastectomy

Stage I and II breast cancer		
Treatment (References)	Mastectomy (%)	BCT (%)
NSABP B-06 [61]	47	46
NCI [62]	58	54
Milan [58]	59	58
IGR (Paris) [63]	65	73
EORTC [59]	73	71
DBCCG [60]	82	79

Follow-up of 6–20 years
BCT breast conservation therapy; *DBCCG* Danish Breast Cancer Cooperative Group; *EORTC* European Organization for Research and Treatment of Cancer; *IGR* Institute Goustave Roussy; *NCI* National Cancer Institute; *NSABP* National Surgical Adjuvant Breast and Bowel Project

1. Multicentric disease, i.e., disease in separate quadrants of the breast.
2. Diffuse malignant appearing, or indeterminate microcalcifications.
3. Prior radiation treatments to doses that combined with the planned dose will exceed tissue tolerance. This may happen in women who have received radiation at younger age for lymphoma, particularly Hodgkin's disease.
4. Inability to obtain negative surgical margins following attempts for breast-conserving surgery. Negative excision margins appear to be the most important factor impacting on local control. If the margins are positive, the risk of local recurrence is increased [8, 82, 83]. Focally positive margins can be controlled with radiation, but more extensively involved margins are usually an indication for reexcision. However, data are also emerging, demonstrating that by increasing the boost dose, the local recurrences are similar to the local recurrences in women with negative margins of excision [8, 83].
5. Pregnancy is a contraindication for breast-conserving therapy because of the concerns on the effects of radiation on the fetus. Sometimes, surgery can be done during the third trimester and followed with radiation after delivery. This latter is to be done only after careful consideration because chances for cure ought not to be compromised for cosmetic reasons.

Relative contraindications for breast conservation include:

1. Tumor size: size of the tumor as compared to the breast size may pose some challenge from the cosmetic outcome perspective. Majority of the randomized trials of breast-conserving therapy included women whose tumors were ≤4 cm. But, the tumor size is mainly a consideration as it relates to the cosmetic outcome. Breast conservation should only be attempted if an acceptable cosmetic outcome can be achieved. If the tissue deficit because of the size of the tumor is large in relation to the breast size, then it is preferable to perform a mastectomy followed by breast reconstruction. The ratio between tumor size and patient's breast size determines the advisability of breast-conserving therapy.
2. Tumor location: tumor location in the vicinity of the nipple may require excision of the nippleareola complex. This may result in less than optimal cosmesis but does not impact on outcome. Many women will opt for breast preservation even if the nipple is removed because it still leaves behind most of the breast tissue and native skin.
3. Breast size: there are some technical difficulties in the radiation treatment of women with large breasts, but if adequate immobilization can be devised and adequate dose homogeneity can be achieved, breast conservation is preferable to a mastectomy that would result in major asymmetry.
4. History of collagen vascular disease: individuals with history of collagen vascular disease, particularly lupus or scleroderma, are reported to be at significantly increased risk of complications, particularly soft tissue and bone necrosis, most likely because of compromised microvasculature. Other criteria such as patient age, family history, and positive axillary lymph nodes are not contraindications for breast-conserving therapy.

Although breast cancer appears to be more aggressive in very young women, there is no clear evidence that if the currently used criteria for breast-conserving therapy are followed, breast conservation should be denied to young women. Very young women aged 35 or less may have more aggressive disease and they are at higher risk of both distant and local recurrences. Some have been advocating mastectomy for these women; however, to date, there has been no documented benefit in survival to mastectomy. At the other end of the age spectrum, although the perception may be that cancer is less aggressive and that older women are not as interested in breast preservation, the studies do not support this contention. Several reports have in fact shown that survival and disease-free survival from breast cancer are lower in older women [84–86]. There are also no indications that elderly women have significantly more problems tolerating radiation compared to younger women.

A challenging question is whether mutations in the two genes that predispose to breast cancer, BRCA1 and BRCA2, are a contraindication for radiation and thus breast-conserving treatment. Hypothesis yet to be proven is whether radiation to the remaining breast tissue, or scatter radiation to the contralateral breast increases the risk of a second breast cancer, or conversely, radiation is more effective in patients with known mutations because the normal function of the genes is DNA repair and the mutations could prevent the tumor cells escape from the effects of radiation. If unable to repair the damaged DNA, the effects of controlling the tumor with radiation may be enhanced. In a case control study of women treated with breast-conserving surgery and radiation, early results showed that following radiation, there is no increased risk of events in the ipsilateral breast in patients with known BRCA mutations compared to those with no mutations [87]. A subsequent update with additional follow-up shows that BRCA1/2 mutations are independent predictors of local recurrence. In women with BRCA1/2 mutations who also underwent oophorectomy, the local recurrence rate following breast-conserving surgery and radiation was 8 % compared to 10 % in women with sporadic breast cancer [88]. Interestingly, the 10-year risk of contralateral breast cancer in the BRCA1/2 carriers was 16 % despite the oophorectomy. In a different study, when patients with local recurrence following radiation were matched with a group without local recurrence, mutations were found to be more common in patients with recurrences and they occurred primarily in younger women, in different quadrants than the index tumor, and occurred late, most likely representing new primaries [89]. There is currently no evidence that women with mutations in BRCA1 or BRCA2 or with a family history of breast cancer have worst survival rates if offered breast-conserving therapy, including radiation [90, 91], particularly if they also undergo oophorectomy and receive adjuvant systemic therapy [88].

Several studies have attempted to define a subpopulation of patients who may not need radiation (Table 17.2). They vary in length of follow-up, inclusion criteria, and details of therapy. In studies from Sweden and from Canada, the investigators tried to determine whether in patients with small tumors, radiation could be omitted. Thus, they limited their studies to patients with ≤2-cm node-negative tumors [92, 93]. These trials showed a significant decrease in local failures when radiation was given but no significant difference in survival. Nevertheless, there was a trend toward overall survival benefit in the group receiving radiation [93, 95]. None of the trials were powered with sufficient number of patients to detect <10 % benefits in survival. In a prospective single institution study, attempts were made to select the most favorable patients with lowest risk of recurrence and enroll them in a study of only breast-conserving surgery without radiation [94]. The criteria for inclusion were tumor size ≤2 cm, negative axillary nodes, absence of lymphatic invasion, absence of extensive intraductal component, at least 1-cm margin of normal breast tissue around the tumor, and the breast easy to follow mammographically. The median tumor size was 6 mm. Even in this very favorable group, the failure rate was 24 % at 7 years. The trial was closed prematurely because the observed failure rate exceeded the expected rate predetermined by the trial stopping rules. This study highlights the difficulty in selecting the patients in whom radiation treatments can be eliminated.

Chemotherapy or tamoxifen may contribute to local control but by themselves are not sufficient. For example, in the NSABP-06 trial, the local failure in patients undergoing only local excision without radiation was approximately 32 %. In those who underwent local excision and also received chemotherapy, it was close to 40 %, demonstrating that chemotherapy did not decrease the local failure rates. However, in the comparable group who after local excision were receiving both chemotherapy and radiation, the cumulative risk at 12 years was only 5 % [95], while in those receiving radiation only, the local failure rates were 12 %. This demonstrates that radiation decreases the local recurrence rates and is further decreased when also combined with chemotherapy. Other studies have also confirmed better local control rates with the addition of chemotherapy to radiation [96, 97]. Even the very high doses of chemotherapy alone that were given as part of bone marrow transplant programs were not sufficient for local control [98].

To increase the feasibility of breast-conserving therapy, neoadjuvant chemotherapy has been attempted with satisfactory results. Some women who would not be candidates for breast conservation because of tumor size may become candidates for breast conservation if they first receive chemotherapy and the tumor shrinks, without impacting on their survival [99].

Table 17.2 Local recurrence (%) following local excision compared with local excision and radiation in stage I breast cancer

	Excision	Excision and radiation	Follow-up (years)
Liljergen et al. [92]	24	8	10
Clark et al. [93]	35	11	8
Lim et al. [94]	23	N/A	7

N/A not applicable

Many women who undergo breast-conserving therapy are also receiving adjuvant chemotherapy, and in these women, the sequencing of chemotherapy and radiation needs to be decided. One prospective randomized trial and several retrospective studies had somewhat conflicting results. Some studies show that giving chemotherapy first before radiation increases the risk of local failure, while others show that giving chemotherapy first does not significantly increase local failure rates and it may result in better distant disease-free survival and overall survival [100–102]. If local excision with negative margins is achieved and the patient is a candidate for breast conservation, it is unlikely that her survival will be impacted by delay in radiation because of initial chemotherapy, particularly with the shorter dose dense chemotherapy regimens. Thus, in general, women complete their chemotherapy before proceeding with the radiation treatments. In some instances, concomitant chemotherapy and radiation therapy have been given. However, this may increase the risk of side effects and jeopardize the cosmetic outcome without demonstrated benefit in outcome.

Depending on the clinical situation, radiation is delivered to the draining lymphatics that include axilla, supraclavicular nodes, and IMNs. Radiation to the draining lymphatics improves distal disease-free survival and decreases the locoregional recurrence rate [103, 104]. Axillary radiation is indicated if the axilla has not been dissected, if a limited dissection or SNB was done and it includes positive nodes, or if gross disease was found, particularly in the apex of the axilla close to the axillary vein. Communication between the surgeon and the radiation oncologist regarding the findings at surgery is of great importance. The undissected axillary apex nodes and supraclavicular nodal areas are treated if the axilla has been dissected and positive nodes were found. Attempts should be made in this situation to eliminate the dissected portion of the axilla from the path of the beam. With the advent of CT-based 3D treatment planning and IMRT, the treatment to the draining lymphatics can be individually tailored to the anatomy and the extent of the disease. Treatment to the IMN is given mostly if the primary lesion is medially or centrally located and the axillary lymph nodes are positive with metastatic breast cancer. CT-based 3D treatment planning and, in selected patients, IMRT planning are of advantage, particularly for left-sided lesions where further care needs to be undertaken to minimize the amount of treated heart. Treatment with DIBH can be used to further reduce the radiation due to the heart. Treatment with DIBH significantly increases the treatment complexity. Emphasis needs to be given to ensure the reproductively of the patient positions during the treatment. Treatment of the regional lymphatics in addition to the tangential fields also adds technical complexity to the treatments. If multiple beam angles are needed, overlap or underdose should be avoided. Use of IMRT in these situations may eliminate the need to match fields.

Good disease control in the axilla with minimum morbidity can be obtained from radiation to axilla without dissection [105] when the axilla is clinically negative. Thus, axillary dissection is indicated if the results would change the planned therapy. In patients who undergo sentinel node biopsy if the sentinel node has no disease, radiation to the axilla is omitted. If 1–2 nodes are positive, complete dissection or radiation to the axilla are likely to be of equivalent efficacy [24, 105–107].

Close follow-up after breast conservation is essential to detect local recurrences, new primaries, and contralateral disease. In general, true local recurrences occur earlier while disease in other quadrants develops later, i.e., 5 years or longer after therapy. Although institutional policies for mammographic follow-up vary, a reasonable policy would be routine yearly mammograms.

Postmastectomy Radiation

Postmastectomy, the risk of local recurrence varies depending on the number of positive nodes in the axilla, size of the tumor, length of follow-up, and how the local recurrences are being scored. As number of nodes with metastatic disease in the axilla increases, the risk of chest wall recurrences increases. In fact, the number of positive axillary lymph nodes has more impact on the rate of chest wall recurrence than the size of the tumor. The length of follow-up and how the recurrences are being scored are also important. Frequently, if a patient develops metastatic disease, there is a tendency to overlook a local recurrence. Most local-regional recurrences occur in the first 3–5 years following mastectomy, but disease may recur even 10–15 years postmastectomy [108, 109]. Thus, long-term follow-up is important in evaluating the risk of recurrences [110]. Local recurrences impact on survival and also have a significant impact on the quality of life. Chest wall recurrences may ulcerate and become malodorous and painful. Radiation can significantly decrease the risk of local recurrences postmastectomy. The benefit is proportional to the risk. Once clinically manifested, the likelihood of controlling a recurrence is only 50–60 %. There is some disagreement regarding who should be receiving postmastectomy irradiation. Most are in agreement when it comes to patients with four or more positive nodes in the axilla or a tumor more than 5 cm in size. But, the dilemma starts with a woman for example with 3.5–4 cm tumor and three positive nodes, particularly if she is young? Do we have sufficient information to counsel these younger women when the potential life expectancy is 20–30 years? Data on sufficient cohorts of women with the various combinations of tumor size, number of positive axillary lymph nodes, and long enough follow-up are difficult to come by, particularly for those who also receive chemotherapy. Recht et al. reviewed the local failure rates in patients treated with mastectomy and chemotherapy without radiation in the various Eastern Cooperative Group

Table 17.3 Percent cumulative incidence of LRF (10 years) following mastectomy and chemotherapy

Node positive	Size (cm)					
	≤1	1.1–2	2.1–3	3.1–4	4.1–5	≥5
1	3	11	12	10	6	27
2	8	14	12	20	14	31
3	20	18	11	8	14	36
4	19	17	22	26	37	33
5–6	22	23	27	25	22	47
7–9	12	33	30	32	32	41
≥10	39	30	31	36	35	31

LRF local regional failure

Source Reprinted with permission. ©1999 American Society of Clinical Oncology. All rights reserved. Recht et al. [111]

trials [111]. Their results are shown in Table 17.3. Arriagada et al. reported the cumulative rates of chest wall failure in patients not receiving chemotherapy to be up to 30–35 % in women with four or more positive nodes, and 25–30 % if one to three nodes are positive [112].

The impact of chest wall radiation on survival had been controversial because the natural history of breast cancer is long, the techniques of radiation are continuously improving, allowing better coverage of the target with less morbidity, and because currently in majority of the women, chemotherapy is also given. older meta-analyses and reports from pre-3D treatment era showed that radiation decreases breast cancer deaths, but in some studies, an increase in the risk of cardiovascular disease was noted [10, 113, 114]. Very few of the studies included in these meta-analyses used 3D radiation therapy planning or gave chemotherapy. The capability currently exists to design CT-guided plans tailored to individual's anatomy. When treatments are designed with CT-guided planning, the exact target location can be determined and the volume of lung and heart in the treatment field minimized, thus decreasing the risk of long-term side effects. Image-guided radiation techniques and respiratory gating have the potential to further decrease the long-term sequelae or radiation.

Two contemporary randomized studies from Denmark and Canada in which women were treated with chemotherapy show better disease-free and overall survival in patients who also received radiation therapy to the chest wall and draining nodes in addition to systemic therapy (Table 17.4) [110, 115–117]. The benefit from radiation therapy on survival was in fact equivalent to the benefit women achieved from chemotherapy [118]. These studies reignited the discussions regarding the benefits of postmastectomy radiation particularly, the benefits in women with one to three positive nodes. The question posed was could the finding be extrapolated to the practice in the USA, since in some women in the Danish Breast Cancer Cooperative Group trial, the median number of lymph nodes dissected was only seven. Some argued that usually in the USA, the axillary node dissections are more extensive. The investigators reanalyzed their data separately for women with one to three positive nodes and also in those with ten or more nodes dissected. They confirmed the significant benefit in survival in women with one to three positive nodes and also in those who had the more extensive axillary dissection [117]. A second criticism of the Danish and Canadian trials was that the chemotherapy used was cyclophosphamide, methotrexate, and 5-fluorouracil (CMF). This regimen is much less frequently used. Contemporary regimens are more dose intense and the question has been raised whether the benefits of radiation therapy are maintained with more intense regimens. There are no randomized trials to answer this question. However, an elegant analysis done by Ragaz et al. shows that at all chemotherapy dose intensity level, radiation therapy significantly decreases the risk of recurrence [110]. Radiation therapy to decrease the local recurrences was needed even following the very high doses of chemotherapy used in bone marrow transplant studies [98]. These results were further confirmed in the most recent update of the Early Breast Cancer Trialists Collaborative Group [34, 75] showing that for every four local recurrences prevented one breast cancer death can be avoided

Table 17.4 Impact of postmastectomy radiation therapy on overall survival in patients also receiving systemic therapy

Overall survival (%)				
	Follow-up (year)	CMF and radiation	CMF	*p* value
Overgaard et al. [115]	18	39	29	0.015
Ragaz et al. [110]	20	52 TAM and radiation	43 TAM	0.02
Overgaard et al. [116]	10	45	36	0.03

CMF cytoxan, methotrexate, 5 fluorouracil; *TAM* tamoxifen

[34, 74]. A trial in the USA was initiated to answer specifically the question of the benefit of postmastectomy radiation in women with one to three positive nodes. However, the trial had to be closed due to low accrual rates. Since in both the Canadian and Danish trials, and in the trials included in the meta-analysis from EBCTCG [75], women were also treated to their IMN, this question also has received renewed interest. Radiation therapy to the IMN may benefit all the women but particularly those with medial or central lesion in whom multiple axillary nodes are positive. Inclusion of the IMN, in left-side breast cancer, will undoubtedly increase the volume of heart treated, and depending on the technique used may possibly increase the dose to the esophagus. Thus, if the IMNs are to be included, treatments should be done with CT-based planning so that the IMN can be localized and the volume of lung, heart, and esophagus minimized. Two recently published randomized trials addressing nodal irradiation [103, 104] did not specifically address the question of IMN irradiation. The only contemporary randomized trial available demonstrates no benefit in OS to IMN irradiation [119].

The management of locoregional breast cancer recurrences depends on the prior therapy. Disease that recurs after breast-conserving surgery and radiation therapy is usually treated with mastectomy. There have been attempts in patients in whom a very early recurrence is found to only perform an excision with satisfactory results. However, the number of patients treated in this manner is low and the follow-up is too short to realize the full impact of this management strategy [120]. A full course of radiation for the second time is difficult to deliver because of the risk of long-term complications. The breast may become fibrotic and cosmetically unappealing. However, recently some data have been emerging regarding the feasibility of retreatment, particularly if there has been a long interval since prior therapy and if only partial breast treatment is done. If feasible, a recurrence that occurs postmastectomy should be excised with negative margins. Radiation, particularly if not previously given, will decrease the risk of further recurrences. The radiation fields need to encompass the chest wall and regional lymphatics, not only the area of recurrence, because it seems that if only a small radiation field is used, recurrences may appear just outside the irradiated area [121].

Radiation and Breast Reconstruction

Many women who undergo mastectomy also opt for breast reconstruction. The techniques of reconstructive surgery have been changing. There is a significant decrease in the use of silicone or saline implants in favor of autologous tissue with pedicle or microanastomosis. The reconstructed, vascularized tissue is of great advantage in minimizing the risk of complications from radiation. The reported risk of complications in patients undergoing reconstruction and radiation varies anywhere from 18 to 51 %. In the more recent publications, the risk of complications is at the lower end of range, probably because of improvement in the techniques of both surgery and radiation. The optimal sequencing of radiation and reconstructive surgery is not well established; thus, multiple factors need to be considered, and because a general consensus is lacking, good communication between all the members of the oncologic team is essential. The issue under consideration is the operation in a previously irradiated field if the reconstruction is being done following radiation. The concerns are less with the techniques that are using autologous vascularized tissues. On the other hand, if the reconstruction is done immediately after mastectomy and this is followed with the radiation, there are concerns regarding the cosmesis, firming, and fat necrosis after radiating the reconstruction, and the possible obscuring of a recurrence. However, there are data showing that the great majority of the recurrences are not obscured by the myocutaneous flap [122]. In general, good to excellent cosmesis is being achieved in the majority of the women who have radiation to the reconstructed breast. If there are no other contraindications, breast cancer occurring in an augmented breast can be treated with breast conservation. There may be some complications such as scaring or fat necrosis, but the risk seems to be low [123] and the cosmetic outcome very good; thus, the augmentation does not need to be removed prior to the radiation. In the minority of patients in whom complications will later develop, the reconstruction may have to be revised or removed. This treatment strategy would leave the majority of women with the breast augmentation spared.

17.3 Locally Advanced Breast Cancer

Locally advanced and inflammatory breast cancers, stage III disease, pose a major management challenge. Because of the very high risk of local and distant failure, no single modality is satisfactory in controlling the disease; thus, all three treatment modalities, i.e., chemotherapy, radiation therapy, and surgery, need to be incorporated in a management plan. Since this disease presentation is not very common and because its definition encompasses a spectrum of diseases from large primary tumors with some skin edema, or small, limited skin ulceration to huge necrotic masses or global inflammatory changes, large randomized trials to define the standard of care are lacking. If the patient is a candidate for mastectomy, surgery may be performed upfront followed by adjuvant systemic therapy and radiation. Radiation alone as the local treatment modality in patients with large tumors is suboptimal. Control of the disease can only be obtained, at most in 50 % of the patients and large doses are needed, which may result in long-term sequelae, including fibrosis and tissue necrosis [124]. However, postmastectomy radiation is very effective in reducing the local failure rates. The microscopic residual disease can be well controlled with 50–60 Gy and failure rates would decrease from 30–40 to 10–15 %. Because the risk of metastatic disease is very high, there is general consensus for the need for systemic therapy despite the fact that several small randomized trials failed to demonstrate benefit for chemotherapy, probably because the patient numbers were low and the disease is very heterogeneous. Retrospective studies show significant benefits compared to historical controls [125, 126].

Despite the general consensus that there is need for aggressive control of both local and distant disease, there are some controversies regarding the sequencing of the various therapies and the need for both radiation and surgery for local control. In most situations, even if the patients are technically operable, neoadjuvant chemotherapy is given first. Response rates to neoadjuvant chemotherapy are usually good, and complete clinical response can be achieved in up to 30 % of the patients. Patients with the best response have also the best chances for survival. If a good response to chemotherapy is obtained, then mastectomy is undertaken followed with additional chemotherapy and radiation. Comprehensive radiation fields are used to include the chest wall and draining lymphatics tailored to the anatomy and clinical situation. If there is no response to initial chemotherapy, a switch to radiation or different chemotherapy regimen is needed. Although not clearly established, retrospective reviews indicate that the local control is better if both surgery and radiation are given than with either modality alone [127].

Inflammatory breast cancer has a very high risk of metastatic disease and also very high risk of local failure if surgery alone is performed. Because of the involvement of dermal lymphatics, the disease is much more extensive than can be clinically appreciated; therefore, even if negative margins can be obtained, the disease soon recurs. Historically, because of its systemic nature, the 5-year survival rates were at most 10 %. However, with the combination of chemotherapy, surgery, and radiation, the 5-year survival rates are approaching 30–50 % [126, 128, 129]. The sequencing of treatments depends on response to therapy. Neoadjuvant chemotherapy is initiated as soon as possible and response assessed after each cycle. If good response is obtained, surgery is being performed followed with additional chemotherapy and radiation to the chest wall and draining lymphatics. If, however, response to chemotherapy is poor, radiation is added in order to bring the patient to a stage of operability. Because of the competing risks of both local and distant disease, concomitant chemotherapy and radiation protocols have been attempted with promising preliminary results [130–132]. The challenge is to concomitantly give sufficient chemotherapy to be therapeutically effective for metastatic disease as well as sufficient dose of radiation to control local disease, all this without severe complications. Currently, targeting inflammatory mediators and associated signaling pathways is studied to develop new treatment strategies. For instance, a Notch inhibitor RO4929097 has shown to down-regulate the expression of inflammatory cytokines IL-6 and IL-8 and reduce self-renewal properties of inflammatory breast cancer stem cells [133].

17.4 Radiation as Palliation

Radiation treatments are frequently an integral component of the palliative management plan for advanced and metastatic disease. Painful, weeping, malodorous chest wall recurrences can be controlled with radiation, thus significantly contributing to quality of life and the ability to resume normal lifestyle. The symptomatic effects of brain, bone, spinal cord, brachial plexus, choroidal, and liver metastases can be palliated with radiation and the effects can be durable for the lifetime of the patient. Single brain metastases or few metastases in the same proximity can be treated with stereotactic radiosurgery, significantly improving the outcome, particularly if the disease at the primary site is controlled, or there is no evidence of disease elsewhere. When the goal is palliation, decisions regarding dose, fractionation, and length of therapy are determined based on the life expectancy and quality of life considerations. It is important to always keep in mind that the goals are palliation; thus, the side effects should be kept to a minimum and the treatment course kept as short as possible.

The role of locoregional therapy in the patient with metastatic diseases is being studied in an ongoing randomized trial. Retrospective studies have shown better prognosis if optimal locoregional therapy is given [134, 135].

17.5 Summary

Radiation therapy is an integral part of the management of breast cancer in all stages of the disease from DCIS to metastatic disease. Treatments should be tailored to each patient's clinical situation and anatomy to obtain the best disease control with minimum side effects. The new and developing technologies such as 3D treatment planning, IMRT, and image-guided techniques provide us with the tools to accomplish this goal.

References

1. Moulin Dd. A short history of breast cancer. Boston: Martinus Nijhoff; 1983.
2. Harsolia A, Kestin L, Grills I, Wallace M, Jolly S, Jones C, et al. Intensity-modulated radiotherapy results in significant decrease in

clinical toxicities compared with conventional wedge-based breast radiotherapy. Int J Radiat Oncol Biol Phys. 2007;68(5):1375–80.
3. Pignol J, Olivotto I, Rakovitch E, Gardner S, Ackerman I, Sixel K, et al. Plenary 1. Int J Radiat Oncol Biol Phys 66(3):S1.
4. Woo TC, Pignol JP, Rakovitch E, Vu T, Hicks D, O'Brien P, et al. Body radiation exposure in breast cancer radiotherapy: impact of breast IMRT and virtual wedge compensation techniques. Int J Radiat Oncol Biol Phys. 2006;65(1):52–8.
5. Whelan TJ, Pignol JP, Levine MN, Julian JA, MacKenzie R, Parpia S, et al. Long-term results of hypofractionated radiation therapy for breast cancer. N Eng J Med. 2010;362(6):513–20.
6. Haviland JS, Owen JR, Dewar JA, Agrawal RK, Barrett J, Barrett-Lee PJ, et al. The UK Standardisation of Breast Radiotherapy (START) trials of radiotherapy hypofractionation for treatment of early breast cancer: 10-year follow-up results of two randomised controlled trials. Lancet Oncol. 2013;14(11):1086–94.
7. MacDonald SM, Patel SA, Hickey S, Specht M, Isakoff SJ, Gadd M, et al. Proton therapy for breast cancer after mastectomy: early outcomes of a prospective clinical trial. Int J Radiat Oncol Biol Phys. 2013;86(3):484–90.
8. Heimann R, Powers C, Halpem HJ, Michel AG, Ewing CA, Wyman B, et al. Breast preservation in stage I and II carcinoma of the breast. The University of Chicago experience. Cancer. 1996;78(8):1722–30.
9. Lingos TI, Recht A, Vicini F, Abner A, Silver B, Harris JR. Radiation pneumonitis in breast cancer patients treated with conservative surgery and radiation therapy. Int J Radiat Oncol Biol Phys. 1991;21(2):355–60.
10. Cuzick J, Stewart H, Rutqvist L, Houghton J, Edwards R, Redmond C, et al. Cause-specific mortality in long-term survivors of breast cancer who participated in trials of radiotherapy. J Clinic Oncol Off J Am Soc Clinic Oncol. 1994;12(3):447–53.
11. Rutqvist LE, Lax I, Fornander T, Johansson H. Cardiovascular mortality in a randomized trial of adjuvant radiation therapy versus surgery alone in primary breast cancer. Int J Radiat Oncol Biol Phys. 1992;22(5):887–96.
12. Vallis KA, Pintilie M, Chong N, Holowaty E, Douglas PS, Kirkbride P, et al. Assessment of coronary heart disease morbidity and mortality after radiation therapy for early breast cancer. J Clinic Oncol Off J Am Soc Clinic Oncol. 2002;20(4):1036–42.
13. Giordano SH, Kuo YF, Freeman JL, Buchholz TA, Hortobagyi GN, Goodwin JS. Risk of cardiac death after adjuvant radiotherapy for breast cancer. J Natl Cancer Inst. 2005;97(6):419–24.
14. Pierce SM, Recht A, Lingos TI, Abner A, Vicini F, Silver B, et al. Long-term radiation complications following conservative surgery (CS) and radiation therapy (RT) in patients with early stage breast cancer. Int J Radiat Oncol Biol Phys. 1992;23(5):915–23.
15. Stewart JR, Fajardo LF, Gillette SM, Constine LS. Radiation injury to the heart. Int J Radiat Oncol Biol Phys. 1995;31(5):1205–11.
16. Seddon B, Cook A, Gothard L, Salmon E, Latus K, Underwood SR, et al. Detection of defects in myocardial perfusion imaging in patients with early breast cancer treated with radiotherapy. Radiother Oncol J Eur Soc Ther Radiol Oncol. 2002;64(1):53–63.
17. Taylor CW, Nisbet A, McGale P, Darby SC. Cardiac exposures in breast cancer radiotherapy: 1950s–1990s. Int J Radiat Oncol Biol Phys. 2007;69(5):1484–95.
18. McGale P, Darby SC, Hall P, Adolfsson J, Bengtsson NO, Bennet AM, et al. Incidence of heart disease in 35,000 women treated with radiotherapy for breast cancer in Denmark and Sweden. Radiother Oncol J Eur Soc Ther Radiol Oncol. 2011;100(2):167–75.
19. Darby SC, Ewertz M, McGale P, Bennet AM, Blom-Goldman U, Bronnum D, et al. Risk of ischemic heart disease in women after radiotherapy for breast cancer. N Eng J Med. 2013;368(11):987–98.
20. Chen MH, Chuang ML, Bornstein BA, Gelman R, Harris JR, Manning WJ. Impact of respiratory maneuvers on cardiac volume within left-breast radiation portals. Circulation. 1997;96(10):3269–72.
21. Lu HM, Cash E, Chen MH, Chin L, Manning WJ, Harris J, et al. Reduction of cardiac volume in left-breast treatment fields by respiratory maneuvers: a CT study. Int J Radiat Oncol Biol Phys. 2000;47(4):895–904.
22. Sixel KE, Aznar MC, Ung YC. Deep inspiration breath hold to reduce irradiated heart volume in breast cancer patients. Int J Radiat Oncol Biol Phys. 2001;49(1):199–204.
23. Warren LE, Miller CL, Horick N, Skolny MN, Jammallo LS, Sadek BT, et al. The impact of radiation therapy on the risk of lymphedema after treatment for breast cancer: a prospective cohort study. Int J Radiat Oncol Biol Phys. 2014;88(3):565–71.
24. Donker M, van Tienhoven G, Straver ME, Meijnen P, van de Velde CJ, Mansel RE, et al. Radiotherapy or surgery of the axilla after a positive sentinel node in breast cancer (EORTC 10981-22023 AMAROS): a randomised, multicentre, open-label, phase 3 non-inferiority trial. Lancet Oncol. 2014;15(12):1303–10.
25. Neugut AI, Weinberg MD, Ahsan H, Rescigno J. Carcinogenic effects of radiotherapy for breast cancer. Oncology (Williston Park, NY). 1999;13(9):1245–56; discussion 57, 61–5.
26. Boice JD Jr, Harvey EB, Blettner M, Stovall M, Flannery JT. Cancer in the contralateral breast after radiotherapy for breast cancer. N Eng J Med. 1992;326(12):781–5.
27. Gao X, Fisher SG, Emami B. Risk of second primary cancer in the contralateral breast in women treated for early-stage breast cancer: a population-based study. Int J Radiat Oncol Biol Phys. 2003;56(4):1038–45.
28. Storm HH, Andersson M, Boice JD Jr, Blettner M, Stovall M, Mouridsen HT, et al. Adjuvant radiotherapy and risk of contralateral breast cancer. J Natl Cancer Inst. 1992;84(16):1245–50.
29. Abdalla I, Thisted RA, Heimann R. The impact of contralateral breast cancer on the outcome of breast cancer patients treated by mastectomy. Cancer J (Sudbury, Mass). 2000;6(4):266–72.
30. Inskip PD, Stovall M, Flannery JT. Lung cancer risk and radiation dose among women treated for breast cancer. J Natl Cancer Inst. 1994;86(13):983–8.
31. Neugut AI, Murray T, Santos J, Amols H, Hayes MK, Flannery JT, et al. Increased risk of lung cancer after breast cancer radiation therapy in cigarette smokers. Cancer. 1994;73(6):1615–20.
32. Taghian A, de Vathaire F, Terrier P, Le M, Auquier A, Mouriesse H, et al. Long-term risk of sarcoma following radiation treatment for breast cancer. Int J Radiat Oncol Biol Phys. 1991;21(2):361–7.
33. Curtis RE, Boice JD Jr, Stovall M, Bernstein L, Greenberg RS, Flannery JT, et al. Risk of leukemia after chemotherapy and radiation treatment for breast cancer. N Eng J Med. 1992;326(26):1745–51.
34. Clarke M, Collins R, Darby S, Davies C, Elphinstone P, Evans V, et al. Effects of radiotherapy and of differences in the extent of surgery for early breast cancer on local recurrence and 15-year survival: an overview of the randomised trials. Lancet. 2005;366(9503):2087–106.

35. Kirova YM, Gambotti L, De Rycke Y, Vilcoq JR, Asselain B, Fourquet A. Risk of second malignancies after adjuvant radiotherapy for breast cancer: a large-scale, single-institution review. Int J Radiat Oncol Biol Phys. 2007;68(2):359–63.
36. Page DL, Dupont WD, Rogers LW, Jensen RA, Schuyler PA. Continued local recurrence of carcinoma 15–25 years after a diagnosis of low grade ductal carcinoma in situ of the breast treated only by biopsy. Cancer. 1995;76(7):1197–200.
37. Betsill WL Jr, Rosen PP, Lieberman PH, Robbins GF. Intraductal carcinoma. Long-term follow-up after treatment by biopsy alone. JAMA. 1978;239(18):1863–7.
38. Siegel RL, Miller KD, Jemal A. Cancer statistics, 2015. CA Cancer J Clin. 2015;65(1):5–29.
39. Frykberg ER, Bland KI. Overview of the biology and management of ductal carcinoma in situ of the breast. Cancer. 1994;74(1 Suppl):350–61.
40. Hillner BE, Desch CE, Carlson RW, Smith TJ, Esserman L, Bear HD. Trade-offs between survival and breast preservation for three initial treatments of ductal carcinoma-in-situ of the breast. J Clinic Oncol Off J Am Soc Clinic Oncol. 1996;14(1):70–7.
41. Fisher B, Dignam J, Wolmark N, Mamounas E, Costantino J, Poller W, et al. Lumpectomy and radiation therapy for the treatment of intraductal breast cancer: findings from National Surgical Adjuvant Breast and Bowel Project B-17. J Clinic Oncol Off J Am Soc Clinic Oncol. 1998;16(2):441–52.
42. Fisher ER, Costantino J, Fisher B, Palekar AS, Redmond C, Mamounas E. Pathologic findings from the National Surgical Adjuvant Breast Project (NSABP) Protocol B-17. Intraductal carcinoma (ductal carcinoma in situ). The National Surgical Adjuvant Breast and Bowel Project Collaborating Investigators. Cancer. 1995;75(6):1310–9.
43. Fisher ER, Dignam J, Tan-Chiu E, Costantino J, Fisher B, Paik S, et al. Pathologic findings from the National Surgical Adjuvant Breast Project (NSABP) eight-year update of Protocol B-17: intraductal carcinoma. Cancer. 1999;86(3):429–38.
44. Wapnir IL, Dignam JJ, Fisher B, Mamounas EP, Anderson SJ, Julian TB, et al. Long-term outcomes of invasive ipsilateral breast tumor recurrences after lumpectomy in NSABP B-17 and B-24 randomized clinical trials for DCIS. J Natl Cancer Inst. 2011;103(6):478–88.
45. Fisher ER, Leeming R, Anderson S, Redmond C, Fisher B. Conservative management of intraductal carcinoma (DCIS) of the breast. Collaborating NSABP investigators. J Surg Oncol. 1991;47(3):139–47.
46. Bijker N, Meijnen P, Peterse JL, Bogaerts J, Van Hoorebeeck I, Julien JP, et al. Breast-conserving treatment with or without radiotherapy in ductal carcinoma-in-situ: ten-year results of European Organisation for Research and Treatment of Cancer randomized phase III trial 10853–a study by the EORTC Breast Cancer Cooperative Group and EORTC Radiotherapy Group. J Clinic Oncol Off J Am Soc Clinic Oncol. 2006;24(21):3381–7.
47. Omlin A, Amichetti M, Azria D, Cole BF, Fourneret P, Poortmans P, et al. Boost radiotherapy in young women with ductal carcinoma in situ: a multicentre, retrospective study of the Rare Cancer Network. Lancet Oncol. 2006;7(8):652–6.
48. Sahoo S, Recant WM, Jaskowiak N, Tong L, Heimann R. Defining negative margins in DCIS patients treated with breast conservation therapy: The University of Chicago experience. Breast J. 2005;11(4):242–7.
49. Fisher B, Dignam J, Wolmark N, Wickerham DL, Fisher ER, Mamounas E, et al. Tamoxifen in treatment of intraductal breast cancer: National Surgical Adjuvant Breast and Bowel Project B-24 randomised controlled trial. Lancet. 1999;353(9169):1993–2000.
50. Silverstein MJ, Lagios MD, Craig PH, Waisman JR, Lewinsky BS, Colburn WJ, et al. A prognostic index for ductal carcinoma in situ of the breast. Cancer. 1996;77(11):2267–74.
51. Silverstein MJ, Lagios MD, Groshen S, Waisman JR, Lewinsky BS, Martino S, et al. The influence of margin width on local control of ductal carcinoma in situ of the breast. N Eng J Med. 1999;340(19):1455–61.
52. Heimann R, Karrison T, Hellman S. Treatment of ductal carcinoma in situ. N Eng J Med. 1999;341(13):999–1000.
53. Macdonald HR, Silverstein MJ, Lee LA, Ye W, Sanghavi P, Holmes DR, et al. Margin width as the sole determinant of local recurrence after breast conservation in patients with ductal carcinoma in situ of the breast. Am J Surg. 2006;192(4):420–2.
54. Wong JS, Kaelin CM, Troyan SL, Gadd MA, Gelman R, Lester SC, et al. Prospective study of wide excision alone for ductal carcinoma in situ of the breast. J Clinic Oncol Off J Am Soc Clinic Oncol. 2006;24(7):1031–6.
55. McCormick B, Winter K, Hudis C, Kuerer HM, Rakovitch E, Smith BL, et al. RTOG 9804: a prospective randomized trial for good-risk ductal carcinoma in situ comparing radiotherapy with observation. J Clinic Oncol Off J Am Soc Clinic Oncol. 2015;33(7):709–15.
56. Hughes LL, Wang M, Page DL, Gray R, Solin LJ, Davidson NE, et al. Local excision alone without irradiation for ductal carcinoma in situ of the breast: a trial of the Eastern Cooperative Oncology Group. J Clinic Oncol Off J Am Soc Clinic Oncol. 2009;27(32):5319–24.
57. NIH Consensus Development Conference statement on the treatment of early-stage breast cancer. Oncology (Williston Park, NY). 1991;5(2):120–4.
58. Veronesi U, Cascinelli N, Mariani L, Greco M, Saccozzi R, Luini A, et al. Twenty-year follow-up of a randomized study comparing breast-conserving surgery with radical mastectomy for early breast cancer. N Eng J Med. 2002;347(16):1227–32.
59. van Dongen JA, Bartelink H, Fentiman IS, Lerut T, Mignolet F, Olthuis G, et al. Randomized clinical trial to assess the value of breast-conserving therapy in stage I and II breast cancer, EORTC 10801 trial. J Natl Cancer Inst Monogr. 1992;11:15–8.
60. Blichert-Toft M, Rose C, Andersen JA, Overgaard M, Axelsson CK, Andersen KW, et al. Danish randomized trial comparing breast conservation therapy with mastectomy: six years of life-table analysis. Danish Breast Cancer Cooperative Group. J Natl Cancer Inst Monogr. 1992(11):19–25.
61. Fisher B, Anderson S, Bryant J, Margolese RG, Deutsch M, Fisher ER, et al. Twenty-year follow-up of a randomized trial comparing total mastectomy, lumpectomy, and lumpectomy plus irradiation for the treatment of invasive breast cancer. N Eng J Med. 2002;347(16):1233–41.
62. Poggi MM, Danforth DN, Sciuto LC, Smith SL, Steinberg SM, Liewehr DJ, et al. Eighteen-year results in the treatment of early breast carcinoma with mastectomy versus breast conservation therapy: the National Cancer Institute Randomized Trial. Cancer. 2003;98(4):697–702.
63. Arriagada R, Le MG, Rochard F, Contesso G. Conservative treatment versus mastectomy in early breast cancer: patterns of failure with 15 years of follow-up data. Institut Gustave-Roussy Breast Cancer Group. J Clinic Oncol Off J Am Soc Clinic Oncol 1996;14(5):1558–64.
64. Hwang ES, Lichtensztajn DY, Gomez SL, Fowble B, Clarke CA. Survival after lumpectomy and mastectomy for early stage invasive breast cancer. Cancer. 2013;119(7):1402–11.
65. Farrow DC, Hunt WC, Samet JM. Geographic variation in the treatment of localized breast cancer. N Eng J Med. 1992;326(17):1097–101.

66. Nattinger AB, Goodwin JS. Geographic and Hospital Variation in the Management of Older Women With Breast Cancer. Cancer Control J Moffitt Cancer Center. 1994;1(4):334–8.
67. Lazovich DA, White E, Thomas DB, Moe RE. Underutilization of breast-conserving surgery and radiation therapy among women with stage I or II breast cancer. JAMA. 1991;266(24):3433–8.
68. Lazovich D, Solomon CC, Thomas DB, Moe RE, White E. Breast conservation therapy in the United States following the 1990 National Institutes of Health Consensus Development Conference on the treatment of patients with early stage invasive breast carcinoma. Cancer. 1999;86(4):628–37.
69. Hiotis K, Ye W, Sposto R, Goldberg J, Mukhi V, Skinner K. The importance of location in determining breast conservation rates. Am J Surg. 2005;190(1):18–22.
70. Hiotis K, Ye W, Sposto R, Skinner KA. Predictors of breast conservation therapy: size is not all that matters. Cancer. 2005;103(5):892–9.
71. Morrow M, Bucci C, Rademaker A. Medical contraindications are not a major factor in the underutilization of breast conserving therapy. J Am Coll Surg. 1998;186(3):269–74.
72. Joslyn SA. Radiation therapy and patient age in the survival from early-stage breast cancer. Int J Radiat Oncol Biol Phys. 1999;44 (4):821–6.
73. Whelan TJ, Julian J, Wright J, Jadad AR, Levine ML. Does locoregional radiation therapy improve survival in breast cancer? A meta-analysis. J Clinic Oncol Off J Am Soc Clinic Oncol. 2000;18(6):1220–9.
74. Punglia RS, Morrow M, Winer EP, Harris JR. Local therapy and survival in breast cancer. N Eng J Med. 2007;356(23):2399–405.
75. McGale P, Taylor C, Correa C, Cutter D, Duane F, Ewertz M, et al. Effect of radiotherapy after mastectomy and axillary surgery on 10-year recurrence and 20-year breast cancer mortality: meta-analysis of individual patient data for 8135 women in 22 randomised trials. Lancet. 2014;383(9935):2127–35.
76. Holland R, Veling SH, Mravunac M, Hendriks JH. Histologic multifocality of Tis, T1-2 breast carcinomas. Implications for clinical trials of breast-conserving surgery. Cancer. 1985;56 (5):979–90.
77. Kurtz JM, Amalric R, Brandone H, Ayme Y, Jacquemier J, Pietra JC, et al. Local recurrence after breast-conserving surgery and radiotherapy. Frequency, time course, and prognosis. Cancer. 1989;63(10):1912–7.
78. Recht A, Silen W, Schnitt SJ, Connolly JL, Gelman RS, Rose MA, et al. Time-course of local recurrence following conservative surgery and radiotherapy for early stage breast cancer. Int J Radiat Oncol Biol Phys. 1988;15(2):255–61.
79. Winchester DP, Cox JD. Standards for breast-conservation treatment. CA Cancer J Clin. 1992;42(3):134–62.
80. Winchester DP, Cox JD. Standards for diagnosis and management of invasive breast carcinoma. American College of Radiology. American College of Surgeons. College of American Pathologists. Society of Surgical Oncology. CA Cancer J Clin. 1998;48(2):83–107.
81. Park CC, Mitsumori M, Nixon A, Recht A, Connolly J, Gelman R, et al. Outcome at 8 years after breast-conserving surgery and radiation therapy for invasive breast cancer: influence of margin status and systemic therapy on local recurrence. J Clinic Oncol Off J Am Soc Clinic Oncol. 2000;18(8):1668–75.
82. Jones H, Antonini N, Colette L, Fourquet A, Hoogenraad WJ, Van den Bogaert W, et al. The impact of boost dose and margins on the local recurrence rate in breast conserving therapy: results from the EORTC boost-no boost trial. Int J Radiat Oncol Biol Phys. (2007);69(3):S2–S3.
83. Jones HA, Antonini N, Hart AA, Peterse JL, Horiot JC, Collin F, et al. Impact of pathological characteristics on local relapse after breast-conserving therapy: a subgroup analysis of the EORTC boost versus no boost trial. J Clinic Oncol Off J Am Soc Clinic Oncol. 2009;27(30):4939–47.
84. Mueller CB, Ames F, Anderson GD. Breast cancer in 3,558 women: age as a significant determinant in the rate of dying and causes of death. Surgery. 1978;83(2):123–32.
85. Yancik R, Ries LG, Yates JW. Breast cancer in aging women. A population-based study of contrasts in stage, surgery, and survival. Cancer. 1989;63(5):976–81.
86. Singh R, Hellman S, Heimann R. The natural history of breast carcinoma in the elderly: implications for screening and treatment. Cancer. 2004;100(9):1807–13.
87. Pierce LJ, Strawderman M, Narod SA, Oliviotto I, Eisen A, Dawson L, et al. Effect of radiotherapy after breast-conserving treatment in women with breast cancer and germline BRCA1/2 mutations. J Clinic Oncol Off J Am Soc Clinic Oncol. 2000;18 (19):3360–9.
88. Pierce LJ, Levin AM, Rebbeck TR, Ben-David MA, Friedman E, Solin LJ, et al. Ten-year multi-institutional results of breast-conserving surgery and radiotherapy in BRCA1/2-associated stage I/II breast cancer. J Clinic Oncol Off J Am Soc Clinic Oncol. 2006;24(16):2437–43.
89. Turner BC, Harrold E, Matloff E, Smith T, Gumbs AA, Beinfield M, et al. BRCA1/BRCA2 germline mutations in locally recurrent breast cancer patients after lumpectomy and radiation therapy: implications for breast-conserving management in patients with BRCA1/BRCA2 mutations. J Clinic Oncol Off J Am Soc Clinic Oncol. 1999;17(10):3017–24.
90. Hellman S. The key and the lamppost. J Clinic Oncol Off J Am Soc Clinic Oncol. 1999;17(10):3007–8.
91. Pierce LJ, Phillips KA, Griffith KA, Buys S, Gaffney DK, Moran MS, et al. Local therapy in BRCA1 and BRCA2 mutation carriers with operable breast cancer: comparison of breast conservation and mastectomy. Breast Cancer Res Treat. 2010;121(2):389–98.
92. Liljegren G, Holmberg L, Bergh J, Lindgren A, Tabar L, Nordgren H, et al. 10-Year results after sector resection with or without postoperative radiotherapy for stage I breast cancer: a randomized trial. J Clinic Oncol Off J Am Soc Clinic Oncol. 1999;17(8):2326–33.
93. Clark RM, Whelan T, Levine M, Roberts R, Willan A, McCulloch P, et al. Randomized clinical trial of breast irradiation following lumpectomy and axillary dissection for node-negative breast cancer: an update. Ontario Clinical Oncology Group. J Natl Cancer Inst. 1996;88(22):1659–64.
94. Lim M, Bellon JR, Gelman R, Silver B, Recht A, Schnitt SJ, et al. A prospective study of conservative surgery without radiation therapy in select patients with Stage I breast cancer. Int J Radiat Oncol Biol Phys. 2006;65(4):1149–54.
95. Fisher B, Anderson S, Redmond CK, Wolmark N, Wickerham DL, Cronin WM. Reanalysis and results after 12 years of follow-up in a randomized clinical trial comparing total mastectomy with lumpectomy with or without irradiation in the treatment of breast cancer. N Eng J Med. 1995;333(22):1456–61.
96. Fisher B, Dignam J, Bryant J, DeCillis A, Wickerham DL, Wolmark N, et al. Five versus more than five years of tamoxifen therapy for breast cancer patients with negative lymph nodes and estrogen receptor-positive tumors. J Natl Cancer Inst. 1996;88 (21):1529–42.
97. Fisher B, Dignam J, Mamounas EP, Costantino JP, Wickerham DL, Redmond C, et al. Sequential methotrexate and fluorouracil for the treatment of node-negative breast cancer patients with estrogen receptor-negative tumors: eight-year results from National Surgical Adjuvant Breast and Bowel Project (NSABP) B-13 and first report of findings from NSABP

B-19 comparing methotrexate and fluorouracil with conventional cyclophosphamide, methotrexate, and fluorouracil. J Clinic Oncol Off J Am Soc Clinic Oncol. 1996;14(7):1982–92.

98. Carter DL, Marks LB, Bean JM, Broadwater G, Hussein A, Vredenburgh JJ, et al. Impact of consolidation radiotherapy in patients with advanced breast cancer treated with high-dose chemotherapy and autologous bone marrow rescue. J Clinic Oncol Off J Am Soc Clinic Oncol. 1999;17(3):887–93.
99. Fisher B, Bryant J, Wolmark N, Mamounas E, Brown A, Fisher ER, et al. Effect of preoperative chemotherapy on the outcome of women with operable breast cancer. J Clinic Oncol Off J Am Soc Clinic Oncol. 1998;16(8):2672–85.
100. McCormick B, Begg CB, Norton L, Yao TJ, Kinne D. Timing of radiotherapy in the treatment of early-stage breast cancer. J Clinic Oncol Off J Am Soc Clinic Oncol. 1993;11(1):191–3.
101. Heimann R, Powers C, Fleming G, Halpern HJ, Rubin SJ, Ewing C, et al. Does the sequencing of radiotherapy and chemotherapy affect the outcome in earlystage breast cancer: a continuing question. Int J Radiat Oncol Biol Phys 30:243.
102. Recht A, Come SE, Henderson IC, Gelman RS, Silver B, Hayes DF, et al. The sequencing of chemotherapy and radiation therapy after conservative surgery for early-stage breast cancer. N Eng J Med. 1996;334(21):1356–61.
103. Whelan TJ, Olivotto IA, Parulekar WR, Ackerman I, Chua BH, Nabid A, et al. Regional nodal irradiation in early-stage breast cancer. N Eng J Med. 2015;373(4):307–16.
104. Poortmans PM, Collette S, Kirkove C, Van Limbergen E, Budach V, Struikmans H, et al. Internal mammary and medial supraclavicular irradiation in breast cancer. N Eng J Med. 2015;373(4):317–27.
105. Fisher B, Redmond C, Fisher ER, Bauer M, Wolmark N, Wickerham DL, et al. Ten-year results of a randomized clinical trial comparing radical mastectomy and total mastectomy with or without radiation. N Eng J Med. 1985;312(11):674–81.
106. Giuliano AE, Hunt KK, Ballman KV, Beitsch PD, Whitworth PW, Blumencranz PW, et al. Axillary dissection vs no axillary dissection in women with invasive breast cancer and sentinel node metastasis: a randomized clinical trial. JAMA. 2011;305(6):569–75.
107. Jagsi R, Chadha M, Moni J, Ballman K, Laurie F, Buchholz TA, et al. Radiation field design in the ACOSOG Z0011 (Alliance) Trial. J Clinic Oncol Off J Am Soc Clinic Oncol. 2014;32(32):3600–6.
108. Heimann R, Hellman S. Clinical progression of breast cancer malignant behavior: what to expect and when to expect it. J Clinic Oncol Off J Am Soc Clinic Oncol. 2000;18(3):591–9.
109. Sugg SL, Ferguson DJ, Posner MC, Heimann R. Should internal mammary nodes be sampled in the sentinel lymph node era? Ann Surg Oncol. 2000;7(3):188–92.
110. Ragaz J, Olivotto IA, Spinelli JJ, Phillips N, Jackson SM, Wilson KS, et al. Locoregional radiation therapy in patients with high-risk breast cancer receiving adjuvant chemotherapy: 20-year results of the British Columbia randomized trial. J Natl Cancer Inst. 2005;97(2):116–26.
111. Recht A, Gray R, Davidson NE, Fowble BL, Solin LJ, Cummings FJ, et al. Locoregional failure 10 years after mastectomy and adjuvant chemotherapy with or without tamoxifen without irradiation: experience of the Eastern Cooperative Oncology Group. J Clinic Oncol Off J Am Soc Clinic Oncol. 1999;17(6):1689–700.
112. Arriagada R, Rutqvist LE, Mattsson A, Kramar A, Rotstein S. Adequate locoregional treatment for early breast cancer may prevent secondary dissemination. J Clinic Oncol Off J Am Soc Clinic Oncol. 1995;13(12):2869–78.
113. Effects of Radiotherapy and Surgery in Early Breast. Cancer—an overview of the randomized trials. N Engl J Med. 1995;333(22):1444–56.
114. Correa CR, Litt HI, Hwang WT, Ferrari VA, Solin LJ, Harris EE. Coronary artery findings after left-sided compared with right-sided radiation treatment for early-stage breast cancer. J Clinic Oncol Off J Am Soc Clinic Oncol. 2007;25(21):3031–7.
115. Nielsen HM, Overgaard M, Grau C, Jensen AR, Overgaard J. Study of failure pattern among high-risk breast cancer patients with or without postmastectomy radiotherapy in addition to adjuvant systemic therapy: long-term results from the Danish Breast Cancer Cooperative Group DBCG 82 b and c randomized studies. J Clinic Oncol Off J Am Soc Clinic Oncol. 2006;24(15):2268–75.
116. Overgaard M, Jensen MB, Overgaard J, Hansen PS, Rose C, Andersson M, et al. Postoperative radiotherapy in high-risk postmenopausal breast-cancer patients given adjuvant tamoxifen: Danish Breast Cancer Cooperative Group DBCG 82c randomised trial. Lancet. 1999;353(9165):1641–8.
117. Overgaard M, Nielsen HM, Overgaard J. Is the benefit of postmastectomy irradiation limited to patients with four or more positive nodes, as recommended in international consensus reports? A subgroup analysis of the DBCG 82 b&c randomized trials. Radiother Oncol J Eur Soc Ther Radiol Oncol. 2007;82(3):247–53.
118. Hellman S. Stopping metastases at their source. N Eng J Med. 1997;337(14):996–7.
119. Hennequin C, Bossard N, Servagi-Vernat S, Maingon P, Dubois JB, Datchary J, et al. Ten-year survival results of a randomized trial of irradiation of internal mammary nodes after mastectomy. Int J Radiat Oncol Biol Phys. 2013;86(5):860–6.
120. Salvadori B, Marubini E, Miceli R, Conti AR, Cusumano F, Andreola S, et al. Reoperation for locally recurrent breast cancer in patients previously treated with conservative surgery. Br J Surg. 1999;86(1):84–7.
121. Halverson KJ, Perez CA, Kuske RR, Garcia DM, Simpson JR, Fineberg B. Isolated local-regional recurrence of breast cancer following mastectomy: radiotherapeutic management. Int J Radiat Oncol Biol Phys. 1990;19(4):851–8.
122. Slavin SA, Love SM, Goldwyn RM. Recurrent breast cancer following immediate reconstruction with myocutaneous flaps. Plast Reconstr Surg. 1994;93(6):1191–204; discussion 205-7.
123. Ryu J, Yahalom J, Shank B, Chaglassian TA, McCormick B. Radiation therapy after breast augmentation or reconstruction in early or recurrent breast cancer. Cancer. 1990;66(5):844–7.
124. Spanos WJ Jr, Montague ED, Fletcher GH. Late complications of radiation only for advanced breast cancer. Int J Radiat Oncol Biol Phys. 1980;6(11):1473–6.
125. Touboul E, Lefranc JP, Blondon J, Ozsahin M, Mauban S, Schwartz LH, et al. Multidisciplinary treatment approach to locally advanced non-inflammatory breast cancer using chemotherapy and radiotherapy with or without surgery. Radiother Oncol J Eur Soc Ther Radiol Oncol. 1992;25(3):167–75.
126. Hortobagyi GN. Multidisciplinary management of advanced primary and metastatic breast cancer. Cancer. 1994;74(1 Suppl):416–23.
127. Perez CA, Graham ML, Taylor ME, Levy JF, Mortimer JE, Philpott GW, et al. Management of locally advanced carcinoma of the breast. I. Noninflammatory. Cancer. 1994;74(1 Suppl):453–65.
128. Gonzalez-Angulo AM, Hennessy BT, Broglio K, Meric-Bernstam F, Cristofanilli M, Giordano SH, et al. Trends for inflammatory breast cancer: is survival improving? Oncologist. 2007;12(8):904–12.
129. Hance KW, Anderson WF, Devesa SS, Young HA, Levine PH. Trends in inflammatory breast carcinoma incidence and survival:

the surveillance, epidemiology, and end results program at the National Cancer Institute. J Natl Cancer Inst. 2005;97(13):966–75.
130. Masters GM, Heimann R, Skoog L. Concomitant chemoradiotherapy with vinorelbine and paclitaxel with filgrastim(G-CSF) support in patients with unresectable breast cancer. Breast Cancer Res Treat. 1997;46(75).
131. Formenti SC, Symmans WF, Volm M, Skinner K, Cohen D, Spicer D, et al. Concurrent paclitaxel and radiation therapy for breast cancer. Seminars Radiat Oncol. 1999;9(2 Suppl 1):34–42.
132. Kao J, Conzen SD, Jaskowiak NT, Song DH, Recant W, Singh R, et al. Concomitant radiation therapy and paclitaxel for unresectable locally advanced breast cancer: results from two consecutive phase I/II trials. Int J Radiat Oncol Biol Phys. 2005;61(4):1045–53.
133. Debeb BG, Cohen EN, Boley K, Freiter EM, Li L, Robertson FM, et al. Pre-clinical studies of Notch signaling inhibitor RO4929097 in inflammatory breast cancer cells. Breast Cancer Res Treat. 2012;134(2):495–510.
134. Fields RC, Jeffe DB, Trinkaus K, Zhang Q, Arthur C, Aft R, et al. Surgical resection of the primary tumor is associated with increased long-term survival in patients with stage IV breast cancer after controlling for site of metastasis. Ann Surg Oncol. 2007;14(12):3345–51.
135. Harris E, Barry M, Kell MR. Meta-analysis to determine if surgical resection of the primary tumour in the setting of stage IV breast cancer impacts on survival. Ann Surg Oncol. 2013;20(9):2828–34.

Adjuvant Systemic Treatment for Breast Cancer: An Overview

18

Rachel Nirsimloo and David A. Cameron

It has long been recognized that breast cancer is not always cured by loco regional treatment alone. To reduce the risk of local and distant recurrence, patients are usually offered adjuvant systemic treatment. The aim of adjuvant systemic therapy is thought to principally be elimination of clinically undetectable micrometastatic disease. The decision to offer this treatment is based on the estimated five- and ten-year risks of recurrence-free survival and overall survival. This risk is estimated using pathological factors such as tumour size, grade of tumour, receptor status, nodal involvement and biological factors such as patient age and co-morbidities along with a multidisciplinary recommendation. The estimated benefits must be balanced against the acute and chronic toxicities of the proposed treatment and an informed decision made with the patient. Increasingly, multi-parametric tests such as Oncotype Dx or MammaPrint are also used to help in this decision process. Systemic treatment includes the use of endocrine therapy, chemotherapy, antibody treatment, and more latterly immunotherapy.

18.1 Aims of Adjuvant Therapy

18.1.1 Micro-Metastatic Disease

The main aim of adjuvant systemic therapy is thought to be the eradication of micro-metastatic disease which otherwise is the cause of relapse in the future. Studies have shown that cancer cells can lie dormant for many years despite radical treatment and cause recurrent disease which is often metastatic by the time it is diagnosed. The difficulty is "proving" who has residual disease when there is no way clinically of detecting it. Understandably, this can be a difficult concept for patients to understand. Currently there is no gold standard algorithm or molecular test to determine the need or not of adjuvant treatment, but the chance of relapse is estimated using the aforementioned prognostic features, individualized to each of the patients. Inevitably by this selection process, some patients will receive chemotherapy inappropriately, gaining no survival benefit, but potentially suffering acute and chronic side effects from the treatment. Even if we could prove that an individual patient did have micro-metastatic disease, could we then prove the treatment will work? Some patients will have chemorefractory or resistant disease and again go through months of unnecessary treatment. Resistance can be acquired or intrinsic to the cancer and this is explained by the molecular complexity of tumours and intramural heterogeneity. Genetic mutations, the microenvironment and the presence of cancer stem cells all enable tumours to develop resistance [1].

18.1.2 Cancer Stem Cells

Cancer stem cells were first demonstrated in haematological malignancies but now are recognized in solid tumours such as breast cancer [2]. Cancer stem cells are able to self-heal, reproduce endlessly and randomly mutate leading to tumour heterogeneity, which is what makes treatment complex [2]. There is some evidence that traditional chemotherapy targets the tumour bulk but not the cancer stem cells, which can produce new clones resistant to treatment. Ongoing studies to evaluate efficacy of targeted molecular therapies to cancer stem cells is a challenging but promising development in the treatment of cancer.

R. Nirsimloo (✉)
Edinburgh Cancer Centre, NHS LOTHIAN, Crewe Road South, Edinburgh, EH4 2XU, UK
e-mail: Rachel.nirsimloo@nhslothian.scot.nhs.uk

D.A. Cameron (✉)
Edinburgh Cancer Research Centre, Western General Hospital, University of Edinburgh, Crewe Road South, Edinburgh, EH4 2XU, UK
e-mail: d.cameron@ed.ac.uk

I. Jatoi and A. Rody (eds.), *Management of Breast Diseases*, DOI 10.1007/978-3-319-46356-8_18

18.1.3 Immunogenicity

Immunogenic cancers such as melanoma have been proven to innately initiate an anticancer T-cell response that can result in tumour death. Due to genetic alterations, cancer cells have many different antigens present in their cell surface [3]. These lead to binding of peptides with major histocompatibility complex class 1 (MHC1) which distinguish cancer cells from normal cells. These complexes can be recognized by CD8 + T cells which are produced in cancer patients [4]. This could lead to immunity or cell death but infrequently does. Many ways of trying to exploit this natural response including vaccines, immune checkpoint therapy and monoclonal antibodies have all gained FDA approval. Based on the success seen in melanoma, trials have been quickly established to evaluate efficacy in other solid tumour types. Breast cancer was long thought to be non–immunogenic; however, many studies have now established that the presence of CD8 + T cells—particularly in the HER2+ and triple negative groups—does translate into a reduction of relative risk of death from the disease [5–8]. Whilst not the current focus of adjuvant systemic treatment in breast cancer, the use of immunotherapy for all solid tumour types is likely to expand into the adjuvant setting over the next few decades.

18.2 Adjuvant Chemotherapy: The Evidence

Over the years many, trials have been done to try and establish the optimal drug or drug combinations, doses and duration of adjuvant chemotherapy. The Early Breast Cancer Trialists' Collaborative Group (EBCTCG) was set up in the mid-1980s with the aim of performing a systematic review of all existing randomized control trials every five years in order to provide the most comprehensive evidence base [9].

18.2.1 Single Agent or Combination Chemotherapy

Adjuvant cytotoxic chemotherapy in breast cancer began with trials of single alkylating agents which then led to trials of combination therapy with anthracyclines and taxanes. Prior to this radical surgery was the gold standard; however, subsequent trials showed that distal recurrence remained a huge issue despite initial radical surgery [10, 11]. The National Surgical Adjuvant Breast Project (NSABP) was the organization behind the first trial to report in 1968 that the alkylating agent thiotepa reduced risk of recurrence after radical surgery in pre-menopausal node positive patients [12]. Similarly, the alkylating agent L-Phenylalanine mustard that had been developed during the Second World War was found to have similar efficacy in reducing disease recurrence when given adjuvantly [13].

Combination chemotherapy in breast cancer was first explored in the 1960s [14]. Cyclophosphamide, methotrexate and 5-fluorouracil (CMF) was the first combination to be trialled for adjuvant breast cancer patients at Istituto Nazionale Tumori in Milan, Italy, with increasingly positive results [15]. Initially the trials targeted node positive pre-menopausal women but as they expanded similar positive results were found in postmenopausal and/or node negative patients [16, 17]. Subsequently, six cycles were found to be as effective as 12 cycles of adjuvant CMF [18].

18.2.2 Anthracyclines

Anthracyclines were initially introduced to try and reduce the duration and emetogenis of the classical CMF regimen. The first widely used regime was doxorubicin and cyclophosphamide (AC). Although there was no apparent advantage in efficacy over CMF [19], thus started the era of trials to find the most efficacious adjuvant regime. In 2001, the National Institute of Health recommended adjuvant chemotherapy as standard practice in locally advanced breast cancer patients [20].

The first meta-analyses of combination chemotherapy (focusing mainly on anthracycline regimes) were done by the EBCTCG in 2005 [21]. They included 194 randomized trials with a total of almost 150,000 patients. From their analyses, there was clear evidence that single agent chemotherapy regimens reduced rates of recurrence; however, combination treatments reduced not only recurrence, but also mortality [10]. Not separating the data for age, the annual rates of recurrence were reported as 0.86 for single agents and 0.77 for combination. Mortality reductions rates were 0.96 for single agents and 0.83 for combination [21].

With both single agent and combination chemotherapy, there were greater benefits established in the younger population (<50 years old) but both for recurrence and mortality the age standardized effects of single versus combination regimens were superior for combination treatments [21]. Of note (as is common in trial populations), there were few patients included aged >70 years.

Figure 18.1 shows the 15-year recurrence and mortality rates split into age groups of <50 and 50–69, all of which show a statistically significant ($2p < 0.00001$) benefit with adjuvant combination regimens [21].

For women aged <50, the absolute 15-year reduction in recurrence-free survival (RFS) was 12.3 % with a 10 % reduction in mortality. In women aged 50–69, the 15-year benefits for RFS and mortality were more modest at 4.1 and 3 %, respectively. This benefit remained significant regardless of axillary lymph node involvement, so this may not be

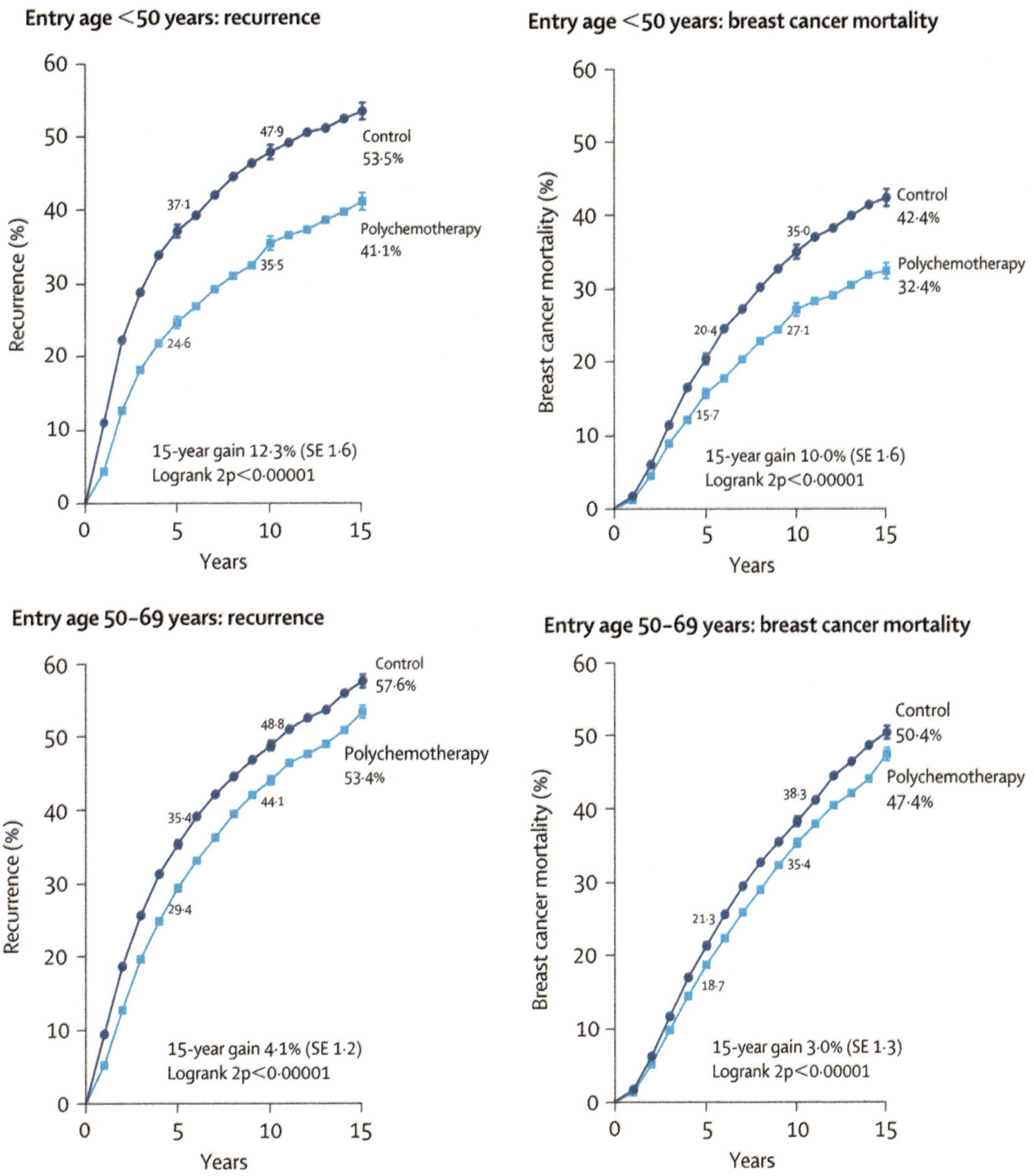

Fig. 18.1 Polychemotherapy versus not, by entry age <50 or 50–69: 15-year probabilities of recurrence and of breast cancer mortality. Younger women, 35 % node positive; older women 70 % node positive. Error bars are 1SE. Reprinted from The Lancet, Vol. 365, Early Breast Cancer Trialists' Collaborative Group (EBCTCG), Effects of chemotherapy and hormonal therapy for early breast cancer on recurrence and 15-year survival: An overview of the randomised trials, pp. 1687–1717, © 2005, with permission from Elsevier

of relevance to the proportional reduction in either age group. For the women aged <50, the 5-year gains in RFS were 9.9 % ($2p < 0.00001$) for node negative patients and 14.6 % ($2p < 0.00001$) for node positive. For the age group 50–69 and node negative, the 5-year RFS improvement was 5.3 % ($2p < 0.00001$) and 5.9 % ($2p < 0.00001$) for node positive patients [21].

Separating the data for age and ER status showed the greatest benefit in RFS was in ER poor patients when treated with adjuvant chemotherapy. For women <50 with ER poor tumours (20 % node positive), RFS improvement at 5 years was 13.2 % ($2p < 0.00001$) and for the same age group but ER positive (34 % node positive) it was 7.6 % ($2p < 0.00001$). For the age group 50–69 who were ER poor (66 % node positive), RFS gain at 5 years was 9.6 % ($2p < 0.00001$) and for the same age group ER positive (73 % node positive) RFS improvement was 4.9 % ($2p < 0.00001$) [21]. In the ER positive group, the arms were combination chemotherapy plus tamoxifen versus tamoxifen alone for both age groups.

For the CMF regimen trials, duration of treatment varied from 6, 9 or 12 months with no statistical difference being observed for longer treatment. The anthracycline-based trials on average had a treatment duration of 6 months but they did change between doxorubicin and epirubicin as the anthracycline used (FAC or FEC) [21].

For ER positive women with breast cancer aged <50, anthracycline regimens studied in this meta-analyses reduced the annual mortality rate by 38 % and for women aged 50–69 by 20 %. This does not include, but added to, the additional benefit of adjuvant endocrine therapy which will be evaluated later in this chapter. These results were significantly more effective than CMF regimens ($2p = 0.0001$ for both recurrence and $2p < 0.00001$ mortality) [21].

In 2008, the EBCTCG published a further view of combination chemotherapy in ER poor patients who appeared to be the subset gaining the biggest survival advantage from adjuvant combination chemotherapy [22]. Ninety-six trials were included in this meta-analysis. In women <50 years old, the 10-year reduction in RFS with the addition of chemotherapy was 12 % ($p < 0.00001$) and reduction in mortality was 8 % ($p = 0.0002$). In women aged 50–69, the 10-year reduction in RFS with the addition of adjuvant chemotherapy was 10 % ($p < 0.00001$) and reduction in mortality was 6 % ($p = 0.0009$) [22].

In 2011, EBCTCG published further analyses of overall survival for adjuvant CMF versus no adjuvant chemotherapy. Adjuvant CMF reduced the risk of recurrence by 30 % at 10 years ($p < 0.0001$) which translates to an absolute gain of 10.2 %. The 10-year mortality was reduced by 16 % ($p < 0.0004$) which translates to an absolute gain of 4.7 % at 10 years [23].

An alternative regimen was to incorporate an anthracycline into the classical CMF treatment which was known as a block-sequential design. Bonadona et al. were the first to use this in a trial of women with breast cancer with more than three positive lymph nodes. They either received sequential doxorubicin then CMF or alternating cycles of doxorubicin and CMF. OS at ten years was 58 % in the sequential arm versus 44 % in the alternating arm ($p = 0.002$) favouring sequential sequencing [24]. The NEAT trial allocated four cycles of epirubicin followed by four cycles of CMF (E-CMF) and in 2008 reported a 28 % benefit for RFS and 30 % advantage in OS compared to standard CMF alone [25]. Overall toxicity in the E-CMF arm was low but unsurprisingly higher than the CMF alone arm. Interestingly, more deaths during treatment occurred on the CMF arm and any deaths on the ECMF arm all occurred during CMF administration [25].

18.2.3 Taxanes

In the 1970s, taxanes became the first new cytotoxic drugs to be developed for decades. Having been shown to be of value in the metastatic setting, the next step was to establish if they would add to the efficacy of adjuvant chemotherapy [26].

Concurrent administration of doxorubicin and paclitaxel enhanced the effect of the anthracycline rendering the regimen too cardiotoxic [27]. Theories suggested that sequential administration may be preferable and result in more anti-tumour activity [28, 29]. Docetaxel, however, does not effect the pharmacokinetics of doxorubicin.

In the CALGB 9344 trial which escalated doses of doxorubicin in combination with cyclophosphamide followed by 4 cycles of paclitaxel in node positive patients, RFS (HR 0.83 $p = 0.0023$) and OS were improved (HR 0.82 $p = 0.006$) [30].

In the NSABP B-28 trial, an additional 4 cycles of paclitaxel after to 4 cycles of doxorubicin and cyclophosphamide (AC) in node positive patients improved RFS but not OS [31]. These two trials differed in trial design as the CALGB 9344 trial gave endocrine therapy after completion of chemotherapy, whereas NSABP B-28 gave it concurrently [32].

As part of the same review in 2011, the EBCTCG meta-analysis reviewed the addition of taxanes to combination chemotherapy to address the question of how much benefit could be gained. Treatments varied by the taxane used (paclitaxel or docetaxel), dose and schedule (3 weekly or weekly). All but two trials compared a taxane plus anthracycline regimen to an anthracycline control arm. The results were grouped into those which added four extra cycles of a taxane to a standard regimen or those which gave the same duration of chemotherapy in all arms [23].

In the trials which gave additional cycles of a taxane after a standard regimen, RFS over 8 years was reduced by 4.6 % ($2p < 0.00001$) and OS by 3.2 % ($2p = 0.0002$), whereas in those trials that tested the benefit of additional taxanes but without prolonging the duration of therapy, the improvement in RFS at 5 years was by 2.9 % ($2p < 0.00001$) and for OS it was 1.2 % ($2p = 0.008$) [23].

AC has also been directly compared to docetaxel and cyclophosphamide (TC) by the US oncology research group. This is one of the few trials that included an arm with no anthracycline. With an average follow-up of 84 months, RFS (HR 0.74 $p = 0.033$) and OS (HR 0.69 $p = 0.0032$) were improved in the TC arm. These data suggest we should consider taxane only therapies as a suitable alternative, especially amongst those patients who may have pre-existing cardiac issues [33, 34].

As mentioned earlier, docetaxel does not have the same pharmacokinetics as paclitaxel when given concurrently with doxorubicin. Trials have compared docetaxel, doxorubicin and cyclophosphamide (TAC) to FAC. The Breast Cancer International Research Group (BCIRG) trial 0001 and GEICAM 9805 saw a definite benefit in RFS (28 % in BCIRG 001) and a trend towards improved OS (BCIRG 0001 did demonstrate a statically significant improvement in

OS but GEICAM did not) [35, 36]. TAC was, however, undoubtedly more toxic in both trials.

So far the question has not been answered as to whether it is the addition of the taxane that improves outcomes or the prolonged duration of adjuvant chemotherapy. PACS01 compared 6 3-weekly cycles of FEC to 3 3-weekly cycles of FEC followed by 3 3-weekly cycles of docetaxel in 1999 node positive patients [37]. RFS (HR 0.85 $p = 0.036$) and OS (HR 0.75 $p = 0.007$) were improved in the taxane arm with median follow-up of 93 months [38].

The UK TACT study also included high-risk node negative patients and had over 4000 patients in the study to ensure it was sufficiently powered. Each arm was extended to include 8 cycles of treatment. The randomization was between a research arm of 4 3-weekly cycles of FEC followed by 4 3-weekly cycles of docetaxel versus control arm of physicians' choice of 8 3-weekly cycles of FEC or 8 3-weekly cycles of E-CMF. No statistical difference was found between either arm after 62 months of follow-up [39].

Chemotherapy can be given in fixed doses at fixed intervals or as smaller doses on a more frequent basis (dose dense regimen). The ECOG E1199 trial was designed to answer whether sequential dose dense taxane administration was superior to a 3-weekly regime [40]. There was no superiority seen between docetaxel and paclitaxel given 3 weekly or weekly, respectively. RFS (HR 0.73 $p = 0.0006$) and OS (HR 0.68 $P = 0.01$) were superior, however, when paclitaxel was given weekly over 12 weeks as opposed to 3 weekly for 4 cycles. [40] The final analysis after 12.1 years of follow-up showed that RFS and OS were improved for weekly paclitaxel (HR 0.84 $p = 0.011$ and HR 0.87 $p = 0.09$) and 3-weekly docetaxel (HR 0.79 $p = 0.001$ and HR 0.86 p = 0.054) in comparison with the standard arm of 4 cycles of 3-weekly paclitaxel [41].

18.3 Adjuvant Endocrine Therapy

It is widely acknowledged that the only patients to gain benefit from adjuvant endocrine treatment are those who have oestrogen receptor (ER) positive breast cancer [42]. The EBCTCG meta-analyses concluded that there was a significant reduction in rate of recurrence and breast cancer mortality when ER positive patients were given 5 years of tamoxifen. This was a clearer benefit than was seen in earlier studies where patients had only been given 1–2 years of tamoxifen [21]. For these women, the annual rate of recurrence was halved and breast cancer mortality reduced by a third. Most of the effect on recurrence is in those 5 years whilst on treatment but the effects on mortality last beyond this time period.

The 15-year gain in patients with ER positive disease after 5 years of tamoxifen for recurrence is 11.8 % ($2p < 0.00001$) and 9.2 % ($2p < 0.00001$) for breast cancer mortality [21]. The risk reduction appears to be independent of patient age, nodal status or whether the patient received adjuvant chemotherapy. The absolute risk reduction is similar in all age groups but is more significant in the node positive population [21].

The NSABP B-14 trial randomized ER positive, node negative patients to five years of tamoxifen versus 5 years of placebo. 10-year follow-up showed improved RFS (69 % vs. 57 % $p < 0.0001$) and OS (80 % vs. 76 % $p = 0.02$) [43]. Again these results were consistent regardless of age and also showed a reduction in the risk of contra-lateral breast cancer (4.0 % vs. 5.8 % $p = 0.007$) [43]. Attempting to address the question of optimum duration of adjuvant endocrine therapy, participants at the end of the trial who had received tamoxifen (and were alive with no recurrence) were randomized to a further 5 years of tamoxifen or 5 years of placebo [43]. Results showed no additional benefit and in fact favoured stopping after 5 years. RFS was 82 % for the placebo group versus 78 % ($p = 0.03$) and OS was 94 % for the placebo group and 91 % for ten years tamoxifen ($P = 0.07$) [44]. These data seemed to support stopping adjuvant endocrine therapy at 5 years; however, subsequent larger trials showed this to be erroneous.

In the ATLAS trial, 12 894 women were randomized to 5 or 10 years of adjuvant tamoxifen. There results show a survival benefit for 10 years of adjuvant treatment which even extended past the 10-year point of stopping treatment [45]. The cumulative risk of recurrence years 5–14 was 21.4 % for those on 10 years of tamoxifen versus 25.1 % control group. Mortality rates from breast cancer years 5–14 were 12.2 and 15 %, respectively. That equals an absolute mortality reduction of 2.8 % [45].

In the aTTom study, women continuing tamoxifen for 10 years had a 25 % lower recurrence rate and a 23 % lower breast cancer mortality rate compared to those who stopped at 5 years. Non-breast cancer mortality was not significantly affected but there were increased incidences of endometrial cancer [46].

18.3.1 Aromatase Inhibitors

The ATAC trial compared the aromatase inhibitor (AI) anastrazole to tamoxifen in postmenopausal women each taken for five years. RFS was improved in the ER positive group who received anastrazole (HR 0.86 $p = 0.003$) but there was no statistical significance in OS. The benefit persisted past the initial 5 years. When further analysed, the greatest benefit was seen in those patients who were ER positive but PGR negative. Whilst on active treatment the risk of fractures was higher in the group receiving AI but after discontinuation there was no difference in risk between groups. Interestingly, however, treatment-related serious adverse events were more common in the tamoxifen arm whilst on active treatment [47]. The BIG 1–98 trial also confirmed RFS was significantly improved in the postmenopausal women randomized to letrozole who had ER positive tumours (HR 0.82 $p = 0.007$) [48].

This led to aromatase inhibitors being recommended as standard adjuvant treatment in many/most postmenopausal women with ER positive breast cancer.

The ARNO 95 study looked at whether postmenopausal ER positive women could gain benefit after 2 years of tamoxifen by switching to the AI anastrazole. RFS (HR 0.66 $P = 0.049$) and OS (HR 0.53 $P = 0.045$) were improved by switching to the AI [49]. This showed RFS is improved for the postmenopausal ER positive subgroup either by having an AI as their standard treatment or sequentially post-tamoxifen.

Similar results were shown with the steroidal AI exemestane with RFS (HR 0.76 $p = 0.0001$) in the intergroup exemestane study [50].

The National Institute of Canada (NCIC) MA17 trial evaluated the efficacy of adding five years of letrozole after completing 5 years of tamoxifen compared to placebo [51]. For node negative patients and node positive patients, RFS was improved (HR 0.47, HR 0.60, respectively). In the node positive subset, this was the first time a benefit in OS had been demonstrated with letrozole (HR 0.61). Most benefit seemed to be in the ER+/PGR+ subset although this was a subset analysis [52].

Based on these trials, current ASCO guidelines recommend that women who have hormone receptor positive breast cancer and are pre- or peri-menopausal after 5 years of adjuvant tamoxifen should be offered to extend treatment to a total of 10 years [53]. If they are postmenopausal, they should be offered the choice of continuing tamoxifen or switching to an aromatase inhibitor to complete ten years of adjuvant endocrine therapy [53]. What remains unknown, although trial results are awaited, is the optimum strategy after 5 years' aromatase inhibition: whether further endocrine therapy is effective, and if so which is optimal, tamoxifen or continued aromatase inhibition.

18.4 Monoclonal Antibodies

Over expression of HER2/neu oncogene occurs in 15–20 % breast cancers and has prognostic implications with shorter RFS and OS [54]. Trastuzumab is a humanized monoclonal antibody against HER2 which has been proven to improve survival for this subset of patients. It does have a risk of cardiac toxicity which is amplified when combined with anthracyclines which form the base of many adjuvant regimens so the risk/benefit ratio has to be evaluated in the adjuvant population.

The NSABP-31 trial and N9831 trial were designed to evaluate the efficacy of adjuvant trastuzumab in node positive HER2 positive breast cancers. The NSABP-31 trial compared doxorubicin and cyclophosphamide followed by 3-weekly paclitaxel versus the same regimen with the addition of trastuzumab with the 1st paclitaxel dose continuing for 52 weeks. N9831 had an additional arm where trastuzumab was given sequentially for 52 weeks after completing paclitaxel [55]. As the two trials were similar in design, joint statistical analysis was performed to derive the estimated survival benefit. The relative improvement in OS was 37 % (HR 0.63 $p < 0.001$) giving an 8.8 % increase in OS at 10 years. RFS was also improved with a relative reduction of 40 % (HR 0.60 $p < 0.001$) and an increase in 10-year RFS 11.5 % [55].

Subsequent analyses evaluated cardiac function in node positive HER2 patients who had completed surgery and were either allocated to AC and then 3-weekly paclitaxel or the same regime but adding trastuzumab concurrently with the paclitaxel cycles. Overall there was a 4.1 % incidence of class III or IV congestive heart failure (CHF) and an overall incidence of any degree of CHF of 19 % [56].

The standard of care has been 1 year of antibody therapy. The HERA trial looked at whether survival could be improved with longer treatment duration, so it additionally compared 1 versus 2 years of trastuzumab to observation only, with all trastuzumab being commenced after completion of the chemotherapy. Severe cardiac toxicity was lower in the HERA trial than in the North American trials where the trastuzumab was commenced 3 weeks after the last dose of anthracycline and was similar at around 1 % in the 1- and 2-year arms. However, less severe cardiac toxicity was higher in the arm who received 2 years of treatment but with no improvement in DFS or OS. As expected, 1 year of trastuzumab was better than observation with DFS (HR 0.76 $p < 0.001$) and OS (HR 0.76 $p = 0.0005$) [57].

There are ongoing studies to evaluate whether 6 months of treatment may be adequate and reduce the incidence of cardiac toxicity. Preliminary data from the PHARE trial suggest 12-month treatment is superior so this still remains standard of care [58]. The Fin Her study (which was a much smaller trial) allocated patients to docetaxel or vinorelbine for 3 cycles followed by 3 FEC and then the HER2 positive patients were randomized to 9 weeks of trastuzumab [59]. Interestingly, RFS was improved even after 9 weeks of treatment from 78 % to 89 % after three years [59].

The BCIRG 006 study tested for HER2 status by FISH amplification in all patients, and like HERA, also included node negative patients [60]. It compared AC and docetaxel (T) trastuzumab (H) with, on the one hand, docetaxel and carboplatin and trastuzumab (TCH), and on the other hand, AC–T. RFS at 5 years was significantly better in the trastuzumab arms—AC–T 75 %, AC–TH 84 % and TCH 81 %. The rates of cardiac toxicity were higher in the anthracycline and trastuzumab arms [60].

18.5 Adjuvant Bisphosphonates

Bisphosphonates have been used in the metastatic setting to treat hypercalcaemia, bone pain and reduce fracture incidence for many years; however, there is increasing evidence that they may be of value in the adjuvant setting. The ABCSG-12 and AZURE trials generated the hypothesis that menopausal status might be the biggest predictor of response to adjuvant bisphosphonates with bone recurrence and breast cancer mortality being reduced in those who were postmenopausal or undergoing ovarian suppression [61, 62]. Previous trials in this area have mixed results but a subsequent individual patient meta-analysis of over 18,000 patients by the Early Breast Cancer Trialist's Collaborative Group provided level one evidence of a bisphosphonate class effect when used in this indication [63]. The meta-analyses included data on 18,766 women from 24 trials. In all women, regardless of menopausal status there was a definite reduction in bone recurrence RR 0.83, 95 % CI 0.73–0.94; $2p = 0.004$. Subanalysis amongst postmenopausal women showed a reduction in overall recurrence RR 0.86, 95 % CI 0.78–0.94; $2p = 0.002$, distant recurrence RR 0.82, 95 % CI 0.74–0.92; $2p = 0.003$, bone recurrence RR 0.72, 95 % CI 0.60–0.86; $2p = 0.0002$ and breast cancer mortality RR 0.82, 95 % CI 0.73–0.93; $2p = 0.002$. Another important effect was the significant reduction in bone fractures (RR 0.85, 95 % CI 0.75–0.97; $2p = 0.02$) [63].

The absolute gain from treatment at 10 years was 3.3 % for breast cancer mortality (95 % CI 0.8–5.7) and 2.2 % for bone recurrence (95 % CI 0.6–3.8). This was independent of ER status, nodal involvement, grade of tumour or concomitant chemotherapy. There was also no significant effect of class of bisphosphonate used or duration of treatment [63]. Despite these data, the use of adjuvant bisphosphonates as standard of care remains controversial and is not a licensed/approved use of these agents.

18.6 Ovarian Suppression

Ovarian ablation as a treatment in breast cancer was first published by George Beatson in the Lancet in 1896 [64]. Although at that time the mechanism was not well understood it remains an integral part of treatment in the modern setting. Nowadays surgical castration is not always needed given the advent of chemical suppression by gonadotropin-releasing agonists which results in down-regulation of oestrogen production.

In 1996, the EBCTCG published an overview in the Lancet of the randomized trials of those allocated to ovarian ablation with the addition of long-term follow-up data. From over 2000 women <50 years old, 15-year survival was increased amongst those who received ovarian ablation (52.4 vs. 46.1 % $2p = 0.001$) as was RFS (45 % vs. 39 % $2p = 0.0007$). The benefit was independent of nodal status but did appear smaller in those women who received chemotherapy as well as ovarian ablation [65].

In meta-analyses of 11 906 premenopausal women across 16 randomized control trials, LHRH agonists as single adjuvant therapy did not significantly reduce recurrence or death [66]. Combination with tamoxifen, chemotherapy or both reduced risk of recurrence by 12 % ($p = 0.02$) and death by 15.1 % ($p = 0.03$) and LHRH agonists were ineffective in hormone receptor negative cancers. LHRH agonists showed similar efficacy to chemotherapy as there was no significant difference when comparing the two arms for recurrence (HR 1.04 $P > 0.25$) or death (HR 0.89 $p > 0.37$). It is important to note, however, that none of the studies included taxanes so it can only be concluded that LHRH efficacy is similar to that of anthracycline-based systemic treatment [66].

We have established that adjuvant therapy with an AI improves outcomes in postmenopausal women with ER positive breast cancer. If ovarian function could be suppressed, would premenopausal women get enhanced benefit from an AI rather than tamoxifen? The TEXT and SOFT trials set out to investigate this randomizing ER positive premenopausal woman to the AI exemestane with ovarian suppression versus tamoxifen with ovarian suppression for a period of five years [67]. Ovarian function could be switched off chemically using gonadotropin-releasing hormone agonist triptorelin, surgically with oophorectomy or with ovarian irradiation. DFS was 91.1 % at 5 years in the group who got an AI + OS and 87.3 % with tamoxifen + OS. OS did not differ significantly and adverse events were similar in both arms [67].

18.7 Genomic Testing

There are several genomic tests for breast cancer and the most validated of these is Oncotype Dx. This analyses the expression in the primary tumour of 21 genes using reverse transcription polymerase chain reaction (RT-PCR) on RNA isolated from paraffin-embedded breast cancer tissue, generating a score for risk of recurrence which aids clinicians and patients in their decision as to whether they should pursue adjuvant systemic therapy. A low score predicts better outcomes, with some evidence that this group of patients' gains little additional benefit from adjuvant chemotherapy. It is thus prognostic and also estimates the likelihood of response to chemotherapy, thus avoiding chemotherapy in those patients who would receive no clinical benefit [68]. In a retrospective planned analysis of 367 specimens in ER positive, node positive postmenopausal women (SWOG 8814 trial which showed survival benefit for adjuvant cyclophosphamide, doxorubicin and fluorouracil (CAF) prior to tamoxifen), the recurrence score was prognostic in the tamoxifen alone group ($p = 0.006$; hazard ratio [HR] 2.64, 95 % CI 1.33–5.27, for a 50-point difference in recurrence score). There was no benefit of CAF if patients had a low recurrence score regardless of nodal involvement (<18; log-rank $p = 0.97$; HR 1.02, 0.54–1.93) but an improvement in RFS for a high recurrence score adjusting for the number of positive nodes (score > or = 31; log-rank $p = 0.033$; HR 0.59, 0.35–1.01) [68]. Oncotype Dx is included in the American Society of Clinical Oncology and National Comprehensive Cancer Network, ESMO and St Gallen guidelines as an adjunct to clinician decision-making regarding adjuvant chemotherapy [69–72].

The MammaPrint assay uses microarray technology to analyse a 70-gene expression profile to identify those at risk of developing metastatic disease [73]. This test was used on T1 tumours to identify how many would be at risk of distant recurrence without adjuvant treatment. The MammaPrint signature was an independent prognostic factor for breast cancer-specific survival (BCSS) at 10 years (HR 3.25 $P < 0.001$) and predicted distant disease-free survival (DDFS) at 10 years for 139 patients with T1a/b cancers (HR 3.45 $p = 0.04$) [74].

In a study designed to assess the predictive value of the MammaPrint assay for adjuvant chemotherapy prior to endocrine treatment, results were pooled from study series [75]. The test classified 253 patients as low risk and 289 as high risk. In the low-risk group, BCSS at 5 years was 97 % for the group on adjuvant endocrine therapy and 99 % for those allocated adjuvant chemotherapy prior to endocrine therapy (HR 0.58 $p = 0.62$). DDFS was 93 % versus 99 % (HR 0.26 $p = 0.20$). In the high-risk group, BCSS was 81 and 94 %, respectively, at 5 years (HR 0.21 $p < 0.01$) and DDFS was 76 % versus 88 % (HR 0.35 $p < 0.01$). This estimates significant survival benefit from adjuvant chemotherapy in the high-risk patients and no significant benefit in the low-risk patients [75].

The prospective RASTER study reported those classified as low risk by the MammaPrint assay (of whom 85 % did not receive adjuvant chemotherapy) had a 5-year distant-free recurrence of 97 % [76]. The FDA has approved the MammaPrint signature to help evaluate whether patients are deemed low or high risk but not to estimate their benefit from adjuvant chemotherapy.

The Prediction Analysis of Microarray 50 (PAM50) generates a risk recurrence score to predict prognosis in ER positive postmenopausal women by separating intrinsic breast cancer subtypes (luminal A, luminal B, HER2 positivity and basal-like). In a study comparing PAM50 with Oncotype Dx, more patients were scored high risk and fewer as intermediate risk by PAM50, suggesting it provided more prognostic information and better differentiation between high- and intermediate-risk patients [77].

So, should intermediate-risk patients still get adjuvant chemotherapy? The TAILORx trial is attempting to answer this question by randomizing those calculated as being intermediate risk to chemotherapy or not. The study is prospectively testing the use of Oncotype Dx to select for patients who can avoid chemotherapy [78]. So far results have only been released for the low-risk group, in which their good prognosis without chemotherapy has been confirmed [79].

The MINDACT trial is comparing the 70-gene signature with the pathological factors we commonly use to make clinical decisions regarding adjuvant chemotherapy. Again this is looking at those deemed intermediate risk and also further evaluating the predictive effect of the MammaPrint assay [80].

This is clearly an evolving area and one that is likely to dramatically influence clinical practice and decision-making over the next few years. So far all of these tests seem to be good prognostic tools but what has not yet been proven is their ability to safely identify patients who do not need chemotherapy. So far no single test has been validated as superior to the others available on the market.

18.8 Trials in Older Patients

An area that is beginning to be explored is incorporating or designing trials where the aim is to establish efficacy in the over 70 population. Many patients now fall into this age category and are fit for systemic treatment; however, we have little evidence of the efficacy of these drugs in this population. Historically, there has been reluctance to include this cohort in trials given potential co-morbidities, decline in organ function and perceived increased susceptibility to toxic side effects. The few studies that have included older women found a comparable incidence of complications in women both older and younger than 65 years of age [81–83]. These older patients, however, appear to have been selected by fitness and their lack of other health problems meaning they do not truly represent the older population as a whole. Hardly any of these trials have included women over 80 meaning we have no reliable information regarding tolerability or efficacy in this cohort [84]. There is increasing thought that geriatricians should be involved from the initial oncology consultation to perform a comprehensive geriatric assessment to aid the decision process and allow adjustments for age-related co-morbidities [85].

The data reviewed in this chapter clearly show that patients' outcomes are improved with adjuvant systemic treatment. The choice of which therapy or combinations of therapies to use depends on the tumour biology, patient characteristics and an evaluation of the relative benefits and deficits.

References

1. Dawood S, Austin L, Cristofanilli M. Cancer stem cells: implications for cancer therapy. Oncology (Williston Park) 2014;28 (12):1101–7, 1110.
2. Zhang S, Balch C, Chan MW, et al. Identification and characterization of ovarian cancer-initiating cells from primary human tumors. Cancer Res. 2008;68:4311–20.
3. Tian T, Olson S, Whitacre JM, Harding A. The origins of cancer robustness and evolvability. Integr Biol (Camb). 2011;3:17–30.
4. Boon T, Cerottini JC, Van den Eynde B, et al. Tumor antigens recognized by T lymphocytes. Annu Rev Immunol. 1994;12:337–65.
5. Adams S, Gray RJ, Demaria S, et al. Prognostic value of tumor-infiltrating lymphocytes in triple-negative breast cancers from two phase III randomized adjuvant breast cancer trials: ECOG 2197 and ECOG 1199. J Clin Oncol. 2014;32(27):2959–66.
6. Ali HR, Provenzano E, Dawson SJ, et al. Association between CD8 + T-cell infiltration and breast cancer survival in 12,439 patients. Ann Oncol. 2014;25(8):1536–43.
7. Loi S, Michiels S, Salgado R, et al. Tumor infiltrating lymphocytes are prognostic in triple negative breast cancer and predictive for trastuzumab benefit in early breast cancer: results from the FinHER trial. Ann Oncol. 2014;25(8):1544–50.
8. Loi S, Sirtaine N, Piette F, et al. Prognostic and predictive value of tumor-infiltrating lymphocytes in a phase III randomized adjuvant breast cancer trial in node-positive breast cancer comparing the addition of docetaxel to doxorubicin with doxorubicin-based chemotherapy: BIG 02-98. J Clin Oncol. 2013;31(7):860–7.
9. Anon. Review of mortality results in randomized trials in early breast cancer. Lancet 1984; 2:1205.
10. Fisher B, Jeong JH, Anderson S, et al. Twenty-five year follow-up of a randomized trial comparing radical mastectomy, total mastectomy, and total mastectomy followed by irradiation. N Engl J Med. 2002;347:567–75.
11. Fisher B, Anderson S, Bryant J, et al. Twenty-year follow-up of a randomized trial comparing total mastectomy, lumpectomy, and lumpectomy plus irradiation for the treatment of invasive breast cancer. N Engl J Med. 2002;347:1233–41.
12. Fisher B, Ravdin RG, Ausman RK, et al. Surgical adjuvant chemotherapy in cancer of the breast: results of a decade of cooperative investigation. Ann Surg. 1968;168:337–56.
13. Fisher B, Carbone P, Economou SG, et al. 1-Phenylalanine mustard (L-PAM) in the management of primary breast cancer. A report of early findings. N Engl J Med. 1975;292:117–22.
14. Greenspan EM, Fieber M, Lesnick G, Edelman S. Response of advanced breast cancer to the combination of the anti-metabolite methotrexate and the alkylating agent thiotepa. J Mt Sinai Hosp. 1963;30:246–67.
15. Bonadonna G, Brusamolino E, Valagussa P, et al. Combination chemotherapy as an adjuvant treatment in operable breast cancer. N Engl J Med. 1976;294:405–10.
16. Albain KS, Barlow WE, Ravdin PM, et al. Breast Cancer Intergroup of North America. Adjuvant chemotherapy and timing of tamoxifen in postmenopausal patients with endocrine-responsive, node-positive breast cancer: a phase 3, open-label, randomised controlled trial. Lancet Oncol. 2009;374:2055–63.
17. Mansour EG, Gray R, Shatila AH, et al. Efficacy of adjuvant chemotherapy in high-risk node-negative breast cancer. An intergroup study. N Engl J Med. 1989;320:485–90.
18. Tancini G, Bonadonna G, Valagussa P, et al. Adjuvant CMF in breast cancer: comparative 5-year results of 12 versus 6 cycles. J Clin Oncol. 1983;1:2–10.
19. Fisher B, Brown AM, Dimitrov NV, et al. Two months of doxorubicin-cyclophosphamide with and without interval reinduction therapy compared with 6 months of cyclophosphamide, methotrexate, and fluorouracil in positive-node breast cancer patients with tamoxifen-nonresponsive tumors: results from the National Surgical Adjuvant Breast and Bowel Project B-15. J Clin Oncol. 1990;8:1483–96.
20. Abrams JS. Adjuvant therapy for breast cancer–results from the USA consensus conference. Breast Cancer. 2001;8:298–304.
21. Early Breast Cancer Trialists' Collaborative Group. Effects of chemotherapy and hormonal therapy for early breast cancer on recurrence and 15-year survival: an overview of the randomised trials. Lancet Oncol. 2005;365:1687–717.
22. Early Breast Cancer Trialists' Collaborative Group. Adjuvant chemotherapy in oestrogen receptor poor breast cancer: patient level meta-analyses of randomized trials. Lancet Oncol. 2008;371 (9606):29–40.
23. Early Breast Cancer Trialists' Collaborative Group. Comparisons between different polychemotherapy regimens for early breast cancer: meta-analyses of long-term outcome among 100,000 women in 123 randomised trials. Lancet Oncol. 2012;379:432–44.
24. Bonadonna G, Zambetti M, Valagussa P. Sequential or alternating doxorubicin and CMF regimens in breast cancer with more than three positive nodes. Ten year results. JAMA. 1995;273(7):542–7.
25. Earl HM, Hiller L, Dunn JA, et al. NEAT: National Epirubicin Adjuvant Trail—toxicity, delivered dose intensity and quality of life. Br J Cancer. 2008;99:1226–31.
26. Wani MC, Taylor HL, Wall ME, et al. Plant antitumor agents VI. Isolation and structure of taxol, a novel antileukemic and antitumour agent from taxus brevifolia. J Am Chem Sco 1971 96: 2325–7.
27. Sparano JA. Doxorubicin/taxane combinations: cardiac toxicity and pharmacokinetics. Semin Oncol. 1999;26:14–9.
28. Norton L. Theoretical concepts and the emerging role of taxanes in adjuvant therapy. Oncologist. 2001;6:30–5.
29. Simon R, Norton L. The Norton-Simon hypothesis: designing more effective and less toxic chemotherapeutic regimens. Nat Clin Pract Oncol. 2006;3:406–7.
30. Henderson IC, Berry DA, Demetri GD, et al. Improved outcomes from adding sequential Paclitaxel but not from escalating Doxorubicin dose in an adjuvant chemotherapy regimen for patients with node-positive primary breast cancer. J Clin Oncol. 2003;21:976–83.
31. Mamounas EP, Bryant J, Lembersky B, et al. Paclitaxel after doxorubicin plus cyclophosphamide as adjuvant chemotherapy for node-positive breast cancer: results from NSABP B-28. J Clin Oncol. 2005;23:3686–96.
32. Anampa J, Makower D. Sparano J Progress in adjuvant chemotherapy for breast cancer: an overview. BMC Med. 2015;13:195.

33. Jones S, Holmes FA, O'Shaughnessy J et al. Extended follow up and analysis by age of the US Oncology Adjuvant Trial 9735: docetaxel/cyclophosphamide is associated with an overall survival benefit compared to doxorubicin/cyclophosphamide and is well tolerated in women 65 or older. Breast Cancer Res Treat. 2007: 106(suppl 1).
34. Jones S, Holmes FA, O'Shaughnessy J, et al. Docetaxel with cyclophosphamide is associated with an overall survival benefit compared with doxorubicin and cyclophosphamide: 7-year follow up of US Oncology Research Trial 9735. J Clin Oncol. 2009;27:1177–83.
35. Martin M, Pienkowski T, Mackey J, et al. Breast Cancer International Research Group 001 Investigators. Adjuvant docetaxel for node-positive breast cancer. N Engl J Med. 2005;352:2302–13.
36. Martin M, Seguí MA, Antón A, et al. GEICAM 9805 Investigators. Adjuvant docetaxel for high-risk, node-negative breast cancer. N Engl J Med. 2010;363:2200–10.
37. Roche H, Fumoleau P, Spielmann M, et al. Sequential adjuvant epirubicin-based and docetaxel chemotherapy for node-positive breast cancer patients: the FNCLCC PACS 01 Trial. J Clin Oncol. 2006;24:5664–71.
38. Coudert B, Asselain B, Campone M, et al. UNICANCER Breast Group. Extended benefit from sequential administration of docetaxel after standard fluorouracil, epirubicin, and cyclophosphamide regimen for node-positive breast cancer: the 8-year follow-up results of the UNICANCER-PACS01 trial. Oncologist. 2012;17:900–9.
39. Ellis P, Barrett-Lee P, Johnson L, et al. TACT Trial Management Group; TACT Trialists. Sequential docetaxel as adjuvant chemotherapy for early breast cancer (TACT): an open-label, phase III, randomised controlled trial. Lancet Oncol. 2009;373:1681–92.
40. Sparano JA, Wang M, Martino S, et al. Weekly paclitaxel in the adjuvant treatment of breast cancer. N Engl J Med. 2008;358:1663–71.
41. Sparano JA, Zhao F, Martino S, et al. Long-term follow-up of the E1199 phase III trial evaluating the role of taxane and schedule in operable breast cancer. J Clin Oncol. 2015;20,33(21):2353–60.
42. Early Breast Cancer Trialists' Collaborative Group. Tamoxifen for early breast cancer: an overview of the randomised trials. Lancet Oncol. 1998;351:1451–67.
43. Fisher B, Dignam J, Bryant J, et al. Five versus more than five years of tamoxifen therapy for breast cancer patients with negative lymph nodes and estrogen receptor-positive tumors. J Natl Cancer Inst. 1996;88:1529–42.
44. Fisher B, Dignam J, Bryant J, et al. Five versus more than five years of tamoxifen for lymph node-negative breast cancer: updated findings from the National Surgical Adjuvant Breast and Bowel Project B-14 randomized trial. J Natl Cancer Inst. 2001;93:684–90.
45. Davies C, Pan H, Godwin J, et al. Long term effects of continuing adjuvant tamoxifen to 10 years versus stopping at 5 years after diagnosis of oestrogen receptor-postitive breast cancer: ATLAS, a randomised trial. Lancet Oncol. 2013;381(9869):805–16.
46. Gray R, Rea D, Handley K et al. aTTom: long-term effects of continuing adjuvant tamoxifen to 10 years versus stopping at 5 years in 6,953 women with early breast cancer. J Clin Oncol, 2013 ASCO Annual Meeting Abstracts. Vol 31, No 18_suppl (June 20 Supplement), 2013:5.
47. Cuzick J, Sestak I, Baum M, et al. Effect of anastrozole and tamoxifen as adjuvant treatment for early-stage breast cancer: 10-year analysis of the ATAC trial. Lancet Oncol. 2010;11 (12):1135–41.
48. Mourisden H, Gershanovich M, Sun Y et al. Superior efficacy of letrozole versus tamoxifen as first line therapy for post menopausal women with advanced breast cancer: results of a phase III study of the International Letrozole Breast Cancer Group. J Clin Oncol. 200119 (10): 2596–606.
49. Kaufmann M, Jonat W, Hilfrich JJ, et al. Improved overall survival in postmenopausal women with early breast cancer after anastrozole initiated after treatment with tamoxifen compared with continued tamoxifen: the ARNO 95 study. J Clin Oncol. 2007;25(19):2664–70.
50. Coombes RC, Kilburn LS, Snowdon CF et al. Survival and safety of exemestane versus tamoxifen after 2–3 years' tamoxifen treatment (Intergroup Exemestane Study): a randomised controlled trial. Lancet Oncol. 2007;369(9561):559–570.
51. Goss PE, Ingle JN, Martino S, et al. A randomised trial of letrozole in postmenopausal women after five years of tamoxifen therapy for early stage breast cancer. N Engl J Med. 2003;349(19):1793–802.
52. Goss P, Ingle JN, Martino S, et al. Randomized trial of letrozole following tamoxifen as extended adjuvant therapy in receptor-positive breast cancer: updated findings from NCIC CTG MA.17. J Natl Cancer Inst. 2005;97(17):1262–71.
53. Burstein HJ, Temin S, Anderson A, et al. Adjuvant endocrine therapy for women with hormone receptor–positive breast cancer: American society of clinical oncology clinical practice guideline focused update. J Clin Oncol. 2014;32(21):2255–69.
54. Slamon DJ, Clark GM, Wong SG. Human breast cancer: correlation of relapse and survival with amplification of the HER-2/neu oncogene. Science. 1987;235:177–82.
55. Perez EA, Romond EH, Suman VJ, et al. Trastuzumab plus adjuvant chemotherapy for human epidermal growth factor receptor 2–positive breast cancer: planned joint analysis of overall survival from NSABP B-31 and NCCTG N9831. J Clin Oncol. 2014;32(33):3744–52.
56. Tan-Chiu E, Yothers G, Romond E et al. Assessment of cardiac dysfunction in a randomized trial comparing doxorubicin and cyclophosphamide followed by paclitaxel, with or without trastuzumab as adjuvant therapy in node-positive, human epidermal growth factor receptor 2–overexpressing breast cancer: NSABP B-31 J Clin Oncol. 23(31):7811–9.
57. Goldhirsch A, Gelber RD, Piccart-Gebhart MJ, et al. 2 years versus 1 year of adjuvant trastuzumab for HER2-positive breast cancer (HERA): an open-label, randomised controlled trial. Lancet Oncol. 2013;382(9897):1021–8.
58. Pivot X, Romieu G, Debled M, et al 6 months versus 12 months of adjuvant trastuzumab for patients with HER2-positive early breast cancer (PHARE): a randomised phase 3 trial. Lancet Oncol. 2013;14(8):741–48.
59. Joensuu H, Kellokumpu-Lehtinen P-L, Bono P. Adjuvant docetaxel or vinorelbine with or without trastuzumab for breast cancer. N Engl J Med 2006;354:809–820.
60. Slamon D, Eiermann W, Robert N. Phase III randomized trial comparing doxorubicin and cyclophosphamide followed by docetaxel (ACT) with doxorubicin and cyclophosphamide followed by docetaxel and trastuzumab (AC TH) with docetaxel, carboplatin and Trastuzumab (TCH) in HER2 positive early breast cancer patients: BCIRG 006 study. Cancer Res. 2009; 69–62.
61. Gnant M, Mlineritsch B, Schippinger W, et al. Endocrine therapy plus zoledronic acid in premenopausal breast cancer. N Engl J Med. 2009;360:679–91.
62. Coleman R, Cameron D, Dodwell D, et al. Adjuvant zoledronic acid in patients with early breast cancer: final efficacy analysis of the AZURE (BIG 01/04) randomised open-label phase 3 trial. Lancet Oncol. 2014;15(9):997–1006.
63. Early Breast Cancer Trialists' Collaborative Group. Adjuvant bisphosphonate treatment in early breast cancer: meta-analyses of individual patient data from randomised trials. Lancet Oncol. 2015;386(10001):1353–61.

64. Beatson GT. On the treatment of inoperable cases of carcinoma of the mamma: suggestions for a new method of treatment with illustrative cases. Lancet Oncol. 1896;2:104–7.
65. Breast Cancer Trialists' Collaborative Group. Ovarian ablation in early breast cancer: overview of the randomised trials. Lancet Oncol. 1996;348(9036):1189–96.
66. Cuzick J, Ambrosine L davidosn N et al. Use of luteinising-hormone-releasing hormone agonists as adjuvant treatment in premenopausal patients with hormone-receptor-positive breast cancer: a meta-analysis of individual patient data from randomised adjuvant trials. Lancet Oncol. 2007;369(9574):1711–23.
67. Pagani O, Regan MM, Walley BA, et al. Adjuvant exemestane with ovarian suppression in premenopausal breast cancer. N Engl Med. 2014;371:107–18.
68. Albain KS, Barlow WE, Shak S, et al. Prognostic and predictive value of the 21-gene recurrence score assay in postmenopausal women with node positive, oestrogen receptor positive breast cancer on chemotherapy: a retrospective planned analysis of a randomised trial. Lancet Oncol. 2010;11:55–65.
69. Harris L, Fritsche H, Mennel R, et al. American Society of Clinical Oncology 2007 update recommendations for the use of tumour markers in breast cancer. J Clin Oncol. 2007;25:5287–312.
70. NCCN Clinical Practice Guidelines in Oncology Breast Cancer (version 1 2011). http://www.nccn.org/professionals/physician_gls/PDF/breast.pdf. Accessed 15 Jan 2016.
71. Aebi S, Davidson T, Gruber G, Castiglione M. Primary breast cancer: ESMO Clinical Practice Guidelines for diagnosis, treatment and follow up. Ann Oncol. 21(suppl 5):v9–v14.
72. Goldhirsch A, Wood WC, Coates AS, et al. Strategies for subtypes —dealing with the diversity of breast cancer: highlight of the St Gallen international expert consensus on the primary therapy of early breast cancer. Ann Oncol. 2011;22(8):1736–47.
73. Glas AM, Floore A, Delahaye LJMJ, et al. Converting a breast cancer microarray signature into a high-throughput diagnostic test. BMC Genom. 2006;7:278.
74. Mook S, Knauer M, Bueno-de-Mesquita JM, et al. Metastatic potential of T1 breast cancer can be predicted by the 70-gene MammaPrint signature. Ann Surg Oncol. 2010;17:1406–13.
75. Knauer M, Mook S, Rutgers EJ, et al. The predictive value of the 70-gene signature for adjuvant chemotherapy in early breast cancer. Breast Cancer Res Treat. 2010;120:655–61.
76. Drukker CA, Bueno-de-Mesquita JM, Retel VP, et al. A prospective evaluation of a breast cancer prognosis signature in the observational RASTER study. Int J Cancer. 2013;133:929–36.
77. Dowsett M, Sestak I, Lopez-Knowles E, et al. Comparison of PAM50 risk of recurrence score with onctotype DX and IHC4 for predicting risk of distant recurrence after endocrine therapy. J Clin Oncol. 2013;31:2783–90.
78. Hormone Therapy with or without combination chemotherapy in treating women who have undergone surgery for node negative breast cancer (The TAILORx trial. Clinical Trial ID: NCTT00310180.
79. Sparano JA, Gray RJ, Makower DF, et al. Prospective Validation of a 21-gene expression assay in breast cancer. N Engl J Med. 2015;2015(373):2005–14.
80. MINDACT (Microarray in node negative and 1 to 3 positive lymph node disease may avoid chemotherapy): A prospective, randomized study to compare the 70-gene signature assay with the common clinical-pathological criteria in selecting patients for adjuvant chemotherapy in breast cancer. Clinical Trial ID: NCT00433589.
81. Gelman RS, Taylor SG. Cyclophosphamide, methotrexate and 5-fluorouracil chemotherapy in women more than 65 years old with advanced breast cancer: the elimination of age trends in toxicity by using doses based on creatinine clearance. J Clin Oncol. 1984;2:1404–13.
82. Christman K, Muss HB, Case LD, Stanley V. Chemotherapy of metastatic breast cancer in the elderly. JAMA. 1992;268:57–62.
83. Ibrahim N, Buzdar A, Frye D, Hortobagyi G. Should age be a determinant factor in treating breast cancer patients with combination chemotherapy? Proc Am Soc Clin Oncol. 1993;12:A74.
84. Balducci L, Phillips DM. Breast Cancer in older women. Am Fam Physician. 1998 Oct 1;58(5):1163–72.
85. Markopoulos C, Van de Water W. Older patients with breast cancer; is there bias in the treatment they receive? Adv Med Oncol. 2012;4(6):321–7.

19 Endocrine Therapy

Olivia Pagani and Rosaria Condorelli

Abbreviations

BC	Breast cancer
ET/ETs	Endocrine therapy/endocrine therapies
ER+	Oestrogen receptor-positive
PR+	Progesterone receptor-positive
EBCTCG	Early Breast Cancer Trialists' Collaborative Group
RR	Relative risk
OFS	Ovarian function suppression
GnRHa	Gonadotropin-releasing hormone analogues
IBCSG	International Breast Cancer Study Group
SOFT	Suppression of Ovarian Function Trial
DSF	Disease-free survival
HR	Hazard ratio
CI	Confidence interval
AI/AIs	Aromatase inhibitor/aromatase inhibitors
TEXT	Tamoxifen and Exemestane Trial
OS	Overall survival
HR−	Hormone receptor-negative
DDFS	Distant DFS
ER−	Oestrogen receptor-negative
HER2+	Human epidermal growth factor receptor 2-positive
pCR	Pathologic complete response
NeoCENT	Neoadjuvant Chemotherapy versus ENdocrine Therapy
BCS	Breast conservative surgery
ORR	Overall response rate
PEPI	Preoperative endocrine prognostic index
RFS	Relapse-free survival
PROACT	Preoperative Arimidex Compared to Tamoxifen
LABC	Locally advanced breast cancer
ABC	Advanced breast cancer

O. Pagani (✉)
Institute of Oncology and Breast Unit of Southern Switzerland, Ospedale San Giovanni, 6500 Bellinzona, Ticino, Switzerland
e-mail: Olivia.Pagani@eoc.ch; opagani@bluewin.ch

R. Condorelli
Department of Medical Oncology, Institute of Oncology of Southern Switzerland, via Ospedale, 6500 Bellinzona, Switzerland
e-mail: Rosaria.Condorelli@eoc.ch

I. Jatoi and A. Rody (eds.), *Management of Breast Diseases*, DOI 10.1007/978-3-319-46356-8_19

TTP	Time to progression
OA	Ovarian ablation
CBR	Clinical benefit rate
LD	Low-dose
HD	High-dose
HR+	Hormone receptor-positive
mTOR	PI3K/Akt/mammalian target of rapamycin
NSAI	Non-steroidal aromatase inhibitor
CDK4 and CDK6	Cyclin-dependent kinases 4 and 6

19.1 Introduction

Breast cancer (BC) is a heterogeneous disease with different immunohistochemical and molecular characteristics associated with different risk profiles and outcomes.

Endocrine responsive BC is the most represented subtype both in pre- and postmenopausal women, overall accounting for 65 % of cases [1]. This implies a wide use of endocrine therapy (ET) across ages in all disease phases.

We will summarize the indications and efficacy of ET in pre- and postmenopausal women in the neo/adjuvant and metastatic disease settings.

19.2 Adjuvant Therapy

In any case of endocrine responsiveness, defined as ≥1 % of oestrogen (ER+) and/or progesterone (PR+) receptor-positive tumour cells, there is indication for adjuvant ET, irrespective of the use of chemotherapy and/or targeted therapy.

The choice among different ETs depends on menopausal status, risk of recurrence, comorbidities, potential drug toxicity and patient's preferences, and should be discussed individually in a dedicated breast unit.

19.2.1 Premenopausal Patients

19.2.1.1 Tamoxifen

In the last decades, 5 years of tamoxifen have been the gold and unique standard.

Tamoxifen competes with oestrogens at the receptor site, inhibiting the growth of oestrogen-dependent BC. In addition, tamoxifen has a partial oestrogen-agonistic effect that is beneficial, for example, in preventing bone demineralization, but also detrimental in increasing the risk of uterine cancer and thromboembolic events. The updated Early Breast Cancer Trialists' Collaborative Group (EBCTCG) overview, conducted only in ER+ tumours, concluded that 5 years of adjuvant tamoxifen reduces the annual BC mortality rate by 31 % irrespective of age, the use of chemotherapy and nodal status [2]. The effect is maintained over time (years 0–4 and 5–14), confirming the previously reported carry-over data (years 0–9). The meta-analysis also reinforced that 5 years of tamoxifen were significantly more effective than 1–2 years in terms of BC recurrence and mortality.

The optimal duration of tamoxifen in the individual patient is still not completely clarified. In the ATLAS randomized trial, 12.894 pre- and postmenopausal women who had completed 5 years of adjuvant tamoxifen were randomized to continue for additional 5 years or to stop treatment. The analysis of the 6.846 women with ER+ disease showed a statistically significant reduction in the risk of BC recurrence (21.4 % vs. 25.1 %), BC mortality (12.2 % vs. 15 %) and overall mortality in the arm of longer assumption. Patients on extended therapy experienced more drug-related side effects with a relative risk (RR) of endometrial cancer of 1.74 and of pulmonary embolism of 1.87 [3]. The aTTom trial confirms, in 2.755 women with ER+ disease, a reduction in both BC recurrence and mortality [4]. Taken together with the results of 5 years of tamoxifen versus no therapy, these data indicate that 10 years of adjuvant tamoxifen, compared with no tamoxifen, can reduce BC mortality by about one-third in the first 10 years following diagnosis and by a half subsequently. This evidence can be of particular interest for patients at high risk of relapse and younger women, the largest population likely to consider 10 years of treatment, despite only 9 % of patients in the ATLAS study and an unspecified proportion in the aTTom study were premenopausal at enrolment.

19.2.1.2 Ovarian Function Suppression (OFS)

In premenopausal women, the main source of circulating oestrogens is by ovarian aromatization of exogenous and endogenous androgens: OFS by surgical castration or irradiation has been the oldest ever ET, being progressively replaced by the administration of gonadotropin-releasing hormone analogues (GnRHa). Surgical castration represents still today a low-cost option in developing countries and a valid alternative in BC patients harbouring a BRCA 1/2 mutation who completed family planning. The chronic administration of a GnRHa, binding to the receptors in the pituitary gland, first induces a flare of FSH and LH secretion and subsequently a fall of gonadotropins and sex steroids to values similar to surgical castration.

The role of OFS as part of ET in premenopausal women has been investigated with contrasting results. The 2007 EBCTCG meta-analysis of 16 randomized trials, including 11.906 women, studied the effects of GnRHa alone, GnRHa plus tamoxifen versus tamoxifen alone, GnRHa plus chemotherapy versus chemotherapy alone and GnRHa plus chemotherapy plus tamoxifen versus chemotherapy plus tamoxifen. The GnRHa duration ranged from 18 months up to 5 years. The analysis showed that GnRHa alone did not significantly reduce recurrence or death after recurrence but when added to tamoxifen, chemotherapy or both achieved a 12.7 % reduction in recurrence and a 15.1 % reduction in death after recurrence [5]. The benefit was especially evident in women ≤40 years after adjuvant chemotherapy, either alone or in addition to tamoxifen, possibly related to the lack of permanent amenorrhoea with chemotherapy alone in this subgroup of patients.

The recently available results of the International Breast Cancer Study Group (IBCSG)-led Suppression of Ovarian Function Trial (SOFT), a comparison between 5 years of tamoxifen plus OFS versus tamoxifen alone, after a median follow-up of 67 months, showed, overall, a disease-free survival (DFS) of 86.6 % in the tamoxifen plus OFS arm and of 84.7 % in the tamoxifen arm (hazard ratio [HR] 0.83; 95 % confidence interval [CI] 0.66–1.04; $p = 0.10$). However, in the pre-planned subgroup analysis of the cohort of patients receiving adjuvant chemotherapy, there was a significant benefit of tamoxifen plus OFS versus tamoxifen alone in terms of reduction in BC recurrences at 5 years (82.5 % vs. 78.0 %, HR 0.78; 95 % CI 0.60–1.02); these patients were at higher risk of relapse than the ones in the no chemotherapy cohort (younger with larger tumours of intermediate-high grade and more frequently node-positive). This result was confirmed in the subset of very young patients (<35 years) who achieved the highest benefit from the addition of OFS over tamoxifen alone (78.9 and 67.7 %, respectively), suggesting that in patients at higher risk of recurrence, the addition of OFS can improve outcomes [6], as acknowledged in all the most recent consensus guidelines [7–10].

The optimal duration of adjuvant GnRHa has not been established. In different trials, GnRHa were given for 2, 3 or 5 years, with no direct comparison. On the basis of the available data, duration should not exceed 5 years and should also take into account side effects, patient preferences and family plans.

19.2.1.3 Aromatase Inhibitors (AIs)

AIs act inhibiting or inactivating aromatase, the enzyme responsible for the synthesis of oestrogens from androgenic substrates, thus almost completely suppressing plasma oestrogen levels in postmenopausal women. In premenopausal women, AIs cannot be used alone, because of the risk of indirect ovarian stimulation via the pituitary loop, with a paradoxical increase in circulating oestrogens.

In premenopausal women, the use of the AI Exemestane in combination with OFS, as compared to tamoxifen plus OFS, has been investigated in 4.690 patients in the combined analysis of TEXT (Tamoxifen and Exemestane Trial) and SOFT. After a median follow-up of 68 months, a DFS of 91.1 % was achieved in the Exemestane group compared with 87.3 % in the tamoxifen group (HR 0.72; 95 % CI 0.60–0.85; $p < 0.001$) with a 3.8 % absolute gain, comparable to the benefit of AIs in postmenopausal women. There was no difference in overall survival (OS) but a longer follow-up is needed in this population of patients who can develop late relapses. Overall, the incidence of adverse events of any grade was similar in the two treatment groups, with a different toxicity profile consistent with the specific class of drugs. Patients under tamoxifen reported more hot flushes, vaginal discharge and sweats, whereas patients who received Exemestane had more bone/joint pain, vaginal dryness and greater loss of sexual interest [11]. Nonetheless, during the treatment period, changes in global quality of life from baseline were similar between the two treatment groups [12].

Different results were reported in the ABCSG-12 trial in 1.803 women randomized to 3 years of OFS plus tamoxifen or plus the AI Anastrozole, with or without Zoledronic acid. After 94.4 months of median follow-up, no DFS difference between treatments was reported, but a higher risk of death for Anastrozole-treated patients was observed (HR 1.63; 95 % CI 1.05–1.45; $p = 0.03$) [13].

These divergent results can be partly explained by some differences between ABCSG-12 and SOFT/TEXT: lower number of patients and smaller statistical power in the Austrian trial, low-risk population (only 5 % of patients receiving neo/adjuvant chemotherapy), shorter treatment duration (only 3 years) and the use of Zoledronic acid.

At present, the results of SOFT and TEXT support the use of the AI Exemestane plus OFS, as a new treatment option in premenopausal women with early, ER + breast cancer for whom OFS is indicated.

19.2.2 GnRHa for Ovarian Protection

Different studies and meta-analyses tried to explore the role of GnRHa as prevention of ovarian failure during adjuvant chemotherapy with contrasting results, mainly due to non-homogeneous definition of ovarian failure and selection of patients.

Recently, the randomized POEMS trial assigned 257 premenopausal women with hormone receptor-negative (HR −) BC to receive standard chemotherapy, with or without the GnRHa Goserelin. After 2 years, the ovarian failure rate was 8 % in the Goserelin group and 22 % in the chemotherapy-alone group. Among the 218 evaluable patients, pregnancy occurred in more women in the Goserelin group than in the chemotherapy-alone group (21 % vs. 11 %) [14].

Despite lack of universal consensus, we suggest to individually discuss this strategy with patients, balancing the adverse effects and benefits of this therapy.

19.2.3 Postmenopausal Women

AIs (both non-steroidal and steroidal) and tamoxifen represent valid adjuvant therapies for postmenopausal, endocrine responsive, early BC, with AIs showing overall a significant benefit in DFS and a slight improvement in OS across different trials.

The BIG 1-98, a randomized phase III double-blind trial, compared 5 years of tamoxifen or letrozole as monotherapy or their sequential administration (2 years of one drug followed by 3 years of the other). At median follow-up of 8.7 years, letrozole monotherapy was significantly better than tamoxifen monotherapy for both the primary DFS endpoint (HR 0.82) and the secondary OS (HR 0.79) distant recurrence-free interval (HR 0.79) and BC-free interval (HR 0.80) endpoints. On the contrary, at median follow-up of 8.0 years, there was no statistically significant difference in any endpoint between sequential therapies and letrozole monotherapy, sequential strategies being therefore a valid option in case of toxicity [15].

Likewise, the ATAC trial compared Anastrozole with tamoxifen, both for 5 years. At median follow-up of 120 months, both in the overall study population and particularly in ER+ patients, there were significant improvements in the Anastrozole group compared with the tamoxifen group, in terms of DFS (HR 0.86), time to recurrence (HR 0.79) and time to distant recurrence (HR 0.85). In ER+ patients, absolute differences in time to recurrence between Anastrozole and tamoxifen increased over time (2.7 % at 5 years, 4.3 % at 10 years) and recurrence rates remained significantly lower with Anastrozole as compared to tamoxifen after treatment completion (HR 0.81), although the carryover benefit decreased after 8 years. Fewer deaths after recurrence were reported with Anastrozole compared with tamoxifen in the ER+ subgroup (HR 0.87) but there was little difference in overall mortality (HR 0.95) [16].

Several other large randomized trials have compared one of the three third-generation AIs (Anastrozole, letrozole or Exemestane) with 5 years of tamoxifen, generally reporting reduced recurrence rates in the AIs treated groups but not a clear-cut reduction in BC mortality.

The latest EBCTCG meta-analysis included data on 31.920 women from randomized trials of different schedules as follows: 5 years of an AI versus 5 years of tamoxifen; 5 years of an AI versus 2–3 years of tamoxifen then the AI to year 5; 2–3 years of tamoxifen then an AI to year 5 versus 5 years of tamoxifen.

In the comparison of 5 years of an AI versus 5 years of tamoxifen, the recurrence rate ratios significantly favoured AIs during treatment (years 0–1 RR 0.64, years 2–4 RR 0.80) but non-significantly thereafter. The 10-year BC mortality was also lower with AIs than with tamoxifen (12.1 % vs. 14.2 %, RR 0.85). In the comparison of 5 years of an AI versus 2–3 years of tamoxifen then the AI to year 5, the recurrence rate ratios significantly favoured AIs when treatment differed (years 0–1 RR 0.74) but not when both groups received the AI (years 2–4), or thereafter; the BC mortality reduction was not significant (RR 0.89). In the comparison of 2–3 years of tamoxifen then an AI to year 5 versus 5 years of tamoxifen, the recurrence rate ratios significantly favoured AIs during years 2–4 when patients received the AI (RR 0.56) but not subsequently, and the 10-year BC mortality was lower when switching to the AI than when keeping on tamoxifen (8.7 % vs. 10.1 %). In summary, aggregating the three schedule comparisons, recurrence rate ratios favoured AIs when treatments differed (RR 0.70) but not significantly thereafter (RR 0.93). The BC mortality was also significantly reduced while treatments differed (RR 0.79), less subsequently (RR 0.89) and for all periods combined (RR 0.86).

The meta-analysis concluded that AIs reduce recurrence rates by about 30 % (proportionately) compared with tamoxifen while treatments differ, but not thereafter. Five years of an AI reduce the 10-year BC mortality rate by about 15 % compared with 5 years of tamoxifen, hence by about 40 % (proportionately) compared with no ET [17]. According to all most recent guidelines [7, 9], AIs should be therefore included at some point during adjuvant treatment.

Integration of AIs and tamoxifen, their upfront or sequential administration has therefore to be individually discussed and planned.

Also in postmenopausal women, the optimal duration of ET is still matter of debate.

The EBCTCG meta-analysis excluded trials comparing an AI after 5 years of tamoxifen versus stopping ET. This sequence has been investigated in the MA.17 trial, a double-blind, placebo-controlled trial designed to determine the effectiveness of 5 years of letrozole after completing 5 years of tamoxifen. The primary endpoint was DFS; secondary endpoints included OS, distant DFS (DDFS) and incidence of contralateral tumours. The trial was stopped early after an interim analysis showed that letrozole improved outcomes: after a median follow-up of 30 months, women in the letrozole arm had statistically significantly better DFS, DDFS and contralateral BC incidence than women in the placebo arm. OS was the same in both arms except in women with node-positive disease who had an improved OS with letrozole. The conclusion from the MA.17 trial was that letrozole after tamoxifen improves both DFS and DDFS but not OS, except in node-positive patients [18, 19].

Considering also the results of the previously mentioned ATLAS trial [3], it is appropriate discussing with patients at sufficient risk of relapse the extension of adjuvant ET beyond 5 years, always bearing in mind drugs' toxicity and patients' preference. The recent results of the phase III, randomized, placebo-controlled MA.17R trial, showed a significantly higher 5-year DFS in patients receiving additional 5 years of letrozole after 4.5–6 years of adjuvant AI, preceded in most patients (79 %) by tamoxifen, than in those under placebo (95 % versus 91 %, HR 0.66; P = 0.01) with the greatest reduction achieved in contralateral BC. The rate of OS was not higher between treatments (HR 0.97; P = 0.83). The superiority of letrozole was observed in all subgroups, with no signs of treatment interaction and the incidence of most toxic effects similar in the two groups, with the exception of bone related toxic effects, more common in the letrozole group. While waiting for the results of ongoing trials, 10 years of adjuvant AIs can represent a reasonable option to discuss in high-risk patients.

19.2.4 Neoadjuvant Therapy

Neoadjuvant chemotherapy trials have consistently reported lower response rates in ER+ BC when compared with ER− or human epidermal growth factor receptor 2-positive (HER2+) patients [20]. The German Breast Group demonstrated pathologic complete response (pCR) rates of 6.2 and 22.8 % for ER+ and ER- tumours, respectively (p = 0.0001) [21]. In addition, in 6.377 patients enrolled in 7 randomized trials of anthracycline–taxane-based chemotherapy, pCR showed to be a good DFS surrogate endpoint for patients with luminal B/HER2-negative, HER2-positive (non-luminal) and triple-negative disease but not for those with luminal A tumours [22]. Direct comparisons of neoadjuvant chemotherapy against ET are rare. In the GEICAM/2006-03 phase II trial, 95 patients were randomized to 8 cycles of chemotherapy (EC-T) or ET (Exemestane 25 mg daily combined with Goserelin in premenopausal patients) for 24 weeks. Overall, the clinical response rate was higher with chemotherapy (66 % vs. 48 %; p = 0.075). In an unplanned exploratory subgroup analysis based on Ki-67 levels (10 % cut-off), similar clinical response was achieved in both treatment groups in patients with low Ki-67 (chemotherapy 63 %, ET 58 %; p = 0.74), while patients with high Ki-67 had a better response with chemotherapy (67 % vs. 42 %; p = 0.075). These results seem to suggest patients with low proliferation index could potentially avoid neoadjuvant chemotherapy [23]. The Neoadjuvant Chemotherapy versus ENdocrine Therapy (NeoCENT) feasibility trial, comparing letrozole for 18–23 weeks to 6 cycles of FEC100, met the recruitment and tissue collection primary endpoints, but despite both treatments showed to be equally effective, a larger phase III trial was deemed unfeasible due to slow accrual [24]. ET can therefore be an attractive alternative to chemotherapy as neoadjuvant therapy at least for some women with ER+ locally advanced primary BC. As neoadjuvant ET usually takes longer to achieve tumour response, treatment should continue for at least 4–8 months or until maximal response [7].

19.2.5 Premenopausal Patients

Little evidence is available in premenopausal patients with locally advanced ER+ BC, for whom the main goal of neoadjuvant therapy is to allow breast conservative surgery (BCS).

The STAGE trial is the only phase III, randomized, multicenter study, randomly assigning patients to receive monthly Goserelin plus either Anastrozole or tamoxifen for 24 weeks before surgery. The primary endpoint was best overall tumour response (complete or partial response). Among the 185 patients who completed the 24-week treatment period, more patients in the Anastrozole group had a complete or partial response than those in the tamoxifen group (70.4 % vs. 50.5 %, respectively). The authors concluded that given its favourable risk–benefit profile, the combination of Anastrozole plus Goserelin could represent an alternative neoadjuvant treatment option for premenopausal women [25]. Despite these encouraging results, data are insufficient to recommend this strategy outside of clinical trials [8].

19.2.6 Postmenopausal Patients

In postmenopausal patients, several randomized trials demonstrated the superiority of AIs over tamoxifen.

The P024 study, a large multinational double-blind trial comparing letrozole versus tamoxifen, showed a significantly better overall response rate (ORR) (55 % vs. 36 %, respectively, $p < 0.001$) and BCS rate (45 % vs. 35 %) with letrozole than with tamoxifen. letrozole was also significantly more effective than tamoxifen in reducing tumour proliferation, measured by Ki-67 immunohistochemistry ($p = 0.0009$) [26]. In addition, at a median follow-up of 61.2 months, patients with pathological stage 1 or 0 and a low-risk biomarker profile in the surgical specimen (Preoperative Endocrine Prognostic Index [PEPI] score 0) had an extremely low risk of relapse (100 % relapse-free survival [RFS]) compared with higher stages ($p < 0.001$) therefore unlikely to benefit from additional adjuvant chemotherapy [27]. On the contrary, a non-statistically significant difference was found between Anastrozole and tamoxifen in the Preoperative Arimidex Compared to Tamoxifen (PROACT) randomized, multicenter trial in women with large, operable (T2-3, N0-2, M0), or potentially operable (T4b, N0-2, M0) BC. Patients received Anastrozole or tamoxifen, with or without chemotherapy for 12 weeks. Objective responses (by ultrasound) were achieved in 39.5 and 35.4 % of patients under Anastrozole and tamoxifen, respectively. In ET-only treated patients, surgery became feasible in 47.2 % of patients receiving Anastrozole and 38.3 % of those receiving tamoxifen ($p = 0.15$) [28].

The IMPACT trial randomized women with ER+ operable or locally advanced BC (LABC) to Anastrozole, tamoxifen, or a combination of tamoxifen and Anastrozole for 12 weeks. Objective response rates, measured either by clinical examination or ultrasound, were not statistically significantly different between treatment arms. A trend towards an improved rate of BCS was observed for patients receiving Anastrozole over tamoxifen (44 % vs. 31 %), which was also not statistically significant ($p = 0.23$). A meta-analysis of these trials supported the notion that an AI is more effective than tamoxifen for promoting breast conservation [29].

Another randomized, double-blind, multicenter study was conducted to compare the anti-tumour activity of letrozole versus tamoxifen. After 4 months of treatment, the overall objective response rate by palpation was significantly superior in the letrozole group compared with tamoxifen (55 % vs. 36 %, $p < 0.001$). The secondary endpoints of ultrasound and mammographic response and BCS rate confirmed letrozole to be significantly superior [30].

In the randomized phase II ACOSOG Z1031 trial, women with clinical stage II-III ER+ BC were randomly assigned to receive neoadjuvant Exemestane, letrozole or Anastrozole for 16 weeks. The primary endpoint was clinical response; secondary endpoints included BCS and Ki-67 changes. Although higher clinical response rates were reported with letrozole and Anastrozole compared with Exemestane, no differences in surgical outcome or Ki-67 changes were detected [31].

On the basis of all these data, it can be concluded that either AI is more effective than tamoxifen in decreasing tumour size and facilitating conservative surgery.

19.3 Metastatic Therapy

Approximately, 10 % of newly diagnosed BC patients have locally advanced and/or metastatic disease and 30 % of women with early BC develop advanced disease during their disease history. As reported in the ABC2 ESO-ESMO international consensus guidelines, ET should be the first-choice therapy in ER+/HER2− disease, also in presence of visceral metastases [32]. Several sequential ETs can be given until disease progression, unacceptable toxicity or development of symptomatic visceral disease. The sequential use of ETs with different mechanisms of action may prolong the duration of response, reduce the risk of resistance and delay the need for chemotherapy [33]. Chemotherapy should be preferred only in case of high disease burden, life-threatening conditions requiring a rapid disease response or in presence of endocrine resistance. Endocrine resistance has been defined as follows: (1) primary endocrine resistance when a relapse occurs during the first two years of adjuvant ET, or a disease progression develops within the first six months of first-line ET for advanced breast cancer (ABC) and (2) secondary (or acquired) resistance when a relapse occurs after the first two years while on adjuvant ET, within 12 months of completing adjuvant ET, or progressive disease develops at least six months after initiating ET for ABC [32].

The selection of the most appropriate ET should take into account the menopausal status of the patient, the type of adjuvant ET received, any past medical history or comorbidities and patient's wishes. The concomitant use of chemotherapy and ET is not recommended, despite an increased ORR or time to progression (TTP) shown in some trials, as potentially antagonistic, but clinical trials in this area, with the newer classes of ETs and chemotherapy regimens/approaches, are lacking.

19.3.1 Premenopausal Patients

In premenopausal women, OFS/ablation combined with oral ET is the first-choice therapy; tamoxifen is the standard oral ET unless tamoxifen resistance is proven [8].

Ovarian ablation (OA) has long been established as an effective therapy for premenopausal women with ABC, with response rates ranging from 14 to 70 % in several studies. Both the presence and degree of HR expression are strongly predictive of response to endocrine manipulations, with responses seen in approximately 60 % of women having both ER+ and PR+ tumours, compared with 30 % in patients with either ER+ or PR+ disease alone [34].

After the introduction of GnRHa, several phase II trials investigated their efficacy in pre- and perimenopausal women with ABC. A meta-analysis of phase II trials with monthly Goserelin in 228 patients reported a median survival of 26.5 months, an ORR of 36 % (44 % in ER+ patients) and a median duration of response of 44 weeks, comparable to the outcomes historically obtained with oophorectomy in similar patient populations [35]. OA by laparoscopic bilateral oophorectomy ensures definitive oestrogen suppression and contraception, avoids potential initial tumour flare with GnRHa and represents a cost-effective alternative particularly in middle-low income countries. Patients should be informed on the options of OFS/OA and decision should be made on a case by case basis.

The comparison between combined ET (tamoxifen plus GnRHa) and single agent ET has been summarized in a meta-analysis of 4 clinical trials randomizing a total of 506 women with ABC to GnRHa alone or GnRHa plus tamoxifen. With a median follow-up of 6.8 years, the combination was superior to monotherapy for all endpoints, with significant benefits in mortality (22 % relative reduction), disease progression (30 % relative reduction), objective clinical response (39 % vs. 30 %) rates as well as response duration (19 months vs. 11 months) [36].

Little data are available on the association of GnRHa and AIs as first- and second-line therapy.

Two small phase II trials evaluated the efficacy of Goserelin plus Anastrozole in women with advanced or recurrent BC. The JMTO BC08-01 trial enrolled 37 patients after failure to standard GnRHa plus tamoxifen; the primary endpoint was objective response rate; secondary endpoints included PFS, OS, clinical benefit rate (CBR, defined as disease response plus disease stabilization ≥6 months) and safety. The objective response rate was 18.9 %, the CBR was 62.2 % and the median PFS was 7.3 months. Eight patients had adverse drug reactions but none resulted in treatment discontinuation [37]. The second phase II study was a prospective, single-arm, multicenter trial in which 35 patients were treated with monthly Goserelin and Anastrozole, the latter starting 21 days after the first GnRHa injection. Patients continued on treatment until disease progression or unacceptable toxicity. One patient (3.1 %) experienced a complete response, 11 (34.4 %) a partial response and 11 (34.4 %) a stable disease lasting at least 6 months, translating in a CBR of 71.9 %. Median TTP was 8.3 months and median survival was not reached at time of publication. As expected, the most common adverse events were fatigue (50 %), arthralgia (53 %) and hot flashes (59 %); no grade 4–5 toxicities were reported [38].

Similar results derive from a single-institution, retrospective analysis of Goserelin plus letrozole in a total of 52 patients as first- (n = 36) or second-line (n = 16) ET. The median treatment duration was 11 months and the median follow-up 31 months. The objective response rate was 21.1 %, including two complete responses (3.8 %) and nine partial responses (17.3 %); the CBR was 50.0 % for an overall clinical benefit of 71.1 % and the PFS was 10 months. Therapy was well tolerated; no grade 3–4 toxicities were reported [39].

Little data are also available on the association of GnRHa and Fulvestrant in this setting. In a small study (n = 26), patients eligible for ET received low-dose (LD) Fulvestrant (250 mg/monthly) and monthly Goserelin as first- to fourth-line therapy. The primary endpoint was CBR. Eighty-one per cent of patients were pre-treated with tamoxifen and 69 % had received prior AIs in combination with Goserelin. The majority of patients (69 %) presented with visceral metastases. The CBR was 58 %, median TTP was 6 months and OS 32 months [40]. Although the drug does appear to be active in this setting, it would deserve further evaluation, made difficult by the forthcoming patent expiration.

19.3.2 Postmenopausal Patients

In postmenopausal patients, the main ET options include the following: AIs, tamoxifen, high-dose (HD) Fulvestrant (i.e. 500 mg monthly) and megestrol acetate. The choice is based mainly on previous ETs received either in the adjuvant and/or advanced disease settings.

In first line, the superiority of AIs over tamoxifen has been tested in several trials [41–44]. A meta-analysis of 6 eligible trials (2.560 patients) showed a significant difference favouring AIs over tamoxifen in ORR (HR 1.56; 95 % CI 1.17–2.07; p = 0.002) and clinical benefit (HR 1.70; 95 % CI 1.24–2.33; p = 0.0009) and a non-significant trend towards an improved OS (HR 1.95; 95 % CI 0.88–4.30; p = 0.10). Toxicities did not differ significantly except for increased vaginal bleeding and thromboembolic events associated with tamoxifen [45]. In the FIRST phase II study [46], HD Fulvestrant proved to be superior to Anastrozole in terms of OS (median OS 54.1 months vs. 48.4 months; HR 0.70; 95 % CI 0.50–0.98; p = 0.04). These data need to be interpreted cautiously as the OS analysis was not originally planned and not all patients had OS follow-up: confirmation is awaited in the larger phase III FALCON trial

(NCT01602380). The combination of a non-steroidal AI and LD Fulvestrant showed discordant results in 2 phase III trials with similar designs [47, 48]. Subset analysis in the successful SWOG study suggests a benefit in PFS and OS for the combination therapy only in patients without prior adjuvant tamoxifen to whom this strategy can be offered. In this study, the addition of Fulvestrant to Anastrozole significantly decreased Anastrozole concentrations in a subset of patients treated with the combination, potentially affecting treatment efficacy [49].

Beyond first line, the optimal sequence of endocrine agents is uncertain and depends on which drugs were used in the neo/adjuvant and first-line ABC settings.

All trials comparing Fulvestrant to AIs in this setting were conducted with LD Fulvestrant. Both treatments are effective and well tolerated with a different toxicity profile which can guide treatment choice in the individual patient; joint disorders (i.e. arthralgia, arthrosis and arthritis), occurring more frequently in patients receiving AIs, are the only significant difference [50–52]. A potential advantage of Fulvestrant over AIs is the monthly parenteral administration, which can enhance long-term adherence at least in selected patients [53].

In the CONFIRM multicenter phase III study, 736 patients were randomly assigned to either HD or LD monthly Fulvestrant based on the observation from preoperative trials that both clinical and biological effects (ER/PR receptor and Ki-67 downregulation) could be dose-dependent. The HD schedule resulted in a significantly longer PFS, corresponding to a 20 % reduction in risk of progression. Fulvestrant 500 mg was well tolerated with no dose-dependent adverse events [54]. Median OS was 26.4 months for HD and 22.3 months for LD Fulvestrant (HR ratio 0.81; 95 % CI 0.69–0.96; nominal $p = 0.02$), corresponding to a 19 % reduction in the risk of death. Type of first subsequent therapy and objective responses to first subsequent therapy were well balanced between the two treatment groups [55].

19.3.3 Hormone Receptor Positive/Human Epidermal Growth Factor Receptor 2-Positive Breast Cancer (HR+/HER2+)

Approximately, 20 % of BC harbours an overexpression/amplification of HER2 and nearly 50 % of these tumours are also ER+ and/or PR+. The co-activation of both HR and HER2 pathways involves a different disease natural history and patients' outcome if compared with both HR−/HER2+ and HR+/HER2− tumours. In particular, prospective studies demonstrated different patterns of recurrence with more early relapses (instead of late) and brain metastases (instead of bone) as first site of relapse in HR−/HER2+ tumours compared with HR+/HER2+ tumours.

Moreover, the co-expression of HR and HER2 pathways seems to influence treatment efficacy: HER2 overexpression usually correlates with low HR expression and low response to ET, and it has been demonstrated that HER2 pathway activation may contribute to the development of endocrine resistance [56].

In the *adjuvant* setting, poorer outcomes have been shown in patients with HR+/HER2+ tumours compared with HR+/HER2− tumours.

Retrospective analysis of the ATAC and BIG1-98 trials reported worse clinical outcomes in postmenopausal HER2+ patients regardless of treatment type, confirmed the overall benefit of AIs over tamoxifen in this subgroup but failed to demonstrate a clear correlation between HER2 status, ET and long-term outcomes, in women frequently not exposed to HER2-targeted therapy due to enrolment periods [57, 58]. In premenopausal women enrolled in SOFT [11], the addition of OFS to tamoxifen appeared to be beneficial over tamoxifen alone (HR 0.78; 95 % CI, 0.62–0.98; $p = 0.03$) in HER2+ patients as previously reported by others [59]. On the other hand, in the combined TEXT–SOFT analysis [11], in the presence of OFS, Exemestane did not confer any advantage over tamoxifen (DFS HR 1.25; 95 % CI 0.80–1.94). HER2 central assessment and further analysis are, however, needed before HER2 status is used for oral ET selection in premenopausal women.

In the *advanced* setting, a retrospective analysis demonstrated better responses to chemotherapy plus anti-HER2 therapy in HR- tumours, whereas in HR+/HER2+ patients a significant benefit in PFS was achieved if maintenance ET was added to trastuzumab after chemotherapy [60]. On the contrary, in a retrospective observational study including patients with HER2+ disease treated with trastuzumab-based first-line therapy, a better long-term clinical benefit was observed in HR+ patients, probably because they received trastuzumab maintenance and/or ET after first-line treatment [61].

A prospective observational study in more than 1.000 HER2+ BC showed prolonged PSF and OS in HR+/HER2+ patients treated with dual targeting therapies (ET and anti-HER2 drugs, with or without chemotherapy), in comparison with patients treated with anti-HER2 therapy only [62].

All these data suggest the combination of ET with anti-HER2 therapies might represent a strategy to overcome both endocrine and anti-HER2 resistance in patients with advanced HR+/HER2+ BC. The TAnDEM trial was the first randomized phase III study to compare ET alone (Anastrozole) and ET plus HER2-targeted therapy (Anastrozole plus trastuzumab). The study showed an improved TTP for the combination over ET alone (2.4 months and 4.8 months respectively, $p = 0.0016$), with a median PFS of 3.8 months versus 5.6 months, an ORR of 7 % versus 20 % and a CBR of 28 % versus 43 %, respectively [63].

The eLEcTRA trial investigated letrozole versus the combination letrozole-trastuzumab. The results were in favour of the combination with a PFS of 14.1 months versus 3.3 months, ORR of 27 % versus 13 % and CBR of 65 % versus 39 % [64]. An additional phase III trial randomized 1.286 postmenopausal women to letrozole plus placebo or Lapatinib (1500 mg once daily) as first-line therapy [65]. In the subgroup of women with HR+/HER2+ disease ($n = 219$), after a median follow-up of 1.8 years, the combination was superior to letrozole alone in terms of median PFS (8.2 and 3.0 months, respectively, HR 0.71; 95 % CI 0.53–0.96, $p = 0.019$) and CBR (48 % vs. 29 %). There was no significant improvement in OS; however, less than 50 % of OS events had occurred at time of reporting.

Even though none of these trials demonstrated a clear benefit in OS, the ABC guidelines recommend the combination of trastuzumab or Lapatinib with an AIs as first-line therapy in postmenopausal women with HR+/HER2+ BC if chemotherapy is not clearly indicated [32].

19.4 Overcoming Endocrine Resistance

The main studied mechanisms of endocrine resistance refer to ER alterations, such as mutations, amplifications or translocations, and/or to upregulation of alternative pathways, such as the PI3K/Akt/mammalian target of rapamycin (mTOR) pathway.

The phase III BOLERO-2 trial investigated the role of everolimus in postmenopausal ER+ patients. Patients previously treated with a non-steroidal AI (NSAI) in the adjuvant setting or progressing under a NSAI in the metastatic setting were randomized to everolimus (10 mg daily) plus Exemestane (25 mg daily) versus placebo plus Exemestane. Previous therapy also included tamoxifen (48 %), LD Fulvestrant (16 %) and chemotherapy (68 %). At the first interim analysis, based on central disease evaluation, the median PFS favoured the combination versus placebo (10.6 vs. 4.1 months, respectively, HR 0.36, $p < 0.001$). At final analysis, with a median 18-month follow-up, the median PFS remained significantly longer with everolimus plus Exemestane versus placebo plus Exemestane (central review: 11.0 vs. 4.1 months, respectively, HR 0.38, $p < 0.0001$) in the overall population and in all prospectively defined subgroups, including patients with visceral metastases. The most common grade 3–4 adverse events in the everolimus arm were stomatitis, anaemia, dyspnea, hyperglycaemia, fatigue and pneumonitis. The OS analysis (secondary endpoint) did not confirm a statistically significant improvement in the everolimus arm (median OS of 31.0 months compared with 26.6 months in the placebo arm, HR 0.89, $p = 0.14$) [66–68].

Everolimus has been also investigated in combination with tamoxifen in a small randomized phase II trial in postmenopausal patients with metastatic BC resistant to AIs. Patients were randomized to tamoxifen 20 mg daily plus everolimus 10 mg daily or tamoxifen alone. The primary endpoint was CBR: the 6-month CBR was 61 % with tamoxifen plus everolimus and 42 % with tamoxifen alone. TTP also increased from 4.5 months to 8.6 months with tamoxifen plus everolimus, corresponding to a 46 % reduction in the risk of progression (HR 0.54). The risk of death was reduced by 55 % with the combination (HR 0.81). The main toxicities associated with tamoxifen plus everolimus were fatigue, stomatitis, rash, anorexia and diarrhoea [69].

Recently, evidence has been collected on the role of cyclin-dependent kinases 4 and 6 (CDK4-6) in the growth of ER + BC, based on their role in promoting progression from the G1 to the S phase of the cell cycle. The randomized phase I/II PALOMA-1 study showed a significant PFS improvement in patients treated with the combination of the CDK4/6 inhibitor Palbociclib and letrozole compared with letrozole alone as first-line treatment (20.2 months vs. 10.2 months, HR 0.488, $p = 0.0004$). The preliminary OS analysis suggested a non-statistically significant trend towards increased OS (37.5 months vs. 33.3 months, HR 0.813, $p = 0.2105$) in the combination arm. Based on these results, the FDA granted Palbociclib-accelerated approval as first-line treatment for postmenopausal women with HR+/HER2− ABC and the drug is going to become commercially available also in European countries [70]. The double-blind phase III PALOMA3 trial randomized 521 patients, regardless of menopausal status, who relapsed or progressed during prior ET, to receive Palbociclib plus HD Fulvestrant or HD Fulvestrant plus placebo. Premenopausal or perimenopausal women also received Goserelin. The primary endpoint was investigator-assessed PFS. Secondary endpoints included OS, objective response, CBR, patient-reported outcomes and safety. The median PFS was 9.2 months with Palbociclib-Fulvestrant and 3.8 months with placebo-Fulvestrant (HR 0.42). Of note, the relative difference in PFS was independent of menopausal status, providing a new treatment option also for young patients with ER+ ABC. Overall objective response was 10.4 % with Palbociclib-Fulvestrant and 6.3 % with placebo-Fulvestrant ($p = 0.16$). CBR at the interim analysis was 34.0 % with Palbociclib-Fulvestrant and 19.0 % with placebo-Fulvestrant ($p < 0.001$). At the time of the interim analysis, OS data were immature, with a total of 28 deaths: 19 patients (5.5 %) in the Palbociclib-Fulvestrant group and 9 (5.2 %) in the placebo-Fulvestrant group. The most common grade 3–4 adverse events in the Palbociclib-Fulvestrant group were neutropenia, leukopenia, anaemia, thrombocytopenia and fatigue [71].

19.5 New Perspectives

Additional mechanisms of ET resistance are under active investigation. An increased genetic heterogeneity has been demonstrated in metastatic tumour cells in comparison with the primary. Many hypotheses could explain this finding: the selection pressure favouring a resistant subclone, altered gene expression profile secondary to treatment exposure and stochastic mutations owing to genetic instability. While studying the most common pathways involved in these mechanisms of resistance, efforts are also directed to the identification of biomarkers predictive of response.

Phase II and III studies are ongoing further exploring the cost-effectiveness of mTOR inhibitors (also in the neoadjuvant setting), and the role of different CDK4-6 inhibitors (ribociclib, Abemaciclib), histone deacetylase inhibitors (entinostat), PI3K inhibitors (pictilisib, buparlisib). Such efforts could hopefully lead to an improvement in understanding and overcoming the mechanisms of resistance to ET. It is currently unknown how the different combinations of ET+ biological agents compare with each other and with single agent chemotherapy and whether a targeted agent should only be combined with ET to restore endocrine sensitivity or whether it may also prevent or delay the development of such a resistance [72]. Appropriate patient selection based on prior treatment history and disease characteristics will become increasingly important in maximizing the potential incremental benefit from these new agents combined with standard ET.

References

1. Bentzon N, Düring M, Rasmussen B, et al. Prognostic effect of estrogen receptor status across age in primary breast cancer. Int J Cancer. 2008;122:1089–94.
2. Early Breast Cancer Trialists' Collaborative Group. Effects of chemotherapy and hormonal therapy for early breast cancer on recurrence and 15-year survival: an overview of the randomised trials. Lancet. 2005;365:1687–717.
3. Davies C, Pan H, Godwin J, et al. Long-term effects of continuing adjuvant tamoxifen to 10 years versus stopping at 5 years after diagnosis of oestrogen receptor-positive breast cancer: ATLAS, a randomised trial. Lancet. 2013;381:805–15.
4. Gray R, Rea D, Handley K, et al. aTTom: long-term effects of continuing adjuvant tamoxifen to 10 years versus stopping at 5 years in 6,953 women with early breast cancer. J Clin Oncol. 2013; 31(suppl; abstr 5).
5. Cuzick J, Ambroisine L, et al. Use of luteinizing-hormone-releasing hormone agonists as adjuvant treatment in premenopausal patients with hormonereceptor-positive breast cancer: a meta-analysis of individual patient data from randomised adjuvant trials. Lancet. 2007;369:1711–23.
6. Francis P, Regan M, Fleming G, et al. Adjuvant ovarian suppression in premenopausal breast cancer. N Engl J Med. 2015;372:436–46.
7. Coates A, Winer E, Goldhirsch A, et al. Tailoring therapies-improving the management of early breast cancer: St Gallen International Expert Consensus on the Primary Therapy of Early Breast Cancer 2015. Ann Oncol. 2015;26(8):1533–46.
8. Paluch-Shimon S, Pagani O, Partridge A, et al. Second international consensus guidelines for breast cancer in young women (BCY2). Breast. 2016;26:87–99.
9. Burstein H, Lacchetti C, Anderson H, et al. Adjuvant endocrine therapy for women with hormone receptor-positive breast cancer: American Society of clinical oncology clinical practice guideline update on ovarian suppression. J Clin Oncol. 2016;pii:JCO659573.
10. Gradishar W, Anderson B, Balassanian R, et al. Invasive breast cancer version 1.2016, NCCN clinical practice guidelines in oncology. J Natl Compr Canc Netw. 2016;3(14):324–54.
11. Pagani O, Regan M, Walley B, et al. Adjuvant exemestane with ovarian suppression in premenopausal breast cancer. N Engl J Med. 2014;371:107–18.
12. Bernhard J, Luo W, Ribi K, et al. Patient-reported outcomes with adjuvant exemestane versus tamoxifen in premenopausal women with early breast cancer undergoing ovarian suppression (TEXT and SOFT): a combined analysis of two phase 3 randomised trials. Lancet Oncol. 2015;16:848–58.
13. Gnant M, Mlineritsch B, Stoeger H, et al. Zoledronic acid combined with adjuvant endocrine therapy of tamoxifen versus anastrozol plus ovarian function suppression in premenopausal early breast cancer: final analysis of the Austrian Breast and Colorectal Cancer Study Group Trial 12. Ann Oncol. 2015;26 (2):313–20.
14. Moore H, Unger J, Phillips K, et al. Goserelin for ovarian protection during breast-cancer adjuvant chemotherapy. N Engl J Med. 2015;372:923–32.
15. Regan M, Neven P, Giobbie-Hurder A, et al. Assessment of letrozole and tamoxifen alone and in sequence for postmenopausal women with steroid hormone receptor-positive breast cancer: the BIG 1–98 randomised clinical trial at 8.1 years median follow-up. Lancet Oncol. 2011;12:1101–8.
16. Cuzick J, Sestak I, Baum M, et al. Effect of anastrozole and tamoxifen as adjuvant treatment for early-stage breast cancer: 10-year analysis of the ATAC trial. Lancet Oncol. 2010;11:1135–41.
17. Dowsett M, Forbes J, Bradley R, et al. Aromatase inhibitors versus tamoxifen in early breast cancer: patient-level meta-analysis of the randomised trials. Early Breast Cancer Trialists' Collaborative Group (EBCTCG). Lancet. 2015;386(10001):1341–52.
18. Goss P, Ingle J, Martino S, et al. A randomized trial of letrozole in postmenopausal women after five years of tamoxifen therapy for early-stage breast cancer. N Engl J Med. 2003;349:1793–802.
19. Goss P, Ingle J, Martino S, et al. Randomized trial of letrozole following tamoxifen as extended adjuvant therapy in receptor-positive breast cancer: updated findings from NCIC CTG MA.17. J Natl Cancer Inst. 2005;97(17):1262–71.
20. von Minckwitz G, Untch M, Nüesch E, et al. Impact of treatment characteristics on response of different breast cancer phenotypes: pooled analysis of the German neo-adjuvant chemotherapy trials. Breast Cancer Res Treat. 2011;125(1):145–56.
21. von Minckwitz G, Raab G, Caputo A, et al. Doxorubicin with cyclophosphamide followed by docetaxel every 21 days compared with doxorubicin and docetaxel every 14 days as preoperative treatment in operable breast cancer: the GEPARDUO study of the German Breast Group. J Clin Oncol. 2005;23:2676–85.

22. von Minckwitz G, Untch M, Blohmer J, et al. Definition and impact of pathologic complete response on prognosis after neoadjuvant chemotherapy in various intrinsic breast cancer subtypes. J Clin Oncol. 2012;30(15):1796–804.
23. Alba E, Calvo L, Albanell J, et al. Chemotherapy (CT) and hormonotherapy (HT) as neoadjuvant treatment in luminal breast cancer patients: results from the GEICAM/2006-03, a multicenter, randomized, phase-II study. Ann Oncol. 2012;23(12):3069–74.
24. Palmieri C, Cleator S, Kilburn L, et al. NEOCENT: a randomised feasibility and translational study comparing neoadjuvant endocrine therapy with chemotherapy in ER-rich postmenopausal primary breast cancer. Breast Cancer Res Treat. 2014;148(3):581–90.
25. Masuda N, Sagara Y, Kinoshita T, et al. Neoadjuvant anastrozole versus tamoxifen in patients receiving goserelin for premenopausal breast cancer (STAGE): a double-blind, randomised phase 3 trial. Lancet Oncol. 2012;13:345–52.
26. Ellis M, Ma C. Letrozole in the neoadjuvant setting: the P024 trial. Breast Cancer Res Treat. 2007;105(Suppl 1):33–43.
27. Ellis M, Tao J, Luo J, et al. Outcome prediction for estrogen receptor-positive breast cancer based on postneoadjuvant endocrine therapy tumor characteristics. J Natl Cancer Inst. 2008;100 (19):1380–8.
28. Cataliotti L, Buzdar A, Noguchi S, et al. Comparison of anastrozole versus tamoxifen as preoperative therapy in postmenopausal women with hormone receptor-positive breast cancer: the pre-operative 'Arimidex' compared to tamoxifen (PROACT) trial. Cancer. 2006;106:2095–103.
29. Seo J, Kim Y, Kim J, et al. Meta-analysis of pre-operative aromatase inhibitor versus tamoxifen in postmenopausal woman with hormone receptor-positive breast cancer. Cancer Chemother Pharmacol. 2009;63:261–6.
30. Eiermann W, Paepke S, Appfelstaedt J, et al. Preoperative treatment of postmenopausal breast cancer patients with letrozole: a randomized double blind multicenter study. Ann Oncol. 2001;12:1527–32.
31. Ellis M, Suman V, Hoog J, et al. Randomized phase II neoadjuvant comparison between letrozole, anastrozole, and exemestane for postmenopausal women with estrogen receptor-rich stage 2 to 3 breast cancer: clinical and biomarker outcomes and predictive value of the baseline PAM50-based int. J Clin Oncol. 2011;29:2342–9.
32. Cardoso F, Costa A, Norton L, et al. ESO-ESMO 2nd international consensus guidelines for advanced breast cancer (ABC2). Breast. 2014;23(5):489–502.
33. Gluck S. Extending the clinical benefit of endocrine therapy for women with hormone receptor-positive metastatic breast cancer: differentiating mechanisms of action. Clin Breast Cancer. 2014;14:75–84.
34. Prowell T, Davidson N. What is the role of ovarian ablation in the management of primary and metastatic breast cancer today? Oncologist. 2004;9:507–17.
35. Blamey R, Jonat W, Kaufmann M, et al. Goserelin depot in the treatment of premenopausal advanced breast cancer. Eur J Cancer. 1992;28A:810–4.
36. Klijn J, Blamey R, Boccardo F, et al. Combined tamoxifen and luteinizing hormone-releasing hormone (LHRH) agonist versus LHRH agonist alone in premenopausal advanced breast cancer: a meta-analysis of four randomized trials. J Clin Oncol. 2001;19:343–53.
37. Nishimura R, Anan K, Yamamoto Y, et al. Efficacy of goserelin plus anastrozole in premenopausal women with advanced or recurrent breast cancer refractory to an LH-RH analogue with tamoxifen: results of the JMTO BC08-01 phase II trial. Oncol Rep. 2013;29:1707–13.
38. Carlson R, Theriault R, Schurman C, et al. Phase II trial of anastrozole plus goserelin in the treatment of hormone receptor-positive, metastatic carcinoma of the breast in premenopausal women. J Clin Oncol. 2010;28:3917–21.
39. Yao S, Xu B, Li Q, et al. Goserelin plus letrozole as first- or second-line hormonal treatment in premenopausal patients with advanced breast cancer. Endocr J. 2011;58(6):509–16.
40. Bartsch R, Bago-Horvath Z, Berghoff A, et al. Ovarian function suppression and fulvestrant as endocrine therapy in premenopausal women with metastatic breast cancer. Eur J Cancer. 2012;48 (13):1932–8.
41. Mouridsen H, Gershanovich M, Sun Y, et al. Phase III study of letrozole versus tamoxifen as first-line therapy of advanced breast cancer in postmenopausal women: analysis of survival and update of efficacy from the International Letrozole Breast Cancer Group. J Clin Oncol. 2003;21:2101–9.
42. Paridaens R, Dirix L, Beex L, et al. Phase III study comparing exemestane with tamoxifen as first-line hormonal treatment of metastatic breast cancer in postmenopausal women: the European Organisation for Research and Treatment of Cancer Breast Cancer Cooperative Group. J Clin Oncol. 2008;26:4883–90.
43. Bonneterre J, Thürlimann B, Robertson J, et al. Anastrozole versus tamoxifen as first-line therapy for advanced breast cancer in 668 postmenopausal women: results of the Tamoxifen or Arimidex Randomized Group Efficacy and Tolerability study. J Clin Oncol. 2000;18:3748–57.
44. Nabholtz J, Buzdar A, Pollak M, et al. Anastrozole is superior to tamoxifen as first-line therapy for advanced breast cancer in postmenopausal women: results of a North American multicenter randomized trial. J Clin Oncol. 2000;18:3758–67 (Arimidex Study Group).
45. Xu H, Liu Y, Li L. Aromatase inhibitor versus tamoxifen in postmenopausal woman with advanced breast cancer: a literature-based meta-analysis. Clin Breast Cancer. 2011;11 (4):246–51.
46. Ellis M, Llombart-Cussac A, Feltl D, et al. Fulvestrant 500 mg versus Anastrozole 1 mg for the first-line treatment of advanced breast cancer: overall survival analysis from the phase II FIRST study. J Clin Onco. 2015;133(32):3781–7.
47. Johnston S, Kilburn L, Ellis P, et al. Fulvestrant plus Anastrozole or placebo versus exemestane alone after progression on non-steroidal aromatase inhibitors in postmenopausal patients with hormone-receptor-positive locally advanced or metastatic breast cancer (SoFEA): a composite, multicentr. Lancet Oncol. 2013;14(10):989–98.
48. Mehta R, Barlow W, Albain K, et al. Combination Anastrozole and Fulvestrant in metastatic breast cancer. N Engl J Med. 2012;367(5):435–44.
49. Hertz D, Barlow W, Kidwell K, et al. Fulvestrant decreases Anastrozole drug concentrations when taken concurrently by patients with metastatic breast cancer treated on SWOG study S0226. Br J Clin Pharmacol. 2016;. doi:10.1111/bcp.12904.
50. Robertson J, Osborne C, Howell A, et al. Fulvestrant versus Anastrozole for the treatment of advanced breast carcinoma in postmenopausal women: a prospective combined analysis of two multicenter trials. Cancer. 2003;98(2):229–38.
51. Howell A, Pippen J, Elledge R, et al. Fulvestrant versus Anastrozole for the treatment of advanced breast carcinoma: a prospectively planned combined survival analysis of two multicenter trials. Cancer. 2005;104(2):236–9.
52. Chia S, Gradishar W, Mauriac L, et al. Double-blind, randomized placebo controlled trial of Fulvestrant compared with exemestane after prior nonsteroidal aromatase inhibitor therapy in postmenopausal women with hormone receptor-positive, advanced

breast cancer: results from EFECT. J Clin Oncol. 2008;26 (10):1664–70.
53. Ciruelos E, Pascual T, Arroyo Vozmediano M, et al. The therapeutic role of Fulvestrant in the management of patients with hormone receptor-positive breast cancer. Breast. 2014;23 (3):201–8.
54. Di Leo A, Jerusalem G, Petruzelka L, et al. Results of the CONFIRM phase III trial comparing Fulvestrant 250 mg with Fulvestrant 500 mg in postmenopausal women with estrogen receptor-positive advanced breast cancer. J Clin Oncol. 2010;28 (30):4594–600.
55. Di Leo A, Jerusalem G, Petruzelka L, et al. Final overall survival: Fulvestrant 500 mg vs 250 mg in the randomized CONFIRM trial. J Natl Cancer Inst. 2014; 106(1):djt337.
56. Schettini F, Buono G, Cardalesi C, et al. Hormone receptor/human epidermal growth factor receptor 2-positive breast cancer: where we are now and where we are going. Cancer Treat Rev. 2016;1 (46):20–6.
57. Dowsett M, Allred C, Knox J, et al. Relationship between quantitative estrogen and progesterone receptor expression and human epidermal growth factor receptor 2 (HER-2) status with recurrence in the Arimidex, Tamoxifen, alone or in combination trial. J Clin Oncol. 2008;26:1059–65.
58. Rasmussen B, Regan M, Lykkesfeldt A, et al. Adjuvant letrozole versus tamoxifen according to centrally-assessed ERBB2 status for postmenopausal women with endocrine-responsive early breast cancer: supplementary results from the BIG 1–98 randomised trial. Lancet Oncol. 2008;9:23–8.
59. Love R, Duc N, Havighurst T, et al. Her-2/neu overexpression and response to oophorectomy plus tamoxifen adjuvant therapy in estrogen receptor-positive premenopausal women with operable breast cancer. J Clin Oncol. 2003;21:453–7.
60. Montemurro F, Rossi V, Cossu Rocca M, et al. Hormone-receptor expression and activity of trastuzumab with chemotherapy in HER2-positive advanced breast cancer patients. Cancer. 2012;118:17–26.
61. Vaz-Luis I, Seah D, Olson E, et al. Clinicopathological features among patients with advanced human epidermal growth factor-2-positive breast cancer with prolonged clinical benefit to first- line trastuzumab-based therapy: a retrospective cohort study. Clin Breast Cancer. 2013;12:254–63.
62. Tripathy D, Kaufman P, Brufsky A, et al. First-line treatment patterns and clinical outcomes in patients with HER2-positive and hormone receptorpositive metastatic breast cancer from registHER. Oncologist. 2013;18:501–10.
63. Kaufman B, Mackey J, Clemens M, et al. Trastuzumab plus Anastrozole versus Anastrozole alone for the treatment of postmenopausal women with human epidermal growth factor receptor 2-positive, hormone receptor-positive metastatic breast cancer: results from the randomized phase III TAnDEM study. J Clin Oncol. 2009;27(33):5529–37.
64. Huober J, Fasching P, Barsoum M, et al. Higher efficacy of letrozole in combination with trastuzumab compared to letrozole monotherapy as firstline treatment in patients with HER2-positive, hormone-receptor-positive metastatic breast cancer—results of the eLEcTRA trial. Breast. 2012;21(1):27–33.
65. Johnston S, Pippen P, Pivot X, et al. Lapatinib combined with letrozole versus letrozole and placebo as first-line therapy for postmenopausal hormone receptor-positive metastatic breast cancer. J Clin Oncol. 2009;27:5538–46.
66. Baselga J, Campone M, Piccart M, et al. Everolimus in postmenopausal hormone receptor-positive advanced breast cancer. N Engl J Med. 2012;366(6):520–9.
67. Yardley D, Noguchi S, Pritchard K, et al. Everolimus plus exemestane in postmenopausal patients with HR+ breast cancer: BOLERO-2 final progression free survival analysis. Adv Ther. 2013;30:870–84.
68. Piccart M, Hortobagyi G, Campone M, et al. Everolimus plus exemestane for hormone receptor-positive, human epidermal growth factor receptor-2-negative advanced breast cancer: overall survival results from BOLERO-2. Ann Oncol. 2014;25 (12):2357–62.
69. Bachelot T, Bourgier C, Cropet C, et al. Randomized phase II trial of everolimus in combination with tamoxifen in patients with hormone receptor-positive, human epidermal growth factor receptor 2-negative metastatic breast cancer with prior exposure to aromatase inhibitors: a GINECO study. J Clin Oncol. 2012;30 (22):2718–24.
70. Finn R, Crown J, Lang I, et al. The cyclin-dependent kinase 4/6 inhibitor palbociclib in combination with letrozole versus letrozole alone as first-line treatment of oestrogen receptor-positive, HER2-negative, advanced breast cancer (PALOMA-1/TRIO-18): a randomised phase 2 study. Lancet Oncol. 2015;16(1):25–35.
71. Turner N, Ro J, André F, et al. Palbociclib in hormone-receptor-positive advanced breast cancer. N Engl J Med. 2015;373(3):209–19.
72. Jerusalem J, Bachelot T, Barrios C, et al. A new era of improving progression-free survival with dual blockade in postmenopausal HR(+), HER2(−) advanced breast cancer. Cancer Treat Rev. 2015;41(2):94–104.

Systemic Therapy

20

Frederik Marmé

20.1 Cytotoxic Agents

Cytotoxic agents still have to be considered as an important backbone in the treatment for many patients with breast cancer in the adjuvant as well as the metastatic setting; especially those who are not considered hormone-sensitive or who have developed endocrine resistance. The following overview addresses drugs that are registered and/or currently used in breast cancer.

20.1.1 Topoisomerase II Inhibitors

20.1.1.1 Anthracyclines

The biological functions of topoisomerase II (Top2) are complex and include a critical role in DNA replication and transcription as well as chromosome segregation. Top2 uses hydrolysis of ATP to cut the DNA double helix and is involved in the unwinding of DNA for transcription and replication.

Broadly, Top2-targeting drugs fall into two classes, so-called Top2 poisons and Top2 catalytic inhibitors. The first class of Top2 poisons comprises most of the clinically active agents, like anthracyclines, etoposide, and mitoxantrone. Their precise mode of action leading to clinical activity is not fully understood and the dominant effects likely differ from agent to agent. Top2 poisons lead to an accumulation of high levels of persistent covalent trapping of Top2 in DNA cleavage complexes.

Anthracyclines stabilize the topoisomerase II complex after it has broken the DNA chain for replication, preventing the DNA double helix from being resealed and thereby preventing the progress of replication. Top2 poisons cause DNA damage including DNA double strand breaks and proteins covalently bound to DNA. In addition, anthracyclines and mitoxantrone function as intercalators whereas etoposide is a non-intercalating Top2 poison. The induction of DNA double strand breaks rapidly leads to a DNA damage response, as reflected by ATM phosphorylation, γH2AX and RAD51 foci formation. Anthracyclines also elicit a variety of Top2 independent effects, including formation of free radicals, membrane damage and DNA–Protein crosslinks [1]. Anthracyclines belong to the most active agents in the treatment of breast cancer. The most commonly used anthracylines are epirubicin and doxorubicin (Table 20.1). In Europe anthracyclines have been used for the treatment of metastatic breast cancer since the 1980s, whereas in the U.S. their approval by the Food and Drug Administration (FDA) followed somewhat later in 1990. The optimal dose of anthracyclines has not been fully established; however, there is an agreement that the therapeutic window is between 20 and 25 mg/m^2/week for doxorubicin and 30–40 mg/m^2/week for epirubicin. Schedules using lower doses have shown significantly lower efficacy and schedules using higher doses, especially of doxorubicin, have shown no increase in efficacy but higher toxicity.

In metastatic disease anthracyclines are nowadays mostly used as monotherapy since the sequential use of single agents is generally regarded as the standard. The use of combination chemotherapy should be restricted to visceral crisis situations, rapid disease progression or strong symptomatic burden [2]. However, as many patients have been pretreated with anthracyclines as they have become standard of care in the adjuvant setting, the use in the metastatic disease has decreased considerably. Anthracycline rechallenge is complicated by their maximum cumulative dose.

In the (neo)adjuvant setting, as per label, anthracyclines originally were approved for primary, node-positive breast cancer, regardless of hormone receptor (HR) or HER2 status. However, since decisions on adjuvant chemotherapy today are more dependent on tumor biology than on stage, they are also routinely used in node-negative primary breast cancer as long as chemotherapy is indicated and there are no relevant comorbidities or cardiac risks.

F. Marmé (✉)
Department of Gynecologic Oncology, National Center of Tumor Diseases, Heidelberg University Hospital, Heidelberg, Germany
e-mail: frederik.marme@med.uni-heidelberg.de

I. Jatoi and A. Rody (eds.), *Management of Breast Diseases*, DOI 10.1007/978-3-319-46356-8_20

Table 20.1 A summary of selected topoisomerase II inhibitors in breast cancer

Medication	Trade name® (examples)	Dosing (mg/m² BSA)	Precautions	Selected interactions	Selected side effects
Epirubicin	Farmorubicin	90–120 q3w in adjuvant regimens 20–30 q1w as a single agent, e.g., in MBC	Save IV application (severe tissue necrosis may occur in case of extravasation); monitor cardiac function; do not exceed maximum cumulative dose; dose reduction in case of liver impairment	Inhibitors and inducers of CYP3A4 and p-GP, Interferone, H2-antihistaminics (e.g., cimetidine)	left ventricular dysfunction, chronic heart failure, acute cardiac toxicity in form of arrhythmias, myelosuppression AML/MDS, mucositis, severe tissue damage/necrosis, thrombophlebitis/phlebosclerosis vomiting, alopecia
Doxorubicin	Adriamycin, Adriblastin	Single agent 60–75 q3w 40–60 in combinations regimens	Save IV application, (severe tissue necrosis may occur in case of extravasation); monitor cardiac function; do not exceed maximum cumulative dose; dose reduction in case of liver impairment	Inhibitors and inducers of CYP3A4 and p-GP, Interferone, H2-antihistaminics (e.g., cimetidine)	left ventricular dysfunction, chronic heart failure, acute cardiac toxicity in form of arrhythmias, myelosuppression AML/MDS, mucositis, severe tissue damage/necrosis, thrombophlebitis/phlebosclerosis, vomiting, alopecia
Pegylated liposomal doxorubicin	Caelyx, Doxil	40–50 q4w	Monitor cardiac function		Myelosuppression, mucositis, nausea and vomiting, left ventricular dysfunction, and chronic heart failure (lower risk compared to non-liposomal formulations), local tissue toxicity, dermatologic toxicity, palmar-plantar erythrodysesthesia/ (hand–foot-skin syndrome), hypersensitivity reaction
Mitoxantrone		12–14 IV q3w	Do not exceed maximum cumulative dose (160–200 mg/m²) Dose modifications according to myelotoxicity and liver impairment Monitor cardiac function if anthracycline-pretreated or cardiovascular risk factors		Myelosuppression, congestive heart failure, secondary leukemia, transient ECG alterations, local tissue damage in case of paravasation, nausea and vomiting, mucositis, alopecia, blue discoloration of urine, and sclerea Cumulative max dose 160–200 mg/m²
Liposomal doxorubicin	Myocet	60–75 q3w in combination with cyclophosphamide (600) q3w	monitor cardiac function; dose reduction in case of liver impairment		Myelosuppression, febrile neutropenia, cardiotoxicity, nausea and vomiting, mucositis, elevation of liver enzymes, hypersensitivity reactions, local tissue toxicity, alopecia, asthenia/fatigue

These highlights do not include all the information needed to use the respective drugs safely and effectively. See full prescribing information for all information needed to use these agents safely. We do not take responsibility for the correctness of the content

For (neo)adjuvant therapy, they are used as part of combination regimens, most frequently in combination with cyclophosphamide, followed by the sequential administration of taxanes or in three drug combinations with 5-fluorouracil and cyclophosphamide or docetaxel and cyclophosphamide (Table 20.2).

Historically, anthracyclines substituted the adjuvant CMF regimen not based on superiority. Two National Surgical Adjuvant Breast and Bowel Project (NSABP) studies (B-15 and B-23) showed that 4 cycles of AC (doxorubicin [60 mg/m²], cyclophosphamide [600 mg/m²]) were equivalent to six cycles CMF with regard to disease-free survival (DFS) and overall survival (OS). Significantly shorter duration of therapy, less frequent applications, and improved tolerability supported the use of AC instead of CMF [3, 4]. In the Cancer and Leukemia Group B (CALGB) 9344 trial, dose escalations of doxorubicin from 60 to up 90 mg/m² in combination with cyclophosphamide (600 mg/m²) did not improve efficacy of the AC combination any further [5]. Subsequently, several studies have demonstrated superiority

Table 20.2 Selected (neo)adjuvant chemotherapy regimens recommended by the NCCN and/or the German AGO guidelines [305, 306] and regimens of commonly used

Setting	Regimen		Cytotoxic agents	Dosing (mg/m^2)	Schedule, cycles
HER2-negative	AC-T_w	AC followed by weekly Paclitaxel	Doxorubicin Cyclophosphamide	60 600	q3w × 4
			Paclitaxel	80	qw × 12
	EC-T_w	EC followed by weekly Paclitaxel	Epirubicin Cyclophosphamide	90 600	
			Paclitaxel	80	qw × 12
	AC-Doc	AC followed by weekly Docetaxel	Doxorubicin Cyclophosphamide	60 600	q3w × 4
			Docetaxel	100	q3w × 4
	EC-Doc	EC followed by weekly Docetaxel	Epirubicin Cyclophosphamide	90 600	q3w × 4
			Docetaxel	100	q3w × 4
	TAC (DAC)	Docetaxel/Doxorubicin/Cyclophosphamide	Docetaxel Doxorubicin Cyclophosphamide	75 50 500	q3w × 6
	ddAC-ddT	Dose-dense AC followed by dose-dense Paclitaxel	Doxorubicin Cyclophosphamide	60 600	q2w × 4
			Paclitaxel	175	q2w × 4
	ddEC-ddT	Dose-dense EC followed by dose-dense Paclitaxel	Epirubicin Cyclophosphamide	90 600	q2w × 4
			Paclitaxel	175	q2w × 4
	ddAC-T_w	Dose-dense AC followed by weekly Paclitaxel	Doxorubicin Cyclophosphamide	60 600	q2w × 4
			Paclitaxel	80	qw × 12
	ddEC-T_w	Dose-dense AC followed by weekly Paclitaxel	Epirubicin Cyclophosphamide	90 600	q2w × 4
			Paclitaxel	80	qw × 12
	DC	Docetaxel/cyclophosphamide	Docetaxel Cyclophosphamide	75 600	q3w × 4
	Classic CMF	CMF	Cyclophosphamide Methotrexat 5-Fluorouracil	600 IV d 1 + 8 or 100 p.o. d 1–14 40 IV d 1 + 8 600 i.v. d 1 + 8	q4w × 6
	FEC-DOC	FEC followed by Docetaxel	5-Fluorouracil Epirubicin Cyclophosphamide	500 100 500	q3w × 3
			Docetaxel	100	q3w × 3
	iddETC	Dose-intense, dose-dense epirubicin followed sequentially by paclitaxel and cyclophosphamide	Epirubicin Paclitaxel Cyclophosphamide	150 225 2000	q2w × 3, q2w × 3, q2w × 3

(continued)

Table 20.2 (continued)

Setting	Regimen		Cytotoxic agents	Dosing (mg/m²)	Schedule, cycles
HER2-positive	AC − T + Tras	EC followed by paclitaxel** + trastuzumab	Doxorubicin Cyclophosphamide	60 600	q3w × 4
			Paclitaxel Trastuzumab	80 2 (4)[a] mg/kg (6 mg/kg)	qw × 12 qw × 12 (q3w to complete 1 year)
	EC − T + Tras	EC followed by paclitaxel** + trastuzumab	Epirubicin Cyclophosphamide	90 600	q3w × 4
			Paclitaxel Trastuzumab	80 2 (4)[a] mg/kg (6 mg/kg)	qw × 12 qw × 12 (q3w to complete 1 year)
	AC − T + Tras + Per*	AC followed by paclitaxel** + trastuzumab + pertuzumab*	Doxorubicin Cyclophosphamide	60 600	q3w × 4
			Paclitaxel Trastuzumab (Pertuzumab)*	80 2 (4[a]) mg/kg (6 mg/kg) 420 mg absolute (840 mg[a]) [a]*loading dose*	qw × 12 qw × 12 (q3w to complete 1 year) q3w during neoadjuvant therapy
	EC − T/Tras ±Per*	EC followed by paclitaxel** + trastuzumab + pertuzumab*	Epirubicin Cyclophosphamide	90 600	q3w × 4
			Paclitaxel Trastuzumab (Pertuzumab)*	80 2 (4[a]) mg/kg (6 mg/kg) 420 mg absolute (840 mg[a]) [a]*loading dose*	qw × 12 qw × 12 (q3w to complete 1 year) q3w during neoadjuvant therapy
	TCH ± pertuzumab	Docetaxel/Carboplatin/Trastuzmab/±Pertuzumab	Docetaxel Carboplatin Trastuzumab (Pertuzumab)*	75 AUC6 2 (4[a]) mg/kg (6 mg/kg) 420 mg absolute (840 mg[a]) [a]*loading dose*	q3w q3w qw × 12 (q3w to complete 1 year) q3w during neoadjuvant therapy
	Paclitaxel + trastuzumab	Paclitaxel/Trastuzumab	Paclitaxel Trastuzumab	80 2 (4)* mg/kg (6 mg/kg)	qw × 12 qw × 12 (q3w to complete 1 year)

*Pertuzumab is currently only approved for *neoadjuvant* therapy in patients with HER2-positive breast cancer at high risk of recurrence. **Paclitaxel might be substituted by docetaxel. These highlights do not include all the information needed to use the respective drugs safely and effectively. See full prescribing information for all information needed to use these agents safely. We do not take responsibility for the correctness of the content

of anthracycline-containing combination regimens over CMF, most using higher doses or longer treatment schedules. The Canadian MA.5 study, which compared six cycles of $FE_{120}C$ (colloquially known as "Canadian FEC") with an administration of epirubicin (60 mg/m^2) and 5-FU (500 mg/m^2) both on day 1 and 8 and oral cyclophosphamide (75 mg/m^2) per day through days 1–14 in a 28-day cycle to classical CMF demonstrated a 5-year event-free survival of 63 % for patients treated with FEC in comparison to 53 % for patients treated with CMF ($p < 0.009$). The corresponding overall survival rates were 77 and 70 %, respectively, ($p < 0.03$) [6]. The benefit was maintained with longer follow-up [7]. The NEAT and BR9601 trial, two phase III trials from the U.K., investigated the efficacy of epirubicin (100 mg/m^2) given for four cycles (q3w) followed by four cycles of CMF compared to six and eight cycles of CMF, respectively. The epirubicin-containing regimens demonstrated an improved relapse-free and overall survival at 5 years in a combined analysis (76 % vs. 69 % and 82 % vs. 75 %; both $p < 0{,}001$, respectively) [8]. In a phase III trial conducted by the Spanish Breast Cancer Research Group (GEICAM), six cycles of FAC q3w (500/50/500) proved to be superior to six cycles CMF in terms of DFS and OS, an effect predominantly seen in node-negative patients [9].

The French Adjuvant Study Group (FASG) investigated the effect of dose intensity of epirubicin in their randomized phase III FASG05 trial. They compared six cycles of $FE_{50}C$ to six cycles of $FE_{100}C$. Patients receiving $FE_{100}C$ had a significantly improved DFS and OS (5-year OS rates: 77.4 % vs. 65.3 %, $p = 0.007$) [10, 11]. A similar dose–response relationship was seen in 2 phase III trials in metastatic breast cancer (MBC) with improved response rates, time to progression and DFS for $FE_{100}C$ [12, 13]. Prior to the taxane era, $FE_{100}C$, also known as "French FEC," was a popular standard regimen for adjuvant chemotherapy of early breast cancer (EBC) in Europe. Epirubicin doses of 50 mg/m^2 in adjuvant combination regimens are considered underdosed.

Overall, trials comparing anthracycline-based chemotherapy to CMF regimens have been heterogeneous in terms of dose intensity, cumulative anthracycline dose as well as in terms of results. The Early Breast Cancer Trialists' Collaborative Group (EBCTCG) performed an individual patient data meta-analysis of randomized adjuvant trials including over 14,000 patients in trials comparing anthracycline-based regimens to standard CMF. In this meta-analysis four cycles of standard AC were equivalent to standard CMF (overall mortality RR 0.97, $p = 0.55$). However, anthracycline-based regimens with higher cumulative dosages than standard 4 × AC (epirubicin ≥ 90 mg/m^2 per cycles or a cumulative dose of >360 mg/m^2 and doxorubicin ≥60 mg/m^2 per cycle or a cumulative dose of >240 mg/m^2; e.g., FEC or FAC) were significantly more effective in reducing breast cancer and overall mortality (OS RR 0.84 $p = 0.0002$). The superiority was seen independent of age, hormone receptor (HR) status, differentiation, tamoxifen use, or lymph node status [14]. Prior to the implementation of taxane-based regimens, FAC and FEC were considered as widely accepted standard therapies. However, considering the proven benefit of taxanes in adjuvant therapy today, anthracycline-based, non-taxane-containing regimens are only used in exceptions. Table 20.2 gives a summary of the recommended and most frequently used adjuvant chemotherapy regimens.

Anthracycline-related toxicities

Anthracyclines can cause severe tissue necrosis if extravasation occurs. Therefore, careful intravenous administration is a prerequisite. If extravasation is suspected, administration needs to be stopped and close observation and plastic surgery consultation are recommended. If blistering or ulceration occurs, wide excision with split-thickness skin grafting is indicated. Intermittent application of ice for 15 min. q.i.d. for three days may be helpful. The role of local administration of drugs (e.g., dexrazosan [Savene®, Totect™]) has not been clearly established. The most frequent acute toxicity is neutropenia with a risk of febrile neutropenia that is usually below the threshold of 20 %, which is the threshold for primary G-CSF prophylaxis in most guidelines in the absence of patient-related risk factors. Only the three drug combination TAC has a febrile neutropenia rate of above 20 % and mandates primary G-CSF (and potentially antibiotics) prophylaxis [15]. Alopecia, mucositis, nausea and vomiting, and thrombophlebitis/phlebosclerosis are further acute toxicities observed with anthracyclines.

Long-term toxicities of anthracyclines have long been recognized and remain of concern. They include congestive heart failure and acute myeloid leukemia (AML) and myelodysplastic syndromes (MDS).

Cardiotoxicity

Cardiac toxicity of anthracyclines is attributed to the generation of free radicals and death of cardiomyocytes as a result of oxidative stress. This so-called type I cardiotoxicity is distinct from trastuzumab-related type 2 cardiotoxicity, which in contrast is generally considered reversible and dose independent. The risk of systolic dysfunction and congestive heart failure is directly related to the lifetime cumulative dose with an estimated risk of congestive heart failure of around 1 % for present standard doses of doxorubicin of 240 mg/m^2 (e.g., 4 cycles of AC) but increasing to around 5 % for cumulative doses of 400 mg/m^2 to near to 15 and 25 % for doses of 500 and 550 mg/m^2, respectively [16]. At equimolar doses, epirubicin is less cardiotoxic than doxorubicin [17]. In a pooled analysis of eight FASG trials, the rate of congestive heart failure after 7 years was 1.4 % for epirubicin-treated patients at a cumulative dose of about 300 mg/m^2 as compared to 0.2 % in CMF treated patients or controls [18]. However, cumulative doses administered in adjuvant epirubicin-containing regimens are considerably higher and the same dose effect as for doxorubicin also applies to epirubicin. At a cumulative dose of 900 mg/m^2, the expected rate of congestive heart failure is 4 %, which rises to 15 % for doses of 1000 mg/m^2 [19]. In the MA.5 trial with a cumulative dose of epirubicin of 720 mg/m^2 [given as 60 mg/m^2 on day 1 and 8 of each of cycles (q4w)] per protocol, the rate of congestive heart failure was 1.1 % compared to 0.3 % in the CMF group [7] Long-term follow-up of the FASG05 trial reported congestive heart failure in 2.3 % of patients available for evaluation and treated with a cumulative dose of epirubicin of 600 mg/m^2 and 0 % in the FE$_{50}$C arm [20]. Rates of systolic dysfunction (without signs of CHF) measured as a decrease of LVEF of more than 10–15 % or below or near to 50 % are reported to be higher. However, the clinical relevance of these observations is unclear. Risk of cardiotoxicity is increased by additional risk factors such as age, prior mediastinal radiation (e.g., Mantel field for Hodgkin lymphoma), hypertension, diabetes, and other cardiovascular risk factors. In addition to the risk of type 1 cardiotoxicity, prior therapy with anthracyclines also increases the risk of trastuzumab-related type 2 toxicity [21].

Maximum cumulative doses of 450 mg/m^2 for doxorubicin and 900 mg/m^2 are usually given according to different sources including manufacturers. However, the best option to minimize cardiotoxicity is to restrict cumulative doses to 360 and 720 mg/m^2, respectively, and be cautious when treating patients older than 65 and with borderline LVEF (50–55 %) where anthracycline-free alternatives should be considered. Reassuringly, all contemporary and widely used anthracycline-containing adjuvant regimens remain well below these strict thresholds and yield CHF rates of 1–2 % or less in patients without risk factors.

AML, MDS

The second long-term toxicity, which causes concern, is a low but increased risk of secondary acute myelogeneous leukemia (AML) and myelodysplastic syndromes (MDS). Treatment-associated AML/MDS occurring after chemotherapy is associated with complex cytogenetics, high-risk karyotypes, and a poorer prognosis compared to de novo AML [22]. Like in congestive heart failure, the risk is proportional to the dose of anthracyclines used. In addition, the cumulative risk of AML/MDS is also related to the dose of cyclophosphamide given, a drug frequently combined with anthracyclines in the adjuvant treatment of primary breast cancer (PBC) [23].

A review of follow-up data of almost 10,000 patients from 19 trials in an effort to investigate the rate of AML/MDS after epirubicin chemotherapy demonstrated an 8-year cumulative risk of 0.55 % in patients treated with epirubicin-containing regimens. Nearly all had also received cyclophosphamide. In patients with cumulative doses of epirubicin and cyclophosphamide equal or less then contemporary (at that time) regimens (E: $\leq$ 720 mg/m^2; C: $\leq$ 6300 mg/m^2) the cumulative risk was only 0.37 % and near to that of patients treated with tamoxifen alone or epirubicin-free chemotherapy. In contrast, the risk increased to up to 4.97 % in patients receiving substantially higher doses of both drugs [24]. In a combined analysis of six NSABP trials investigating different intensities of AC, patients treated with four cycles of standard AC (60/600) had a 5-year cumulative rate of AML/MDS of 0.21 %. Similarly to the data for epirubicin, the risk increased with increasing doses of cyclophosphamide (up to 1 %) and the use of breast irradiation [23]. Wolff et al. reported 51 patients who developed acute leukemia after breast cancer amongst 20,000 patients with stage I-III breast cancer treated within Centers of the National Comprehensive Cancer Network. The 5- and 10-year incidence of marrow neoplasm in patients treated with surgery only was 0.05 and 0.2 % but 0.27 and 0.49 % in patients who received adjuvant chemotherapy. Rates for patients receiving adjuvant chemotherapy plus radiation were similar (0.32 and 0.51 %, respectively) [25]. In an observational study based on data from the Surveillance, Epidemiology, and End Results (SEER) database including almost 65,000 women with nonmetastatic breast cancer of whom about 10,000 received adjuvant chemotherapy, the 10-year absolute risk of AML as identified by claims for its treatment was 1.8 % as compared to 1.2 % in those not treated with adjuvant chemotherapy. Radiotherapy in this study did not increase the risk of AML [26]. The study has its limitations as it only included patients over the age of 66 and data on the drug schedules and dosages used were not available and the diagnoses of AML and chemotherapy use were deducted from Medicare claims. MDS for example cannot be identified by claims. In Europe, dose-dense, dose-intensified adjuvant regimens are considered a possible standard for patients with high nodal stage. The regimen developed by Moebus et al. provided a 10 % OS benefit at 10 years for patients with four or more involved lymph nodes. After a median follow-up of 62 months, the trial reported four AML cases in the 658 patients (0.61 %) treated with the intensified regimen (cumulative dose of epirubicin: 450 mg/m^2 and cyclophosphamide: 7500 mg/m^2) versus none in the conventionally scheduled arm (cum. dose of epirubicin: 360 mg/m^2 and cyclophosphamide: 2400 mg/m^2). The background lifetime risk of AML is estimated to be 0.4 %. Therefore, contemporary adjuvant anthracycline-based chemotherapy regimens add only little to this absolute risk and the benefits of adjuvant chemotherapy, if indicated wisely, outweigh these risks largely [27].

Continuing role of anthracyclines in adjuvant chemotherapy and alternative anthracycline-free regimens

The compelling efficacy and routine use of taxanes in PBC combined with concerns about the long-term anthracycline-related toxicities (AML, MDS and congestive heart failure, etc.) started a debate if anthracyclines are still indispensable in the adjuvant chemotherapy for early stage breast cancer. Two prominent randomized trials have addressed this question in both HER2-negative as well as HER2-positive disease. The US Oncology 9735 phase III trial (n = 1016) demonstrated superior disease-free as well as overall survival for four cycles of TC (docetaxel, cyclophosphamide) over four cycles of AC (doxorubicin, cyclophosphamide) [28]. Most patients in the trial had HR-positive disease, half were node-negative, and only a minority (11 %) had four or more involved lymph nodes. Thus, applicability of the results cannot confidently be extended to patients with high-risk breast cancer. However, the trial was not designed to investigate the efficacy of a non-anthracycline-containing regimen compared to an anthracycline/taxane combination. Shulman et al. failed to prove non-inferiority of four or six cycles weekly paclitaxel to AC in a large randomized phase III trial in patients with none to three involved axillary lymph nodes (n = 3871) [29]. A second trial provides support for anthracycline-free adjuvant chemotherapy in HER2-positive disease. The Breast Cancer International Research Group 006 phase III trial (BCIRG006; n = 3222) [21, 30] randomized patients to either AC-T (without trastuzumab), AC-T with trastuzumab (AC-TH) or TCbH (Docetaxel, Carboplatin, and Trastuzumab). Both trastuzumab containing regimens were superior to AC-T in terms of DFS. There was a small non-significant numerical difference in DFS events between AC-TH and TCbH in favor of AC-TH, however, this was counterbalanced by a fivefold increase of congestive heart failure at 10 years (n = 21 vs. n = 4) and an increased risk of treatment-associated leukemia (n = 8 vs. n = 1) for the AC-TH arm [30]. Subgroup analysis stratified by nodal status suggests a similar efficacy in of AC-TH and TCbH in patients with four or more involved lymph nodes. The trial was not powered to detect differences between the AC-TH and TCbH arm. Trastuzumab may also be added to other non-anthracycline-based regimens like TC [31, 32] or weekly paclitaxel, however, so far there are only data from single-arm trials. Trastuzumab is very effective in HER2-positive disease and optimizing the chemotherapy backbone in this setting might not be of such importance. Hence, these results cannot be generalized to HER2-negative disease in which effective targeted therapies (other than endocrine) are not available. Robust evidence supports the use of anthracycline- **and** taxane-based combinations, and cumulative anthracycline doses used in contemporary regimens convey a low risk of long-term toxicity. However, the data support the omission of anthracyclines in patients at risk of anthracycline toxicity, e.g., older patient or those with risk factors for CHF or patients at the lower end of the spectrum of recurrence risk [27]. In fact in the U.S. the use of anthracyclines has substantially decreased over the last years [33, 34]. Evidence of superiority or non-inferiority of an anthracycline-free taxane-based regimen over an anthracycline and taxane combination is needed before anthracyclines could be omitted across all patient subgroups. Ongoing trials like the WSG PlanB trial (NCT01049425) and the US Oncology "TIC/TAC" trial (NCT00493870), both comparing TC to TAC will answer this question but results are still pending. Until these data are available, anthracyclines remain an integral part of adjuvant chemotherapy for many women with PBC.

Liposomal anthracyclines

Anthracyclines are considered among the most effective drugs for the treatment of breast cancer. Yet, their use is limited by a cumulative (cardio-) toxicity. This is a major limitation of treatment for metastatic breast cancer and often precludes anthracycline rechallenge which is not uncommon practice for taxanes for example. Nonetheless, liposomal formulations of doxorubicin are available, which exhibit a significantly reduced cardiotoxicity and differ considerably from nonencapsulated doxorubicin in their toxicity profile and pharmacokinetics. Pegylated liposomal doxorubicin (PLD; Doxil/Caelyx®) has been licensed in Europe for the treatment of metastatic breast cancer in patients at increased cardiac risk based on a phase III trial demonstrating comparable efficacy to doxorubicin but a significantly reduced cardiotoxicity even at higher cumulative doses [35]. PLD is also characterized by lower rates of alopecia and myelosuppression but higher rates of mucositis and palmar-plantar erythrodysesthesia (see Table 20.1). Due to the relatively high rate of PPE, PLD is frequently used at a dose of 40 mg/m^2 as opposed to the 50 mg/m^2 in the label [36]. In the U.S. as well as in Europe it is also approved for the treatment of recurrent ovarian cancer, AIDS-related Kaposi's sarcoma, and multiple myeloma. Non-pegylated liposomal doxorubicin (Myocet®) has been approved in Europe and Canada as a first-line treatment of metastatic breast cancer in combination with cyclophosphamide based on superior TTP in a phase III trial [37]. Like PLD, it is associated with a significantly reduced cardiotoxicity but due to its different pharmacokinetic profile, it produces less PPE [38]. Although data are limited, liposomal formulations of doxorubicin appear to be more effective in patients previously treated with anthracyclines and there is a rationale for a rechallenge with liposomal anthracyclines in some circumstances [38].

Mitoxantrone and other topoisomerase II inhibitors

In some European countries like Germany, mitoxantrone is approved for the treatment of metastatic breast cancer as well as for the treatment of hormone-refractory prostate cancer and in combination regimens for acute nonlymphocytic leukemia, whereas the FDA label only includes prostate cancer and acute leukemia. In early trials mitoxantrone as a single agent has been shown to be similarly active or at most only marginally less active when directly compared to single agent doxorubicin (n = 325) as a second-line therapy [39] or compared to $FE_{50}C$ in the first-line setting ($n = 260$) [40], however, with significantly reduced toxicity in terms of nausea and vomiting, mucositis, alopecia as well as cardiotoxicity (Table 20.1). The most frequent toxicity is myelosuppression and infections. Cardiotoxicity, even if less frequent when compared to doxorubicin and epirubicin, can occur and cumulative doses of >160 mg/m^2 should be avoided. Special caution should be taken in anthracycline-pretreated patients and patients with cardiovascular disease or risk factors. Despite its proven activity against and approval at least in parts of the world, mitoxantrone hardly has a role in the treatment of metastatic breast cancer mostly due to the frequent anthracycline use in the adjuvant setting and the availability of several drugs with proven single agent activity and favorable toxicity profiles. Etoposide and other topoisomerase II inhibitors are not approved for the treatment of breast cancer.

20.1.2 Tubulin Inhibitors

Tubulin inhibitors are a class of drugs that bind to tubulin. A- and β-tubulin are the main components of microtubules, which are key components of the cytoskeleton and exert important functions in eukaryotic cells. They build up the mitotic spindle and is important for intracellular organelle transport, axonal transport, and cell motility. By binding to β-tubulin, tubulin inhibitors interfere with either microtubule polymerization or depolymerization, which interrupts proper function of the mitotic spindle. The first tubulin-binding drug, colchicine, was isolated from the autumn crocus but is not used in cancer therapy.

Vinca alkaloids, taxanes, epothilones, and halichondrins represent the tubulin inhibitors currently used as cytotoxic agents. They have originally all been isolated from plants or microorganisms and differ in their binding sites and exact mode of action in inhibiting microtubule dynamics.

20.1.2.1 Taxanes

Taxane-based chemotherapeutic agents lead to the inhibition of the mitotic progress (M-phase) by the stabilization of microtubuli during mitosis, resulting in a cell cycle arrest at the G2 phase. This prevents further cell proliferation or maturation [41].

Until the early 1990s, taxanes were mainly isolated from the bark (paclitaxel) and the needles (docetaxel) of the pacific yew tree (*Taxus brevifolia*). Meanwhile, a semi-synthetic production method has been adopted, avoiding shortages in supply as a result of the limitation of natural resources. Due to the hydrophobic behavior of both substances, lipid-based solvents are needed (Cremophor EL, Triton), along with special IV (intravenous) infusion tubes. This can induce hypersensitivity reactions, which are manageable when corticosteroids and antihistamines are given as premedication before and after the start of taxane-based chemotherapy.

Nab-paclitaxel is a polyethoxylated castor oil-free albumin-bound paclitaxel and does not require this premedication. Paclitaxel and docetaxel are approved for the treatment of patients with primary and metastatic breast cancer (MBC), nab-paclitaxel currently only for MBC.

Docetaxel and Paclitaxel

In primary breast cancer (PBC), paclitaxel- and docetaxel-containing regimes can be regarded as the preferred (neo-)adjuvant treatment options if chemotherapy is indicated, regardless of nodal status and hormone receptor status. They are either used as single agents in sequential regimes after anthracyclines (e.g., combined with cyclophosphamide), e.g., EC-D (epirubicin/cyclophosphamide—docetaxel), A(E) C-P (epirubicin or doxorubicin/cyclophosphamide—paclitaxel) or concurrently in combination with anthracyclines and/or cyclophosphamide (TC, TAC; Table 20.2). Dose-dense schedules mainly use paclitaxel based on a better tolerability.

Several large randomized trials in node-positive and node-negative EBC as well as the result from several meta-analyses have provided solid evidence for the benefit of taxanes in the adjuvant therapy for breast cancer. In the PACS-01 study, conducted in node-positive disease, three cycles of $FE_{100}C$ followed by three cycles of docetaxel (100 mg/m^2) were associated with an 18 % reduction of the relative risk of relapse ($p = 0.012$) as well as a 27 % reduction of the relative risk of death ($p = 0.017$) compared to a control arm consisting of six cycles of $FE_{100}C$. The effect was mainly seen in the subgroup of patients who were 50 years or older [42].

BCIRG-001 compared six cycles of $FA_{50}C$ to six cycles of DAC (75/50/500 mg/m^2) in node-positive PBC. After 10 years of follow-up the docetaxel-containing regimen demonstrated a 7 % absolute improvement in both disease-free (HR 0.8, $p = 0.004$) and overall survival (HR 0.74, $p = 0.002$) [43, 44]. Similarly, the GEICAM9805 study, comparing the same regimens in node-negative, high-risk EBC, demonstrated a 6 % improvement from 82 to 88 % for DAC versus FAC at a median follow-up of 77 months (HR 0.68, $p = 0.01$). GEICAM9805 has not yet been able to demonstrate a significant OS benefit, but at the time, the results were reported, the number of events was small and a numerical trend in favor of DAC could be observed (OS events: DAC 24, FAC 36) [45]. In the WSG-AGO EC-Doc trial, the sequential EC-Doc regimen provided improved EFS and OS compared to six cycles of $FE_{100}C$ in intermediate risk node-positive breast cancer (pN1): 5-year EFS: 89.8 % versus 87.3 % ($p = 0.038$); 5-year OS: 94.5 % versus 92.8 % ($p = 0.034$). These differences appear marginal. However, a subgroup analysis stratified by centrally determined Ki-67 (at a cut-off of 20 %) demonstrated a significantly greater benefit in luminal B-like tumors with an EFS benefit of 89 % versus 74 % (HR 0.39, 95 % CI 0.18—0.80), whereas luminal A-like tumors did not derive any benefit at all. The test for interaction between treatment and Ki-67 was positive [46].

In the BCIRG005 study, which directly compared EC-Doc to DAC in node-positive EBC, both regimens proved equally effective in terms of DFS and OS (estimated 5-year disease-free survival rates were 79 % in both groups (HR 1.0; 95 % CI, 0.86–1.16; $p = 0.98$), and 5-year overall survival rates were 88 % and 89 %, respectively (HR, 0.91; 95 % CI, 0.75–1.11; $p = 0.37$). Results were similar in subgroups stratified by numbers of involved lymph nodes or hormone receptor status. However, both regimens differed in their toxicity profiles with DAC being more myelosuppressive and EC-Doc resulting in higher rates of peripheral polyneuropathy.

The Eastern Cooperative Oncology Group (ECOG) trial E1199 addressed the issue which taxane and schedule would be the most beneficial. For this purpose, patients were randomized after four cycles of AC to either paclitaxel or docetaxel, both given every 3 weeks for four cycles or in a weekly fashion for 12 applications. After a median follow-up of 12 years, both weekly paclitaxel and three-weekly docetaxel significantly improved DFS (HR 0.84, $p = 0.011$ and HR 0.79, $p = 0.001$, respectively) and marginally improved OS (HR 0.87, $p = 0.09$ and HR 0.86, $p = 0.054$, respectively) as compared to three-weekly paclitaxel. An exploratory subgroup analysis suggests substantial benefit from weekly paclitaxel within the subgroup of triple-negative patients in terms of DFS (HR 0.69, $p = 0.01$) and OS (HR 0.69, $p = 0.02$) [47].

Thus, when paclitaxel is used as a single agent sequentially to anthracyclines in adjuvant therapy it appears to be more effective when administered in a weekly fashion as compared to three-weekly paclitaxel. On the other hand, three-weekly docetaxel seems more effective compared to weekly docetaxel [47]. Similar results have been demonstrated for metastatic disease [48, 49].

An exploratory subgroup analysis of the CALGB-9344 study [5, 50] questioned if estrogen receptor-positive, HER2-negative patients benefited from taxanes as the investigators were unable to demonstrate any benefit in this subgroup. Other trials like GEICAM 9805, BCIRG-001, and the PACS-01 studies, however, were able to demonstrate a benefit regardless of ER status [51]. In the WSG-AGO EC-Doc study the taxane benefit in the ER-positive population was restricted to patients with luminal B-like tumors as determined by Ki-67 staining (>20 %) [46]. It can be reasonably argued that low-risk luminal A-like tumors, which are likely not to benefit from chemotherapy at all, will in turn also not benefit from the addition of taxanes.

Two large meta-analyses provide evidence that the benefit from the addition of taxanes in the adjuvant therapy for EBC is independent of node and hormone receptor status [52, 53]. The meta-analysis conducted by the Early Breast Cancer Trialists' Collaborative Group (EBCTCG) confirms the benefit in ER-positive patients [14].

Thus, taxane-containing combinations or sequential regimens constitute the preferred therapy for early node-negative and -positive breast cancer if adjuvant chemotherapy is indicated. The pivotal question is to define the subgroup of patients with estrogen receptor-positive tumors which should receive adjuvant chemotherapy. The distinction between luminal A- and B-like tumors either by multigene signatures or a combination of grading and Ki-67 is currently recommended by the St. Gallen international consensus expert panel for this purpose [54]. Patients thought to benefit from adjuvant chemotherapy on this basis should be offered taxane (and anthracycline)-based regimens.

Today, docetaxel is also commonly used in alternative anthracycline-free adjuvant regimens both in HER2-negative and -positive EBC, especially in patients with cardiovascular disease or risk factors who are at higher risk of cardiotoxicity (see Table 20.1). The US Oncology 9735 phase III trial provides evidence that four cycles of a combination of docetaxel and cyclophosphamide lead to an improved overall survival compared to four cycles of AC. However, so far, DC has not been compared to a contemporary anthracycline and taxane-containing regimen. In Her2-positive EBC the combination of docetaxel, carboplatin, and trastuzumab, explored in BCIRG 006, offers a similarly efficacious anthracycline-free option with significantly reduced cardiotoxicity and fewer cases of secondary leukemia.

The side effects of taxanes are shown in Table 20.3. They include myelosuppression, mucositis/stomatitis, hand–foot skin reaction, nail disorders, arthralgia, elevated liver enzymes, diarrhea and obstipation, and fluid retention. One of the most compromising side effects is peripheral polyneuropathy, which occurs in more than 10 % (more than 20 % for Paclitaxel in E1199, [55]). However, severe grade 3/4 PNP is relatively rare and occurs in only 0–8 % of patients [55, 56]. In most cases polyneuropathy resolves after stopping taxane-based chemotherapy but unfortunately, this can take several months or even years. However, formal long time follow-up of PNP in large randomized trials has not been reported and the proportion of underreported yet relevant long-lasting PNP might be considerable.

Similarly to the adjuvant setting, weekly administration of paclitaxel is the preferred regimen for metastatic disease because it has demonstrated superior DFS and OS when compared to 3-weekly paclitaxel [49]. Docetaxel given every 3 weeks has also demonstrated superiority over 3-weekly paclitaxel and remains the most widely used schedule for docetaxel [28]. Several trials have investigated a diverse range of taxane-based combinations. O'Shaughnessy et al. have even demonstrated a superior overall survival for the combination of docetaxel and capecitabine when compared to docetaxel alone [57]. However, few patients in the monotherapy arm received capecitabine as a post-study treatment [58]. In addition, the combination causes considerable toxicity and its use has not been widely adopted into clinical practice. Similar results have been demonstrated for the combination of paclitaxel and gemcitabine [59]. Today it is widely accepted that taxanes, like other agents used in the metastatic setting, should be used as single agents. So far, no trial has been able to demonstrate superiority of a combination regimen over the sequential use of the same drugs in terms of survival. Combinations provide higher response rates and longer PFS, but also have an inferior therapeutic index and should be reserved for situations of rapidly progressive, life-threatening disease when a rapid remission and high response rates are the main goal [2].

Nab-Paclitaxel

Unlike conventional paclitaxel, this solvent-free formulation of nanoparticle albumin bound paclitaxel is thought to utilize the natural albumin binding and transport pathways, specifically gp60 and caveolin-mediated transcytosis, to achieve enhanced drug delivery to the tumor [59, 60].

A phase III trial compared *nab*-paclitaxel to conventional paclitaxel in patients with MBC. 454 patients were randomly assigned to either *nab*-paclitaxel 260 mg/m^2 intravenously (q3w) without premedication (n = 229) or standard paclitaxel 175 mg/m^2 intravenously (q3w) with premedication (n = 225). Results showed that response rates were significantly higher (33 vs. 19 %, $P > 0.001$) and time to progression was significantly longer (23.0 vs. 16.9 weeks; HR 0.75, $P > 0.006$) in the *nab*-paclitaxel group compared to conventional solvent-based paclitaxel. Although the dosage of *nab*-paclitaxel was 49 % higher than standard paclitaxel, the incidence of grade 4 neutropenia was significantly lower for nab-paclitaxel (9 vs. 22 %, $P < 0.001$). Grade 3 sensory neuropathy was more common in the nab-paclitaxel arm than in the standard paclitaxel arm (10 vs. 2 %, $P < 0.001$), but improved rapidly (median, 22 days). No hypersensitivity reactions occurred with *nab*-paclitaxel despite the absence of premedication and shorter administration time [61]. *Nab*-paclitaxel was approved by the FDA in 2005 as monotherapy for patients with advanced breast cancer after failure of combination chemotherapy for metastatic disease or relapse within 6 months of adjuvant chemotherapy. Prior therapy should have included an anthracycline unless clinically contraindicated. In Europe, the EMA (European Medicines Agency) approved *nab*-paclitaxel in 2008 as monotherapy after failure of first-line chemotherapy. Patients should have received prior anthracyclines. Based on the observation that conventional paclitaxel is more effective when administered in a weekly schedule [49] as well as on emerging phase II data [62], *nab*-paclitaxel is frequently used in a weekly schedule despite the fact that this has not been confirmed in a phase III trial. There is some debate on the ideal weekly dosage, but practical- and evidence-based considerations suggest doses between 100 and 125 mg/m^2 given on 3 out of 4 weeks [63]. In the recent randomized neoadjuvant phase III GeparSepto trial, *nab*-Paclitaxel (12 × 125 mg/m^2 weekly) followed by four cycles of EC led to a significantly higher pCR rate (38 %, ypT0 ypN0) compared to standard solvent-based weekly paclitaxel (29 %, $p = 0.001$), an effect that was even more pronounced in triple-negative disease, further supporting the superior efficacy of *nab*-paclitaxel [64, 65].

20.1.2.2 Epothilones (Ixabepilone)

Another tubulin-targeted agent is ixabepilone, a semi-synthetic analog of epothilone B. Similar to taxanes, it leads to microtubule stabilization. However, taxanes and ixabepilone are structurally unrelated and bind to tubulin in a distinct manner and at distinct binding sites. Ixabepilone can retain activity in taxane-resistant tumor cells.

Two large phase III trials of ixabepilone in combination with capecitabine compared to single agent capecitabine demonstrated significantly superior response rates (35 % vs. 14 % and 43 % vs. 29 %, respectively) as well as PFS (5.8 vs. 4.2 months and 6.2 vs. 4.2 months, respectively). However, the combination did not lead to an improved OS and was associated with significantly increased toxicity, including 70 % grade 3/4 neutropenia and 20–24 % of grade 3/4 peripheral neuropathy. Furthermore, slightly more treatment-associated deaths were observed in the combination arms (3 % vs. 1 %) [66, 67]. Other commonly observed toxicities were anemia, leucopenia, thrombocytopenia, fatigue/asthenia, myalgia/arthralgia, alopecia, nausea, vomiting, stomatitis/mucositis, diarrhea, and musculoskeletal pain [67–70].

In October 2007, the FDA approved ixabepilone for the treatment of aggressive metastatic or locally advanced breast cancer no longer responding to currently available chemotherapy regimes. Ixabepilone is indicated in combination with capecitabine or as monotherapy for the treatment of patients with metastatic or locally advanced breast cancer resistant to treatment with an anthracycline and a taxane or as monotherapy in patients resistant to anthracycline, taxanes, and capecitabine. In contrast, the EMA has refused a marketing authorization for ixabepilone because of its unfavorable therapeutic index [71].

Table 20.3 Summary of selected tubulin-targeted cytotoxic agents in breast cancer

Medication	Trade name® (examples)	Dosing (mg/m^2 BSA)	Precautions	Interactions	Selected side effects
Paclitaxel	Taxol	135–250 q3w; 80–90* weekly. *e.g., in combination with bevacizumab. Paclitaxel is then given at days 1, 8, 15 q4w	Premedication to prevent severe hypersensitivity reactions including corticosteroids, diphenhydramine and H2-antagonists; use PVC free IV lines, etc.; dose reductions in case of liver function impairment	Interaction with inhibitors and inducer of CYP3A4 and CYP2C8	Polyneuropathy, dysgeusia, myelosuppression, stomatitis/mucositis, palmar-plantar erythrodysesthesia (hand–foot-skin syndrome), fatigue, arthralgia, nausea, vomiting, diarrhea, musculoskeletal pain, pulmonary toxicity (interstitial pneumonitis, pulmonary fibrosis, ARDS), hepatotoxicity (hyperbilirubinemia, elevated transaminases), hypersensitivity reaction (can be severe), skin and nail changes, alopecia, injection site reactions, fluid retention
Docetaxel	Taxotere	75–100 q3w	Premedication to prevent severe hypersensitivity reactions including corticosteroids, diphenhydramine and H2-antagonists; use PVC free IV lines, etc.; dose reductions in case of liver function impairment	Interaction with inhibitors and inducer of CYP3A4	Polyneuropathy, dysgeusia, myelosuppression, febrile neutropenia, stomatitis/mucositis, palmar-plantar erythrodysesthesia (hand–foot-skin syndrome), pulmonary toxicity (interstitial pneumonitis, pulmonary fibrosis, ARDS), hepatotoxicity (hyperbilirubinemia, elevated transaminases), fatigue, arthralgia, nausea, vomiting, diarrhea, musculoskeletal pain, hypersensitivity reaction (can be severe), skin and nail changes, alopecia, injection site reactions, fluid retention
Nab-Paclitaxel	Abraxane	260 q3w; weekly schedules are widely used (dose range 100–150 q3/4w)	Dose reductions in case of liver function impairment	Interaction with inhibitors and inducer of CYP3A4 and CYP2C8	Polyneuropathy, dysgeusia, myelosuppression, stomatitis/mucositis, hand–foot-skin syndrome, pulmonary toxicity (interstitial pneumonitis, pulmonary fibrosis, ARDS), hepatotoxicity (hyperbilirubinemia, elevated transaminases), fatigue, arthralgia, nausea, vomiting, diarrhea, musculoskeletal pain, hypersensitivity reaction (significantly less frequent than with pacli- and docetaxel), skin and nail changes, alopecia, fluid retention, injection site reactions

(continued)

Table 20.3 (continued)

Medication	Trade name® (examples)	Dosing (mg/m^2 BSA)	Precautions	Interactions	Selected side effects
Ixabepilone	Imprexa	40 q3w	Premedication with an H1-and H2-antagonists, dose reductions in case of liver function impairment; dose should be capped at 2.2 m2 BSA; Must not be used in patients with hypersensitivity against drugs formulated with cremophor (e.g., paclitaxel) patients with AST or ALT > 2.5 × ULN or bilirubin > 1 × ULN must not be treated with ixabepilone in combination with capecitabine	Interaction with inhibitors and inducer of CYP3A4	Peripheral neuropathy, myelosuppression, stomatitis/mucositis, hand–foot syndrome fatigue/asthenia, alopecia, nausea, vomiting, diarrhea, musculoskeletal pain (myalgia/arthralgia), anorexia, abdominal pain, nail disorder, hypersensitivity reactions
Vinorelbine	Navelbine	30 weekly	Save IV application, dose reduction in case of liver function impairment	Interaction with inhibitors and inducer of CYP3A4	myelosuppression, polyneuropathy, nausea and vomiting, constipation, elevated liver enzymes, mucositis, injections site reactions and local tissue damage (including necrosis), pulmonary toxicity (interstitial pneumonitis, ARDS, bronchospasm)
Eribulin	Halaven	1.23 mg/m^2 d1, 8 q3w (equivalent to eribulin mesylate: 1,4 mg/m^2 d1, 8 q3w)	Dose reductions in case of impaired liver and renal function ECG monitoring in patients with heart disease	Interaction with drugs that prolong QT interval	Neutropenia, peripheral neuropathy, fatigue/asthenia, alopecia, nausea

These highlights do not include all the information needed to use the respective drugs safely and effectively. See full prescribing information for all information needed to use these agents safely. We do not take responsibility for the correctness of the content

20.1.2.3 Vinca Alkaloids (Vinorelbine)

Vinca alkaloids are a class of drugs originally isolated from the Madagascar periwinkle plant (*Catharanthus roseus, syn. Vinca rosea*).

Vinblastine, vincristine, vinorelbine, vindesine, and vinflunin are the most widely used members of this class of drugs. Vinorelbine is the only vinca alkaloid currently approved for the treatment of breast cancer (in the EU). Vinca alkaloids bind tubulin at a different binding site compared to taxanes. Unlike taxanes, which prevent tubulin depolymerization, vinca alkaloids inhibit tubulin polymerization, thereby preventing microtubule formation and the proper function of the mitotic spindle.

Single agent vinorelbine has demonstrated activity against advanced breast cancer in a range of single-arm phase II trials including 45–157 patients each. In the first-line setting, vinorelbine, given at a dose of 30 mg/m^2 (qw), demonstrated objective response rates between 35 and 50 % with a time to treatment failure ranging from 5 to 6 months and a median duration of response of 9 months. Median overall survival in trials reporting OS was between 15 and 18 months [72–76]. In more heavily pretreated patients, response rates ranged from 16 to 36 % with a median duration of response of 5–8.5 months and a median overall survival of 14.5–16 months [73, 77, 78].

The number of randomized trials investigating the role of vinorelbine in breast cancer in any setting is very limited. A randomized phase III trial comparing vinorelbine to melphalan in 183 anthracycline-pretreated patients run in the early 1990s demonstrated vinorelbine to be superior to melphalan with a response rate of 16 % versus 9 % and a significantly improved TTP and OS [79]. A large randomized phase III trial compared single agent vinorelbine to a combination of vinorelbine and gemcitabine. Single agent vinorelbine had a significantly shorter PFS of 4 versus 6 months (p = 0.0028) and a numerically smaller response rate of 26 % versus 36 % (p = 0.09). However, overall survival did not differ between both treatment arms (V: 16.4 months and VG: 15.6, p = 0.8) [80]. A trial directly comparing vinorelbine to capecitabine was prematurely closed after inclusion of only 46 patients, but efficacy was similar for the two drugs with significantly different toxicity profiles [81]. Unlike in Europe, where vinorelbine is approved for the treatment of non-small-cell lung cancer (NSCLC) and metastatic breast cancer after failure of anthracyclines or taxanes in the 1990s, vinorelbine has only gained approval for NSCLC in the US.

The main dose-limiting toxicity of vinorelbine is neutropenia, which can occur as grade 3/4 in more than 50 % of patients if vinorelbine is used as a single agent. Peripheral neuropathy is usually mild and only rarely occurs as grade 3/4 in about 3 % of patients (single agent). Vinorelbine can cause phlebitis and inflammation at the injection site. Care has to be taken to correctly position the IV catheter or needle as severe local tissue necrosis may occur in rare cases. Rarer side effects include interstitial pulmonary disease (in rare cases severe ARDS), bronchospasm, cardiac ischemia, and diarrhea. Vinorelbine rarely causes apparent alopecia. An oral formulation, which has demonstrated activity, has been marketed and registered in Europe for the same settings [82, 83]. Vinorelbine is mostly used as second- or third-line therapy. In addition, vinorelbine has shown good efficacy in combination with trastuzumab [84].

20.1.2.4 Eribulin

Eribulin is a structurally modified synthetic analog of halinchondrin B, a natural compound isolated from a rare Japanese marine sponge (Halichondria okadai). Like most tubulin-targeted agents, it impairs the proper function of the mitotic spindle leading to a G2-M cell cycles arrest and inhibiting cell proliferation. However, unlike other antimitotic drugs such as taxanes and vinca alkaloids which inhibit microtubule growth and shortening, eribulin predominantly inhibits microtubule polymerization and leads to the sequestration of tubulin into nonproductive aggregates. Microtubule shortening remains largely unaffected [85].

Eribulin was first approved as a monotherapy by the FDA in 2010 and the EMA in 2011 for the treatment of metastatic breast cancer in women who have received two or more prior chemotherapies for advanced disease. Prior therapy should have included anthracyclines and a taxane, either in the adjuvant or metastatic setting. The approval was based on results from the EMBRACE study (study 305; NCT00388726), a randomized phase III trial that included patients with 2–5 prior lines of chemotherapy for advanced disease and compared eribulin to treatment of physician's choice (TPC). The study demonstrated a significant improvement in overall survival (HR 0.81; $p = 0.041$) in favor of eribulin [86]. A second large phase III trial directly compared eribulin to capecitabine as first- to third–line therapy for metastatic breast cancer previously treated with anthracyclines and taxanes. This study (E301; NCT00337103) failed to demonstrate a superiority of eribulin over capecitabine (OS HR 0.88; $p = 0.056$). Neither PFS nor ORR differed between the two therapies [87]. A pooled analysis of the two trials confirmed the OS benefit of eribulin versus control and suggested a more pronounced benefit in HER2-negative and triple-negative subgroups [88]. In the EU, the indication for eribulin has been expanded to patients with only one prior line of chemotherapy in the advanced/metastatic setting. The most common side effects of eribulin are neutropenia, fatigue/asthenia, alopecia, peripheral neuropathy, and nausea.

20.1.3 Alkylating Agents

20.1.3.1 Cyclophosphamide

Cyclophosphamide is a widely used anticancer drug and is listed on the World Health Organization's List of Essential Medicines. It is a member of the oxazaphosphorine family of mustard-alkylating agents and was first synthesized in 1958 by Norbert Brock and has since been used to treat a range of diseases [89]. Cyclophosphamide itself is a prodrug that needs to be activated by the cytochrome P450 in the liver. The resulting metabolite is called 4-hydroxy-cyclophosph amide (4-OH-CPA). It has to undergo β-elimination to yield phosphoramide mustard and acrolein. Phosphoramide mustard alkylates both DNA and proteins and forms DNA crosslinks both between and within DNA strands at guanine N-7 positions. These inter- and intrastrand crosslinks are irreversible and finally lead to apoptosis [90]. The intracellular release of the active alkylating agent also leads to direct inhibition of DNA polymerases [91]. Cyclophosphamide is one of the best known agents of this class and has a long history in the treatment of all kinds of cancers. Even today, more than 50 years after its introduction, it is one of the most widely used chemotherapeutic agents. Cyclophosphamide is nowadays part of the majority of chemotherapeutic regimes in the treatment of breast cancer in the adjuvant and neoadjuvant setting but is less frequently used in the metastatic setting. It is also used in the treatment of other types of cancers such as leukemia, multiple myeloma, or retinoblastoma. When used as a single agent in the treatment of breast cancer, response rates between 10 and 50 % were observed.

Cyclophosphamide is one of the agents that made up the first successfully implemented adjuvant chemotherapy regimen consisting of cyclophosphamide, methotrexate, and 5-fluoruracil, the CMF regimen, which significantly reduced the risk of recurrence and improved overall survival, compared to observation [92, 93]. CMF is rarely used today and cyclophosphamide is usually given as part of combination regimes, mostly together with anthracyclines, e.g., doxorubicin (AC) or epirubicin (EC) followed by a taxane but also

Table 20.4 Selected alkylating agents used in the treatment of breast cancer

Medication	Trade name® (examples)	Dosing (mg/m^2 BSA)	Precautions	Interactions	Selected side effect
Cyclophosphamide	Endoxan	Varies between several different adjuvant regimens., e.g., 500 mg/m^2 IV q3w, as part of the "CAF" protocol or 600 mg/m^2 IV d1, 8 q4w as part of the "CMF" regimen. And up to as high as 2000 mg/m^2 in dose-intensified, dose-dense ETC (see Table 20.2) Or 50 mg p.o. daily as part of a oral metronomic therapy in combination with methotrexate (2 × 2.5 mg p. o. d 1, 2 q1w)	>1000 mg/m^2: uroprotection with MESNA, sufficient hydration, exclude urinary obstruction	Several. Refer to prescribing information	Myelosuppression, immunosuppression, amenorrhea, ovarian failure, infertility, alopecia, nausea, vomiting, mucositis, hemorrhagic cystitis, nephrotoxicity, cardiotoxicity (e.g., hemorrhagic perimyocarditis), pulmonary toxicity, secondary malignancies (e.g., AML/MD and bladder cancer). Can cause fetal harm.
Bendamustin	Ribomustin	120–150 mg/m^2 IV day 1, 2 q4w; no standard dose/schedule defined for breast cancer. Bendamustin is not approved for the treatment of breast cancer	None	None	Myelosurppression, mucositis, stomatistis, nausea, vomiting, alopecia. Can cause fetal harm

These highlights do not include all the information needed to use the respective drugs safely and effectively. See full prescribing information for all information needed to use these agents safely. We do not take responsibility for the correctness of the content

in combination with docetaxel (see Table 20.4) [4, 31, 94, 95].

Cyclophosphamide also plays a role in metronomic chemotherapeutic regimens, often in combination with methotrexate. In heavily pretreated patients, such metronomic regimens (CM) provide response rates of around 20 % [96]. Recently, the same regimen given for 12 months as maintenance therapy in a randomized phase trial (IBCSG 22-00) after adjuvant chemotherapy has demonstrated some signs of activity at least in the high-risk subpopulation of node-positive, triple-negative patients within the trial [97]. For these low-dose cyclophosphamide regimens, alternative modes of action are proposed and low-dose cyclophosphamide is rather thought to induce beneficial immunomodulatory effects, e.g., by eliminating regulatory T cells and in metronomic dosing schedules also antiangiogenic effects [89, 98]. In addition, high-dose cyclophosphamide is also used as an immunosuppressant to treat severe and refractory autoimmune diseases like lupus because high doses cause general lymphodepletion.

Side effects of cyclophosphamide include nausea and vomiting, bone marrow suppression, alopecia, fatigue, amenorrhea, hemorrhagic cystitis, nephrotoxicity, and secondary malignancies. The urotoxic effect of cyclophosphamide is caused by acrolein, one of its metabolites. The risk can be minimized by securing adequate hydration, excluding urinary tract obstruction, avoiding night time dosage and the administration of MESNA at higher doses of cyclophosphamide. MESNA (sodium 2-mercaptoethan sulfonate) binds and neutralizes acrolein [99]. As cyclophosphamide significantly increases the risk of premature menopause and infertility, younger patients in the adjuvant setting need to be offered counseling on fertility preservation (as with all adjuvant chemotherapy regimens) prior to the start of therapy. Cyclophosphamide also has procarcinogenic effects and can lead to secondary malignancies including leukemia, MDS, skin cancer, bladder cancer, and other malignancies. The risk of treatment-related AML (t-AML) appears to be dose dependent, but is also influenced by additional factors including other agents, e.g., anthracyclines which can also increase the risk. T-AML is often preceded by MDS and often associated with complex cytogenetics and a worse prognosis compared to de novo AML. Cyclophosphamide at high doses can also induce cardiac toxicity, which can manifest as a range of conditions, including hemorrhagic perimyocarditis.

20.1.3.2 Bendamustine

Another substance of this group is bendamustine (Table 20.4), which has structural similarities to both alkylating agents and purine analogs. Its function is not yet entirely clear, but it has demonstrated to be noncross resistant with other alkylating drugs [100].

It is a long-known cytotoxic agent, which was once widely used in the former German Democratic Republic for a variety of cancers types. It is mainly indicated for hematological malignancies like Hodgkin's, non-Hodgkin's disease, multiple myeloma, but there are promising results for bendamustine in breast cancer patients as second- or third-line chemotherapy [101]. In a phase III trial, the combination of bendamustine, cyclophosphamide, and 5-fluorouracil was compared with conventional CMF as first-line treatment for MBC and achieved a longer progression-free survival [102]. Current ongoing studies are evaluating new schedules, doses, and the management of toxicities and combinations with other cytotoxic agents (e.g., NCT00661739, NCT00705250) to optimize cancer therapy with bendamustine. Bendamustine seems to have a favorable range of side effects, especially for heavily pretreated patients with metastasized breast cancer. In a phase II study, the main side effects reported were myelosuppression, infection, mucositis, and diarrhea. Those events mostly occurred within grade 1–2 and were well manageable [100, 103]. However, due to a range of alternative effective drugs and several other reasons, bendamustine is currently not frequently used in the treatment of breast cancer and has not been approved for this indication either.

20.1.4 Platinum-Based Chemotherapeutic Agents

Cisplatin and carboplatin are widely used drugs to treat various types of cancers, including sarcomas, a range of carcinomas (e.g., small cell lung cancer, and ovarian cancer), lymphomas, and germ cell tumors as well as breast cancer (Table 20.5). Platinum-based agents form complexes within the cells, which induce intra- and interstrand crosslinks, which result in double strand breaks during replication and ultimately the induction of apoptosis.

The activity of platinum salts in breast cancer was first demonstrated in the 1980s in several small trials, with cisplatin achieving response rates of 47–54 % in previously untreated patients. However, a considerably lower activity (RR ~ 10 %) was observed in more heavily pretreated patients [104–109]. These data suggest a dose and pretreatment-dependent activity. With the introduction of anthracyclines and taxanes as effective but less toxic therapies, interest in platinum therapies for breast cancer decreased. Investigators regained interest in platinum salts for breast cancer when in the 2000s several preclinical studies reported an outstanding efficacy of platinum in BRCA-mutated cancer cells and in addition, new regimens to manage toxicities have been established.

The strong interest in platinum-based therapies that mainly focused on TNBC were based on phenotypic similarities between BRCA1-associated breast cancer and triple-negative disease or more precisely the basal-like subtype. Roughly 80 % of BRCA1-associated tumors are basal like. However, the majority of basal-like tumors are not BRCA-associated but sporadic. Yet, the shared phenotype led to the speculation that sporadic basal-like tumors might also share defects in homologous recombination (HR) with their BRCA-associated counterparts, yet, caused by different mechanisms and might therefore have a similar sensitivity to platinum salts [110]. The double strand breaks induced by platinum salts during replication require homologous recombination (HR) as an error-free DNA repair mechanism. If cells harbor HR defects, error-prone compensatory repair mechanisms step in and lead to a high degree of genomic instability, finally resulting in the death of the tumor cell. Preclinical data pointed to an extraordinary sensitivity to platinum agents of BRCA-associated breast and ovarian cancers. However, it took a long time until randomized trials provided first evidence that at least a subgroup of TNBC patients might specifically benefit from platinum-based chemotherapy. Several studies in unselected TNBCs revealed discouraging results [111–113]. Finally, the TNT trial randomized 376 patients with metastatic TNBC to either carboplatin or docetaxel as a head-to-head comparison. There were no significant differences in terms of ORR, PFS, and OS in the overall study population. However, an exploratory analysis revealed a significant benefit from carboplatin over docetaxel in *BRCA1/2* mutation carriers, with an ORR of 68 % versus 33 % and a PFS of 6.8 months versus 4.8 months. A test for interaction between BRCA status and therapy was positive, providing evidence that BRCA mutations but not TNBC status or basal-like subtype predicts benefit from platinum salts in breast cancer [114].

Several trials have investigated the role of carboplatin in the neoadjuvant setting in patients with TNBC. With one exception, they have all demonstrated increased pathologic complete response (pCR) rates for the platinum-based regimens. The GeparSixto trial and the CALGB 40603 trial reported an increase in pCR rates (ypT0/is ypN0) of 10.5 and 13 % by the addition of carboplatin to anthracycline- and taxane-based combinations in TNBC [115, 116]. Recently, carboplatin, when added to four cycles of neoadjuvant *nab*-paclitaxel, increased pCR rates by 17.2 % compared to gemcitabine in TNBC [117]. So far, only the GeparSixto and CALGB 40603 have reported preliminary survival data. In GeparSixto, the addition of carboplatin led to a 10 % improvement in 3-year DFS (HR 0.56; $p = 0.035$) [118], whereas in the CALGB 40603 the increased pCR rates did not result in an improved survival [119]. In the GeparSixto trial, the benefit from the addition of carboplatin in terms of pCR and event-free survival was not restricted to BRCA-mutated Patients but seen in BRCA wild-type patients as well [118]. The use of carboplatin against TNBC in the (neo)adjuvant setting cannot be regarded as a standard until additional data on survival are available. Thus far, in the (neo)adjuvant setting, carboplatin is only used as a

Table 20.5 Platinum-based cytotoxic agents used in the treatment of breast cancer

Medication	Trade name® (examples)	Dosing	Precautions	Interactions	Selected adverse effects
Cisplatin		30–75 mg/m^2, e.g., q3w, various regimens	Dose reduction according to GFR. Ensure sufficient hydration prior to and after cisplatin infusion (1000–2000 ml each)	Avoid further nephrotoxic drugs	Myelosuppression, renal toxicity, alopecia, marked nausea and vomiting, neurotoxicity, ototoxicity, electrolyte disturbances, allergic/anaphylactic reactions
Carboplatin		Area under the curve (AUC), e.g., as calculated by the "Calvert formula": Total dose (mg) = (target AUC) × (GFR + 25), e.g., AUC 4–6 q3w or AUC 2 q1w as a single agent or in combination	Dose reduction according to GFR	None	Myelosuppression, renal toxicity (less than cisplatin), alopecia, nausea, vomiting, neurotoxicity and ototoxicity (less than cisplatin), electrolyte disturbances, allergic/anaphylactic reactions

These highlights do not include all the information needed to use the respective drugs safely and effectively. See full prescribing information for all information needed to use these agents safely. We do not take responsibility for the correctness of the content

standard treatment option in HER2-positive breast cancer in combination with docetaxel and trastuzumab (and pertuzumab).

There is no data to suggest that in breast cancer either *cis*- or carboplatin was superior to the other. However, due to the reduced toxicity, particularly with regard to renal and ototoxicity, carboplatin is often preferred over cisplatin. The adverse reactions of carboplatin and cisplatin consist of myelosuppression affecting all lineages, including the risk of severe thrombopenia, nephrotoxicity, neurotoxicity, ototoxicity, nausea and vomiting, allergic, and anaphylactic reactions.

In addition to the significantly reduced nephrotoxicity and ototoxicity of carboplatin, nausea, and vomiting are also less severe and more easily controlled, compared to cisplatin. In turn, myelosuppression appears to be more severe with carboplatin including higher rates of grade 3/4 thrombopenia.

20.1.5 Antimetabolites

Methotrexate, 5-FU, capecitabine, and gemcitabine are antimetabolites frequently used in the treatment of metastatic breast cancer (Table 20.6).

20.1.5.1 Methotrexate (MTX)

Methotrexate (MTX) is a widely used antimetabolite with a wide range of indications including the therapy of several cancer types, like breast cancer, trophoblast diseases, leukemia, lymphomas, and as an intrathecal application to treat meningeal carcinomatosis or primary CNS lymphomas. In addition, it is also used for the conservative management of extrauterine pregnancy, severe forms of rheumatoid arthritis and psoriasis. It is available as IV, IT, IM as well as oral formulations.

MTX competitively inhibits dihydrofolate reductase (DHFR), an enzyme involved in tetrahydrofolate synthesis [120]. Folic acid is a crucial enzyme in the de novo synthesis of thymidine, which is essential for DNA synthesis. Folate is also essential for the synthesis of purine and pyrimidine bases. MTX therefore inhibits DNA as well as RNA synthesis.

In breast cancer it has mostly been used in combination with cyclophosphamide and 5-fluorouracil (CMF), in the metastatic as well as the adjuvant setting. Adjuvant CMF was the first adjuvant therapy to be successfully established for the therapy of primary breast cancer. It has been replaced by "standard" AC or EC not based on superiority but rather due to the shorter duration and better tolerability of the latter regimens. Subsequently, anthracycline-containing regimens with higher cumulative doses and longer duration proved to be more effective, which is reflected by the EBCTCG meta-analysis [14]. The CMF regimen today is infrequently used as an anthracycline-free option.

MTX has also demonstrated some activity as part of a metronomic regimen consisting of oral cyclophosphamide (50 mg per day continuously) and oral MTX (5 mg on day 1 and 2, qw). It is not used as monotherapy.

To prevent excessive bone marrow and gastrointestinal toxicity from higher doses of MTX (>100 mg/m^2 BSA), folinic acid (leucovorin rescue) has to be given at the appropriate time after the administration of MTX.

Table 20.6 Antimetabolites used in the treatment of breast cancer

Medication	Trade name® (examples)	Dosing (mg/m^{2}BSA)	Precautions	Interactions (selected examples)	Selected side effects
Methotrexate		E.g., 40 mg/m^2 IV on days 1 and 8 of each cycle as part of the classic CMF protocol in combination with cyclophosphamide and 5-FU or as part of a metronomic therapy at a dose 5 mg/d on day 1 and 2, q1w, in combination with continuous oral cyclophosphamide (50 mg/d)	Dose reduction in case of renal impairment, MTX elimination also impaired in patients with ascites and pleural effusion. leucovorin rescue (calcium folinate) is mandatory at higher doses (>100 mg/m^2)	Unexpectedly severe bone marrow suppression, aplastic anemia, and gastrointestinal toxicity have been reported with concomitant administration of some nonsteroidal anti-inflammatory drugs (NSAIDs)	Myelosuppression, mucositis, stomatitis, diarrhea, hepatotoxicity, pulmonary toxicity (including. interstitial pneumonitis), skin toxicity, renal failure Can cause fetal damage or death
5-Fluorouracil		As part of the classic CMF protocol: 600 mg/m^2 IV in combination with cyclophosphamide and MTX q4w As part of the FAC or FEC regimen: 500 mg/m^2 in combination with doxorubicin or epirubicin and cyclophosphamide, q3w Several other dosing schedules are used in the treatment for other malignancies		Methotrexate, leucovorin (calcium folinate) increases efficacy and toxicity. Brivudin und Sorivudin. 5-FU may lead to unexpected severe toxicity in patients with dihydropyrimidindehydrogenase (DPD) deficiency	Myelosuppression, palmar-plantar erythrodysesthesia, alopecia, nail changes, mucositis, stomatitis, diarrhea, nausea, vomiting, CNS toxicity, allergic reactions, cardiac toxicity including ECG changes, hepatotoxicity
Capecitabine	Xeloda	2 × 1000–1250 daily p. o. d1-14 q3w	Dose reductions for renal impairment (GFR 30–50 ml/min.), contraindicated in patients with a GFR < 30 ml/min	Methotrexate, Leucovorin, coumarin-type anticoagulants May lead to unexpected severe toxicity in patients with dihydropyrimidindehydrogenase (DPD) deficiency	Myelosuppression, palmar-plantar erythrodysesthesia, diarrhea, dehydration, cardiotoxicity, renal impairment
Gemcitabine	Gemzar	Approved for breast cancer at a dose of 1250 mg/m^2 on days 1 and 8 of each cycle in combination with paclitaxel (175 mg/m^2 given on day 1) q3w. Other dosing regimens, not officially approved in breast cancer include gemcitabine monotherapy at a does of 1000 mg/m^2 d 1, 8, 15 q4w or at doses from 750 mg/m^2 d 1, 8 q3w, e.g., in combination with cisplatin		Cisplatin, radiosensitizer	Myelosuppression, nausea and vomiting, pulmonary toxicity (including cases of ARDS), hepatotoxicity, hemolytic uremic syndrome, skin rash, capillary leak syndrome, peripheral edema, posterior reversible encephalopathy. Gemcitabine may exacerbate toxicity of radiotherapy

These highlights do not include all the information needed to use the respective drugs safely and effectively. See full prescribing information for all information needed to use these agents safely. We do not take responsibility for the correctness of the content

20.1.5.2 Capecitabine, 5-Fluourouracil (5-FU)

Capecitabine is a prodrug which is enzymatically converted to 5-FU by carboxyesterase, cytidine deaminase, and thymidine phosphorylase in the liver and in tumor cells. 5-FU (and capecitabine) exerts it cytotoxic effects via the inhibition of thymidylate synthase, blocking the synthesis of the pyrimidine thymidine, a nucleoside required for DNA replication.

5-FU has a long history in breast cancer and has been used as part of an adjuvant regimen consisting of 5-FU, epi- or doxorubicin, and cyclophosphamide (FEC, FAC). Recently, a large randomized phase III trial (GIM-2), however, demonstrated, that 5-FU did not add any benefit to the combination of epirubicin and cyclophosphamide followed by paclitaxel [121]. It has now been replaced by modern anthracycline-/taxane-based regimens (Table 20.6).

Capecitabine has been approved based on a series of phase II/III trials as monotherapy for metastatic breast cancer after failure of anthracycline- and taxane-containing therapies. Response rates for capecitabine monotherapy range between 14 and 29 %, with a TTP and OS of 3.1–7.9 and 10.1–29.4 months, respectively across all settings [122–124]. Based on a randomized phase III trial in the first-line setting, capecitabine has also been approved in combination with docetaxel after prior anthracycline-based therapies. This trial is one of the few chemotherapy trials for MBC which have demonstrated a significant overall survival for the combination over docetaxel monotherapy. However, the regimen produces considerable toxicity, including high rates of febrile neutropenia, and there are some questions about subsequent therapies [57, 58]. Therefore, it mainly remains a valuable option in situations which require rapid responses, otherwise sequential monotherapies are generally preferred due to their better therapeutic index.

In the US, capecitabine is also approved in combination with ixabepilone in otherwise resistant metastatic breast cancer. However, due to an unfavorable therapeutic index and risk of severe toxicities, this combination has not been approved by the EMA in Europe. In contrast, capecitabine in Europe but not the US has been granted approval as first-line therapy for MBC in combination with bevacizumab. Further, capecitabine is used in combination with lapatinib or trastuzumab for the treatment of HER2-positive breast cancer. It is also used to treat colorectal cancer and gastric cancer.

Capecitabine has also been investigated in the adjuvant setting as an adjunct to anthracycline- and taxane-based regimens. However, none of these regimens provided evidence of a benefit from the addition of capecitabine in unselected patients [125–128]. Some studies suggest that there might be a role for capecitabine in selected patients with primary breast cancer. The GeparTrio trial demonstrated a survival benefit from switching to a noncross-resistant regimen consisting of capecitabine and vinorelbine in patients with luminal type breast cancers not responding to two cycles of neoadjuvant docetaxel, doxorubicin, and cyclophosphamide (TAC) [129]. Very recently, a phase III trial in the post-neoadjuvant setting demonstrated an overall survival benefit of 6 months; thanks to capecitabine in Asian patients not achieving a pCR after anthracycline- and taxane- containing neoadjuvant chemotherapy [130]. If this effect can be extrapolated in other ethnicities is unclear.

One of the most frequent and compromising side effect is hand–foot syndrome (HFS, Palmar-plantar erythrodysesthesia) with an incidence of up to 20 %, and diarrhea. HFS can become very painful and significantly impair daily activities and quality of life. An association between hand–foot syndrome and efficacy has been suspected but is still unproven. In general, the side effects are manageable with dose interruptions or reductions and a complete termination of therapy is rarely necessary. Diarrhea can be severe and potentially life-threatening in rare cases, especially if capecitabine is given in combination with lapatinib. Useful guidelines for management of chemotherapy-induced diarrhea have been developed by the American Society of Clinical Oncology (ASCO) [131]. Other adverse events include myelosuppression, stomatitis, nausea and vomiting, abdominal pain, dehydration, and hyperbilirubinemia.

Capecitabine is metabolized and inactivated by dihydro-pyrimidin-dehydrogenase (DPD). Polymorphisms within this gene can result in DPD-deficiency and patients are at risk of severe, potentially life-threatening toxicities. Use of capecitabine should be avoided in patients with known DPD-deficiency.

20.1.5.3 Gemcitabine

Gemcitabine is another chemotherapeutic agent which acts as an antimetabolite. It is a nucleoside analog (2″,2′-difluoro-deoxycytidine; dFdC) that is phosphorylated intracellularly [132–134] by deoxycytidine kinases and interferes with DNA replication. The diphosphate inhibits ribonucleotide reductase that is crucial for the production of deoxynucleotide triphosphates needed for normal DNA synthesis, whereas the triphosphate is incorporated into the DNA instead of deoxycytidine triphosphate [132–134].

A series of phase II studies, none including more than 41 evaluable patients, has investigated the activity of gemcitabine as monotherapy for MBC. In chemotherapy-naïve patients, response rates vary between 14.3 and 37 %, whereas in anthracycline- and taxane-pretreated patients, response rates between 0 and 23 % where observed. In pretreated patients, activity as single agent is modest, but the toxicity profile is favorable [135].

Due to the lack of overlapping toxicities and the expectation of noncross resistance, gemcitabine has been investigated in combination regimens, e.g., with taxanes. In a registrational phase III first-line trial, Albain et al. compared paclitaxel as a single agent (175 mg/m^2, q3w) to the combination of paclitaxel and gemcitabine (175 mg/m^2, d1/1250 mg/m^2, d1, 8; q3w). The trial demonstrated a significant 3-month improvement in OS, the trial's primary endpoint (18.6 vs. 15.8 months, $p = 0.048$) as well as response rates (41.4 vs. 26.2 %, $p < 0.001$) and TTP [59, 136]. Toxicity, mainly in terms of myelosuppression was also significantly increased. Today, three-weekly paclitaxel can no longer be considered a standard, as weekly schedules have demonstrated significantly improved response rates, TTP, and overall survival [49]. In a head-to-head comparison of docetaxel plus gemcitabine versus docetaxel plus capecitabine, a regimen which has provided a significantly improved OS over single agent docetaxel, no significant differences in terms of efficacy or toxicity could be discovered [136, 137]. Based on the phase III trial, gemcitabine has been approved by the FDA and EMA in combination with paclitaxel for the first-line treatment of metastatic breast cancer after failure of prior adjuvant anthracycline-containing therapy, unless anthracyclines are contraindicated (Table 20.6). In addition, gemcitabine is used in the treatment of ovarian cancer, pancreatic cancer, and non-small-cell lung cancer.

Trials trying to demonstrate a benefit from the addition of gemcitabine to adjuvant regimens have failed thus far.

Side effects of gemcitabine include nausea and vomiting, myelosuppression, pulmonary toxicity including ARDS, hepatotoxicity (transaminitis), haematuria, rash, hemolytic uremic syndrome (HUS), capillary leak syndrome, and posterior reversible encephalopathy. Gemcitabine exacerbates toxicity of radiotherapy and administration should be avoided within 7 days of radiotherapy.

20.2 Targeted Therapies

20.2.1 Human Epidermal Growth Factor Receptor 2 (HER2)-Targeted Therapies

20.2.1.1 Trastuzumab

The Human Epidermal Growth Factor Receptor 2 gene (HER2), a member of the erbB epidermal growth factor receptor tyrosine kinase family, has been independently described by several groups in the mid 1980s [138–141] (Table 20.7).

HER2 is also referred to as HER2/neu or ErbB-2. Shortly thereafter, Slamon and colleagues provided evidence that the HER2 gene was overexpressed and amplified in 20–30 % of patients with EBC. They further found HER2 overexpression/amplification to be a strong and independent prognostic factor in this setting [142, 143]. Several groups, including researchers at Genetech Inc. have developed murine monoclonal antibodies against the extracellular domain of HER2, which proved to be potent inhibitors of cell growth in HER2 overexpressing human breast cancer xenografts. The most potent of these antibodies, muMAB 4D5, was in turn humanized to minimize the generation of human anti-mouse immune responses possibly neutralizing its effects in humans. The resulting chimeric antibody was called trastuzumab and entered clinical trials. Since then an unprecedented success story in the therapy of breast cancer has begun [144].

In a multinational phase II trial 222 patients who had received one or two chemotherapies for MBC were treated with trastuzumab monotherapy. The response rate was 15 % with a median duration of response of 9.1 months within the intention to treat population. However, in patients with HER2 ampflification the response rate was 19 % compared to 0 % in patients who were found to be negative by fluorescence in situ hybridization (FISH) [145]. In a phase II study carried out in the first-line setting the response rate for single agent trastuzumab amounted to 26 % (35 % in HER2 amplified) [146].

A pivotal first-line phase III trial randomized 469 HER2 overexpressing patients to either chemotherapy alone or in combination with trastuzumab. Patients who had received anthracyclines in the adjuvant setting received paclitaxel 175 mg/m^2 three-weekly, the remaining were mainly treated with doxorubicin/cyclophosphamide, both for six cycles. The addition of trastuzumab significantly improved response rates (32 % vs. 50 %, $p < 0.001$), PFS (4.6 months vs. 7.4 months, $p < 0.001$) and overall survival (20.3 months vs. 25.1 months, $p = 0.046$). Over 70 % of patients received open-label trastuzumab as one of the subsequent therapies, which might have obscured the real survival benefit from trastuzumab. In the subgroup of patients treated with paclitaxel combined with trastuzumab, response rates were increased from 17 to 41 % and PFS from 3 months to 6.9 months [147]. An additional phase II study ($n = 186$) provided further evidence of the efficacy of trastuzumab in combination with docetaxel. The addition of trastuzumab to docetaxel in the first-line treatment of patients with HER2-positive breast cancer improved response rates from 34 to 61 % ($p = 0.0002$) as well as overall survival from 22.7 to 31.2 months. This OS benefit was observed despite 57 % crossing over to trastuzumab upon progression as part of the trial. In fact, OS in patients who did not cross over to trastuzumab was merely 16.6 months [148]. The combination of trastuzumab and vinorelbine proved equally effective as trastuzumab plus docetaxel in the randomized phase III HERNATA trial, of which the first has a favorable tolerability [84]. This combination has not been approved by the FDA or EMA.

Table 20.7 HER2-directed therapies

Anti-Her2 Agent	Trade name® (examples)	Mode of action	Dosing	Interactions	Selected side effects
Trastuzumab	Herceptin	Humanized monoclonal antibody targeting the extracellular domain of the HER2 protein Inhibition of HER2-signalling, antibody-dependent cellular cytotoxicity (ADCC)	2 mg/kg body weight per week after a loading dose of 4 mg/kg or 6 mg/kg body weight per week after a loading dose of 8 mg/kg; 600 mg absolute as a 5 min subcutaneous injection (EMA, EU)		Cardiotoxicity, infusion reactions, skin rash, flu-like symptoms, headache, diarrhea, nausea, vomiting, fatigue, abdominal pain, pulmonary toxicity including cough, dyspnea, interstitial pneumonitis, ARDS, exacerbation of chemotherapy-induced neutropenia, anemia, myalgia Trastuzumab can cause fetal harm (e.g., oligohydramnion, pulmonary hypoplasia, etc.)
Lapatinib	Tykerb (USA), Tyverb (EU)	HER-1 and HER-2 receptor tyrosine kinase inhibitor (TKI) Inhibits autophosphorylation of HER1 (EGFR) and HER2 and downstream signalling	1250 mg daily p.o. in combination with capecitabine (2000 mg/m^2 d 1–14, q3w); 1500 mg p.o. daily in combination with letrozol 1000 mg p.o. daily in combination with trastuzumab	Interaction with inhibitors and inducer of CYP3A4 and CYP2C8	Diarrhea, nausea, vomiting, skin rash, erythema multiforme, fatigue, arthralgia, cardiotoxicity, headache, abdominal pain, loss of weight, hepatotoxicity, e.g., elevation of liver enzymes, interstitial lung disease, paronychia Lapatinib can cause fetal harm Lapatinib should be administered with caution to patients who have or may develop prolongation of QTc
Pertuzumab	Perjeta	Humanized monoclonal antibody directed against the dimerization domain of HER2. Pertuzumab inhibits the interaction of HER2 with other HER family members. Ligand-activated signaling from HER2:HER1 and HER2: HER3 heterodimers is thereby inhibited	420 mg pertuzumab (absolute) q3w following a loading dose of 840 mg (absolute)		Cardiotoxicity (left ventricular dysfunction), infusion reactions, anaphylactic reactions, diarrhea, nausea, vomiting, fatigue, skin rash, loss of weight, neutropenia, febrile neutropenia, elevated liver enzymes
Trastuzumab-Emtansin (T-DM1)	Cadcyla	Antibody–drug conjugate consisting of the humanized monoclonal antibody trastuzumab, directed against HER2 covalently linked to emtansine (DM-1), a potent anti-microtubule agent. T-DM1 is internalized upon binding to the HER2 receptor on HER2 overexpressing cells and the cytotoxic agents is released intracellularly	3.6 mg/kg body weight q3w	CYP3A4 inhibitors	Thrombocytopenia, hepatotoxicity, elevation of liver enzymes, hyperbilirubinemia, nodular regenerative hyperplasia, pulmonary toxicity (e.g., interstitial lung disease, pneumonitis), infusion related reactions, anaphylaxis, cardiotoxicity, peripheral neuropathy Can cause embryofetal death or birth defects
Afatinib	Giotrif, Gilotrif		40 mg p.o./d (max. 50 mg/d) Currently approved for lung cancer only. Phase II/III trials in breast cancer negative	P-gp inhibitors	Diarrhea, interstitial lung disease, bullous and exfoliative skin disorders, hepatoxicity, hepatic toxicity, keratitis Embryofetal toxicity

These highlights do not include all the information needed to use the respective drugs safely and effectively. See full prescribing information for all information needed to use these agents safely. We do not take responsibility for the correctness of the content

As a result of these trials trastuzumab has been approved by the FDA in 1998 for the first-line therapy of HER2-positive breast cancer in combination with paclitaxel or as a single agent as second or third-line therapy. In Europe trastuzumab was approved by the EMA in 2000 and is now registered for first-line therapy in combination with paclitaxel and docetaxel or as a single agent after two prior chemotherapies for metastatic disease including anthracyclines and taxanes. In Europe, trastuzumab has consecutively also been approved for the treatment of metastatic disease in combination with anastrozol in HER2- and HR-positive disease for patients without prior trastuzumab therapy for MBC (see below), as well as in combination with lapatinib, a TKI directed against epidermal growth factor receptor (EGFR) and HER2 for patients with HER2-positive and HR-negative disease having failed prior therapy with trastuzumab in combination with chemotherapy [149, 150].

A randomized phase III trial compared the combination of anastrozol and trastuzumab to anastrozol alone in trastuzumab-naïve patients who have had no prior therapy for metastatic HER2- and ER-positive breast cancer. Response rates as well as PFS were significantly improved in the combination arm, however, at a low level. The ORR was 20.3 % in the combination arm compared to 6.8 % in the monotherapy arm ($p = 0.018$) and PFS was 4.8 months compared to 2.8 months ($p = 0.0016$), respectively. OS did not show a significant improvement (23.9 vs. 28.5, $p = 0.33$) [150].

Several strategies have been investigated for patients progressing on or after treatment with trastuzumab. In a phase II trial ($n = 156$) conducted by the German Breast Group, patients who had progressed after prior first-line therapy containing taxane and trastuzumab were randomized to either capecitabine alone or in combination with trastuzumab. The trial was prematurely closed due to slow accrual. However, the "treatment beyond progression" arm demonstrated significantly higher response rates (48 % vs. 27 %, $p = 0.01$) and a prolonged TTP (8.5 months vs. 5.8 months, HR 0.69; $p = 0.03$). The OS was longer in patients treated with capecitabine plus trastuzumab. However, this observation did not reach statistical significance (25.5 months vs. 20.4 months, $p = 0.26$) [151].

There is further evidence for the strategy to continue treatment with trastuzumab after disease progression from a phase III trial investigating the combination of trastuzumab and lapatinib versus lapatinib alone in this setting. An overall survival benefit was seen in patients with HER2-positive and HR-negative disease [149, 152].

Further treatment options for patients progressing on or after treatment with trastuzumab will be discussed in subsequent sections on lapatinib, pertuzumab and T-DM1.

Based on its activity against metastatic HER2-positive breast cancer, several studies analyzed the benefit of trastuzumab in the (neo)adjuvant setting.

In early randomized neoadjuvant trials, like the NOAH trial, pathologic complete response rates showed a twofold increase due to trastuzumab, resulting in unprecedented pCR rates, which were confirmed in additional neoadjuvant trials, like TECHNO and GeparQuattro [153–157]. The achievement of a pCR was strongly correlated with survival in those trials, which have reported survival.

One of the pivotal trials in the adjuvant setting was the HERA trial ($n = 5099$). It started in 2001 as an international multicenter trial and randomized patients to either 1 or 2 years of trastuzumab or to observation alone after completion of standard neoadjuvant or adjuvant chemotherapy in women with HER2-positive, node-positive, or high-risk node-negative breast cancer (NCT00045032). It was shown that after a median follow-up of 8 years the addition of one year of trastuzumab significantly reduced the relative risk for death by 24 % (82.7 % vs. 77.4 %%; HR 0.76, $p = 0.0005$) in the intention to treat population. 8-year DFS was 71.2 % versus 64.8 % (HR 0.76, $p < 0.0001$) in the ITT analysis. These benefits were observed despite 52.1 % of patients in the observation arm crossing over to trastuzumab prior to a DFS event after the first results of the trial were released [158, 159]. In contrast, continuing trastuzumab for 2 years instead of one did not improve outcomes any further [159].

At the same time, two large randomized adjuvant trials in North America investigated the efficacy of 12 months of trastuzumab, added to a sequential adjuvant regimen consisting of doxorubicin/cyclophosphamide (AC) followed by paclitaxel. Trastuzumab was either started concomitantly to weekly[1] or three-weekly[2] paclitaxel or sequentially after completion of chemotherapy[3] and compared to the same adjuvant regimens without trastuzumab. The trials were very similar in design and the FDA and National Cancer Institute (NCI) allowed a joint efficacy analysis of both trials. The definitive OS analysis showed that adjuvant trastuzumab led to a relative reduction in mortality by 37 %, accompanied by a relative improvement in DFS by 40 %. 10-year OS rates improved from 75.2 to 84 % (HR 0.63, $p < 0.001$) and DFS rates from 62.2 to 73.7 % (HR0.60, $p < 0.001$), respectively [160, 161]. The N9831 trial also compared concomitant (starting with paclitaxel) to sequential adjuvant trastuzumab. The concomitant arm revealed a 5-year DFS rate of 84.4 % compared to 80.1 % in the sequential arm (HR 0.77, $p = 0.02$). However, this did not meet the prespecified statistical criteria to be significant in this interim analysis [162]. Today, the concomitant administration of trastuzumab to paclitaxel in sequential regimens is a common practice and a standard of care based on these results.

[1]in NCCTG N9831 and NSABP B31.
[2]in NSABP B31.
[3]in N9831.

The Breast Cancer International Research Group 006 phase III trial (BCIRG 006; $n = 3222$) randomized patients to either AC-T with (AC-TH) or without trastuzumab (AC-T) or TCbH (Docetaxel, Carboplatin and trastuzumab) [21]. Both trastuzumab containing regimens were superior to AC-T in terms of DFS. There was a small nonsignificant numerical difference in DFS events between AC-TH and TCbH in favor of AC-TH. However, this was counterbalanced by a fivefold increase of congestive heart failure at 10 years (21 vs. 4) and an increased risk of treatment-associated leukemia (8 vs. 1) in the AC-TH arm. [21, 30] The trial was not powered to detect differences between the AC-TH and the TCbH arm.

In the FinHer trial HER2-positive patients ($n = 232$) were randomized to receive trastuzumab or not for 9 weeks in parallel to either three cycles of docetaxel or vinorelbine, followed by $FE_{100}C$ as adjuvant therapy. Despite the short duration of therapy, the addition of trastuzumab led to an improvement in DFS from 78 to 89 % at 3 years (HR 0.42, $p = 0.01$) and a nonsignificant improvement of 3-year OS from 89.7 to 96.3 % (HR 0.41, $p = 0.07$) [163].

The French PHARE trial investigated whether a shorter duration of trastuzumab was enough. In this non-inferiority trial 6 months of trastuzumab failed to meet the criteria to prove non-inferiority compared to 1 year of adjuvant trastuzumab, which remains the current standard of care [164]. The HERA trial additionally compared one versus 2 years of adjuvant trastuzumab. No significant benefit was seen from continuing trastuzumab beyond 1 year [165]. As a consequence of these data, the FDA first granted approval to adjuvant trastuzumab in 2006. It is currently labeled as part of a regimen consisting of doxorubicin, cyclophosphamide, either paclitaxel, or docetaxel or in combination with docetaxel and carboplatin or as a single agent following multimodality anthracycline-based therapy. In 2006, trastuzumab was approved as adjuvant therapy for HER2+ EBC in Europe. In addition, the EMA recently approved a subcutaneous formulation of a fixed dose of trastuzumab based on the neoadjuvant phase III HannaH trial [166].

One of the main side effects of trastuzumab is cardiac dysfunction. Trastuzumab-related cardiotoxicity is distinct from type 1 cardiotoxicity observed with anthracyclines, in such a way that there is no dose/effect relationship and it is mostly reversible upon discontinuation of therapy. HER2 is also expressed on cardiomyocytes and is thought to be implicated in the repair of cell damage.

The definition of cardiac events slightly differed within the large randomized adjuvant trials. However, the trials report results within the same order of magnitude. After 8-years of follow-up the HERA trial reported rates of severe congestive heart failure (CHF, NYHA III & IV) of 0.8 % in the trastuzumab containing arms (1- and 2-years, sequentially) versus 0 % in the control arm. The rate of confirmed significant drops in LVEF (>10 % and below 50 %) was 7.2 % for 2 years, and 4.1 % versus 0.9 % in the 1 year and control group, respectively. Acute recovery occurred in more than 80 % of patients [167]. In a long-term safety analysis NSABP B31 and N9831 reported cardiac events mainly defined as NYHA III & IV CHF in 4.0 and 3.4 % for the concomitant arms compared to 1.3 and 0.6 % in the control arms, again with a high rate of spontaneous recovery upon cessation of trastuzumab [168, 169]. One point worthy of note is that 6.9 % of patients in NSABP B31 had unacceptably low post-AC LFEV measurements, precluding the start of trastuzumab therapy altogether [168]. The rate of cardiac death within the trials was very low and did not significantly differ between experimental and control arms. It is mandatory to assess left ventricular ejection fraction (LVEF) prior to initiation of trastuzumab and at regular intervals during treatment.

Apart from infrequent infusion reactions, which are easily controlled, trastuzumab is well tolerated, and especially, hematologic toxicities are negligible. Another rare but potentially serious adverse reaction is pulmonary toxicity, e.g., in the form of interstitial pneumonitis.

20.2.1.2 Lapatinib

Lapatinib is a small molecule dual tyrosine kinase inhibitor (TKI) directed against epidermal growth factor receptor (EGFR) and HER2. Lapatinib inhibits receptor signaling by binding to the ATP-binding pocket of the EGFR/HER2 protein kinase domain, preventing self-phosphorylation and subsequent activation of the signal cascade. Therefore, it could potentially abrogate signaling from constitutively active HER2 receptors, e.g., caused by shedding of the extracellular domain of the HER2 receptor, which cannot be inhibited by trastuzumab and in addition from HER1/HER2 heterodimers.

In a phase III study, the combination of lapatinib and capecitabine compared to capecitabine alone resulted in a prolonged TTP of 6.2 versus 4.3 months (HR 0.57, $p < 0.001$) and an increased response rate of 23.7 % compared to 13.9 % (OR 1.9, $p = 0.017$). OS in the ITT population was not significantly improved, however, the trial was stopped early as it met prespecified criteria for superiority and crossover to the combination was offered to patients in the control arm. The benefit was achieved without an increase in serious toxic effects or symptomatic cardiac events in patients with normal left ventricular ejection fraction at baseline [170–172]. Based on this trial, lapatinib was approved in combination with capecitabine in 2006 for the treatment of patients with advanced or metastatic HER2-positive breast cancer, who had received prior therapies, including anthracyclines, taxanes, and trastuzumab (second or third line). In a direct comparison of capecitabine plus either lapatinib or trastuzumab as part of a large randomized phase III trial (CEREBEL), however, the lapatinib-based combination was inferior to trastuzumab plus capecitabine [173]. An attempt to prove benefit of lapatinib in patients with HER2-negative MBC in a large randomized phase III trial based on the inhibition of EGFR in addition to HER2 failed [174].

Subsequently, the indication for lapatinib has been expanded in the US and Europe to include the combination of lapatinib and letrozol in HER2- and HR-positive patients. However, the underlying phase III trial was run in the first-line setting and patients had neither been pretreated with trastuzumab nor an aromatase inhibitor [175, 176]. The combination of lapatinib plus letrozol was tested against letrozol alone and demonstrated a significantly improved PFS and ORR, yet, without an improvement in OS. There are no comparisons of lapatinib (or trastuzumab) plus an AI versus trastuzumab plus chemotherapy, for which a clear survival benefit has been demonstrated in first-line therapy. This combination might be an alternative for patients who are not candidates for chemotherapy or with a very low disease burden, although the efficacy is lower than the combination of trastuzumab and chemotherapy. In Europe, the indication for lapatinib has also been expanded to include the combination of lapatinib and trastuzumab for trastuzumab refractory HER2-positive, HR-negative patients. A randomized phase III trial showed a significant improvement in OS from 9.5 to 14 months (HR 0.74, $p = 0.026$), which was restricted to the HR-negative subgroup (HR 0.68, $p = 0.012$) [149, 152]. However, today there are other compelling treatment options after progression on or after treatment with trastuzumab (see below).

The most common side effect, which leads to a discontinuation of lapatinib is diarrhea. Skin rash and elevation of liver enzymes are further common side effects of lapatinib. Although rarely life-threatening, the physical and psychosocial distress associated with these dermatologic reactions may reduce compliance with EGFR inhibitors [177–179]. There are data suggesting that the occurrence and severity of rash might correlate with clinical response [180], but the final confirmation of this correlation is still pending. Cardiac toxicity is a major concern in drugs targeting HER2 based on the data from trastuzumab. Perez et al. analyzed cardiac toxicity in 3689 patients treated with lapatinib within phase I–III trials. There was a 1.3 % incidence of symptomatic and asymptomatic decreases in LVEF in patients treated with lapatinib compared to 0.7 % in patients from comparator arms within these trials [181]. Thus, the cardiac toxicity of lapatinib appears to be comparably small [182].

In the neoadjuvant setting, the NeoALTTO study demonstrated promising results for lapatinib in combination with trastuzumab and chemotherapy. The dual HER2 blocking strategy lead to an almost twofold increase in pCR rates compared to chemotherapy plus trastuzumab alone [181, 183]. In its adjuvant counterpart, the ALTTO trial ($n > 8000$), however, the dual inhibition of HER2 by trastuzumab and lapatinib disappointingly did not significantly improve DFS or OS [184]. The experimental arm investigating chemotherapy and lapatinib as the single anti-HER2 agent was closed early due to inferiority to the standard arm of chemotherapy plus trastuzumab, an observation in keeping with results from several neoadjuvant trials [183, 185–187].

20.2.1.3 Pertuzumab

Pertuzumab (Perjeta®) is a fully humanized monoclonal antibody directed against the dimerization domain of HER2, preventing homo- as well as heterodimerization of HER2 with other HER family members, including the EGFR, HER3, and HER4 [188]. As a result, pertuzumab inhibits downstream signaling of two key signal pathways regulating cell growth and survival: the mitogen-activated protein kinase (MAPK) pathway and the phosphatidylinositol-3-kinase (PI3K) pathway. Inhibition of these signaling pathways can result in cell growth arrest and apoptosis [189]. In addition, it is thought to contribute to antibody-dependent cell-mediated cytotoxicity (ADCC).

The efficacy and safety of pertuzumab have been investigated in two phase II and one phase III trial in MBC. The phase II trials included patients who had received at least three prior lines of chemotherapy and had progressed on trastuzumab. Patients received pertuzumab plus trastuzumab without chemotherapy. In BO17929 ($n = 66$), the combination demonstrated significant antitumor activity with a response rate of 24.2 % and a median PFS of 5.5 months [190]. To determine if the observed effect was a result of the combination of pertuzumab and trastuzumab or mainly pertuzumab alone, a second cohort was recruited which was initially treated with single agent pertuzumab with trastuzumab added in upon progression of disease. Results for the monotherapy with pertuzumab were disappointing (ORR 3.4 %) but activity could be recovered by the addition of trastuzumab (ORR 17.9 %), providing solid evidence that the clinical benefit is only obtained by the combination of the two antibodies [191].

The main evidence for the efficacy of pertuzumab plus trastuzumab was obtained from the pivotal CLEOPATRA trial. In this large randomized, placebo-controlled phase III trial, patients were randomized to docetaxel plus trastuzumab and either pertuzumab or placebo as first-line therapy for HER2-positive breast cancer. Patients were allowed to have received prior (neo)adjuvant chemotherapy with or without trastuzumab if the disease-free interval was more than 12 months. Response rates in the pertuzumab group were significantly increased from 69.3 to 80.2 % ($p = 0.001$) as was median PFS (Δ 6.1 months; HR 0.62, $p < 0.001$). The effect size observed in patients who had received prior trastuzumab was identical. However, even more striking was an unprecedented improvement of OS by 15.7 months from 40.8 to 56.6 months (HR 0.68, $p < 0.001$) [192–194]. These results have clearly defined the new standard for the first-line treatment of HER2-positive metastatic breast cancer. In Europe and the US, pertuzumab has been approved in combination with docetaxel and trastuzumab for the treatment of patients with HER2-positive advanced breast cancer, who have not received prior anti-HER2 or chemotherapy for metastatic disease.

In addition, two neoadjuvant phase II trials, the NeoSphere and the TRYPHAENA trial demonstrated superior pCR rates for the dual blockade with pertuzumab and trastuzumab. Taken together with the large survival benefit in metastatic disease, these data have led to the approval of pertuzumab in combination with trastuzumab and chemotherapy in the neoadjuvant setting, based on pCR as a possible surrogate for survival.

In the Neosphere trial, 417 patients with HER2 + primary breast cancer and tumors larger than 2 cm were randomized to four cycles of docetaxel in combination with either trastuzumab or pertuzumab alone or the combination of both. A chemotherapy-free treatment option consisting of the combination of trastuzumab and pertuzumab was also investigated. Patients receiving docetaxel in combination with pertuzumab and trastuzumab achieved a pCR rate of 45.8 %, which was significantly higher than that in the docetaxel/trastuzumab group (29 %; $p = 0.0063$). The chemotherapy-free treatment arm achieved a pCR rate of 16.8 % (31 % for HER2+/HR− patients) and the docetaxel/pertuzumab combination 23 % [195].

The TRYPHAENA trial was designed to evaluate the safety and tolerability of trastuzumab and pertuzumab in combination with either anthracycline-based or carboplatin-based neoadjuvant chemotherapy. 225 patients were randomized to three cycles of FEC followed by three cycles of docetaxel and either trastuzumab and pertuzumab concurrently with the entire adjuvant chemotherapy or beginning with docetaxel. The third arm received a combination of docetaxel (75 mg/m^2), carboplatin (AUC5), trastuzumab, and pertuzumab. PCR rates (ypT0 ypN0) ranged from 45.3 to 51.9 %, with the highest pCR rate observed in the anthracycline-free treatment arm. The FDA and EMA have now approved pertuzumab in combination with chemotherapy for neoadjuvant therapy in HER2-positive patients with a high risk of recurrence [196].

The main adverse reactions observed with pertuzumab (in combination with trastuzumab and chemotherapy) are diarrhea, neutropenia, febrile neutropenia, and asthenia. Cardiac safety is a main concern in HER2-directed therapy, especially in dual HER2-blockade. However, the addition of pertuzumab to trastuzumab in the available trials only marginally increased the rates of cardiac events. In the CLEOPATRA trial, the rate of symptomatic congestive heart failure was 1.8 % in the combination group compared to 1.0 % in patients only receiving trastuzumab. The rate of decline of LVEF by more than 10 % and below the 50 % threshold was also slightly higher (6.6 % vs. 3.8 %), however, the majority of patients recovered spontaneously after cessation of treatment with pertuzumab and trastuzumab [197, 198].

20.2.1.4 Ado-Trastuzumab Emtansine, T-DM1

T-DM1 (Kadcyla®) is a novel antibody–drug conjugate composed of emtansine covalently linked to trastuzumab. Emtansine, a maytansine derivative, is a highly potent anti-microtubule agent. Trastuzumab specifically directs the linked emtansine against HER2-overexpressing cells, thereby minimizing exposure of normal tissue and increasing the therapeutic window.

The EMILIA trial randomized 991 patients, who had previously been treated with a taxane and trastuzumab, to either lapatinib/capecitabine or T-DM1. Compared to capecitabine and lapatinib, T-DM1 significantly prolonged the median PFS from 6.4 to 9.6 months (HR 0.65, $p < 0.001$) as well as overall survival from 25.1 to 30.9 months (HR 0.68, $p < 0.001$). Moreover, T-DM1 also demonstrated a lower overall toxicity and was generally well tolerated. Rates of adverse events of grade ⩾3 were higher for lapatinib/capecitabine than for patients treated with T-DM1 (57 % vs. 41 %) [199, 200]. Based on the EMILIA study, the FDA and EMA granted T-DM1 approval in 2013 for the treatment of patients with HER2-positive metastatic breast cancer who have previously been treated with a taxane and trastuzumab. Patients must have received prior therapy for metastatic disease or must have relapsed within 6 months after completing adjuvant therapy.

An additional large phase III trial (TH3RESA) comparing T-DM1 to a physician's choice of treatment in patients, who had previously been treated with at least two lines of HER2-directed therapies for advanced disease, including trastuzumab, lapatinib, and a taxane provides further evidence for the efficacy and tolerability of T-DM1. In this heavily pretreated population, with more than half of patients having received at least three prior lines of therapy for advanced disease, T-DM1 significantly prolonged PFS from 3.3 to 6.2 months (HR 0.528, $p < 0.0001$) as well as OS from 15.8 to 22.78 months (HR 0.68, $p = 0.0007$) [201, 202].

The most prominent grade 3/4 adverse events of T-DM1 are thrombocytopenia and elevated liver enzymes. Cardiac events were low in both trials.

Based on data from EMILIA and TH3RESA, T-DM1 is now the standard of care as second-line therapy of HER2-positive MBC, as well as in later lines if prior therapy did not include T-DM1 [203].

T-DM1 does also appear to have some activity in CNS metastasis. A subgroup analysis of the EMILIA trial focusing on patients with brain metastasis at baseline demonstrated a longer OS in patients treated with T-DM1 (26.8 vs. 12.9 months; HR 0.38, $p = 0.008$) [204]. In addition, several case series document response of brain metastases to T-DM1 [205, 206].

Given the benefit from the addition of pertuzumab to trastuzumab plus docetaxel observed in CLEOPATRA, a large randomized phase III trial, the MARIANNE trial, set to investigate the combination of T-DM1 and pertuzumab in the first-line setting. MARIANNE randomized 1095 women with HER2-positive MBC to either trastuzumab plus a taxane or to T-DM1 plus either placebo or pertuzumab. Surprisingly, none of the treatment arms showed a significantly improved PFS (13.7, 14.1, and 15.2 months, respectively) [207] and OS data are still immature. Thus, standards for first and second-line treatment choices remain unaffected.

The role of T-DM1 in the (neo)adjuvant setting is currently scrutinized in several trials. The ADAPT trial recently reported a pCR rate (ypT0/is ypN0) of 41 % in HER2- and HR-positive patients treated with only four cycles of T-DM1 (± endocrine therapy) [208].

20.2.1.5 New HER2-Directed Agents and Combinations Under Investigation

Currently a new generation of HER2-directed TKIs is under investigation. The most extensively studied members are neratinib and afatinib, both irreversible inhibitors, neratinib directed against HER1, −2 and −4, and afatinib a pan-HER inhibitor. For both agents, diarrhea is a main dose-limiting toxicity [199].

Afatinib has failed to demonstrate a benefit in phase II and III trials in breast cancer (LUX-Breast 1 and 3) and is unlikely to gain approval for HER2-positive MBC [209, 210].

Neratinib has yielded some positive data in clinical trials and has recently demonstrated to prolong invasive disease-free survival (iDFS) in the ExteNET trial (NCT00878709), which randomized patients with HER2-positive PBC within 1 year after completion of adjuvant trastuzumab to either 1 year of neratinib or placebo. IDFS was significantly improved in the group treated with neratinib (HR 0.73, $p = 0.023$), an effect that was exclusively observed in the HR-positive subgroup (HR 0.57, $p = 0.004$) [211]. These data are in contrast to data from the extended (2 years) trastuzumab arm in the HERA trial [159].

Based on the hypothesis, that downstream activation of the PI3K-Akt-mTOR pathway can be responsible for trastuzumab resistance, preclinical data have demonstrated that resistance to trastuzumab can be reversed by the addition of everolimus, an oral mTOR inhibitor blocking the PI3K pathway (Table 20.8) [212]. The combination of chemotherapy, trastuzumab, and everolimus has been investigated in two phase III trials for MBC, BOLERO-1, and BOLERO-3. The two trials demonstrated no or only a marginal benefit in terms of DFS [213, 214]. Nonetheless, it was indicated that HR-negative patients might derive more benefit from adding everolimus to trastuzumab. However, at this point there is no role for everolimus in the therapy of HER2-positive metastatic breast cancer. Several PIK3CA inhibitors such as BYL719, taselisib, and pilaralisib are currently being investigated in HER2+ breast cancer [65]. The addition of bevacizumab, a recombinant humanized monoclonal antibody against VEGF, to trastuzumab and chemotherapy has not improved outcomes in early or metastatic breast cancer in two large randomized phase III trials (AVAREL, BETH) [80, 81].

20.2.2 Antiangiogenic Agents

Neo-angiogenesis is one of the hallmarks of cancer implicated in tumor growth, invasion, and metastasis. It is a prerequisite for the progression of solid tumors. Inhibition of tumor angiogenesis is therefore regarded as an attractive therapeutic target. Table 20.9 summarizes antiangiogenic therapies used or investigated in breast cancer.

20.2.2.1 Bevacizumab

Bevacizumab (Avastin®) is a recombinant humanized monoclonal IgG1 antibody that binds to vascular endothelial growth factor A (VEGF-A), one of the most potent pro-angiogenic factors and inhibits its biologic activity in vitro and in vivo assay systems [215]. Bevacizumab prevents the interaction of VEGF with its receptors (Flt-1 and KDR) on the surface of endothelial cells, which normally leads to endothelial cell proliferation and new blood vessel formation. Administration of bevacizumab to xenotransplant models of colon cancer in mice caused reduction of microvascular growth and inhibition of metastatic disease progression. Therapies that inhibit VEGF may have multiple effects on angiogenesis and tumor growth, most importantly, reducing the tumor's blood supply, preventing the development of new blood vessels in the tumor and facilitating the delivery of chemotherapy to the tumor cells, which can be explained by the concept of "normalization of tumor vasculature" [216–218].

Based on preclinical findings demonstrating activity of bevacizumab in breast cancer, bevacizumab was tested in MBC initially as monotherapy. Cobleigh et al. evaluated the safety and efficacy in a phase I/II dose escalation trial in patients with previously treated MBC [219]. The overall response rate was 9.3 % (confirmed response rate, 6.7 %) and the median duration of confirmed response was

Table 20.8 Endocrine therapies and targeted agents used in combination with endocrine therapy

Agent	Trade name® (examples)	Mode of action	Dosing	Interactions	Selected adverse effects
Tamoxifen	Nolvadex	Selective estrogen receptor modulator. Tamoxifen is a prodrug that needs to be metabolized into several active metabolites including endoxifen	20 mg daily p.o.	Interaction with inhibitors of CYP2D6 Strong inhibitors of CYP2D6 should be avoided as they might lead to significantly reduced levels of active metabolites May increase anticoagulant effects if used in combination with coumarin-type anticoagulants	thromboembolic events, raised blood triglyceride levels, vaginal bleeding, endometrium hyperplasia, endometrial polyps and endometrial cancer, headache, vaginal discharge and dryness, pruritus vulvae, fluid retention, hot flushes, menopausal symptoms, hair thinning, mood disturbances, visual disturbances, including corneal changes, retinal vein thrombosis, retinopathy and cataracts, fatigue, elevation of liver enzymes, fatty liver may cause fetal harm
Exemestan Anastrozol Letrozol	Aromasin Arimidex Femara	Steroidal irreversible aromatase inhibitor Nonsteroidal AI Nonsteroidal AI	25 mg daily p.o. 1 mg daily p.o. 2.5 mg daily p.o.	CYP450 enzymes	Loss of bone mineral density, osteoporosis, fractures, fatigue, raised blood triglyceride, hypercholesterinemia, vaginal dryness, vaginal bleeding, headache, hot flushes, increased sweating, night sweats, menopausal symptoms, arthralgia, headache, nausea, vomiting, skin rash, hair thinning, elevation of liver enzymes
Goserelin Leuprorelin	Zoladex Enantone Gyn	GnRH (gonadotropin-releasing hormone)- agonist	3.6 mg q4w s.c. (the 10.8 mg q12w dose is only approved for the treatment of prostate cancer) 3.75 mg q4w s.c. or IM (not US)	None	Fatigue, hot flushes, increased sweating, loss of bone mineral density, osteoporosis, hypertension, hypotension, headache, arthralgia, menopausal symptoms, decreased libido, vaginitis, seborrhea, peripheral edema, emotional lability, depression, hypersensitivity reactions
Fulvestrant	Faslodex	Selective estrogen receptor downregulator	500 mg q4w IM with an additional dose on day 15 of the first cycle	None	Nausea, vomiting, constipation, diarrhea, abdominal pain, headache, back pain, hot flushes, sore throat, vaginal bleeding, thromboembolic events Due to its intramuscular injection, fulvestrant should be used with great caution in patients with bleeding disorders, thrombocytopenia or taking anticoagulants
Everolimus	Afinitor	An oral mTOR inhibitor targeting mTORC1, one of the two mTOR complexes	10 mg daily p.o.	CYP3A4, p-GP;inhibitors and inducers should be avoided	Hyperglycemia, hypertriglycerinemia, hypercholesterinemia, noninfectious pneumonitis, infections, infestations, oral ulcerations, renal impairment, anemia, lymphopenia, neutropenia, thrombocytopenia, impaired wound healing. Avoid live vaccines and close contact with those who have received live vaccines. Can cause fetal harm

(continued)

Table 20.8 (continued)

Agent	Trade name® (examples)	Mode of action	Dosing	Interactions	Selected adverse effects
Palbociclib	Ibrance	an oral cdk4/6 inhibitor	125 mg once daily taken 21 days followed by 7 days off-treatment	CYP3A inhibitors and inducers (should be avoided)	neutropenia, leukopenia, infections, febrile neutropenia, fatigue, nausea, anemia, stomatitis, headache, diarrhea, thrombocytopenia, constipation, alopecia, vomiting, rash, and decreased appetite, pulmonary embolism can cause fetal harm

These highlights do not include all the information needed to use the respective drugs safely and effectively. See full prescribing information for all information needed to use these agents safely. We do not take responsibility for the correctness of the content

Table 20.9 Antiangiogenic agents

Agent	Trade name	Mode of action	Dosing	Interactions	Selected adverse effects
Bevacizumab	Avastin	Humanized monoclonal anti-VEGF a monoclonal IgG1 antibody	10 mg/kg q2w or 15 mg/kg q3w IV (for breast cancer) in combination with paclitaxel or capecitabine as first-line treatment of MBC EMA approval, not approved for breast or ovarian cancer by the FDA		Proteinuria, hypertension, hypertensive crisis, hemorrhage, arterial and venous thromboembolic events, surgery and wound healing complications, gastrointestinal perforations and fistulae, reversible posterior leukoencephalopathy syndrome (RPLS), fatigue, nausea, vomiting, mucositis, stomatitis, fatigue, congestive heart failure, may increase risk of osteonecrosis of the jaw. Bevacizumab may cause fetal harm.
Sorafenib	Nexavar	Multi-tyrosine kinase inhibitor with antiproliferative (RAF, c-KIT, Flt-3) and anti-angio-genic (VEGFR-2, PDGFR-β) effects	800 mg/d (400 mg twice daily) p.o. Not approved for breast cancer, has failed to provide evidence of efficacy in phase II/III trials	Interaction with inhibitors and inducer of CYP3A4	Palmar-plantar erythrodysesthesia, skin rash, severe skin toxicity, hypertension, (hypertensive crisis), hemorrhage, nausea, vomiting, diarrhea, drug induced hepatitis (monitor liver enzymes), myelosuppression, electrolyte disturbances including hypophosphatemia, QT prolongation, cataract, arterial and venous thrombosis, gastrointestinal perforations. Can cause fetal harm
Sunitinib	Sutent	Multi-tyrosine kinase inhibitor with antiproliferative (c-KIT, CSF1R) and anti-angio-genic (VEGFR-R, PDGFR) effects	GIST and RCC: 50 mg orally once daily, with or without food, 4 weeks on treatment followed by 2 weeks off. pNET: 37.5 mg orally once daily, with or without food, continuously without a scheduled off-treatment period. Not approved for the treatment of breast cancer. Negative findings from phase II/III trials	Interaction with inhibitors and inducer of CYP3A4	Hepatotoxicity, proteinuria, hemorrhage, QT interval prolongation, hypertension, wound healing and surgical complications, left ventricular dysfunction, thyroid dysfunction, hypoglycemia, dermatologic toxicities including erythema multiforme and Stevens–Johnson syndrome, osteonecrosis of the jaw, thromboembolic events Sunitinib can cause fetal harm

(continued)

Table 20.9 (continued)

Agent	Trade name	Mode of action	Dosing	Interactions	Selected adverse effects
Aflibercept (VEGF-Trap)	Zaltrap	Fully human soluble VEGF receptor fusion protein targeting vascular endothelial growth factor (VEGF)	4 mg/kg body weight q2w IV in combination with FOLFIRI approved for mCRC Not approved for breast cancer		Proteinuria, hypertension (hypertensive crisis), fatigue, nausea, vomiting, mucositis, stomatitis, hemorrhage, epistaxis, wound healing disturbances, gastrointestinal perforations and fistulae, arterial and venous thromboembolic events, neutropenia (in combination with chemotherapy), infusion and hypersensitivity reactions, reversible posterior leukoencephalopathy syndrome (RPLS) May cause fetal harm.
Ramucirumab	Cymraza	fully human monoclonal antibody directed against the extracellular domain of VEGFR-2 which blocks the interaction between VEGF A, C, D and VEGFR-2	8 mg/kg q2w IV as single agent or in combination with weekly paclitaxel Approved for metastatic gastric cancer not approved for breast cancer		Hypertension, arterial and venous thromboembolic events, hemorrhage, gastrointestinal perforations and fistulae, impaired wound healing, infusion reactions, reversible posterior leukoencephalopathy syndrome (RPLS), clinical deterioration of liver Child-Pugh B or C liver cirrhosis. May cause fetal harm

These highlights do not include all the information needed to use the respective drugs safely and effectively. See full prescribing information for all information needed to use these agents safely. We do not take responsibility for the correctness of the content

5.5 months (range 2.3–13.7 months) with an overall survival of 10.2 months. Bevacizumab was well tolerated; the main side effects were headache, nausea and vomiting, hypertension, minor bleeding (epistaxis), venous thromboembolic events, and proteinuria. The dose-limiting toxicity was headache associated with nausea and vomiting. This was neither caused by hypertension nor by brain metastases.

Several phase III trials have subsequently investigated the efficacy of bevacizumab in combination with chemotherapy. The pivotal open-label randomized phase III trial, ECOG 2100, demonstrated that the addition of bevacizumab to paclitaxel increased median PFS from 5.9 to 11.8 months (HR 0.6, $p < 0.001$) and doubled the response rates (25.2 % vs. 49.2 %, $p < 0.001$) in first-line unselected metastatic breast cancer. However, there was no significant improvement in OS [220, 221].

In 2008, the FDA granted accelerated approval for bevacizumab to be used in combination with first-line paclitaxel for metastatic HER2-negative breast cancer, based on these results. Approval by the EMA followed in 2009.

Consistent with E2100, all of the phase III trials in the first-line setting (AVADO, Ribbon-1) as well as later lines (Ribbon-2), demonstrated significantly improved overall response rates as well as progression-free survival, even if at a considerably lower level, but failed to provide evidence that bevacizumab in combination with first-line chemotherapy prolongs overall survival [123, 222–224]. The efficacy of bevacizumab in addition to weekly paclitaxel could further be confirmed by identical results observed for the combination in the TURANDOT study (PFS 11 months, ORR 44 %) and CALGB 40502 study (PFS 10.6 months) [225, 226].

Subsequently, a pooled analysis of the three randomized phase III first-line trials including 2447 patients also failed to demonstrate any indication of an overall survival benefit from bevacizumab [227]. Triple-negative breast cancer is associated with a significantly higher expression and more frequent amplification of VEGF-A [228–230]. This has led to the hypothesis of a specifically higher activity of antiangiogenic agents in TNBC. Yet, neither of the individual trials nor the combined analyses found a sign of a more pronounced or even OS benefit from bevacizumab in triple-negative MBC. The combined analysis included 621 patients with TNBC from these trials and confirmed the increased ORR (42 % vs. 23 %) and PFS (8.1 vs. 5.4 months; HR 0.63; $p < 0.0001$), however, without a trend for an improved OS (18.9 vs. 17.5 months; HR 0.96; ns) [227].

In November 2011, the FDA revoked its accelerated approval for bevacizumab for the treatment of breast cancer based on the findings from the confirmatory trials. Thus, bevacizumab is no longer approved for the treatment of metastatic breast cancer in the US. Other indications remained untouched from this decision. In contrast, bevacizumab remains approved in the EU by the EMA for first-line treatment of HER2-negative metastatic breast cancer in combination with paclitaxel and capecitabine.

The role of bevacizumab in early breast cancer has also been investigated in several phase II and III trials. Data from neoadjuvant trials provide evidence for a moderate improvement of pCR rates from the addition of bevacizumab to anthracycline- and taxane-based neoadjuvant chemotherapy. In the German neoadjuvant GeparQuinto trial ($n = 1948$), adding bevacizumab significantly improved pCR rates (ypT0/is ypN0) from 16.5 to 20.5 % ($p = 0.03$). This effect was completely driven by patients with TNBC (27.9 vs. 39.3 %, $p = 0.003$) [231]. In GeparQuinto, bevacizumab was only given during the neoadjuvant treatment phase. Thus, effects of longer adjuvant bevacizumab maintenance could not be investigated. The trial reported no trends for improved survival (DFS and OS), neither in the overall study population nor in the TNBC subgroup [232]. At the same time, the NSABP B40 phase III trial reported a numerical but insignificant increase of pCR by the addition of bevacizumab, from 23 to 27.9 % ($p = 0.08$) [233]. In contrast to GeparQuinto, a significant difference in pCR rates was observed within the HR-positive subgroup (11.1 % vs. 16.8 %, $p = 0.03$). Recently, a randomized neoadjuvant trial exclusively conducted in triple-negative disease, the CALGB 40603 (Alliance) trial ($n = 443$), reported a marginal increase in pCR (ypT0/is ypN0) from 44 to 52 % ($p = 0.057$) for patients randomized to bevacizumab [116]. Thus, data from the neoadjuvant trials remain inconclusive.

It is still a matter of debate how far pCR rates can be regarded a surrogate for survival and moreover, how large the increment in pCR rates has to be in order to translate into a survival benefit. Thus, data from adjuvant trials have to be regarded as more informative in this respect. To date, two large adjuvant randomized phase III trials have reported survival data in addition to the neoadjuvant NSABP B40 in which patients received adjuvant bevacizumab maintenance therapy [234]. BEATRICE ($n = 2591$) exclusively included patients with triple-negative disease. The trial randomized patients after standard adjuvant chemotherapy to either 12 months of adjuvant bevacizumab maintenance or observation [235]. After a median follow-up of 32 months, there was no significant difference in invasive DFS (iDFS), the primary endpoint. 3-year iDFS was 82.7 in the observation arm versus 83.7 % in patients randomized to receive bevacizumab (HR 0.87, $p = 0.18$). Based on the number of events in this triple-negative population a signal of efficacy could have been expected if there was any clinically meaningful difference, despite the relatively short follow-up. The second large randomized phase III trial investigating the adjuvant role of bevacizumab, the ECOG 5103 trial ($n = 4950$), also included all HR-positive patients. Patients either received standard chemotherapy consisting of AC followed by weekly paclitaxel alone or in combination with bevacizumab concomitantly to the chemotherapy-only or for an additional maintenance phase [236]. There was no significant difference in iDFS between the chemotherapy-only arm and the bevacizumab maintenance arm. 5-year iDFs was 77 % for chemotherapy-only and 80 % for patients receiving bevacizumab maintenance (HR 0.87, $p = 0.17$). 5-year OS rates were identical between the two arms (90 %). In patients with triple-negative disease, there seemed to be a trend for a better iDFS in patients receiving bevacizumab (HR 0.77, 95 % CI 0.58–1.03). In NSABP B40, which also included patients with HR-positive disease, bevacizumab led to a significant improvement in OS (HR 0.68, $p = 0.004$). The effect, however, was more pronounced in the HR-positive subset. Thus, the data on bevacizumab in the adjuvant setting are inconsistent and bevacizumab does not play a role in the treatment of primary breast cancer.

To date, there is no clinically useful validated predictive biomarker for the benefit of bevacizumab, precluding the possibility to define a subgroup of patients with clearer benefit from bevacizumab and possibly an OS improvement. Retrospective analyses of several prospective trials have suggested that plasma VEGF-A levels might provide such a biomarker for patient selection. The prospective MERIDIAN trial (NCT01663727) was designed to validate the predictive value of plasma VEGF-A. Patients were randomized to paclitaxel plus either placebo or bevacizumab as first-line therapy, stratified by baseline plasma VEGF-A. The trial confirmed the well-recognized PFS benefit from bevacizumab (HR 0.68, $p = 0.0007$) but failed to demonstrate any meaning of pVEGF-A as a predictive biomarker. There was no differential benefit from bevacizumab comparing the pVEGF-A high versus low group. The results have only been presented in abstract form at the ESMO meeting 2015 [237].

Due to the only modest benefit associated with bevacizumab, the ESO-ESMO 2nd international consensus guidelines for advanced breast cancer (ABC2) state that this is only an option in selected cases for first- (and second-) line therapy [2]. This might apply, e.g., to situations in which a fast response is of importance (e.g., heavy disease burden, visceral crisis) and in which combination chemotherapy regimens might otherwise be considered.

The most important bevacizumab-associated side effects are hypertension, proteinuria, thromboembolic events, bleeding, surgery and wound healing complications, bowel perforations, fistulae, and reversible posterior leukoencephalopathy syndrome (RPLS) as a very rare but serious complication. Bevacizumab has also been suspected to increase the risk of osteonecrosis of the jaw when combined with bisphosphonates and also to increase the risk of symptomatic congestive heart failure.

20.2.2.2 Antiangiogenic Tyrosine Kinase Inhibitors (TKIs) and Other Agents, Sorafenib, Sunitinib

In addition to monoclonal antibodies, a series of tyrosine kinase inhibitors (TKIs) against pro-angiogenic kinases like VEGF- and PDGF-receptors has been developed, including Sunitinib, Sorafenib, and Pazopanib. As a result of the increased off-target effects of these TKIs, combination with chemotherapeutic agents has proven difficult. Their efficacy as monotherapy in MBC is limited with ORRs ranging from 0 to 11 % [238–241]. Sunitinib and Sorafenib have been developed in phase IIb/III programs.

Sunitinib (SUTENT®)

Sunitinib is an oral multi-targeted antiangiogenic tyrosine kinase inhibitor (TKI). It inhibits vascular endothelial growth factor receptor (VEGFR), platelet-derived growth factor receptor (PDGFR), stem cell factor receptor (KIT), and colony-stimulating factor-1 receptor (CSF1R). Currently, it is approved in the US and EU as a single agent for the treatment of gastrointestinal stromal tumors (GIST), advanced renal cell carcinoma (RCC) and pancreatic neuroendocrine tumors (pNET). Sunitinib demonstrated an overall response rate of 11 % in a single-arm phase II trial in patients with metastatic breast cancer who were pretreated with anthracycline and taxane [242]. It has been extensively investigated in a series of phase III clinical trials, but failed to prove any benefit both as monotherapy and in combination with chemotherapy. However, it caused considerable additional toxicity [238, 243–245]. Further development of sunitinib in breast cancer has been discontinued.

Sorafenib (NEXAVAR®)

Sorafenib is an oral inhibitor of multiple tyrosine kinases, currently indicated for hepatocellular carcinoma, advanced renal cell carcinoma, and differentiated thyroid carcinoma. It inhibits RAF kinases, c-KIT, and Flt-3, VEGFR-2 as well as PDGFR-β and has antiproliferative as well as antiangiogenic effects, targeting both tumor and endothelial cells [246, 247]. It has been hypothesized that this broader spectrum of activity might help bypass some of the resistance mechanisms observed with bevacizumab which prevent greater efficacy of the anti-VEGF-mAB. Sorafenib demonstrated activity in a phase IIb study in combination with either capecitabine or gemcitabine in patients who had received prior therapy with bevacizumab, though accompanied by a high rate of palmar-plantar erythema (45 % grade 3) [248, 249]. However, in the confirmatory placebo-controlled phase III trial, sorafenib, when combined with capecitabine, failed to improve PFS (HR 0.97, $p = 0.46$) or OS (HR 1.19, $p = 0–93$), but expectedly caused extensive toxicities [250]. Other randomized trials investigating the combination of sorafenib and docetaxel also failed to demonstrate efficacy of sorafenib in chemotherapy combinations [251, 252]. Based on the available data, further investigations of the role of sorafenib in breast cancer do not seem warranted.

Several other antiangiogenic multi-tyrosine kinase inhibitors, like pazopanib (VOTRIENT®) and cediranib, have been investigated in breast cancer [253–256]. In the light of their modest activity but considerable toxicity none of these antiangiogenic TKIs will play a role in the treatment of MBC.

20.2.2.3 Aflibercept, VEGF-Trap (ZALTRAP®)

Aflibercept (VEGF-Trap) is a fully human soluble VEGF receptor fusion protein with a unique mechanism of action. It is a potent inhibitor of angiogenesis that binds to VEGF-A with higher affinity than monoclonal antibodies. It blocks all VEGF-A and -B isoforms plus placental growth factor (PIGF), another pro-angiogenic factor involved in tumor angiogenesis. VEGF-Trap exerts its antiangiogenic effects through regression of tumor vasculature, remodeling, or normalization of surviving vasculature and inhibition of new tumor vessel growth. VEGF-Trap has a relatively long half-life of approximately 2 weeks. Based on a significant prolongation of OS in a randomized phase III trial, it has been approved in combination with FOLFIRI for the treatment of metastatic colorectal cancer (mCRC) after prior therapy with oxaliplatin [257, 258]. The North Central Cancer Treatment Group (NCCTG) N0573 2-stage phase II trial explored the efficacy of single agent aflibercept in metastatic breast cancer after prior therapy with anthracyclines and taxanes and could only demonstrate minor activity with an overall response rate of 4.8 % and a median PFS of 2.4 months. As the trial did not meet its primary efficacy goals, the study was terminated after the inclusion of 21 patients [259]. Toxicity was as expected for an anti-VEGF therapy. There is currently no further development of aflibercept in breast cancer.

20.2.2.4 Ramucirumab (CYRAMZA®)

Ramucirumab is a fully human monoclonal antibody directed against the extracellular domain of VEGFR-2 which blocks the interaction between VEGF and VEGFR-2. It has demonstrated improvements in OS in metastatic gastric cancer and advanced non-small-cell lung cancer [260, 261]. Ramucirumab is currently approved for the treatment of metastatic gastric cancer. In breast cancer, ramucirumab has been investigated in a large randomized phase III trial (TRIO-012; $n = 1144$) in the first-line setting. Patients were randomly assigned to either docetaxel plus placebo or ramucirumab. The addition of ramucirumab did not lead to a meaningful improvement of clinical outcome (PFS: HR 0.88, $p = 0.08$; OS HR 1.01, $p = 0.92$) [262]. There are currently no ongoing trials for the clinical development of ramucirumab in breast cancer.

20.2.2.5 Trebananib (AMG386)

Apart from VEGF and its receptors, a second key regulatory pathway, the angiopoetin axis, is involved in the induction and regulation of tumor angiogenesis. Angiopoetin-1 and Angiopoetin-2 (Ang-1, Ang-2) regulate the vasculature by binding to their proprietary receptor tyrosine kinase tie-2. Vascular remodeling is regulated by the balance between Ang-1 and Ang-2. Ang-1, predominantly secreted by vascular smooth muscle cell and pericytes, leads to vessel normalization, whereas Ang-2 increases vessel destabilization and endothelial cell migration [263–266]. Although both pathways, VEGF/VEGFR and angiopoetin/Tie-2, are distinct they interact and block both pathways simultaneously which may lead to a more complete control of tumor growth than blocking just one. Trebananib is a novel recombinant peptide-Fc fusion protein (peptibody) selectively targeting the interaction of Ang1 and Ang2 with the Tie2 receptor. In preclinical studies, the combination of bevacizumab and trebananib showed enhanced antitumor activity compared to each drug alone. In a randomized phase III trial (TRINOVA-1, $n = 919$) in recurrent ovarian cancer, trebananib (15 mg/kg) demonstrated activity when added to weekly paclitaxel with a significantly prolonged median PFS (HR 0.66, $p < 0.0001$). At the interim analysis there was no significant difference in overall survival [267]. Generalized or localized edema as well as pleural effusions and ascites account for the most striking toxicity specifically associated with trebananib. In breast cancer, the efficacy of trebananib was investigated in a large randomized phase II trial. Patients with metastatic, HER2-negative breast cancer received weekly paclitaxel in combination with bevacizumab plus two different doses of trebananib or in combination with either bevacizumab or trebananib alone. The trial was unable to demonstrate a significant prolongation of PFS from the addition of trebananib to paclitaxel and bevacizumab [268].

20.2.3 Endocrine Therapy (ET)

About 60–80 % of breast cancers are hormone receptor (HR) positive. The concept of endocrine therapy in the treatment of breast cancer was already introduced in 1896 when George Beatson reported surgical removal of the ovaries (now known as the major source of estrogen) could benefit women with inoperable breast cancer. However, at that time neither estrogens nor their receptors and functions were known. See Table 20.8 for a summary of antihormonal agents and targeted agents used in combination with endocrine therapy.

20.2.3.1 Selective Estrogen Receptor Modulators (SERMs), Tamoxifen

Selective estrogen receptor modulators (SERMs), in contrast to complete estrogen receptor (ER) antagonists, exert differential tissue selective, mixed agonist–antagonist effects. These tissue selective effects vary between the different members of the class. Upon dimerization, estrogen receptors are translocated into the cell nucleus and exert most of their function as transcription factors. Further, nongenomic functions of ER have been described but are not very well understood yet.

Most SERMs exhibit anti-estrogenic effects on breast tissue and some members of this class of drugs have proven to be effective chemopreventive agents against breast cancer. However, several SERMs, e.g., tamoxifen exhibit agonistic activity in the endometrium, which in the case of tamoxifen leads to a significantly (two- to threefold) increased risk of endometrial cancer, which has been observed in many trials. In contrast, raloxifen does not seem to have any relevant stimulatory effects on the endometrium. In addition, SERMs generally exhibit tissue selective agonist activity on the bone, which in the case of raloxifen, has been clinically exploited to prevent and treat osteoporosis [269]. These tissue selective agonistic activities are not observed with therapies purely leading to estrogen deprivation like aromatase inhibitors (AIs), which explains their detrimental effects on bone mineral density and unchanged risk of endometrial cancer. Although not fully understood, most of the tissue-specific antagonist–agonist activity of SERMs is explained by three interactive mechanisms: differential expression of ERα and ERβ in different target tissues, a differential conformational change upon ligand binding, and differential expression and binding of ER co-regulatory proteins.

Tamoxifen

Tamoxifen has been the most commonly used drug for the treatment of breast cancer for decades. It is currently used for the treatment of HR-positive advanced and early breast cancer, irrespective of stage and menopausal status. Tamoxifen is the standard endocrine treatment for male breast cancer as well.

Tamoxifen itself is considered a prodrug with relatively weak affinity for ER and is subject to extensive metabolism. For the conversion of tamoxifen into its clinically active metabolites 4-hydroxy-tamoxifen and endoxifen (4-hydroxy-*N*-desmethyltamoxifen), the cytochrome P450 enzyme CYP2D6 in the liver is the rate limiting step. The active metabolites have a 30–100-fold greater affinity for ER and endoxifen is regarded as the most clinically active metabolite. CYP2D6 is a highly polymorphic gene, and it has been suggested that patients carrying variants with lower enzymatic activity (poor metabolizers) might derive less benefit from tamoxifen. Endoxifen blood levels do vary according to CYP2D6 genotype and are influenced by the concomitant use of CYP2D6 inhibitors like paroxetine. In addition, some retrospective studies have demonstrated reduced clinical activity of tamoxifen in poor metabolizers [270–274]. However, several subsequent clinical investigations have produced conflicting results [275]. A retrospective analysis of CYP2D6 variants in two large randomized phase III trials of adjuvant endocrine therapy (BIG 1-98 and ATAC) failed to provide any evidence of a predictive role of CYP2D6 genetic testing with regards to benefit from tamoxifen [276, 277]. Therefore, currently there is no role of CYP2D6 testing to tailor endocrine therapy for breast cancer.

Tamoxifen first reported activity as an endocrine therapy option for the treatment of breast cancer in 1971 with a response rate of 22 % [278]. Of note, early trials have not been conducted exclusively in HR-positive patients but in unselected populations [279]. Compared to other endocrine treatment options available at the time, tamoxifen had a favorable toxicity profile. Subsequent trials have confirmed the clinical activity of tamoxifen in metastatic breast cancer and a meta-analysis including more than 5000 patients from clinical trials demonstrated a response rate of 30–34 % with an additional 19 % of patients achieving a stable disease for more than six months [279, 280]. Higher doses than 20 mg per day did not provide improved efficacy [281–283].

Tamoxifen was first approved by the FDA in 1977 and subsequently also in Europe for the treatment of advanced breast cancer and later for the treatment of early breast cancer for both pre- and postmenopausal women as well. According to the Early Breast Cancer Trialists' Collaborative Group (EBCTCG) meta-analysis, 5-years of adjuvant tamoxifen reduces breast cancer mortality by about a third (HR 0.68, $p < 0.00001$), largely independent of age, progesterone receptor (PR) status and use of chemotherapy. 5-years of tamoxifen were significantly more effective in reducing the risk of recurrence and breast cancer deaths than 1–2 years of tamoxifen. In ER-positive disease the annual breast cancer mortality rates are similar during years 0–4 and 5–15 as is the proportional risk reduction by tamoxifen during these years. As a result of this carry-over effect the cumulative risk reduction is more than twice as big after 15 years as at year 5 [283, 284]. Recently, two large randomized phase III trials, ATTOM and ATLAS, have demonstrated a significant benefit from 10 years of tamoxifen compared to 5 years. The absolute reduction of breast cancer mortality seen in these trials 15 years after starting adjuvant endocrine therapy was about 3 % and deaths from endometrial cancer or pulmonary embolism were significantly increased. Thus, the expected gain in the individual patient has to be weighed against the risk of potentially fatal adverse events [285, 286].

In the US, tamoxifen has also been approved for women with DCIS to reduce the risk of invasive cancer in later life and as a prophylaxis for women at high risk for breast cancer based on results from the NSABP B24 and the NSABP P1 trial [283, 287–289].

Tamoxifen is a well tolerated and accepted drug; however, there are some side effects, which may interfere with compliance and some which are potentially fatal. Adverse events include hot flashes, vaginal discharge, vaginal dryness, pruritus vulvae, headaches, dizziness, mood alterations/depression, hair thinning and/or partial hair loss, fluid retention/edema, visual disturbances (e.g., cataracts, corneal disturbances, and retinopathy), elevation of liver enzymes, elevation of triglyceride levels, hypercalcemia, and loss of appetite. The potentially dangerous side effects of tamoxifen include deep vein thrombosis, pulmonary embolism, and endometrial cancer. The risk of endometrial cancer is increased by a factor of 2–7 and is explained by the tissue-specific agonistic effect of tamoxifen on the endometrium. These cancers occur almost exclusively in postmenopausal women and become clinically evident by postmenopausal bleeding. Serial ultrasound scans for the detection of endometrial thickening is not helpful, as many patients develop subendometrial edema, induced by tamoxifen, which cannot be discriminated from malignant growth.

20.2.3.2 Aromatase Inhibitors

Whereas in premenopausal women, estrogen is mostly produced by the ovaries, in the postmenopausal setting estrogen synthesis mainly occurs in peripheral tissues through the conversion of androgens produced in the adrenal gland into estrogen by an enzyme called aromatase. This can effectively and specifically be inhibited by third-generation aromatase inhibitors (AIs). There are three third-generation aromatase inhibitors in clinical use for the treatment of breast cancer today, namely: anastrozol, exemestane, and letrozol. In contrast to nonsteroidal AIs (letrozole and anastrozol), exemestane, a steroidal AI, covalently binds to the enzyme leading to an irreversible inhibition. Third-generation AIs, the most potent and specific as well as least toxic AIs, can reduce serum estrogen levels by more than 95 % [290].

Several randomized phase III trials have investigated the efficacy of the three AIs compared to tamoxifen in the first-line treatment of HR-positive advanced breast cancer in postmenopausal women. At the time, the trials were conducted and only a minority of patients in these trials had received prior adjuvant endocrine therapy (14–19 %) [291–293]. In all of these trials AIs compared favorably to tamoxifen with objective response rates (ORR) from 30 to 46 % and time to progression (TTP) ranging from 9.4 to

10.7 months. In addition, aromatase inhibitors have also demonstrated clinical activity after the failure of tamoxifen [294]. In turn, letrozol, anastrozole, and exemestane have been approved for the treatment of HR-positive metastatic breast cancer in postmenopausal women and have largely replaced tamoxifen as the first-line therapy. Whereas steroidal and nonsteroidal aromatase inhibitors seem not to be completely cross-resistant, there is no evidence to suggest that any of these agents are superior to the others [295, 296].

The role of aromatase inhibitors in the adjuvant setting has been investigated in a series of phase III trials pursuing several strategies, including upfront aromatase inhibitors, switching to an AI after 2–3 years of tamoxifen or extended therapy with an AI after completion of 5 years of tamoxifen. All of these trials demonstrate a superiority of AIs over tamoxifen alone in the adjuvant treatment of postmenopausal HR-positive breast cancer [297–302]. BIG 1-98 directly compared 5 years of letrozole to 5 years of tamoxifen and demonstrated a significant overall survival advantage for letrozole at an 8-year follow-up, both for the ITT population and an analysis adjusting for crossover (IPCW) [IIT: HR 0.87; $p = 0.048$; IPCW: HR 0.79; $p = 0.0006$] [299].

In a large patient-level meta-analysis from the EBCTCG including 31, 920 women from 9 randomized trials, patients treated with 5 years of an aromatase inhibitor compared to 5 years of tamoxifen had a significantly improved DFS (HR 0.8; $p < 0.0001$) and OS (HR 0.89; $p = 0.1$), with absolute 10-year gains of 3.6 % for DFS and 2.7 % for OS. In contrast, 5 years of an AI were only marginally better in terms of DFS (RR 0.9; $p = 0.045$—absolute difference 0.7 %) but not OS (RR 0.96; $p = 0.45$) if compared to tamoxifen for 2–3 years followed by an AI. The sequencing strategy, however, was significantly more effective compared to 5 years of tamoxifen (DFS RR 0.82; $p = 0.0001$ and OS RR 0.82; $p = 0.0002$) [303]. There is no evidence to suggest superiority of one AI over the others in the adjuvant therapy. Based on the available data, it is generally recommended in international guidelines (e.g., NCCN, ASCO, AGO, St. Gallen), that adjuvant endocrine therapy for postmenopausal women should include an AI (if tolerated) [54, 304–306]. However, the optimal sequence and duration remains elusive.

It is also a widely accepted concept that giving an AI upfront to high-risk patients (e.g., with axillary lymph node involvement) might be beneficial. However, switching to tamoxifen after 2–3 years of AI can be considered in case of intolerability since there was no statistically significant difference in DFS among patients who received 5 years of AI compared to 2–3 years of AI followed by tamoxifen [307]. This concept is mainly supported by results from BIG 1-98, which has also investigated an inverse sequence of letrozole followed by tamoxifen.

As more than half of breast cancer recurrences occur more than 5 years after the initial diagnosis and after completion of tamoxifen, several trials have investigated the strategy of extended endocrine therapy with AIs (MA.17, ABCSG 6a, NSABP B33) [308–311]. All of these trials have shown a reduction of breast cancer recurrence (HR 0.60–0.68). MA.17, the largest of these trials, comparing 5 years of letrozole to placebo after completion of 5 years of tamoxifen, also provided evidence for an OS benefit in node-positive patients (HR 0.61, $p = 0.04$) [308, 309, 312].

Aromatase inhibitors are generally well tolerated. Their toxicity profile substantially differs from tamoxifen. In contrast to tamoxifen AIs are not associated with an increased risk of endometrial cancer and venous thromboembolic events. Instead, they lead to a more pronounced bone loss and a higher rate of fractures as well as musculoskeletal symptoms like arthralgias and osteoarthritis. Musculoskeletal symptoms are estimated to occur in up to 50 % of patients and lead to a treatment discontinuation in 20 % [313]. Further common side effects are vasomotor symptoms (hot flushes), increased sweating, depression, edema, increases in cholesterol levels, and an increased risk of cardiac ischemic events (myocardial infarction, angina). It is advisable to monitor bone mineral density regularly in women who take AIs [307].

In premenopausal women the inhibition of the aromatase does not significantly decrease the production and the amount of circulating estrogen, but the initial slight decrease in estrogen levels activates the hypothalamus and pituitary axis to increase gonadotropin secretion, which in turn increases the FSH and LH levels. Aromatase inhibitors are contraindicated for premenopausal women.

20.2.3.3 Fulvestrant—Selective Estrogen Receptor Downregulator (SERD)

Fulvestrant is a selective estrogen receptor downregulator (SERD), which are directed against estrogen receptors and exert purely antagonistic effects. Fulvestrant is the only representative of the class of drugs currently in clinical use. It competitively binds to estrogen receptors with a binding affinity 100 times greater than that of tamoxifen [314]. Upon binding, it blocks ER dimerization and DNA binding, inhibits nuclear uptake, and increases the turnover and degradation of ER leading to inhibition of estrogen signaling.

Clinically, fulvestrant was first developed at a dose of 250 mg given as a monthly intramuscular injection. Fulvestrant$_{250}$ was shown to be equally effective as anastrozole in patients who had progressed on endocrine therapy (mostly tamoxifen) [294]. Based on these results, fulvestrant received approval as a further option for HR-positive advanced breast cancer by the FDA in 2002 and in Europe in 2004 for the treatment of hormone receptor-positive metastatic breast cancer in postmenopausal women with disease progression following anti-estrogen therapy.

A randomized neoadjuvant phase trial (NEWEST) pointed to a greater biologic activity of fulvestrant at a dose of

500 mg compared to 250 mg, including a significantly higher reduction of Ki67 labeling index [315]. This and further data prompted several trials to investigate the clinical efficacy of this higher dose.

The FIRST trial, a randomized phase II trial, compared fulvestrant$_{500}$ to anastrozole as first-line therapy for metastatic breast cancer. Although there was no difference in clinical benefit rate (primary end point) or response, the TTP was significantly longer in the fulvestrant arm (23.5 vs. 13.1 months; HR 0.66; $p = 0.01$) as well as overall survival (54.1 vs. 48.4 months; HR 0.7; $p = 0.04$) [316, 317]. Results of the ongoing confirmatory phase III FALCON trial are expected in 2016 (NCT01602380). The CONFIRM trial (phase III) randomized patients with HR-positive metastatic breast cancer, who experienced progression after prior endocrine therapy with tamoxifen or an AI to either fulvestrant 500 mg q4w or 250 mg q4w. Patients treated with 500 mg of fulvestrant had significantly longer PFS (6.5 vs. 5.5 months; HR 0.81; $p = 0.0006$) as well as OS (26.4 vs. 22.3 months; HR 0.81; $p = 0.016$) [318, 319].

Fulvestrant has a similar tolerability profile as anastrozole and AIs, but with a significantly lower incident of musculoskeletal symptoms like arthralgia. Like the AIs, fulvestrant lacks the increased risk of endometrial cancer and thromboembolism observed with tamoxifen, because it is void of any estrogenic effects. In current clinical trials, fulvestrant has turned into a preferred endocrine combination partner due to its efficacy and tolerability.

20.2.3.4 Combination of Endocrine Therapies

As the currently available endocrine drugs have different modes of actions and are partially noncross-resistant, several trials set out to investigate combinations of endocrine therapies to improve efficacy of ET. However, conflicting results have been reported from the comparison of the combination of fulvestrant (250 mg) with anastrozole versus anastrozole as a single agent. The FACT trial demonstrated no advantage from the combination, whereas the SWOG S0226 trial showed a benefit in terms of TTP and OS [320, 321]. Furthermore, the SoFEA trial provided similar efficacy for the combination of fulvestrant and anastrozole compared with fulvestrant or exemestane alone as second-line endocrine therapy. Therefore, until there is further evidence, combinations of endocrine therapies should not be adopted into routine clinical practice [296, 322].

20.2.3.5 Gonadotropin-Releasing Hormone (GnRH) Analogs

Synthetic GnRH or luteinizing hormone (LHRH) analogs differ from native GnRH by a 100–200-fold stronger binding affinity to GnRH receptors on pituitary gonadotroph cells. Synthetic GnRH/LHRH analogs lead to an initial intense release of stored luteinizing hormone (LH) and follicle-stimulating hormone (FSH) called flare-up effect, resulting in a transient raise in serum estradiol in women. A prolonged application of these agents, as opposed to the pulsatile secretion that occurs naturally, however, leads to a desensitization of gonadotropin producing cells caused by downregulation of GnRH/LHRH receptors and a dysregulation of intracellular signaling [323]. This leads to an inhibition of LH/FSH secretion and ultimately the production of estradiol. GnRH/LHRH analogs are administered as depot injections. In contrast, GnRH/LHRH antagonists, which are not in clinical use against breast cancer, inhibit gonadotropin secretion by direct competitive receptor blockade without receptor downregulation.

After the first description of this therapeutic principle by Beatson in 1896[324], ovarian ablation, either by means of oophorectomy or radioablation remained the gold standard for the treatment of premenopausal patients with advanced breast cancer for decades. Subsequently, GNRH/LHRH analogs have demonstrated similar efficacy, providing an alternative. In early trials, tamoxifen has demonstrated comparable efficacy to ovarian ablation [325, 326]. Later trials as well as a meta-analysis proved that the combination of tamoxifen and GnRH/LHRH analogs was superior than either agent alone in terms of PFS and OS [327, 328]. Hence, the combination of tamoxifen with ovarian ablation is the standard recommended by current international guidelines (ABC2 consensus; National Comprehensive Cancer Network [NCCN], Guidelines, breast cancer, version 1.2016; AGO, v2016.1) [2, 305, 306]. After progression on or after tamoxifen and with an indication for further endocrine therapy, it is currently recommended for pre- and perimenopausal patients to be treated by ovarian ablation (either by GnRH-A or through surgical oophorectomy) and then treated as if they were postmenopausal [2, 296, 305].

Data on the adjuvant use of GnRH analogs are more inconclusive. Adding tamoxifen to goserelin after six cycles of CAF as adjuvant treatment of breast cancer in premenopausal women significantly improves DFS [329].

However, for many years, evidence from randomized trials to demonstrate benefit from the addition of goserelin to tamoxifen in the adjuvant setting was lacking and a patient-level meta-analysis provided only very limited information [330]. Recently, data from a randomized phase III trial (SOFT) demonstrated that the addition of ovarian ablation (by means of GnRH analogs, radioablation, or oophorectomy) did not significantly improve DFS in the overall study population [331]. However, a subgroup analysis showed that for women at sufficient risk of recurrence to warrant adjuvant chemotherapy, ovarian function suppression improved outcomes but at the cost of tolerability [331]. Based on these data, the use of GnRH analogs in the adjuvant endocrine treatment of premenopausal patients remains an option for selected individual patients after weighing risk of recurrence, expected benefit, tolerability, and QoL [332].

Side effects include hot flushes, sweating, emotional lability, depression, anxiety, loss of bone mineral density, dizziness, headache, arthralgia, musculoskeletal symptoms, amenorrhea, seborrhea, decreased libido, vaginitis, dyspareunia, breast atrophy, peripheral edema, weight gain, and tiredness.

Currently, goserelin (Zoladex®) is the only agent approved for the palliative treatment of advanced breast cancer in pre- and perimenopausal women in the US as well as Europe. In addition, leuprorelin has received approval for metastatic breast cancer in Europe. Several additional GnRH/LHRH analogs are available for the treatment of advanced prostate cancer. Based on their mode of action there is no rationale for the use of GNRH analog in postmenopausal patients. GnRH/LHRH analogs are also used for several gynecologic diseases as well as in assisted reproduction.

20.2.3.6 Further Targeted Agents Used in Combination with Endocrine Therapies

Some patients with HR-positive MBC show primary resistance to endocrine therapy and the remaining patients will ultimately develop secondary resistance and progress. Furthermore, since most patients today receive adjuvant endocrine therapy, some even for an extended duration of 10 years, patients we treat in the first-line setting today, differ substantially from those included in the large phase III trials on AIs and fulvestrant in first-line, which included predominantly ET naïve patients. They are likely to develop endocrine resistance more quickly. Endocrine resistance therefore presents a major clinical problem.

A huge effort has been undertaken to target mechanisms of endocrine resistance such as the PIK3CA/AKT/mTOR pathway, the cell cycle machinery, and the cross talk between HR and growth factor receptor signaling by combining endocrine therapies with novel targeted agents to restore endocrine sensitivity. With everolimus, an mTORC1 inhibitor, and palbociclib, a cdk4/6 inhibitor, two such agents have received approval and document the progress made.

mTOR and PIK3CA Inhibitors

Preclinical studies provide evidence that growth factor receptor signaling pathways, particularly those that converge on phosphatidylinositol 3-kinase (PI3K) and mitogen-activated protein kinase (MAPK/ERK), are involved in resistance to endocrine therapy [333, 334]. PI3K is the most frequently altered pathway in breast cancer. PI3K activation, experimentally, is associated with de novo and acquired endocrine resistance and blocking the pathway can restore endocrine sensitivity. Based on this rational several agents blocking the PI3K-Akt-mTOR at different levels have been developed and are in clinical testing.

Everolimus (Afinitor)

Everolimus is an oral mTOR inhibitor targeting mTORC1, one of the two mTOR complexes (mTORC1 & 2). Based on results from the randomized, double-blind phase III BOLERO-2 trial (n = 724), everolimus has been approved for the treatment of postmenopausal women with HR-positive MBC in combination with exemestane after failure of a nonsteroidal AI. In BOLERO-2, patients randomized to the combination of exemestane and everolimus had a significantly longer PFS (6.9 vs. 2.8 months; HR 0.43; $p < 0.001$) [335]. However, OS was not significantly improved (31.0 vs. 26.6 months; HR, 0.89; $p = 0.1426$) [336]. Supporting data come from a randomized phase II trial (TAMRAD), comparing tamoxifen plus everolimus to tamoxifen alone, providing a significant improvement in time to progression (TTP) from 4.5 to 8.6 months (HR 0.54) [337].

However, the toxicity profile of everolimus can be challenging. In BOLERO-2, the rate of grade 3/4 adverse events was significantly higher in patients receiving everolimus compared to placebo (55 % vs. 33 %) as was the proportion of patients who discontinued treatment due to adverse events (29 % vs. 5 %) [336]. Side effects of everolimus include stomatitis and oral ulcerations, noninfectious pneumonitis, increased risk of infections, hyperglycemia, elevation of blood lipid levels, elevation of liver enzymes, renal failure, hematologic toxicity including anemia, neutropenia, lymphopenia, thrombopenia, impaired wound healing, rash, fatigue, and gastrointestinal disturbances amongst others. Patients should avoid live vaccines and close contact to those who have received live vaccines.

Ongoing translational research has been trying to investigate predictive biomarkers, however, thus far has failed to do so. For example, activating PIK3CA mutations, major candidates, at least if tested mainly on primary tumor tissue did not provide any predictive information [338].

PIK3CA Inhibitors

Alterations in PIK3CA are the most frequent molecular alterations in HR-positive breast cancer and are identified in 45 and 29 % of luminal A and B tumors, respectively [296]. However, the role of PIK3CA mutations in luminal breast cancers is complex and still not entirely understood. Their implications might in fact play distinctive roles in early versus advanced breast cancer. In primary breast cancer the presence of PIK3CA mutations is consistently associated with good prognosis luminal A-like breast cancers (lower grade, less lymph node involvement, and progesterone receptor positivity) [339]. In advanced ER-positive breast cancers selected by primary endocrine therapy, PIK3CA mutations may behave as a mechanism of endocrine resistance that merits combined therapy [340]. In fact, in vitro, the combination of estrogen deprivation and PI3K inhibition acts synergistically [341]. PI3K therefore constitutes an attractive target in combination with endocrine therapy in breast cancer.

Several PI3K inhibitors are currently in clinical development programs, ranging from unspecific pan-PI3K inhibitors (e.g., buparlisib) to modern third generation, α isoform specific PIK3CA inhibitors (e.g., alpelisib, taselisib), sparing off-target effects, and as hoped, unnecessary toxicity. Most activation mutations affect hot spot regions within PIK3CA [342].

First clinical data have emerged from randomized trials. In a randomized phase II trial (FERGI), pictilisib, a pan-PI3K inhibitor, when added to fulvestrant, was associated with a nonsignificant PFS improvement from 5.1 to 6.6 months (HR 0.74; $p = 0.095$). PIK3CA mutation status did not predict outcome [343]. The BELLE-2 trial, a randomized, double-blind, placebo-controlled phase III trial, randomized postmenopausal patients who progressed after or on an AI, to fulvestrant plus either placebo or buparlisib (BKM120), a pan-Class I PI3K inhibitor, that targets all four PI3K isoforms. The trial met its primary endpoint by increasing PFS in the full study population by 1.9 months from 5.0 to 6.9 months (HR 0.78; $p < 0.001$). PI3K activation, determined by PI3K mutations (mostly in the primary tumor) and PTEN loss, did not predict PFS benefit from buparlisib, a coprimary endpoint in the trial. However, PIC3CA mutations determined in circulating tumor DNA (ctDNA) at the time of entering the trial was a significant predictive factor for activity of buparlisib. In patients with PIC3CA ctDNA mutations there was a PFS improvement from 3.2 to 7.0 months (HR 0.58; $p < 0.001$), whereas in patients without ctDNA PIK3CA mutations there was no difference in PFS by treatment (6.8 months in both arms) [344]. Buparlisib was associated with considerable toxicities and grade 3/4 AEs were significantly more frequent with buparlisib (77.3 % vs. 32 %). The safety profile was mainly characterized by elevation of liver enzymes, rash, hyperglycemia, and mood disorders like depression and anxiety [344]. The PFS benefit in the ITT population is modest at best. The ctDNA PIK3CA mutant subgroup may derive a clinically meaningful benefit, if this predictive biomarker is validated. Future will tell if this will outweigh the toxicity associated with this pan-PI3K class I inhibitor. It is likely, however, that clinical development will move to another class of PI3K inhibitors.

There is hope that PI3Kα-selective inhibitors might offer an improved therapeutic index, with greater activity and less toxicity. Alpelisib (BYL719) and Taselisib (GDC0032) are examples of this class of drugs. Currently, large randomized phase III trials investigating their role are ongoing and will provide more definitive answers concerning the future of PIK3CA inhibitors in HR+ breast cancer (SOLAR [Alpelisib], NCT02437318; SANDPIPER [Taselisib], NCT02340221).

Palbociclib (Ibrance™) and Cdk4/6 Inhibitors

Translational research points to a profound deregulation of the cyclin D1/CDK4/6/retinoblastoma (Rb) pathway in HR-positive breast cancer, with frequent cyclin D1 amplifications, gains in CDK4 and overexpression of Rb [345, 346]. The activation of CDK4/6 by cyclin D leads to Rb phosphorylation and progression of the cell cycle into S phase and is associated with resistance to endocrine therapy [296, 347]. In vitro studies showed that luminal ER-positive cell lines (including those, which are HER2 amplified) were most sensitive to palbociclib, an orally active, highly selective inhibitor of the cyclin D kinases (CDK)4 and CDK6, whereas non-luminal/basal-like cell lines were most resistant. Palbociclib preclinically demonstrates synergy with endocrine therapies [348]. These observations served as a rationale to develop palbociclib primarily in HR+ breast cancer. In the randomized phase II PALOMA-1 trial, palbociclib in combination with letrozole as first-line therapy for HR+ MBC in postmenopausal patients, significantly improved PFS from 10.2 to 20.2 months in comparison to letrozole alone (HR 0.48; $p = 0.0004$) [349]. Based on these results, the FDA granted palbociclib in combination with letrozole in the first-line setting accelerated approval in 2015. Approval for Europe by the EMA is currently outstanding, but is expected in 2016. Subsequently, data from the randomized, double-blind, placebo-controlled phase III trial (PALOMA-2) confirmed the activity. In contrast to PALOMA-1, PALOMA-2 recruited patients with advanced HR-positive, HER2-negative breast cancer who had relapsed or progressed during prior endocrine therapy. Patients were randomized to fulvestrant in combination with either palbociclib or placebo. The median progression-free survival was increased from 3.8 months in the placebo arm to 9.2 months with palbociclib (HR 0.42; $P < 0.001$). Turner et al. [350] Palbociclib is very well tolerated, with a rate of treatment discontinuation due to AEs of only 2.6 %. Hematologic toxicities, predominantly neutropenia and lymphopenia, make up for the most frequent grade 3/4 toxicities. However, despite the rate of grade 3/4 neutropenia of 62 % febrile neutropenia was a rare event in PALOMA-2 (0.6 %) and was not different when compared to the placebo arm [350]. Other common side effects of palbociclib are leukopenia, anemia, thrombopenia, fatigue, hair loss, and stomatitis.

Based on these results the FDA has extended the indication of palbociclib to the combination with fulvestrant in women progressing after or on prior endocrine therapy.

Due to a favorable toxicity profile compared to everolimus in daily clinical practice, palbociclib is often used in earlier lines. Apart from palbociclib, two further cdk4/6 inhibitors, ribociclib (LEE011), and abamaciclib (LY2853219), are being investigated in phase III clinical trials (MONALEESA-2; MONARCH-2). In addition, large randomized phase III trials are currently recruiting patients with HR-positive primary breast cancer to investigate the role of palbociclib in the post-neoadjuvant (PENELOPE–NCT01864746) and adjuvant setting (PALLAS–NCT02513394).

20.2.4 PARP-Inhibitors

Homologous recombination (HR) represents an important error-free DNA repair mechanism for double strand breaks. HR uses the homologous sequence of the sister chromatid which is used to precisely repair the double strand break. The BRCA1 and BRCA2 genes are important components of the HR machinery. In *BRCA*-associated tumors, the nonmutated *BRCA1/2* allele is inactivated. In turn, these tumors accumulate double strand breaks and are characterized by genomic instability. The inhibition of base excision repair in such cells leads to the accumulation of double strand breaks during replication, which cannot be repaired accurately due to the HR deficiency. Poly-(Adenosine-Diphosphate)-Ribose-Polymerase (PARP) is an enzyme centrally involved in BER. Inhibiting PARP in HR deficient cells leads to specific synthetic lethality [351].

Phenotypic similarities between basal-like subtype and *BRCA*-associated breast cancers have lead to the strategy to select patients for PARP-inhibition by their TNBC phenotype. An alternative strategy is to restrict the development of PARP inhibitors to *BRCA*-associated breast cancer types. Currently several PARP inhibitor such as Olaparib, Veliparib, Rucaparib, Niraparib, Talazoparib (BMN673), and others are undergoing clinical development. Olaparib was the first PARP inhibitor to be granted regulatory approval of recurrent high-grade serous ovarian cancer by the FDA and the EMEA. Olaparib was first developed in a single-arm phase II study recruiting patients with *BRCA*-associated breast cancer in two consecutive cohorts treated with 100 mg bid and 400 mg bid, respectively. This trial demonstrated a promising dose-dependent ORR of 22 % (100 mg bid) and 41 % (400 mg bid) with a median PFS of 5.7 months for the higher dose [352]. Similar results were observed for *BRCA*-associated ovarian cancer [353].

Gelmon et al. studied the efficacy of Olaparib in unselected TNBC. However, they were unable to demonstrate any confirmed responses among 26 patients included which was in contrast to the efficacy observed in ovarian cancer in the same trial [354]. A recent study including several *BRCA*-associated solid tumors demonstrated a discouraging ORR of only 12.9 % with a PFS of only 3.7 months in the 62 *BRCA*-associated breast cancers included. The ORR seemed to be higher in breast cancer patients without prior platinum chemotherapy (20 % vs. 9.5 %). However, again results were more promising in the ovarian cancer cohort. Overall, these data suggest that PARP-inhibition at least by Olaparib is more effective in (BRCA associated) ovarian cancer than in *BRCA* associated breast cancer.

As part of the I-Spy 2 trial the combination of Carboplatin and Veliparib added to weekly Paclitaxel and followed by Doxorubicin/Cyclophosphamide led to a doubling of the pCR rate in the triple-negative study population from 26 to 52 %. Trial statistics predict a probability of 90 % of success for this combination in a phase III trial [355]. Currently several PARP inhibitors are in clinical development for breast cancer in the adjuvant, neoadjuvant, and metastatic setting. Table 20.10 summarizes current phase III trials investigating PARP inhibitors in breast cancer. Olaparib is usually well tolerated, with moderate side effects including, nausea, vomiting as well as anorexia and fatigue. Of more concern are long-term adverse events which include increased rates of treatment-associated MDS and AML especially when these drugs are used in the adjuvant setting.

20.2.5 Bone-Targeted Agents

Breast cancer patients are at risk of several skeletal complications, including treatment-induced bone loss leading to osteoporosis and an increased fracture risk. In addition, the majority of patients with advanced breast cancer will develop bone metastases, which can lead to pain, dysfunction, fractures, and hypercalcemia as an oncologic emergency. Bone-targeted agents are used to prevent or treat these conditions. In addition, there is data suggesting potential role of bone-targeted agents in the adjuvant setting to prevent recurrences and decrease mortality (Table 20.11).

20.2.5.1 Bisphosphonates

Bisphosphonates (BPs) are synthetic analogs of naturally occurring pyrophosphates of the bone matrix. They are subdivided into nonnitrogenous and nitrogenous (amino) bisphosphonates, which differ partly in their mode of action by which they inhibit osteoclasts and in their capacity to inhibit bone absorption [356, 357]. Bisphosphonates are clinically used for the treatment of osteoporosis, osteitis deformans (Paget's disease of the bone), bone metastases, malignancy-associated hypercalcemia, and multiple myeloma.

Table 20.10 Current Phase III trials of PARP inhibitors in breast cancer (modified after [110])

Sponsor	ClinicalTrial.gov Identifier	Trial	Treatment	Population	Biomarker
Abbvie	NCT02032277	Brightness	Carboplatin-based NAC + Veliparib/Palcebo	Triple-negative early breast cancer	–
AstraZeneca	NCT02032823	OlympiA	Maintainance Olaparib/Placebo	HER2-early breast cancer	BRCA1/2 mutation
AstraZeneca	NCT02000622	OlympiaD	Olaparib versus Physician's choice	Advanced/metastatic HER2-breast cancer	BRCA1/2 mutation
Abbvie	NCT02163694	Brocade	Carboplatin/Paclitaxel plus Veliparib/Placebo	Advanced/metastatic HER2-breast cancer	BRCA1/2 mutation
Tesaro	NCT01905592	BRAVO	Niraparib versus Physician's choice	Advanced/metastatic HER2-breast cancer	BRCA1/2 mutation
BioMarin	NCT01945775	EMBRACA	Talazoparib versus Physician's choice	Advanced/metastatic HER2-breast cancer	BRCA1/2 mutation

Source Marmé and Schneeweiss [393]. Epub 2015 Jun 24. Copyright © 2015 Karger Publishers, Basel, Switzerland
Abbreviations: *NAC* neoadjuvant chemotherapy

Table 20.11 Bone-targeted agents

Agent	Trade name® (selection)	Mode of action	Dosing	Interactions	Selected adverse events and precautions
Zoledronate	Zometa®	Inhibition of osteoclasts	4 mg q4w (q3w) IV	Absorption reduced if taken together with calcium, Mg, Fe containing substances or antacids	Acute phase reactions with flu-like symptoms and musculoskeletal pain, electrolyte disturbances including hypocalcemia, hypophosphatemia, hypomagnesenemia, renal failure, edema, osteonecrosis of the jaw and atypical femoral fractures. Stomach pain, dyspepsia, inflammation and erosions of the esophagus and diarrhea predominantly for oral BPs Precaution sufficient hydration! Substitution of vitamin D and calcium p.o. according to specific label Can cause fetal harm.
Ibandronate	Bondronate®		6 mg q4w (q3w) IV or 50 mg daily p.o.		
Clodronate	Bonefos®		1,600 mg daily p.o.		
Pamidronate	Aredia®		90 mg q4w (q3w) i.v.		
Denosumab	Xgeva® Prolia® (for the treatment and prevention of osteoporosis only)	Fully human monoclonal IgG2-anti-RANKL antibody	Xgeva: 120 mg s. c. q4w Prolia: 60 mg s.c. q6 m	None	Osteonecrosis of the jaw, hypocalcemia (severe and fatal cases reported), hypophosphatemia, acute phase reactions, atypical fractures, fatigue/asthenia Supplementation of calcium and vitamin D required to prevent severe hypocalcemia Can cause fetal harm

These highlights do not include all the information needed to use the respective drugs safely and effectively. See full prescribing information for all information needed to use these agents safely. We do not take responsibility for the correctness of the content

Nonnitrogenous Bisphosphonates

BPs are taken up by osteoclasts via endocytosis and then further metabolized to compounds that replace the terminal pyrophosphate moiety of adenosine triphosphate (ATP), forming a nonfunctional molecule that competes with ATP in the cellular energy metabolism. Accumulation of these metabolites inhibits the absorption capacity and induces apoptosis by inhibiting ATP-dependent enzymes. This leads to an overall decrease in bone absorption [356, 357].

Nitrogenous Bisphosphonates (Amino-bisphosphonates)

Second- and third-generation, nitrogen-containing BPs, furthermore block farnesyl diphosphate (FPP) synthase, a key enzyme of the mevalonate pathway. Loss of FPP synthesis and its metabolites prevents posttranslational modifications of small GTPases (Ras, Rab, Rho, and Rac), which are crucial in the regulation of various processes important for osteoclast function. The disruption of the mevalonate pathway leads to the accumulation of isopentenyl pyrophosphate (IPP) in osteoclasts, which is converted to a cytotoxic ATP analog [356]. The potency of amino-BPs, e.g., zoledronic acid, in preclinical experiments is substantially higher than that of first generation bisphosphonates like clodronate (Table 20.12) [358].

The clinical activity of BPs to prevent so-called skeletal-related events (SREs) in patients with bone metastases, defined as pathological fractures, hypercalcemia, spinal cord compression, or the need for surgical intervention or radiotherapy has been demonstrated in several phase III trials as well as a meta-analysis [359–366]. They are also effective in reducing bone pain and improving global quality of life [359, 362]. In a randomized phase III trial comparing zoledronic acid (ZA) to placebo, ZA significantly delayed the time-to-first-SRE and reduced the overall rate of SRE by 41 % (HR 0.59, $p = 0.019$) compared with placebo [359].

In keeping with preclincal data, zoledronic acid has demonstrated the highest efficacy in reducing the risk of skeletal complications when compared to other BPs [367–370]. It is the most commonly used BP in the oncologic setting, however, risk of related adverse events like osteonecrosis of the jaw (ONJ) might also be higher compared to less potent BPs.

Zoledronate, clodronate, ibandronate, and pamidronate are approved for the therapy of (bone-) metastasized breast cancer, whereas alendronate is only approved for osteoporosis in postmenopausal women. Recommended agents for the use in the United States are zoledronate (4 mg IV every 3–4 weeks) and pamidronate (90 mg IV every 3–4 weeks) as indicated by the National Comprehensive Cancer Network guideline, breast cancer version 1.2016. In addition to zoledronate and pamidronate, ibandronate and clodronate are recommended for the treatment of bone metastases in Europe.

According to its label, zoledronate is administered as a 4 mg intravenous infusion every 3–4 weeks with concomitant substitution of calcium and vitamin D. Recent evidence suggests that prolonging dosing intervals to 12 weeks after a year of 3–4 weekly dosing does not compromise efficacy, but might have fewer side effects [356, 371].

The toxicity profile of bisphosphonates is favorable, with the most frequent side effects being acute phase reactions, manifesting as fever, chills, and mylagias. They can be observed in up to 55 % of patients [372] and usually occur within 24 h of the first infusions and are short lived. Antipyretics and anti-inflammatory drugs can successfully alleviate symptoms. Not all BPs are associated with the same frequency of acute phase reactions. Zoledronate has a higher tendency compared to other BPs. Furthermore, two infrequent but serious adverse events are of major concern: renal toxicity and osteonecrosis of the jaw (ONJ). ONJ is a rare but severe event, which is reported in approximately 1.3 % of patients treated with zoledronate in randomized trials as therapy for bone metastases [373, 374]. The risk for developing ONJ is considerably higher during intravenous amino-bisphosphonate therapy than in patients on oral BPs. Most affected patients present with specific risk factors like poor oral hygiene, history of dental extractions, preexisting dental or paradontal disease, use of dental appliances, radiotherapy, and concomitant administration of antiangiogenic agents [374]. Prior to the start of IV BP therapy, patients should be referred to a dentist or dental surgeon for an examination. If required, dental surgical procedures should ideally be completed before the start of the treatment and if dental extractions become necessary during BP therapy, special measures have to be taken. Other risk factors for ONJ are corticosteroid use, diabetes mellitus, smoking, as well as the potency of the bisphosphonate, and the duration of use. Patient education about these serious side effects is crucial.

Table 20.12 Summary of different classes of bisphosphonates and their relative potencies

Nonnitrogenous bisphosphonates		Potency in relation to etidronate [358]
First generation	Etidronate	1
	Clodronate	10
	Tiludronate	10
Nitrogen-containing bisphosphonates		
Second generation	Pamidronate	100
	Neridronate	100
	Alendronate	500
	Ibandronate	1000
Third generation	Risedronate	2000
	Zoledronate	10,000

Renal toxicity is a further major concern with (IV) BPs. Increased creatinine levels from baseline are seen in about 10 % of patients under BP therapy. The rates vary between the individual BPs. Monitoring of serum creatinine levels and creatinine clearance is crucial during IV BP therapy and additional nephrotoxic drugs should be avoided if possible. Of note, patients with metastatic cancer are at risk of kidney failure as a result of numerous predisposing factors like frequent administration of contrast media, analgesics, and last but not least nephrotoxic cytotoxic agents. The use of denosumab for this indication avoids this problem. Further side effects include edema and electrolyte imbalances, including hypophosphatemia, hypocalcemia and hypomagnesemia, and atypical fractures. Prophylactic substitution of vitamin D and calcium is therefore recommended during BP therapy [372]. Oral administration of BPs like ibandronate or clodronate can also provoke dyspepsia and gastroesophageal irritation as well as diarrhea [356].

20.2.5.2 Rank Ligand (RANKL) Inhibitors

Denosumab

Denosumab is a fully human monoclonal IgG2 antibody that specifically targets a ligand known as RANKL (Receptor Activator of NF-κB Ligand), which is a key mediator of osteoclast formation, function, and survival. RANKL is naturally expressed by osteoblasts and counterbalanced by osteoprotegrin, its natural inhibitor to keep bone turnover in balance. Tumor cells within the bone can secrete cytokines (e.g., TNF, IL-1, TGF-β) which stimulate the expression and secretion of RANKL in osteoblast. Upon binding to its receptor (RANK), which is expressed on immature osteoclasts, RANKL leads to osteoclast differentiation, activation, and survival, thereby inducing bone absorption. Denosumab mimics the endogenous function of osteoprotegrin to prevent bone resorption.

The clinical activity of denosumab to prevent SREs has been evaluated in three phase III registrational trials, with identical study design, comparing denosumab (120 mg s.c. q28d) to IV zoledronate, the most potent BP in clinical use, in patients with bone metastases. In the phase III trial, investigating the use of denosumab in breast cancer metastasized to the bone ($n = 2046$), denosumab was superior to zoledronic acid and significantly delayed the time-to-first SRE (HR 0.82; $p = 0.01$), the primary endpoint, as well as the time-to-first and subsequent SRE (RR 0.77, $p = 0.001$) [375]. Consistent results were reported for patients with bone metastases from solid tumors in the other trials. However, denosumab did not show superiority in patients with multiple myeloma [376–378]. An integrated analysis demonstrated that denosumab was also significantly superior in preventing bone pain and improving quality of life [378, 379].

Denosumab 120 mg s.c., q28d (XGeva®) has been approved for the prevention of SRE in patients with bone metastases from solid tumors by the FDA in 2010 and the EMA for Europe in 2011.

Based on a large randomized phase III trial, denosumab 60 mg s.c. (Prolia®) given every 6 months, in the US is also indicated to increase bone mass in women at high risk for fracture receiving adjuvant aromatase inhibitor therapy for breast cancer [380]. In addition, in the US as well as in Europe, denosumab 60 mg s.c. given every 6 months has received approval for the treatment of postmenopausal women with osteoporosis at high risk for fracture. In a large randozimed phase III trial, denosumab reduced the risk of new vertebral fractures by 68 % (RR 0.32; $p < 0.001$) [381].

As denosumab can induce severe and potentially life-threatening hypocalcemia, supplementation of calcium and vitamin D is essential, as is the monitoring of serum calcium levels and the education about associated signs and symptoms. Other relevant adverse effects include ONJ, which occurred in 1.8 % of patients within the phase III trials in patients with bone metastases [373], acute phase reactions, fatigue/asthenia, hypophosphatemia, and nausea. Atypical fractures of the femur neck are further rare events.

20.2.5.3 Adjuvant Use of Bone-Targeted Agents

Adjuvant Bisphosphonates

In addition to their ability to inhibit bone resorption in bone metastases, preclinical data from animal models and early clinical data suggested that bisphosphonates might also play a role in preventing bone metastases [382]. As a consequence, bisphosphonates have been investigated as adjuvant therapies for early breast cancer. Several adjuvant trials have reported improved bone metastases-free, disease-free, and overall survival for oral clodronate and intravenous zoledronic acid [383, 384]. However, other trials failed to demonstrate similar benefits from adjuvant bisphosphonates [385–387]. Prespecified and exploratory subgroup analyses in these trials suggested that benefits are restricted to postmenopausal or older patients [388].

Finally, a large individual patient data-based meta-analysis carried out by the Early Breast Cancer Trialists' Collaborative Group (EBCTCG), including 18766 patients treated within 26 clinical trials addressed the question of the role of adjuvant bisphosphonate therapy. In this meta-analysis significant effects on recurrences, distant recurrences, bone metastases, and breast cancer mortality were observed but proved to be small and of borderline significance in the overall population. However, among the 11,767 postmenopausal patients within these trials, a highly statistically significant reduction in recurrences (RR 0.86,

$p = 0.002$), distant recurrences (0.82, $p = 0.0003$), bone recurrences (0.72, $p = 0.0002$) and breast cancer mortality (0.82, $p = 0.002$) was observed, whereas mortality from other causes was unchanged. Further subgroup analysis did not demonstrate a differential effect by type or schedule of bisphosphonate, duration of therapy, and hormone receptor status [389]. In contrast, no benefit from adjuvant bisphosphonates was seen in premenopausal patients.

Although possible explanations, why this effect is only seen in postmenopausal women remain hypothetical, there is some preclinical data from mouse models that support the validity of this observation. In a mouse model, zoledronate only inhibited the formation of bone metastases in ovariectomized animals [390].

The data on adjuvant bisphosphonates are controversially perceived and discussed amongst experts, due to the conflicting results of the individual trials. The current 2016 version of the American National Comprehensive Cancer Network (NCCN) guidelines does not give a statement regarding the use of BPs in the adjuvant setting, whereas the most recent (2016) yearly updated treatment guideline by the "Arbeitsgemeinschaft Gynäkologische Onkologie" (AGO) recommends the use of adjuvant BPs in postmenopausal patients. Finally, the Panel of the 2015 St. Gallen International Expert Consensus on the Primary Therapy of Early Breast Cancer was divided on this question, with a small majority supporting the adjuvant use of BPs in postmenopausal patients and only a minority supporting their use in premenopausal patients receiving LHRH plus tamoxifen.

Adjuvant Denosumab

Recently, a randomized, placebo-controlled phase III trial (ABCSG-18, NCT00556374), investigating the role of adjuvant denosumab (60 mg s.c. q6 m) reported data on the prevention of clinical bone fractures during adjuvant aromatase inhibitor therapy, its primary endpoint. The addition of denosumab led to a 50 % relative reduction in clinical fractures [391]. The substantial difference in the primary endpoint led the independent data monitoring committee to recommend that patients should be offered unblinding and cross over to denosumab in case they received placebo. As a result, a time-driven, "premature" DFS analysis (secondary endpoint) was recommended and performed. The results of the DFS analysis were presented at the San Antonio Breast Cancer Symposium in December 2015. The intention to treat analysis showed a borderline significant improvement in DFS (HR 0.816, $p = 0.051$), which reached significance in a sensitivity analysis, censoring at crossover (HR 0.81, $p = 0.042$) as well as in a subgroup analysis of patients with a tumor size larger than 2 cm (HR 0.66, $p = 0.017$) [392]. Due to the limitations mentioned above, the adjuvant use of denosumab 60 mg s.c. q6 m, cannot be recommended, as yet. It does, however, represent a valuable treatment option to prevent fractures and bone loss in patients at risk. For a general recommendation of denosumab as adjuvant therapy in breast cancer, results from the randomized, placebo-controlled phase III D-Care trial (NCT01077154) have to be awaited. This trial investigates the efficacy of denosumab (given at higher doses of 120 mg s.c.) to reduce recurrences in patients with early breast cancer at high risk of recurrence.

Until further data are available, recommendations for individual patients have to be made on an individual basis, taking into account, bone mineral density, the risk of fractures, adjuvant therapy, menopausal status, risk of recurrence as well as potential adverse effects of bisphosphonates and denosumab.

References

1. Nitiss JL. Targeting DNA topoisomerase II in cancer chemotherapy. Nat Rev Cancer. 2009;9(5):338–50.
2. Cardoso F, Costa A, Norton L, Senkus E, Aapro M, Andre F, et al. ESO-ESMO 2nd international consensus guidelines for advanced breast cancer (ABC2)dagger. Ann Oncol (Official Journal of the European Society for Medical Oncology/ESMO). 2014;25(10):1871–88.
3. Fisher B, Anderson S, Tan-Chiu E, Wolmark N, Wickerham DL, Fisher ER, et al. Tamoxifen and chemotherapy for axillary node-negative, estrogen receptor-negative breast cancer: findings from National Surgical Adjuvant Breast and Bowel Project B-23. J Clin Oncol (Official Journal of the American Society of Clinical Oncology). 2001;19(4):931–42.
4. Fisher B, Brown AM, Dimitrov NV, Poisson R, Redmond C, Margolese RG, et al. Two months of doxorubicin-cyclophosphamide with and without interval reinduction therapy compared with 6 months of cyclophosphamide, methotrexate, and fluorouracil in positive-node breast cancer patients with tamoxifen-nonresponsive tumors: results from the National Surgical Adjuvant Breast and Bowel Project B-15. J Clin Oncol (Official Journal of the American Society of Clinical Oncology). 1990;8(9):1483–96.
5. Henderson IC, Berry DA, Demetri GD, Cirrincione CT, Goldstein LJ, Martino S, et al. Improved outcomes from adding sequential Paclitaxel but not from escalating Doxorubicin dose in an adjuvant chemotherapy regimen for patients with node-positive primary breast cancer. J Clin Oncol (Official Journal of the American Society of Clinical Oncology). 2003;21(6):976–83.
6. Levine MN, Bramwell VH, Pritchard KI, Norris BD, Shepherd LE, Abu-Zahra H, et al. Randomized trial of intensive cyclophosphamide, epirubicin, and fluorouracil chemotherapy compared with cyclophosphamide, methotrexate, and fluorouracil in premenopausal women with node-positive breast cancer. National Cancer Institute of Canada Clinical Trials Group. J Clin Oncol (Official Journal of the American Society of Clinical Oncology). 1998;16(8):2651–8.
7. Levine MN, Pritchard KI, Bramwell VH, Shepherd LE, Tu D, Paul N. Randomized trial comparing cyclophosphamide, epirubicin, and fluorouracil with cyclophosphamide, methotrexate, and

fluorouracil in premenopausal women with node-positive breast cancer: update of National Cancer Institute of Canada Clinical Trials Group Trial MA5. J Clin Oncol (Official Journal of the American Society of Clinical Oncology). 2005;23(22):5166–70.
8. Poole CJ, Earl HM, Hiller L, Dunn JA, Bathers S, Grieve RJ, et al. Epirubicin and cyclophosphamide, methotrexate, and fluorouracil as adjuvant therapy for early breast cancer. N Engl J Med. 2006;355(18):1851–62.
9. Martin M, Villar A, Sole-Calvo A, Gonzalez R, Massuti B, Lizon J, et al. Doxorubicin in combination with fluorouracil and cyclophosphamide (i.v. FAC regimen, day 1, 21) versus methotrexate in combination with fluorouracil and cyclophosphamide (i.v. CMF regimen, day 1, 21) as adjuvant chemotherapy for operable breast cancer: a study by the GEICAM group. Ann Oncol (Official Journal of the European Society for Medical Oncology/ESMO). 2003;14(6):833–42.
10. FASG fasg. Benefit of a high-dose epirubicin regimen in adjuvant chemotherapy for node-positive breast cancer patients with poor prognostic factors: 5-year follow-up results of French Adjuvant Study Group 05 randomized trial. J Clin Oncol (Official Journal of the American Society of Clinical Oncology). 2001;19(3):602–11.
11. Bonneterre J, Roche H, Kerbrat P, Bremond A, Fumoleau P, Namer M, et al. Epirubicin increases long-term survival in adjuvant chemotherapy of patients with poor-prognosis, node-positive, early breast cancer: 10-year follow-up results of the French Adjuvant Study Group 05 randomized trial. J Clin Oncol (Official Journal of the American Society of Clinical Oncology). 2005;23(12):2686–93.
12. Brufman G, Colajori E, Ghilezan N, Lassus M, Martoni A, Perevodchikova N, et al. Doubling epirubicin dose intensity (100 mg/m^2 versus 50 mg/m^2) in the FEC regimen significantly increases response rates. An international randomised phase III study in metastatic breast cancer. The Epirubicin High Dose (HEPI 010) Study Group. Ann Oncol (Official Journal of the European Society for Medical Oncology/ESMO). 1997;8(2):155–62.
13. Focan C, Andrien JM, Closon MT, Dicato M, Driesschaert P, Focan-Henrard D, et al. Dose-response relationship of epirubicin-based first-line chemotherapy for advanced breast cancer: a prospective randomized trial. J Clin Oncol (Official Journal of the American Society of Clinical Oncology). 1993;11(7):1253–63.
14. EBCTCG EBCTC, Group, Peto R, Davies C, Godwin J, Gray R, Pan HC, et al. Comparisons between different polychemotherapy regimens for early breast cancer: meta-analyses of long-term outcome among 100,000 women in 123 randomised trials. Lancet. 2012;379(9814):432–44.
15. von Minckwitz G, Kummel S, du Bois A, Eiermann W, Eidtmann H, Gerber B, et al. Pegfilgrastim ± ciprofloxacin for primary prophylaxis with TAC (docetaxel/doxorubicin/cyclophosphamide) chemotherapy for breast cancer. Results from the GEPARTRIO study. Ann Oncol (Official Journal of the European Society for Medical Oncology/ESMO). 2008;19(2):292–8.
16. Swain SM, Whaley FS, Ewer MS. Congestive heart failure in patients treated with doxorubicin: a retrospective analysis of three trials. Cancer. 2003;97(11):2869–79.
17. Bird BR, Swain SM. Cardiac toxicity in breast cancer survivors: review of potential cardiac problems. Clin Cancer Rese (an Official Journal of the American Association for Cancer Research). 2008;14(1):14–24.
18. Fumoleau P, Roche H, Kerbrat P, Bonneterre J, Romestaing P, Fargeot P, et al. Long-term cardiac toxicity after adjuvant epirubicin-based chemotherapy in early breast cancer: French Adjuvant Study Group results. Ann Oncol (Official Journal of the European Society for Medical Oncology/ESMO). 2006;17(1):85–92.
19. Ryberg M, Nielsen D, Cortese G, Nielsen G, Skovsgaard T, Andersen PK. New insight into epirubicin cardiac toxicity: competing risks analysis of 1097 breast cancer patients. J Natl Cancer Inst. 2008;100(15):1058–67.
20. Bonneterre J, Roche H, Kerbrat P, Fumoleau P, Goudier MJ, Fargeot P, et al. Long-term cardiac follow-up in relapse-free patients after six courses of fluorouracil, epirubicin, and cyclophosphamide, with either 50 or 100 mg of epirubicin, as adjuvant therapy for node-positive breast cancer: French adjuvant study group. J Clin Oncol (Official Journal of the American Society of Clinical Oncology). 2004;22(15):3070–9.
21. Slamon D, Eiermann W, Robert N, Pienkowski T, Martin M, Press M, et al. Adjuvant trastuzumab in HER2-positive breast cancer. N Engl J Med. 2011;365(14):1273–83.
22. Nardi V, Winkfield KM, Ok CY, Niemierko A, Kluk MJ, Attar EC, et al. Acute myeloid leukemia and myelodysplastic syndromes after radiation therapy are similar to de novo disease and differ from other therapy-related myeloid neoplasms. J Clin Oncol (Official Journal of the American Society of Clinical Oncology). 2012.
23. Smith RE, Bryant J, DeCillis A, Anderson S. Acute myeloid leukemia and myelodysplastic syndrome after doxorubicin-cyclophosphamide adjuvant therapy for operable breast cancer: the National Surgical Adjuvant Breast and Bowel Project Experience. J Clin Oncol (Official Journal of the American Society of Clinical Oncology). 2003;21(7):1195–204.
24. Praga C, Bergh J, Bliss J, Bonneterre J, Cesana B, Coombes RC, et al. Risk of acute myeloid leukemia and myelodysplastic syndrome in trials of adjuvant epirubicin for early breast cancer: correlation with doses of epirubicin and cyclophosphamide. J Clin Oncol (Official Journal of the American Society of Clinical Oncology). 2005;23(18):4179–91.
25. Wolff AC, Blackford AL, Visvanathan K, Rugo HS, Moy B, Goldstein LJ, et al. Risk of marrow neoplasms after adjuvant breast cancer therapy: the national comprehensive cancer network experience. J Clin Oncol (Official Journal of the American Society of Clinical Oncology). 2015;33(4):340–8.
26. Patt DA, Duan Z, Fang S, Hortobagyi GN, Giordano SH. Acute myeloid leukemia after adjuvant breast cancer therapy in older women: understanding risk. J Clin Oncol (Official Journal of the American Society of Clinical Oncology). 2007;25(25):3871–6.
27. Turner N, Biganzoli L, Di Leo A. Continued value of adjuvant anthracyclines as treatment for early breast cancer. Lancet Oncol. 2015;16(7):e362–9.
28. Jones S, Holmes FA, O'Shaughnessy J, Blum JL, Vukelja SJ, McIntyre KJ, et al. Docetaxel with cyclophosphamide is associated with an overall survival benefit compared with doxorubicin and cyclophosphamide: 7-year follow-up of US Oncology Research Trial 9735. J Clin Oncol (Official Journal of the American Society of Clinical Oncology). 2009.
29. Shulman LN, Berry DA, Cirrincione CT, Becker HP, Perez EA, O'Regan R, et al. Comparison of doxorubicin and cyclophosphamide versus single-agent paclitaxel as adjuvant therapy for breast cancer in women with 0 to 3 positive axillary nodes: CALGB 40101 (Alliance). J Clin Oncol (Official Journal of the American Society of Clinical Oncology). 2014;32(22):2311–7.
30. Slamon D, Eiermann W, Robert N, Giermek J, Martin M, Jasiowka M, et al. Abstract S5-04: Ten year follow-up of BCIRG-006 comparing doxorubicin plus cyclophosphamide followed by docetaxel (AC → T) with doxorubicin plus cyclophosphamide followed by docetaxel and trastuzumab (AC → TH) with docetaxel, carboplatin and trastuzumab

(TCH) in HER2 + early breast cancer. Cancer Res. 2016;76(4 Suppl):S5-04.

31. Jones SE, Collea R, Paul D, Sedlacek S, Favret AM, Gore I Jr, et al. Adjuvant docetaxel and cyclophosphamide plus trastuzumab in patients with HER2-amplified early stage breast cancer: a single-group, open-label, phase 2 study. Lancet Oncol. 2013;14 (11):1121–8.
32. Tolaney SM, Barry WT, Dang CT, Yardley DA, Moy B, Marcom PK, et al. Adjuvant paclitaxel and trastuzumab for node-negative, HER2-positive breast cancer. N Engl J Med. 2015;372(2):134–41.
33. Giordano SH, Lin YL, Kuo YF, Hortobagyi GN, Goodwin JS. Decline in the use of anthracyclines for breast cancer. J Clin Oncol (Official Journal of the American Society of Clinical Oncology). 2012;30(18):2232–9.
34. Li S, Blaes AH, Liu J, Hu Y, Hernandez RK, Stryker S, et al. Trends in the use of adjuvant anthracycline- and taxane-based chemotherapy regimens in early-stage breast cancer, by surgery type. ASCO Meet Abstr. 2014;32(15 suppl):e12017.
35. O'Brien MER. Reduced cardiotoxicity and comparable efficacy in a phase III trial of pegylated liposomal doxorubicin HCl (CAELYX™/Doxil®) versus conventional doxorubicin for first-line treatment of metastatic breast cancer. Ann Oncol. 2004;15(3):440–9.
36. Al-Batran SE, Meerpohl HG, von Minckwitz G, Atmaca A, Kleeberg U, Harbeck N, et al. Reduced incidence of severe palmar-plantar erythrodysesthesia and mucositis in a prospective multicenter phase II trial with pegylated liposomal doxorubicin at 40 mg/m^2 every 4 weeks in previously treated patients with metastatic breast cancer. Oncology. 2006;70(2):141–6.
37. Chan S, Davidson N, Juozaityte E, Erdkamp F, Pluzanska A, Azarnia N, et al. Phase III trial of liposomal doxorubicin and cyclophosphamide compared with epirubicin and cyclophosphamide as first-line therapy for metastatic breast cancer. Ann Oncol (Official Journal of the European Society for Medical Oncology/ESMO). 2004;15(10):1527–34.
38. Batist G, Harris L, Azarnia N, Lee LW, Daza-Ramirez P. Improved anti-tumor response rate with decreased cardiotoxicity of non-pegylated liposomal doxorubicin compared with conventional doxorubicin in first-line treatment of metastatic breast cancer in patients who had received prior adjuvant doxorubicin: results of a retrospective analysis. Anticancer Drugs. 2006;17(5):587–95.
39. Henderson IC, Allegra JC, Woodcock T, Wolff S, Bryan S, Cartwright K, et al. Randomized clinical trial comparing mitoxantrone with doxorubicin in previously treated patients with metastatic breast cancer. J Clin Oncol (Official Journal of the American Society of Clinical Oncology). 1989;7(5):560–71.
40. Heidemann E. Is first-line single-agent mitoxantrone in the treatment of high-risk metastatic breast cancer patients as effective as combination chemotherapy? No difference in survival but higher quality of life were found in a multicenter randomized trial. Ann Oncol. 2002;13(11):1717–29.
41. Rowinsky EK. Clinical pharmacology of Taxol. J Natl Cancer Inst Monogr. 1993;15:25–37.
42. Roche H, Fumoleau P, Spielmann M, Canon JL, Delozier T, Serin D, et al. Sequential adjuvant epirubicin-based and docetaxel chemotherapy for node-positive breast cancer patients: the FNCLCC PACS 01 Trial. J Clin Oncol (Official Journal of the American Society of Clinical Oncology). 2006;24(36):5664–71.
43. Martin M, Pienkowski T, Mackey J, Pawlicki M, Guastalla JP, Weaver C, et al. Adjuvant docetaxel for node-positive breast cancer. N Engl J Med. 2005;352(22):2302–13.
44. Mackey JR, Martin M, Pienkowski T, Rolski J, Guastalla JP, Sami A, et al. Adjuvant docetaxel, doxorubicin, and cyclophosphamide in node-positive breast cancer: 10-year follow-up of the phase 3 randomised BCIRG 001 trial. Lancet Oncol. 2013;14(1):72–80.
45. Martin M, Segui MA, Anton A, Ruiz A, Ramos M, Adrover E, et al. Adjuvant docetaxel for high-risk, node-negative breast cancer. N Engl J Med. 2010;363(23):2200–10.
46. Nitz U, Gluz O, Huober J, Kreipe HH, Kates RE, Hartmann A, et al. Final analysis of the prospective WSG-AGO EC-Doc versus FEC phase III trial in intermediate-risk (pN1) early breast cancer: efficacy and predictive value of Ki67 expressiondagger. Ann Oncol (Official Journal of the European Society for Medical Oncology/ESMO). 2014;25(8):1551–7.
47. Sparano JA, Zhao F, Martino S, Ligibel JA, Perez EA, Saphner T, et al. Long-term follow-up of the E1199 Phase III trial evaluating the role of taxane and schedule in operable breast cancer. J Clin Oncol (Official Journal of the American Society of Clinical Oncology). 2015;33(21):2353–60.
48. Jones SE, Erban J, Overmoyer B, Budd GT, Hutchins L, Lower E, et al. Randomized phase III study of docetaxel compared with paclitaxel in metastatic breast cancer. J Clin Oncol (Official Journal of the American Society of Clinical Oncology). 2005;23(24):5542–51.
49. Seidman AD, Berry D, Cirrincione C, Harris L, Muss H, Marcom PK, et al. Randomized phase III trial of weekly compared with every-3-weeks paclitaxel for metastatic breast cancer, with trastuzumab for all HER-2 overexpressors and random assignment to trastuzumab or not in HER-2 nonoverexpressors: final results of Cancer and Leukemia Group B protocol 9840. J Clin Oncol (Official Journal of the American Society of Clinical Oncology). 2008;26(10):1642–9.
50. Hayes DF, Thor AD, Dressler LG, Weaver D, Edgerton S, Cowan D, et al. HER2 and response to paclitaxel in node-positive breast cancer. N Engl J Med. 2007;357(15):1496–506.
51. Andre F, Broglio K, Roche H, Martin M, Mackey JR, Penault-Llorca F, et al. Estrogen receptor expression and efficacy of docetaxel-containing adjuvant chemotherapy in patients with node-positive breast cancer: results from a pooled analysis. J Clin Oncol (Official Journal of the American Society of Clinical Oncology). 2008;26(16):2636–43.
52. De Laurentiis M, Cancello G, D'Agostino D, Giuliano M, Giordano A, Montagna E, et al. Taxane-based combinations as adjuvant chemotherapy of early breast cancer: a meta-analysis of randomized trials. J Clin Oncol (Official Journal of the American Society of Clinical Oncology). 2008;26(1):44–53.
53. Jacquin JP, Jones S, Magne N, Chapelle C, Ellis P, Janni W, et al. Docetaxel-containing adjuvant chemotherapy in patients with early stage breast cancer. Consistency of effect independent of nodal and biomarker status: a meta-analysis of 14 randomized clinical trials. Breast Cancer Res Treat. 2012;134(3): 903–13.
54. Coates AS, Winer EP, Goldhirsch A, Gelber RD, Gnant M, Piccart-Gebhart M, et al. Tailoring therapies-improving the management of early breast cancer: St Gallen International Expert Consensus on the Primary Therapy of Early Breast Cancer 2015. Ann Oncol (Official Journal of the European Society for Medical Oncology/ESMO). 2015;26(8):1533–46.
55. Sparano JA, Wang M, Martino S, Jones V, Perez EA, Saphner T, et al. Weekly paclitaxel in the adjuvant treatment of breast cancer. N Engl J Med. 2008;358(16):1663–71.
56. Eiermann W, Pienkowski T, Crown J, Sadeghi S, Martin M, Chan A, et al. Phase III study of doxorubicin/cyclophosphamide with concomitant versus sequential docetaxel as adjuvant treatment in patients with human epidermal growth factor receptor 2-normal, node-positive breast cancer: BCIRG-005 trial. J Clin Oncol (Official Journal of the American Society of Clinical Oncology). 2011;29(29):3877–84.

57. O'Shaughnessy J, Miles D, Vukelja S, Moiseyenko V, Ayoub JP, Cervantes G, et al. Superior survival with capecitabine plus docetaxel combination therapy in anthracycline-pretreated patients with advanced breast cancer: phase III trial results. J Clin Oncol (Official Journal of the American Society of Clinical Oncology). 2002;20(12):2812–23.
58. Miles D, Vukelja S, Moiseyenko V, Cervantes G, Mauriac L, Van Hazel G, et al. Survival benefit with capecitabine/docetaxel versus docetaxel alone: analysis of therapy in a randomized phase III trial. Clin Breast Cancer. 2004;5(4):273–8.
59. Albain KS, Nag SM, Calderillo-Ruiz G, Jordaan JP, Llombart AC, Pluzanska A, et al. Gemcitabine plus Paclitaxel versus Paclitaxel monotherapy in patients with metastatic breast cancer and prior anthracycline treatment. J Clin Oncol (Official Journal of the American Society of Clinical Oncology). 2008;26 (24):3950–7.
60. Desai N, Trieu V, Yao Z, Louie L, Ci S, Yang A, et al. Increased antitumor activity, intratumor paclitaxel concentrations, and endothelial cell transport of cremophor-free, albumin-bound paclitaxel, ABI-007, compared with cremophor-based paclitaxel. Clin Cancer Res (An Official Journal of the American Association for Cancer Research). 2006;12(4):1317–24.
61. Gradishar WJ, Tjulandin S, Davidson N, Shaw H, Desai N, Bhar P, et al. Phase III trial of nanoparticle albumin-bound paclitaxel compared with polyethylated castor oil-based paclitaxel in women with breast cancer. J Clin Oncol (Official Journal of the American Society of Clinical Oncology). 2005;23 (31):7794–803.
62. Gradishar WJ, Krasnojon D, Cheporov S, Makhson AN, Manikhas GM, Clawson A, et al. Significantly longer progression-free survival with nab-paclitaxel compared with docetaxel as first-line therapy for metastatic breast cancer. J Clin Oncol (Official Journal of the American Society of Clinical Oncology). 2009;27(22):3611–9.
63. Gebhart G, Gamez C, Holmes E, Robles J, Garcia C, Cortes M, et al. 18F-FDG PET/CT for early prediction of response to neoadjuvant lapatinib, trastuzumab, and their combination in HER2-positive breast cancer: results from Neo-ALTTO. J Nucl Med (Official Publication, Society of Nuclear Medicine). 2013;54 (11):1862–8.
64. Untch M, Jackisch C, Schneeweiß A, Conrad B, Aktas B, Denkert C, et al. Abstract S2-07: a randomized phase III trial comparing neoadjuvant chemotherapy with weekly nanoparticle-based paclitaxel with solvent-based paclitaxel followed by anthracyline/cyclophosphamide for patients with early breast cancer (GeparSepto); GBG 69. Cancer Res. 2015;75(9 Suppl):S2-07.
65. von Minckwitz G, Untch M, Jakisch C, Schneeweiss A, Conrad B, Aktas B, et al. Abstract P1–14-11: nab-paclitaxel at a dose of 125 mg/m^2 weekly is more efficacious but less toxic than at 150 mg/m^2. Results from the neoadjuvant randomized GeparSepto study (GBG 69). Cancer Res. 2016;76(4 Suppl):P1-14-1.
66. Sparano JA, Vrdoljak E, Rixe O, Xu B, Manikhas A, Medina C, et al. Randomized phase III trial of ixabepilone plus capecitabine versus capecitabine in patients with metastatic breast cancer previously treated with an anthracycline and a taxane. J Clin Oncol (Official Journal of the American Society of Clinical Oncology). 2010;28(20):3256–63.
67. Thomas ES, Gomez HL, Li RK, Chung HC, Fein LE, Chan VF, et al. Ixabepilone plus capecitabine for metastatic breast cancer progressing after anthracycline and taxane treatment. J Clin Oncol (Official Journal of the American Society of Clinical Oncology). 2007;25(33):5210–7.
68. Baselga J, Zambetti M, Llombart-Cussac A, Manikhas G, Kubista E, Steger GG, et al. Phase II genomics study of ixabepilone as neoadjuvant treatment for breast cancer. J Clin Oncol (Official Journal of the American Society of Clinical Oncology). 2009;27(4):526–34.
69. Thomas ES. Ixabepilone plus capecitabine for metastatic breast cancer progressing after anthracycline and taxane treatment. J Clin Oncol (Official Journal of the American Society of Clinical Oncology). 2008;26(13):2223.
70. Perez EA, Lerzo G, Pivot X, Thomas E, Vahdat L, Bosserman L, et al. Efficacy and safety of ixabepilone (BMS-247550) in a phase II study of patients with advanced breast cancer resistant to an anthracycline, a taxane, and capecitabine. J Clin Oncol (Official Journal of the American Society of Clinical Oncology). 2007;25 (23):3407–14.
71. EMEA. Questions and answers on the withdrawal of the marketing authorisation for Ixempra 2009. Available from http://www.ema.europa.eu/docs/en_GB/document_library/Medicine_QA/2010/01/WC500062428.pdf.
72. Vogel C, O'Rourke M, Winer E, Hochster H, Chang A, Adamkiewicz B, et al. Vinorelbine as first-line chemotherapy for advanced breast cancer in women 60 years of age or older. Ann Oncol (Official Journal of the European Society for Medical Oncology/ESMO). 1999;10(4):397–402.
73. Weber BL, Vogel C, Jones S, Harvey H, Hutchins L, Bigley J, et al. Intravenous vinorelbine as first-line and second-line therapy in advanced breast cancer. J Clin Oncol (Official Journal of the American Society of Clinical Oncology). 1995;13(11): 2722–30.
74. Romero A, Rabinovich MG, Vallejo CT, Perez JE, Rodriguez R, Cuevas MA, et al. Vinorelbine as first-line chemotherapy for metastatic breast carcinoma. J Clin Oncol (Official Journal of the American Society of Clinical Oncology). 1994;12(2):336–41.
75. Garcia-Conde J, Lluch A, Martin M, Casado A, Gervasio H, De Oliveira C, et al. Phase II trial of weekly IV vinorelbine in first-line advanced breast cancer chemotherapy. Ann Oncol (Official Journal of the European Society for Medical Oncology/ESMO). 1994;5(9):854–7.
76. Fumoleau P, Delgado FM, Delozier T, Monnier A, Gil Delgado MA, Kerbrat P, et al. Phase II trial of weekly intravenous vinorelbine in first-line advanced breast cancer chemotherapy. J Clin Oncol (Official Journal of the American Society of Clinical Oncology). 1993;11(7):1245–52.
77. Gasparini G, Caffo O, Barni S, Frontini L, Testolin A, Guglielmi RB, et al. Vinorelbine is an active antiproliferative agent in pretreated advanced breast cancer patients: a phase II study. J Clin Oncol (Official Journal of the American Society of Clinical Oncology). 1994;12(10):2094–101.
78. Degardin M, Bonneterre J, Hecquet B, Pion JM, Adenis A, Horner D, et al. Vinorelbine (navelbine) as a salvage treatment for advanced breast cancer. Ann Oncol (Official Journal of the European Society for Medical Oncology/ESMO). 1994;5(5):423–6.
79. Jones S, Winer E, Vogel C, Laufman L, Hutchins L, O'Rourke M, et al. Randomized comparison of vinorelbine and melphalan in anthracycline-refractory advanced breast cancer. J Clin Oncol (Official Journal of the American Society of Clinical Oncology). 1995;13(10):2567–74.
80. Martin M, Ruiz A, Munoz M, Balil A, Garcia-Mata J, Calvo L, et al. Gemcitabine plus vinorelbine versus vinorelbine monotherapy in patients with metastatic breast cancer previously treated with anthracyclines and taxanes: final results of the phase III Spanish Breast Cancer Research Group (GEICAM) trial. Lancet Oncol. 2007;8(3):219–25.
81. Pajk B, Cufer T, Canney P, Ellis P, Cameron D, Blot E, et al. Anti-tumor activity of capecitabine and vinorelbine in patients with anthracycline- and taxane-pretreated metastatic breast

cancer: findings from the EORTC 10001 randomized phase II trial. Breast. 2008;17(2):180–5.
82. Baweja M, Suman VJ, Fitch TR, Mailliard JA, Bernath A, Rowland KM, et al. Phase II trial of oral vinorelbine for the treatment of metastatic breast cancer in patients > or = 65 years of age: an NCCTG study. Ann Oncol (Official Journal of the European Society for Medical Oncology/ESMO). 2006;17 (4):623–9.
83. Freyer G, Delozier T, Lichinister M, Gedouin D, Bougnoux P, His P, et al. Phase II study of oral vinorelbine in first-line advanced breast cancer chemotherapy. J Clin Oncol (Official Journal of the American Society of Clinical Oncology). 2003;21 (1):35–40.
84. Andersson M, Lidbrink E, Bjerre K, Wist E, Enevoldsen K, Jensen AB, et al. Phase III randomized study comparing docetaxel plus trastuzumab with vinorelbine plus trastuzumab as first-line therapy of metastatic or locally advanced human epidermal growth factor receptor 2-positive breast cancer: the HERNATA study. J Clin Oncol (Official Journal of the American Society of Clinical Oncology). 2011;29(3):264–71.
85. Okouneva T, Azarenko O, Wilson L, Littlefield BA, Jordan MA. Inhibition of centromere dynamics by eribulin (E7389) during mitotic metaphase. Mol Cancer Ther. 2008;7(7):2003–11.
86. Cortes J, O'Shaughnessy J, Loesch D, Blum JL, Vahdat LT, Petrakova K, et al. Eribulin monotherapy versus treatment of physician's choice in patients with metastatic breast cancer (EMBRACE): a phase 3 open-label randomised study. Lancet. 2011;377(9769):914–23.
87. Kaufman PA, Awada A, Twelves C, Yelle L, Perez EA, Velikova G, et al. Phase III open-label randomized study of eribulin mesylate versus capecitabine in patients with locally advanced or metastatic breast cancer previously treated with an anthracycline and a taxane. J Clin Oncol (Official Journal of the American Society of Clinical Oncology). 2015;33(6):594–601.
88. Twelves C, Cortes J, Vahdat L, Olivo M, He Y, Kaufman PA, et al. Efficacy of eribulin in women with metastatic breast cancer: a pooled analysis of two phase 3 studies. Breast Cancer Res Treat. 2014;148(3):553–61.
89. Madondo MT, Quinn M, Plebanski M. Low dose cyclophosphamide: mechanisms of T cell modulation. Cancer Treat Rev. 2016;42:3–9.
90. Hall AG, Tilby MJ. Mechanisms of action of, and modes of resistance to, alkylating agents used in the treatment of haematological malignancies. Blood Rev. 1992;6(3):163–73.
91. Brock N. Oxazaphosphorine cytostatics: past-present-future. Seventh Cain Memorial Award Lecture. Cancer Res. 1989;49 (1):1–7.
92. Bonadonna G, Moliterni A, Zambetti M, Daidone MG, Pilotti S, Gianni L, et al. 30 years' follow up of randomised studies of adjuvant CMF in operable breast cancer: cohort study. BMJ. 2005;330(7485):217.
93. Bonadonna G, Valagussa P, Moliterni A, Zambetti M, Brambilla C. Adjuvant cyclophosphamide, methotrexate, and fluorouracil in node-positive breast cancer: the results of 20 years of follow-up. N Engl J Med. 1995;332(14):901–6.
94. Piccart MJ, Di Leo A, Beauduin M, Vindevoghel A, Michel J, Focan C, et al. Phase III trial comparing two dose levels of epirubicin combined with cyclophosphamide with cyclophosphamide, methotrexate, and fluorouracil in node-positive breast cancer. J Clin Oncol (Official Journal of the American Society of Clinical Oncology). 2001;19(12):3103–10.
95. Fisher B, Redmond C, Legault-Poisson S, Dimitrov NV, Brown AM, Wickerham DL, et al. Postoperative chemotherapy and tamoxifen compared with tamoxifen alone in the treatment of positive-node breast cancer patients aged 50 years and older with tumors responsive to tamoxifen: results from the National Surgical Adjuvant Breast and Bowel Project B-16. J Clin Oncol (Official Journal of the American Society of Clinical Oncology). 1990;8(6):1005–18.
96. Colleoni M. Low-dose oral methotrexate and cyclophosphamide in metastatic breast cancer: antitumor activity and correlation with vascular endothelial growth factor levels. Ann Oncol. 2002;13(1):73–80.
97. Colleoni M, Gray KP, Gelber SI, Lang I, Thurlimann BJK, Gianni L, et al. Low-dose oral cyclophosphamide-methotrexate maintenance (CMM) for receptor-negative early breast cancer (BC). ASCO Meet Abstr. 2015;33(15 suppl):1002.
98. Sistigu A, Viaud S, Chaput N, Bracci L, Proietti E, Zitvogel L. Immunomodulatory effects of cyclophosphamide and implementations for vaccine design. Semin Immunopathol. 2011;33 (4):369–83.
99. Emadi A, Jones RJ, Brodsky RA. Cyclophosphamide and cancer: golden anniversary. Nat Rev Clin Oncol. 2009;6(11):638–47.
100. Cheson BD, Rummel MJ. Bendamustine: rebirth of an old drug. J Clin Oncol (Official Journal of the American Society of Clinical Oncology). 2009;27(9):1492–501.
101. Pirvulescu C, von Minckwitz G, Loibl S. Bendamustine in metastatic breast cancer: an old drug in new design. Breast care. 2008;3(5):333–9.
102. von Minckwitz G, Chernozemsky I, Sirakova L, Chilingirov P, Souchon R, Marschner N, et al. Bendamustine prolongs progression-free survival in metastatic breast cancer (MBC): a phase III prospective, randomized, multicenter trial of bendamustine hydrochloride, methotrexate and 5-fluorouracil (BMF) versus cyclophosphamide, methotrexate and 5-fluorouracil (CMF) as first-line treatment of MBC. Anticancer Drugs. 2005;16(8):871–7.
103. Reichmann U, Bokemeyer C, Wallwiener D, Bamberg M, Huober J. Salvage chemotherapy for metastatic breast cancer: results of a phase II study with bendamustine. Ann Oncol (Official Journal of the European Society for Medical Oncology/ESMO). 2007;18(12):1981–4.
104. Decatris MP, Sundar S, O'Byrne KJ. Platinum-based chemotherapy in metastatic breast cancer: current status. Cancer Treat Rev. 2004;30(1):53–81.
105. Kolaric K, Roth A. Phase II clinical trial of cis-dichlorodiammine platinum (cis-DDP) for antitumorigenic activity in previously untreated patients with metastatic breast cancer. Cancer Chemother Pharmacol. 1983;11(2):108–12.
106. Sledge GW Jr, Loehrer PJ Sr, Roth BJ, Einhorn LH. Cisplatin as first-line therapy for metastatic breast cancer. J Clin Oncol (Official Journal of the American Society of Clinical Oncology). 1988;6(12):1811–4.
107. Yap HY, Salem P, Hortobagyi GN, Bodey GP Sr, Buzdar AU, Tashima CK, et al. Phase II study of cis-dichlorodiammineplatinum(II) in advanced breast cancer. Cancer Treat Rep. 1978;62(3):405–8.
108. Forastiere AA, Hakes TB, Wittes JT, Wittes RE. Cisplatin in the treatment of metastatic breast carcinoma: a prospective randomized trial of two dosage schedules. Am J Clin Oncol. 1982;5 (3):243–7.
109. Martino S, Samal BA, Singhakowinta A, Yoshida S, Mackenzie M, Jain J, et al. A phase II study of cis-diamminedichloroplatinum II for advanced breast cancer. Two dose schedules. J Cancer Res Clin Oncol. 1984;108(3):354–6.
110. Marme F, Schneeweiss A. Targeted therapies in triple-negative breast cancer. Breast care. 2015;10(3):159–66.
111. Baselga J, Gomez P, Greil R, Braga S, Climent MA, Wardley AM, et al. Randomized phase II study of the anti-epidermal

growth factor receptor monoclonal antibody cetuximab with cisplatin versus cisplatin alone in patients with metastatic triple-negative breast cancer. J Clin Oncol (Official Journal of the American Society of Clinical Oncology). 2013;31(20):2586–92.
112. Carey LA, Rugo HS, Marcom PK, Mayer EL, Esteva FJ, Ma CX, et al. TBCRC 001: randomized phase II study of cetuximab in combination with carboplatin in stage IV triple-negative breast cancer. J Clin Oncol (Official Journal of the American Society of Clinical Oncology). 2012;30(21):2615–23.
113. Isakoff SJ, Mayer EL, He L, Traina TA, Carey LA, Krag KJ, et al. TBCRC009: a multicenter phase II clinical trial of platinum monotherapy with biomarker assessment in metastatic triple-negative breast cancer. J Clin Oncol (Official Journal of the American Society of Clinical Oncology). 2015;33(17):1902–9.
114. Tutt A, Ellis P, Kilburn L, Gilett C, Pinder S, Abraham J, et al. Abstract S3-01: the TNT trial: a randomized phase III trial of carboplatin (C) compared with docetaxel (D) for patients with metastatic or recurrent locally advanced triple negative or BRCA1/2 breast cancer (CRUK/07/012). Cancer Res. 2015;75 (9 Suppl):S3–4.
115. von Minckwitz G, Schneeweiss A, Loibl S, Salat C, Denkert C, Rezai M, et al. Neoadjuvant carboplatin in patients with triple-negative and HER2-positive early breast cancer (GeparSixto; GBG 66): a randomised phase 2 trial. Lancet Oncol. 2014;15(7):747–56.
116. Sikov WM, Berry DA, Perou CM, Singh B, Cirrincione CT, Tolaney SM, et al. Impact of the addition of carboplatin and/or bevacizumab to neoadjuvant once-per-week paclitaxel followed by dose-dense doxorubicin and cyclophosphamide on pathologic complete response rates in stage II to III triple-negative breast cancer: CALGB 40603 (Alliance). J Clin Oncol (Official Journal of the American Society of Clinical Oncology). 2015;33(1):13–21.
117. Gluz O, Nitz U, Liedtke C, Christgen M, Sotlar K, Grischke E, et al. Abstract S6-07: comparison of 12 weeks neoadjuvant Nab-paclitaxel combined with carboplatinum vs. gemcitabine in triple- negative breast cancer: WSG-ADAPT TN randomized phase II trial. Cancer Res. 2016;76(4 Suppl):S6-07.
118. von Minckwitz G, Loibl S, Schneeweiss A, Salat C, Rezai M, Zahm D-M, et al. Abstract S2-04: early survival analysis of the randomized phase II trial investigating the addition of carboplatin to neoadjuvant therapy for triple-negative and HER2-positive early breast cancer (GeparSixto). Cancer Res. 2016;76(4 Suppl): S2-04.
119. Sikov W, Berry D, Perou C, Singh B, Cirrincione C, Tolaney S, et al. Abstract S2-05: event-free and overall survival following neoadjuvant weekly paclitaxel and dose-dense AC ± carboplatin and/or bevacizumab in triple-negative breast cancer: outcomes from CALGB 40603 (Alliance). Cancer Res. 2016;76(4 Suppl): S2-05.
120. Goodsell DS. The molecular perspective: methotrexate. Oncologist. 1999;4(4):340–1.
121. Del Mastro L, De Placido S, Bruzzi P, De Laurentiis M, Boni C, Cavazzini G, et al. Fluorouracil and dose-dense chemotherapy in adjuvant treatment of patients with early-stage breast cancer: an open-label, 2 × 2 factorial, randomised phase 3 trial. Lancet. 2015;385(9980):1863–72.
122. O'Shaughnessy JA, Kaufmann M, Siedentopf F, Dalivoust P, Debled M, Robert NJ, et al. Capecitabine monotherapy: review of studies in first-line HER-2-negative metastatic breast cancer. Oncologist. 2012;17(4):476–84.
123. Robert NJ, Dieras V, Glaspy J, Brufsky AM, Bondarenko I, Lipatov ON, et al. RIBBON-1: randomized, double-blind, placebo-controlled, phase III trial of chemotherapy with or without bevacizumab for first-line treatment of human epidermal growth factor receptor 2-negative, locally recurrent or metastatic breast cancer. J Clin Oncol (Official Journal of the American Society of Clinical Oncology). 2011;29(10):1252–60.
124. Chan A, Verrill M. Capecitabine and vinorelbine in metastatic breast cancer. Eur J Cancer. 2009;45(13):2253–65.
125. Joensuu H, Kellokumpu-Lehtinen PL, Huovinen R, Jukkola-Vuorinen A, Tanner M, Asola R, et al. Adjuvant capecitabine in combination with docetaxel and cyclophosphamide plus epirubicin for breast cancer: an open-label, randomised controlled trial. Lancet Oncol. 2009;10(12): 1145–51.
126. Joensuu H, Gligorov J. Adjuvant treatments for triple-negative breast cancers. Ann Oncol (Official Journal of the European Society for Medical Oncology/ESMO). 2012;23 Suppl 6:vi40–vi5.
127. J O'Shaughnessy. First efficacy results of a randomized, open-label, phase III study of adjuvant doxorubicin plus cyclophosphamide, followed by docetaxel with or without capecitabine, in high-risk early breast cancer. Cancer Res. 2010;72(24 suppl):S2-4.
128. Jiang Y, Yin W, Zhou L, Yan T, Zhou Q, Du Y, et al. First efficacy results of capecitabine with anthracycline- and taxane-based adjuvant therapy in high-risk early breast cancer: a meta-analysis. PLoS ONE. 2012;7(3):e32474.
129. von Minckwitz G, Blohmer JU, Costa SD, Denkert C, Eidtmann H, Eiermann W, et al. Response-guided neoadjuvant chemotherapy for breast cancer. J Clin Oncol (Official Journal of the American Society of Clinical Oncology). 2013;31(29):3623–30.
130. Toi M, Lee S-J, Lee E, Ohtani S, Im Y-H, Im S-A, et al. Abstract S1-07: a phase III trial of adjuvant capecitabine in breast cancer patients with HER2-negative pathologic residual invasive disease after neoadjuvant chemotherapy (CREATE-X, JBCRG-04). Cancer Res. 2016;76(4 Suppl):S1-07.
131. Benson AB 3rd, Ajani JA, Catalano RB, Engelking C, Kornblau SM, Martenson JA Jr, et al. Recommended guidelines for the treatment of cancer treatment-induced diarrhea. J Clin Oncol (Official Journal of the American Society of Clinical Oncology). 2004;22(14):2918–26.
132. Seidman AD. The evolving role of gemcitabine in the management of breast cancer. Oncology. 2001;60(3):189–98.
133. Seidman AD. Gemcitabine as single-agent therapy in the management of advanced breast cancer. Oncology. 2001;15(2 Suppl 3):11–4.
134. Hertel LW, Boder GB, Kroin JS, Rinzel SM, Poore GA, Todd GC, et al. Evaluation of the antitumor activity of gemcitabine (2′,2′-difluoro-2′-deoxycytidine). Cancer Res. 1990;50(14):4417–22.
135. Ferrazzi E, Stievano L. Gemcitabine: monochemotherapy of breast cancer. Ann Oncol (Official Journal of the European Society for Medical Oncology/ESMO). 2006;17(Suppl 5):v169–72.
136. Gudena V, Montero AJ, Gluck S. Gemcitabine and taxanes in metastatic breast cancer: a systematic review. Ther Clin Risk Manag. 2008;4(6):1157–64.
137. Chan S, Romieu G, Huober J, Delozier T, Tubiana-Hulin M, Schneeweiss A, et al. Phase III study of gemcitabine plus docetaxel compared with capecitabine plus docetaxel for anthracycline-pretreated patients with metastatic breast cancer. J Clin Oncol (Official Journal of the American Society of Clinical Oncology). 2009;27(11):1753–60.
138. Schechter AL, Hung MC, Vaidyanathan L, Weinberg RA, Yang-Feng TL, Francke U, et al. The neu gene: an

erbB-homologous gene distinct from and unlinked to the gene encoding the EGF receptor. Science. 1985;229(4717):976–8.
139. Coussens L, Yang-Feng TL, Liao YC, Chen E, Gray A, McGrath J, et al. Tyrosine kinase receptor with extensive homology to EGF receptor shares chromosomal location with neu oncogene. Science. 1985;230(4730):1132–9.
140. Schechter AL, Stern DF, Vaidyanathan L, Decker SJ, Drebin JA, Greene MI, et al. The neu oncogene: an erb-B-related gene encoding a 185,000-Mr tumour antigen. Nature. 1984;312 (5994):513–6.
141. Shih C, Padhy LC, Murray M, Weinberg RA. Transforming genes of carcinomas and neuroblastomas introduced into mouse fibroblasts. Nature. 1981;290(5803):261–4.
142. Slamon DJ, Godolphin W, Jones LA, Holt JA, Wong SG, Keith DE, et al. Studies of the HER-2/neu proto-oncogene in human breast and ovarian cancer. Science. 1989;244(4905):707–12.
143. Slamon DJ, Clark GM, Wong SG, Levin WJ, Ullrich A, McGuire WL. Human breast cancer: correlation of relapse and survival with amplification of the HER-2/neu oncogene. Science. 1987;235(4785):177–82.
144. Harries M, Smith I. The development and clinical use of trastuzumab (Herceptin). Endocr Relat Cancer. 2002;9(2):75–85.
145. Cobleigh MA, Vogel CL, Tripathy D, Robert NJ, Scholl S, Fehrenbacher L, et al. Multinational study of the efficacy and safety of humanized anti-HER2 monoclonal antibody in women who have HER2-overexpressing metastatic breast cancer that has progressed after chemotherapy for metastatic disease. J Clin Oncol (Official Journal of the American Society of Clinical Oncology). 1999;17(9):2639–48.
146. Vogel CL, Cobleigh MA, Tripathy D, Gutheil JC, Harris LN, Fehrenbacher L, et al. Efficacy and safety of trastuzumab as a single agent in first-line treatment of HER2-overexpressing metastatic breast cancer. J Clin Oncol (Official Journal of the American Society of Clinical Oncology). 2002;20(3):719–26.
147. Slamon DJ, Leyland-Jones B, Shak S, Fuchs H, Paton V, Bajamonde A, et al. Use of chemotherapy plus a monoclonal antibody against HER2 for metastatic breast cancer that overexpresses HER2. N Engl J Med. 2001;344(11):783–92.
148. Marty M, Cognetti F, Maraninchi D, Snyder R, Mauriac L, Tubiana-Hulin M, et al. Randomized phase II trial of the efficacy and safety of trastuzumab combined with docetaxel in patients with human epidermal growth factor receptor 2-positive metastatic breast cancer administered as first-line treatment: the M77001 study group. J Clin Oncol (Official Journal of the American Society of Clinical Oncology). 2005;23(19):4265–74.
149. Blackwell KL, Burstein HJ, Storniolo AM, Rugo HS, Sledge G, Aktan G, et al. Overall survival benefit with lapatinib in combination with trastuzumab for patients with human epidermal growth factor receptor 2-positive metastatic breast cancer: final results from the EGF104900 study. J Clin Oncol (Official Journal of the American Society of Clinical Oncology). 2012;30 (21):2585–92.
150. Kaufman B, Mackey JR, Clemens MR, Bapsy PP, Vaid A, Wardley A, et al. Trastuzumab plus anastrozole versus anastrozole alone for the treatment of postmenopausal women with human epidermal growth factor receptor 2-positive, hormone receptor-positive metastatic breast cancer: results from the randomized phase III TAnDEM study. J Clin Oncol (Official Journal of the American Society of Clinical Oncology). 2009;27 (33):5529–37.
151. von Minckwitz G, du Bois A, Schmidt M, Maass N, Cufer T, de Jongh FE, et al. Trastuzumab beyond progression in human epidermal growth factor receptor 2-positive advanced breast cancer: a german breast group 26/breast international group 03-05 study. J Clin Oncol (Official Journal of the American Society of Clinical Oncology). 2009;27(12):1999–2006.
152. Blackwell KL, Burstein HJ, Storniolo AM, Rugo H, Sledge G, Koehler M, et al. Randomized study of Lapatinib alone or in combination with trastuzumab in women with ErbB2-positive, trastuzumab-refractory metastatic breast cancer. J Clin Oncol (Official Journal of the American Society of Clinical Oncology). 2010;28(7):1124–30.
153. Gianni L, Eiermann W, Semiglazov V, Lluch A, Tjulandin S, Zambetti M, et al. Neoadjuvant and adjuvant trastuzumab in patients with HER2-positive locally advanced breast cancer (NOAH): follow-up of a randomised controlled superiority trial with a parallel HER2-negative cohort. Lancet Oncol. 2014;15 (6):640–7.
154. Buzdar AU, Ibrahim NK, Francis D, Booser DJ, Thomas ES, Theriault RL, et al. Significantly higher pathologic complete remission rate after neoadjuvant therapy with trastuzumab, paclitaxel, and epirubicin chemotherapy: results of a randomized trial in human epidermal growth factor receptor 2-positive operable breast cancer. J Clin Oncol (Official Journal of the American Society of Clinical Oncology). 2005;23(16):3676–85.
155. Buzdar AU, Valero V, Ibrahim NK, Francis D, Broglio KR, Theriault RL, et al. Neoadjuvant therapy with paclitaxel followed by 5-fluorouracil, epirubicin, and cyclophosphamide chemotherapy and concurrent trastuzumab in human epidermal growth factor receptor 2-positive operable breast cancer: an update of the initial randomized study population and data of additional patients treated with the same regimen. Clin Cancer Res (An Official Journal of the American Association for Cancer Research). 2007;13(1):228–33.
156. Untch M, Fasching PA, Konecny GE, Hasmuller S, Lebeau A, Kreienberg R, et al. Pathologic complete response after neoadjuvant chemotherapy plus trastuzumab predicts favorable survival in human epidermal growth factor receptor 2-overexpressing breast cancer: results from the TECHNO trial of the AGO and GBG study groups. J Clin Oncol (Official Journal of the American Society of Clinical Oncology). 2011;29(25): 3351–7.
157. Untch M, Rezai M, Loibl S, Fasching PA, Huober J, Tesch H, et al. Neoadjuvant treatment with trastuzumab in HER2-positive breast cancer: results from the GeparQuattro study. J Clin Oncol (Official Journal of the American Society of Clinical Oncology). 2010;28(12):2024–31.
158. Piccart-Gebhart MJ, Procter M, Leyland-Jones B, Goldhirsch A, Untch M, Smith I, et al. Trastuzumab after adjuvant chemotherapy in HER2-positive breast cancer. N Engl J Med. 2005;353 (16):1659–72.
159. Goldhirsch A, Gelber RD, Piccart-Gebhart MJ, de Azambuja E, Procter M, Suter TM, et al. 2 years versus 1 year of adjuvant trastuzumab for HER2-positive breast cancer (HERA): an open-label, randomised controlled trial. Lancet. 2013;382 (9897):1021–8.
160. Perez EA, Romond EH, Suman VJ, Jeong JH, Sledge G, Geyer CE Jr, et al. Trastuzumab plus adjuvant chemotherapy for human epidermal growth factor receptor 2-positive breast cancer: planned joint analysis of overall survival from NSABP B-31 and NCCTG N9831. J Clin Oncol (Official Journal of the American Society of Clinical Oncology). 2014;32(33):3744–52.
161. Romond EH, Perez EA, Bryant J, Suman VJ, Geyer CE Jr, Davidson NE, et al. Trastuzumab plus adjuvant chemotherapy for operable HER2-positive breast cancer. N Engl J Med. 2005;353 (16):1673–84.
162. Perez EA, Suman VJ, Davidson NE, Gralow JR, Kaufman PA, Visscher DW, et al. Sequential versus concurrent trastuzumab in adjuvant chemotherapy for breast cancer. J Clin Oncol (Official

Journal of the American Society of Clinical Oncology). 2011;29 (34):4491–7.
163. Joensuu H, Kellokumpu-Lehtinen PL, Bono P, Alanko T, Kataja V, Asola R, et al. Adjuvant docetaxel or vinorelbine with or without trastuzumab for breast cancer. N Engl J Med. 2006;354(8):809–20.
164. Pivot X, Romieu G, Debled M, Pierga J-Y, Kerbrat P, Bachelot T, et al. 6 months versus 12 months of adjuvant trastuzumab for patients with HER2-positive early breast cancer (PHARE): a randomised phase 3 trial. Lancet Oncol. 2013;14(8):741–8.
165. Goldhirsch A, Gelber RD, Piccart-Gebhart MJ, de Azambuja E, Procter M, Suter TM, et al. 2 years versus 1 year of adjuvant trastuzumab for HER2-positive breast cancer (HERA): an open-label, randomised controlled trial. Lancet. 2013.
166. Ismael G, Hegg R, Muehlbauer S, Heinzmann D, Lum B, Kim S-B, et al. Subcutaneous versus intravenous administration of (neo)adjuvant trastuzumab in patients with HER2-positive, clinical stage I-III breast cancer (HannaH study): a phase 3, open-label, multicentre, randomised trial. Lancet Oncol. 2012;13 (9):869–78.
167. de Azambuja E, Procter MJ, van Veldhuisen DJ, Agbor-Tarh D, Metzger-Filho O, Steinseifer J, et al. Trastuzumab-associated cardiac events at 8 years of median follow-up in the Herceptin Adjuvant trial (BIG 1-01). J Clin Oncol (Official Journal of the American Society of Clinical Oncology). 2014;32(20):2159–65.
168. Romond EH, Jeong JH, Rastogi P, Swain SM, Geyer CE Jr, Ewer MS, et al. Seven-year follow-up assessment of cardiac function in NSABP B-31, a randomized trial comparing doxorubicin and cyclophosphamide followed by paclitaxel (ACP) with ACP plus trastuzumab as adjuvant therapy for patients with node-positive, human epidermal growth factor receptor 2-positive breast cancer. J Clin Oncol (Official Journal of the American Society of Clinical Oncology). 2012;30(31):3792–9.
169. Advani PP, Ballman KV, Dockter TJ, Colon-Otero G, Perez EA. Long-term cardiac safety analysis of NCCTG N9831 (Alliance) adjuvant trastuzumab trial. J Clin Oncol (Official Journal of the American Society of Clinical Oncology). 2015.
170. Geyer CE, Forster J, Lindquist D, Chan S, Romieu CG, Pienkowski T, et al. Lapatinib plus capecitabine for HER2-positive advanced breast cancer. N Engl J Med. 2006;355(26):2733–43.
171. Cameron D, Casey M, Oliva C, Newstat B, Imwalle B, Geyer CE. Lapatinib plus capecitabine in women with HER-2-positive advanced breast cancer: final survival analysis of a phase III randomized trial. Oncologist. 2010;15(9): 924–34.
172. Cameron D, Casey M, Press M, Lindquist D, Pienkowski T, Romieu CG, et al. A phase III randomized comparison of lapatinib plus capecitabine versus capecitabine alone in women with advanced breast cancer that has progressed on trastuzumab: updated efficacy and biomarker analyses. Breast Cancer Res Treat. 2008;112(3):533–43.
173. Pivot X, Manikhas A, Zurawski B, Chmielowska E, Karaszewska B, Allerton R, et al. CEREBEL (EGF111438): a phase III, randomized, open-label study of lapatinib plus capecitabine versus trastuzumab plus capecitabine in patients with human epidermal growth factor receptor 2-positive metastatic breast cancer. J Clin Oncol (Official Journal of the American Society of Clinical Oncology). 2015;33(14):1564–73.
174. Di Leo A, Gomez HL, Aziz Z, Zvirbule Z, Bines J, Arbushites MC, et al. Phase III, double-blind, randomized study comparing lapatinib plus paclitaxel with placebo plus paclitaxel as first-line treatment for metastatic breast cancer. J Clin Oncol (Official Journal of the American Society of Clinical Oncology). 2008;26(34):5544–52.
175. Schwartzberg LS, Franco SX, Florance A, O'Rourke L, Maltzman J, Johnston S. Lapatinib plus letrozole as first-line therapy for HER-2+ hormone receptor-positive metastatic breast cancer. Oncologist. 2010;15(2):122–9.
176. Johnston S, Pippen J Jr, Pivot X, Lichinitser M, Sadeghi S, Dieras V, et al. Lapatinib combined with letrozole versus letrozole and placebo as first-line therapy for postmenopausal hormone receptor-positive metastatic breast cancer. J Clin Oncol (Official Journal of the American Society of Clinical Oncology). 2009;27(33):5538–46.
177. Mukherjee A, Dhadda AS, Shehata M, Chan S. Lapatinib: a tyrosine kinase inhibitor with a clinical role in breast cancer. Expert Opin Pharmacother. 2007;8(13):2189–204.
178. Montemurro F, Valabrega G, Aglietta M. Lapatinib: a dual inhibitor of EGFR and HER2 tyrosine kinase activity. Expert Opin Biol Ther. 2007;7(2):257–68.
179. Dhillon S, Wagstaff AJ. Lapatinib. Drugs. 2007;67(14):2101–8; discussion 9–10.
180. Burris HA 3rd, Hurwitz HI, Dees EC, Dowlati A, Blackwell KL, O'Neil B, et al. Phase I safety, pharmacokinetics, and clinical activity study of lapatinib (GW572016), a reversible dual inhibitor of epidermal growth factor receptor tyrosine kinases, in heavily pretreated patients with metastatic carcinomas. J Clin Oncol (Official Journal of the American Society of Clinical Oncology). 2005;23(23):5305–13.
181. de Azambuja E, Holmes AP, Piccart-Gebhart M, Holmes E, Di Cosimo S, Swaby RF, et al. Lapatinib with trastuzumab for HER2-positive early breast cancer (NeoALTTO): survival outcomes of a randomised, open-label, multicentre, phase 3 trial and their association with pathological complete response. Lancet Oncol. 2014;15(10):1137–46.
182. Perez EA, Koehler M, Byrne J, Preston AJ, Rappold E, Ewer MS. Cardiac safety of lapatinib: pooled analysis of 3689 patients enrolled in clinical trials. Mayo Clin Proc. 2008;83(6):679–86.
183. Baselga J, Bradbury I, Eidtmann H, Di Cosimo S, de Azambuja E, Aura C, et al. Lapatinib with trastuzumab for HER2-positive early breast cancer (NeoALTTO): a randomised, open-label, multicentre, phase 3 trial. Lancet. 2012;379(9816):633–40.
184. Piccart-Gebhart MJ, Holmes AP, Baselga J, De Azambuja E, Dueck AC, Viale G, et al. First results from the phase III ALTTO trial (BIG 2-06; NCCTG [Alliance] N063D) comparing one year of anti-HER2 therapy with lapatinib alone (L), trastuzumab alone (T), their sequence (T → L), or their combination (T + L) in the adjuvant treatment of HER2-positive early breast cancer (EBC). ASCO Meet Abstr. 2014;32(18 suppl):LBA4.
185. Untch M, Loibl S, Bischoff J, Eidtmann H, Kaufmann M, Blohmer JU, et al. Lapatinib versus trastuzumab in combination with neoadjuvant anthracycline-taxane-based chemotherapy (GeparQuinto, GBG 44): a randomised phase 3 trial. Lancet Oncol. 2012;13(2):135–44.
186. Guarneri V, Frassoldati A, Piacentini F, Jovic G, Giovannelli S, Oliva C, et al. Preoperative chemotherapy plus lapatinib or trastuzumab or both in HER2-positive operable breast cancer (CHERLOB Trial). Clin Breast Cancer. 2008;8(2):192–4.
187. Robidoux A, Tang G, Rastogi P, Geyer CE Jr, Azar CA, Atkins JN, et al. Lapatinib as a component of neoadjuvant therapy for HER2-positive operable breast cancer (NSABP protocol B-41): an open-label, randomised phase 3 trial. Lancet Oncol. 2013;14(12):1183–92.
188. Adams CW, Allison DE, Flagella K, Presta L, Clarke J, Dybdal N, et al. Humanization of a recombinant monoclonal antibody to produce a therapeutic HER dimerization inhibitor, pertuzumab. Cancer Immunol Immunother (CII). 2006;55(6):717–27.
189. Attard G, Kitzen J, Blagden SP, Fong PC, Pronk LC, Zhi J, et al. A phase Ib study of pertuzumab, a recombinant humanised

antibody to HER2, and docetaxel in patients with advanced solid tumours. Br J Cancer. 2007;97(10):1338–43.

190. Baselga J, Gelmon KA, Verma S, Wardley A, Conte P, Miles D, et al. Phase II trial of pertuzumab and trastuzumab in patients with human epidermal growth factor receptor 2-positive metastatic breast cancer that progressed during prior trastuzumab therapy. J Clin Oncol (Official Journal of the American Society of Clinical Oncology). 2010;28(7):1138–44.
191. Cortes J, Fumoleau P, Bianchi GV, Petrella TM, Gelmon K, Pivot X, et al. Pertuzumab monotherapy after trastuzumab-based treatment and subsequent reintroduction of trastuzumab: activity and tolerability in patients with advanced human epidermal growth factor receptor 2-positive breast cancer. J Clin Oncol (Official Journal of the American Society of Clinical Oncology). 2012;30(14):1594–600.
192. Swain SM, Baselga J, Kim SB, Ro J, Semiglazov V, Campone M, et al. Pertuzumab, trastuzumab, and docetaxel in HER2-positive metastatic breast cancer. N Engl J Med. 2015;372(8): 724–34.
193. Swain SM, Kim SB, Cortes J, Ro J, Semiglazov V, Campone M, et al. Pertuzumab, trastuzumab, and docetaxel for HER2-positive metastatic breast cancer (CLEOPATRA study): overall survival results from a randomised, double-blind, placebo-controlled, phase 3 study. Lancet Oncol. 2013;14(6):461–71.
194. Baselga J, Cortes J, Kim SB, Im SA, Hegg R, Im YH, et al. Pertuzumab plus trastuzumab plus docetaxel for metastatic breast cancer. N Engl J Med. 2012;366(2):109–19.
195. Gianni L, Pienkowski T, Im YH, Roman L, Tseng LM, Liu MC, et al. Efficacy and safety of neoadjuvant pertuzumab and trastuzumab in women with locally advanced, inflammatory, or early HER2-positive breast cancer (NeoSphere): a randomised multicentre, open-label, phase 2 trial. Lancet Oncol. 2012;13 (1):25–32.
196. Schneeweiss A, Chia S, Hickish T, Harvey V, Eniu A, Hegg R, et al. Pertuzumab plus trastuzumab in combination with standard neoadjuvant anthracycline-containing and anthracycline-free chemotherapy regimens in patients with HER2-positive early breast cancer: a randomized phase II cardiac safety study (TRYPHAENA). Ann Oncol (Official Journal of the European Society for Medical Oncology/ESMO). 2013;24(9):2278–84.
197. Moya-Horno I, Cortes J. The expanding role of pertuzumab in the treatment of HER2-positive breast cancer. Breast Cancer (Dove Med Press). 2015;7:125–32.
198. Swain SM, Ewer MS, Cortes J, Amadori D, Miles D, Knott A, et al. Cardiac tolerability of pertuzumab plus trastuzumab plus docetaxel in patients with HER2-positive metastatic breast cancer in CLEOPATRA: a randomized, double-blind, placebo-controlled phase III study. Oncologist. 2013;18(3):257–64.
199. Jiang H, Rugo HS. Human epidermal growth factor receptor 2 positive (HER2+) metastatic breast cancer: how the latest results are improving therapeutic options. Ther Adv Med Oncol. 2015;7 (6):321–39.
200. Verma S, Miles D, Gianni L, Krop IE, Welslau M, Baselga J, et al. Trastuzumab emtansine for HER2-positive advanced breast cancer. N Engl J Med. 2012;367(19):1783–91.
201. Krop IE, Kim S-B, González-Martín A, LoRusso PM, Ferrero J-M, Smitt M, et al. Trastuzumab emtansine versus treatment of physician's choice for pretreated HER2-positive advanced breast cancer (TH3RESA): a randomised, open-label, phase 3 trial. Lancet Oncol. 2014.
202. Wildiers H, Kim S-B, Gonzalez-Martin A, LoRusso P, Ferrero J-M, Yu R, et al. Abstract S5-05: trastuzumab emtansine improves overall survival versus treatment of physician's choice in patients with previously treated HER2-positive metastatic breast cancer: Final overall survival results from the phase 3 TH3RESA study. Cancer Res. 2016;76(4 Suppl):S5–6.
203. Hurvitz SA, Dirix L, Kocsis J, Bianchi GV, Lu J, Vinholes J, et al. Phase II randomized study of trastuzumab emtansine versus trastuzumab plus docetaxel in patients with human epidermal growth factor receptor 2-positive metastatic breast cancer. J Clin Oncol (Official Journal of the American Society of Clinical Oncology). 2013;31(9):1157–63.
204. Krop IE, Lin NU, Blackwell K, Guardino E, Huober J, Lu M, et al. Trastuzumab emtansine (T-DM1) versus lapatinib plus capecitabine in patients with HER2-positive metastatic breast cancer and central nervous system metastases: a retrospective, exploratory analysis in EMILIA. Ann Oncol (Official Journal of the European Society for Medical Oncology/ESMO). 2015;26 (1):113–9.
205. Bartsch R, Berghoff AS, Preusser M. Breast cancer brain metastases responding to primary systemic therapy with T-DM1. J Neurooncol. 2014;116(1):205–6.
206. de Vries CL, Linn SC, Brandsma D. Response of symptomatic brain metastases from HER-2 overexpressing breast cancer with T-DM1. J Neurooncol. 2016.
207. Ellis PA, Barrios CH, Eiermann W, Toi M, Im Y-H, Conte PF, et al. Phase III, randomized study of trastuzumab emtansine (T-DM1) {±} pertuzumab (P) vs trastuzumab + taxane (HT) for first-line treatment of HER2-positive MBC: Primary results from the MARIANNE study. ASCO Meet Abstr. 2015;33(15 suppl):507.
208. Harbeck N, Gluz O, Christgen M, Braun M, Kuemmel S, Schumacher C, et al. Abstract S5-03: final analysis of WSG-ADAPT HER2+/HR+ phase II trial: efficacy, safety, and predictive markers for 12-weeks of neoadjuvant TDM1 with or without endocrine therapy versus trastuzumab + endocrine therapy in HER2-positive hormone-receptor-positive early breast cancer. Cancer Res. 2016;76(4 Suppl):S5–03.
209. Cortés J, Dieras V, Ro J, Barriere J, Bachelot T, Hurvitz S, et al. Abstract P5-19-07: randomized phase II trial of afatinib alone or with vinorelbine versus investigator's choice of treatment in patients with HER2-positive breast cancer with progressive brain metastases after trastuzumab and/or lapatinib-based therapy: LUX-Breast 3. Cancer Res. 2015;75(9 Suppl):P5-19-07.
210. Harbeck N, Huang C-S, Hurvitz S, Yeh D-C, Shao Z, Im S-A, et al. Abstract P5-19-01: randomized phase III trial of afatinib plus vinorelbine versus trastuzumab plus vinorelbine in patients with HER2-overexpressing metastatic breast cancer who had progressed on one prior trastuzumab treatment: LUX-Breast 1. Cancer Res. 2015;75(9 Suppl):P5-19-01.
211. Chan A, Delaloge S, Holmes F, Moy B, Iwata H, Harker G, et al. Abstract S5-02: neratinib after trastuzumab-based adjuvant therapy in early-stage HER2+ breast cancer: 3-year analysis from a phase 3 randomized, placebo-controlled, double-blind trial (ExteNET). Cancer Res. 2016;76(4 Suppl):S5–6.
212. Lu CH, Wyszomierski SL, Tseng LM, Sun MH, Lan KH, Neal CL, et al. Preclinical testing of clinically applicable strategies for overcoming trastuzumab resistance caused by PTEN deficiency. Clin Cancer Res (An Official Journal of the American Association for Cancer Research). 2007;13(19):5883–8.
213. Hurvitz SA, Andre F, Jiang Z, Shao Z, Mano MS, Neciosup SP, et al. Combination of everolimus with trastuzumab plus paclitaxel as first-line treatment for patients with HER2-positive advanced breast cancer (BOLERO-1): a phase 3, randomised, double-blind, multicentre trial. Lancet Oncol. 2015;16(7):816–29.
214. Andre F, O'Regan R, Ozguroglu M, Toi M, Xu B, Jerusalem G, et al. Everolimus for women with trastuzumab-resistant, HER2-positive, advanced breast cancer (BOLERO-3): a

randomised, double-blind, placebo-controlled phase 3 trial. Lancet Oncol. 2014;15(6):580–91.
215. Presta LG, Chen H, O'Connor SJ, Chisholm V, Meng YG, Krummen L, et al. Humanization of an anti-vascular endothelial growth factor monoclonal antibody for the therapy of solid tumors and other disorders. Cancer Res. 1997;57(20):4593–9.
216. Jain RK, Duda DG, Clark JW, Loeffler JS. Lessons from phase III clinical trials on anti-VEGF therapy for cancer. Nat Clin Pract Oncol. 2006;3(1):24–40.
217. Kerbel R, Folkman J. Clinical translation of angiogenesis inhibitors. Nat Rev Cancer. 2002;2(10):727–39.
218. Jain RK. Normalizing tumor vasculature with anti-angiogenic therapy: a new paradigm for combination therapy. Nat Med. 2001;7(9):987–9.
219. Cobleigh MA, Langmuir VK, Sledge GW, Miller KD, Haney L, Novotny WF, et al. A phase I/II dose-escalation trial of bevacizumab in previously treated metastatic breast cancer. Semin Oncol. 2003;30(5 Suppl 16):117–24.
220. Gray R, Bhattacharya S, Bowden C, Miller K, Comis RL. Independent review of E2100: a phase III trial of bevacizumab plus paclitaxel versus paclitaxel in women with metastatic breast cancer. J Clin Oncol (Official Journal of the American Society of Clinical Oncology). 2009;27(30):4966–72.
221. Miller K, Wang M, Gralow J, Dickler M, Cobleigh M, Perez EA, et al. Paclitaxel plus bevacizumab versus paclitaxel alone for metastatic breast cancer. N Engl J Med. 2007;357(26):2666–76.
222. Miles DW, Chan A, Dirix LY, Cortes J, Pivot X, Tomczak P, et al. Phase III study of bevacizumab plus docetaxel compared with placebo plus docetaxel for the first-line treatment of human epidermal growth factor receptor 2-negative metastatic breast cancer. J Clin Oncol (Official Journal of the American Society of Clinical Oncology). 2010;28(20):3239–47.
223. Brufsky A, Valero V, Tiangco B, Dakhil S, Brize A, Rugo HS, et al. Second-line bevacizumab-containing therapy in patients with triple-negative breast cancer: subgroup analysis of the RIBBON-2 trial. Breast Cancer Res Treat. 2012;133(3):1067–75.
224. Brufsky AM, Hurvitz S, Perez E, Swamy R, Valero V, O'Neill V, et al. RIBBON-2: a randomized, double-blind, placebo-controlled, phase III trial evaluating the efficacy and safety of bevacizumab in combination with chemotherapy for second-line treatment of human epidermal growth factor receptor 2-negative metastatic breast cancer. J Clin Oncol (Official Journal of the American Society of Clinical Oncology). 2011;29 (32):4286–93.
225. Lang I, Brodowicz T, Ryvo L, Kahan Z, Greil R, Beslija S, et al. Bevacizumab plus paclitaxel versus bevacizumab plus capecitabine as first-line treatment for HER2-negative metastatic breast cancer: interim efficacy results of the randomised, open-label, non-inferiority, phase 3 TURANDOT trial. Lancet Oncol. 2013;14(2):125–33.
226. Rugo HS, Barry WT, Moreno-Aspitia A, Lyss AP, Cirrincione C, Leung E, et al. Randomized phase III trial of paclitaxel once per week compared with nanoparticle albumin-bound nab-paclitaxel once per week or ixabepilone with bevacizumab as first-line chemotherapy for locally recurrent or metastatic breast cancer: CALGB 40502/NCCTG N063H (Alliance). J Clin Oncol (Official Journal of the American Society of Clinical Oncology). 2015;33(21):2361–9.
227. Miles DW, Dieras V, Cortes J, Duenne AA, Yi J, O'Shaughnessy J. First-line bevacizumab in combination with chemotherapy for HER2-negative metastatic breast cancer: pooled and subgroup analyses of data from 2447 patients. Ann Oncol (Official Journal of the European Society for Medical Oncology/ESMO). 2013;24 (11):2773–80.
228. Andre F, Job B, Dessen P, Tordai A, Michiels S, Liedtke C, et al. Molecular characterization of breast cancer with high-resolution oligonucleotide comparative genomic hybridization array. Clin Cancer Res (An Official Journal of the American Association for Cancer Research). 2009;15(2):441–51.
229. Linderholm BK, Hellborg H, Johansson U, Elmberger G, Skoog L, Lehtio J, et al. Significantly higher levels of vascular endothelial growth factor (VEGF) and shorter survival times for patients with primary operable triple-negative breast cancer. Ann Oncol (Official Journal of the European Society for Medical Oncology/ESMO). 2009;20(10):1639–46.
230. Linderholm BK, Gruvbreger-Saal S, Ferno M, Bendahl PO, Malmstrom P. Vascular endothelial growth factor is a strong predictor of early distant recurrences in a prospective study of premenopausal women with lymph-node negative breast cancer. Breast. 2008;17(5):484–91.
231. von Minckwitz G, Eidtmann H, Rezai M, Fasching PA, Tesch H, Eggemann H, et al. Neoadjuvant chemotherapy and bevacizumab for HER2-negative breast cancer. N Engl J Med. 2012;366 (4):299–309.
232. von Minckwitz G, Loibl S, Untch M, Eidtmann H, Rezai M, Fasching PA, et al. Survival after neoadjuvant chemotherapy with or without bevacizumab or everolimus for HER2-negative primary breast cancer (GBG 44-GeparQuinto)dagger. Ann Oncol (Official Journal of the European Society for Medical Oncology/ESMO). 2014;25(12):2363–72.
233. Bear HD, Tang G, Rastogi P, Geyer CE Jr, Robidoux A, Atkins JN, et al. Bevacizumab added to neoadjuvant chemotherapy for breast cancer. N Engl J Med. 2012;366(4):310–20.
234. Bear HD, Tang G, Rastogi P, Geyer CE, Liu Q, Robidoux A, et al. Neoadjuvant plus adjuvant bevacizumab in early breast cancer (NSABP B-40 [NRG Oncology]): secondary outcomes of a phase 3, randomised controlled trial. Lancet Oncol. 2015;16 (9):1037–48.
235. Cameron D, Brown J, Dent R, Jackisch C, Mackey J, Pivot X, et al. Adjuvant bevacizumab-containing therapy in triple-negative breast cancer (BEATRICE): primary results of a randomised, phase 3 trial. Lancet Oncol. 2013;14(10):933–42.
236. Miller K, O'Neill AM, Dang CT, Northfelt DW, Gradishar WJ, Goldstein LJ, et al. Bevacizumab (Bv) in the adjuvant treatment of HER2-negative breast cancer: final results from Eastern Cooperative Oncology Group E5103. ASCO Meet Abstr. 2014;32(15 suppl):500.
237. David Miles LF, Yan V. Wang, Joyce O'Shaughnessy. MERiDiAN: a phase III, randomized, double-blind study of the efficacy, safety, and associated biomarkers of bevacizumab plus paclitaxel compared with paclitaxel plus placebo, as first-line treatment of patients with HER2-negative metastatic breast cancer. J Clin Oncol (Official Journal of the American Society of Clinical Oncology). 2013;31(suppl; abstr TPS1142).
238. Barrios CH, Liu MC, Lee SC, Vanlemmens L, Ferrero JM, Tabei T, et al. Phase III randomized trial of sunitinib versus capecitabine in patients with previously treated HER2-negative advanced breast cancer. Breast Cancer Res Treat. 2010;121 (1):121–31.
239. Moreno-Aspitia A, Morton RF, Hillman DW, Lingle WL, Rowland KM Jr, Wiesenfeld M, et al. Phase II trial of sorafenib in patients with metastatic breast cancer previously exposed to anthracyclines or taxanes: North Central Cancer Treatment Group and Mayo Clinic Trial N0336. J Clin Oncol (Official Journal of the American Society of Clinical Oncology). 2009;27(1):11–5.
240. Bianchi G, Loibl S, Zamagni C, Salvagni S, Raab G, Siena S, et al. Phase II multicenter, uncontrolled trial of sorafenib in patients with metastatic breast cancer. Anticancer Drugs. 2009;20 (7):616–24.

241. Taylor SK, Chia S, Dent S, Clemons M, Agulnik M, Grenci P, et al. A phase II study of pazopanib in patients with recurrent or metastatic invasive breast carcinoma: a trial of the Princess Margaret Hospital phase II consortium. Oncologist. 2010;15 (8):810–8.
242. Burstein HJ, Elias AD, Rugo HS, Cobleigh MA, Wolff AC, Eisenberg PD, et al. Phase II study of sunitinib malate, an oral multitargeted tyrosine kinase inhibitor, in patients with metastatic breast cancer previously treated with an anthracycline and a taxane. J Clin Oncol (Official Journal of the American Society of Clinical Oncology). 2008;26(11):1810–6.
243. Crown JP, Dieras V, Staroslawska E, Yardley DA, Bachelot T, Davidson N, et al. Phase III trial of sunitinib in combination with capecitabine versus capecitabine monotherapy for the treatment of patients with pretreated metastatic breast cancer. J Clin Oncol (Official Journal of the American Society of Clinical Oncology). 2013;31(23):2870–8.
244. Bergh J, Bondarenko IM, Lichinitser MR, Liljegren A, Greil R, Voytko NL, et al. First-line treatment of advanced breast cancer with sunitinib in combination with docetaxel versus docetaxel alone: results of a prospective, randomized phase III study. J Clin Oncol (Official Journal of the American Society of Clinical Oncology). 2012;30(9):921–9.
245. Robert NJ, Saleh MN, Paul D, Generali D, Gressot L, Copur MS, et al. Sunitinib plus paclitaxel versus bevacizumab plus paclitaxel for first-line treatment of patients with advanced breast cancer: a phase III, randomized, open-label trial. Clin Breast Cancer. 2011;11(2):82–92.
246. Wilhelm SM, Adnane L, Newell P, Villanueva A, Llovet JM, Lynch M. Preclinical overview of sorafenib, a multikinase inhibitor that targets both Raf and VEGF and PDGF receptor tyrosine kinase signaling. Mol Cancer Ther. 2008;7(10):3129–40.
247. Wilhelm SM, Carter C, Tang L, Wilkie D, McNabola A, Rong H, et al. BAY 43-9006 exhibits broad spectrum oral antitumor activity and targets the RAF/MEK/ERK pathway and receptor tyrosine kinases involved in tumor progression and angiogenesis. Cancer Res. 2004;64(19):7099–109.
248. Schwartzberg LS, Tauer KW, Hermann RC, Makari-Judson G, Isaacs C, Beck JT, et al. Sorafenib or placebo with either gemcitabine or capecitabine in patients with HER-2-negative advanced breast cancer that progressed during or after bevacizumab. Clin Cancer Res (An Official Journal of the American Association for Cancer Research). 2013;19(10):2745–54.
249. Baselga J, Segalla JG, Roche H, Del Giglio A, Pinczowski H, Ciruelos EM, et al. Sorafenib in combination with capecitabine: an oral regimen for patients with HER2-negative locally advanced or metastatic breast cancer. J Clin Oncol (Official Journal of the American Society of Clinical Oncology). 2012;30 (13):1484–91.
250. Baselga J, Zamagni C, Gomez P, Bermejo B, Nagai S, Melichar B, et al. LBA8A PHASE III RANDOMIZED, DOUBLE-BLIND, TRIAL COMPARING SORAFENIB PLUS CAPECITABINE VERSUS PLACEBO PLUS CAPECITABINE IN THE TREATMENT OF LOCALLY ADVANCED OR METASTATIC HER2-NEGATIVE BREAST CANCER (RESILIENCE). Ann Oncol. 2014;25(suppl 4).
251. Marme F, Gerber B, Schmidt M, Moebus VJ, Foerster FG, Grischke E-M, et al. Sorafenib (SOR) plus docetaxel (DOC) as first-line therapy in patients with HER2-negative metastatic breast cancer (MBC): a randomized, placebo-controlled phase II trial. ASCO Meet Abstr. 2014;32(15 suppl):1072.
252. Mariani G, Burdaeva O, Roman L, Staroslawska E, Udovitsa D, Driol P, et al. A double-blind, randomized phase lib study evaluating the efficacy and safety of sorafenib (SOR) compared to placebo (pl) when administered in combination with docetaxel and/or letrozole in patients with metastatic breast cancer (MBC): FM-B07-01 trial. Eur J Cancer. 47:10.
253. Tan AR, Johannes H, Rastogi P, Jacobs SA, Robidoux A, Flynn PJ, et al. Weekly paclitaxel and concurrent pazopanib following doxorubicin and cyclophosphamide as neoadjuvant therapy for HER-negative locally advanced breast cancer: NSABP Foundation FB-6, a phase II study. Breast Cancer Res Treat. 2015;149(1):163–9.
254. Hyams DM, Chan A, de Oliveira C, Snyder R, Vinholes J, Audeh MW, et al. Cediranib in combination with fulvestrant in hormone-sensitive metastatic breast cancer: a randomized Phase II study. Invest New Drugs. 2013;31(5):1345–54.
255. Amiri-Kordestani L, Tan AR, Swain SM. Pazopanib for the treatment of breast cancer. Expert Opin Investig Drugs. 2012;21 (2):217–25.
256. Taylor SK, Chia S, Dent S, Clemons M, Agulnik M, Grenci P, et al. A phase II study of pazopanib in patients with recurrent or metastatic invasive breast carcinoma: a trial of the Princess Margaret Hospital phase II consortium. Oncologist. 2010;15 (8):810–8.
257. Tabernero J, Van Cutsem E, Lakomy R, Prausova J, Ruff P, van Hazel GA, et al. Aflibercept versus placebo in combination with fluorouracil, leucovorin and irinotecan in the treatment of previously treated metastatic colorectal cancer: prespecified subgroup analyses from the VELOUR trial. Eur J Cancer. 2014;50(2):320–31.
258. Van Cutsem E, Tabernero J, Lakomy R, Prenen H, Prausova J, Macarulla T, et al. Addition of aflibercept to fluorouracil, leucovorin, and irinotecan improves survival in a phase III randomized trial in patients with metastatic colorectal cancer previously treated with an oxaliplatin-based regimen. J Clin Oncol (Official Journal of the American Society of Clinical Oncology). 2012;30(28):3499–506.
259. Sideras K, Dueck AC, Hobday TJ, Rowland KM Jr, Allred JB, Northfelt DW, et al. North central cancer treatment group (NCCTG) N0537: phase II trial of VEGF-trap in patients with metastatic breast cancer previously treated with an anthracycline and/or a taxane. Clin Breast Cancer. 2012;12(6):387–91.
260. Fuchs CS, Tomasek J, Yong CJ, Dumitru F, Passalacqua R, Goswami C, et al. Ramucirumab monotherapy for previously treated advanced gastric or gastro-oesophageal junction adenocarcinoma (REGARD): an international, randomised, multicentre, placebo-controlled, phase 3 trial. Lancet. 2014;383(9911):31–9.
261. Garon EB, Ciuleanu TE, Arrieta O, Prabhash K, Syrigos KN, Goksel T, et al. Ramucirumab plus docetaxel versus placebo plus docetaxel for second-line treatment of stage IV non-small-cell lung cancer after disease progression on platinum-based therapy (REVEL): a multicentre, double-blind, randomised phase 3 trial. Lancet. 2014;384(9944):665–73.
262. Mackey JR, Ramos-Vazquez M, Lipatov O, McCarthy N, Krasnozhon D, Semiglazov V, et al. Primary results of ROSE/TRIO-12, a randomized placebo-controlled phase III trial evaluating the addition of ramucirumab to first-line docetaxel chemotherapy in metastatic breast cancer. J Clin Oncol (Official Journal of the American Society of Clinical Oncology). 2015;33 (2):141–8.
263. Augustin HG, Koh GY, Thurston G, Alitalo K. Control of vascular morphogenesis and homeostasis through the angiopoietin-Tie system. Nat Rev Mol Cell Biol. 2009;10 (3):165–77.
264. Falcon BL, Hashizume H, Koumoutsakos P, Chou J, Bready JV, Coxon A, et al. Contrasting actions of selective inhibitors of angiopoietin-1 and angiopoietin-2 on the normalization of tumor blood vessels. Am J Pathol. 2009;175(5):2159–70.

265. Reiss Y, Knedla A, Tal AO, Schmidt MH, Jugold M, Kiessling F, et al. Switching of vascular phenotypes within a murine breast cancer model induced by angiopoietin-2. J Pathol. 2009;217 (4):571–80.
266. Thomas M, Augustin HG. The role of the Angiopoietins in vascular morphogenesis. Angiogenesis. 2009;12(2):125–37.
267. Monk BJ, Poveda A, Vergote I, Raspagliesi F, Fujiwara K, Bae D-S, et al. Anti-angiopoietin therapy with trebananib for recurrent ovarian cancer (TRINOVA-1): a randomised, multicentre, double-blind, placebo-controlled phase 3 trial. Lancet Oncol. 2014;15(8):799–808.
268. Dieras V, Wildiers H, Jassem J, Dirix LY, Guastalla JP, Bono P, et al. Trebananib (AMG 386) plus weekly paclitaxel with or without bevacizumab as first-line therapy for HER2-negative locally recurrent or metastatic breast cancer: a phase 2 randomized study. Breast. 2015;24(3):182–90.
269. Mirkin S, Pickar JH. Selective estrogen receptor modulators (SERMs): a review of clinical data. Maturitas. 2015;80(1):52–7.
270. Lim HS, Ju Lee H, Seok Lee K, Sook Lee E, Jang IJ, Ro J. Clinical implications of CYP2D6 genotypes predictive of tamoxifen pharmacokinetics in metastatic breast cancer. J Clin Oncol (Official Journal of the American Society of Clinical Oncology) 2007;25(25):3837–45.
271. Jin Y, Desta Z, Stearns V, Ward B, Ho H, Lee KH, et al. CYP2D6 genotype, antidepressant use, and tamoxifen metabolism during adjuvant breast cancer treatment. J Natl Cancer Inst. 2005;97(1):30–9.
272. Stearns V, Johnson MD, Rae JM, Morocho A, Novielli A, Bhargava P, et al. Active tamoxifen metabolite plasma concentrations after coadministration of tamoxifen and the selective serotonin reuptake inhibitor paroxetine. J Natl Cancer Inst. 2003;95(23):1758–64.
273. Goetz MP, Rae JM, Suman VJ, Safgren SL, Ames MM, Visscher DW, et al. Pharmacogenetics of tamoxifen biotransformation is associated with clinical outcomes of efficacy and hot flashes. J Clin Oncol (Official Journal of the American Society of Clinical Oncology). 2005;23(36):9312–8.
274. Schroth W, Antoniadou L, Fritz P, Schwab M, Muerdter T, Zanger UM, et al. Breast cancer treatment outcome with adjuvant tamoxifen relative to patient CYP2D6 and CYP2C19 genotypes. J Clin Oncol (Official Journal of the American Society of Clinical Oncology). 2007;25(33):5187–93.
275. Higgins MJ, Stearns V. Pharmacogenetics of endocrine therapy for breast cancer. Annu Rev Med. 2011;62:281–93.
276. Regan MM, Leyland-Jones B, Bouzyk M, Pagani O, Tang W, Kammler R, et al. CYP2D6 genotype and tamoxifen response in postmenopausal women with endocrine-responsive breast cancer: the breast international group 1-98 trial. J Natl Cancer Inst. 2012;104(6):441–51.
277. Rae JM, Drury S, Hayes DF, Stearns V, Thibert JN, Haynes BP, et al. CYP2D6 and UGT2B7 genotype and risk of recurrence in tamoxifen-treated breast cancer patients. J Natl Cancer Inst. 2012;104(6):452–60.
278. Cole MP, Jones CT, Todd ID. A new anti-oestrogenic agent in late breast cancer. An early clinical appraisal of ICI46474. Br J Cancer. 1971;25(2):270–5.
279. Fossati R, Confalonieri C, Torri V, Ghislandi E, Penna A, Pistotti V, et al. Cytotoxic and hormonal treatment for metastatic breast cancer: a systematic review of published randomized trials involving 31,510 women. J Clin Oncol (Official Journal of the American Society of Clinical Oncology). 1998;16(10): 3439–60.
280. Litherland S, Jackson IM. Antioestrogens in the management of hormone-dependent cancer. Cancer Treat Rev. 1988;15(3):183–94.
281. Bratherton DG, Brown CH, Buchanan R, Hall V, Kingsley Pillers EM, Wheeler TK, et al. A comparison of two doses of tamoxifen (Nolvadex) in postmenopausal women with advanced breast cancer: 10 mg bd versus 20 mg bd. Br J Cancer. 1984;50 (2):199–205.
282. Osborne CK. Tamoxifen in the treatment of breast cancer. N Engl J Med. 1998;339(22):1609–18.
283. EBCTCG. Effects of chemotherapy and hormonal therapy for early breast cancer on recurrence and 15-year survival: an overview of the randomised trials. Lancet. 2005;365 (9472):1687–717.
284. Davies C, Godwin J, Gray R, Clarke M, Cutter D, Darby S, et al. Relevance of breast cancer hormone receptors and other factors to the efficacy of adjuvant tamoxifen: patient-level meta-analysis of randomised trials. Lancet. 2011;378(9793):771–84.
285. Davies C, Pan H, Godwin J, Gray R, Arriagada R, Raina V, et al. Long-term effects of continuing adjuvant tamoxifen to 10 years versus stopping at 5 years after diagnosis of oestrogen receptor-positive breast cancer: ATLAS, a randomised trial. Lancet. 2012.
286. Gray RG, Rea D, Handley K, Bowden SJ, Perry P, Earl HM, et al. aTTom: long-term effects of continuing adjuvant tamoxifen to 10 years versus stopping at 5 years in 6,953 women with early breast cancer. ASCO Meet Abstr. 2013;31(15 suppl):5.
287. Cuzick J, Sestak I, Pinder SE, Ellis IO, Forsyth S, Bundred NJ, et al. Effect of tamoxifen and radiotherapy in women with locally excised ductal carcinoma in situ: long-term results from the UK/ANZ DCIS trial. Lancet Oncol. 2011;12(1):21–9.
288. Fisher B, Costantino JP, Wickerham DL, Cecchini RS, Cronin WM, Robidoux A, et al. Tamoxifen for the prevention of breast cancer: current status of the National Surgical Adjuvant Breast and Bowel Project P-1 study. J Natl Cancer Inst. 2005;97 (22):1652–62.
289. Fisher B, Dignam J, Wolmark N, Wickerham DL, Fisher ER, Mamounas E, et al. Tamoxifen in treatment of intraductal breast cancer: National Surgical Adjuvant Breast and Bowel Project B-24 randomised controlled trial. Lancet. 1999;353(9169):1993–2000.
290. Altundag K, Ibrahim NK. Aromatase inhibitors in breast cancer: an overview. Oncologist. 2006;11(6):553–62.
291. Bonneterre J, Buzdar A, Nabholtz JM, Robertson JF, Thurlimann B, von Euler M, et al. Anastrozole is superior to tamoxifen as first-line therapy in hormone receptor positive advanced breast carcinoma. Cancer. 2001;92(9):2247–58.
292. Mouridsen H, Gershanovich M, Sun Y, Perez-Carrion R, Boni C, Monnier A, et al. Superior efficacy of letrozole versus tamoxifen as first-line therapy for postmenopausal women with advanced breast cancer: results of a phase III study of the International Letrozole Breast Cancer Group. J Clin Oncol (Official Journal of the American Society of Clinical Oncology). 2001;19(10):2596–606.
293. Paridaens RJ, Dirix LY, Beex LV, Nooij M, Cameron DA, Cufer T, et al. Phase III study comparing exemestane with tamoxifen as first-line hormonal treatment of metastatic breast cancer in postmenopausal women: the European Organisation for Research and Treatment of Cancer Breast Cancer Cooperative Group. J Clin Oncol (Official Journal of the American Society of Clinical Oncology). 2008;26(30):4883–90.
294. Robertson JF, Osborne CK, Howell A, Jones SE, Mauriac L, Ellis M, et al. Fulvestrant versus anastrozole for the treatment of advanced breast carcinoma in postmenopausal women: a prospective combined analysis of two multicenter trials. Cancer. 2003;98(2):229–38.
295. Miller WR, Bartlett J, Brodie AM, Brueggemeier RW, di Salle E, Lonning PE, et al. Aromatase inhibitors: are there differences

between steroidal and nonsteroidal aromatase inhibitors and do they matter? Oncologist. 2008;13(8):829–37.
296. Reinert T, Barrios CH. Optimal management of hormone receptor positive metastatic breast cancer in 2016. Ther Adv Med Oncol. 2015;7(6):304–20.
297. Cuzick J, Sestak I, Baum M, Buzdar A, Howell A, Dowsett M, et al. Effect of anastrozole and tamoxifen as adjuvant treatment for early-stage breast cancer: 10-year analysis of the ATAC trial. Lancet Oncol. 2010;11(12):1135–41.
298. Breast International Group 1-98 Collaborative G, Thurlimann B, Keshaviah A, Coates AS, Mouridsen H, Mauriac L, et al. A comparison of letrozole and tamoxifen in postmenopausal women with early breast cancer. N Engl J Med 2005;353 (26):2747–57.
299. Regan MM, Neven P, Giobbie-Hurder A, Goldhirsch A, Ejlertsen B, Mauriac L, et al. Assessment of letrozole and tamoxifen alone and in sequence for postmenopausal women with steroid hormone receptor-positive breast cancer: the BIG 1-98 randomised clinical trial at 8.1 years median follow-up. Lancet Oncology. 2011;12(12):1101–8.
300. Bliss JM, Kilburn LS, Coleman RE, Forbes JF, Coates AS, Jones SE, et al. Disease-related outcomes with long-term follow-up: an updated analysis of the intergroup exemestane study. J Clin Oncol (Official Journal of the American Society of Clinical Oncology). 2012;30(7):709–17.
301. Jakesz R, Jonat W, Gnant M, Mittlboeck M, Greil R, Tausch C, et al. Switching of postmenopausal women with endocrine-responsive early breast cancer to anastrozole after 2 years' adjuvant tamoxifen: combined results of ABCSG trial 8 and ARNO 95 trial. Lancet. 2005;366(9484):455–62.
302. Kaufmann M, Jonat W, Hilfrich J, Eidtmann H, Gademann G, Zuna I, et al. Improved overall survival in postmenopausal women with early breast cancer after anastrozole initiated after treatment with tamoxifen compared with continued tamoxifen: the ARNO 95 Study. J Clin Oncol (Official Journal of the American Society of Clinical Oncology). 2007;25(19):2664–70.
303. EBCTCG. Aromatase inhibitors versus tamoxifen in early breast cancer: patient-level meta-analysis of the randomised trials. Lancet. 2015;386(10001):1341–52.
304. Burstein HJ, Temin S, Anderson H, Buchholz TA, Davidson NE, Gelmon KE, et al. Adjuvant endocrine therapy for women with hormone receptor-positive breast cancer: american society of clinical oncology clinical practice guideline focused update. J Clin Oncol (Official Journal of the American Society of Clinical Oncology). 2014;32(21):2255–69.
305. National Comprehensive Cancer Network N. breast cancer 2016. Available from http://www.nccn.org/professionals/physician_gls/f_guidelines.asp.
306. Arbeitsgemeinschaft Gynaekologische Onkologie OM. Guidelines Breast Version 2016.1 2016. Available from http://www.ago-online.de/de/infothek-fuer-aerzte/leitlinienempfehlungen/mamma/.
307. Chumsri S. Clinical utilities of aromatase inhibitors in breast cancer. Int J Womens Health. 2015;7:493–9.
308. Goss PE, Ingle JN, Martino S, Robert NJ, Muss HB, Livingston RB, et al. Impact of premenopausal status at breast cancer diagnosis in women entered on the placebo-controlled NCIC CTG MA17 trial of extended adjuvant letrozole. Ann Oncol (Official Journal of the European Society for Medical Oncology/ESMO). 2013;24(2):355–61.
309. Jin H, Tu D, Zhao N, Shepherd LE, Goss PE. Longer-term outcomes of letrozole versus placebo after 5 years of tamoxifen in the NCIC CTG MA.17 trial: analyses adjusting for treatment crossover. J Clin Oncol (Official Journal of the American Society of Clinical Oncology). 2012;30(7):718–21.
310. Mamounas EP, Jeong JH, Wickerham DL, Smith RE, Ganz PA, Land SR, et al. Benefit from exemestane as extended adjuvant therapy after 5 years of adjuvant tamoxifen: intention-to-treat analysis of the National Surgical Adjuvant Breast And Bowel Project B-33 trial. J Clin Oncol (Official Journal of the American Society of Clinical Oncology). 2008;26(12):1965–71.
311. Jakesz R, Greil R, Gnant M, Schmid M, Kwasny W, Kubista E, et al. Extended adjuvant therapy with anastrozole among postmenopausal breast cancer patients: results from the randomized Austrian Breast and Colorectal Cancer Study Group Trial 6a. J Natl Cancer Inst. 2007;99(24):1845–53.
312. Goss PE, Ingle JN, Martino S, Robert NJ, Muss HB, Piccart MJ, et al. Randomized trial of letrozole following tamoxifen as extended adjuvant therapy in receptor-positive breast cancer: updated findings from NCIC CTG MA.17. J Natl Cancer Inst. 2005;97(17):1262–71.
313. Niravath P. Aromatase inhibitor-induced arthralgia: a review. Ann Oncol (Official Journal of the European Society for Medical Oncology/ ESMO). 2013;24(6):1443–9.
314. Wakeling AE, Dukes M, Bowler J. A potent specific pure antiestrogen with clinical potential. Cancer Res. 1991;51 (15):3867–73.
315. Kuter I, Gee JM, Hegg R, Singer CF, Badwe RA, Lowe ES, et al. Dose-dependent change in biomarkers during neoadjuvant endocrine therapy with fulvestrant: results from NEWEST, a randomized Phase II study. Breast Cancer Res Treat. 2012;133 (1):237–46.
316. Ellis MJ, Llombart-Cussac A, Feltl D, Dewar JA, Jasiowka M, Hewson N, et al. Fulvestrant 500 mg versus anastrozole 1 mg for the first-line treatment of advanced breast cancer: overall survival analysis from the phase II FIRST study. J Clin Oncol (Official Journal of the American Society of Clinical Oncology). 2015;33 (32):3781–7.
317. Robertson JF, Lindemann JP, Llombart-Cussac A, Rolski J, Feltl D, Dewar J, et al. Fulvestrant 500 mg versus anastrozole 1 mg for the first-line treatment of advanced breast cancer: follow-up analysis from the randomized 'FIRST' study. Breast Cancer Res Treat. 2012;136(2):503–11.
318. Di Leo A, Jerusalem G, Petruzelka L, Torres R, Bondarenko IN, Khasanov R, et al. Final overall survival: fulvestrant 500 mg vs 250 mg in the randomized CONFIRM trial. J Natl Cancer Inst. 2014;106(1):djt337.
319. Di Leo A, Jerusalem G, Petruzelka L, Torres R, Bondarenko IN, Khasanov R, et al. Results of the CONFIRM phase III trial comparing fulvestrant 250 mg with fulvestrant 500 mg in postmenopausal women with estrogen receptor-positive advanced breast cancer. J Clin Oncol (Official Journal of the American Society of Clinical Oncology). 2010;28(30):4594–600.
320. Mehta RS, Barlow WE, Albain KS, Vandenberg TA, Dakhil SR, Tirumali NR, et al. Combination anastrozole and fulvestrant in metastatic breast cancer. N Engl J Med. 2012;367(5): 435–44.
321. Bergh J, Jonsson PE, Lidbrink EK, Trudeau M, Eiermann W, Brattstrom D, et al. FACT: an open-label randomized phase III study of fulvestrant and anastrozole in combination compared with anastrozole alone as first-line therapy for patients with receptor-positive postmenopausal breast cancer. J Clin Oncol (Official Journal of the American Society of Clinical Oncology). 2012;30(16):1919–25.
322. Migliaccio I, Malorni L, Hart CD, Guarducci C, Di Leo A. Endocrine therapy considerations in postmenopausal patients with hormone receptor positive, human epidermal growth factor receptor type 2 negative advanced breast cancers. BMC Med. 2015;13:46.

323. Rody A, Loibl S, von Minckwitz G, Kaufmann M. Use of goserelin in the treatment of breast cancer. Expert Rev Anticancer Ther. 2005;5(4):591–604.
324. Beatson. On the treatment of inoperable cases of carcinoma of the mamma: suggestions for a new method of treatment, with illustrative cases. Lancet. 1896;148(3802).
325. Boccardo F, Rubagotti A, Perrotta A, Amoroso D, Balestrero M, De Matteis A, et al. Ovarian ablation versus goserelin with or without tamoxifen in pre-perimenopausal patients with advanced breast cancer: results of a multicentric Italian study. Ann Oncol (Official Journal of the European Society for Medical Oncology/ESMO). 1994;5(4):337–42.
326. Buchanan RB, Blamey RW, Durrant KR, Howell A, Paterson AG, Preece PE, et al. A randomized comparison of tamoxifen with surgical oophorectomy in premenopausal patients with advanced breast cancer. J Clin Oncol (Official Journal of the American Society of Clinical Oncology). 1986;4(9):1326–30.
327. Klijn JG, Blamey RW, Boccardo F, Tominaga T, Duchateau L, Sylvester R, et al. Combined tamoxifen and luteinizing hormone-releasing hormone (LHRH) agonist versus LHRH agonist alone in premenopausal advanced breast cancer: a meta-analysis of four randomized trials. J Clin Oncol (Official Journal of the American Society of Clinical Oncology). 2001;19 (2):343–53.
328. Klijn JG, Beex LV, Mauriac L, van Zijl JA, Veyret C, Wildiers J, et al. Combined treatment with buserelin and tamoxifen in premenopausal metastatic breast cancer: a randomized study. J Natl Cancer Inst. 2000;92(11):903–11.
329. Davidson NE, O'Neill AM, Vukov AM, Osborne CK, Martino S, White DR, et al. Chemoendocrine therapy for premenopausal women with axillary lymph node-positive, steroid hormone receptor-positive breast cancer: results from INT 0101 (E5188). J Clin Oncol (Official Journal of the American Society of Clinical Oncology). 2005;23(25):5973–82.
330. Cuzick J, Ambroisine L, Davidson N, Jakesz R, Kaufmann M, Regan M, et al. Use of luteinising-hormone-releasing hormone agonists as adjuvant treatment in premenopausal patients with hormone-receptor-positive breast cancer: a meta-analysis of individual patient data from randomised adjuvant trials. Lancet. 2007;369(9574):1711–23.
331. Francis PA, Regan MM, Fleming GF, Lang I, Ciruelos E, Bellet M, et al. Adjuvant ovarian suppression in premenopausal breast cancer. N Engl J Med. 2014.
332. Hershman DL. Perfecting breast-cancer treatment–incremental gains and musculoskeletal pains. N Engl J Med. 2015;372 (5):477–8.
333. Miller TW, Balko JM, Arteaga CL. Phosphatidylinositol 3-kinase and antiestrogen resistance in breast cancer. J Clin Oncol (Official Journal of the American Society of Clinical Oncology). 2011;29 (33):4452–61.
334. Lauring J, Park BH, Wolff AC. The phosphoinositide-3-kinase-Akt-mTOR pathway as a therapeutic target in breast cancer. J Natl Compr Canc Netw. 2013;11 (6):670–8.
335. Baselga J, Campone M, Piccart M, Burris HA 3rd, Rugo HS, Sahmoud T, et al. Everolimus in postmenopausal hormone-receptor-positive advanced breast cancer. N Engl J Med. 2012;366(6):520–9.
336. Piccart M, Hortobagyi GN, Campone M, Pritchard KI, Lebrun F, Ito Y, et al. Everolimus plus exemestane for hormone-receptor-positive, human epidermal growth factor receptor-2-negative advanced breast cancer: overall survival results from BOLERO-2dagger. Ann Oncol (Official Journal of the European Society for Medical Oncology/ESMO). 2014;25 (12):2357–62.
337. Bachelot T, Bourgier C, Cropet C, Ray-Coquard I, Ferrero JM, Freyer G, et al. Randomized phase II trial of everolimus in combination with tamoxifen in patients with hormone receptor-positive, human epidermal growth factor receptor 2-negative metastatic breast cancer with prior exposure to aromatase inhibitors: a GINECO study. J Clin Oncol (Official Journal of the American Society of Clinical Oncology). 2012;30 (22):2718–24.
338. Hortobagyi GN, Chen D, Piccart M, Rugo HS, Burris HA, Pritchard KI, et al. Correlative analysis of genetic alterations and everolimus benefit in hormone receptor-positive, human epidermal growth factor receptor 2-negative advanced breast cancer: results from BOLERO-2. J Clin Oncol. 2015.
339. Sabine VS, Crozier C, Brookes CL, Drake C, Piper T, van de Velde CJ, et al. Mutational analysis of PI3K/AKT signaling pathway in tamoxifen exemestane adjuvant multinational pathology study. J Clin Oncol (Official Journal of the American Society of Clinical Oncology). 2014;32(27):2951–8.
340. Mayer IA, Arteaga CL. PIK3CA activating mutations: a discordant role in early versus advanced hormone-dependent estrogen receptor-positive breast cancer? J Clin Oncol (Official Journal of the American Society of Clinical Oncology). 2014;32(27):2932–4.
341. Crowder RJ, Phommaly C, Tao Y, Hoog J, Luo J, Perou CM, et al. PIK3CA and PIK3CB inhibition produce synthetic lethality when combined with estrogen deprivation in estrogen receptor-positive breast cancer. Cancer Res. 2009;69(9):3955–62.
342. Engelman JA. Targeting PI3K signalling in cancer: opportunities, challenges and limitations. Nat Rev Cancer. 2009;9(8):550–62.
343. Krop I, Johnston S, Mayer IA, Dickler M, Ganju V, Forero-Torres A, et al. Abstract S2-02: The FERGI phase II study of the PI3K inhibitor pictilisib (GDC-0941) plus fulvestrant vs fulvestrant plus placebo in patients with ER+, aromatase inhibitor (AI)-resistant advanced or metastatic breast cancer—Part I results. Cancer Res. 2015;75(9 Suppl):S2-02.
344. Baselga J, Im S-A, Iwata H, Clemons M, Ito Y, Awada A, et al. Abstract S6-01: PIK3CA status in circulating tumor DNA (ctDNA) predicts efficacy of buparlisib (BUP) plus fulvestrant (FULV) in postmenopausal women with endocrine-resistant HR +/HER2− advanced breast cancer (BC): first results from the randomized, Phase III BELLE-2 trial. Cancer Res. 2016(Supplement):S6-01.
345. Cadoo KA, Gucalp A, Traina TA. Palbociclib: an evidence-based review of its potential in the treatment of breast cancer. Breast Cancer (Dove Med Press). 2014;6:123–33.
346. Ma CX, Ellis MJ. The Cancer Genome Atlas: clinical applications for breast cancer. Oncology. 2013;27(12):1263–9, 74–9.
347. Thangavel C, Dean JL, Ertel A, Knudsen KE, Aldaz CM, Witkiewicz AK, et al. Therapeutically activating RB: reestablishing cell cycle control in endocrine therapy-resistant breast cancer. Endocr Relat Cancer. 2011;18(3):333–45.
348. Finn RS, Dering J, Conklin D, Kalous O, Cohen DJ, Desai AJ, et al. PD 0332991, a selective cyclin D kinase 4/6 inhibitor, preferentially inhibits proliferation of luminal estrogen receptor-positive human breast cancer cell lines in vitro. Breast Cancer Res (BCR). 2009;11(5):R77.
349. Finn RS, Crown JP, Lang I, Boer K, Bondarenko IM, Kulyk SO, et al. The cyclin-dependent kinase 4/6 inhibitor palbociclib in combination with letrozole versus letrozole alone as first-line treatment of oestrogen receptor-positive, HER2-negative, advanced breast cancer (PALOMA-1/TRIO-18): a randomised phase 2 study. Lancet Oncol. 2015;16(1):25–35.
350. Turner NC, Ro J, Andre F, Loi S, Verma S, Iwata H, et al. Palbociclib in Hormone-receptor-positive advanced breast cancer. N Engl J Med. 2015.

351. Farmer H, McCabe N, Lord CJ, Tutt AN, Johnson DA, Richardson TB, et al. Targeting the DNA repair defect in BRCA mutant cells as a therapeutic strategy. Nature. 2005;434 (7035):917–21.
352. Tutt A, Robson M, Garber JE, Domchek SM, Audeh MW, Weitzel JN, et al. Oral poly(ADP-ribose) polymerase inhibitor olaparib in patients with BRCA1 or BRCA2 mutations and advanced breast cancer: a proof-of-concept trial. Lancet. 2010;376(9737):235–44.
353. Audeh MW, Carmichael J, Penson RT, Friedlander M, Powell B, Bell-McGuinn KM, et al. Oral poly(ADP-ribose) polymerase inhibitor olaparib in patients with BRCA1 or BRCA2 mutations and recurrent ovarian cancer: a proof-of-concept trial. Lancet. 2010;376(9737):245–51.
354. Gelmon KA, Tischkowitz M, Mackay H, Swenerton K, Robidoux A, Tonkin K, et al. Olaparib in patients with recurrent high-grade serous or poorly differentiated ovarian carcinoma or triple-negative breast cancer: a phase 2, multicentre, open-label, non-randomised study. Lancet Oncol. 2011;12(9):852–61.
355. Rugo H, Olopade O, DeMichele A, van 't Veer L, Buxton M, Hylton N, et al. Abstract S5-02: Veliparib/carboplatin plus standard neoadjuvant therapy for high-risk breast cancer: First efficacy results from the I-SPY 2 TRIAL. Cancer Res. 2013;73 (24 Suppl):S5-02.
356. Gampenrieder SP, Rinnerthaler G, Greil R. Bone-targeted therapy in metastatic breast cancer—all well-established knowledge? Breast Care. 2014;9(5):323–30.
357. Van Acker HH, Anguille S, Willemen Y, Smits EL, Van Tendeloo VF. Bisphosphonates for cancer treatment: mechanisms of action and lessons from clinical trials. Pharmacol Ther. 2016;158:24–40.
358. Coleman RE. Metastatic bone disease: clinical features, pathophysiology and treatment strategies. Cancer Treat Rev. 2001;27 (3):165–76.
359. Kohno N, Aogi K, Minami H, Nakamura S, Asaga T, Iino Y, et al. Zoledronic acid significantly reduces skeletal complications compared with placebo in Japanese women with bone metastases from breast cancer: a randomized, placebo-controlled trial. J Clin Oncol (Official Journal of the American Society of Clinical Oncology). 2005;23(15):3314–21.
360. Rosen LS, Gordon DH, Dugan W Jr, Major P, Eisenberg PD, Provencher L, et al. Zoledronic acid is superior to pamidronate for the treatment of bone metastases in breast carcinoma patients with at least one osteolytic lesion. Cancer. 2004;100(1):36–43.
361. Rosen LS, Gordon D, Tchekmedyian NS, Yanagihara R, Hirsh V, Krzakowski M, et al. Long-term efficacy and safety of zoledronic acid in the treatment of skeletal metastases in patients with nonsmall cell lung carcinoma and other solid tumors: a randomized, Phase III, double-blind, placebo-controlled trial. Cancer. 2004;100(12):2613–21.
362. Wong MH, Stockler MR, Pavlakis N. Bisphosphonates and other bone agents for breast cancer. Cochrane database of systematic reviews. 2012;2:CD003474.
363. Tripathy D, Lichinitzer M, Lazarev A, MacLachlan SA, Apffelstaedt J, Budde M, et al. Oral ibandronate for the treatment of metastatic bone disease in breast cancer: efficacy and safety results from a randomized, double-blind, placebo-controlled trial. Ann Oncol (Official Journal of the European Society for Medical Oncology/ESMO). 2004;15(5):743–50.
364. Body JJ, Diel IJ, Lichinitzer M, Lazarev A, Pecherstorfer M, Bell R, et al. Oral ibandronate reduces the risk of skeletal complications in breast cancer patients with metastatic bone disease: results from two randomised, placebo-controlled phase III studies. Br J Cancer. 2004;90(6):1133–7.
365. Lipton A, Theriault RL, Hortobagyi GN, Simeone J, Knight RD, Mellars K, et al. Pamidronate prevents skeletal complications and is effective palliative treatment in women with breast carcinoma and osteolytic bone metastases: long term follow-up of two randomized, placebo-controlled trials. Cancer. 2000;88(5):1082–90.
366. Theriault RL, Lipton A, Hortobagyi GN, Leff R, Gluck S, Stewart JF, et al. Pamidronate reduces skeletal morbidity in women with advanced breast cancer and lytic bone lesions: a randomized, placebo-controlled trial. Protocol 18 Aredia Breast Cancer Study Group. J Clin Oncol (Official Journal of the American Society of Clinical Oncology). 1999;17(3):846–54.
367. Rosen LS, Gordon D, Tchekmedyian S, Yanagihara R, Hirsh V, Krzakowski M, et al. Zoledronic acid versus placebo in the treatment of skeletal metastases in patients with lung cancer and other solid tumors: a phase III, double-blind, randomized trial–the Zoledronic Acid Lung Cancer and Other Solid Tumors Study Group. J Clin Oncol (Official Journal of the American Society of Clinical Oncology). 2003;21(16):3150–7.
368. Rosen LS, Gordon D, Kaminski M, Howell A, Belch A, Mackey J, et al. Long-term efficacy and safety of zoledronic acid compared with pamidronate disodium in the treatment of skeletal complications in patients with advanced multiple myeloma or breast carcinoma: a randomized, double-blind, multicenter, comparative trial. Cancer. 2003;98(8):1735–44.
369. Barrett-Lee P, Casbard A, Abraham J, Hood K, Coleman R, Simmonds P, et al. Oral ibandronic acid versus intravenous zoledronic acid in treatment of bone metastases from breast cancer: a randomised, open label, non-inferiority phase 3 trial. Lancet Oncology. 2014;15(1):114–22.
370. Major P, Lortholary A, Hon J, Abdi E, Mills G, Menssen HD, et al. Zoledronic acid is superior to pamidronate in the treatment of hypercalcemia of malignancy: a pooled analysis of two randomized, controlled clinical trials. J Clin Oncol (Official Journal of the American Society of Clinical Oncology). 2001;19 (2):558–67.
371. Ibrahim MF, Mazzarello S, Shorr R, Vandermeer L, Jacobs C, Hilton J, et al. Should de-escalation of bone-targeting agents be standard of care for patients with bone metastases from breast cancer? A systematic review and meta-analysis. Ann Oncol (Official Journal of the European Society for Medical Oncology/ESMO). 2015;26(11):2205–13.
372. Mortimer JE, Pal SK. Safety considerations for use of bone-targeted agents in patients with cancer. Semin Oncol. 2010;37(Suppl 1):S66–72.
373. XXX
374. Saad F, Brown JE, Van Poznak C, Ibrahim T, Stemmer SM, Stopeck AT, et al. Incidence, risk factors, and outcomes of osteonecrosis of the jaw: integrated analysis from three blinded active-controlled phase III trials in cancer patients with bone metastases. Ann Oncol (Official Journal of the European Society for Medical Oncology/ESMO). 2012;23(5):1341–7.
375. Stopeck AT, Lipton A, Body JJ, Steger GG, Tonkin K, de Boer RH, et al. Denosumab compared with zoledronic acid for the treatment of bone metastases in patients with advanced breast cancer: a randomized, double-blind study. J Clin Oncol (Official Journal of the American Society of Clinical Oncology). 2010;28 (35):5132–9.
376. Henry DH, Costa L, Goldwasser F, Hirsh V, Hungria V, Prausova J, et al. Randomized, double-blind study of denosumab versus zoledronic acid in the treatment of bone metastases in patients with advanced cancer (excluding breast and prostate cancer) or multiple myeloma. J Clin Oncol (Official Journal of the American Society of Clinical Oncology). 2011;29(9):1125–32.

377. Fizazi K, Carducci M, Smith M, Damiao R, Brown J, Karsh L, et al. Denosumab versus zoledronic acid for treatment of bone metastases in men with castration-resistant prostate cancer: a randomised, double-blind study. Lancet. 2011;377(9768):813–22.
378. Henry D, Vadhan-Raj S, Hirsh V, von Moos R, Hungria V, Costa L, et al. Delaying skeletal-related events in a randomized phase 3 study of denosumab versus zoledronic acid in patients with advanced cancer: an analysis of data from patients with solid tumors. Support Care Cancer (Official Journal of the Multinational Association of Supportive Care in Cancer). 2014;22 (3):679–87.
379. von Moos R, Body JJ, Egerdie B, Stopeck A, Brown JE, Damyanov D, et al. Pain and health-related quality of life in patients with advanced solid tumours and bone metastases: integrated results from three randomized, double-blind studies of denosumab and zoledronic acid. Support Care Cancer Official Journal of the Multinational Association of Supportive Care in Cancer). 2013;21(12):3497–507.
380. Ellis GK, Bone HG, Chlebowski R, Paul D, Spadafora S, Smith J, et al. Randomized trial of denosumab in patients receiving adjuvant aromatase inhibitors for nonmetastatic breast cancer. J Clin Oncol (Official Journal of the American Society of Clinical Oncology). 2008;26(30):4875–82.
381. Cummings SR, San Martin J, McClung MR, Siris ES, Eastell R, Reid IR, et al. Denosumab for prevention of fractures in postmenopausal women with osteoporosis. N Engl J Med. 2009;361(8):756–65.
382. Hall DG, Stoica G. Effect of the bisphosphonate risedronate on bone metastases in a rat mammary adenocarcinoma model system. J Bone Miner Res. 1994;9(2):221–30.
383. Gnant M, Mlineritsch B, Stoeger H, Luschin-Ebengreuth G, Knauer M, Moik M, et al. Zoledronic acid combined with adjuvant endocrine therapy of tamoxifen versus anastrozol plus ovarian function suppression in premenopausal early breast cancer: final analysis of the Austrian Breast and Colorectal Cancer Study Group Trial 12. Ann Oncol (Official Journal of the European Society for Medical Oncology/ESMO). 2014.
384. Gnant M, Eidtmann H. The anti-tumor effect of bisphosphonates ABCSG-12, ZO-FAST and more. Crit Rev Oncol/Hematol. 2010;74(Suppl 1):S2-6.
385. Paterson AH, Anderson SJ, Lembersky BC, Fehrenbacher L, Falkson CI, King KM, et al. Oral clodronate for adjuvant treatment of operable breast cancer (National Surgical Adjuvant Breast and Bowel Project protocol B-34): a multicentre, placebo-controlled, randomised trial. Lancet Oncol. 2012.
386. von Minckwitz G, Mobus V, Schneeweiss A, Huober J, Thomssen C, Untch M, et al. German adjuvant intergroup node-positive study: a phase III trial to compare oral ibandronate versus observation in patients with high-risk early breast cancer. J Clin Oncol (Official Journal of the American Society of Clinical Oncology). 2013.
387. Coleman R, Cameron D, Dodwell D, Bell R, Wilson C, Rathbone E, et al. Adjuvant zoledronic acid in patients with early breast cancer: final efficacy analysis of the AZURE (BIG 01/04) randomised open-label phase 3 trial. Lancet Oncol. 2014;15(9):997–1006.
388. Knauer M, Thurlimann B. Adjuvant bisphosphonates in breast cancer treatment. Breast Care. 2014;9(5):319–22.
389. Coleman R. Adjuvant bisphosphonate treatment in early breast cancer: meta-analyses of individual patient data from randomised trials. Lancet. 2015;386(10001):1353–61.
390. Ottewell PD, Wang N, Brown HK, Reeves KJ, Fowles CA, Croucher PI, et al. Zoledronic acid has differential antitumor activity in the pre- and postmenopausal bone microenvironment in vivo. Clin Cancer Res (An Official Journal of the American Association for Cancer Research). 2014;20(11):2922–32.
391. Gnant M, Pfeiler G, Dubsky PC, Hubalek M, Greil R, Jakesz R, et al. Adjuvant denosumab in breast cancer (ABCSG-18): a multicentre, randomised, double-blind, placebo-controlled trial. Lancet. 2015;386(9992):433–43.
392. Gnant M, Pfeiler G, Dubsky P, Hubalek M, Greil R, Jakesz R, et al. Abstract S2-02: the impact of adjuvant denosumab on disease-free survival: Results from 3,425 postmenopausal patients of the ABCSG-18 trial. Cancer Res. 2016;76(4 Suppl):S2-02.
393. Marmé F, Schneeweiss A. Targeted therapies in triple-negative breast cancer. Breast Care (Basel). 2015;10(3):159–66. doi:10.1159/000433622.

HER2-Targeted Therapy

21

Phuong Dinh and Martine J. Piccart

21.1 Introduction

In 1987, the initial description of the HER2 proto-oncogene was described as a poor prognostic factor in breast cancer. In 2001, the first randomized trial of a monoclonal antibody directed against HER2 in combination with chemotherapy for the treatment of metastatic HER2-positive (HER2+) breast cancer was published. In 2005, the dramatic benefit of trastuzumab in the adjuvant setting was presented in multiple presentations at the American Society of Clinical Oncology (ASCO)—which significantly impacted clinical practice worldwide. The HER2+ landscape, since, has not stopped to evolve with research continuing in neoadjuvant strategies and the development of new molecules for dual inhibition of HER family of receptors.

The HER2+ subtype of breast cancer represents less than 25 % of incident breast cancers, and traditionally has been regarded as having the more aggressive phenotype, higher recurrence rates and reduced survival [1, 2]. The remarkable progress in anti-HER2 therapeutics, over the last decades, has undoubtedly improved long-term outcomes for HER2+ patients. Nonetheless, a proportion of these patients still do poorly, and treatment resistance remains a problem. Deciphering the resistance mechanisms will facilitate better tailoring of therapy to individual patient tumors and further improve patient outcomes.

This chapter will discuss the evolution of HER2-targeted therapy, beginning with the initial success of trastuzumab to the controversies that remain, and from there, to the discussion of newer anti-HER2 approaches currently under investigation.

P. Dinh
Westmead Hospital, Hawkesbury Road, Westmead, NSW 2145, Australia

M.J. Piccart (✉)
Medicine Department, Institut Jules Bordet, 1, rue Heger-Bordet, 1000 Bruxelles, Belgium
e-mail: martine.piccart@bordet.be

21.2 Targeting the HER2 Receptor

HER2 belongs to the human epidermal growth factor receptor family of tyrosine kinases consisting of EGFR (HER1; erbB1), HER2 (erbB2, HER2/*neu*), HER3 (erbB3), and HER4 (erbB4). All these receptors have an extracellular ligand-binding region, a single membrane-spanning region, and a cytoplasmic tyrosine-kinase-containing domain, the last being absent in HER3. Ligand binding to the extracellular region results in homo- and heterodimer activation of the cytoplasmic kinase domain and phosphorylation of a specific tyrosine [3], leading to the activation of various intracellular signaling pathways involved in cell proliferation and survival.

HER2 was first identified as an oncogene activated by a point mutation in chemically induced rat neuroblastomas [4], and soon after, found to be amplified in breast cancer cell lines [5]. In the clinic, patients with HER2 gene amplified tumors were shown to represent less than 25 % of the human breast population, having poorer disease-free survival [1, 6–8], and also displaying resistance to certain chemotherapeutic agents [9–11].

With the accumulating body of evidence supporting the HER2 oncogene hypothesis, the HER2 receptor represented an ideal target for anticancer therapy. By targeting HER2 receptors, either intracellularly or extracellularly, downstream pathways could be indirectly inhibited to induce cell cycle arrest, apoptosis, as well as inhibition of tumor cell invasion and metastases [12].

Up until recently, trastuzumab and lapatinib had been the mainstays of anti-HER2 treatment in combination with chemotherapy. Trastuzumab (Herceptin; Genentech, South San Francisco) is a recombinant, humanized anti-HER2 monoclonal antibody that exerts its action through several mechanisms including (1) induction of receptor downregulation/degradation, (2) prevention of HER2 ectodomain cleavage, (3) inhibition of HER2 kinase signal transduction via ADCC, and (4) inhibition of angiogenesis. Lapatinib is a small molecule tyrosine kinase inhibitor which

I. Jatoi and A. Rody (eds.), *Management of Breast Diseases*, DOI 10.1007/978-3-319-46356-8_21

is capable of dual receptor inhibition of both EGFR and HER2. It is an ATP mimetic that competitively binds to the ATP-binding cleft at the activation loop of target kinases, thereby inhibiting both kinase activities.

More recently, two additional HER2-directed therapies have been approved for HER2+ breast cancer. Pertuzumab is a recombinant, humanized, monoclonal antibody directed against the extracellular dimerization domain (subdomain II) of HER2, preventing dimerization of HER2 with other members of the HER family, such as HER3, HER1, and HER4. This results in inhibited downstream signaling of two key pathways that regulate cell survival and growth (the mitogen-activated protein kinase [MAPK] pathway, and the phosphoinositide 3-kinase [PI3 K] pathway), in addition to mediating antibody-dependent cell-mediated cytotoxicity [13]. Ado-trastuzumab emtansine (T-DM1) is a human epidermal growth factor receptor 2 (HER2)-targeted antibody-drug conjugate composed of trastuzumab, a stable linker (MCC), and the cytotoxic agent DM1 (derivative of maytansine; mertansine). T-DM1 retains the mechanisms of action of trastuzumab, but also acts as a, selectively delivered, tubulin inhibitor. Following antigen-mediated binding to the tumor cell, T-DM1 is endocytosed and intracellularly catabolized resulting in the release of its cytotoxic moiety [14].

21.2.1 ASCO/CAP Updated Recommendations for HER2 Testing

A HER2 positive status is not only an adverse prognostic marker in breast cancer but also a positive predictive marker of response to anti-HER2 therapies. Tailored treatment requires proper identification of these patients who are most likely to derive benefit, and least likely to experience unnecessary toxicity. Recently, the American Society of Clinical Oncology and the College of American Pathologists have updated their 2007 clinical practice guidelines for HER2 testing in breast cancer with the 2013 version [15]. The update not only provides guidelines for the test performance parameters, with the aim of improving test accuracy, reproducibility, and precision, but also provides comprehensive recommendations on the post-analytical interpretation of the results, and requires improved communication among healthcare providers. Notably, for in situ hybridization interpretation, the 2013 guidelines returned to the prior threshold of a HER2/CEP17 ratio of 2.0 or greater for positive and eliminated 1.8–2.2 as the equivocal range. Also, the HER2 signal/nucleus ratio was accounted for, with 6.0 or greater for positive and 4.0 to less than 6.0 for equivocal, even in cases with a HER2/CEP17 ratio less than 2.0.

HER2 status is thus reported as an algorithm of positive, equivocal, negative, or indeterminate. The HER2 test is reported as positive if: (a) IHC 3+ positive or (b) ISH positive using either a single probe ISH or dual-probe ISH. The HER2 test is reported equivocal if: (a) IHC 2+ equivocal or (b) ISH equivocal using single probe ISH or dual probe ISH. For equivocal cases, a reflex test should be ordered on the same specimen using the alternative test. The HER2 test is reported as negative if a single test (or all tests) performed in a tumor specimen show: (a) IHC 1+ negative or IHC 0 negative or (b) ISH negative using single probe ISH or dual probe ISH. The HER2 test is reported as indeterminate if technical issues prevent one or both tests (IHC and ISH) performed in a tumor specimen from being reported as positive, negative, or equivocal. This may occur if specimen handling was inadequate, if artifacts (crush or edge artifacts) make interpretation difficult, or if the analytic testing failed.

21.3 Trastuzumab in the Metastatic Setting

Since the first reports of trastuzumab's activity in HER2+ MBC, many studies have been conducted to investigate the optimum schedule in this patient group, both as single-agent therapy and in combination.

21.3.1 Single-Agent Therapy in Heavily Pretreated Patients

In an early trial evaluating weekly trastuzumab efficacy in 222 women with HER2+ MBC that had progressed after one or two chemotherapy regimens [16], the response rate (RR) was 15 % in the intent-to-treat population and was significantly higher in strong HER2+ overexpressers (18 % vs. 6 % for those with 3+ and 2+ IHC, respectively). The median response duration was 9.1 months. Cardiac dysfunction was the most common adverse event, occurring in 5 % of treated patients, many of whom had received prior doxorubicin. The alternative 3-weekly schedule of trastuzumab was investigated in a phase II study [17] of 105 patients where comparable results were achieved (overall RR of 19 % and clinical benefit rate of 33 %). Median time to progression (TTP) was 3.4 months (range 0.6–23.6 months).

21.3.2 First-Line Single-Agent Therapy

The benefit of first-line trastuzumab monotherapy was studied in 114 women with HER2+ MBC [18] randomized to receive first-line treatment with trastuzumab 4 mg/kg loading dose, followed by 2 mg/kg weekly, or a higher 8 mg/kg loading dose, followed by 4 mg/kg weekly. RRs in 111 assessable patients with 3+ and 2+ HER2 overexpression by IHC were 35 % (95 % CI 24.4–44.7 %) and none

(95 % CI, 0–15.5 %), respectively. The RRs in 108 assessable patients with and without HER2 gene amplification by FISH analysis were 34 % (95 % CI 23.9–45.7 %) and 7 % (95 % CI 0.8–22.8 %), respectively. Interestingly, overall RR was nearly double that reported for previously treated patients [19]. There was no clear evidence of a dose–response relationship for response, survival, or adverse events.

21.3.3 Trastuzumab in Combination with Chemotherapy

21.3.3.1 Trastuzumab and Taxanes

Preclinical studies have shown additive or synergistic interactions between trastuzumab and multiple cytotoxic agents, including platinum analogs, taxanes, anthracyclines, vinorelbine, gemcitabine, capecitabine, and cyclophosphamide [19]. The pivotal randomized combination trials of trastuzumab [20] demonstrated that trastuzumab plus a taxane is associated with a clinical benefit that is superior to that of a taxane alone.

The first trial enrolled 469 HER2+ MBC patients who had not received prior treatment for advanced disease. For those patients who had previously received anthracyclines in the adjuvant setting or who were not suitable to receive anthracyclines ($n = 188$), randomization took place between paclitaxel with or without trastuzumab. All other patients ($n = 281$) were randomized to receive an anthracycline plus cyclophosphamide with or without trastuzumab. The addition of trastuzumab to chemotherapy was associated with a longer TTP (median 7.4 vs. 4.6 months; $P < 0.001$), a higher rate of objective RR (50 % vs. 32 %, $P < 0.001$), a longer duration of response (median 9.1 vs. 6.1 months; $P < 0.001$), a lower rate of death at 1 year (22 % vs. 33 %, $P = 0.008$), and longer survival (median survival 25.1 vs. 20.3 months; $P = 0.01$ and 20 % relative reduction in the risk of death overall) [21]. However, cardiotoxicity was more common with combined treatment, especially with AC plus trastuzumab (27 %), leading to the recommendation that anthracyclines and trastuzumab should not be combined.

In a phase II study of 95 HER2-normal and HER2+ MBC patients evaluating weekly trastuzumab and paclitaxel therapy [21], the overall RR was 56.8 % (95 % CI 47–67 %). In those with HER2+ tumors, the overall RR was higher than those with HER2-normal tumors (range of 67–81 % compared with range of 41–46 %). Treatment was associated with grade 3/4 neutropenia in 6 %, and 3 patients had severe cardiac complications.

In the M77001 trial which investigated the combination of weekly trastuzumab plus weekly or 3-weekly docetaxel in 188 MBC patients, the median overall survival (OS) was 22.7 months with docetaxel alone and 31.2 months with trastuzumab plus docetaxel. Median TTP (10.6 vs. 5.7 months) was superior for trastuzumab plus docetaxel versus docetaxel alone [22].

In a multicenter phase II trial with 101 HER2+ MBC patients randomized between combination therapy trastuzumab plus docetaxel and sequential therapy of single-agent trastuzumab followed at disease progression by docetaxel alone as first-line chemotherapy [23], the median PFS was 9.4 versus 9.9 months and the 1-year PFS rates were 44 % versus 35 %, respectively. The overall response rates (RRs) were 79 % versus 53 %, ($P = 0.016$), and overall survival was 30.5 versus 19.7 months, ($P = 0.11$). In the sequential group, RRs to monotherapy trastuzumab and subsequent docetaxel were 34 and 39 %, respectively, with a median PFS during single-agent trastuzumab of 3.9 months. The incidence and severity of neuropathy were significantly higher in the combination group. Retrospective analysis of trastuzumab treatment beyond progression (applied in 46 % of patients in the combination group and 37 % in the sequential group) showed a correlation with longer overall survival in both treatment arms (36.0 vs. 18.0 months and 30.3 vs. 18.6 months, respectively). Thus, first-line treatment with sequential trastuzumab, then docetaxel resulted in a similar PFS compared with combination trastuzumab and docetaxel, but the RR was lower and the overall survival nonsignificantly shorter.

21.3.3.2 Trastuzumab and Platinum Salts

In addition to a possible synergistic interaction [24], in vitro data suggests that trastuzumab may also reverse primary platinum resistance by modulating HER2 activity [25]. The benefit of adding platinum salts to trastuzumab-based combination therapy was shown in a phase III trial comparing trastuzumab and paclitaxel with and without carboplatin in 194 women with HER2+ MBC [26]. The addition of carboplatin to paclitaxel and trastuzumab significantly improved RR (52 % vs. 36 %) and median PFS (10.7 vs. 7.1 months). Although the triple therapy was associated with higher rates of grade 3/4 hematologic toxicity, there was no difference in the rates of neurologic, cardiopulmonary, or febrile complications.

In contrast, a lack of benefit for adding carboplatin to trastuzumab plus a taxane was shown in the BCIRG 007 trial [27], in which 263 previously untreated patients with HER2 FISH+ MBC were randomly assigned to trastuzumab plus 8 courses of either docetaxel alone (TH) (100 mg/m^2 every 3 weeks) or docetaxel (75 mg/m^2 every 3 weeks) plus carboplatin (TCH) (AUC of 6). There was no significant difference in terms of the primary endpoint, time to progression (medians of 11.1 and 10.4 months, respectively; hazard ratio, 0.914; 95 % CI, 0.694–1.203; $P = 0.57$), RR (72 % for both groups), or overall survival (medians of 37.1 and 37.4 months, respectively; $P = 0.99$). Rates of grades 3 or 4 adverse effects for doublet versus triplet therapy respectively, were neutropenic-related complications, 29 and 23 %; thrombocytopenia, 2 and 15 %; anemia, 5 and 11 %; sensory neuropathy, 3 and 0.8 %; fatigue, 5 and 12 %; peripheral edema, 3.8 and 1.5 %; and diarrhea, 2 and 10 %. Adding carboplatin, therefore, did not enhance docetaxel–trastuzumab antitumor activity.

21.3.3.3 Trastuzumab Plus Vinorelbine

Trastuzumab and vinorelbine constitute effective and well-tolerated first-line treatment for HER2+ MBC. In a multicentre phase II study evaluating this combination in 54 women [28], the RR was 68 % (95 % CI 54–80 %). Two patients experienced cardiotoxicity in excess of grade 1; one patient experienced symptomatic heart failure. This combination was also shown to be effective in patients who had progressed while receiving anthracyclines and taxanes [29–31]. The combination of trastuzumab with vinorelbine was well tolerated in all of these trials. There was no evidence that this combination resulted in more cardiac events compared with trastuzumab alone.

21.3.3.4 Trastuzumab with Capecitabine

Several studies have demonstrated that trastuzumab and the 5-fluorouracil prodrug, capecitabine, have at least additive antitumor activity in human breast cancer models [32], and this has been supported by several clinical studies. In a phase II trial of 27 MBC patients refractory to anthracyclines and taxanes who received capecitabine (1250 mg/m^2 twice daily for 14 of every 21 days) plus weekly trastuzumab, there were 12 objective responses (45 %) with 4 complete responses [33]. Nine additional patients (33 %) had disease stabilization for at least 9 weeks, and the median PFS was 6.7 months. There was a low incidence of grade 3 or 4 adverse events. This high RR was mirrored in a phase II study of first line trastuzumab–capecitabine therapy, in which an objective RR of 76 % (5 CR, 14 PR) was recorded [34]. In both phase II studies, the combination of trastuzumab plus capecitabine was generally well tolerated. There was no evidence of greater cardiotoxicity with this combination.

21.3.3.5 Trastuzumab Plus Gemcitabine

Trastuzumab plus gemcitabine was evaluated in a phase II study [35] with 64 patients where the majority (95 %) had been treated with prior anthracyclines and taxanes. Gemcitabine (1200 mg/m^2 weekly Day 1, 8 in a 21-day cycle) plus weekly doses of trastuzumab was administered until disease progression. The objective RR was 38 % in the intent-to-treat population (23 of 61) and 44 % among the 39 patients with HER2 3+ expression. The median response duration was 5.8 months, median OS was 14.7 months, and median TTP was 5.8 months. Trastuzumab plus gemcitabine was well tolerated with no cases of clinical congestive heart failure.

21.3.3.6 Trastuzumab and Eribulin

Eribulin mesylate [36] is a non-taxane inhibitor of microtubule dynamics in the halichondrin class of antineoplastic drugs. Eribulin has a novel mode of action that is distinct from those of other tubulin-targeting agents; it only binds to the growing positive ends, inhibiting the microtubule growth phase without affecting the shortening phase and causing tubulin sequestration into nonproductive aggregates.

In a multicenter, phase II, single arm study of 52 patients [37] with recurrent or metastatic HER2+ breast cancer, eribulin mesylate at 1.4 mg/m^2 was administered intravenously (I.V.) on days 1 and 8 of each 21-day cycle with an initial trastuzumab dose of 8 mg/kg I.V. on day 1, followed by 6 mg/kg of trastuzumab on day 1 of each subsequent cycle. The overall RR was 71.2 % (n = 37) with median TTR of 1.3 months, DOR of 11.1 months, and PFS of 11.6 months. The most common grade 3/4 treatment-emergent adverse events were neutropenia in 20 (38.5 %) patients, peripheral neuropathy in 14 (26.9 %; all Grade 3) patients, fatigue in 4 (7.7 %) patients, and febrile neutropenia in 4 (7.7 %) patients. Because of the high overall RR, prolonged median PFS, and acceptable safety profile, combination eribulin/trastuzumab is an acceptable treatment option for locally recurrent or metastatic HER2+ breast cancer.

A Phase II study is currently being conducted to look at the combination of eribulin, trastuzumab, and pertuzumab in metastatic, unresectable locally advanced, or locally recurrent HER2+ breast cancer [38].

21.3.3.7 Trastuzumab with Polychemotherapy

Trastuzumab has also been added to combination chemotherapy for MBC. Several studies have shown that triple combinations are effective and produce high RRs [27, 39–44], although overlapping toxicities must be carefully considered.

21.3.4 Trastuzumab in Combination with Hormonal Therapy

In the estrogen receptor (ER) positive patient populations, the rate of HER2 positivity is between 11 and 35 % [45–47]. Resistance to hormonal therapy, particularly tamoxifen, appears to be a characteristic of ER+, HER2+ tumors [48], and it has been hypothesized that the addition of trastuzumab to hormonal therapy may overcome this relative resistance. In preclinical studies, the combination of tamoxifen with anti-HER2 antibodies can produce a greater inhibitory effect on cell growth than either agent alone [49, 50]. There is also some evidence that compared with tamoxifen, aromatase inhibitors may elicit a greater response in HER2+ tumors [51]. Taken together, these findings provide a clear rationale for combining trastuzumab with hormonal agents in patients with HER2+/ER+ MBC.

In a multicenter, open-label, phase II trial assessing the combination of letrozole and trastuzumab in 31 evaluable patients with HER2+/ER+ MBC [52], a RR of 26 %, including 1 CR, was reported. An additional 8 patients had stable disease. Two patients withdrew from the study due to toxicity (1 patient had grade 3 arthralgia and 1 patient developed congestive heart failure).

The international, multicenter, randomized, phase III TAnDEM trial evaluated anastrozole with or without trastuzumab in the first- and second-line treatment of postmenopausal women with HER2+/ER+ MBC [53], and allowed for crossover at the time of progression. A total of 208 patients were randomized (103 patients received trastuzumab plus anastrozole; 104 received anastrozole alone). Patients in the trastuzumab plus anastrozole arm experienced significant improvements in PFS compared with patients receiving anastrozole alone (hazard ratio = 0.63; 95 % CI, 0.47–0.84; median PFS, 4.8 vs. 2.4 months; log-rank $P = 0.0016$). In patients with centrally confirmed hormone receptor positivity ($n = 150$), median PFS was 5.6 and 3.8 months in the trastuzumab plus anastrozole and anastrozole alone arms, respectively (log-rank $P = 0.006$). Overall survival in the overall and centrally confirmed hormone receptor-positive populations showed no statistically significant treatment difference; however, 70 % of patients in the anastrozole alone arm crossed over to receive trastuzumab after progression on anastrozole alone. Incidence of grade 3 and 4 adverse events was 23 and 5 %, respectively, in the trastuzumab plus anastrozole arm, and 15 and 1 %, respectively, in the anastrozole alone arm; one patient in the combination arm experienced New York Heart Association class II congestive heart failure.

21.3.5 Trastuzumab After Disease Progression

An important clinical question is whether trastuzumab should be continued after progression on a first-line trastuzumab-containing regimen. Preclinical data and retrospective analysis of clinical trials support the hypothesis that continuing treatment with trastuzumab after disease progression may provide patient benefit [54–56].

An extension study of the pivotal phase III trial of trastuzumab combined with chemotherapy as first-line treatment evaluated the safety of continuing the biological agent monotherapy beyond disease progression [53]. Although not designed to evaluate efficacy, the RR to second-line trastuzumab was similar for patients who initially received chemotherapy alone and for those who initially received chemotherapy plus trastuzumab (14 and 11 % respectively), as was median response duration (about 7 months). In another retrospective analysis, trastuzumab alone or combined with a different chemotherapy was continued beyond disease progression in 80 patients with HER2+ MBC [54]. Continued trastuzumab appeared safe, and 32 responses were noted (4 complete responses).

In a study of 105 patients with HER2+ MBC who had received two or more trastuzumab-containing regimens [55], RRs were, in fact, similar for second line as compared to first-line therapy, with some first-line nonresponders eventually achieving a response in second-line treatment. Nonfatal cardiac events were reported in 22 patients and most patients were able to continue trastuzumab.

Two prospective trials looking at this issue prematurely closed. The first was the US Intergroup study randomizing patients who had progressed on taxanes plus trastuzumab to vinorelbine versus vinorelbine plus trastuzumab. This trial closed early due to low accrual. The other was the BIG 3-05 study [57] which randomized 152 patients who had progressed on trastuzumab to either capecitabine or capecitabine plus trastuzumab. This trial also closed early due to slow accrual but the preplanned interim analysis of 119 patients showed a longer TTP favoring the combination arm (33 vs. 24 weeks, $P = 0.178$), and no difference in serious adverse events.

In a pooled analyses [58] of 2618 patients treated with trastuzumab beyond progression in 29 studies (4 randomized controlled phase III trials, 2 observational studies, 8 prospective nonrandomized trials, and 15 retrospective case series), the median RR, TTP, and OS obtained from the selected articles were 28.7 %, 7, and 24 months. This pooled analysis confirms that continuing trastuzumab beyond the first progression continues to be 1 of the effective and preferred choices in HER2+ MBC, failing a trastuzumab-based first-line regimen.

In a large German observational study of 1843 trastuzumab-treated patients [59], a sub-cohort of 418 fulfilled the selection criteria for the trastuzumab beyond progression analysis with 261 continuing trastuzumab and 157 discontinuing. Survival from progression was significantly longer in those patients continuing trastuzumab treatment beyond disease progression (median 22.1 months vs. 14.9 months; HR = 0.64; $P = 0.00021$).

21.3.6 Trastuzumab and New Drugs

21.3.6.1 Lapatinib

Lapatinib is a small molecule tyrosine kinase inhibitor which is capable of dual receptor inhibition of both EGFR and HER2. It is an ATP mimetic that competitively binds to the

ATP-binding cleft at the activation loop of target kinases, thereby inhibiting both kinase activities. Lapatinib also has the advantage of being able to bind and inhibit p95HER2, which is the truncated form of HER2 lacking an extracellular domain but possessing greater kinase activity than wild-type HER2. Because trastuzumab is unable to neither bind nor inhibit p95HER2, its resistance may be mediated at least, in part, through the expression of p95HER2 in disease progression.

In single-agent phase I/II studies, lapatinib has resulted in objective responses between 4.3 and 7.8 % in HER2+ patients who had progressed on multiple trastuzumab-containing regimens [60], with a substantial number having stable disease at 4 months (34–41 %) and 6 months (18–21 %).

A randomized study of lapatinib alone or in combination with trastuzumab in 296 women [61] with HER2+ trastuzumab-refractory metastatic breast cancer was conducted to investigate a chemotherapy-free option. The combination of lapatinib with trastuzumab was superior to lapatinib alone for PFS (hazard ratio [HR] = 0.73; 95 % CI, 0.57–0.93; $P = 0.008$) and CBR (24.7 % in the combination arm vs. 12.4 % in the monotherapy arm; $P = 0.01$). A trend for improved OS in the combination arm was observed (HR = 0.75; 95 % CI, 0.53–1.07; $P = 0.106$). There was no difference in overall RR (10.3 % in the combination arm vs. 6.9 % in the monotherapy arm; $P = 0.46$). The most frequent adverse events were diarrhea, rash, nausea, and fatigue; diarrhea was higher in the combination arm ($P = 0.03$). The incidence of symptomatic and asymptomatic cardiac events was low (combination therapy = 2 and 3.4 %; monotherapy = 0.7 and 1.4 %, respectively).

In the updated analyses of the combination study EGF10151, which was a phase III randomized comparison of lapatinib plus capecitabine versus capecitabine alone in 399 women with advanced HER2+ breast cancer that had progressed on trastuzumab, the addition of lapatinib prolonged TTP with a hazard ratio (HR) of 0.57 (95 % CI, 0.43–0.77; $P < 0.001$) and provided a trend toward improved overall survival (HR: 0.78, 95 % CI: 0.55–1.12, $P = 0.177$), and fewer cases with CNS involvement at first progression (4 vs. 13, $P = 0.045$) [62].

A multicenter phase II study of lapatinib in 242 patients with brain metastases from HER2+ breast cancer [63] demonstrated objective responses to lapatinib in 6 % of patients. In an exploratory analysis, 21 % of patients experienced a ≥20 % volumetric reduction in their CNS lesions. An association was observed between volumetric reduction and improvement in progression-free survival and neurologic signs and symptoms. Of the 50 evaluable patients who entered the lapatinib plus capecitabine extension, 20 % experienced a CNS objective response and 40 % experienced a ≥20 % volumetric reduction in their CNS lesions. This study confirmed the modest CNS antitumor activity of lapatinib, with additional responses observed with the combination of lapatinib and capecitabine.

21.3.6.2 Pertuzumab

In preclinical models, pertuzumab inhibits the growth of HER2-overexpressing cell lines in vitro and potent synergy is observed with the combination of trastuzumab and pertuzumab. Tumor regression also occurs when pertuzumab is added after progression on trastuzumab alone [64, 65].

In a phase II single arm clinical trial, 66 patients with HER2+ MBC who had progressed on trastuzumab were treated with trastuzumab and pertuzumab. Trastuzumab was given either as an 8 mg/kg IV loading dose followed by 6 mg/kg q3 weeks or as a 4 mg/kg loading dose followed by 2 mg/kg IV weekly, and pertuzumab was given as an 840 mg IV loading dose followed by 420 mg IV q3 weeks. An objective RR of 24.2 % with a clinical benefit rate (CBR) of 50 % was seen including 5 (7.6 %) complete responses (CR), 11 (16.7 %) PR, and 17 (25.8 %) SD lasting 6 months or greater [66].

These results led to the phase III randomized, double-blind trial called CLEOPATRA [67], which was a study of 808 patients with HER2+ MBC who had not received prior trastuzumab therapy in the metastatic setting. These patients were randomized to receive docetaxel and trastuzumab with either pertuzumab (THP) or placebo (TH). Only 11 % of patients had received trastuzumab in the adjuvant or neoadjuvant setting, thus this study primarily tested the activity of dual HER2 monoclonal antibody therapy in a trastuzumab-naïve population. Median PFS was 12.4 months with placebo and 18.5 months with pertuzumab [hazard ratio (HR) 0.62 (95 % CI: 0.51–0.75), $P < 0.0001$]. At the time of the independent assessment of PFS, the interim analysis of OS showed a trend in favor of the pertuzumab group, but this was not significant. After a follow-up of 30 months, the results showed a statistically significant improvement in OS favoring the pertuzumab-containing arm, with a 34 % reduction in the risk of death (HR: 0.66; 95 % CI: 0.52–0.84; $P = 0.0008$). At median follow-up of 50 months, the statistically significant improvement in OS in favor of the pertuzumab group was maintained (HR: 0.68; 95 % CI: 0.56–0.84; $P = 0.0002$). The median OS was 40.8 months in the control group and 56.5 months in the pertuzumab group, with difference of 15.7 months. The objective RR in the CLEOPATRA trial was 69.3 % in the control group and 80.2 % in the pertuzumab group. The difference in RR was 10.8 percentage points (95 % CI: 4.2–17.5; $P = 0.001$). As OS at the interim analysis did not cross the stopping boundary for significance, the statistical test result for objective RR was considered to be exploratory. An analysis of the incidence and time to development of CNS metastases

[68] in patients from the CLEOPATRA trial showed that the proportion of patients developing CNS as first site of disease progression was similar between the control group (51 of 406, 12.6 %) and the pertuzumab group (55 of 402, 13.7 %). The median time to progression in the CNS was 11.9 months in the control group and 15.0 months in the pertuzumab group (HR: 0.58; 95 % CI: 0.39–0.85; $P = 0.0049$). Median OS in patients who developed CNS metastases showed a trend in favor of the pertuzumab group, being 26.3 months versus 34.4 months in the control and pertuzumab groups, respectively (HR: 0.66; 95 % CI: 0.39–1.11). The difference observed was not statistically significant for the log-rank test ($P = 0.1139$) but was significant for the Wilcoxon test ($P = 0.0449$). In June 2012, the FDA approved pertuzumab in combination with trastuzumab and docetaxel for HER2+ MBC in patients who had not received prior HER2-directed therapy or chemotherapy for metastatic disease. The European Medicines Agency (EMA) gave its approval in March 2013.

Several studies with pertuzumab are ongoing. In the frontline metastatic setting, PHEREXA (NCT01026142) will evaluate pertuzumab, trastuzumab with capecitabine in improving PFS in 452 patients. PERUSE (NCT01572038) will evaluate the combination of pertuzumab, trastuzumab and taxane in the first-line treatment of 1438 HER2+ patients. PERTAIN (NCT01491737) is a phase II study randomizing 250 patients, studying the combination of pertuzumab, trastuzumab and an aromatase Inhibitor in ER+ and HER2+ MBC. VELVET (NCT01565083) is evaluating pertuzumab, trastuzumab and vinorelbine in a single arm phase II study of first line metastatic or locally advanced HER2+ breast cancer.

21.3.6.3 Ado-Trastuzumab Emtansine (T-DM1)

T-DM1 is an ADC consisting of DM1, a maytansinoid antimicrotubule agent, bound to trastuzumab through nonreducible thioether bonds. T-DM1 delivers this highly potent cytotoxic agent specifically to HER2-expressing cells. Once T-DM1 binds to HER2 on the cell surface, the T-DM1-HER2 complex is internalized and the antibody component is proteolytically degraded, releasing the DM1 into the cytoplasm [69]. Importantly, T-DM1 retains the biologic activity of trastuzumab (i.e., HER2 signaling blockade and induction of ADCC) [70].

Given the promising activity seen in phase I studies, several phase II studies have been completed with the 3.6 mg/kg q3-week dosing schedule. In the single arm proof-of-concept study that enrolled 112 patients with HER2+ MBC who progressed on HER2-directed therapy [71] (median of 8 prior therapies, with prior trastuzumab and almost two-thirds (66/112) had received prior lapatinib), the objective RR was 25.9 % (95 % CI: 18.4–34.4 %). Of 75 patients who had previously discontinued trastuzumab due to progression, 21 achieved objective responses (ORR 28.0 %, 95 % CI: 18.2–38.9 %). Of the 66 patients who previously had received lapatinib, the objective RR was 24.2 % (95 % CI: 14.5–36.0 %). The median PFS was 4.6 months (95 % CI: 3.9–8.6 months).

In a confirmatory phase II study of T-DM1 in 110 patients who previously received chemotherapy and two HER2-directed therapies including lapatinib and trastuzumab [72], the objective RR was 32.7 % (95 % CI: 24.1–42.1 %) and median PFS 7.2 months.

In the frontline setting, T-DM1 was compared head-to-head with trastuzumab plus docetaxel (HT) in a randomized phase II trial for the treatment of HER2+ locally advanced or MBC [73] with 137 patients who had not received chemotherapy for metastatic disease and if they were ≥6 months from prior chemotherapy in the adjuvant setting. Sixty-seven patients were treated with T-DM1, compared to 70 patients treated with HT. The median PFS was 14.2 months for T-DM1 versus 9.2 months for HT (HR 0.59; 95 % CI: 0.36–0.97; $P = 0.035$). There were three CRs in the HT arm and seven CRs in the T-DM1 arm ($P = 0.453$). For patients who received T-DM1, the ORR was 64.2 % (95 % CI: 51.8–74.8 %) compared to 58.0 % (95 % CI: 45.5–69.2 %) for HT. OS was similar between the two arms, although at the time of reporting, only 13 deaths had occurred. Compared to HT, fewer grade 3/4 AEs were seen in the T-DM1 arm (46.4 % vs. 90.9 % for TDM-1 and HT, respectively). Overall, T-DM1 treatment resulted in fewer treatment discontinuations (7.2 %) compared to for HT (34.8 %) and fewer serious AEs (20.3 % vs. 25.8 %).

The phase III randomized EMILIA trial unequivocally demonstrated the efficacy of T-DM1 in patients with HER2+, trastuzumab-pretreated MBC [74]. A total of 991 subjects with HER2+ advanced breast cancer, previously treated with taxane and trastuzumab were randomized to receive TDM-1 or lapatinib plus capecitabine. A statistically significant improvement in ORR was seen with T-DM1 compared with lapatinib and capecitabine (43.6 % vs. 30.8 %, $P < 0.001$). Median PFS was 9.6 months for T-DM1 vs. 6.4 months with lapatinib and capecitabine (HR 0.65; 95 % CI: 0.55–0.77; $P < 0.001$), and median OS at the second interim analysis was 30.9 versus 25.1 months (HR 0.68; 95 % CI: 0.55–0.85; $P < 0.001$). Fewer grade 3 or greater toxicities were seen with T-DM1 compared to lapatinib and capecitabine, with rates of 41 and 57 %, respectively. Thrombocytopenia and elevated transaminases were more common with T-DM1, while diarrhea, nausea, vomiting, palmar-plantar dysesthesia were more common in the lapatinib and capecitabine arm. Based on this seminal result, both the FDA and EMA have licensed T-DM1 as monotherapy for HER2+ MBC in patients who had previously received taxane and trastuzumab-based therapy [75].

TH3RESA [76] was a randomized, open-label trial evaluating T-DM1 versus treatment of physician's choice in patients who had previously received two or more HER2-directed therapies, including trastuzumab and lapatinib as well as taxane chemotherapy. A total of 602 patients were enrolled: 404 received T-DM1 and 198 patients received therapy per physician's choice. For the T-DM1 arm, median PFS was 6.2 months, compared to 3.3 months for TPC (stratified HR 0.528, 0.422–0.661, $P < 0.001$). Interim OS data also demonstrated a trend toward improvement in the T-DM1 arm (HR 0.552, 95 % CI: 0.369–0.826, $P = 0.0034$). T-DM1 treatment resulted in fewer grade 3 or greater AE compared to TPC: 32 % versus 43 %, respectively. Grade 3 thrombocytopenia was the only AE more frequently seen with T-DM1 and was seen in 5 % of patients treated with T-DM1, compared with 2 % in the control arm. Grade 3 neutropenia, diarrhea and febrile neutropenia were all more common for TPC than for T-DM1 arm.

There are several ongoing phase II and III studies with T-DM1. MARIANNE (NCT01120184) is a three-arm phase III study randomly assigning 1095 patients with progressed or recurrent locally advanced or previously untreated metastatic HER2+ breast cancer to receive T-DM1 plus pertuzumab (363 patients), T-DM1 plus placebo (367 patients), or HT (docetaxel or paclitaxel; 365 patients). At the time the trial was initiated, the control arm represented the standard of care for this patient population. After a median follow-up of 35 months [77], both T-DM1—containing regimens showed non-inferior PFS, but not superiority, over HT. The median PFS was 15.2 months in the T-DM1 plus pertuzumab arm (hazard ratio [HR] 0.87, 95 % CI [0.69, 1.08]; $P = 0.14$), 14.1 months with T-DM1 alone (HR 0.91, 95 % CI [0.73, 1.13]; $P = 0.31$) compared with 13.7 months with HT. The overall survival data were not yet reached. The objective response rate was 64.2, 59.7, and 67.9 % among the T-DM1 plus pertuzumab, T-DM1 alone, and HT arms, respectively. However, the median duration of response was 21.2 months (95 % CI [15.8, 29.3]) in the T-DM1 plus pertuzumab arm, 20.7 months (95 % CI [14.8, 25.0]) in the T-DM1 alone arm, and 12.5 months (95 % CI [10.5, 16.6]) in the HT arm. Rates of grade 3/4 neutropenia, febrile neutropenia, and diarrhea were lower in the T-DM1—containing arms. Rates of alopecia were also substantially lower with T-DM1, as were health-related quality of life outcomes as assessed by patient-reported physical and functional well-being. The median time to a five-point or more decrease from baseline in the Health-Related Quality of Life score ranged from 7.7 months with T-DM1 and 9.0 months with T-DM1 plus pertuzumab to 3.6 months with HT.

21.3.7 The Algorithm for Treating Metastatic HER2+ Breast Cancers (ASCO 2014 Guidelines)

21.3.7.1 First-Line Therapy

HER2-targeted therapy in combination with chemotherapy in the first-line setting is associated with improvements in RR, PFS, TTP and OS, when compared with chemotherapy alone. The recommended regimen is a combination of trastuzumab, pertuzumab, and a taxane-based primarily on the results of CLEOPATRA [64].

For patients who had disease recurrence greater than 12 months of trastuzumab-based adjuvant treatment, clinicians should follow the first-line therapy recommendation—i.e., offer pertuzumab/trastuzumab/taxane.

For patients who had disease recurrence within 12 months of trastuzumab-based adjuvant treatment, clinicians should follow the second-line therapy recommendation—i.e., offer T-DM1.

21.3.7.2 Second-Line Therapy

If a patient's HER2+ advanced breast cancer has progressed during or after first-line HER-2 targeted therapy, clinicians should recommend T-DMI as a second line treatment-based primarily on the results of EMILIA [74].

21.3.7.3 Third-Line Therapy and Beyond

If a patient's HER2+ advanced breast cancer has progressed during or after second-line or greater HER2-targeted treatment, clinicians should recommend further HER-2 targeted therapy. If the patient has not received TDM-1 or pertuzumab, then clinicians should offer TDM-1 (EMILIA [74]) or pertuzumab (informal consensus) respectively. If the patient has received both TDM-1 and pertuzumab, options include: lapatinib and capecitabine, as well as other combinations of chemotherapy and trastuzumab, lapatinib and trastuzumab, or hormonal therapy (in ER+ and HER2+ patients only).

21.4 Trastuzumab in the Adjuvant Setting

21.4.1 Adjuvant Trastuzumab Trials—Efficacy Results

Current clinical guidelines clearly state that standard of care in 2015 recommends the use of the monoclonal anti-HER2 antibody, trastuzumab, in combination with or after adjuvant chemotherapy in medically fit patients diagnosed with Stage I to III HER2+ breast cancer. The four landmark randomized trials investigating the benefit of adjuvant trastuzumab National Surgical Adjuvant Breast and Bowel Project [NSABP] B-31 and North Central Cancer Treatment Group [NCCTG] N9831 [78], HERA [79] and Breast Cancer International Research Group [BCIRG] 006 [80] in their initial analyses reported outcomes with median follow-ups of 24–36 months. With enrollment of over 13,000 women, the range in benefit in disease-free survival (DFS) in favor of trastuzumab was with hazard ratios (HRs) between 0.48 and 0.67 ($P < 0.0001$), and the range in benefit in overall survival (OS) was between 0.59 and 0.67 (P = NS to $P = 0.015$). Absolute improvements in DFS ranged from 6 to 11 %, with corresponding absolute differences in OS of 1–2.5 %.

With longer follow-up from these trials (8-year median follow-up from HERA [79] and from the combined analyses of NSABP B-31 and NCCTG N9831 [78]), there continues to be statistically and clinically significant improvements in DFS and OS. Though the magnitude of benefit, as measured by HRs, appears to have lessened slightly over time as more events (both relapses and deaths) occur, absolute gains in overall survival are larger now than in earlier analyses. Relapses unfortunately continue to occur at a relatively constant rate over time in the trastuzumab-treated arm(s)—with an estimated 10-year DFS of 73.7 % from the combined analyses of NSABP B-31 and NCCTG N9831 [78] (Tables 21.1 and 21.2).

21.4.2 Adjuvant Trastuzumab Trials: Safety Results

Hypersensitivity was the most common adverse effect of trastuzumab, and occurred mainly with the first infusion. Unexpected short-term side effects did not emerge in any of the trials, with the exception of 9 cases of interstitial pneumonitis in B-31 and N9831 [78], though the relationship to trastuzumab is still not clearly defined. Cardiotoxicity remains the most important adverse effect of trastuzumab. Across the adjuvant trials, the definitions for cardiac events, the schedules for cardiac monitoring, analyses of cardiac endpoints and follow-up times all differed.

Nonetheless, it appeared that the incidence of cardiac events with trastuzumab was not high, with initial reports ranging from 0.4 % in the BCIRG 006 trial [80] and 4.1 % in the B-31 [78] trial. Within the control arms of all studies, the incidence of cardiac events ranged from 0 to 0.8 %. With longer follow-up, the cumulative incidence of cardiac adverse events plateaus, with cardiac events rarely occurring following completion of trastuzumab treatment. In the HERA [79] study, at 8-year follow-up, only 4.1 % of patients experienced NYHA Class I/II cardiac dysfunction with a left ventricular ejection fraction (LVEF) drop of 10 % or more below baseline and to an absolute LVEF of 50 % or less. The majority of cardiac events secondary to trastuzumab were reversible in nature.

Table 21.1 Initial reports from the large adjuvant trastuzumab trials

Trial	Herceptin duration	Median F/U	Treatment arms	No. patients	HR for DFS (95 % CI)	2–3 year DFS (%)	HR for OS (95 % CI)	2 year OS (%)
HERA [79]	1 year	24 months	Chemo	1698		77.4		95.1
			Chemo → H	1703	0.64 (0.64 − 0.76)	85.8	0.66 (0.47 − 0.91)	96.0
NSABP B-31 [78]	1 year	24 months	AC → P	1679		75.4		91.7
NCCTG N9831			AC → P→H	1672	0.48 (0.39 − 0.59)	87.1	0.67 (0.48 − 0.93)	94.3
BCIRG 006 [80]	1 year	36 months	AC → T	1073		81		N/A
			AC → TH	1074	0.61 (0.46 − 0.76)	88	0.59 (0.42 − 0.85)	N/A
			TcarboH	1075	0.67 (0.54 − 0.83)	87	0.66 (0.47 − 0.93)	N/A

Abbreviations: *HR* hazard ratio; *DFS* disease-free survival; *OS* overall survival; *H* trastuzumab; *NSABP* National Surgical Adjuvant Breast and Bowel Project; *A* doxorubicin; *C* cyclophosphamide; *P* paclitaxel; *NCCTG* National Central Cancer Treatment Group; *BCIRG* Breast Cancer International Research Group; *T* docetaxel; *carbo* carboplatin

Table 21.2 Longer term follow-up from the large adjuvant trastuzumab trials

Trial	Median F/U	Treatment arms	HR for DFS (95 % CI)	DFS (%)	HR for OS (95 % CI)	OS (%)
HERA [79]	8 year	Chemo		76.0		N/A
		Chemo → H	0.76 (0.67 − 0.86)		0.76 (0.65 − 0.88)	N/A
NSABP B-31 [78]	8.4 year	AC → P		62.2		75.2
NCCTG N9831		AC → P→H	0.60 (0.53 − 0.68)	73.7	0.63 (0.54 − 0.73)	84.0
BCIRG 006 [80]	5.5 year	AC → T		75		87
		AC → TH	0.64 (0.53 − 0.78)	84	0.63 (0.48 − 0.81)	92
		TcarboH	0.67 (0.54 − 0.83)	81	0.77 (0.60 − 0.99)	91

Abbreviations: *HR* hazard ratio; *DFS*, disease-free survival; *OS* overall survival; *H* trastuzumab; *NSABP* National Surgical Adjuvant Breast and Bowel Project; *A* doxorubicin; *C* cyclophosphamide; *P* paclitaxel; *NCCTG* National Central Cancer Treatment Group; *BCIRG* Breast Cancer International Research Group; *T* docetaxel; *carbo* carboplatin

21.4.3 The Sequencing and Timing of Adjuvant Trastuzumab Treatment

In the 4 adjuvant trials, the timing of trastuzumab initiation varied considerably. In HERA [79], trastuzumab was delayed for a median time of 8 months after surgery; for 4 months in the combined B-31 and N9831 [78] group, and for 1 month in the platinum-taxane arm of BCIRG 006 [80]. In the NCCTG N9831 study, an unplanned, premature analysis directly comparing arms C (concurrent) and B (sequential) showed a numerical increase in DFS (84.4 % vs. 80.1 %), favoring the concurrent arm, although it did not meet statistical significance. There was no difference in toxicity between the two arms either. Despite these results, for convenience and earlier completion of therapy, it may be overall advantageous to deliver the trastuzumab concurrent with the taxane [81].

21.4.4 The Duration of Adjuvant Trastuzumab Treatment

At present, the standard of care is for 1 year of adjuvant trastuzumab therapy. The FinHer [82] was a phase III randomized adjuvant trial of 1010 breast cancer patients, of which 232 had HER2+ tumors. In the HER2+ cohort, patients were randomly assigned to 9 weeks of trastuzumab versus 12 months of trastuzumab, with chemotherapy. The shorter trastuzumab treatment in FinHer produced comparable hazard ratios for 3-year RFS (0.42) and OS (0.41), although, the confidence intervals were wide for both (95 % CI 0.21–0.83, $P = 0.001$ and 95 % CI 0.16–1.08, $P = 0.07$ respectively). This may, in part, be explained by the upfront use of trastuzumab within a synergistic chemotherapy combination with vinorelbine or docetaxel, or the efficacious administration of FEC itself. Furthermore, synergism between FEC and trastuzumab may have occurred, due to the long half-life of trastuzumab exerting its action several weeks after the last administration [83]. This group of investigators has successfully completed recruitment of 2168 patients in November 2014 into a trial directly comparing the 9-weeks of trastuzumab therapy to 52-weeks—the SOLD trial (NCT00593697)—and results are awaited.

Other studies including PHARE [84] (Protocol of Herceptin Adjuvant with Reduced Exposure) and PERSEPHONE (no longer recruiting; results awaited), also compared shorter duration trastuzumab (6 months) versus 1 year of standard treatment. PHARE is an open-label, randomized, phase III trial with 1691 patients randomly assigned to receive 12 months of trastuzumab and 1693 to receive 6 months of trastuzumab. After a median follow-up of 42.5 months, 175 disease-free survival events were noted in the 12-month group and 219 in the 6-month group. A 2-year disease-free survival was 93.8 % (95 % CI 92.6–94.9) in the 12-month group and 91.1 % (89.7–92.4) in the 6-month group (hazard ratio 1.28, 95 % CI 1.05–1.56; $P = 0.29$). 119 (93 %) of the 128 cardiac events (clinical or based on assessment of left ventricular ejection fraction) occurred while patients were receiving trastuzumab. Significantly more patients in the 12-month group experienced a cardiac event than did those in the 6-month group (96 [5.7 %] of 1690 patients vs. 32 [1.9 %] of 1690 patients, $P < 0.0001$). The study failed to meet its no-inferiority endpoint to show that 6 months of treatment with trastuzumab was non-inferior to 12 months of trastuzumab.

In the HERA study [79], the comparison of 2 years versus 1 year of trastuzumab treatment involved a landmark analysis of 3105 patients who were disease-free 12 months after randomisation to one of the trastuzumab groups, and was planned after observing at least 725 disease-free survival events. 367 events of disease-free survival in 1552 patients in the 1 year group and 367 events in 1553 patients in the 2-year group (hazard ratio [HR] 0.99, 95 % CI 0.85–1.14, $P = 0.86$). HRs for a comparison of 1 year of trastuzumab treatment versus observation were 0.76 (95 % CI 0.67–0.86, $P < 0.0001$) for disease-free survival and 0.76 (0.65–0.88, $P = 0.0005$) for overall survival, despite crossover of 884 (52 %) patients from the observation group to trastuzumab therapy. Thus, the updated HERA results confirmed that 1 year of treatment provides a significant disease-free and overall survival benefit compared with observation, and that 2 years of trastuzumab did not produce any additional benefit compared with 1 year of trastuzumab [85].

21.4.5 Avoiding Anthracyclines

BCIRG 006 [80] was interesting in its suggestion that a non-anthracycline regimen, combined with trastuzumab may be adequate to treat HER2+ early breast cancer patients. The study randomly assigned 3222 women with HER2+ early-stage breast cancer to receive doxorubicin and cyclophosphamide followed by docetaxel every 3 weeks (AC-T), the same regimen plus 52 weeks of trastuzumab (AC-T plus trastuzumab), or docetaxel and carboplatin plus 52 weeks of trastuzumab (TCH). At a median follow-up of 65 months [86], with 656 events, the estimated disease-free survival rates at 5 years were 75 % among patients receiving AC-T, 84 % among those receiving AC-T plus trastuzumab, and 81 % among those receiving TCH. Estimated rates of overall survival were 87, 92, and 91 %, respectively. No significant differences in efficacy (disease-free or overall survival) were found between the two trastuzumab regimens, whereas both were superior to AC-T. The rates of congestive heart failure and cardiac dysfunction were significantly higher in the group receiving AC-T plus trastuzumab than in the TCH group ($P < 0.001$). Eight cases of acute leukemia were reported: seven in the groups receiving the anthracycline-based regimens and one in the TCH group subsequent to receiving an anthracycline outside the study. The addition of 1 year of adjuvant trastuzumab significantly improved disease-free and overall survival among women with HER2-positive breast cancer. The authors argued that the risk—benefit ratio favored the non-anthracycline TCH regimen over AC-T plus trastuzumab, given its similar efficacy, fewer acute toxic effects, and lower risks of cardiotoxicity and leukemia.

21.4.6 Small HER2+ Tumors

In the four phase 3 randomized trials involving more than 8000 patients [78–80], trastuzumab when administered in combination with or after chemotherapy, resulted in recurrence risk reduction by approximately 50 %, with improvement in overall survival. However, all of these trials focused largely on patients with stage II or stage III HER2+ breast cancers, with limited information to guide optimal treatment of T1a–bN0 HER2+ breast cancers. Currently, no single standard treatment regimen is recommended for patients with stage I HER2+ breast cancer.

Several studies have examined the risk of disease recurrence in small HER2+ breast cancer patients who have not received trastuzumab or, in most cases, chemotherapy. The largest of the studies focused on 520 patients in the NCCN [87] database who had small HER2+ breast cancers (≤1 cm). The 5-year rate of DFS was 94 % for patients with T1bN0 ER− tumors, 93 % for T1aN0 ER− tumors, and 94–96 % for patients with T1a–bN0 ER+ disease. A study from the M.D. Anderson Cancer Center [88] suggested that among 98 patients with T1a–bN0 HER2-positive tumors, the 5-year rate of recurrence-free survival was 77.1 %, and the 5-year rate of survival free from distant recurrence was 86.4 %. In a study of 117 node-negative, HER2-positive tumors measuring up to 2 cm in a tumor registry in British Columbia, Canada [89], the 10-year rate of relapse-free survival was 68.3 % among patients with hormone-receptor-negative tumors and 77.5 % among patients with hormone-receptor-positive tumors. Although recurrence rates vary across these studies, the rates range from approximately 5 to 30 %, with distant recurrences occurring in as many as 20 % of patients with tumors measuring up to 1 cm. The studies consistently suggest that the risk of recurrence, at least in the first 5 years, is higher in the ER- group than in the ER+ group.

Although patients with stage I HER2+ tumors are expected to derive a smaller absolute benefit from adjuvant therapy than those with larger or node-positive tumors, the data suggest that they remain at more than minimal risk for a recurrence of breast cancer, and therefore, adjuvant trastuzumab should be actively considered for these smaller tumors.

In an uncontrolled, single group, multicenter, investigator-initiated study of adjuvant paclitaxel and trastuzumab [90] in 406 early HER2+ breast cancer patients (tumors ≤3 cm), patients received weekly treatment with paclitaxel and trastuzumab for 12 weeks, followed by 9 months of trastuzumab monotherapy. With a median follow-up period of 4.0 years, the 3-year rate of DFS was 98.7 % (95 % CI 97.6–99.8). A total of 13 patients (3.2 %; 95 % CI, 1.7–5.4) reported at least one episode of grade 3 neuropathy, and 2 had symptomatic congestive heart failure (0.5 %; 95 % CI, 0.1–1.8), both of whom had normalization of the left ventricular ejection fraction after discontinuation of trastuzumab. A total of 13 patients had significant asymptomatic declines in ejection fraction (3.2 %; 95 % CI, 1.7–5.4), as defined by the study, but 11 of these patients were able to resume trastuzumab therapy after a brief interruption.

21.4.7 Trastuzumab and/or Other Targeted Therapies

21.4.7.1 Lapatinib

The ALTTO (Adjuvant Lapatinib and/or Trastuzumab Treatment Optimisation) trial [91] was a four-arm randomized adjuvant study comparing trastuzumab for 12 months (T), lapatinib for 12 months (L), trastuzumab for 12 weeks followed sequentially by lapatinib for 34 weeks (T → L), and the combination of trastuzumab and lapatinib for 12 months (TL). It randomly assigned 8381 patients, of whom 40 % had node-negative disease and 57 % had hormone receptor-positive disease. Although the study was powered for 850 DFS events, the study was analyzed at 4.5 years (median) of follow-up as per protocol stipulation but with only 555 DFS events. At the first efficacy interim analysis, the comparison of L to T crossed the futility boundary, and as such, the L arm was crossed over to a recommended course of trastuzumab for 12 months. At the time of reporting of the efficacy of the primary endpoint at the 2014 ASCO Annual Meeting, the 4-year DFS for the T, T → L, and TL arms were 86, 87 and 88 %, respectively. The HR comparing TL and T was 0.84 (0.70–1.02; $P \leq 0.048$), which was not significant, for a $P \leq 0.025$ was required for statistical significance. The interaction test for hormone receptor status and for schedule of anti-HER2 therapy was not significant. However, numerically, the sequential administration of anti-HER2 therapy arms had some difference (T vs. T → L 4-year DFS of 83 % vs. 86 %, respectively), whereas the combination arms did not (T vs. TL 4-year DFS of 90 % vs. 90 %, respectively). Lapatinib was also associated with a greater rate of adverse events, which subsequently led to only 60–78 % of patients in the lapatinib treatment arms receiving at least 85 % of the intended dose intensity of L.

TEACH (Tykerb® Evaluation After Chemotherapy) was a placebo-controlled, multicentre, randomized phase 3 trial which evaluated the effectiveness of 12 months of lapatinib versus placebo, given as either immediate or delayed therapy, in HER2+ early breast cancer [92]. 3161 women were enrolled and 3147 were assigned to lapatinib ($n = 1571$) or placebo ($n = 1576$). After a median follow-up of 47.4 months (range 0.4–60.0) in the lapatinib group and 48.3 (0.7–61.3) in the placebo group, 210 (13 %) disease-free survival events had occurred in the lapatinib group versus 264 (17 %) in the placebo group (hazard ratio [HR] 0.83, 95 % CI 0.70–1.00; $P = 0.053$). Central review of HER2 status showed that only 2490 (79 %) of the randomized women were HER2+. 157 (13 %) of 1230 confirmed HER2+ patients in the lapatinib group and in 208 (17 %) of 1260 in the placebo group had a disease-free survival event (HR 0.82, 95 % 0.67–1.00; $P = 0.04$). Serious adverse events occurred in 99 (6 %) of 1573 patients taking lapatinib and 77 (5 %) of 1574 patients taking placebo, with higher incidences of grade 3-4 diarrhea (97 [6 %] vs. nine [<1 %]), rash (72 [5 %] vs. three [<1 %]), and hepatobiliary disorders (36 [2 %] vs. one [<1 %]). This study did not show any significant difference in disease-free survival between groups when analyzed in the intention-to-treat population.

21.4.7.2 Pertuzumab

APHINITY (NCT0135887—Adjuvant Pertuzumab and Herceptin IN IniTial therapY of breast cancer) is a large adjuvant study that randomized 4800 patients with stage I-III HER2+ breast cancer to standard chemotherapy (non-anthracycline- or anthracycline-based) concurrent with pertuzumab/trastuzumab, or to standard chemotherapy concurrent with trastuzumab. In both arms, the same HER2-targeted therapy is administered postchemotherapy to complete 1 year of therapy. Recruitment has completed and the results are awaited. Indeed, if these results were to be positive, the addition of pertuzumab to chemotherapy/trastuzumab in the adjuvant setting will likely become standard of care.

21.4.7.3 Neratinib

Neratinib is an orally available, 6,7-disubstituted-4-anilinoquinoline-3-carbonitrile irreversible inhibitor of the HER-2 receptor tyrosine kinase with potential antineoplastic activity. Neratinib binds to the HER-2 receptor irreversibly, thereby reducing autophosphorylation in cells, apparently by targeting a cysteine residue in the ATP-binding pocket of the receptor. Treatment of cells with this agent results in inhibition of downstream signal transduction events and cell cycle regulatory pathways; arrest at the G1-S (Gap 1/DNA synthesis)-phase transition of the cell division cycle; and ultimately decreased cellular proliferation. Neratinib also inhibits the epidermal growth factor receptor (EGFR) kinase and the proliferation of EGFR-dependent cells [93].

ExteNET is a double-blind phase III trial of neratinib (240 mg orally once daily) versus placebo in 2821 women with early-stage HER2+ (local confirmation) breast cancer after adjuvant treatment with trastuzumab, the primary endpoint being iDFS. At 24 months [94], patients who received neratinib had an iDFS rate of 93.9 % compared to 91.6 % in the placebo group (hazard ratio [HR] 0.67, 95 % CI [0.50, 0.91]; $P = 0.009$). There were 73 distant recurrences (5.1 %) in the placebo group, and 52 (3.7 %) in the neratinib group. Patients with hormone receptor-positive disease were observed to derive an even greater benefit with neratinib therapy, and the iDFS rates were 95.4 % for neratinib and 91.2 % for placebo ($P = 0.001$). There was no significant difference in the patients with hormone receptor-negative disease (92.0 % vs. 92.2 %). Diarrhea was the most common adverse event with neratinib; grade 3/4 diarrhea occurred in 39.9 % of patients compared with 1.6 % of patients who received placebo. Overall survival data are still needed before neratinib could be considered a new standard, and questions remain about which populations will benefit from this therapy.

21.4.7.4 Bevacizumab

In HER2+ breast cancer, preclinical models have demonstrated that HER2 amplification is associated with an increase in VEGF gene expression [95]. The vascular endothelial growth factor (VEGF) receptor family plays an essential role in angiogenesis, and therefore, in cancer metastases dissemination [96]. The principal agent targeting VEGF is bevacizumab, a humanized monoclonal antibody directed against VEGF which can reduce tumor angiogenesis [97] and the tumor interstitial fluid pressure, leading to a better delivery of large therapeutic molecules into solid tumors.

The addition of bevacizumab (Avastin) to adjuvant chemotherapy did not improve invasive disease-free survival or overall survival in patients with high-risk HER2-positive breast cancer in the large randomized phase III BETH trial [98]. BETH enrolled 3509 women with HER2+ node-positive or high-risk node-negative breast cancer in two cohorts. Cohort 1 included 3231 patients randomly assigned to receive the non-anthracycline regimen TCH (docetaxel, carboplatin, and trastuzumab) or TCH plus bevacizumab. In cohort 2, 278 patients were randomly assigned to anthracycline-based therapy with T-FEC-H (docetaxel, fluorouracil, epirubicin, cyclophosphamide, plus trastuzumab) with or without bevacizumab.

At a median follow-up of 38 months, the rate of invasive disease-free survival in cohort 1 was 92 % in both TCH arms (with and without bevacizumab), and in cohort 2, 89 % in the anthracycline-containing arms without bevacizumab versus 91 % with bevacizumab. This difference between the anthracycline and non-anthracycline-containing arms was not statistically significant.

21.5 Neoadjuvant HER2+ Approaches

21.5.1 Neoadjuvant Trastuzumab

The standard clinical use of neoadjuvant chemotherapy today can be categorized into two populations of patients: the locally advanced breast cancers (LABC) and the primary operable breast cancers (POBC). The defined purpose for the use of neoadjuvant chemotherapy for LABC is to convert a baseline inoperable condition to an operable state. In POBC, neoadjuvant chemotherapy has the potential to downstage a tumor and thus convert a baseline mastectomy candidate into a breast conservation candidate. Other advantages of delivery in the neoadjuvant setting include the ability to study new agents with the utility of a surrogate endpoint for outcome; the ability to obtain tumor tissue for pharmacodynamic assessment, understanding of biology and discovery of predictive biomarkers; earlier initiation of systemic therapies; and the ability to monitor response. There remains an ongoing debate regarding the correlation of pCR status and long-term clinical outcomes such as DFS, EFS, and OS. Multiple studies have repeatedly demonstrated a prognostic effect for the cohort of patients achieving a pCR—particularly those achieving a pCR in breast and lymph nodes (tpCR). Recently, a pooled analysis of 12 large trials of 11,955 patients treated with preoperative chemotherapy with available data on pCR and at least 3-year follow-up data on EFS and OS was performed by the FDA (CTNeoBC pooled analysis) [99]. The analysis demonstrated that the association between pCR and long-term outcomes was strongest in triple negative breast cancer and HER2+/ER− breast cancers treated with trastuzumab. The German Breast Group also performed a similar analysis with seven of their trials involving 6366 patients [100]. They found similar results to the CTNeoBC pooled analyses (Table 21.3).

The first landmark trial investigating the benefit of neoadjuvant trastuzumab in the LABC setting was the NOAH trial [101]. NOAH randomly selected 228 patients with HER2+ disease to receive a neoadjuvant regimen consisting of doxorubicin, paclitaxel, cyclophosphamide, methotrexate, and 5-fluorouracil (CMF) with or without concurrent trastuzumab (throughout the entire chemotherapeutic regimen). This is the largest randomized trial of a true locally advanced and inflammatory population to date. The trastuzumab-treated cohort demonstrated a significantly superior rate of pCR in breast and nodes (total pCR [tpCR]; 38 % vs. 19 %; $P \leq 0.001$), which ultimately translated to an improved 3-year event-free survival (EFS; 71 % vs. 56 %, HR 0.59; 95 % CI, 0.38–0.90). Although the use of the specific chemotherapy regimen from NOAH is not likely to be common, the concept of neoadjuvant trastuzumab concurrent with chemotherapy now is.

21.5.2 Lapatinib-Based Neoadjuvant Regimens

The GeparQuinto study [102] compared trastuzumab (8 mg/kg loading dose followed by 6 mg/kg every 3 weeks given concurrently with chemotherapy during the preoperative period) with lapatinib (1250 mg/day continuously for 12 weeks) added to a backbone of four cycles of epirubicin (90 mg/m^2) and cyclophosphamide (600 mg/m^2) followed

Table 21.3 Neoadjuvant trials of dual HER2 targeted therapies

Trial	No. of patients	Treatment arms	Pcr (breast and nodes) (%)	*p*	3-year EFS (%)
GeparQuinto	309	ECH → TH	31.3	$P < 0.05$	N/A
	311	ECL→	21.7		N/A
NeoALTTO	149	H → HP	27.6		76
	154	L → LP	20.0	$P = 0.13$	78
	152	HL → HLP	46.9	$P = 0.001$	84
CHER-LOB	36	HP → FECH	25		N/A
	39	LP → FECL	26.3		N/A
	46	HLP → FECHL	46.7		N/A
NSABP B-41	177	AC → HP	52.5 (breast)		N/A
	171	AC → LP	53.2 (breast)	$P = 0.9852$	N/A
	171	AC → HLP	62.0 (breast)	$P = 0.095$	N/A
CALGB 40601	120	HP	40 (breast)		N/A
	67	LP	32 (breast)		N/A
	118	HLP	51 (breast)	$P = 0.11$	N/A
NeoSphere	107	TH	29.0 (breast)		N/A
	107	PerHT	45.8 (breast)	$P = 0.0141$	N/A
	107	PerH	24.0 (breast)		N/A
	96	PerT	16.8 (breast)		N/A
Tryphena	73	PerHFEC → PerTH	61.6 (breast)		N/A
	75	FEC → PerTH	57.3 (breast)		N/A
	77	TcarboHPer	66.2 (breast)		N/A

Abbreviations: *pCR* pathologic complete response; *EFS* event-free survival; *E* epirubicin; *C* cyclophosphamide; *H* trastuzumab; *T* docetaxel; *L* lapatinib; *P* paclitaxel; *F* 5-fluorouracil; *NSABP* National Surgical Adjuvant Breast and Bowel Project; *A* doxorubicin; *CALGB* Cancer and Leukemia Group B; *Per* pertuzumab; *carbo* carboplatin

by four of docetaxel (100 mg/m^2) in 615 patients with HER2 + disease. A significantly higher tpCR rate (breasts and nodes) was seen in the trastuzumab arm (30.3 % vs. 22.7 %; odds ratio 0.68; 95 % CI, 0.47–0.97; $P \leq 0.04$). Furthermore, in this study, dose reductions were required in nearly one-third of patients receiving lapatinib, prompting a protocol amendment reducing the lapatinib dose to 1000 mg/m^2. The smaller CHER-LOB study [103] was conducted using a chemotherapy backbone of weekly paclitaxel (80 mg/m^2) for 12 weeks followed by three-weekly 5-fluorouracil, epirubicin, cyclophosphamide (FEC; 500/75/500 mg/m^2, respectively) with either weekly trastuzumab (4 mg/kg loading dose followed by 2 mg/kg weekly) or lapatinib (1250 mg daily) given concurrently with chemotherapy. This study also examined the efficacy of a trastuzumab-lapatinib doublet with dose-adjusted lapatinib (750 mg/day). Dual HER2 targeting substantially improved pCR (breast and nodes) over either trastuzumab or lapatinib alone. pCR rates were 46 % (90 % CI, 34.4–58.9 %), 25 % (90 % CI, 13.1–36.9 %), and 26.3 % (90 % CI, 14.5–38.1 %), respectively. As was seen in the GeparQuinto trial, gastrointestinal toxicity with lapatinib was a significant adverse event. More than 50 % of those receiving lapatinib experienced diarrhea of grade 1 or higher, even after a protocol amendment directing a dose reduction from 1500 to 1250 mg/day in the single-agent arm, and from 1000 to 750 mg/day in the doublet arm. The NeoAdjuvant Lapatinib and/or Trastuzumab Optimization (NeoALTTO) trial [104] was a three-armed study addressing the comparative efficacy of single compared with dual HER2 blockade using trastuzumab (4 mg/kg loading dose followed by 2 mg/kg weekly), lapatinib (1500 mg daily), or a combination (trastuzumab standard dose and lapatinib 1000 mg daily), alongside weekly paclitaxel (80 mg/m^2) chemotherapy. This trial scheduled a 6-week lead in period of targeted therapy alone before introduction of paclitaxel for a further 12 weeks of therapy. Dual HER2 targeting induced tpCR (breast and nodes) rates in 46.8 % of patients compared with 27.6 % in the trastuzumab alone arm ($P \leq 0.0007$). There was no statistically significant difference in pCR rates between the trastuzumab alone and lapatinib alone arms (27.6 and 20 %; $P \leq 0.13$). The NSABP B-41 study [105] randomly selected 529 patients with HER2+ disease to receive doxorubicin (60 mg/m^2) and cyclophosphamide (600 mg/m^2) every 3 weeks for four cycles, followed by weekly paclitaxel (80 mg/m^2) for a further 12 weeks with either concurrent weekly trastuzumab (4 mg/kg loading dose followed by 2 mg/kg weekly), 1250 mg of lapatinib daily, or weekly trastuzumab plus lapatinib (750 mg/day). pCR was achieved for 62 % of patients receiving combination HER2 targeting compared with 52.5 % in the trastuzumab arm ($P \leq 0.095$). There was no significant difference between the trastuzumab and lapatinib alone arms (52.5 % vs. 53.2 %; $P \leq 0.990$). The Cancer and Leukemia Group B 40601, a neoadjuvant phase III trial of weekly paclitaxel (T) and trastuzumab (H) with and without lapatinib (L) in HER2-positive breast cancer, was presented at the 2013 ASCO Annual Meeting [106]. This trial randomly selected 305 patients, of which two-thirds had clinical stage II disease. The pCR rates in the breast alone were 51 % (42–60 %) THL, 40 % (32–49 %) TH, 32 % (22–44 %) TL. The combination arm of THL was not significantly different from the standard arm of trastuzumab and paclitaxel ($P \leq 0.11$).

21.5.3 Pertuzumab-Based Neoadjuvant Regimens

In the NeoSphere trial [107], 417 women with HER2+ POBC/LABC disease were randomly selected to receive either four cycles of neoadjuvant trastuzumab (8 mg/kg loading dose, followed by 6 mg/kg every 3 weeks), docetaxel (75 mg/m^2 escalating to 100 mg/m^2 as tolerated) and pertuzumab (loading dose 840 mg, followed by 420 mg every 3 weeks), or trastuzumab plus docetaxel, or pertuzumab and trastuzumab without chemotherapy, or pertuzumab plus docetaxel. The combination of dual-HER2 targeting and docetaxel induced a pCR (breast) for 45.8 % (95 % CI, 36.1–55.7) compared with 29 % of those randomly assigned to trastuzumab and docetaxel (95 % CI, 20.6–38.5; $P \leq 0.0141$). After surgery, all patients received three cycles of FEC and the remainder of 1 year of trastuzumab. pCR was achieved for 24.0 % of those receiving pertuzumab and docetaxel and 16.8 % of women who were treated with dual HER2 targeted therapy in the absence of chemotherapy. Neither short nor long-term clinical outcomes (EFS and OS) have been reported yet from NeoSphere.

TRYPHENA [108] was a phase II trial with cardiac safety as the primary endpoint. All 225 participants received dual HER2 targeting with trastuzumab and pertuzumab. The three study arms were randomly assigned to 500 mg 5-fluorouracil, 100 mg epirubicin, and 500 mg/m^2 cyclophosphamide (FEC100) for three cycles, followed by docetaxel (75 mg/m^2) with concurrent with trastuzumab and pertuzumab; FEC for three cycles followed by docetaxel with trastuzumab and pertuzumab given only alongside docetaxel; or six cycles of docetaxel, carboplatin, trastuzumab, and pertuzumab. In this trial, pCR (breast) was a secondary endpoint, with rates ranging between 57.3 and 66.2 %, in keeping with results published in other studies. The lack of an arm without pertuzumab limits the extrapolation of these results to other studies and to standard clinical practice. In September 2013, the U.S. Food and Drug Administration (FDA) granted accelerated approval to pertuzumab in combination with trastuzumab and chemotherapy as a neoadjuvant treatment regimen in patients with HER2+ locally advanced, inflammatory, or early-stage disease (tumor size <2 cm or with positive lymph nodes).

21.5.4 Neratinib-Based Neoadjuvant Regimens

Neratinib has been studied in a neoadjuvant manner as part of the I-SPY 2 program, as well as in an extended manner in a placebo-controlled trial in a population of patients following 1 year of standard adjuvant trastuzumab-based therapy. In the I-SPY 2 trial, neratinib was given in combination with weekly paclitaxel (80 mg/m^2 for 12 weeks) in both the HER2+ and HER2− cohorts [109]. All patients subsequently received sequential doxorubicin (60 mg/m^2) and cyclophosphamide (600 mg/m^2) for four cycles without neratinib or trastuzumab before proceeding to definitive surgery. In the HER2+ signature cohort, the pCR rate was 39 % in the neratinib plus paclitaxel arm, compared to 23 % in the trastuzumab plus paclitaxel arm. The magnitude of improvement in pCR was similar regardless of the hormone receptor status in the HER2+ cohort. No significant difference in pCR rates was seen in the HER2− signature cohort. A significant rate of grade 2–3 diarrhea was seen, however, in the neratinib arms resulting in dose reductions/holds in 65 % of cases for neratinib (vs. 15 % in the control arm).

21.6 Other Exploratory Anti-HER2 Blockade Strategies

The main mechanisms for resistance to anti-HER2 therapy with trastuzumab include redundancy, reactivation and escape. Redundancy within the HER receptor layer refers to the ability of the pathway to continue to signal despite being partially inhibited because of redundant ligands and receptors that enable alternative dimerization patterns. Reactivation, on the other hand refers to the ability to reactivate pathway signaling at or downstream of the receptor layer such as with activating HER or downstream mutations, or loss of downstream pathway negative-regulating mechanisms. Escape refers to the use of other pathways, which may preexist or be acquired at the time of resistance, but are not usually driving the cancer cell when HER2 is uninhibited [110, 111].

Multiple other pathways and mechanisms involved in intrinsic and acquired resistance to HER-targeted therapy have been suggested, including various receptor and cellular tyrosine kinases (e.g., MET, IGFR-1, c-SRC, and EphA2) [112–114], mucins [115], regulators of cell cycle and apoptosis [116–118] and various elements of the tumor microenvironment and the host immune system [119–121].

21.7 Conclusion

HER2 is a redundant, robust and powerful signaling pathway and understanding the mechanisms mediating resistance to HER2 blockade has opened new therapeutic avenues which have resulted in significant improvements in patient outcomes. Different combinations of anti-HER2 therapies have been explored and the next challenge is to find predictive biomarkers to identify cohorts of patients that may need differential combinations and/or durations of anti-HER2 therapies. HER2+ breast cancer has, indeed, come a long way, and trastuzumab has revolutionized the HER2+ subtype from being one with the worst prognosis to one arguably with the best long-term outcomes. The evolution continues as the mechanisms of HER2 resistance get further unraveled.

References

1. Slamon DJ, Clark GM, Wong SG, et al. Human breast cancer: correlation of relapse and survival with amplification of the HER-2/neu oncogene. Science. 1987;235:177–82.
2. Slamon DJ, Godolphin W, Jones LA, et al. Studies of the HER-2/neu proto-oncogene in human breast and ovarian cancer. Science. 1989;244:707–12.
3. Yarden Y. The EGFR family and its ligands in human cancer: signalling mechanisms and therapeutic opportunities. Eur J Cancer. 2001;37(Suppl 4):S3–8.
4. Schechter AL, Stern DF, Vaidyanathan L, et al. The neu oncogene: an erb-B-related gene encoding a 185,000-M, tumour antigen. Nature. 1984;312:513–6.
5. King CR, Kraus MH, Aaronsen SA. Amplification of a novel v-erb-related gene in a human mammary carcinoma. Science. 1985;229:974–6.
6. Depowski P, Mulford D, Minot P, et al. Comparative analysis of HER-2/neu protein overexpression in breast cancer using paraffin-embedded tissue and cytologic specimens. Mod Pathol. 2002;15:70A.
7. Joensuu H, Isola J, Lundin M, et al. Amplification of erbB2 and erbB2 expression are superior to estrogen receptor status as risk factors for distant recurrence in pT1N0Mo breast cancer: a nationwide population-based study. Clin Cancer Res. 2003; 9:923–30.
8. Press MF, Bernstein PA, Thomas LF, et al. HER-2/neu gene amplification characterized by fluorescence in situ hybridization: poor prognosis in node-negative breast carcinomas. J Clin Oncol. 1997;15:2894–904.
9. Muss HB, Thor AD, Berry DA, et al. c-erbB-2 expression and response to adjuvant therapy in women with node-positive early breast cancer. New Engl J Med. 1994;330:1260–6.
10. Paik S, Bryant J, Park C, et al. erbB-2 and response to doxorubicin in patients with axillary lymph node-positive, hormone receptor-negative breast cancer. J Natl Cancer Inst. 1998;90:1361–70.
11. Thor AD, Berry DA, Budman DR, et al. erbB-2, p53, and efficacy of adjuvant therapy in lymph node-positive breast cancer. J Natl Cancer Inst. 1998;90:1346–60.
12. Mendelsohn J, Baselga J. Status of epidermal growth factor receptor antagonists in the biology and treatment of cancer. J Clin Oncol. 2003;21:2787–99.
13. Franklin MC, Carey KD, Vajdos FF, et al. Insights into ErbB signalling from the structure of the ErbB2-pertuzumab complex. Cancer Cell. 2004;5:317–28.
14. Erickson HK, Park PU, Widdison WC, et al. Antibody-maytansinoid conjugates are activated in targeted cancer cells by lysosomal degradation and linker-dependent intracellular processing. Cancer Res. 2006;66:4426–33.
15. Wolff AC, Hammond ME, Hicks DG, et al. Recommendations for human epidermal growth factor receptor 2 testing in breast cancer: American Society of Clinical Oncology/College of American Pathologists clinical practice guideline update. J Clin Oncol. 2013;31(31):3997–4013.
16. Cobleigh MA, Vogel CL, Tripathy D, et al. Multinational study of the efficacy and safety of humanized anti-HER2 monoclonal antibody in women who have HER2-overexpressing metastatic breast cancer that has progressed after chemotherapy for metastatic disease. J Clin Oncol. 1999;17(9):2639–48.
17. Baselga J, Carbonell X, Castaneda-Soto NJ, et al. Phase II study of efficacy, safety, and pharmacokinetics of trastuzumab monotherapy administered on a 3-weekly schedule. J Clin Oncol. 2005;23(10):2162–71.
18. Vogel CL, Cobleigh MA, Tripathy D, et al. Efficacy and safety of trastuzumab as a single agent in first-line treatment of HER2-overexpressing metastatic breast cancer. J Clin Oncol. 2002;20(3):719–26.
19. Pegram MD, Konecny GE, O'Callaghan C, et al. Rational combinations of trastuzumab with chemotherapeutic drugs used in the treatment of breast cancer. J Natl Cancer Inst. 2004;96 (10):739–49.
20. Slamon DJ, Leyland-Jones B, Shak S, et al. Use of chemotherapy plus a monoclonal antibody against HER2 for metastatic breast cancer that overexpresses HER2. N Engl J Med. 2001;344 (11):783–92.
21. Seidman AD, Fornier MN, Esteva FJ, et al. Weekly trastuzumab and paclitaxel therapy for metastatic breast cancer with analysis of efficacy by HER2 immunophenotype and gene amplification. J Clin Oncol. 2001;19(10):2587–95.
22. Marty M, Cognetti F, Maraninchi D, et al. Randomized phase II trial of the efficacy and safety of trastuzumab combined with docetaxel in patients with human epidermal growth factor receptor 2-positive metastatic breast cancer administered as first-line treatment: the M77001 study group. J Clin Oncol. 2005;23(19):4265–74.
23. Hamberg P1, Bos MM, Braun HJ et al. Randomized phase II study comparing efficacy and safety of combination-therapy trastuzumab and docetaxel vs. sequential therapy of trastuzumab followed by docetaxel alone at progression as first-line chemotherapy in patients with HER2+ metastatic breast cancer: HERTAX trial. Clin Breast Cancer. 2011;11(2):103–13.
24. Pegram MD, Konecny GE, O'Callaghan C, et al. Rational combinations of trastuzumab with chemotherapeutic drugs used

in the treatment of breast cancer. J Natl Cancer Inst. 2004;96 (10):739–49.
25. Pegram MD, Finn RS, Arzoo K, et al. The effect of HER-2/neu overexpression on chemotherapeutic drug sensitivity in human breast and ovarian cancer cells. Oncogene. 1997;15(5):537–47.
26. Robert N, Leyland-Jones B, Asmar L, et al. Randomized phase III study of trastuzumab, paclitaxel, and carboplatin compared with trastuzumab and paclitaxel in women with HER-2-overexpressing metastatic breast cancer. J Clin Oncol. 2006;24(18):2786–92.
27. Valero V1, Forbes J, Pegram MD, et al. Multicenter phase III randomized trial comparing docetaxel and trastuzumab with docetaxel, carboplatin, and trastuzumab as first-line chemotherapy for patients with HER2-gene-amplified metastatic breast cancer (BCIRG 007 study): two highly active therapeutic regimens BCIRG 007. J Clin Oncol. 2011;10;29(2):149–56.
28. Burstein HJ, Harris LN, Marcom PK, et al. Trastuzumab and vinorelbine as first-line therapy for HER2-overexpressing metastatic breast cancer: multicenter phase II trial with clinical outcomes, analysis of serum tumor markers as predictive factors, and cardiac surveillance algorithm. J Clin Oncol. 2003;21 (15):2889–95.
29. Jahanzeb M, Mortimer JE, Yunus F, et al. Phase II trial of weekly vinorelbine and trastuzumab as first-line therapy in patients with HER2(+) metastatic breast cancer. Oncologist. 2002;7(5):410–7.
30. Burstein HJ, Kuter I, Campos SM, et al. Clinical activity of trastuzumab and vinorelbine in women with HER2-overexpressing metastatic breast cancer. J Clin Oncol. 2001;19(10):2722–30.
31. Chan A, Martin M, Untch M, et al. Vinorelbine plus trastuzumab combination as first-line therapy for HER 2-positive metastatic breast cancer patients: an international phase II trial. Br J Cancer. 2006;95(7):788–93.
32. Fujimoto-Ouchi K, Sekiguchi F, Tanaka Y. Antitumor activity of combinations of anti-HER-2 antibody trastuzumab and oral fluoropyrimidines capecitabine/5′-dFUrd in human breast cancer models. Cancer Chemother Pharmacol. 2002;49:211–6.
33. Schaller G, Fuchs I, Gonsch T, et al. Phase II study of capecitabine plus trastuzumab in human epidermal growth factor receptor 2 overexpressing metastatic breast cancer pretreated with anthracyclines or taxanes. J Clin Oncol. 2007;25(22):3246–50.
34. Xu L, Song S, Zhu J, et al. Results of a phase II trial of Herceptin® plus Xeloda® in patients with previously untreated HER2-positive metastatic breast cancer. Breast Cancer Res Treat. 2004;88(suppl 1):S128.
35. O'Shaughnessy JA, Vukelja S, Marsland T, et al. Phase II study of trastuzumab plus gemcitabine in chemotherapy-pretreated patients with metastatic breast cancer. Clin Breast Cancer. 2004;5 (2):142–7.
36. Jordan MA, Kamath K, Manna T, et al. The primary antimitotic mechanism of action of the synthetic halichondrin E7389 is suppression of microtubule growth. Mol Cancer Ther. 2005;4:1086–95.
37. Wilks S, Puhalla S, O'Shaughnessy J, et al. Phase 2, multicenter, single-arm study of eribulin mesylate with trastuzumab as first-line therapy for locally recurrent or metastatic HER2-positive breast cancer. Clin Breast Cancer. 2014;14 (6):405–12.
38. https://clinicaltrials.gov/ct2/show/NCT01912963.
39. Wardley A, Antón-Torres A, Pivot X, et al. Trastuzumab plus docetaxel with or without capecitabine in patients with HER2-positive advanced/metastatic breast cancer: first efficacy results from the Phase II MO16419 (CHAT) study. Breast Cancer Res and Treat. 2006;100:abstract 2063.
40. Perez EA, Suman VJ, Rowland KM, et al. Two concurrent phase II trials of paclitaxel/carboplatin/trastuzumab (weekly or every-3-week schedule) as first-line therapy in women with HER2-overexpressing metastatic breast cancer: NCCTG study 983252. Clin Breast Cancer. 2005;6(5):425–32.
41. Polyzos A, Mavroudis D, Boukovinas J, et al. A multicenter phase II study of docetaxel, gemcitabine and trastuzumab administration as first-line treatment in patients with advanced breast cancer (ABC) overexpressing HER-2. J Clin Oncol (2004 ASCO Annual Meeting Proceedings, Post-Meeting Edition). 2004;22(No 14S):728 (July 15 Supplement).
42. Fountzilas G, Christodoulou C, Tsavdaridis D, et al. Paclitaxel and gemcitabine, as first-line chemotherapy, combined with trastuzumab in patients with advanced breast cancer: a phase II study conducted by the Hellenic Cooperative Oncology Group (HeCOG). Cancer Invest. 2004;22(5):655–62.
43. Venturini M, Bighin C, Monfardini S, et al. Multicenter phase II study of trastuzumab in combination with epirubicin and docetaxel as first-line treatment for HER2-overexpressing metastatic breast cancer. Breast Cancer Res Treat. 2006;95(1):45–53.
44. Yardley DA, Greco FA, Porter LL, et al. First line treatment with weekly docetaxel, vinorelbine, and trastuzumab in HER2 overexpressing metastatic breast cancer (HER2+ MBC): A Minnie Pearl Cancer Research Network phase II trial. J Clin Oncol (ASCO Annual Meeting Proceedings, Post-Meeting Edition). 2004;22(No 14S):643 (July 15 Supplement).
45. Arpino G, Green SJ, Allred DC, et al. HER-2 amplification, HER-1 expression, and tamoxifen response in estrogen receptor-positive metastatic breast cancer: a southwest oncology group study. Clin Cancer Res. 2004;10(17):5670–6.
46. Fornier MN, Seidman AD, Panageas KS, et al. Correlation of ER/PR [immunohistochemistry (IHC)] status to HER2 status by IHC and gene amplification (GA) [fluorescent in-situ hybridization (FISH)], and response rate (RR) for weekly (W) trastuzumab (H) and paclitaxel (T) in metastatic breast cancer (MBC) patients (pts). Proc Am Soc Clin Oncol. 2002;21:56a.
47. Pinto AE, Andre S, Pereira T, et al. C-erbB-2 oncoprotein overexpression identifies a subgroup of estrogen receptor positive (ER+) breast cancer patients with poor prognosis. Ann Oncol. 2001;12:525–33.
48. Lipton A, Ali SM, Leitzel K, et al. Elevated serum Her-2/neu level predicts decreased response to hormone therapy in metastatic breast cancer. J Clin Oncol. 2002;20:1467–72.
49. Benz CC, Scott GK, Sarup JC, et al. Estrogen-dependent, tamoxifen-resistant tumorigenic growth of MCF-7 cells transfected with HER2/neu. Breast Cancer Res Treat. 1993;24:85–95.
50. Mackey JR, Kaufman B, Clemens M, et al. Trastuzumab prolongs progression-free survival in hormone-dependent and HER2-positive metastatic breast cancer. Breast Cancer Res and Treat. 2006;100:abstract 3.
51. Ellis MJ, Coop A, Singh B, et al. Letrozole is more effective neoadjuvant endocrine therapy than tamoxifen for ErbB-1- and/or ErbB-2-positive, estrogen receptor-positive primary breast cancer: evidence from a phase III randomized trial. J Clin Oncol. 2001;19:3808–16.
52. Marcom PK, Isaacs C, Harris L, et al. The combination of letrozole and trastuzumab as first or second-line biological therapy produces durable responses in a subset of HER2 positive and ER positive advanced breast cancers. Breast Cancer Res Treat. 2007;102(1):43–9.
53. Kaufman B1, Mackey JR, Clemens MR, et al. Trastuzumab plus anastrozole versus anastrozole alone for the treatment of postmenopausal women with human epidermal growth factor receptor 2-positive, hormone receptor-positive metastatic breast

cancer: results from the randomized phase III TAnDEM study. J Clin Oncol. 2009;27(33):5529–37.
54. Tripathy D, Slamon DJ, Cobleigh M. Safety of treatment of metastatic breast cancer with trastuzumab beyond disease progression. J Clin Oncol. 2004;22(6):1063–70.
55. Fountzilas G, Razis E, Tsavdaridis D, et al. Continuation of trastuzumab beyond disease progression is feasible and safe in patients with metastatic breast cancer: a retrospective analysis of 80 cases by the hellenic cooperative oncology group. Clin Breast Cancer. 2003;4(2):120–5.
56. Gelmon KA, Mackey J, Verma S. Use of trastuzumab beyond disease progression: observations from a retrospective review of case histories. Clin Breast Cancer. 2004;52–8:discussion 59-62.
57. Von Minckwitz G, Vogel P, Schmidt M, et al. Trastuzumab treatment beyond progression in patients with HER2 positive metastatic breast cancer—the TBP study (GBG 26/BIG 3-05). In: San Antonio breast cancer symposium, San Antonio, 13th–16th Dec 2007; abstract 4056.
58. Petrelli F, Barni S. A pooled analysis of 2618 patients treated with trastuzumab beyond progression for advanced breast cancer. Clin Breast Cancer. 2013;13(2):81–7.
59. Jackisch C, Welslau M, Schoenegg W, et al. Impact of trastuzumab treatment beyond disease progression for advanced/metastatic breast cancer on survival—results from a prospective, observational study in Germany. Breast. 2014;23 (5):603–8.
60. Howard A, Burris HA III. Dual kinase inhibition in the treatment of breast cancer: initial experience with the EGFR/ErbB-2 inhibitor lapatinib. Oncologist. 2004;9(suppl 3):10–5.
61. Blackwell KL1, Burstein HJ, Storniolo AM, et al. Randomized study of lapatinib alone or in combination with trastuzumab in women with ErbB2-positive, trastuzumab-refractory metastatic breast cancer. J Clin Oncol. 2010;28(7):1124–30.
62. Cameron D1, Casey M, Press M, et al. A phase III randomized comparison of lapatinib plus capecitabine versus capecitabine alone in women with advanced breast cancer that has progressed on trastuzumab: updated efficacy and biomarker analyses. Breast Cancer Res Treat. 2008;112(3):533–43.
63. Lin NU1, Diéras V, Paul D, et al. Multicenter phase II study of lapatinib in patients with brain metastases from HER2-positive breast cancer. Clin Cancer Res. 2009;15(4):1452–9.
64. Scheuer W, Friess T, Burtscher H, et al. Strongly enhanced antitumor activity of trastuzumab and pertuzumab combination treatment on HER2-positive human xenograft tumor models. Cancer Res. 2009;69:9330–6.
65. Nahta R, Hung MC, Esteva FJ. The HER-2-targeting antibodies trastuzumab and pertuzumab synergistically inhibit the survival of breast cancer cells. Cancer Res. 2004;64:2343–6.
66. Baselga J, Gelmon KA, Verma S, et al. Phase II trial of pertuzumab and trastuzumab in patients with human epidermal growth factor receptor 2-positive metastatic breast cancer that progressed during prior trastuzumab therapy. J Clin Oncol. 2010;28:1138–44.
67. Swain SM, Kim SB, Cortés J, et al. Pertuzumab, trastuzumab, and docetaxel for HER2-positive metastatic breast cancer (CLEOPATRA study): overall survival results from a randomised, double-blind, placebo-controlled, phase 3 study. Lancet Oncol. 2013;14(6):461–71.
68. Swain SM, Baselga J, Miles D, et al. Incidence of central nervous system metastases in patients with HER2-positive metastatic breast cancer treated with pertuzumab, trastuzumab, and docetaxel: results from the randomized phase III study CLEOPATRA. Ann Oncol. 2014;25(6):1116–21.
69. Erickson HK, Park PU, Widdison WC, et al. Antibody-maytansinoid conjugates are activated in targeted cancer cells by lysosomal degradation and linker-dependent intracellular processing. Cancer Res. 2006;66:4426–33.
70. Lewis Phillips GD, Li G, Dugger DL, et al. Targeting HER2-positive breast cancer with trastuzumab-DM1, an antibody-cytotoxic drug conjugate. Cancer Res. 2008;68:9280–90.
71. Burris HA 3rd, Rugo HS, Vukelja SJ, et al. Phase II study of the antibody drug conjugate trastuzumab-DM1 for the treatment of human epidermal growth factor receptor 2 (HER2)-positive breast cancer after prior HER2-directed therapy. J Clin Oncol. 2011;29:398–405.
72. Krop IE, LoRusso P, Miller KD, et al. A phase II study of trastuzumab emtansine in patients with human epidermal growth factor receptor 2-positive metastatic breast cancer who were previously treated with trastuzumab, lapatinib, an anthracycline, a taxane, and capecitabine. J Clin Oncol. 2012;30:3234–41.
73. Hurvitz SA, Dirix L, Kocsis J, et al. Phase II randomized study of trastuzumab emtansine versus trastuzumab plus docetaxel in patients with human epidermal growth factor receptor 2-positive metastatic breast cancer. J Clin Oncol. 2013;31:1157–63.
74. Verma S, Miles D, Gianni L, et al. Trastuzumab emtansine for HER2-positive advanced breast cancer. N Engl J Med. 2012;367:1783–91.
75. Amiri-Kordestani L, Blumenthal GM, Xu QC, et al. FDA approval: ado-trastuzumab emtansine for the treatment of patients with HER2-positive metastatic breast cancer. Clin Cancer Res. 2014;20:4436–41.
76. Krop IE, Kim SB, González-Martín A, et al. Trastuzumab emtansine versus treatment of physician's choice for pretreated HER2-positive advanced breast cancer (TH3RESA): a randomised, open-label, phase 3 trial. Lancet Oncol. 2014;15:689–99.
77. Paul Anthony Ellis, Carlos H. Barrios, Wolfgang Eiermann et al. Phase III, randomized study of trastuzumab emtansine (T-DM1) ± pertuzumab (P) vs trastuzumab + taxane (HT) for first-line treatment of HER2-positive MBC: primary results from the MARIANNE study. J Clin Oncol. 2015;33(suppl; abstr 507).
78. Romond EH, Perez EA, Bryant J, et al. Trastuzumab plus adjuvant chemotherapy for operable HER2-positive breast cancer. N Engl J Med. 2005;353:1673–84.
79. Slamon D, Eiermann W, Robert N, et al. Adjuvant trastuzumab in HER-2 positive breast cancer. N Engl J Med. 2011;365:1273–83.
80. Slamon D, Eiermann W, Robert N, et al. Adjuvant trastuzumab in HER-2 positive breast cancer. N Engl J Med. 2011;365:1273–83.
81. Perez EA, Suman VJ, Davidson NE, et al. Sequential versus concurrent trastuzumab in adjuvant chemotherapy for breast cancer. J Clin Oncol. 2011;29:4491–7.
82. Joensuu H, Kellokumpu-Lehtinen PL, Bono P, et al. Adjuvant docetaxel or vinorelbine with or without trastuzumab for breast cancer. N Engl J Med. 2006;354:809–0.
83. Leyland-Jones B, Gelmon K, Ayoub JP, et al. Pharmacokinetics, safety, and efficacy of trastuzumab administered every three weeks in combination with paclitaxel. J Clin Oncol. 2003;21:3965–71.
84. Pivot X, Romeiu G, Debled M, et al. 6 months versus 12 months of adjuvant trastuzumab for patients with HER-2 positive early breast cancer (PHARE): a randomised phase 3 trial. Lancet Oncol. 2013;14:741–8.
85. Goldhirsch A, Gelber RD, Piccart-Gebhart MJ, et al. 2 year versus 1 year of adjuvant trastuzumab for HER2 positive breast cancer (HERA): an open label randomised controlled trial. Lancet. 2013;382:1021–8.
86. Slamon D, Eiermann W, Robert N, et al. Adjuvant trastuzumab in HER2-positive breast cancer. N Engl J Med. 2011;365(14):1273–83.

87. Vas-Luis I, Ottesen RA, Hughes ME, et al. Outcomes by tumor subtype and treatment pattern in women with small node negative breast cancer: a multi-institutional study. J Clin Oncol. 2014;32:2142–50.
88. Gonzalez-Angulo AM, Litton JK, Broglio KR, et al. High risk of recurrence for patients with breast cancer who have human epidermal growth factor receptor 2-positive, node-negative tumors 1 cm or smaller. J Clin Oncol. 2009;27:5700–6.
89. Chia S, Norris B, Speers C, et al. Human epidermal growth factor receptor 2 overexpression as a prognostic factor in a large tissue microarray series of node-negative breast cancers. J Clin Oncol. 2008;26:5697–704.
90. Tolaney SM, Barry WT, Dang CT, et al. Adjuvant paclitaxel and trastuzumab for node negative HER2 positive breast cancer. N Engl J Med. 2015;372:134–41.
91. Piccart-Gebhart M, Holmes AP, Baselga J, et al. First results from the phase III ALTTO trial (BIG 02-06; NCCTG 063D) comparing one year of anti-HER2 therapy with lapatinib alone (L), trastuzumab alone (T), their sequence (T then L) or their combination (L & T) in the adjuvant treatment of HER2-positive early breast cancer (EBC). 50th ASCO Annual Meeting. June 2014. Chicago, IL; 2014.
92. Goss PE, Smith IE, O'Shaughnessy J, et al. Adjuvant lapatinib for women with early-stage HER2-positive breast cancer: a randomised, controlled, phase 3 trial. Lancet Oncol. 2013;14 (1):88–96.
93. http://www.cancer.gov/publications/dictionaries/cancer-drug?CdrID=453548.
94. Chan A, Delaloge S, Holmes FA, et al. Neratinib after adjuvant chemotherapy and trastuzumab in HER2-positive early breast cancer: Primary analysis at 2 years of a phase 3, randomized, placebo-controlled trial (ExteNET). J Clin Oncol. 2015;33: (suppl; abstr 508).
95. Petit AM, Rak J, Hung MC, et al. Neutralizing antibodies against epidermal growth factor and ErbB-2/neu receptor tyrosine kinases down-regulate vascular endothelial growth factor production by tumor cells in vitro and in vivo: angiogenic implications for signal transduction therapy of solid tumors. Am J Pathol. 1997;151:1523–30.
96. Folkman J. Angiogenesis in cancer, vascular, rheumatoid and other disease. Nat Med. 1995;1:27–31.
97. Kim KJ, Li B, Winer J, et al. Inhibition of vascular endothelial growth factor-induced angiogenesis suppresses tumour growth in vivo. Nature. 1993;362:841–4.
98. Slamon DL, Swain SM, Buyse M, et al. Primary results from BETH, a phase 3 controlled study of adjuvant chemotherapy and trastuzumab ± bevacizumab in patients with HER2-positive, node-positive, or high-risk node-negative breast cancer. In: 2013 San Antonio breast cancer symposium. Abstract S1-03. Presented 11 Dec 2014.
99. Cortazar P, Zhang L, Untch M, et al. Pathological complete response and long term clinical benefit in breast cancer: the CTNEOBC pooled analysis. Lancet. 2014;384:164–72.
100. Von Minchwitz G, Untch M, Blohmer JU, et al. Definition and impact of pathologic complete response on prognosis after neoadjuvant chemotherapy in various intrinsic breast cancer subtypes. J Clin Oncol. 2012;30:1796–804.
101. Gianni L, Eiermann W, Semiglazov V, et al. Neoadjuvant chemotherapy with trastuzumab followed by adjuvant trastuzumab versus neoadjuvant chemotherapy alone, in patients with HER2-positive locally advanced breast cancer (the NOAH trial): a randomised controlled superiority trial with a parallel HER2-negative cohort. Lancet. 2010;375:377–84.
102. Untch M, Loibl S, Bischoff J, et al. Lapatinib versus trastuzumab in combination with neoadjuvant anthracycline-taxane-based chemotherapy (GeparQuinto, GBG 44): a randomised phase 3 trial. Lancet Oncol. 2012;13:135–44.
103. Guarneri V, Frassoldati A, Bottini A, et al. Preoperative chemotherapy plus trastuzumab, lapatinib, or both in human epidermal growth factor receptor 2-positive operable breast cancer: results of the randomized phase II CHER-LOB study. J Clin Oncol. 2012;30:1989–95.
104. Baselga J, Bradbury I, Eidtmann H, et al. Lapatinib with trastuzumab for HER2-positive early breast cancer (NeoALTTO): a randomised, open label, multicentre, phase 3 trial. Lancet. 2012;379:633–40.
105. Robidoux A, Tang G, Rastogi P, et al. Lapatinib as a component of neo- adjuvant therapy for HER2+ operable breast cancer: NSABP protocol B-41: an open label, randomised phase 3 trial. Lancet Oncol. 2013;14:1183–92.
106. Carey LA, Berry DA, Ollila D, et al. Clinical and translational results of CALGB 40601: a neoadjuvant phase III trial of weekly paclitaxel and trastuzumab with or without lapatinib for HER2-positive breast cancer. J Clin Oncol. 2013;31: (suppl; abstr 500).
107. Gianni L, Pienkowski T, Im YH, et al. Efficacy and safety of neoadjuvant pertuzumab and trastuzumab in women with locally advanced, inflammatory, or early HER2-positive breast cancer (NeoSphere): a randomised multicentre, open-label, phase 2 trial. Lancet Oncol. 2012;13:25–32.
108. Schneeweiss A, Chia S, Hickish T, et al. Pertuzumab plus trastuzumab in combination with standard neoadjuvant anthracycline-containing and anthracycline-free chemotherapy regimens in patients with HER2- positive early breast cancer: a randomized phase II cardiac safety study (TRYPHAENA). Ann Oncol. 2013;24:2278–84.
109. Park JW, Liu MC, Yee D, et al. Neratinib plus standard neoadjuvant therapy for high risk breast cancer: efficacy results from the I-SPY 2 trial. 105th AACR annual meeting 2014, April 2014. San Diego, CA; 2014.
110. Rimawi MF, Schiff R, Osborne CK. Targeting HER2 for the treatment of breast cancer. Annu Rev Med. 2015;66:111–28.
111. Rexer BN, Arteaga CL. Intrinsic and acquired resistance to HER2-targeted therapies in HER2 gene-amplified breast cancer: mechanisms and clinical implications. Crit Rev Oncog. 2012;17:1–16.
112. Lu Y, Zi X, Pollak M. Molecular mechanisms underlying IGF-I-induced attenuation of the growth-inhibitory activity of trastuzumab (Herceptin) on SKBR3 breast cancer cells. Int J Cancer. 2004;108:334–41.
113. Nahta R, Yuan LX, Zhang B, et al. Insulin-like growth factor-I receptor/human epidermal growth factor receptor 2 heterodimerization contributes to trastuzumab resistance of breast cancer cells. Cancer Res. 2005;65:11118–28.
114. Maroun CR, Rowlands T. The Met receptor tyrosine kinase: a key player in oncogenesis and drug resistance. Pharmacol Ther. 2014;142:316–38.
115. Chen AC, Migliaccio I, Rimawi M, et al. Upregulation of mucin4 in ER-positive/HER2-overexpressing breast cancer xenografts with acquired resistance to endocrine and HER2-targeted therapies. Breast Cancer Res Treat. 2012;134: 583–93.
116. Nahta R, Takahashi T, Ueno NT, et al. P27(kip1) down-regulation is associated with trastuzumab resistance in breast cancer cells. Cancer Res. 2004;64:3981–6.
117. Giuliano M, Wang YC, Gutierrez C, et al. Parallel upregulation of Bcl2 and estrogen receptor (ER) expression in HER2+ breast cancer patients treated with neoadjuvant lapatinib. Cancer Res. 2012;72:24s (suppl; abstr S5-8).

118. Xia W, Bacus S, Hegde P, et al. A model of acquired autoresistance to a potent ErbB2 tyrosine kinase inhibitor and a therapeutic strategy to prevent its onset in breast cancer. Proc Natl Acad Sci USA. 2006;103:7795–800.
119. Clynes RA, Towers TL, Presta LG, et al. Inhibitory Fc receptors modulate in vivo cytotoxicity against tumor targets. Nat Med. 2000;6:443–6.
120. Beano A, Signorino E, Evangelista A, et al. Correlation between NK function and response to trastuzumab in metastatic breast cancer patients. J Transl Med. 2008;6:25.
121. Varchetta S, Gibelli N, Oliviero B, et al. Elements related to heterogeneity of antibody-dependent cell cytotoxicity in patients under trastuzumab therapy for primary operable breast cancer overexpressing Her2. Cancer Res. 2007;67:11991–9.

22 Inflammatory and Locally Advanced Breast Cancer

Tamer M. Fouad, Gabriel N. Hortobagyi, and Naoto T. Ueno

22.1 Introduction

The term locally advanced breast cancer (LABC) includes a variety of breast tumors with different prognoses, ranging from neglected slow-growing tumors to the aggressive inflammatory breast cancer (IBC). These tumors continue to be challenging because of their high rate of relapse and subsequent death. However, with the multidisciplinary approach that includes preoperative systemic therapy, surgery, and radiotherapy, the prognosis for these patients has improved. In general, patients with tumors larger than 5.0 cm in diameter, patient with tumors that involve the skin or the chest wall, or patients with fixed axillary lymph node metastasis, or any supraclavicular, infraclavicular, or internal mammary lymph node metastasis are considered to have LABC. This encompasses a subset of patients with stage IIB disease (T3N0) and stage IIIA to IIIC disease. A distinct subtype of LABC, IBC, is a rapidly progressive disease characterized by the presence of edema and erythema of the skin.

This chapter reviews the epidemiology, staging, diagnosis, prognostic factors, molecular markers, and treatment approaches for these malignancies. IBC, although included in the definition of LABC, will have separate annotations due to its distinct clinical presentation and aggressive behavior.

T.M. Fouad · G.N. Hortobagyi · N.T. Ueno (✉)
Department of Breast Medical Oncology, The University of Texas MD Anderson Cancer Center, 1515 Holcombe Blvd., Unit 1354, Houston, TX 77030, USA
e-mail: nueno@mdanderson.org

T.M. Fouad
e-mail: tamer.fouad@nci.cu.edu.eg

G.N. Hortobagyi
e-mail: ghortoba@mdanderson.org

22.2 Epidemiology

Since the establishment of screening programs with mammography, the rate of patients diagnosed with LABC has significantly declined. Among women who participate in regular mammographic screening programs, less than 5 % have stage III disease [1]. However, national and worldwide rates remain higher, perhaps because many women from underserved populations in the USA and other countries do not have access to screening programs; in consequence, LABC constitutes approximately 8–10 % of women diagnosed with breast cancer in the USA, while in countries with limited resources that figure is closer to 60 % [2–4]. In terms of age distribution, patients diagnosed with stage III constituted the following proportions relative to all patients diagnosed with breast cancer in the USA between 2003 and 2013: 22 % of patients are 29 years or younger, 15 % are 30–39 years, 10 % are 40–49 years, 10 % are 50–59 years, 8 % are 60–69 years, 7 % are 70–79 years, and 20 % are 80 years or older according to the American College of Surgeons National Cancer Data Base statistics [4]. The same source indicates that patients with stage III breast cancer have a 5-year relative survival rate of 54 % and a 10-year relative survival rate of 36 % [4]. However, LABC includes different tumors with important variations in outcome that not only depend on the anatomical stage and biological tumor subtype but are also influenced by socioeconomic and ethnic characteristics.

IBC is a rare, distinct epidemiologic form of LABC. An analysis by Hance et al. of the Surveillance, Epidemiology, and End Results (SEER) database [5] looked at 180, 224 histologically confirmed invasive breast cancer patients diagnosed between the years 1988 and 2000. IBC comprised approximately 2 % of all breast cancer cases in the database. The mean age at diagnosis of IBC was 58.8 years, and these patients were younger than patients with non-IBC LABC, who tended to present at a mean age of 66.2 years ($P < 0.001$). Interestingly, among women with IBC, the median age at diagnosis was younger for African American

I. Jatoi and A. Rody (eds.), *Management of Breast Diseases*, DOI 10.1007/978-3-319-46356-8_22

women than for white women. During this time period, the analysis also showed the incidence rate of IBC increasing by approximately 25 % for white women (2.0–2.5 cases per 100,000 women-years) and 19 % for black women (2.6–3.1 cases per 100,000 women-years) [6]. Differences in IBC incidence rates have also been observed within different states in the USA, and also across different countries, accounting for approximately 6 and 10 % of all breast cancers in Tunisia and Egypt, respectively [7–9]. Due to the rarity of IBC, epidemiological studies that have addressed the etiology of IBC are sparse and mostly retrospective. Factors such as age of menarche, menopausal status, smoking, and alcohol consumption have not been consistently associated with IBC [6, 10]. In a small retrospective study by Chang et al. [10], high body mass index (BMI > 26.65 kg/m^2) was associated with an increased risk of IBC when compared to non-IBC patients (odds ratio >2.40, 95 % CI 1.05–5.73). Clinical and epidemiological studies that have investigated the clinical outcome of patients with IBC have consistently demonstrated a worse outcome when compared to both LABC and non-T4 breast cancer, stage for stage [11–13]. In the SEER study by Hance et al. [5], IBC accounted for 7 % of all breast cancer-specific deaths and had a median survival of 2.9 years compared to 6.4 years for patients with LABC. Anderson et al. [14] showed that the 5-year actuarial survivals for all breast cancer patients who had either estrogen receptor (ER)-positive or ER-negative tumors were 91 % (95 % CI, 90.8–91.2 %) and 77 % (95 % CI, 76.6–77.5 %), respectively, when compared to IBC patients whose corresponding survivals were 48.5 % (95 % CI, 45.2–52.1 %) and 25.3 % (95 % CI, 22.1–28.5 %) for ER-positive and ER-negative tumors, respectively.

22.3 Diagnosis and Staging

Like any breast cancer, LABC can be detected by mammography, but most of the cases are easily palpable and even visible since some of them represent neglected tumors present for a long time before diagnosis. However, some LABC can present without a dominant mass, requiring diagnostic mammographic and sonographic assessment and, on occasions, magnetic resonance imaging (MRI). Core needle biopsy is the preferred method for histologic diagnosis. Incisional biopsies are seldom required. Diagnosis can also be established by fine needle aspirate (FNA). Although this modality cannot differentiate invasive from noninvasive tumors, it provides information about tumor grade, estrogen, progesterone, and HER2/*neu* receptor status, as well as other markers, such as p53 and Ki67. FNA may also be used to confirm the presence of lymph node metastasis when guided by ultrasound. Once the diagnosis of invasive cancer is made, the patient should undergo a full staging evaluation to determine the extent of the disease. A complete physical examination is complemented with baseline biochemical profile and tumor markers. Bilateral mammograms are essential to rule out clinically occult lesions in the same or the contralateral breast. Ultrasonography is useful to measure tumor size but is even more important to assess whether axillary, supraclavicular, or infraclavicular lymph nodes are involved. MRI is used mainly to define the extent of local disease in patients for whom neither mammography nor sonography provides clear bidimensional measurements. Additionally, it is crucial to mark the exact tumor site with titanium clips or other radiopaque material under mammographic or sonographic guidance before administering neoadjuvant therapy, especially given the improved complete clinical and pathological response rates with newer regimens. This procedure is mandatory in patients who are candidates for breast conservation surgery as well as for accurate pathological assessment of the tumor bed [15].

Once the extent of local involvement is established, patients should have evaluation for systemic disease. Chest radiograph, radionuclide bone scan, and computed tomography (CT) of the abdomen are usually obtained to rule out distant metastases. Other tests, such as CT scan of the chest, pelvis, or brain, and body MRI are performed if physical examination or symptoms indicate the need for these examinations. Increasingly, positron emission tomography (PET) is being employed for initial staging of patients with locally advanced breast cancer and to determine the potential malignant nature of solitary masses in other organs [16, 17].

The diagnosis of IBC is clinical. Unlike other forms of invasive breast cancer that usually present with a painless mass, IBC has a variety of clinical presentations, making the diagnosis somewhat difficult. In 1956, Haagensen [18] recognized this problem and established a set of clinical diagnostic criteria that are still in use. Clinical characteristics of IBC include a painful, tender, rapidly enlarging breast, and edema and erythema of the skin of the breast. More often than not, a breast mass is not palpable. Other changes associated with IBC include "peau d'orange" (skin of an orange) appearance of the overlying skin of the breast [19] that represents the exaggerated appearance of hair follicle pits that occurs secondary to skin edema. Flattening, crusting, and retraction of the nipple can also occur as the disease progresses [20]. Unfortunately, most of the clinical characteristics associated with IBC are nonspecific, resulting in a significant number of cases being initially diagnosed as mastitis or breast abscesses. This results in delays in appropriate investigation, and together with the rapid rate of disease progression that is pathognomonic of IBC, a significant proportion of patients present with advanced disease. Multiple reports have shown the high frequency of ipsilateral axillary and supraclavicular lymph node involvement, with up to one-third of patients also presenting with distant metastases at the time of diagnosis compared to non-IBC [5, 11, 13]. Figure 22.1 shows different clinical presentations of IBC. The pathological characteristic of IBC is the presence of dermal lymphatic invasion, and although this frequently correlates with the clinical findings, it is not always the case and therefore it is not considered pathognomonic of IBC but is helpful in confirming the clinical diagnosis. The TNM system from the American Joint Committee on Cancer (AJCC) designates IBC as a T4d tumor that is staged as either IIIB, IIIC or IV, depending on the staging work-up [21].

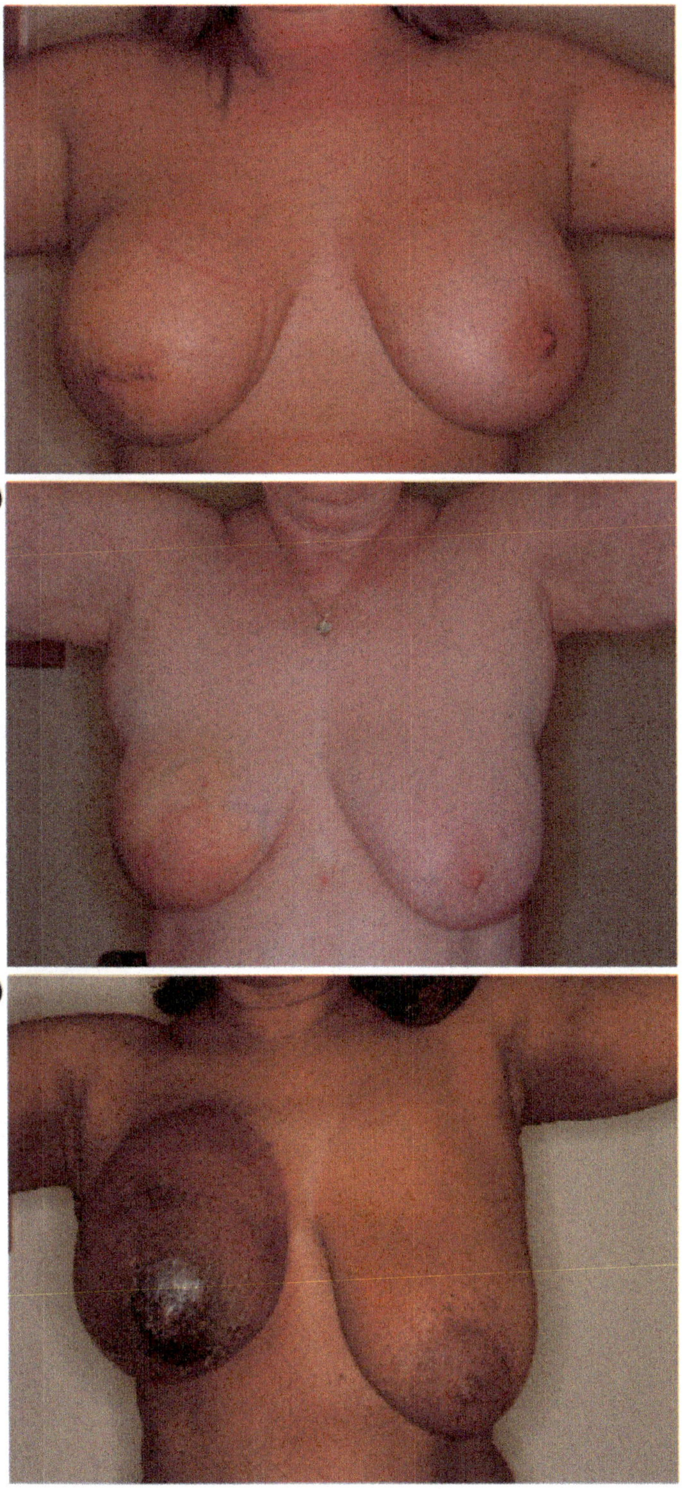

Fig. 22.1 Different presentations of inflammatory breast cancer: mild erythema and edema **a**, skin discoloration **b**, classic "*peau d'orange*" (skin of an *orange*), flattening, crusting, and retraction of the nipple can also occur as the disease progresses **c**

As with LABC, histologic diagnosis of invasive breast cancer can be made by core biopsy or FNA, although two additional skin punch biopsies are highly recommended. Baseline assessment is the same recommended for any LABC; unfortunately, IBC grows to advanced stages without necessarily forming a palpable mass, and this pattern of growth, which infiltrates in sheaths, as opposed to forming masses explains why many IBCs are difficult to image with conventional mammography. However, new imaging techniques are being studied for the diagnosis and follow-up of this disease. In an 80-patient study at the MD Anderson Cancer Center, MRI was the most accurate imaging technique in detecting a primary breast parenchymal lesion in IBC patients. Sonography was useful in diagnosing regional nodal disease. PET/CT provided additional information on distant metastasis [22]. Figure 22.2 shows a case of IBC imaged by MRI and PET scan.

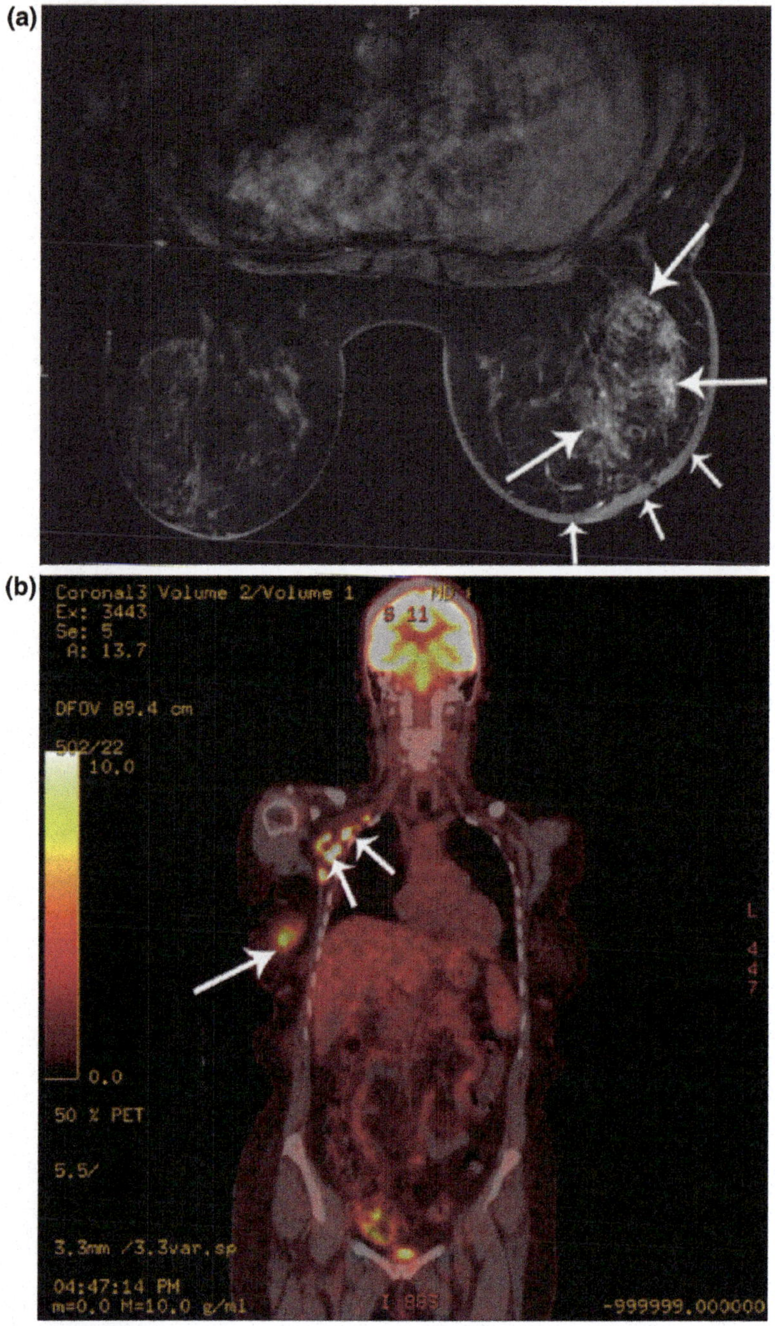

Fig. 22.2 Contrast-enhanced T1-weighted fat-saturated axial image shows asymmetric nonmass-like enhancement in the *right* breast (*long arrows*), with marked global skin thickening (*short arrows*) **a**. Coronal PET/CT in a different plane shows hypermetabolic *right* breast mass (*long arrows*), and *right* subpectoral adenopathy (*short arrows*) **b**

22.4 Management

LABC and IBC should be treated by a multidisciplinary team, where all interested specialists (radiologists, pathologists, medical oncologists, surgeons, and radiation oncologists) examine the patient, review the diagnostic tests, and together determine the best type and sequence of treatments before they are implemented.

22.5 Systemic Therapy

Preoperative systemic therapy (chemotherapy, HER2-directed therapy, or hormonal therapy) is advantageous since it has the potential of in vivo assessment of tumor response and of reducing the extent of the primary tumor and regional lymphatic disease to make breast conservation an option. The selection of the appropriate preoperative therapy should be carefully considered on a case-by-case basis.

22.5.1 Neoadjuvant Chemotherapy

22.5.1.1 Preoperative Anthracycline and Taxane

The current standard neoadjuvant regimen for the treatment of both LABC and IBC includes anthracycline and taxane [23]. Ever since the first clinical trials with neoadjuvant chemotherapy were reported in the 1970s [24], several randomized trials as well as in a large meta-analysis have demonstrated that neoadjuvant and adjuvant chemotherapy produce equivalent outcomes in both patients with operable and locally advanced disease.

The National Surgical Adjuvant Breast and Bowel Project (NSABP) B-18 randomized 1523 patients with T1-3, N1-0, and M0 breast cancer to receive either a preoperative or postoperative regimen consisting of four cycles of doxorubicin plus cyclophosphamide (AC) [25]. Overall, a clinical complete response (CR) was seen in 35 % of patients, but only 17 % of patients who had locally advanced disease with a primary tumor greater than 5 cm in diameter had a clinical CR. Rates of response to primary chemotherapy were 75 % for all patients with LABC compared with 81 % for patients with tumors measuring 2–5 cm in diameter and 79 % for patients with tumors less than 2 cm. In this trial, comparison of the adjuvant and neoadjuvant groups revealed no differences in the 5-year rates of disease-free survival (66.3 % vs. 66.7 %) or OS (80.0 % vs. 79.6 %). No survival differences were seen in the subgroup of patients with T3 tumors. However, in an update of the trial results presented at the National Cancer Institute State of the Sciences Meeting, there was significantly higher recurrence-free survival rate for patients treated with neoadjuvant chemotherapy, although this benefit appeared to be restricted to the premenopausal group [25]. Similarly, the NSABP B-27 study included women with T3 or N1 breast tumors. All patients received four cycles of AC preoperatively and were randomized to either no additional preoperative chemotherapy (group 1), four additional cycles of preoperative docetaxel 100 mg/m^2 (group 2), or four additional cycles of docetaxel given after surgery (group 3). All treatment groups showed similar OS and DFS rates [25]. Moreover, a meta-analysis of 9 randomized trials that included patients with stage III showed no differences in terms of mortality, disease progression, or distant disease recurrence between patients who received neoadjuvant and adjuvant treatments for breast cancer [26].

The benefit of adding a taxane to the standard anthracycline-based neoadjuvant regimen for LABC was confirmed in multiple studies. The NSABP-B27 trial, discussed above, demonstrated that preoperative AC followed by docetaxel was associated with equivalent DFS and OS to the postoperative treatment arms. Moreover, the addition of docetaxel was associated with increased pCR rates when compared with preoperative AC alone (26.1 % vs. 13.7 %, $P < 0.0001$) [25]. A similar result was reported in a study from MD Anderson Cancer Center, which showed that paclitaxel followed by fluorouracil, doxorubicin, and cyclophosphamide (FEC) resulted in improved pCR rates from 15.7 to 28.2 % [27]. Taxanes given as a single agent were found to be less effective than either the dose-dense or sequential regimens. The role concurrent versus sequential taxanes and dose-dense chemotherapy was evaluated in more detail in the "GeparDuo" study by the German Gynecologic Oncology Group (AGO) [28]. This phase III study investigated 913 women with untreated operable breast cancer (T2-3, N0-2, and M0) randomly assigned to receive either doxorubicin plus docetaxel (concurrent) every 14 days for four cycles with filgrastim support, or doxorubicin plus cyclophosphamide every 21 days followed by docetaxel every 21 days for four cycles each (sequential). The likelihood of achieving pCR was significantly greater with sequential docetaxel (14.3 %; $n > 63$) than with concurrent (7.0 %; $n > 31$) (odds ratio, 2.22; 90 % CI, 1.52–3.24; $P < 0.001$).

22.5.1.2 Platinum Agents

The addition of carboplatin to neoadjuvant therapy for patients with locally advanced TNBC stems from its activity in the treatment of metastatic TNBC as well as from its proposed role in TNBC associated with BRCA1 mutation carriers. In the German GeparSixto trial, patients received a 3-drug backbone neoadjuvant regimen consisting of paclitaxel and nonpegylated liposomal doxorubicin with bevacizumab and were then randomized to either additional carboplatin (weekly) or no carboplatin [29]. Patients who received additional carboplatin experienced significantly higher pCR rates (53 % vs. 37 %). However, this was also accompanied by a higher rate of toxicity-associated treatment discontinuation (49 % vs. 36 %) in the carboplatin arm. In the CALGB 40603 phase II trial, patients received weekly paclitaxel plus dose-dense AC and were randomly assigned to concurrent carboplatin and/or bevacizumab [30]. The improved pCR rate (54 % vs. 41 %) seen with the addition of carboplatin was again associated with more severe (grade 3/4) toxicity. In this study, only 80 % of patients who were assigned to receive carboplatin were able to complete all four doses due to therapy-related adverse effects. Similarly, improved pCR rates were seen in the adaptive multicohort phase II trial, I-SPY 2, which randomly assigned patients with TNBC to receive dose-dense AC/T plus or minus the combination of carboplatin and an oral PARP inhibitor (veliparib). Whether this improvement was attributed to carboplatin, veliparib, or the combination was not determined [31]. Despite consistently higher pCR rates associated with carboplatin in these trials, it comes at the expense of significant treatment-related toxicity and delays and it is not clear if this translates into long-term benefits. This has led many to express caution regarding the routine incorporation of carboplatin in the treatment of patients with triple-negative disease.

22.5.1.3 Other Noncross-Resistant Agents

The GeparTrio study tested the role of noncross-resistant chemotherapy after no clinical response to two cycles of docetaxel, doxorubicin, and cyclophosphamide (TAC) [32]. Patients with histologically confirmed invasive, unilateral, or bilateral breast cancer were included in the GeparTrio study. LABC was eligible and randomized to a different stratum. Six-hundred and twenty nonresponding patients were randomized to continue TAC or to receive a combination of vinorelbine and capecitabine for four cycles. The pCR rates were similar and quite low in both arms of the study (5.3 % vs. 5.9 %, $P > 0.7$). This study, as well as the Aberdeen neoadjuvant trial [33], shows the low probabilities of pCR in clinical nonresponders to initial chemotherapy. Similar results were confirmed later in the GeparQuinto [34].

22.5.2 Preoperative HER2-Directed Therapy

22.5.2.1 Trastuzumab

Several prospective studies of LABC have addressed the role of trastuzumab in combination with primary systemic chemotherapy in patients with HER2-positive tumors. The first study reported used a combination docetaxel and cisplatin every 3 weeks with weekly trastuzumab for four cycles in 48 patients (including some IBC patients). The pCR rate was 17 % in breast and axilla, and the regimen was well tolerated [35]. A second single-arm study used a combination of docetaxel and trastuzumab in 22 patients. They reported a clinical complete response (CR) rate of 40 %, including nine patients with IBC [36]. The NOAH (NeOAdjuvant Herceptin) trial [37, 38] is the largest international phase III randomized trial of neoadjuvant trastuzumab in combination with chemotherapy in patients with HER2-positive LABC. All patients received neoadjuvant chemotherapy with three cycles of doxorubicin–paclitaxel, 4 cycles of paclitaxel, and 3 cycles of cyclophosphamide/methotrexate/5-fluorouracil. Patients with HER2-positive tumors ($n > 288$) were randomized to receive concomitant trastuzumab or chemotherapy alone. Addition of trastuzumab significantly improved the pCR rate (43 % vs. 23 %, $P > 0.002$). The authors concluded that neoadjuvant trastuzumab in combination with chemotherapy is feasible and highly active in patients with HER2-positive LABC. A pooled analysis of two randomized studies of neoadjuvant trastuzumab, including the NOAH trial above, confirmed the improved pCR rates, lower relapse rates, and a trend toward lower mortality associated with the administration of trastuzumab [37, 39, 40]. The largest benefit was observed in locally advanced patients.

22.5.2.2 Pertuzumab

Pertuzumab is a recombinant, humanized, monoclonal antibody that inhibits dimerization of HER2 and has a complementary mechanism of action to trastuzumab by binding to a different epitope of the HER2 receptor. The combination of pertuzumab with trastuzumab and docetaxel as a neoadjuvant regimen received accelerated approval by the FDA in the neoadjuvant setting for patients with HER2-positive locally advanced tumors. This was based on higher pCR levels seen with the combination in two phase II trials: NeoSphere and TRYPHAENA. Both studies included patients with IBC. The NeoSphere trial randomized patients into one of four groups: trastuzumab plus docetaxel, pertuzumab plus docetaxel, pertuzumab and trastuzumab, or the combination all of three drugs. The combination of pertuzumab plus trastuzumab and docetaxel was associated with higher pCR rates compared to trastuzumab plus docetaxel (45.8 % vs. 29 %; $P = 0.0063$) [41]. A 5-year analysis that was recently published shows overlapping confidence intervals for both PFS and DFS [42]. Similarly, in the TRYPHAENA trial, 223 women with operable, locally advanced, or inflammatory HER2-positive breast cancer were assigned to receive trastuzumab plus pertuzumab and randomly assigned to receive either concurrent FEC followed by concurrent docetaxel, FEC alone followed by concurrent docetaxel or concurrent docetaxel and carboplatin [43]. The incidence of adverse cardiac events was low (≤5 %), and the pCR rates were equivalent across all three arms (62, 57, and 66 %). Surprisingly, both these trials report high pCR rates even when dual HER2-targeted therapy is given without chemotherapy, particularly in patients with ER-negative disease.

22.5.2.3 Lapatinib

Lapatinib is a dual tyrosine kinase inhibitor, which targets the HER2/neu and epidermal growth factor receptor (EGFR) pathways. The GeparQuinto is a phase III trial that compared the addition of either lapatinib or trastuzumab to four cycles of epirubicin/cyclophosphamide followed by docetaxel. The pCR rate was higher in patients who received trastuzumab plus chemotherapy compared to patients who received lapatinib plus chemotherapy (30.3 % vs. 22.7 %, $P = 0.04$) [44]. The lapatinib regimen was less tolerated and, given the inferior results, is not recommended in place of trastuzumab.

Several trials have explored the potential of combining two HER2-targeting therapies in the neoadjuvant setting. The NeoALTTO trial randomized patients into one of 3 arms: lapatinib plus paclitaxel, trastuzumab plus paclitaxel, or the combination of lapatinib and trastuzumab plus paclitaxel [45]. The combination arm was associated with a pCR rate of 51.3 % or an increase of 21.1 % above the trastuzumab arm ($P = 0.0001$), whereas there was no difference between the lapatinib and trastuzumab arms. The combination arm was also associated with higher grade (3/4) toxicity compared to trastuzumab alone. The extraordinary pCR rates reported in the NeoALTTO trial have been the subject of much debate after the results of two trials, the NSABP B-41 and the recently published CALGB 4060, failed to show a statistically significant difference in pCR rates between the combined trastuzumab–lapatinib arms and single-agent HER2-directed therapy [46, 47]. Moreover, a follow-up of the NeoALTTO showed no difference in terms of event-free survival or overall survival between treatment groups [48].

22.5.3 Neoadjuvant Endocrine Therapy

The role of neoadjuvant hormonal therapy for patients with LABC with hormone receptor-positive tumors has been assessed in several small studies. Veronesi et al. [49] treated 46 postmenopausal women with LABC with no inflammatory signs with tamoxifen. At 6 weeks, 17 % of patients had an objective response; with further therapy, 30 % of all patients achieved responses. Although these response rates are somewhat lower than those typically reported for chemotherapy, this study demonstrated that hormonal therapy is a safe and effective alternative in postmenopausal women for whom chemotherapy may not be an option. The MD Anderson Cancer Center experience with neoadjuvant tamoxifen includes a single-arm trial of 47 patients with LABC who either were older than 75 years or had severe comorbid conditions that precluded the use of chemotherapy. After 6 months of therapy, 47 % of patients had achieved an objective response and 6 % of patients had a CR. At a median follow-up of 40 months, 49 % of all patients remained disease-free [50]. More recently, the Grupo Español de Investigación del Cáncer de Mama (GEICAM) conducted a randomized phase II study in which 95 luminal breast cancer patients were assigned to receive either four cycles of neoadjuvant EC followed by four cycles of docetaxel or 24 weeks of exemestane (with LHRH analog in premenopausal patients) [51]. Clinical response rate was higher in the chemotherapy arm (66 % vs. 48 %); however, only 3 patients in the chemotherapy arm achieved pCR and none of the patients in the exemestane arm did. Grade 3 or 4 toxicity was significantly higher in the chemotherapy arm (47 % vs. 9 %) in this study. These results confirm that induction hormonal therapy is less effective than chemotherapy. However, for postmenopausal patients who cannot tolerate or decline chemotherapy, hormonal treatment is a viable alternative.

When it comes to the choice of neoadjuvant endocrine therapy, evidence suggests higher response rates with aromatase inhibitors compared to tamoxifen (55 % vs. 36 %) in patients with hormone receptor-positive breast cancer who were ineligible for breast-conserving surgery [52]. The PROACT trial (PreOperative Anastrozole Compared with Tamoxifen) randomly assigned 451 women with hormone receptor-positive breast cancer to treatment with three months of either neoadjuvant anastrozole or tamoxifen [53]. The study included patients with both operable and inoperable breast cancer. Overall response rates were similar for both treatment options. These studies established the benefit of neoadjuvant hormonal therapy in a subset of patients not treated with chemotherapy. However, for postmenopausal patients who can tolerate chemotherapy, this remains the recommended treatment.

22.5.4 Investigational Therapy

22.5.4.1 Angiogenesis Inhibitors

The benefit of incorporating angiogenesis inhibitors in the preoperative treatment of LABC remains unclear. Data on the use of bevacizumab in the adjuvant setting come from four clinical trials, GeparQuinto, CALGB 40603, NSABP B-40, and the recently published ARTemis. The German GeparQuinto trial randomized patients with breast cancer including those with locally advanced T3 and T4 breast cancer and IBC into one of 5 treatment arms. Initial reports found a significantly higher pCR rate in the bevacizumab arm in patients with hormone receptor-negative disease only [54]. Despite the encouraging results from GeparQuinto, a recent update failed to show an improvement in DFS or OS rates among patients who received bevacizumab [55]. In the CALGB 40603 phase II trial, patients received weekly paclitaxel plus dose-dense AC and were randomly assigned to concurrent carboplatin and/or bevacizumab [30]. The addition of bevacizumab improved pCR rates (59 % vs.

48 %, $P = 0.0089$). However, the CALGB 40603 study did not support the addition of bevacizumab in patients with TNBC when the definition of pCR included the presence of residual tumor in the axilla, and it is not known whether this approach improves survival. Consistent with these results, the phase III ARTemis study also confirmed that the highest pCR rates associated with neoadjuvant bevacizumab were seen among ER-negative and minimally ER-positive patients [56]. In contrast to the other 3 trials, the NSABP B-40 reported the highest pCR rates associated with incorporation of bevacizumab in patients with hormone receptor-positive rather than negative tumors [57]. Results of the secondary outcomes of the NSABP B-40 published in 2015 reported an improved OS associated with bevacizumab, in contradiction to other studies [58]. At this time, it is not clear which patients are most likely to benefit from the addition of angiogenesis inhibitors. Given the high rates of serious adverse events and the regulatory restrictions on its use in the treatment of breast cancer, bevacizumab should only be administered within a well-designed clinical trial.

22.5.4.2 mTOR Inhibitors

The GeparQuinto trial also evaluated the use of the m-TOR inhibitor, everolimus, in combination with paclitaxel in patients who did not respond to neoadjuvant EC with or without bevacizumab. No difference in pCR rates (3.6 % vs. 5.6 %) was reported, and almost 50 % of patients in the combination arm are reported to have terminated therapy due to toxicity [54].

22.5.4.3 PARP Inhibitors

Poly(ADP-ribose) polymerases (PARP) inhibitors cause DNA damage by inhibiting enzymes involved in DNA-damage repair. This is thought to be particularly effective in tumors with defective BRCA1 or BRCA2 genes that are also involved in DNA repair. The role of the oral PARP inhibitor, veliparib, was evaluated in the neoadjuvant treatment of TNBC in the multiple cohort adaptive phase II trial, the I-SPY 2 (Investigation of Serial Studies to Predict Your Therapeutic Response with Imaging and Molecular Analysis 2). Patients with TNBC who received veliparib and carboplatin in addition to neoadjuvant dose-dense AC/T achieved higher pCR rates compared to those who did not (52 % vs. 26 %) [59]. Despite being encouraging, there was no way to determine whether the improved rates were due to carboplatin, the PARP inhibitor, or the combination.

22.5.5 Immunotherapy

Checkpoint inhibitors are antibodies that block immunoinhibitory receptors (e.g., CTLA-4 or PD-1) that are expressed on tumor cells, thus rendering tumors more susceptible to attack by cytotoxic T cells. Since their successful use in advanced melanoma, there has been considerable interest in their role in locally advanced triple-negative and inflammatory breast cancer. The Keynote 173 is an ongoing trial (NCT02622074) of pembrolizumab plus neoadjuvant chemotherapy in locally advanced triple-negative breast cancer. Pembrolizumab is an anti-PD1 antibody, which provides dual ligand blockage of PD-L1 and PD-L2 with recent approval in melanoma and clinical activity reported in multiple tumor types. Similarly, MPDL3280A is a novel PDL-1 inhibitor that is currently being tested in combination with nab-paclitaxel in neoadjuvant treatment of locally advanced TNBC (NCT02530489).

22.5.6 Systemic Therapy in Patients Who Do not Achieve PCR

Additional postoperative chemotherapy is not recommended in patients with LABC or IBC who have completed a full course of neoadjuvant chemotherapy, even in those who have not achieved pCR [60, 61]. Nonetheless, several ongoing trials are designed to assess the efficacy of new agents in patients who do not achieve pCR. These include the KATHERINE trial (NCT01772472), which compares TDM-1 and trastuzumab in patients with HER2-positive tumors who do not show pCR. OLYMPIA (NCT02032823) is a phase II trial that investigates the efficacy of olaparib in patients with TNBC who are BRCA1/2 carriers and have residual tumors after neoadjuvant chemotherapy. PENELOPE (NCT01864746) examines the role of the cyclin D kinase 4/6 inhibitor, palbociclib, when combined with endocrine therapy who have residual cancer in the lymph nodes (Table 22.1 and Fig. 22.3).

22.5.7 Systemic Therapy for Inflammatory Breast Cancer

IBC is a challenging clinical entity characterized by rapid progression and early dissemination. Before the introduction of combination chemotherapy in the treatment paradigm, IBC was a uniformly fatal disease with fewer than 5 % of patients, treated with either surgery and/or radiotherapy, surviving past 5 years, with an expected median survival of less than 15 months [69]. Its management in the last 40 years has evolved [20], with current treatment guidelines emphasizing the use of a multidisciplinary approach [70] using neoadjuvant systemic therapy followed by locoregional treatment, including surgery and RT.

Historically, the use of surgery [71], RT [72], or a combination of the two [73] improved locoregional control rates but had minimal effect on survival, and most patients died of

Table 22.1 Clinical and pathological response for stage III breast carcinoma after combined modality treatment

Authors	Year	Regimen	No. of patients	Pathological CR (%)	Clinical response (%)
NSABP B-18 [26]	2005	ACx4	743	13	79
Estevez [62]	2003	Weekly Doc	56	16	68
Buzdar [63]	1999	Pacx4 versus FACx4	174	8 16	80 80
Aberdeen trial [64]	2002	CVAPx8 CVAPx4 → Docx4	50 47	16 34	66 94
GeparDuo [28]	2005	A + Doc AC → Doc	455 458	8 16	77 87
NSABP B-27 [65]	2003	ACx4 ACx4 → Doc	762 752	9 19	86 91
AGO [66]	2002	E + Pacx4 Ex3 → Pacx4	233 242	N/A	Clinical CR: 10 18
GeparQuattro study [66]		ECx4 → Doc + Cap + Tz	456	19 45	N/A
TECHNO trial [66]		ECx4 → Pac + Tz	217	39	N/A
Coudert [67]	2006	Docx6 + Tz	33	42	88
Penault-Llorca [68]		Various regimen Without trastuzumab	51 287	23 7	N/A
Buzdar [39]	2007	Pacx4 → FECx4 Pacx4 → FECx4 + Tz	42	26 65	N/A
NOAH trial [37, 38]	2010	AP → Pac → CMF AP → Pac → CMF + Tz	235	19 38	N/A
NeoALTTO trial [45, 48]		Lap + Pac Tz + Pac Lap + Tz + Pac	450	24 29 51	53 30 67
NeoSphere [41, 42]	2012	TH THP HP TP	417	29 46 17 24	81 88 66 74
TRYPHAENA [43]	2013	Tz + Pz + FEC → Doc FEC → Doc + Tz + Pz Doc + Carbo + Tz + Pz	225	62 57 66	Clinical CR: 50 28 40

CT chemotherapy; *NA* not available; *RT* radiation therapy; *S* surgery

distant disease. One of the earliest studies that showed the benefit of neoadjuvant chemotherapy in the treatment of IBC was a retrospective analysis of 179 patients with stage III IBC, in which patients who received chemotherapy followed by surgery and RT had a superior 5-year disease-free survival of 40 % compared to 24 % for patients who received surgery and RT, and with 6 % for patients who received radiation alone [74]. Several other studies have confirmed the survival advantage conferred by the addition of neoadjuvant chemotherapy to locoregional therapy, as well as the higher survival outcomes for patients who achieve a clinical CR or a pCR [75, 76].

The use of anthracycline-based chemotherapy is known to improve both disease-free survival and OS in breast cancer patients [76]. The MD Anderson group compared four anthracycline-containing regimens in combination with locoregional therapy in a total of 242 patients with IBC [77–80]. All four regimens had equal efficacy, with an overall response rate of 72 % and a pCR rate of 12 % after neoadjuvant chemotherapy. Patients who achieved either a complete or a partial response had 15-year OS rates of 51 and 31 %, respectively, compared to 7 % for those who achieved minimal response. The addition of taxanes to anthracycline neoadjuvant chemotherapy in the treatment of IBC has also shown benefit. A study from MD Anderson compared FAC

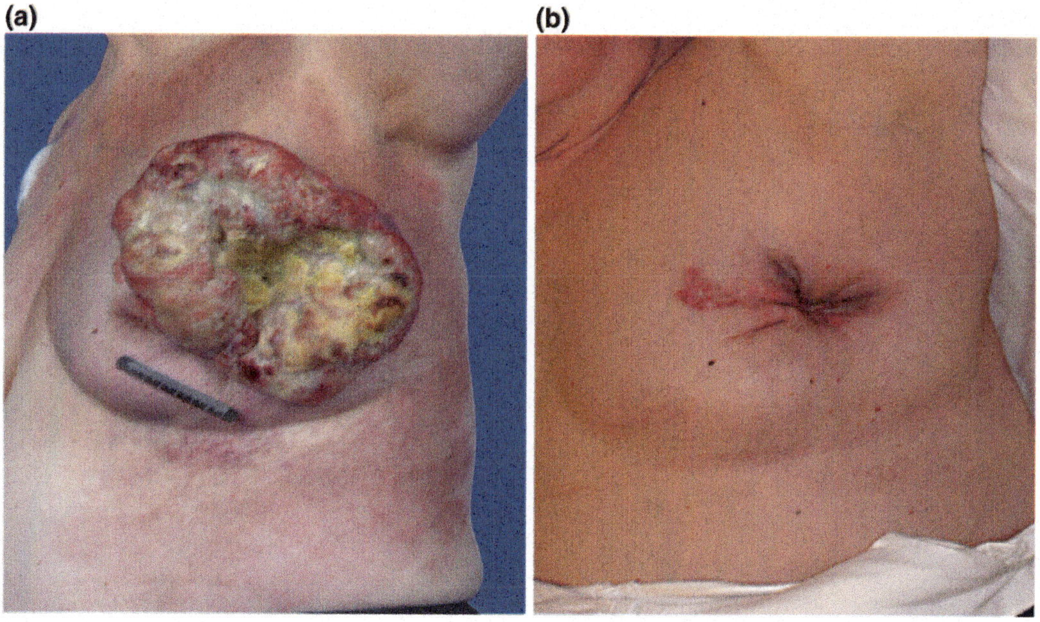

Fig. 22.3 Locally advanced breast cancer that presented with an exophytic mass **a** and follow-up after 4 cycles of 5-FU, doxorubicin, and cyclophosphamide **b**

(fluorouracil/doxorubicin/cyclophosphamide) alone with FAC followed by paclitaxel, in patients with IBC, and showed higher pCR rates (25 % vs. 10 %) and higher median OS and progression-free survival in the group receiving the additional taxane, although the survival differences were limited to the patients with ER-negative tumors [81].

A high incidence of HER2 overexpression has been observed in patients with IBC, suggesting the appropriate setting for the use of trastuzumab. Several prospective studies mentioned above that included patients with IBC have addressed the issue of trastuzumab in combination with neoadjuvant chemotherapy. The first trial, from the University of Miami, used a combination docetaxel and cisplatin every 3 weeks with weekly trastuzumab for four cycles in 33 patients with LABC and IBC, achieving pCR rate of 22 % [35]. A second study, from Baylor College of Medicine in Houston, combined docetaxel with trastuzumab in 22 patients, nine of which had IBC: 40 % of all patients had a complete clinical response [36]. The NOAH trial focused on LABC and included patients with IBC; 235 of them had HER2-positive disease and were randomized to either chemotherapy, or chemotherapy plus concomitant trastuzumab. pCR rates were 38 % in the group that received additional trastuzumab and 19 % in the group that received chemotherapy alone. These results, in combination with the survival advantage seen with the addition of adjuvant trastuzumab [82, 83] in early stage breast cancer patients, indicate an important role for trastuzumab in the treatment of patients with HER2-overexpressed/HER2-amplified IBC. Furthermore, lapatinib, a potent dual (ErbB1 and ErB2) reversible, tyrosine kinase inhibitor, is also being currently studied in patients with HER2-overexpressed IBC. A phase II trial to confirm the sensitivity of IBC to lapatinib and to determine whether response is HER2- or EGFR-dependent was completed by Johnston et al. [84] in 45 patients with recurrent or anthracycline-refractory IBC. There was a 50 % response rate to lapatinib in patients that had HER2-positive tumors; time to progression was not reported. The authors concluded that lapatinib was well tolerated with clinical activity in heavily pretreated HER2-positive, but not EGFR-positive/ HER2-negative IBC. In this study, coexpression of pHER2 and pHER3 in tumors seems to predict for a favorable response to lapatinib. Later on, a phase II trial of 42 patients with newly diagnosed HER2-positive IBC was reported by Boussen et al. [85]. Patients went on to receive lapatinib monotherapy (days 1–14) followed by an additional 12 weeks in combination with weekly paclitaxel. The primary objective was pCR in breast and lymph nodes at the time of definitive surgical resection upon completing 14 weeks of therapy. Of the evaluable patients, 78 % had a clinical response and 18 % had a pCR. Although encouraging results for the dual HER2 blockade with lapatinib–trastuzumab in addition to neoadjuvant chemotherapy were reported in the NeoALTTO study, the use of this combination has become less desirable after two phase III trials failed to show a statistically significant benefit and results from the ALTTO study failed to show an advantage for the use of lapatinib–trastuzumab in addition to chemotherapy in the adjuvant setting. The most exciting development in the treatment of stage III IBC came with the recent accelerated approval of the neoadjuvant combination of pertuzumab with trastuzumab and docetaxel in HER2-positive IBC. The regulatory approval was based on higher pCR levels seen with the combination in two phase II trials: NeoSphere and TRYPHAENA, which are discussed in detail earlier in this chapter.

The role of high-dose chemotherapy with autologous bone marrow transplant has been explored in patients with IBC, but no definitive data have demonstrated improved survival. Arun et al. described a series of 24 patients with IBC who underwent high-dose chemotherapy with autologous stem cell transplantation in addition to standard multidisciplinary treatment. The 2-year OS rate was 73 % [86]. Investigators from Washington University reported the 4-year OS rate of 47 patients treated with high-dose chemotherapy and stem cell transplantation to be at 52 % [87]. Another trial of bone marrow transplantation for IBC from Germany involved 56 patients who had a 3-year survival rate of 72 % [88]. The larger report of this intervention included 120 patients who received conventional dose chemotherapy and surgery and were treated sequentially with single- or tandem-cycle dose-intense chemotherapy regimens. At a median follow-up of 61 months (range, 21–161 months), the estimated 5-year relapse-free survival (RFS) and OS rates were 44 % (95 % CI, 34–53 %) and 64 % (95 % CI, 55–73 %), respectively [89]. The recently published PEGASE 07 trial evaluated the addition of postoperative docetaxel-5FU to dose-intense EC with stem cell support [90]. After a median follow-up of 60 months, identical results in terms of 5-year DFS (55 %) and OS (70 %) were observed in patients who received postoperative docetaxel-5FU. The use of unconventional treatment regimens in both the experimental and control arm makes this study difficult to interpret. Although the survival data from these trials seems encouraging, the patient populations were highly selected, and further research is clearly needed before high-dose chemotherapy with stem cell transplantation is recommended outside the context of a clinical trial.

Other agents that are currently being studied for the treatment of IBC include antiangiogenic agents and Ras pathway inhibitors. IBC tumors are known to be highly vascular tumors that express a number of angiogenic factors such as vascular endothelial growth factor (VEGF) [91]. This has prompted a number of studies looking at the role of anti-VEGF agents such as bevacizumab [92] and sunitinib [93], in combination with chemotherapy, in the treatment of IBC, with promising results. In a study of 21 patients with IBC and LABC, bevacizumab reduced angiogenesis in post-treatment tumor biopsies and dynamic contrast-enhanced MRI [92]. Similarly, a phase I trial of semaxanib (SU5416), a potent tyrosine kinase inhibitor that targets the VEGF pathway, showed the drug may have some clinical activities in patients with IBC [93]. Data on the clinical use of bevacizumab in the neoadjuvant setting come from 4 clinical trials. The GeparQuinto and the ARTemis trials enrolled patients with IBC, while the CALGB 40603 and the NSABP B-40 did not. Both the GeparQuinto and the ARTemis trials report highest pCR rates with the use of neoadjuvant bevacizumab among patients with hormone receptor-negative tumors. However, updated results from the GeparQuinto [55] failed to show an improvement in DFS or OS rates among patients who received bevacizumab.

Tipifarnib, a farnesyl transferase inhibitor (FTIs) that targets RhoC proteins, which are overexpressed in IBC, has entered phase II trials in combination with neoadjuvant chemotherapy for IBC [94, 95]. A phase II study (NCT01036087) exploring the role of panitumumab, nab-paclitaxel, and carboplatin followed by FEC neoadjuvant chemotherapy for patients with primary HER2-negative inflammatory breast cancer reported high pCR rates in triple-negative IBC [96]. Several agents that target the inflammatory pathways, such as chemokine receptor antagonists, prostanoid receptors (EP4) antagonists, and novel selective COX inhibitors (apricoxib, tranilast), are currently under investigation both in the preclinical and in the clinical settings in IBC [97].

22.6 Local Therapy

Historically, patients with locally advanced disease have been treated with radical mastectomy if technically possible. In 1943, Haagensen and Stout, two surgeons at Memorial Hospital in New York, published the results of surgical treatment in patients with breast cancer. They reviewed 1040 women, 61.5 % of them treated with radical mastectomy; of these, 36 % were free of disease at 5 years. Reviewing the cases of the patients whose disease recurred, the authors identified eight factors that were associated with recurrence: distant metastases, inflammatory carcinoma, supraclavicular lymph node involvement, edema of the arm, satellite breast skin nodules, intercostal or parasternal nodules, extensive edema of skin over the breast, and carcinoma that developed during pregnancy or lactation. They concluded that any of these signs of advanced disease made a tumor "categorically inoperable." The authors also defined five "grave signs": skin ulceration, edema of limited extent, fixation of tumor to the chest wall, axillary lymph nodes greater than 2.5 cm in diameter, and fixed axillary lymph nodes. Any patient who had two or more "grave signs" was also considered to have inoperable disease since only one of such patients was without disease recurrence at 5 years. Finally, the authors recommended that surgery not be performed in patients with locally advanced disease who had the worst prognoses [98]. After this publication, fewer patients with LABC were treated with mastectomy, although surgical treatment did not produce high survival rates even in those patients considered to have operable disease under the referenced criteria.

Failure of mastectomy alone to produce good survival rates prompted the use of primary RT for locally advanced tumors, especially those that were considered inoperable. In 1965, Baclesse [99] reported a series of 431 patients that received primary RT. The 5-year survival was 41 % for the 95 patients, who were classified as having Columbia Clinical Classification stage C disease, and 13 % for the 200 patients who had stage D. In a retrospective series of 454 patients with T3, or T4, nonmetastatic breast cancer who underwent primary RT and 133 of whom also underwent mastectomy, the median survival was 2.5 years, and relapse occurred in 45 % of patients within 18 months. The authors concluded that RT alone was inadequate for patients with LABC [100]. For patients who are treated with primary RT, a high dose of radiation is necessary to optimize local control. This was initially described in a retrospective review of 137 patients, by Harris et al. [101], who found that treatment with a total radiation dose greater than 6000 rads was associated with improved local control and improved freedom from distant metastatic relapse. Likewise, Sheldon et al. [102] found that among 192 patients with LABC treated with RT alone, the patients that received total doses greater than 6000 cGy had improved rates of local control (83 % vs. 70 %, $P > 0.06$). However, such higher doses were associated with long-term complications, including chest wall fibrosis, brachial plexopathy, lymphedema, skin ulceration, and rib necrosis [103, 104].

Evidence supports the importance of local control with adequate surgery and RT for LABC. A series of 542 patients treated at MD Anderson Cancer Center with neoadjuvant chemotherapy, mastectomy, and radiation were compared to 134 patients who received similar treatment but without radiation. Irradiated patients had a lower rate of local-regional recurrence (10-year rates: 11 % vs. 22 %, $P > 0.0001$), and radiation reduced local-regional recurrence for patients with clinical T3 or T4 tumors, pathological tumor size greater than 2 cm, or four or more positive nodes ($P < 0.002$ for all comparisons). Radiation improved cause-specific survival in patients with stage equal or greater than IIIB, clinical T4 tumors, and four or more positive nodes ($P < 0.007$ for all comparisons). On multivariate analyzes of cause-specific survival, the hazard ratio (HR) for lack of radiation was 2.0 (95 % CI, 1.4–2.9; $P < 0.0001$). The authors concluded that after neoadjuvant chemotherapy and mastectomy, comprehensive radiation was found to benefit both local control and survival for patients presenting with clinical T3 tumors or stage III disease and for patients with four or more positive nodes [105]. One of the benefits of neoadjuvant chemotherapy for patients with LABC is that it can result in downstaging sufficient enough to allow for breast conservation in patients who otherwise would not be candidates for limited surgery. In a review of 143 patients with stage IIB to IIIC, who had complete or partial response to induction chemotherapy and underwent mastectomy and axillary lymph node dissection at the MD Anderson Cancer Center, the authors applied strict criteria to determine which of these patients might have been candidates for breast conservation. Thirty-three patients (32 %) had complete resolution of skin edema, residual tumor diameter less than 5 cm, and absence of known multicentric disease or extensive lymphatic invasion and would have been eligible for breast conservation surgery [106]. At the time of surgery, 42 % of these patients had a pCR of the primary tumor and 45 % were node-negative; no eligible patients had multicentric disease; and none developed recurrence in the chest wall after mastectomy. At a median follow-up of 34 months, three patients had developed metastatic disease, suggesting that breast-conserving surgery is a reasonable option for carefully selected patients with LABC. Kuerer et al. [107] reviewed the MD Anderson experience of breast-conserving therapy following neoadjuvant chemotherapy in 109 patients with stage II or III breast cancer. Fifty-five percent of patients had a clinical CR and half of them had a pCR. Chemotherapy decreased the median tumor diameter from 4 to 1 cm, and due to the high response rate, the authors recommended that metallic tumor markers be placed in patients if the primary tumor shrinks to 2 cm or less in diameter. Calais et al. [108] treated patients with neoadjuvant chemotherapy followed by mastectomy for tumors at least 3 cm in diameter or lumpectomy for tumors smaller than 3 cm. They reported that 49 % of patients could be treated with breast-conserving therapy and that rates of local failure did not differ for the patients treated with mastectomy versus breast conservation. In 1978, De Lena et al. [24] demonstrated that LABC could be managed effectively with neoadjuvant chemotherapy, RT, and then adjuvant chemotherapy. With this approach, most patients had breast preservation, with a local recurrence rate of 24 %. Other investigators have similarly reported that regimens of induction chemotherapy followed by irradiation permit breast preservation and have associated rates of local relapse rates of 19–24 % [109, 110]. Some authors have recommended that breast conservation via either lumpectomy or irradiation be used only in those patients who respond to induction chemotherapy, reserving mastectomy for patients who do not adequately respond to chemotherapy [111, 112]. Table 22.2 summarizes the MD Anderson Selection Criteria and Contraindications for Breast conservation in patients with LABC. Other investigators have confirmed that with careful patient selection, breast conservation after induction chemotherapy is as effective as mastectomy in 34–81 % of patients with locally advanced disease [113, 114]. In NSABP B-18, patients who were treated with four cycles of neoadjuvant regimen of doxorubicin and

Table 22.2 MD Anderson cancer center selection criteria and contraindications for breast-conserving surgery after primary systemic therapy

Selection criteria
Patient desires breast-conserving therapy
Adequate response to neoadjuvant systemic therapy
Ability to completely excise residual disease with acceptable cosmesis
Availability of RT
Contraindications
Skin edema
Residual tumors ≥5 cm
Skin or chest wall fixation
Extensive lymphovascular invasion
Extensive suspicious microcalcifications
Multicentricity
Medical contraindications to radiation

cyclophosphamide (AC) had a higher rate of breast conservation than did women treated with adjuvant AC (67 % vs. 60 %; $P > 0.002$). However, of the 69 women who were initially recommended for mastectomy but whose tumors were downstaged and treated with lumpectomy after AC therapy, 14.5 % had recurrence in the ipsilateral breast, compared with only 6.9 % of those women who were initially candidates for lumpectomy ($P > 0.04$) [115]. Findings of the EORTC Trial 10902 were similar; 23 % of the patients in the neoadjuvant chemotherapy arm, who were initially candidates only for mastectomy, were able to be treated with lumpectomy instead [116]. In general, the indications for BCT after neoadjuvant therapy are similar to those used for women with newly diagnosed breast cancer who did not receive neoadjuvant therapy. In 2002, the American College of Surgeons, the American College of Radiology, the College of American Pathologists, and the Society of Surgical Oncology published consensus recommendations for the appropriate selection of patients for BCT [117]. Similar guidelines have been developed by the Canadian Steering Committee on Clinical Practice Guidelines for the Care and Treatment of Breast Cancer [118].

The ASCO guidelines recommend against the use of sentinel lymph node biopsy (SLNB) in women with large or locally advanced (T3/T4), or inflammatory breast cancer [119]. For these patients, axillary lymph node dissection remains unavoidable even when the nodes are clinically negative. This is based on the assumption that SLNB would be less reliable in this setting, given that larger tumors are known to have a higher risk of axillary lymph node spread (T3: 68 %; T4: 86 %) [120]. However, several studies have shown to the contrary that performing SLNB in T3 tumors with clinically negative nodes is associated with relatively low false-negative rates [121, 122]. As a result, some surgeons do not recognize performing SLNB in this setting as a contraindication. For women with LABC who wish to undergo breast reconstruction, delayed reconstruction with autologous tissue is preferred for these women especially those who are likely to need postmastectomy radiation, as this produces fewer complications with acceptable cosmetic results (Table 22.2).

The radiation dose and treatment fields used to treat breast cancer do not change with the use of neoadjuvant systemic therapy. Patients treated with breast-conserving surgery should receive postoperative whole-breast irradiation. Likewise, patients who are treated with mastectomy should receive postmastectomy radiation to the chest wall and regional lymph nodes. Although preoperative systemic therapy may cause downstaging of the disease, it should not affect the indications for postoperative radiation and decisions should be based on preoperative clinical stage. The American Society of Therapeutic Radiation Oncology recommends adjuvant RT for postmastectomy patients who had locally advanced disease or four or more positive axillary lymph nodes [123]. Buchholz et al. [124] investigated local recurrence rates in patients treated with neoadjuvant chemotherapy followed by mastectomy without adjuvant radiation. They found that the risk of local recurrence was a function of both the extent of pathological residual disease and the initial clinical stage [124, 125]. For this reason, in our institution, the current recommendation is postmastectomy irradiation for all patients with clinical LABC (any T3, or any N2-3 disease) including those who achieve pCR [126].

IBC is inoperable by definition. The standard management of this entity is multidisciplinary, including neoadjuvant chemotherapy, mastectomy, local-regional radiotherapy, and hormonal therapy for hormone receptor-positive disease. Breast-conserving surgery and SLNB are not an option for women with IBC and all women with operable disease after neoadjuvant treatment should undergo mastectomy with axillary lymph node dissection. In a small report of 26 patients with IBC, who were treated with neoadjuvant chemotherapy, RT, surgery and adjuvant chemotherapy, the authors noted local recurrences in two of ten patients treated with mastectomy and in 7 of 13 patients treated with breast conservation [127].

Immediate reconstruction following surgery should be avoided in patients with IBC given the risk of delaying radiotherapy and the high risk of local recurrence. Subsequent radiation therapy at a total dose of 60 gray (Gy) should follow mastectomy in patients that do not have poor risk factors. For women with IBC who also have risk factors for recurrence, an escalated radiation dose may achieve better locoregional control. Even with optimal local therapy, the rates of local-regional relapse from IBC remain high. In a report of 95 patients from Washington University, the local-regional failure rates were 73 % for patients treated with radiation alone, 27 % for those treated with radiation and surgery, 65 % for patients treated with chemotherapy plus radiation, and 16 % for those treated with chemotherapy, surgery, and radiation [128]. Even with combined modality, most reports show that 14–34 % of patients will experience a local recurrence [79, 128–130]. Some studies have suggested an improvement in local control by using twice-daily fractionated RT [131, 132]. Chu et al. [132] reported that such therapy reduced the rates of local relapse from 69 to 33 %. A second report by Barker et al. [131] showed a reduction from 46 to 27 %. Additional ways of reducing the rates of local-regional failure in IBC using newer techniques of RT are under investigation.

22.7 Molecular Biology of IBC

When compared to noninflammatory LABC, IBC tumors tend to be of high grade, have a negative hormone receptor status [133], and overexpress HER2 [134], all factors that predict for a poorer outcome [5]. Other biological features of IBC include the constitutive activation of major inflammatory signaling pathways, mutation at the p53 suppressor gene, overexpression of E-cadherin, and increased expression of pro-angiogenic factors.

The designation of "inflammatory" in IBC derives from the breast skin changes that resemble an acute inflammatory process. These skin changes are due to invasion of the dermal lymphatic vessels by tumor emboli rather than infiltration of inflammatory cells [135], and it is believed that these invasive tumor emboli create the reservoir for cancer cells that then further disseminate through the body to form distant metastases. However, although a true state of **inflammation** is not present in IBC, there is evidence to suggest the constitutive activation of major inflammatory signaling pathways (JAK/STAT, NF-κB, and COX-2) [97]. In a recent study, the immune-checkpoint blocker, PDL1, was overexpressed in 38 % of IBC samples [136]. This was seen in samples with estrogen receptor-negative status, basal, and ERBB2-enriched aggressive subtypes. PDL1 overexpression was also associated with better pCR rates in response to chemotherapy. Moreover, inflammatory cytokines such as interleukin-6, gamma interferon, TGF-beta, and TNF-α have been linked to tumorigenesis in IBC. This has led to the testing of anti-inflammatory agents such as selective COX-2 inhibitors in IBC [97].

High-throughput methods using **cDNA microarrays** have been used to study the phenotypic features of IBC. Van Laere et al. [137] performed genome-wide expression profiling of 16 IBC and 18 nonstage-matched non-IBC pretreatment samples. Using unsupervised hierarchical clustering, they identified a set of 50 genes that segregated IBC samples from non-IBC samples with an accuracy of 88 %. They observed a high number of nuclear factor kappa B (**NF-kB)-related genes** in the IBC samples compared to the non-IBC samples. NF-kB is an important mediator of cell migration, invasion, and metastasis that may contribute to the aggressive nature of IBC. Bertucci et al. [138] identified a set of **109 genes** (from 81 patients, 31 of which had IBC) that correctly predicted 79 % of IBC specimens and 89 % of non-IBC specimens, and a set of 85 genes that had an 85 % accuracy of predicting for pCR. In an extension of the same study [139], the authors showed that the **subtypes (luminal A and B, basal, ERBB2-overexpressing and normal breast-like)** used to classify non-IBC tumors [140] were also present in their IBC cohort, suggesting that despite the aggressive phenotype of IBC, it may not be distinguishable from other breast cancers. In contrast, Van Laere et al. [137] were able to segregate IBC tumors into basal-like and ErbB2-overexpressing groups that could be distinguished from non-IBC tumors. The discrepancy between the two studies may be explained by the different definitions of IBC used to include patients in both studies and, at the same time, illustrates how this may affect the results and interpretation of any molecular study. Using Affymetrix profile data (HGU133-series), the same group analyzed whole-genome expression data from 137 patients with IBC and 252 patients with non-IBC (nonIBC). Differences in the genomic signature were found to correspond to differences in the proportion of molecular subtypes [141]. Similarly, a separate study that compared microdissected IBC to non-IBC samples using gene expression analysis and comparative genomic hybridization was unable to demonstrate a validated dataset that identifies IBC [142], while a gene expression analysis comparing triple-negative IBC to non-IBC did not report differences in subtype distribution [143].

MicroRNAs (MiRNAs) are a class of small noncoding RNA molecules that have been found to play a role in regulating cellular proliferation, apoptosis, migration, and differentiation. MicroRNA analysis, comparing IBC to non-IBC, revealed lower expression of miRNA-205 which correlated with worse distant metastasis-free survival and overall survival [144]. Another study showed that high serum miR-19a levels were predictive of favorable clinical outcome in patients with metastatic HER2+ IBC [145].

The function of the **p53** gene product is to inhibit tumor growth through cell-cycle arrest or induction of apoptosis. Mutation or absence of the p53 gene is associated with tumor progression, and decreased response to chemotherapy occurs in at least 50 % of sporadic breast cancers; in addition, a high level of p53 protein in the nucleus is associated with poor clinical outcome [146]. In an analysis of 24 patients with IBC, Riou et al. [147] showed that patients with tumors that exhibited a combination of a p53 gene mutation and nuclear expression of the p53 protein had an 8.6-fold higher risk of death when compared to the patients with tumors with wild-type p53. An analysis of 48 patients with IBC at the MD Anderson Cancer Center [148] confirmed these results, showing a lower estimated 5-year progression-free survival and OS for patients with nuclear p53-positive (35 and 55 %, respectively) compared to p53-negative tumors (44 and 54 %, respectively).

E-cadherin, a calcium-regulated, transmembrane glycoprotein expressed in normal breast epithelium, is essential to maintain cell–cell adhesion contact and is considered to be a tumor suppressor. Loss of E-cadherin contributes to increased proliferation and promotes invasion and metastases [149]. Both animal and human IBC tumor models have paradoxically shown an increased expression of E-cadherin compared to non-IBC breast tumors. Tomlinson et al. [150] observed that in the MARY-X xenograft model, E-cadherin was overexpressed 10- to 20-fold and was required for IBC tumor emboli formation in the dermal lymphatics of nude and SCID mice. In addition, the same IBC xenograft model has also been shown to express the **sialyl-Lewis** X/A-deficient MUCI, a glycoprotein that acts as ligand for the cell adhesion receptor E-selectin and that promotes lymphovascular invasion [151]. Kleer et al. [149] confirmed these preclinical findings in patient samples by comparing 20 IBC samples to 22 stage-matched, non-IBC tumor samples. Thus, it appears that the overexpression of E-cadherin and expression of sialyl-Lewis X/A-deficient MUCI is unique to IBC and appears to contribute to the integrity of the tumor emboli as they invade dermal lymphatics.

IBC tumors are known to be highly vascular with associated features of angiolymphatic invasion consisting of increased microvessel density, high endothelial cell proliferation, and expression of **angiogenic factors** (basic fibroblast growth factor [bFGF], VEGF, interleukin-6, and interleukin-8) [91, 133]. The WIBC-9 animal xenograft IBC model overexpresses other angiogenic factors such as Ang-1, Tie-1, and Tie-2, when compared to a noninflammatory breast cancer xenograft (SK-BR3) [152]. Lymphangiogenic factors, including VEGF-C, VEGF-D, VEGFR-3, Prox-1, and lymphatic vessel endothelial receptor 1, have also been shown to be strongly expressed in IBC [153].

The role of **p27kip1, a cyclin-dependent kinase inhibitor** that is thought to be involved in induction of apoptosis, cell adhesion, promotion of cell differentiation, and regulation of drug resistance [154, 155], was studied in IBC by M. D Anderson investigators who evaluated the role of p27kip1 in 38 IBC patients that had received primary systemic chemotherapy [156]. In this study, p27kip1 was downregulated in the majority of patients (84.2 %) and predicted for poor outcome.

A preclinical study directed to identify genetic determinants of IBC was completed by van Golen et al. [157]. The authors found 17 transcripts to be differentially expressed between the IBC cell line **SUM149** and human mammary epithelial cells (HME), nine of which were expressed solely in the tumor cell line. Using in situ hybridization technique, expression patterns of all seventeen transcripts were further confirmed in 20 archival IBC and 30 non-IBC LABC tissue samples. Two genes were found that were uniquely altered in the IBC specimens compared to the non-IBC samples: **Rho C GTPase** was found overexpressed in more than 90 % of IBC tumors compared to 38 % of non-IBC specimens. **WNT-1-induced secreted protein 3 (Wisp 3)** was found lost in more than 80 % of IBC specimens versus only 21 % of non-IBC tumors. The role of both genes in IBC has since been extensively studied [157]. Rho C GTPase, a member of the Ras superfamily of small GTP-binding proteins [158], is thought to contribute to the metastatic characteristic of IBC by promoting cell motility and invasion, disruption of cell–cell junctions, and upregulation of angiogenic factors (VEGF, bFGF) [159, 160]. WISP3, a gene coding for insulin-like growth factor-binding-related protein (IGFBP-rP9), has been shown to be a tumor suppressor gene [161], regulating tumor cell growth, invasion, and angiogenesis. Loss of Wisp 3 protein expression is thought to contribute to the aggressive phenotypic feature of IBC. In vitro evidence also shows that Wisp 3 shares an inverse relationship with Rho C GTPase expression [162].

Evidence also suggests that some IBC tumors may express stem cell surface markers (CD44+/CD24–/low and aldehyde dehydrogenase 1 [ALDH-1] enzyme production) [163]. This was also seen in the SUM149 IBC cell line and the Mary-X preclinical model of IBC and may be associated with poor prognosis [163, 164].

Despite the multitude of studies that have looked at the role of various molecular markers described above, in IBC, a more thorough understanding of the biology of IBC is required. The markers described above are not specific for IBC and their prognostic and predictive roles have been studied in small groups of patients. Therefore, they cannot be considered validated and further studies will be important to distinguish LABC from IBC at the molecular level.

22.8 Prognostic Factors of Locally Advanced Breast Cancer

Several prognostic factors have been described for patients with locally advanced breast cancer who undergo preoperative chemotherapy. These include clinical stage at diagnosis, pathological response to chemotherapy, and hormone receptor and HER2 receptor status [165]. An analysis of 340 patients treated at MD Anderson examined the patterns of local-regional recurrence (LRR) and ipsilateral breast tumor recurrence (IBTR) with neoadjuvant chemotherapy followed by conservative surgery and radiation therapy. More than 40 % of patients had locally advanced disease at diagnosis [166]. Advanced nodal involvement at diagnosis, residual tumor larger than 2 cm, multifocal residual disease, and lymphovascular space invasion was found to predict higher rates of LRR and IBTR.

22.8.1 Pathological Complete Response (pCR)

Despite being widely used as a primary endpoint for the evaluation of neoadjuvant trials, the value of pathological compete response (pCR) as a surrogate for overall survival benefit is not without controversy as higher pCR rates have not always translated into improved outcomes. The prognostic significance of pCR has been evaluated in several meta-analyses, the largest of which was conducted by the Collaborative Trials in Neoadjuvant Breast Cancer (CTNeoBC) working group and included almost 12,000 patients from 12 randomized trials [167]. This study included data from patients with both locally advanced and operable breast cancer. Patients who achieved a pCR were associated with significant improvements in event-free survival (EFS) and overall survival (OS). pCR rates varied by breast cancer subtype. The association between pathological CR and long-term outcomes was strongest in patients with triple-negative breast cancer and in those with HER2-positive and hormone receptor- negative tumors who received trastuzumab. Although the study ended the controversy surrounding the preferred definition of pCR (ypT0/is ypN0), it was unable to validate pathological CR as a surrogate endpoint for improved EFS and OS. The authors suggest that this may be due to the heterogeneous nature of the treatment received by the study population, especially among hormone receptor-positive subsets who tend to receive the most effective treatment (endocrine therapy) after pCR is determined, thus diluting the prognostic effect of pCR.

von Minckwitz et al. [165] also examined the prognostic impact of pCR among various intrinsic breast cancer subtypes in an analysis of 6377 patients who had received neoadjuvant anthracycline- and taxane-based chemotherapy for operable or nonoperable primary breast cancer. In the study, pCR was associated with improved DFS in luminal B/HER2-negative ($P = 0.005$), HER2-positive/nonluminal ($P < 0.001$), and triple-negative ($P < 0.001$) tumors but not in luminal A ($P = 0.39$) or luminal B/HER2-positive ($P = 0.45$) breast cancer.

The controversy about the value of pCR as a surrogate for OS benefit has been reignited after results of the ALTTO trial failed to translate the outstanding pCR rates reported in the NeoALTTO for the use of dual anti-HER2 therapy (trastuzumab and lapatinib) into a survival benefit in the adjuvant setting [168]. Similarly, a meta-regression analysis of 29 studies failed to support the use of pCR as a surrogate endpoint [169].

22.8.2 Prognosis in Patients Who Do not Achieve pCR

In patients who receive neoadjuvant systemic therapy but do not achieve pCR, there are several models currently being evaluated to better define the prognosis of these patients. These include calculation of the residual cancer burden (RCB) score, the breast cancer index (BCI), the clinicopathological stage, and biological markers (CPS-EG) score and for patients treated with preoperative endocrine therapy: the preoperative endocrine prognostic index (PEPI) score [170–172].

The RCB (residual cancer burden) score requires collecting several pathological measurements that are not routinely recorded such as the percent of invasive cancer cells in the residual tumor as well as the size of the largest nodal metastatic deposit [173]. Although the RCB score was found to correlate with outcome in patients who had received neoadjuvant anthracycline- and taxane-based chemotherapy, further validation is required in LABC and IBC before it can be used in routine practice. The RPCB score is an integrated score of RCB and Ki67 and was found to provide more accurate prognosis than when either variable is used alone [174, 175].

22.9 Survival

Patients with LABC cancer are at high risk of relapse and death as a result of metastatic disease. A phase III clinical trial conducted by the National Cancer Institute reported on the long-term survival of patients with stage III IBC and non-IBC who were treated using combined modality therapy [176]. The fifteen-year OS survival was 20 % for IBC (median OS 3.8 years) versus 50 % for stage IIIA and 23 % for stage IIIB non-IBC. Neither pathologic response, nor the presence of dermal lymphatic invasion was found to affect survival in IBC. Similarly, a retrospective analysis from the MD Anderson Cancer Center studied patients categorized into 2 groups on the basis of their clinical diagnosis of IBC or non-IBC LABC. LABC was defined as stage IIB, IIIA, IIIB, or IIIC breast cancer (AJCC system) [21]. A clinical diagnosis of IBC required the presence of diffuse erythema, heat, ridging, or peau d'orange (corresponding to T4d in the AJCC classification system) [21]. The clinical diagnosis was confirmed for all patients by assessment of a multidisciplinary team, and all patients were treated in separate but parallel protocols with similar multidisciplinary approaches consisting of induction chemotherapy, locoregional treatment (surgery and radiotherapy), adjuvant chemotherapy, and hormonal therapy (for ER-positive disease). The median follow-up period was 69 months, and pCR rates were 13.9 and 11.7 % in the IBC and non-IBC LABC groups, respectively ($P > 0.42$). The 5-year estimates of cumulative incidence of recurrence were 64.8 % for IBC and 43.4 % for non-IBC LABC ($P < 0.0001$). Patients with IBC had significantly higher cumulative incidence of local-regional recurrence and distant soft-tissue and bone disease. The 5-year OS rates were 40.5 % for the IBC group (95 % CI, 34.5–47.4 %) and 63.2 % for the non-IBC LABC group (95 % CI, 60.0–66.6 %; $P < 0.0001$) (see Fig. 22.4).

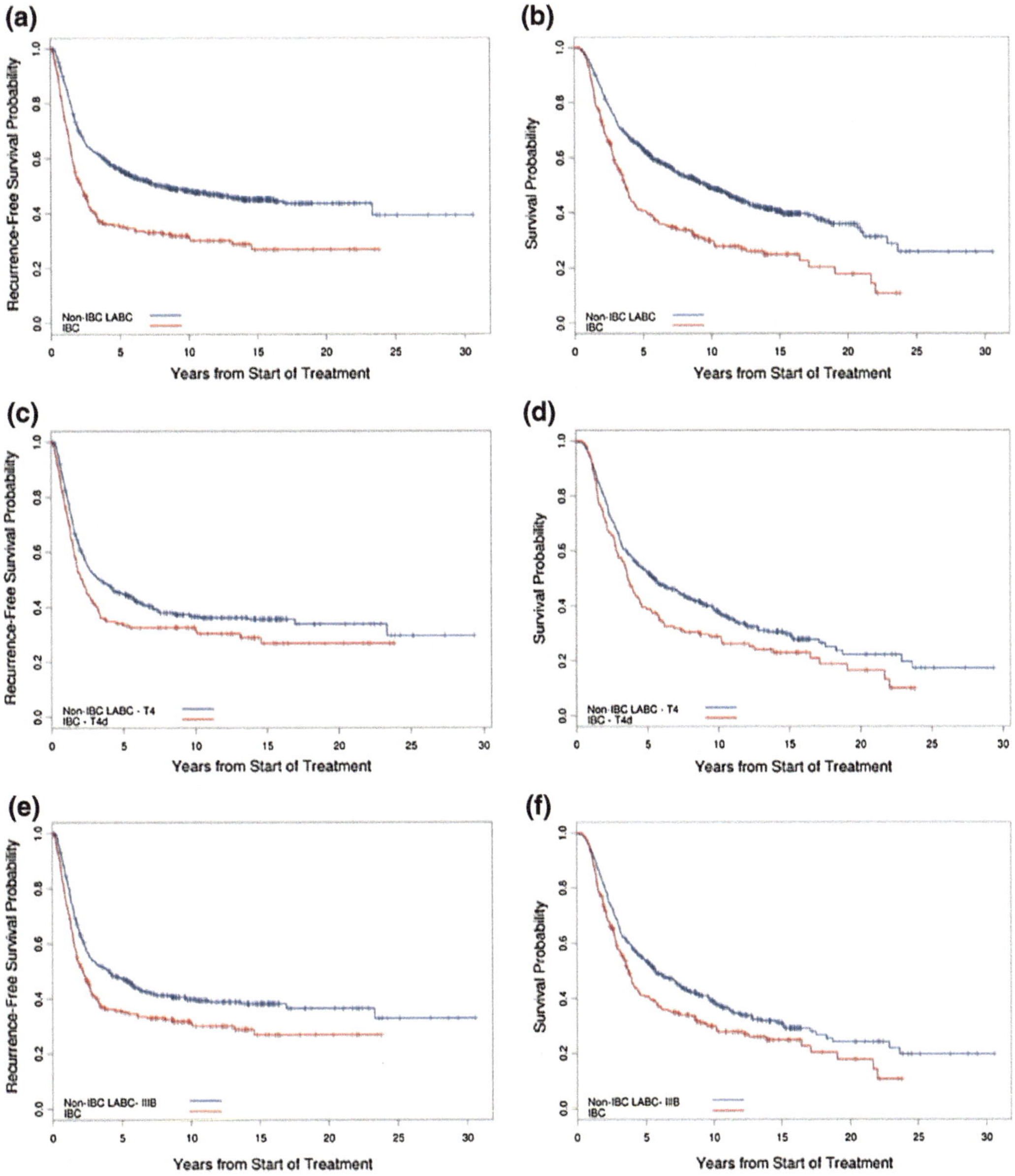

Fig. 22.4 Kaplan–Meier representation of relapse-free survival (*RFS*) rates by patient group: **a** IBC (*red line*) versus LABC (*blue line*); **b** Kaplan–Meier representation of overall survival (*OS*) rates are shown in the same two patient groups. Kaplan–Meier representation of RFS is shown in two patients' groups: **c** IBC versus non-IBC LABC (T4 *only*) and **d** Kaplan–Meier representation of OS rates in the same groups. Kaplan–Meier representation of RFS in two patients' groups is shown for **e** IBC versus non-IBC LABC (stage IIIB) and **f** Kaplan–Meier representation of OS rates in the same groups. From Cristofanilli et al. [11]

The authors concluded that IBC was associated with a worse prognosis and a distinctive pattern of early recurrence compared with LABC [11].

Using data from National Cancer Institute's Surveillance, Epidemiology, and End Results (SEER) program, Schlichting et al. [177] compared the survival of 4441 patients with stage III IBC and 32,867 patients with stage III non-IBC diagnosed between 1990 and 2000. The analysis which again included patients with stage III A (non-IBC) reported a median survival of 4.75 years for stage III IBC versus 13.4 years in patients with stage III non-IBC ($P < 0.0001$). Dawood et al. also analyzed data from SEER to compare the outcome of IBC and non-IBC among stage-matched patients with stage IIIB and IIIC breast cancer diagnosed after the adoption of multidisciplinary management and anthracycline-/taxane-based polychemotherapy as a standard of care (between 2004 and 2007). At 2 years, BCSS was 84 % versus 91 % in IBC versus non-IBC, respectively ($P = 0.008$) [178].

Unfortunately, despite the clear stepwise advances that are being made in the adjuvant treatment of breast cancer with the introduction of novel agents in the treatment of breast cancer (e.g., taxanes, aromatase inhibitors, and HER2-targeting therapy), the impact of such therapies on the outcome of patients with IBC has not been clear [12]. In a study at MD Anderson Cancer Center, 398 patients with IBC were treated between 1974 and 2005 to evaluate whether survival had improved over the past 30 years. Patient outcomes were tabulated and compared among four decades of diagnosis. The study was unable to find a difference in either the risk of recurrence or death between the various decade-of-diagnosis groups (median recurrence-free survival = 2.3 years; median OS = 4.2 years) [12]. Another report from Panades et al. [179] also failed to show breast cancer-specific survival differences when comparing IBC patients treated between 1980 and 1990 with patients treated between 1991 and 2000. The 10-year breast cancer-specific survival rates were 27.4 % (95 % confidence interval [CI], 18.8–36.7 %), and 28.6 % (95 % CI, 20.3–37.5 %), respectively ($P > 0.37$).

In a recent analysis using data from the National Cancer Database, researchers were able to demonstrate nationwide disparities in the use of trimodality therapy in patients with stage III IBC that fluctuated from 58.4 to 73.4 % annually [180]. Patients who received all three treatment modalities had the highest survival rates (5- and 10-years OS = 55.4 and 37.3 %, respectively) compared to those who did not.

Taken together, this evidence demonstrates that IBC should be treated separately from non-IBC LABC and that the use of standard combinations of cytotoxic agents alone will not substantially modify the prognosis of patients with this disease. More sensitive diagnostic interventions and novel therapeutic strategies should be developed to increase the efficacy of systemic treatments (Table 22.3).

Lastly, LABC and IBC, although molecularly heterogeneous, are approached based on the hormone receptor-positive, HER2-positive, and triple-negative groupings. Treatments for these three groups are partially overlapping,

Table 22.3 Outcome for patients with inflammatory breast cancer treated with combined modality treatment

Study	Date range	Stage and study design	Sample size	Survival
Low et al. [176]	1980–1988	Prospective (NCI) Stage III (IBC vs. non-IBC)	Total: 107 IBC: 46 Non-IBC: 61	OS at 15 years: IBC versus non-IBC (IIIB): 20.0 % versus 23.1 %
Cristofanilli et al. [11]	1974–2000	Retrospective (single institution) Stage III (IBC vs. non-IBC)	Total: 1071 IBC: 240 Non-IBC: 831	OS at 5 years: IBC versus non-IBC: 40.5 versus 63.2 ($P < 0.0001$)
Dawood et al. [178]	2004–2007	Retrospective (SEER) Stage III (IBC vs. non-IBC)	Total: 4304 IBC: 828 Non-IBC: 3476	BCSS at 2-years: IBC versus non-IBC: 84 % versus 91 % ($P = 0.008$)
Schlichting [177]	1990–2008	Retrospective (SEER) Stage III (IBC vs. non-IBC)	Stage III: 37,308 IBC: 4441 Non-IBC: 32,867	Median BCSS Stage III, IBC versus non-IBC: 4.75 years versus 13.4 years ($P < 0.0001$)
Rueth et al. [180]	1998–2010	Retrospective (SEER) Stage III IBC	Total: 10,197	5- and 10-year survival: 55.4 and 37.3 %, respectively, in patients who received trimodality therapy

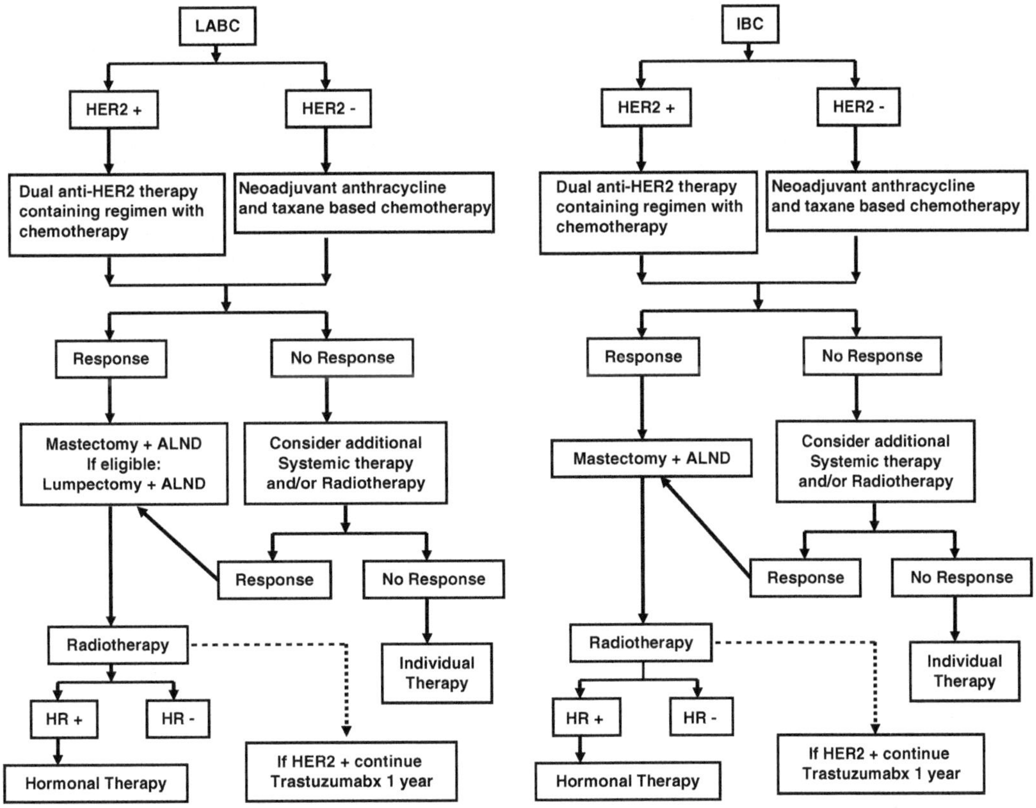

Fig. 22.5 Flow diagram describing the management of LABC and IBC

and the "major" therapeutic intervention is different in the groups, endocrine therapy, HER2-directed therapy, and chemotherapy, respectively, and should be complemented with adequate local-regional therapy and reconstructive surgery (Fig. 22.5).

References

1. Seidman H, Gelb SK, Silverberg E, LaVerda N, Lubera JA. Survival experience in the breast cancer detection demonstration project. CA Cancer J Clin. 1987;37(5):258–90.
2. Eniu A, Carlson RW, Aziz Z, Bines J, Hortobagyi GN, Bese NS, et al. Breast cancer in limited-resource countries: treatment and allocation of resources. Breast J. 2006;12(Suppl 1):S38–53.
3. Lee MC, Newman LA. Management of patients with locally advanced breast cancer. Surg Clin N Am. 2007;87(2):379–98, ix.
4. http://www.facs.org/cancer/publicncdb.html [Internet]. 2013 [cited 16 June 2016].
5. Hance KW, Anderson WF, Devesa SS, Young HA, Levine PH. Trends in inflammatory breast carcinoma incidence and survival: the surveillance, epidemiology, and end results program at the National Cancer Institute. J Natl Cancer Inst. 2005;97(13):966–75.
6. Anderson WF, Schairer C, Chen BE, Hance KW, Levine PH. Epidemiology of inflammatory breast cancer (IBC). Breast Dis. 2005;22:9–23.
7. Soliman AS, Banerjee M, Lo AC, Ismail K, Hablas A, Seifeldin IA, et al. High proportion of inflammatory breast cancer in the population-based Cancer Registry of Gharbiah, Egypt. Breast J. 2009;15(4):432–4.
8. Schairer C, Soliman AS, Omar S, Khaled H, Eissa S, Ayed FB, et al. Assessment of diagnosis of inflammatory breast cancer cases at two cancer centers in Egypt and Tunisia. Cancer Med. 2013;2(2):178–84.
9. Boussen H, Bouzaiene H, Ben Hassouna J, Gamoudi A, Benna F, Rahal K. Inflammatory breast cancer in Tunisia: reassessment of incidence and clinicopathological features. Semin Oncol. 2008;35 (1):17–24.
10. Chang S, Buzdar AU, Hursting SD. Inflammatory breast cancer and body mass index. J Clin Oncol (Official Journal of the American Society of Clinical Oncology). 1998;16(12):3731–5.
11. Cristofanilli M, Valero V, Buzdar AU, Kau SW, Broglio KR, Gonzalez-Angulo AM, et al. Inflammatory breast cancer (IBC) and patterns of recurrence: understanding the biology of a unique disease. Cancer. 2007;110(7):1436–44.
12. Gonzalez-Angulo AM, Hennessy BT, Broglio K, Meric-Bernstam F, Cristofanilli M, Giordano SH, et al. Trends for inflammatory breast cancer: is survival improving? Oncologist. 2007;12(8):904–12.
13. Fouad TM, Kogawa T, Liu DD, Shen Y, Masuda H, El-Zein R, et al. Overall survival differences between patients with inflammatory and noninflammatory breast cancer presenting with distant metastasis at diagnosis. Breast Cancer Res Treat. 2015.
14. Anderson WF, Chu KC, Chang S. Inflammatory breast carcinoma and noninflammatory locally advanced breast carcinoma: distinct clinicopathologic entities? J Clin Oncol (Official Journal of the American Society of Clinical Oncology). 2003;21(12):2254–9.
15. Nadeem R, Chagla LS, Harris O, Desmond S, Thind R, Flavin A, et al. Tumour localisation with a metal coil before the administration of neo-adjuvant chemotherapy. Breast. 2005;14(5):403–7.

16. Niikura N, Liu J, Costelloe CM, Palla SL, Madewell JE, Hayashi N, et al. Initial staging impact of fluorodeoxyglucose positron emission tomography/computed tomography in locally advanced breast cancer. Oncologist. 2011;16(6):772–82.
17. National Comprehensive Cancer Network. NCCN guidelines, version 2.2016, invasive breast cancer 2016 [BINV-14]. Available from: http://www.nccn.org/professionals/physician_gls/pdf/breast.pdf.
18. Haagensen CD. Diseases of the female breast. Trans N Engl Obstet Gynecol Soc. 1956;10:141–56.
19. Robertson FM, Bondy M, Yang W, Yamauchi H, Wiggins S, Kamrudin S, et al. Inflammatory breast cancer: the disease, the biology, the treatment. CA Cancer J Clin. 2010;60(6):351–75.
20. Jaiyesimi IA, Buzdar AU, Hortobagyi G. Inflammatory breast cancer: a review. J clin Oncol (Official Journal of the American Society of Clinical Oncology). 1992;10(6):1014–24.
21. Singletary SE, Allred C, Ashley P, Bassett LW, Berry D, Bland KI, et al. Revision of the American Joint Committee on Cancer staging system for breast cancer. J Clin Oncol (Official Journal of the American Society of Clinical Oncology). 2002;20 (17):3628–36.
22. Yang WT, Le-Petross HT, Macapinlac H, Carkaci S, Gonzalez-Angulo AM, Dawood S, et al. Inflammatory breast cancer: PET/CT, MRI, mammography, and sonography findings. Breast Cancer Res Treat. 2008;109(3):417–26.
23. National Comprehensive Cancer Network. NCCN guidelines, version 2.2016, invasive breast cancer 2016 [BINV-K]. Available from: http://www.nccn.org/professionals/physician_gls/pdf/breast.pdf.
24. De Lena M, Zucali R, Viganotti G, Valagussa P, Bonadonna G. Combined chemotherapy-radiotherapy approach in locally advanced (T3b-T4) breast cancer. Cancer Chemother Pharmacol. 1978;1(1):53–9.
25. Rastogi P, Anderson SJ, Bear HD, Geyer CE, Kahlenberg MS, Robidoux A, et al. Preoperative chemotherapy: updates of national surgical adjuvant breast and bowel project protocols B-18 and B-27. J Clin Oncol (Official Journal of the American Society of Clinical Oncology). 2008;26(5):778–85.
26. Mauri D, Pavlidis N, Ioannidis JP. Neoadjuvant versus adjuvant systemic treatment in breast cancer: a meta-analysis. J Natl Cancer Inst. 2005;97(3):188–94.
27. Green MC, Buzdar AU, Smith T, Ibrahim NK, Valero V, Rosales MF, et al. Weekly paclitaxel improves pathologic complete remission in operable breast cancer when compared with paclitaxel once every 3 weeks. J Clin Oncol (Official Journal of the American Society of Clinical Oncology). 2005;23 (25):5983–92.
28. von Minckwitz G, Raab G, Caputo A, Schutte M, Hilfrich J, Blohmer JU, et al. Doxorubicin with cyclophosphamide followed by docetaxel every 21 days compared with doxorubicin and docetaxel every 14 days as preoperative treatment in operable breast cancer: the GEPARDUO study of the German Breast Group. J Clin Oncol (Official Journal of the American Society of Clinical Oncology). 2005;23(12):2676–85.
29. von Minckwitz G, Schneeweiss A, Loibl S, Salat C, Denkert C, Rezai M, et al. Neoadjuvant carboplatin in patients with triple-negative and HER2-positive early breast cancer (GeparSixto; GBG 66): a randomised phase 2 trial. Lancet Oncol. 2014;15(7):747–56.
30. Sikov WM, Berry DA, Perou CM, Singh B, Cirrincione CT, Tolaney SM, et al. Impact of the addition of carboplatin and/or bevacizumab to neoadjuvant once-per-week paclitaxel followed by dose-dense doxorubicin and cyclophosphamide on pathologic complete response rates in stage II to III triple-negative breast cancer: CALGB 40603 (Alliance). J Clin Oncol (Official Journal of the American Society of Clinical Oncology). 2015;33(1): 13–21.
31. Rugo HS, Olopade O, DeMichele A, van't Veer L, Buxton M, Hylton N, et al., editors. Veliparib/carboplatin plus standard neoadjuvant therapy for high-risk breast cancer: first efficacy results from the I-SPY 2 TRIAL. The 36th annual San Antonio breast cancer symposium, San Antonio, TX, 10–14 Dec 2013.
32. von Minckwitz G, Kummel S, Vogel P, Hanusch C, Eidtmann H, Hilfrich J, et al. Neoadjuvant vinorelbine-capecitabine versus docetaxel-doxorubicin-cyclophosphamide in early nonresponsive breast cancer: phase III randomized GeparTrio trial. J Natl Cancer Inst. 2008;100(8):542–51.
33. Heys SD, Hutcheon AW, Sarkar TK, Ogston KN, Miller ID, Payne S, et al. Neoadjuvant docetaxel in breast cancer: 3-year survival results from the Aberdeen trial. Clin Breast Cancer. 2002;3(Suppl 2):S69–74.
34. Huober J, Fasching PA, Hanusch C, Rezai M, Eidtmann H, Kittel K, et al. Neoadjuvant chemotherapy with paclitaxel and everolimus in breast cancer patients with non-responsive tumours to epirubicin/cyclophosphamide (EC) ± bevacizumab - results of the randomised GeparQuinto study (GBG 44). Eur J Cancer. 2013;49(10):2284–93.
35. Hurley J, Doliny P, Reis I, Silva O, Gomez-Fernandez C, Velez P, et al. Docetaxel, cisplatin, and trastuzumab as primary systemic therapy for human epidermal growth factor receptor 2-positive locally advanced breast cancer. J Clin Oncol (Official Journal of the American Society of Clinical Oncology). 2006;24 (12):1831–8.
36. Van Pelt AE, Mohsin S, Elledge RM, Hilsenbeck SG, Gutierrez MC, Lucci A Jr, et al. Neoadjuvant trastuzumab and docetaxel in breast cancer: preliminary results. Clin Breast Cancer. 2003;4 (5):348–53.
37. Gianni L, Eiermann W, Semiglazov V, Manikhas A, Lluch A, Tjulandin S, et al. Neoadjuvant chemotherapy with trastuzumab followed by adjuvant trastuzumab versus neoadjuvant chemotherapy alone, in patients with HER2-positive locally advanced breast cancer (the NOAH trial): a randomised controlled superiority trial with a parallel HER2-negative cohort. Lancet. 2010;375 (9712):377–84.
38. Gianni L, Eiermann W, Semiglazov V, Lluch A, Tjulandin S, Zambetti M, et al. Neoadjuvant and adjuvant trastuzumab in patients with HER2-positive locally advanced breast cancer (NOAH): follow-up of a randomised controlled superiority trial with a parallel HER2-negative cohort. Lancet Oncol. 2014;15 (6):640–7.
39. Buzdar AU, Valero V, Ibrahim NK, Francis D, Broglio KR, Theriault RL, et al. Neoadjuvant therapy with paclitaxel followed by 5-fluorouracil, epirubicin, and cyclophosphamide chemotherapy and concurrent trastuzumab in human epidermal growth factor receptor 2-positive operable breast cancer: an update of the initial randomized study population and data of additional patients treated with the same regimen. Clin Cancer Res (Official Journal of the American Association for Cancer Research). 2007;13(1):228–33.
40. Petrelli F, Borgonovo K, Cabiddu M, Ghilardi M, Barni S. Neoadjuvant chemotherapy and concomitant trastuzumab in breast cancer: a pooled analysis of two randomized trials. Anticancer Drugs. 2011;22(2):128–35.
41. Gianni L, Pienkowski T, Im YH, Roman L, Tseng LM, Liu MC, et al. Efficacy and safety of neoadjuvant pertuzumab and trastuzumab in women with locally advanced, inflammatory, or early HER2-positive breast cancer (NeoSphere): a randomised multicentre, open-label, phase 2 trial. Lancet Oncol. 2012;13 (1):25–32.

42. Gianni L, Pienkowski T, Im YH, Tseng LM, Liu MC, Lluch A, et al. 5-year analysis of neoadjuvant pertuzumab and trastuzumab in patients with locally advanced, inflammatory, or early-stage HER2-positive breast cancer (NeoSphere): a multicentre, open-label, phase 2 randomised trial. Lancet Oncol. 2016;17 (6):791–800.
43. Schneeweiss A, Chia S, Hickish T, Harvey V, Eniu A, Hegg R, et al. Pertuzumab plus trastuzumab in combination with standard neoadjuvant anthracycline-containing and anthracycline-free chemotherapy regimens in patients with HER2-positive early breast cancer: a randomized phase II cardiac safety study (TRYPHAENA). Ann Oncol (Official Journal of the European Society for Medical Oncology/ESMO). 2013;24(9): 2278–84.
44. Untch M, Loibl S, Bischoff J, Eidtmann H, Kaufmann M, Blohmer JU, et al. Lapatinib versus trastuzumab in combination with neoadjuvant anthracycline-taxane-based chemotherapy (GeparQuinto, GBG 44): a randomised phase 3 trial. Lancet Oncol. 2012;13(2):135–44.
45. Baselga J, Bradbury I, Eidtmann H, Di Cosimo S, de Azambuja E, Aura C, et al. Lapatinib with trastuzumab for HER2-positive early breast cancer (NeoALTTO): a randomised, open-label, multicentre, phase 3 trial. Lancet. 2012;379(9816):633–40.
46. Robidoux A, Tang G, Rastogi P, Geyer CE Jr, Azar CA, Atkins JN, et al. Lapatinib as a component of neoadjuvant therapy for HER2-positive operable breast cancer (NSABP protocol B-41): an open-label, randomised phase 3 trial. Lancet Oncol. 2013;14(12):1183–92.
47. Carey LA, Berry DA, Cirrincione CT, Barry WT, Pitcher BN, Harris LN, et al. Molecular heterogeneity and response to neoadjuvant human epidermal growth factor receptor 2 targeting in CALGB 40601, a randomized phase III trial of paclitaxel plus trastuzumab with or without lapatinib. J Clin Oncol (Official Journal of the American Society of Clinical Oncology). 2016;34 (6):542–9.
48. de Azambuja E, Holmes AP, Piccart-Gebhart M, Holmes E, Di Cosimo S, Swaby RF, et al. Lapatinib with trastuzumab for HER2-positive early breast cancer (NeoALTTO): survival outcomes of a randomised, open-label, multicentre, phase 3 trial and their association with pathological complete response. Lancet Oncol. 2014;15(10):1137–46.
49. Veronesi A, Frustaci S, Tirelli U, Galligioni E, Trovo MG, Crivellari D, et al. Tamoxifen therapy in postmenopausal advanced breast cancer: efficacy at the primary tumor site in 46 evaluable patients. Tumori. 1981;67(3):235–8.
50. Hoff PM, Valero V, Buzdar AU, Singletary SE, Theriault RL, Booser D, et al. Combined modality treatment of locally advanced breast carcinoma in elderly patients or patients with severe comorbid conditions using tamoxifen as the primary therapy. Cancer. 2000;88(9):2054–60.
51. Alba E, Calvo L, Albanell J, De la Haba JR, Arcusa Lanza A, Chacon JI, et al. Chemotherapy (CT) and hormonotherapy (HT) as neoadjuvant treatment in luminal breast cancer patients: results from the GEICAM/2006-03, a multicenter, randomized, phase-II study. Ann Oncol (Official Journal of the European Society for Medical Oncology/ESMO). 2012;23(12):3069–74.
52. Ellis MJ, Ma C. Letrozole in the neoadjuvant setting: the P024 trial. Breast Cancer Res Treat. 2007;105(Suppl 1):33–43.
53. Cataliotti L, Buzdar AU, Noguchi S, Bines J, Takatsuka Y, Petrakova K, et al. Comparison of anastrozole versus tamoxifen as preoperative therapy in postmenopausal women with hormone receptor-positive breast cancer: the Pre-Operative "Arimidex" Compared to Tamoxifen (PROACT) trial. Cancer. 2006;106 (10):2095–103.
54. Gerber B, von Minckwitz G, Eidtmann H, Rezai M, Fasching P, Tesch H, et al. Surgical outcome after neoadjuvant chemotherapy and bevacizumab: results from the GeparQuinto study (GBG 44). Ann Surg Oncol. 2014;21(8):2517–24.
55. von Minckwitz G, Loibl S, Untch M, Eidtmann H, Rezai M, Fasching PA, et al. Survival after neoadjuvant chemotherapy with or without bevacizumab or everolimus for HER2-negative primary breast cancer (GBG 44-GeparQuinto) dagger. Ann Oncol (Official Journal of the European Society for Medical Oncology/ESMO). 2014;25(12):2363–72.
56. Earl HM, Hiller L, Dunn JA, Blenkinsop C, Grybowicz L, Vallier AL, et al. Efficacy of neoadjuvant bevacizumab added to docetaxel followed by fluorouracil, epirubicin, and cyclophosphamide, for women with HER2-negative early breast cancer (ARTemis): an open-label, randomised, phase 3 trial. Lancet Oncol. 2015;16(6):656–66.
57. Bear HD, Tang G, Rastogi P, Geyer CE Jr, Robidoux A, Atkins JN, et al. Bevacizumab added to neoadjuvant chemotherapy for breast cancer. N Engl J Med. 2012;366(4):310–20.
58. Bear HD, Tang G, Rastogi P, Geyer CE Jr, Liu Q, Robidoux A, et al. Neoadjuvant plus adjuvant bevacizumab in early breast cancer (NSABP B-40 [NRG Oncology]): secondary outcomes of a phase 3, randomised controlled trial. Lancet Oncol. 2015;16 (9):1037–48.
59. Rugo HS, Olopade O, DeMichele A, van't Veer L, Buxton M, Hylton N, et al. Veliparib/carboplatin plus standard neoadjuvant therapy for high-risk breast cancer: first efficacy results from the I-SPY 2 TRIAL. The San Antonio breast cancer symposium, San Antonio; 2013.
60. Goldhirsch A, Winer EP, Coates AS, Gelber RD, Piccart-Gebhart M, Thurlimann B, et al. Personalizing the treatment of women with early breast cancer: highlights of the St. Gallen International Expert Consensus on the Primary Therapy of Early Breast Cancer 2013. Ann Oncol (Official Journal of the European Society for Medical Oncology/ESMO). 2013;24(9):2206–23.
61. National Comprehensive Cancer Network. NCCN guidelines, version 2.2016, invasive breast cancer 2016 [BINV-15]. Available from: http://www.nccn.org/professionals/physician_gls/pdf/breast.pdf.
62. Estevez LG, Cuevas JM, Anton A, Florian J, Lopez-Vega JM, Velasco A, et al. Weekly docetaxel as neoadjuvant chemotherapy for stage II and III breast cancer: efficacy and correlation with biological markers in a phase II, multicenter study. Clin Cancer Res (Official Journal of the American Association for Cancer Research). 2003;9(2):686–92.
63. Buzdar AU, Singletary SE, Theriault RL, Booser DJ, Valero V, Ibrahim N, et al. Prospective evaluation of paclitaxel versus combination chemotherapy with fluorouracil, doxorubicin, and cyclophosphamide as neoadjuvant therapy in patients with operable breast cancer. J Clin Oncol (Official Journal of the American Society of Clinical Oncology). 1999;17(11):3412–7.
64. Smith IC, Heys SD, Hutcheon AW, Miller ID, Payne S, Gilbert FJ, et al. Neoadjuvant chemotherapy in breast cancer: significantly enhanced response with docetaxel. J Clin Oncol (Official Journal of the American Society of Clinical Oncology). 2002;20(6):1456–66.
65. Bear HD, Anderson S, Brown A, Smith R, Mamounas EP, Fisher B, et al. The effect on tumor response of adding sequential preoperative docetaxel to preoperative doxorubicin and cyclophosphamide: preliminary results from National Surgical Adjuvant Breast and Bowel Project Protocol B-27. J Clin Oncol (Official Journal of the American Society of Clinical Oncology). 2003;21(22):4165–74.

66. Untch M, von Minckwitz G. Recent advances in systemic therapy: advances in neoadjuvant (primary) systemic therapy with cytotoxic agents. Breast Cancer Res BCR. 2009;11(2):203.
67. Coudert BP, Largillier R, Arnould L, Chollet P, Campone M, Coeffic D, et al. Multicenter phase II trial of neoadjuvant therapy with trastuzumab, docetaxel, and carboplatin for human epidermal growth factor receptor-2-overexpressing stage II or III breast cancer: results of the GETN(A)-1 trial. J Clin Oncol (Official Journal of the American Society of Clinical Oncology). 2007;25 (19):2678–84.
68. Penault-Llorca F, Abrial C, Mouret-Reynier MA, Raoelfils I, Durando X, Leheurteur M, et al. Achieving higher pathological complete response rates in HER-2-positive patients with induction chemotherapy without trastuzumab in operable breast cancer. Oncologist. 2007;12(4):390–6.
69. Bozzetti F, Saccozzi R, De Lena M, Salvadori B. Inflammatory cancer of the breast: analysis of 114 cases. J Surg Oncol. 1981;18 (4):355–61.
70. Shenkier T, Weir L, Levine M, Olivotto I, Whelan T, Reyno L, et al. Clinical practice guidelines for the care and treatment of breast cancer: 15. Treatment for women with stage III or locally advanced breast cancer. CMAJ. 2004;170(6):983–94.
71. Lee BJ, Tannenbaum NE. Inflammatory carcinoma of the breast. Surg Gynecol Obstet. 1924;39:580–95.
72. Atkins HL, Horrigan WD. Treatment of locally advanced carcinoma of the breast with roentgen therapy and simple mastectomy. Am J Roentgenol Radium Ther Nucl Med. 1961;85:860–4.
73. Toonkel LM, Fix I, Jacobson LH, Bamberg N, Wallach CB. Locally advanced breast carcinoma: results with combined regional therapy. Int J Radiat Oncol Biol Phys. 1986;12 (9):1583–7.
74. Perez CA, Graham ML, Taylor ME, Levy JF, Mortimer JE, Philpott GW, et al. Management of locally advanced carcinoma of the breast. I Noninflammatory. Cancer. 1994;74(1 Suppl):453–65.
75. Bauer RL, Busch E, Levine E, Edge SB. Therapy for inflammatory breast cancer: impact of doxorubicin-based therapy. Ann Surg Oncol. 1995;2(4):288–94.
76. Early Breast Cancer Trialists' Collaborative G. Effects of chemotherapy and hormonal therapy for early breast cancer on recurrence and 15-year survival: an overview of the randomised trials. Lancet. 2005;365(9472):1687–717.
77. Ueno NT, Buzdar AU, Singletary SE, Ames FC, McNeese MD, Holmes FA, et al. Combined-modality treatment of inflammatory breast carcinoma: twenty years of experience at MD Anderson Cancer Center. Cancer Chemother Pharmacol. 1997;40(4):321–9.
78. Singletary SE, Ames FC, Buzdar AU. Management of inflammatory breast cancer. World J Surg. 1994;18(1):87–92.
79. Buzdar AU, Singletary SE, Booser DJ, Frye DK, Wasaff B, Hortobagyi GN. Combined modality treatment of stage III and inflammatory breast cancer. M.D. Anderson Cancer Center experience. Surg Oncol Clin N Am. 1995;4(4):715–34.
80. Cristofanilli M, Buzdar AU, Sneige N, Smith T, Wasaff B, Ibrahim N, et al. Paclitaxel in the multimodality treatment for inflammatory breast carcinoma. Cancer. 2001;92(7):1775–82.
81. Cristofanilli M, Gonzalez-Angulo AM, Buzdar AU, Kau SW, Frye DK, Hortobagyi GN. Paclitaxel improves the prognosis in estrogen receptor negative inflammatory breast cancer: the MD Anderson Cancer Center experience. Clin Breast Cancer. 2004;4 (6):415–9.
82. Romond EH, Perez EA, Bryant J, Suman VJ, Geyer CE Jr, Davidson NE, et al. Trastuzumab plus adjuvant chemotherapy for operable HER2-positive breast cancer. N Engl J Med. 2005;353 (16):1673–84.
83. Piccart-Gebhart MJ, Procter M, Leyland-Jones B, Goldhirsch A, Untch M, Smith I, et al. Trastuzumab after adjuvant chemotherapy in HER2-positive breast cancer. N Engl J Med. 2005;353 (16):1659–72.
84. Johnston S, Trudeau M, Kaufman B, Boussen H, Blackwell K, LoRusso P, et al. Phase II study of predictive biomarker profiles for response targeting human epidermal growth factor receptor 2 (HER-2) in advanced inflammatory breast cancer with lapatinib monotherapy. J Clin Oncol (Official Journal of the American Society of Clinical Oncology). 2008;26(7):1066–72.
85. Boussen H, Cristofanilli M, Zaks T, DeSilvio M, Salazar V, Spector N. Phase II study to evaluate the efficacy and safety of neoadjuvant lapatinib plus paclitaxel in patients with inflammatory breast cancer. J Clin Oncol (Official Journal of the American Society of Clinical Oncology). 2010;28(20):3248–55.
86. Arun B, Slack R, Gehan E, Spitzer T, Meehan KR. Survival after autologous hematopoietic stem cell transplantation for patients with inflammatory breast carcinoma. Cancer. 1999;85(1):93–9.
87. Adkins D, Brown R, Trinkaus K, Maziarz R, Luedke S, Freytes C, et al. Outcomes of high-dose chemotherapy and autologous stem-cell transplantation in stage IIIB inflammatory breast cancer. J Clin Oncol (Official Journal of the American Society of Clinical Oncology). 1999;17(7):2006–14.
88. Schwartzberg L, Weaver C, Lewkow L, McAneny B, Zhen B, Birch R, et al. High-dose chemotherapy with peripheral blood stem cell support for stage IIIB inflammatory carcinoma of the breast. Bone Marrow Transplant. 1999;24(9):981–7.
89. Somlo G, Frankel P, Chow W, Leong L, Margolin K, Morgan R Jr, et al. Prognostic indicators and survival in patients with stage IIIB inflammatory breast carcinoma after dose-intense chemotherapy. J Clin Oncol (Official Journal of the American Society of Clinical Oncology). 2004;22(10):1839–48.
90. Goncalves A, Pierga JY, Ferrero JM, Mouret-Reynier MA, Bachelot T, Delva R, et al. UNICANCER-PEGASE 07 study: a randomized phase III trial evaluating postoperative docetaxel-5FU regimen after neoadjuvant dose-intense chemotherapy for treatment of inflammatory breast cancer. Ann Oncol (Official Journal of the European Society for Medical Oncology/ESMO). 2015;26(8):1692–7.
91. Van der Auwera I, Van Laere SJ, Van den Eynden GG, Benoy I, van Dam P, Colpaert CG, et al. Increased angiogenesis and lymphangiogenesis in inflammatory versus noninflammatory breast cancer by real-time reverse transcriptase-PCR gene expression quantification. Clin Cancer Res (Official Journal of the American Association for Cancer Research). 2004;10 (23):7965–71.
92. Wedam SB, Low JA, Yang SX, Chow CK, Choyke P, Danforth D, et al. Antiangiogenic and antitumor effects of bevacizumab in patients with inflammatory and locally advanced breast cancer. J Clin Oncol (Official Journal of the American Society of Clinical Oncology). 2006;24(5):769–77.
93. Overmoyer B, Fu P, Hoppel C, Radivoyevitch T, Shenk R, Persons M, et al. Inflammatory breast cancer as a model disease to study tumor angiogenesis: results of a phase IB trial of combination SU5416 and doxorubicin. Clin Cancer Res (Official Journal of the American Association for Cancer Research). 2007;13(19):5862–8.
94. Johnston SR, Hickish T, Ellis P, Houston S, Kelland L, Dowsett M, et al. Phase II study of the efficacy and tolerability of two dosing regimens of the farnesyl transferase inhibitor, R115777, in advanced breast cancer. J Clin Oncol (Official Journal of the American Society of Clinical Oncology). 2003;21 (13):2492–9.
95. Andreopoulou E, Vigoda IS, Valero V, Hershman DL, Raptis G, Vahdat LT, et al. Phase I-II study of the farnesyl transferase

inhibitor tipifarnib plus sequential weekly paclitaxel and doxorubicin-cyclophosphamide in HER2/neu-negative inflammatory carcinoma and non-inflammatory estrogen receptor-positive breast carcinoma. Breast Cancer Res Treat. 2013;141(3):429–35.
96. Matsuda N, Wang X, Krishnamurthy S, Alvarez RH, Willey JS, Lim B, et al., editors. Phase II study of panitumumab, nab-paclitaxel, and carboplatin followed by FEC neoadjuvant chemotherapy for patients with primary HER2-negative inflammatory breast cancer. American Society of Clinical Oncology; 2016.
97. Fouad TM, Kogawa T, Reuben JM, Ueno NT. The role of inflammation in inflammatory breast cancer. Adv Exp Med Biol. 2014;816:53–73.
98. Haagensen CD, Stout AP. Carcinoma of the breast. II-criteria of operability. Ann Surg. 1943;118(6):1032–51.
99. Baclesse F. Five-year results in 431 breast cancers treated solely by roentgen rays. Ann Surg. 1965;161:103–4.
100. Zucali R, Uslenghi C, Kenda R, Bonadonna G. Natural history and survival of inoperable breast cancer treated with radiotherapy and radiotherapy followed by radical mastectomy. Cancer. 1976;37(3):1422–31.
101. Harris JR, Sawicka J, Gelman R, Hellman S. Management of locally advanced carcinoma of the breast by primary radiation therapy. Int J Radiat Oncol Biol Phys. 1983;9(3):345–9.
102. Sheldon T, Hayes DF, Cady B, Parker L, Osteen R, Silver B, et al. Primary radiation therapy for locally advanced breast cancer. Cancer. 1987;60(6):1219–25.
103. Fletcher GH, Montague ED. Radical irradiation of advanced breast cancer. Am J Roentgenol Radium Ther Nucl Med. 1965;93:573–84.
104. Spanos WJ Jr, Montague ED, Fletcher GH. Late complications of radiation only for advanced breast cancer. Int J Radiat Oncol Biol Phys. 1980;6(11):1473–6.
105. Huang EH, Tucker SL, Strom EA, McNeese MD, Kuerer HM, Buzdar AU, et al. Postmastectomy radiation improves local-regional control and survival for selected patients with locally advanced breast cancer treated with neoadjuvant chemotherapy and mastectomy. J Clin Oncol (Official Journal of the American Society of Clinical Oncology). 2004;22 (23):4691–9.
106. Singletary SE, McNeese MD, Hortobagyi GN. Feasibility of breast-conservation surgery after induction chemotherapy for locally advanced breast carcinoma. Cancer. 1992;69(11):2849–52.
107. Kuerer HM, Singletary SE, Buzdar AU, Ames FC, Valero V, Buchholz TA, et al. Surgical conservation planning after neoadjuvant chemotherapy for stage II and operable stage III breast carcinoma. Am J Surg. 2001;182(6):601–8.
108. Calais G, Descamps P, Chapet S, Turgeon V, Reynaud-Bougnoux A, Lemarie E, et al. Primary chemotherapy and radiosurgical breast-conserving treatment for patients with locally advanced operable breast cancers. Int J Radiat Oncol Biol Phys. 1993;26(1):37–42.
109. Conte PF, Alama A, Bertelli G, Canavese G, Carnino F, Catturich A, et al. Chemotherapy with estrogenic recruitment and surgery in locally advanced breast cancer: clinical and cytokinetic results. Int J Cancer. 1987;40(4):490–4.
110. Hery M, Namer M, Moro M, Boublil JL, LaLanne CM. Conservative treatment (chemotherapy/radiotherapy) of locally advanced breast cancer. Cancer. 1986;57(9):1744–9.
111. Perloff M, Lesnick GJ. Chemotherapy before and after mastectomy in stage III breast cancer. Arch Surg. 1982;117(7):879–81.
112. Touboul E, Lefranc JP, Blondon J, Ozsahin M, Mauban S, Schwartz LH, et al. Multidisciplinary treatment approach to locally advanced non-inflammatory breast cancer using chemotherapy and radiotherapy with or without surgery. Radiother Oncol (Journal of the European Society for Therapeutic Radiology and Oncology). 1992;25(3):167–75.
113. Bonadonna G, Veronesi U, Brambilla C, Ferrari L, Luini A, Greco M, et al. Primary chemotherapy to avoid mastectomy in tumors with diameters of three centimeters or more. J Natl Cancer Inst. 1990;82(19):1539–45.
114. Schwartz GF, Birchansky CA, Komarnicky LT, Mansfield CM, Cantor RI, Biermann WA, et al. Induction chemotherapy followed by breast conservation for locally advanced carcinoma of the breast. Cancer. 1994;73(2):362–9.
115. Powles TJ, Hickish TF, Makris A, Ashley SE, O'Brien ME, Tidy VA, et al. Randomized trial of chemoendocrine therapy started before or after surgery for treatment of primary breast cancer. J Clin Oncol (Official Journal of the American Society of Clinical Oncology). 1995;13(3):547–52.
116. Mauriac L, MacGrogan G, Avril A, Durand M, Floquet A, Debled M, et al. Neoadjuvant chemotherapy for operable breast carcinoma larger than 3 cm: a unicentre randomized trial with a 124-month median follow-up. Institut Bergonie Bordeaux Groupe Sein (IBBGS). Ann Oncol (Official Journal of the European Society for Medical Oncology/ESMO). 1999;10(1): 47–52.
117. Morrow M, Strom EA, Bassett LW, Dershaw DD, Fowble B, Giuliano A, et al. Standard for breast conservation therapy in the management of invasive breast carcinoma. CA Cancer J Clin. 2002;52(5):277–300.
118. Scarth H, Cantin J, Levine M. Steering Committee on Clinical Practice Guidelines for the C, Treatment of Breast C. Clinical practice guidelines for the care and treatment of breast cancer: mastectomy or lumpectomy? The choice of operation for clinical stages I and II breast cancer (summary of the 2002 update). CMAJ. 2002;167(2):154–5.
119. Lyman GH, Temin S, Edge SB, Newman LA, Turner RR, Weaver DL, et al. Sentinel lymph node biopsy for patients with early-stage breast cancer: American Society of Clinical Oncology clinical practice guideline update. J Clin Oncol (Official Journal of the American Society of Clinical Oncology). 2014;32 (13):1365–83.
120. Silverstein MJ, Skinner KA, Lomis TJ. Predicting axillary nodal positivity in 2282 patients with breast carcinoma. World J Surg. 2001;25(6):767–72.
121. Chung MH, Ye W, Giuliano AE. Role for sentinel lymph node dissection in the management of large (> or =5 cm) invasive breast cancer. Ann Surg Oncol. 2001;8(9):688–92.
122. Wong SL, Chao C, Edwards MJ, Tuttle TM, Noyes RD, Carlson DJ, et al. Accuracy of sentinel lymph node biopsy for patients with T2 and T3 breast cancers. Am Surg. 2001;67 (6):522–6; discussion 7–8.
123. Harris JR, Halpin-Murphy P, McNeese M, Mendenhall NP, Morrow M, Robert NJ. Consensus statement on postmastectomy radiation therapy. Int J Radiat Oncol Biol Phys. 1999;44(5): 989–90.
124. Buchholz TA, Tucker SL, Masullo L, Kuerer HM, Erwin J, Salas J, et al. Predictors of local-regional recurrence after neoadjuvant chemotherapy and mastectomy without radiation. J Clin Oncol (Official Journal of the American Society of Clinical Oncology). 2002;20(1):17–23.
125. Buchholz TA, Strom EA, Perkins GH, McNeese MD. Controversies regarding the use of radiation after mastectomy in breast cancer. Oncologist. 2002;7(6):539–46.
126. Buchholz TA, Hunt KK, Whitman GJ, Sahin AA, Hortobagyi GN. Neoadjuvant chemotherapy for breast carcinoma: multidisciplinary considerations of benefits and risks. Cancer. 2003;98(6):1150–60.

127. Brun B, Otmezguine Y, Feuilhade F, Julien M, Lebourgeois JP, Calitchi E, et al. Treatment of inflammatory breast cancer with combination chemotherapy and mastectomy versus breast conservation. Cancer. 1988;61(6):1096–103.
128. Fields JN, Perez CA, Kuske RR, Fineberg BB, Bartlett N. Inflammatory carcinoma of the breast: treatment results on 107 patients. Int J Radiat Oncol Biol Phys. 1989;17(2):249–55.
129. Perez CA, Fields JN. Role of radiation therapy for locally advanced and inflammatory carcinoma of the breast. Oncology (Williston Park). 1987;1(1):81–94.
130. Attia-Sobol J, Ferriere JP, Cure H, Kwiatkowski F, Achard JL, Verrelle P, et al. Treatment results, survival and prognostic factors in 109 inflammatory breast cancers: univariate and multivariate analysis. Eur J Cancer. 1993;29A(8):1081–8.
131. Barker JL, Montague ED, Peters LJ. Clinical experience with irradiation of inflammatory carcinoma of the breast with and without elective chemotherapy. Cancer. 1980;45(4):625–9.
132. Chu AM, Wood WC, Doucette JA. Inflammatory breast carcinoma treated by radical radiotherapy. Cancer. 1980;45(11): 2730–7.
133. Kleer CG, van Golen KL, Merajver SD. Molecular biology of breast cancer metastasis. Inflammatory breast cancer: clinical syndrome and molecular determinants. Breast Cancer Res BCR. 2000;2(6):423–9.
134. Turpin E, Bieche I, Bertheau P, Plassa LF, Lerebours F, de Roquancourt A, et al. Increased incidence of ERBB2 overexpression and TP53 mutation in inflammatory breast cancer. Oncogene. 2002;21(49):7593–7.
135. Gruber G, Ciriolo M, Altermatt HJ, Aebi S, Berclaz G, Greiner RH. Prognosis of dermal lymphatic invasion with or without clinical signs of inflammatory breast cancer. Int J Cancer. 2004;109(1):144–8.
136. Bertucci F, Finetti P, Colpaert C, Mamessier E, Parizel M, Dirix L, et al. PDL1 expression in inflammatory breast cancer is frequent and predicts for the pathological response to chemotherapy. Oncotarget. 2015;6(15):13506–19.
137. Van Laere SJ, Van den Eynden GG, Van der Auwera I, Vandenberghe M, van Dam P, Van Marck EA, et al. Identification of cell-of-origin breast tumor subtypes in inflammatory breast cancer by gene expression profiling. Breast Cancer Res Treat. 2006;95(3):243–55.
138. Bertucci F, Finetti P, Rougemont J, Charafe-Jauffret E, Nasser V, Loriod B, et al. Gene expression profiling for molecular characterization of inflammatory breast cancer and prediction of response to chemotherapy. Cancer Res. 2004;64(23):8558–65.
139. Bertucci F, Finetti P, Rougemont J, Charafe-Jauffret E, Cervera N, Tarpin C, et al. Gene expression profiling identifies molecular subtypes of inflammatory breast cancer. Cancer Res. 2005;65(6):2170–8.
140. Sorlie T, Perou CM, Tibshirani R, Aas T, Geisler S, Johnsen H, et al. Gene expression patterns of breast carcinomas distinguish tumor subclasses with clinical implications. Proc Natl Acad Sci USA. 2001;98(19):10869–74.
141. Van Laere SJ, Ueno NT, Finetti P, Vermeulen P, Lucci A, Robertson FM, et al. Uncovering the molecular secrets of inflammatory breast cancer biology: an integrated analysis of three distinct affymetrix gene expression datasets. Clin Cancer Res (Official Journal of the American Association for Cancer Research). 2013;19(17):4685–96.
142. Woodward WA, Krishnamurthy S, Yamauchi H, El-Zein R, Ogura D, Kitadai E, et al. Genomic and expression analysis of microdissected inflammatory breast cancer. Breast Cancer Res Treat. 2013;138(3):761–72.
143. Masuda H, Baggerly KA, Wang Y, Iwamoto T, Brewer T, Pusztai L, et al. Comparison of molecular subtype distribution in triple-negative inflammatory and non-inflammatory breast cancers. Breast Cancer Res BCR. 2013;15(6):R112.
144. Huo L, Wang Y, Gong Y, Krishnamurthy S, Wang J, Diao L, et al. MicroRNA expression profiling identifies decreased expression of miR-205 in inflammatory breast cancer. Mod Pathol (Official Journal of the United States and Canadian Academy of Pathology, Inc.). 2016;29(4):330–46.
145. Anfossi S, Giordano A, Gao H, Cohen EN, Tin S, Wu Q, et al. High serum miR-19a levels are associated with inflammatory breast cancer and are predictive of favorable clinical outcome in patients with metastatic HER2+ inflammatory breast cancer. PLoS ONE. 2014;9(1):e83113.
146. Faille A, De Cremoux P, Extra JM, Linares G, Espie M, Bourstyn E, et al. p53 mutations and overexpression in locally advanced breast cancers. Br J Cancer. 1994;69(6):1145–50.
147. Riou G, Le MG, Travagli JP, Levine AJ, Moll UM. Poor prognosis of p53 gene mutation and nuclear overexpression of p53 protein in inflammatory breast carcinoma. J Natl Cancer Inst. 1993;85(21):1765–7.
148. Gonzalez-Angulo AM, Sneige N, Buzdar AU, Valero V, Kau SW, Broglio K, et al. p53 expression as a prognostic marker in inflammatory breast cancer. Clin Cancer Res (Official Journal of the American Association for Cancer Research). 2004;10(18 Pt 1):6215–21.
149. Kleer CG, van Golen KL, Braun T, Merajver SD. Persistent E-cadherin expression in inflammatory breast cancer. Mod Pathol (Official Journal of the United States and Canadian Academy of Pathology, Inc.). 2001;14(5):458–64.
150. Tomlinson JS, Alpaugh ML, Barsky SH. An intact overexpressed E-cadherin/alpha, beta-catenin axis characterizes the lymphovascular emboli of inflammatory breast carcinoma. Cancer Res. 2001;61(13):5231–41.
151. Alpaugh ML, Tomlinson JS, Kasraeian S, Barsky SH. Cooperative role of E-cadherin and sialyl-Lewis X/A-deficient MUC1 in the passive dissemination of tumor emboli in inflammatory breast carcinoma. Oncogene. 2002;21(22):3631–43.
152. Shirakawa K, Tsuda H, Heike Y, Kato K, Asada R, Inomata M, et al. Absence of endothelial cells, central necrosis, and fibrosis are associated with aggressive inflammatory breast cancer. Cancer Res. 2001;61(2):445–51.
153. Van der Auwera I, Van den Eynden GG, Colpaert CG, Van Laere SJ, van Dam P, Van Marck EA, et al. Tumor lymphangiogenesis in inflammatory breast carcinoma: a histomorphometric study. Clin Cancer Res (Official Journal of the American Association for Cancer Research). 2005;11(21):7637–42.
154. Katayose Y, Kim M, Rakkar AN, Li Z, Cowan KH, Seth P. Promoting apoptosis: a novel activity associated with the cyclin-dependent kinase inhibitor p27. Cancer Res. 1997;57(24):5441–5.
155. Durand B, Gao FB, Raff M. Accumulation of the cyclin-dependent kinase inhibitor p27/Kip1 and the timing of oligodendrocyte differentiation. EMBO J. 1997;16(2):306–17.
156. Gonzalez-Angulo AM, Guarneri V, Gong Y, Cristofanilli M, Morales-Vasquez F, Sneige N, et al. Downregulation of the cyclin-dependent kinase inhibitor p27kip1 might correlate with poor disease-free and overall survival in inflammatory breast cancer. Clin Breast Cancer. 2006;7(4):326–30.
157. van Golen KL, Davies S, Wu ZF, Wang Y, Bucana CD, Root H, et al. A novel putative low-affinity insulin-like growth factor-binding protein, LIBC (lost in inflammatory breast cancer), and RhoC GTPase correlate with the inflammatory breast cancer phenotype. Clin Cancer Res (Official Journal of the American Association for Cancer Research). 1999;5(9):2511–9.
158. Ridley AJ. The GTP-binding protein Rho. Int J Biochem Cell Biol. 1997;29(11):1225–9.

159. van Golen KL, Wu ZF, Qiao XT, Bao LW, Merajver SD. RhoC GTPase, a novel transforming oncogene for human mammary epithelial cells that partially recapitulates the inflammatory breast cancer phenotype. Cancer Res. 2000;60(20):5832–8.
160. van Golen KL, Wu ZF, Qiao XT, Bao L, Merajver SD. RhoC GTPase overexpression modulates induction of angiogenic factors in breast cells. Neoplasia. 2000;2(5):418–25.
161. Kleer CG, Zhang Y, Pan Q, van Golen KL, Wu ZF, Livant D, et al. WISP3 is a novel tumor suppressor gene of inflammatory breast cancer. Oncogene. 2002;21(20):3172–80.
162. Kleer CG, Zhang Y, Pan Q, Gallagher G, Wu M, Wu ZF, et al. WISP3 and RhoC guanosine triphosphatase cooperate in the development of inflammatory breast cancer. Breast Cancer Res BCR. 2004;6(1):R110–5.
163. Xiao Y, Ye Y, Yearsley K, Jones S, Barsky SH. The lymphovascular embolus of inflammatory breast cancer expresses a stem cell-like phenotype. Am J Pathol. 2008;173(2):561–74.
164. Charafe-Jauffret E, Ginestier C, Iovino F, Tarpin C, Diebel M, Esterni B, et al. Aldehyde dehydrogenase 1-positive cancer stem cells mediate metastasis and poor clinical outcome in inflammatory breast cancer. Clin Cancer Res (Official Journal of the American Association for Cancer Research). 2010;16(1):45–55.
165. von Minckwitz G, Untch M, Blohmer JU, Costa SD, Eidtmann H, Fasching PA, et al. Definition and impact of pathologic complete response on prognosis after neoadjuvant chemotherapy in various intrinsic breast cancer subtypes. J Clin Oncol (Official Journal of the American Society of Clinical Oncology). 2012;30(15):1796–804.
166. Chen AM, Meric-Bernstam F, Hunt KK, Thames HD, Oswald MJ, Outlaw ED, et al. Breast conservation after neoadjuvant chemotherapy: the MD Anderson Cancer Center experience. J Clin Oncol (Official Journal of the American Society of Clinical Oncology). 2004;22(12):2303–12.
167. Cortazar P, Zhang L, Untch M, Mehta K, Costantino JP, Wolmark N, et al. Pathological complete response and long-term clinical benefit in breast cancer: the CTNeoBC pooled analysis. Lancet. 2014;384(9938):164–72.
168. Piccart-Gebhart M, Holmes E, Baselga J, de Azambuja E, Dueck AC, Viale G, et al. Adjuvant lapatinib and trastuzumab for early human epidermal growth factor receptor 2-positive breast cancer: results from the randomized phase III adjuvant lapatinib and/or trastuzumab treatment optimization trial. J Clin Oncol (Official Journal of the American Society of Clinical Oncology). 2016;34(10):1034–42.
169. Berruti A, Amoroso V, Gallo F, Bertaglia V, Simoncini E, Pedersini R, et al. Pathologic complete response as a potential surrogate for the clinical outcome in patients with breast cancer after neoadjuvant therapy: a meta-regression of 29 randomized prospective studies. J Clin Oncol (Official Journal of the American Society of Clinical Oncology). 2014;32(34):3883–91.
170. Mathieu MC, Mazouni C, Kesty NC, Zhang Y, Scott V, Passeron J, et al. Breast Cancer index predicts pathological complete response and eligibility for breast conserving surgery in breast cancer patients treated with neoadjuvant chemotherapy. Ann Oncol (Official Journal of the European Society for Medical Oncology/ESMO). 2012;23(8):2046–52.
171. Jeruss JS, Mittendorf EA, Tucker SL, Gonzalez-Angulo AM, Buchholz TA, Sahin AA, et al. Combined use of clinical and pathologic staging variables to define outcomes for breast cancer patients treated with neoadjuvant therapy. J Clin Oncol (Official Journal of the American Society of Clinical Oncology). 2008;26(2):246–52.
172. Mittendorf EA, Jeruss JS, Tucker SL, Kolli A, Newman LA, Gonzalez-Angulo AM, et al. Validation of a novel staging system for disease-specific survival in patients with breast cancer treated with neoadjuvant chemotherapy. J Clin Oncol (Official Journal of the American Society of Clinical Oncology). 2011;29(15):1956–62.
173. Symmans WF, Peintinger F, Hatzis C, Rajan R, Kuerer H, Valero V, et al. Measurement of residual breast cancer burden to predict survival after neoadjuvant chemotherapy. J Clin Oncol (Official Journal of the American Society of Clinical Oncology). 2007;25(28):4414–22.
174. Jones RL, Salter J, A'Hern R, Nerurkar A, Parton M, Reis-Filho JS, et al. The prognostic significance of Ki67 before and after neoadjuvant chemotherapy in breast cancer. Breast Cancer Res Treat. 2009;116(1):53–68.
175. Sheri A, Smith IE, Johnston SR, A'Hern R, Nerurkar A, Jones RL, et al. Residual proliferative cancer burden to predict long-term outcome following neoadjuvant chemotherapy. Ann Oncol (Official Journal of the European Society for Medical Oncology/ESMO). 2015;26(1):75–80.
176. Low JA, Berman AW, Steinberg SM, Danforth DN, Lippman ME, Swain SM. Long-term follow-up for locally advanced and inflammatory breast cancer patients treated with multimodality therapy. J Clin Oncology (Official Journal of the American Society of Clinical Oncology). 2004;22(20):4067–74.
177. Schlichting JA, Soliman AS, Schairer C, Schottenfeld D, Merajver SD. Inflammatory and non-inflammatory breast cancer survival by socioeconomic position in the Surveillance, Epidemiology, and End Results database, 1990–2008. Breast Cancer Res Treat. 2012;134(3):1257–68.
178. Dawood S, Ueno NT, Valero V, Woodward WA, Buchholz TA, Hortobagyi GN, et al. Differences in survival among women with stage III inflammatory and noninflammatory locally advanced breast cancer appear early: a large population-based study. Cancer. 2011;117(9):1819–26.
179. Panades M, Olivotto IA, Speers CH, Shenkier T, Olivotto TA, Weir L, et al. Evolving treatment strategies for inflammatory breast cancer: a population-based survival analysis. J Clin Oncol (Official Journal of the American Society of Clinical Oncology). 2005;23(9):1941–50.
180. Rueth NM, Lin HY, Bedrosian I, Shaitelman SF, Ueno NT, Shen Y, et al. Underuse of trimodality treatment affects survival for patients with inflammatory breast cancer: an analysis of treatment and survival trends from the National Cancer Database. J Clin Oncol (Official Journal of the American Society of Clinical Oncology). 2014;32(19):2018–24.

Neoadjuvant Systemic Treatment (NST) 23

Cornelia Liedtke and Achim Rody

23.1 Indications for Neoadjuvant Chemotherapy

Systemic treatment before surgical therapy of breast cancer (neoadjuvant or preoperative systemic therapy, NST) has become standard of care particularly among patients whose indication for chemotherapy becomes evident at the time of diagnosis. Neoadjuvant chemotherapy has been demonstrated to result in survival rates comparable to those expectable following adjuvant chemotherapy. This is consequence to the fact that the cytotoxic drugs or schedules used in the neoadjuvant setting should be the same as used for adjuvant treatment. NST carries the potential for adjustment of therapy during treatment based on treatment response, may facilitate surgical approaches due to a reduction in tumor burden and may provide time for genetic testing, thereby enabling patient and physician to adjust the treatment plan accordingly.

Many patients such as those with a non-inflammatory hormone receptor (HR)-positive and HER2-negative, low proliferating breast cancer (luminal A subtype) have no indication for (neoadjuvant) chemotherapy due to low chance for treatment response and therefore should receive endocrine therapy only. In contrast, high-risk HR+, HER2 patients defined by high proliferation rate (Luminal B), high tumor burden (e.g., large tumor size, extensive nodal involvement), or further risk factors (e.g., high-grade molecular testing with high-risk classification) are candidates for cytotoxic therapy. The use of chemotherapy in HER2+ and triple-negative breast cancer (TNBC) is mandatory, and for this reason, neoadjuvant chemotherapy seems to be commonly used in combination with targeted agents such as trastuzumab and pertuzumab or bevacizumab. A lack of expression of estrogen and progesterone receptor (ER, PR), overexpression of HER2, and absence of all receptors (TNBC) and high proliferative activity indicated by poor histopathological grading, high expression of Ki67, or genomic grade index [1] are the most important predictors for treatment response provided that optimal systemic therapy has been performed [2]. Less important predictors are young age, non-lobular tumor type, or early clinical response after treatment initiation [3].

An indication for (neo) adjuvant chemotherapy may result from factors such as:

- Unfavorable intrinsic subtype
- Poor prognosis based on histopathological and molecular parameters
- High tumor burden with inoperable tumor spread
- Presentation of inflammatory breast cancer

suggest an absolute or relative indication for NST. Moreover, an:

- Unfavorable breast-to-tumor relation,

which would require surgery by primary mastectomy might also serve as an indication for neoadjuvant treatment with the goal of downsizing the tumor and enabling breast conservation after sufficient tumor response. Furthermore, it has been shown that reduction in tumor size is associated with a reduced size of excised tumor specimen and thereby may lead to a better cosmetic outcome. Further (in part future) objectives are to:

- individualize treatment according to an evaluation of a midcourse treatment effect
- allow for an assessment of recurrence risk after neoadjuvant therapy and surgery
- introduce post-neoadjuvant treatment concepts.

C. Liedtke · A. Rody (✉)
Department of Obstetrics and Gynecology, University Hospital Schleswig-Holstein/Campus Lübeck, Ratzeburger Allee 160, 23538 Lübeck, Schleswig-Holstein, Germany
e-mail: Achim.rody@uksh.de

C. Liedtke
e-mail: cornelia.liedtke@uksh.de

I. Jatoi and A. Rody (eds.), *Management of Breast Diseases*, DOI 10.1007/978-3-319-46356-8_23

23.2 Pathohistological Complete Remission (pCR) as a Surrogate Marker for Survival

23.2.1 Prognostic Significance of pCR

NST has gained broad acceptance in recent years as an important approach in the treatment of breast cancer. This includes not only clinical and therapeutic aspects, but also specific issues of translational research. Achieving a histopathological complete remission in the preoperative setting is the primary goal of therapy, and numerous studies have shown that the pCR is an independent prognostic marker [4] and thus may serve as a surrogate marker for long-term survival of breast cancer. However, the question is debatable whether achieving a pCR also represents a valid prognostic factor in all (molecular) tumor subgroups since intrinsic subtypes are the major predictors of treatment response [5, 6] with highest pCR rates being observed particularly among patients with triple-negative or with HER2-positive breast cancer. Hence, several large-scale analyses suggest that while pCR is an important outcome parameter among patients with high-risk breast cancer subtypes (such as triple-negative breast cancer (TNBC) or HER2-positive/hormone receptor (HR)-negative breast cancer), other breast cancer subtypes (such as unaggressive hormone receptor-positive (luminal A) breast cancer subtypes) may have a favorable prognosis independent of chemotherapy response. For instance, Cortazar et al. [4] were able to demonstrate in a meta-analysis of 11,955 patients from 12 neoadjuvant studies that overall pCR (defined as ypT0, ypN0, or ypT0/ypN0) is associated with improved overall survival. However, pCR has not been validated as a surrogate endpoint for the event-free survival (EFS) or overall survival (OS). In the analysis of the total cohort, a significant benefit in terms of EFS (HR: 0.48; 95 % CI: 0.4–0.54) and OS (HR: 0.36; 95 % CI: 0.31–0.42) could be shown. In particular, achieving pCR in the subgroup of triple-negative and HER2-positive/hormone receptor-negative subtypes is associated with a significant advantage in terms of EFS (triple-negative: HR 0.42; 95 % CI: 0.18–0.33) and HER2-positive/HR-negative: HR 0.25; 95 % CI: 0.18–0.34. These data have not been confirmed for HR-positive/HER2-negative breast cancer. However, most studies were not able to differentiate tumors in Luminal A and B tumors. Von Minckwitz et al. [7] in a meta-analysis of german neoadjuvant trials were able to demonstrate pCR representing a prognostic factor for disease-free survival only in the group of Luminal B tumors and not in the group of Luminal A tumors.

In the overall analysis of the various studies, Cortazar et al. showed only a weak (and non-numeric) association between increased pCR and improved EFS or OS. Nevertheless, to achieve a pCR is considered to be an important endpoint for regulatory authorities such as the Food and Drug Administration.

23.2.2 Definitions of pCR

Achievement of pCR and its association with an improved survival prognosis in patients with breast cancer is closely related to its definition. The optimal definition of pCR so far seems to be unclear. Furthermore, the question as to whether residual DCIS should be included in the definition of pCR (thereby being rendered prognostically irrelevant or not) is still matter of intense discussion [7, 8]. Similarly, the relevance of axillary metastases is still a matter for debate. Hennessy et al. [9] could demonstrate that the outcome of patients with cytologically proven axillar metastases mainly depends on the treatment response in axillary nodes. Patients who show a complete response in axillary nodes but not in primary tumor have a clinical outcome that is comparable to patients with pathological complete response in both primary tumor axillary nodes.

Also, the simple dichotomy of chemotherapy response as pCR or residual tumor has been frequently criticized since response to chemotherapy may be perceived as a continuum rather than a two tired-score. An optimized quantification of chemotherapy response can be achieved, for example, by use of semiquantitative scoring systems such as the residual cancer burden (RCB) [10]. This index combines the histopathological tumor diameter, tumor cellularity, and the number and diameter of axillary lymph node metastases with a value that reflects the extent of treatment response on a scale of 0–3. These values correlate significantly with the further prognosis of the patient. The RCB score, however, is increasingly used primarily in the US or in the context of studies.

23.3 Biomarkers in Neoadjuvant Systemic Therapy

Given the high prognostic importance of pCR among patients undergoing NST, there is particular and increasing interest in defining factors that may predict for an achievement of pCR. Among the plethora of factors, some are of particular importance such as:

- tumor-infiltrating lymphocytes (TILs)
- individual biomarkers
- parameters reflecting tumor cell proliferation.

23.3.1 Tumor-Infiltrating Lymphocytes

Recent data could demonstrate with a high level of evidence that TILs from patients treated within clinical trials are able to predict treatment response reliably. This parameter has gained particular interest in association with TNBC and response to carboplatin [11]. There is, however, uncertainty as to whether TILs may predict a substance-specific effect or are rather associated with overall chemotherapy sensitivity. Furthermore, before this biomarker justifies introduction to daily clinical routine, hurdles, such as lack of standardization in analysis of TILs, have to be overcome [12].

23.3.2 Individual Molecular Biomarkers of Resistance

Several individual genes have been analyzed with respect to their importance in predicting neoadjuvant treatment response. For instance, while mutations in PIK3CA [13] have not been demonstrated to be predictive in prospective trials, a recent pooled analysis of four different clinical trials (GeparQuattro/GeparQuinto, GeparSixto, NeoALTTO, and CHERLOB) suggests that presence of PIK3CA mutations in HER2+ breast cancer is associated with a significantly lower rate of pCR [14]. PIK3CA mutations in HER2+ tumors constantly are frequently found to be in the range of 20 % irrespective of HR status, and an increase in response rates has not been seen even if using a double blockade of HER2 by treatment combination with lapatinib and trastuzumab.

23.3.3 Tumor Cell Proliferation

The significance of expression of the proliferation marker Ki-67 in particular in the distinction of luminal breast cancer subtypes (luminal A vs. luminal B) is similarly intensely discussed. Hormone receptor-positive breast cancers with an increased expression of Ki-67 (luminal B subtype) are strongly associated with a poor prognosis but show a higher probability of responding to neoadjuvant chemotherapy. Denkert et al. examined the association between the expression of the proliferation marker Ki-67 and the response to neoadjuvant chemotherapy as well as disease prognosis in individual breast cancer subtypes. This analysis was performed on the basis of 1166 pre-cytotoxic tumor biopsies which have been obtained as part of the neoadjuvant GeparTrio trial [15]. Denkert et al. stratified the patients based on the Ki-67 expression in three groups with cutoff values lower than 15 %, 15–35 %, and higher than 35 %, respectively. It was found that Ki-67 has different prognostic and predictive values in different breast cancer subtypes.

For patients with triple-negative breast cancer, for example, a significant correlation between the immunohistochemical expression of Ki-67 and the pathological complete remission rate could be demonstrated. The pCR rates for Ki-67 expression of ≤15, 15–35, and ≥35 % were 15, 22, and 38 % ($p = 0.003$). However, overall survival probabilities in the three groups were not significantly different. In contrast, no significant correlation between the expression of Ki-67 and patients prognosis has been showed. Accordingly, the immunohistochemical expression of Ki-67 is a significant predictive marker in terms of response to neoadjuvant chemotherapy, but not a relevant biomarker for prognosis among patients with TNBC. This should be considered when interpreting surprisingly high Ki-67 expression levels in patients with TNBC.

23.4 Choice of Chemotherapy Regimens in Neoadjuvant Systemic Therapy

When deciding about neoadjuvant chemotherapy regimens, physicians typically chose the same regimen that would have been chosen in case of adjuvant therapy of the same patient. Usually, neoadjuvant treatment regimens consist in combination chemotherapy regimens containing both taxanes and anthracyclins sequentially or simultaneously. However, anthracycline-free chemotherapy regimens may be considered a valuable alternative, particularly in case of cardiotoxicity concerns.

In the German GeparTrio trial, patients with insufficient response after two cycles of TAC chemotherapy were randomised to either continue TAC chemotherapy or switch to a non-cross-resistant chemotherapy with vinorelbine and capecitabine. Although the response rates (i.e., pCR rates) were not different [16], a significant improvement of disease-free survival and overall could be reached (HR 0.71; 95 % Ki 0.60–0.85; $p < 0.001$ and HR 0.79; 95 % Ki 0.63–0.99; $0 < 0.048$, respectively). However, this effect was different among distinct breast cancer subgroups: patients with TNBC did not derive particular benefit (HR 0.87; 95 % Ki 0.61–1.27; $p = 0.464$) whereas patients with hormone receptor-positive disease showed significant improvement of both study endpoints [17].

Response control during NST is an important issue particularly after cycle 2 of PST. Patients not responding to NST and presenting with a tumor progression should stop treatment, and immediate surgery or radiotherapy is indicated.

23.4.1 Choice of Therapy Regimens in HER2-Positive Breast Cancer

In the adjuvant setting, the poor prognosis of this molecular subgroup could be significantly improved by the anti-HER2 therapy with trastuzumab. In numerous neoadjuvant studies, the addition of a HER2-targeted therapy to chemotherapy showed a significant increase in pCR. Furthermore, a positive HER2 status is defined as a predictive marker of response to neoadjuvant chemotherapy.

To date, there are numerous HER2-targeted drugs available—implying the question of the optimal treatment regimen is in this subgroup.

For instance, there is a significant body of evidence regarding the use of lapatinib (alone or in combination with trastuzumab) for use in neoadjuvant therapy in HER2-positive breast cancer. For instance, in the small Phase-2-CHER-LOB trial published by Guarneri et al. [18], a taxane-based chemotherapy was followed by 4 cycles of FEC chemotherapy, accompanied by an anti-HER2-targeted treatment consisting of lapatinib or trastuzumab alone or dual blockade with trastuzumab and lapatinib in combination. The pCR rate for monotherapy with lapatinib or trastuzumab was 25 or 26.3 %, respectively, but was doubled in the combination arm with 46.7 %.

Untch et al. [19] showed in the German GeparQuattro trial that neoadjuvant therapy of HER2-positive breast cancer by combination of chemotherapy with trastuzumab is associated with an increase in pCR rate to 31.7 % compared to 15.7 % in the HER2-negative patient subgroup who did not receive trastuzumab. In this context, it is noteworthy that HER2-positive patients, who showed no response during the first four cycles of EC, could still achieve a pCR rate of 16.6 % by switching to a taxane-containing combination with trastuzumab compared to 3.3 % in the HER2-negative subgroup.

In the German GeparQuinto trial, patients were randomly assigned to receive trastuzumab (ECH-TH group) or lapatinib (ECL-TL group) in addition to EC followed by docetaxel. The rate of pCR was 30.3 % versus 22.7 % in the trastuzumab arm, which was significantly higher compared to the lapatinib arm. However, according to the adverse events, there was 75 % rate of diarrhea in the lapatinib arm with a dropout rate of 33.1 % [20].

Von Minckwitz et al. [21] could demonstrate in the GeparSixto trial that the addition of carboplatin to pegylated liposomal doxorubicin and paclitaxel in combination with lapatinib and trastuzumab in HER2-positive breast cancer is not associated with an improvement of achieving a pCR (32.8 % with carboplatin versus 36.8 % without carboplatin). Thus, the anti-HER2 therapy with trastuzumab in combination with neoadjuvant chemotherapy has provided significant improvement by increasing rate of pCR.

To date, there are two major questions that need to be addressed with regard to neoadjuvant therapy in HER2-positive breast cancer:

- There is yet uncertainty as to under which circumstances (i.e., scale, agents, and patient subgroup) improvements in pCR reliably translate into an improvement of survival.
- Given that in the view of new HER2-targeting compounds evolving and investigated within clinical trials, the optimal HER2-targeted agent to be combined with trastuzumab is still a matter of debate.

One example regarding the association between pCR and prognosis involves the NeoALTTO/ALTTO trials. The NeoALTTO trial [22] (Fig. 23.1) prospectively randomized a total of 455 HER2-positive breast cancer patients in three treatment arms. All patients received preoperative 12 cycles of paclitaxel weekly, either in combination with lapatinib or trastuzumab alone or the combination of both. The combination of lapatinib and trastuzumab yielded the highest rate of pCR (51.3 %) compared to trastuzumab alone with 29.5 % and lapatinib with 24.7 %. The difference between

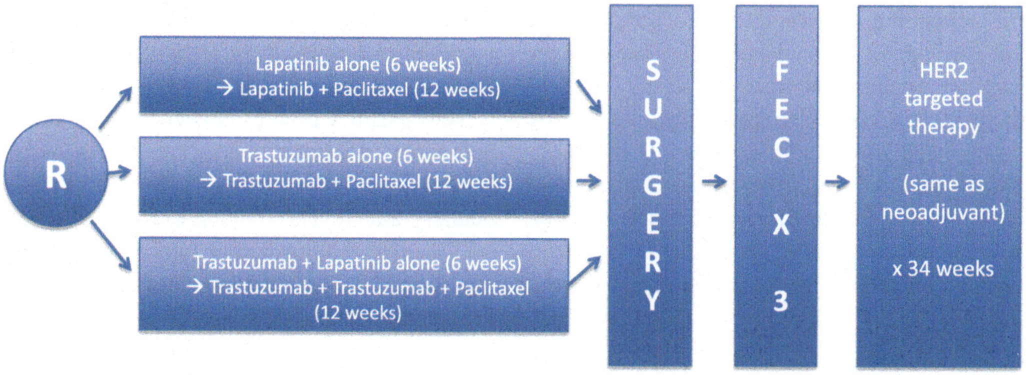

Fig. 23.1 Design of the NeoALTTO trial

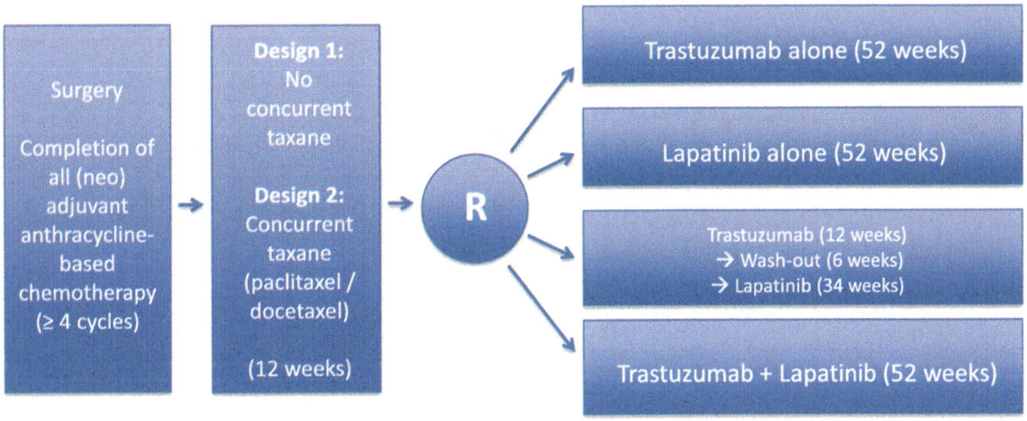

Fig. 23.2 Design of the ALTTO trial

trastuzumab and lapatinib was not of statistically significant. Follow-up data of the NeoALTTO trial suggested superiority of this combination therapy with regard to DFS; however, statistical relevance could not be demonstrated which certainly was a consequence of lack of adequate power regarding a survival endpoint [23]. Furthermore, in the corresponding adjuvant trial (i.e., ALTTO) (Fig. 23.2) among 8381 women with HER2-positive breast cancer, the addition of lapatinib to trastuzumab did not result in a significant increase in DFS compared to standard therapy with trastuzumab (4.5-year DFS 86 % for trastuzumab vs. 88 % for trastuzumab/lapatinib). However, again flaws with regard to study design were held responsible for causing these disappointing results such as inclusion of a large number of patients with low-risk HER2-positive disease, and therefore, lack of an adequate number of DFS-event again leading to a lack of sufficient power.

One of the most promising agents for use in the neoadjuvant setting rather than lapatinib is the HER2 dimerization inhibitor pertuzumab. Gianni et al. [24] recently reported results from NeoSphere trial. In this trial 417, HER2-positive breast cancer patients with a tumor size larger than 2 cm were randomized to four treatment arms: trastuzumab/docetaxel versus pertuzumab/trastuzumab/docetaxel versus pertuzumab/trastuzumab versus pertuzumab/docetaxel. There was a significant increase in pCR by the addition of pertuzumab to trastuzumab and docetaxel (45.8 % vs. 29.0 %). In the subgroup of HER2-positive/HR-negative patients, a pCR rate of 63.2 % has been observed, and there was also an amazing rate of pCR in the chemotherapy-free arm (16.8 % combination of pertuzumab/trastuzumab). Moreover, patients who received docetaxel in addition to trastuzumab and pertuzumab showed a trend in terms of an improved disease-free survival. This meant that pertuzumab has received a label extension for neoadjuvant therapy situation in combination with trastuzumab. Thus, the dual HER2 blockade by pertuzumab and trastuzumab in combination with docetaxel may be defined as a new gold standard.

Figure 23.3 summarizes the results of the most prominent clinical trials addressing the role of dual HER2 blockade in HER2-positive breast cancer.

23.4.2 Choice of Therapy Regimens in Patients with TNBC

TNBC despite carrying an overall unfavorable prognosis is characterized by an increased chance of response to neoadjuvant chemotherapy that is reflected by increased rates of pCR in association with this breast cancer subtype [25–28]. This phenomenon is often referred to as triple-negative paradox in the literature [29] and may be explained primarily by the following observations:

- Patients with TNBC that achieves a pCR have an optimal prognosis which is not significantly inferior to patients with non-TNBC achieving a pCR
- Patients with TNBC not achieving a pCR have a highly unfavorable prognosis that is significantly inferior to that observable among patients with other breast cancer subtypes. This may be explained in part by the fact that the adverse prognosis associated with non-pCR among patients with non-TNBC subtypes may be compensated by additional (post-neoadjuvant/adjuvant) systemic therapy such as HER2-directed agents and/or endocrine therapy.

Therefore, there is an urgent need to optimize efficacy of neoadjuvant chemotherapy and thereby improve prognosis among patients with TNBC through:

NeoSpere (n=417)

	pCR (ypTo)
trastuzumab + docetaxel	29.0%
Pertuzumab + trastuzumab + docetaxel	45.8%
pertuzumab + trastuzumab	16.8%
Pertuzumab + docetaxel	24.0%

Neo-ALTTO (n=455)

	pCR (ypT0/is ypN0)
Trastuzumab → trastuzumab + paclitaxel	29.5%
lapatinib → lapatinib + paclitaxel	24.7%
Trastuzumab/ lapatinib → Trastuzumab/ lapatinib + paclitaxel	51.3%

TRYPHaena (n=225)

	pCR (ypT0/is)	pCR (ypT0 ypN0)
FEC + pertuzumab + trastuzumab × 3 → pertuzumab + trastuzumab + docetaxel × 3	61.6%	50.7%
FEC × 3 → pertuzumab + trastuzumab + docetaxel × 3	57.3%	45.3%
TCbH + pertuzumab ×6	66.2%	51.9%

GeparQuinto (n=620)

	pCR (ypT0 and ypN0)
Epirubicine + cyclophosphamide + trastuzumab → docetaxel + trastuzumab	30·3%
Epirubicine + cyclophosphamide + lapatinib → docetaxel + lapatinib	22·7%

GeparSixto (n=137)

	pCR (ypT0 ypN0)
Weekly paclitaxel + non-pegylated liposomal doxorubicin + trastuzumab + lapatinib x 18	36·8%
Weekly paclitaxel + non-pegylated liposomal doxorubicin + trastuzumab + lapatinib x 18 + Carboplatin	32·8%

GeparSepto (n=1.200)

	pCR (ypT0 ypN0)
Weekly nab-paclitaxel x 12 → 4 x EC + trastuzumab + pertuzumab	74,6 %
Weekly paclitaxel x 12 → 4 x EC + trastuzumab + pertuzumab	66,7 %;

Fig. 23.3 Results of the most prominent clinical trials addressing the role of dual HER2 blockade in HER2-positive breast cancer

- optimization of chemotherapy scheduling (i.e., through dose-dense/dose-intensified regimens) [30]
- use of additional agents in combination with standard combination chemotherapy regimens
- development of novel targeted agents for patients with TNBC
- identification of biomarkers in response to neoadjuvant chemotherapy in TNBC to allow for treatment individualization.

Sequential or simultaneous combination chemotherapy containing both anthracyclins and taxanes has long been regarded as standard neoadjuvant chemotherapy approach for patients with TNBC. Several studies have aimed at increasing chemotherapy efficacy through the addition of novel agents such as capecitabine [31–33] or eribulin [34]; however, solid data and validation studies are lacking despite the fact that subgroups analyses showed a significant benefit in TN breast cancer subgroups by these approaches.

This has changed due to the observation that triple-negative and/or BRCA1-associated breast cancer may derive particular benefit from the addition of platinum-containing agents. While historical data have suggested for several years that platinum-containing chemotherapy may be particularly beneficial to patients with TNBC [35], prospective evidence was lacking until the publication of two important neoadjuvant clinical trials:

- GeparSixto (NCT01426880) by the *German Breast Group* (*GBG*) [31] (Fig. 23.4)
- The CALGB/ALLIANCE-40603 (NCT00861705) by the *Cancer and Leukemia Group B* (*CALGB*) (Fig. 23.5).

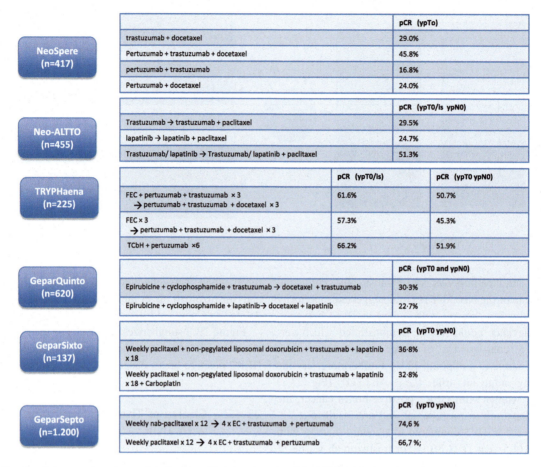

In the first study (GeparSixto) [36], 84 of 158 patients with TNBC (53.2 %; 95 % CI 54.4–60.9) experienced a pCR (defined as ypT0 ypN0) through the addition of carboplatin compared to 58 of 157 patients without carboplatin (36.9 %; 95 % CI 29.4–44.5, $p = 0.005$). Among patients with HER2-positive disease, no significant effect through carboplatin could be observed. In interpretation of these results, there is still an ongoing debate to what extend this was achieved as a part of a substance-specific effect or though introduction of a more intensified regimen. Most importantly, at SABCS 2015, von Minckwitz and colleagues demonstrated that the addition of carboplatin not only led to an increase in pCR, but that this pCR benefit also translated

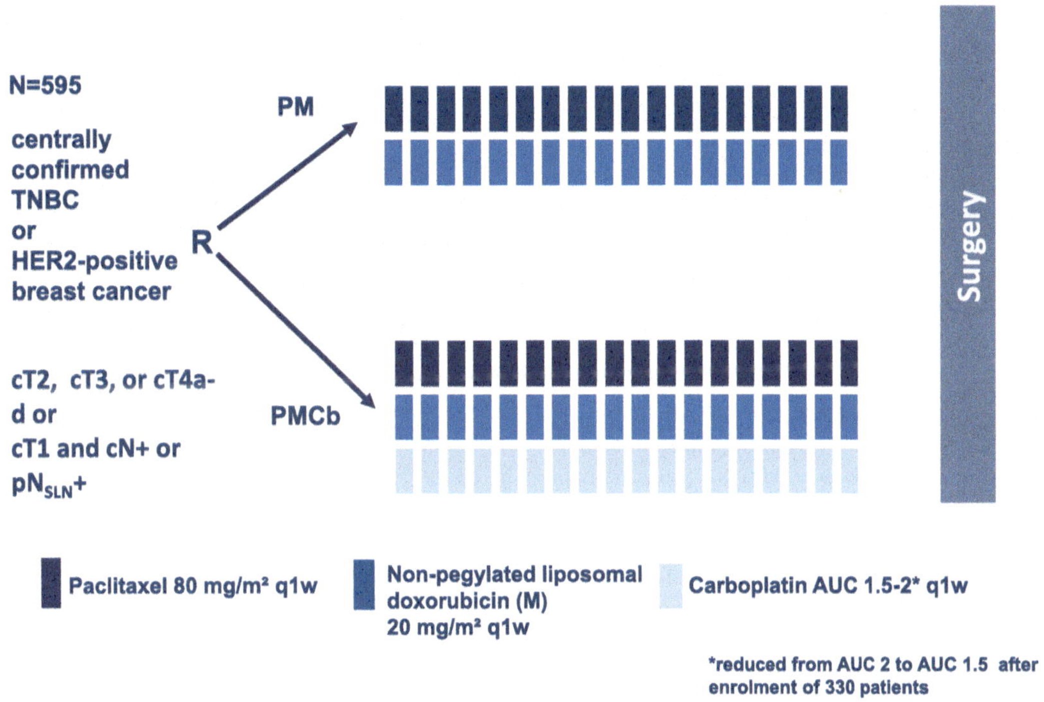

Fig. 23.4 Design of the GeparSixto phase II trial

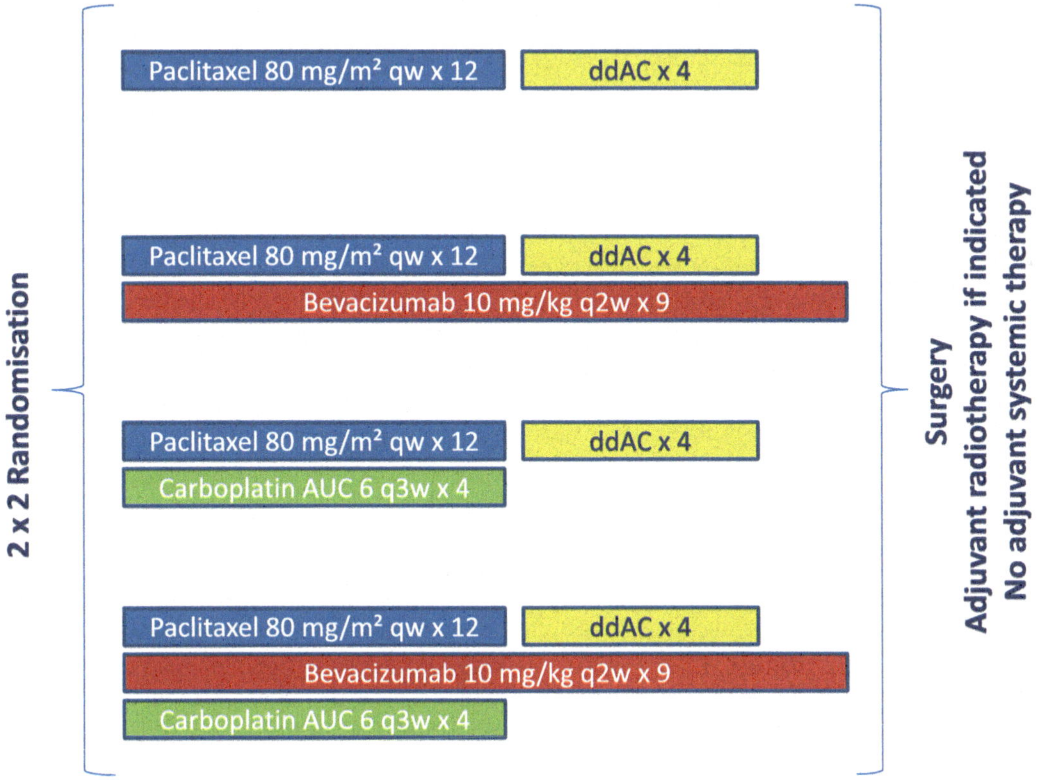

Fig. 23.5 Design of the CALGB 40603 phase II trial

into an improved prognosis among patients with TNBC: After a median follow-up of three years, disease-free survival for patients assigned to carboplatin was 85.5 % compared with 76.1 % for patients assigned no carboplatin. This meant that patients with TNBC who received carboplatin as part of their neoadjuvant chemotherapy regimen were almost half as likely to have had disease relapse at three years after starting the treatment compared with those who did not receive carboplatin, and it was those patients who had a pCR were least likely to have disease relapse [37].

The second study (CALGB40603) analyzed the use of carboplatin (and bevacizumab) among patients with TNBC in addition to a sequential anthracycline/taxane chemotherapy regimen [38]. Again, the addition of carboplatin resulted in an increase in pCR rate 41–54 % ($p = 0.0018$). Since hematologic toxicity and particularly SAEs were less common in association with this latter regimen, the sequential use of carboplatin is regarded by many as a more safely feasible regimen in daily clinical management of patients with TNBC. In contrast to the observations in GeparSixto, CALGB40603 could not demonstrate significant improvement of DFS with the addition of carboplatin with 3-year rates of 74.1 and 83.2 %, respectively. Only an insignificant EFS hazard ratio of 0.84 (95 % CI 0.58–1.22, $P = 0.36$) and a survival hazard of 1.15 (95 % CI 0.74–1.79, $P = 0.53$) were observed [39].

Given that a lack of power might be responsible for the lack of observing a significant effect, both analyses point toward carboplatin playing an important role in the treatment of primary TNBC. Overall, two distinct scenarios regarding the future use of carboplatin among patients with TNBC seem imaginable:

- Use of platinum salts as part of therapy intensification aiming at increase efficacy at the cost of increased toxicity.
- Use of platinum salts as part of therapy de-escalation by replacing taxanes or more importantly anthracyclins to improve the therapeutic index through the improvement of treatment tolerability.

23.4.3 Biomarkers for Prediction of Platinum Efficacy in TNBC

The following aspects may justify hesitation with regard to routine use of platinum salts among patients with TNBC:

- The addition of carboplatin may lead to increase toxicity.
- Many patients (35–40 %) achieve a pCR with anthracyclins and taxane chemotherapy without carboplatin and in case of addition of platinum salts are exposed to unnecessary toxicity.
- Data regarding a translation of the pCR benefit associated with carboplatin into a survival benefit are contradictory.

Therefore, there is a yet unmet need to develop and validate biomarkers that allow for stratification of patients with TNBC into those that do need carboplatin and those that do not.

In vitro data and preclinical analyses suggest a particular sensitivity of BRCA1-associated breast cancers against platinum salts [40]. Since TNBC may commonly observed among patients carrying a BRCA1 mutation and furthermore, share many histological and molecular features with hereditary breast cancer, there has been an intense (and yet unsolved) debate as to whether diagnosis of TNBC or rather diagnosis of hereditary breast cancer (regardless of molecular subtype) represents the optimal predictive factor for the use of carboplatin in a neoadjuvant treatment regimen.

While translational analyses of the GeparSixto study could not confirm a predictive association between BRCA1 mutations and carboplatin efficacy among patients with TNBC [41] analyses derived from patients in the metastatic setting suggest a particular superiority of carboplatin compared to docetaxel in first-line mono-chemotherapy among patients with metastatic TNBC response rates 68 % versus 33.3 % ($p = 0.03$) [42]. Furthermore, given that in the GeparSixto trial, carboplatin was used as an add-on rather than a substitute for standard chemotherapy, one has to acknowledge when analyzing data from that trial that a biomarker that is associated with increased chance of pCR from carboplatin may reflect (i) a platinum-specific effect or (ii) an effect observed by a more intense therapy (irrespective of the type of additional chemotherapy). Trials that compare a carboplatin-based combination regimen to a similarly intensive regimen using an alternative substance may provide a better answer as to whether BRCA predict for platinum efficacy specifically. The German ADAPT TN trial (Fig. 23.6) compares neoadjuvant chemotherapy with carboplatin/nab-paclitaxel to a neoadjuvant regimen of gemcitabine/nab-paclitaxel. pCR rates (ypT0/ypTis ypN0) as reported at SABCS 2015 were 45.9 % versus 28.7 % ($p < 0.001$), respectively [41].

In general, while carboplatin has for sometime been suggested for use only in the presence of a BRCA1/2 mutation, its use is currently not limited to hereditary breast cancer only. Nevertheless, given that the addition of carboplatin is associated with an increase in treatment toxicity, indication of carboplatin should be seen with caution and with a particular regard to the patient's performance status, tumor biology, and competing risks.

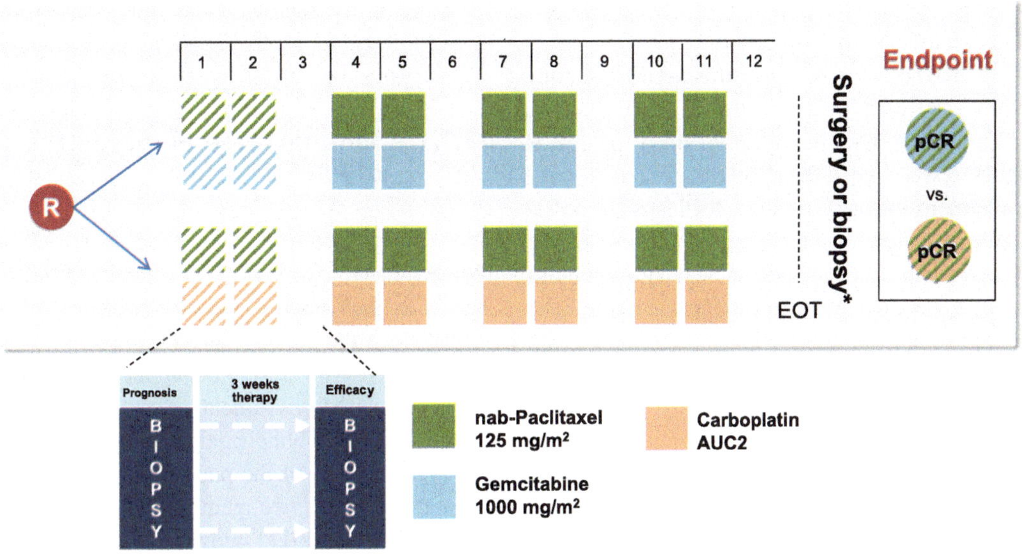

Fig. 23.6 Design of the WSG ADAPT TN phase II trial

23.4.4 Use of Bevacizumab in Neoadjuvant Chemotherapy

Preclinical and translational data have long been regarded to suggest particular benefit by the use of bevacizumab in neoadjuvant systemic therapy particularly among patients with TNBC and/or HER2-positive disease. Therefore, several studies have analyzed the value of an addition of bevacizumab to standard neoadjuvant chemotherapy. These studies, however, have yielded conflicting results regarding (i) the capability of bevacizumab in enhancing pCR rates, (ii) efficacy of bevacizumab in molecular breast cancer subgroups, and (iii) translation of pCR rate alterations into prognostic effects [43, 44].

23.5 Neoadjuvant Endocrine Approaches

Neoadjuvant endocrine therapy is an option mainly for postmenopausal women with highly endocrine-responsive breast cancer and may represent an alternative to neoadjuvant chemotherapy particularly in case of contraindications for chemotherapy. Patients suitable for primary endocrine therapy should present with tumors with high ER/PR sensitivity, low nuclear grade, or low Ki67 [45].

In selected patients, 3 month of preoperative hormonal treatment (anastrozole and exemestane) may be equally effective compared to neoadjuvant taxane-based chemotherapy (i.e., 4 × AT) [46].

However, it has to be acknowledged that pCR rates may not represent the optimal study endpoint in the context of primary endocrine therapy given that pCR rates in the neoadjuvant endocrine setting are commonly very low. For instance, after 3 months of tamoxifen therapy, pCR rates may not exceed 2 %, and even in case of treatment with aromatase, inhibitors may not be significantly higher.

Another critical issue refers to the optimal duration of primary endocrine therapy, since prolonged endocrine therapy (i.e., 4–6 months) has been associated with increased response rates of up to 10 % [47].

In summary, neoadjuvant endocrine treatment approaches may represent an option for those patients who are not suitable candidates for neoadjuvant or adjuvant chemotherapy or carry contraindications for surgery because of comorbidities, a poor general condition or advanced age.

23.6 Novel Therapeutic Concepts: Post-neoadjuvant Therapy, Dynamic Biomarkers, and "Window Studies"

Pathological complete response rates have become a popular study endpoint due to early availability and strict definition.

A major challenge yet, however, has become therapy of patients that do not derive substantial benefit from neoadjuvant multi-agent approaches and left with residual cancer at the time of surgery. For these patents, additional/ alternative treatment approaches are warranted. In this context, post-neoadjuvant therapy might be an additional treatment option. In the case of failure to achieve a pCR, the use of additional non-cross resistant therapies could improve the prognosis of these patients. Recent analyses (Japan) suggest that post-neoadjuvant use of capecitabine might become an option for patients with TNBC and residual tumor following preoperative chemotherapy in the future. In addition to this, a particular focus lies in the introduction of new substances, such as the selective inhibitor of cyclin-dependent kinase (CDK) 4 and 6 in hormone receptor-negative cancers (Penelope B, NCT01864746) or trastuzumab-DM1, among patients with HER2-positive disease (Katherine, NCT01772472). On the other hand, achievement of a pCR mirroring highly responsive disease might also justify the reduction in treatment intensity such as, for instance, cessation of trastuzumab therapy in the post-neoadjuvant setting. Unfortunately, at present there are no sufficient data available. Studies that will investigate such treatment concepts, however, are still recruiting or in preparation.

Other studies use the neoadjuvant window to investigate the biological response of tumor cells to a three-week primary systemic therapy, as for example by determining tumor cell proliferation before and after therapeutic intervention and adjustment of further systemic treatment according to biological behaviour. In the ADAPT study (*Adjuvant Dynamic marker-Adjusted Personalized Therapy Trial optimizing risk assessment and therapy response prediction in early breast cancer*), researchers of the West German Study Group (WSG) analyze how in patients with hormone receptor-positive breast cancer and a significant decrease in Ki-67 expression after can be dispensed with three-week endocrine therapy in adjuvant chemotherapy (http://www.wsg-online.com). Comparable study concepts for patients with other breast cancer subtypes (such as HER2-positive or triple-negative tumors) are ongoing.

23.7 Surgical Considerations in the Context of Neoadjuvant Systemic Therapy

While administering neoadjuvant chemotherapy, clinical response of the tumor should be controlled during the course of treatment. Thus, it is important to document the tumor location accurately and to provide a titanium clip marker in particular for small tumor volume or very good response of tumors to therapy. A clip can be placed under ultrasound control and carried out generously by mammographic control. In case of clinical suspicion of a pCR, preoperative wire localization of the lying clip should be done for intraoperative navigation. In addition to ultrasound and mammography, operative planning can be enhanced by means of MRI particularly in case of breast density of ACR3-4. Furthermore, MRI may increase preoperative estimation whether a pCR may be expected. In case of significant tumor shrinkage during neoadjuvant therapy, excision of the tumor in its new border increases the chance of an optimal cosmetic outcome. Moreover certain situations such as advanced breast cancer with skin infiltration, inflammation, and/or multicentricity, possible breast conservation is considered by some but may be difficult to achieve. Therefore, strict indication and detailed elucidation of the patient are warranted.

23.7.1 Sentinel Node Biopsy in the Context of PST

The removal of the so-called sentinel lymph node (sentinel lymphadenectomy, SLNE) is established as the gold standard of axillary staging in clinically uninvolved lymph nodes (cN0), since the conduction of complete axillary dissection is associated with a significant increase in operative morbidity. Impaired movement of the arm due to iatrogenic nerve lesions or a lymphedema of the affected arm may limit the quality of life of the patient to a large extent.

In the primary treatment setting, the publication of the results of the Z0011 study by the American College of Surgeons Oncology Group (ACOSOG) has for the first time led to a paradigm shift in the implementation of the axillary staging. This trial was able to demonstrate that under certain conditions even if limited lymph node involvement has been detected a complete axillary clearing can be dispensed. In this prospective randomized phase III trial, 445 women received a complete axillary dissection after the detection of involved sentinel nodes, whereas 445 women underwent sentinel node biopsy only, even if this node showed tumor involvement. The prerequisite for this was the presence of a tumor with a cT1 or 2-stage, clinically node-negative axilla (cN0), less than 3 involved lymph nodes as well as the implementation of a breast-conserving therapy with breast radiation and adequate systemic treatment. After a median follow-up of 6.3 years no significant difference between the two groups has been observed according to in-breast recurrences, axillary relapse, disease-free and overall survival. This study is discussed very controversially in terms of several aspects, e.g., this trial has been stopped early because of difficulties in recruiting patients. Moreover, breast radiation was a priori not clearly defined. Nevertheless, in view of these study results and according to the principle "*primum non nocere*," axillary dissection cannot be recommended unequivocally in cases if Z0011 criteria are met. This has found its way into the appropriate guidelines.

Consequently, there is an intense discussion as to the optimal time of axillary dissection in the context of PST in order to similarly reduce the extend of axillary surgery with the goal to reduce treatment-associated morbidity.

Patients with a clinically negative axilla are candidates for SLNE analogous to the primary preoperative setting. If SLNE is performed before systemic therapy (in a systemically untreated axilla), the patient will need to undergo two surgical procedures, i.e., SLNE before and removal of the primary tumor after NST. If SLNE is performed after axillary surgery, there are concerns as to the adequacy of the procedure and as to the loss of the prognostic/predictive information of axillary status prior to NST with respect to tailoring of NST. Data regarding the reliability of axillary staging by SLNE are limited. Classe et al. analyzed 195 patients with advanced breast cancer and found SLNE in patients that were clinically node-negative before NST to be reliable with a detection rate of 94.6 % and a false-negative rate of 9.4 %. Despite additional data not being available yet, SLNE may be carried out following PST among patients that were clinically node-negative before NST in selected cases [48].

More different yet better analyzed is the performance of SLNE among patients that show an axillary conversion from cN+ to ycN0 through NST. If SLNE was as reliable among those patients, these individuals would benefit from an axillary downstaging resulting in less extensive axillary surgery. This optimistic vision is confronted by the concerns regarding an increased false-negative rate of SLNB after NST and the uncertainty as to what extent the clinical lymph node status before PST could be incorporated in the decision for or against a particular (e.g., dose-dense) chemotherapy regimen.

Two clinical trials that have attempted to address the question of the optimal timing of axillary staging in the context of PST are the German SENTINA and the American ACOSOG Z1071.

In the Z1071 study of the American College of Surgeons Oncology Group (ACOSOG) [49], 637 patients were registered with pathological evidence of diseased axillary lymph nodes with neoadjuvant chemotherapy. In all patients, a SLNE was conducted with secondary komplettierender axillary dissection. The detection rate was 92.7 % (95 % CI 90.5–94.6) indicated. Under chemotherapy, a conversion rate of a positive axilla status before chemotherapy was given to a negative lymph node status after primary systemic therapy of 40 %. In 46 patients (7.1 %) an SLN could not be identified, only one SLN was excised in 78 patients (12.6 %). Of the remaining 525 patients with 2 or more SLNs removed, no cancer was identified in the axillary lymph nodes of 215 patients corresponding to a pathological complete nodal response rate of 41.0 %. Among 39 patients, no cancer was identified in the SLNs but was found in lymph nodes obtained in completion ALND, corresponding to an FNR of 12.6 %. However, only a sentinel lymph node was removed, was the false-negative rate of 31.5 %. Before background of these data, the authors of this study concluded that the SLNB would after primary systemic therapy a useful method stage for the event that 2 Sentinel lymph nodes are removed and a dual tracer method (i.e., blue coloring and radio colloid) is used 29th. In this context, the discussion about the optimal time of axillary dissection in the context of PST can be seen.

These observations contradict data from Germany. The SENTINA study [50] investigated the optimal time for performing the axillary staging in the context of the PST and recruited patients in 4 different study arms based on the clinical lymph node status before and after PST (see Chart 4). This corresponded to an arm of the study (see Arm C) largely the study population of ACOSOG Z1071 study and contained 592 patients. This arm showed a conversion rate (i.e., clinically positive axilla prior systemic therapy for clinically negative axilla after systemic therapy) of 52.3 %. The false-negative rate (FNR) in this study arm was estimated at 14.2 % (was carried out, i.e., a re-SLNE). In the study arm in which patients a second SLNB after chemotherapy received prior SLNE before chemotherapy, the FNR was unacceptable 51.6 %. The authors of the study therefore concluded that the FNR was not acceptable for repeated SLNE after PST. The FNR of 14.2 % is well below the rate observed in studies in primary operation (i.e., without prior chemotherapy) in the initial studies on the SLNE.

At the present time, the publication of further results and methodological details of the two studies should be awaited before a final conclusion can be drawn. Before the safety of the axillary staging by SLNE can be demonstrated beyond doubt after neoadjuvant chemotherapy in patients converting from cN+ to ycN0, SLNE after PST SHOULD not be routinely used. In patients with clinically normal axilla (cN0), SLNE should be done before the start of PST.

23.8 Radiotherapy After NST

Retrospective data [51] from 106 non-inflammatory breast cancer patients who achieved a pCR and have been treated with mastectomy and postmastectomy radiation after NST suggest that postmastectomy radiation therapy in patients with advanced stage (stage III) provides a significant clinical benefit in terms of local-regional recurrence and distant metastases.

References

1. Liedtke C, Hatzis C, Symmans WF, et al. Genomic grade index is associated with response to chemotherapy in patients with breast cancer. J Clin Oncol. 2009;27(19):3185–91.
2. Liedtke C, Mazouni C, Hess KR, et al. Response to neoadjuvant therapy and long-term survival in patients with triple-negative breast cancer. J Clin Oncol. 2008;26(8):1275–81.
3. von Minckwitz G, Blohmer JU, Raab G, et al. German Breast Group. In vivo chemosensitivity-adapted preoperative chemotherapy in patients with early-stage breast cancer: the GEPARTRIO pilot study. Ann Oncol. 2005;16(1):56–63.

4. Cortazar P, Zhang L, Untch M, et al. Pathological complete response and long-term clinical benefit in breast cancer: the CTNeoBC pooled analysis. Lancet. 2014;384(9938):164–72.
5. Rouzier R, Perou CM, Symmans WF, et al. Breast cancer molecular subtypes respond differently to preoperative chemotherapy. Clin Cancer Res. 2005;11(16):5678–85.
6. Rody A, Karn T, Solbach C, et al. The erbB2+ cluster of the intrinsic gene set predicts tumor response of breast cancer patients receiving neoadjuvant chemotherapy with docetaxel, doxorubicin and cyclophosphamide within the GEPARTRIO trial. Breast. 2007;16:235–40.
7. von Minckwitz G, Untch M, Blohmer JU, et al. Definition and impact of pathologic complete response on prognosis after neoadjuvant chemotherapy in various intrinsic breast cancer subtypes. J Clin Oncol. 2012;30(15):1796–804.
8. Mazouni C, Peintinger F, Wan-Kau S, et al. Residual ductal carcinoma in situ in patients with complete eradication of invasive breast cancer after neoadjuvant chemotherapy does not adversely affect patient outcome. J Clin Oncol. 2007;25(19):2650–5.
9. Hennessy BT, Hortobagyi GN, Rouzier R, et al. Outcome after pathologic complete eradication of cytologically proven breast cancer axillary node metastases following primary chemotherapy. J Clin Oncol. 2005;23(36):9304–11.
10. Symmans WF, Peintinger F, Hatzis C, et al. Measurement of residual breast cancer burden to predict survival after neoadjuvant chemotherapy. J Clin Oncol. 2007;25(28):4414–22.
11. Denkert C, von Minckwitz G, Brase JC, et al. Tumor-infiltrating lymphocytes and response to neoadjuvant chemotherapy with or without carboplatin in human epidermal growth factor receptor 2-positive and triple-negative primary breast cancers. J Clin Oncol. 2015;33(9):983–91.
12. Salgado R, Denkert C, Demaria S, et al. The evaluation of tumor-infiltrating lymphocytes (TILs) in breast cancer: recommendations by an International TILs Working Group 2014. Ann Oncol. 2015;26(2):259–71.
13. Loibl S, von Minckwitz G, Schneeweiss A, et al. PIK3CA mutations are associated with lower rates of pathologic complete response to anti-human epidermal growth factor receptor 2 (her2) therapy in primary HER2-overexpressing breast cancer. J Clin Oncol. 2014;32(29):3212–20.
14. Loibl S, Majewski I, Guarneri V, et al. Correlation of PIK3CA mutation with pathological complete response in primary HER2-positive breast cancer: combined analysis of 967 patients from three prospective clinical trials. J Clin Oncol. 2015;33(suppl; abstr 511).
15. Denkert C, Loibl S, Müller BM, et al. Ki67 levels as predictive and prognostic parameters in pretherapeutic breast cancer core biopsies: a translational investigation in the neoadjuvant GeparTrio trial. Ann Oncol. 2013;24(11):2786–93.
16. von Minckwitz G, Kümmel S, Vogel P, et al. German Breast Group. Neoadjuvant vinorelbine-capecitabine versus docetaxel-doxorubicin-cyclophosphamide in early nonresponsive breast cancer: phase III randomized GeparTrio trial. J Natl Cancer Inst. 2008;100(8):542–51.
17. von Minckwitz G1, Blohmer JU, Costa SD, et al. Response-guided neoadjuvant chemotherapy for breast cancer. J Clin Oncol. 2013;31(29):3623–30.
18. Guarneri V, Frassoldati A, Bottini A, et al. Preoperative chemotherapy plus trastuzumab, lapatinib, or both in human epidermal growth factor receptor 2-positive operable breast cancer: results of the randomized phase II CHER-LOB study. J Clin Oncol. 2012;30(16):1989–95.
19. Untch M, Rezai M, Loibl S, et al. Neoadjuvant treatment with trastuzumab in HER2-positive breast cancer: results from the GeparQuattro study. J Clin Oncol. 2010;28(12):2024–31.
20. Untch M, Loibl S, Bischoff J, et al. German Breast Group (GBG). Arbeitsgemeinschaft Gynäkologische Onkologie-Breast (AGO-B) Study Group, lapatinib versus trastuzumab in combination with neoadjuvant anthracycline-taxane-based chemotherapy (Gepar-Quinto, GBG 44): a randomised phase 3 trial. Lancet Oncol. 2012;13(2):135–44.
21. von Minckwitz G, Schneeweiss A, Loibl S, et al. Neoadjuvant carboplatin in patients with triple-negative and HER2-positive early breast cancer (GeparSixto; GBG 66): a randomised phase 2 trial. Lancet Oncol. 2014;15(7):747–56.
22. Baselga J, Bradbury I, Eidtmann H, et al. NeoALTTO Study Team. Lapatinib with trastuzumab for HER2-positive early breast cancer (NeoALTTO): a randomised, open-label, multicentre, phase 3 trial. Lancet. 2012;379(9816):633–40.
23. de Azambuja E, Holmes AP, Piccart-Gebhart M, et al. Lapatinib with trastuzumab for HER2-positive early breast cancer (NeoALTTO): survival outcomes of a randomised, open-label, multicentre, phase 3 trial and their association with pathological complete response. Lancet Oncol. 2014;15(10):1137–46.
24. Gianni L, Pienkowski T, Im YH, et al. Efficacy and safety of neoadjuvant pertuzumab and trastuzumab in women with locally advanced, inflammatory, or early HER2-positive breast cancer (NeoSphere): a randomised multicentre, open-label, phase 2 trial. Lancet Oncol. 2012;13(1):25–32.
25. Lee LJ, Alexander B, Schnitt SJ, et al. Clinical outcome of triple negative breast cancer in BRCA1 mutation carriers and noncarriers. Cancer. 2011;117:3093–100.
26. Liedtke C, Mazouni C, Hess KR, et al. Response to neoadjuvant therapy and long-term survival in patients with triple-negative breast cancer. J Clin Oncol. 2008;26:1275–81.
27. Foulkes WD, Smith IE, Reis-Filho JS. Triple-negative breast cancer. N Engl J Med. 2010;363:1938–48.
28. Bulut N, Kilickap S, Sari E, et al. Response to taxanes in triple negative breast cancer. Cancer Chemother Pharmacol. 2008;63:189.
29. Carey LA, Dees EC, Sawyer L, et al. The triple negative paradox: primary tumor chemosensitivity of breast cancer subtypes. Clin Cancer Res. 2007;13:2329–34.
30. Gluz O, Nitz UA, Harbeck N, et al. Triple-negative high-risk breast cancer derives particular benefit from dose intensification of adjuvant chemotherapy: results of WSG AM-01 trial. Ann Oncol. 2008;19:861–70.
31. Joensuu H, Kellokumpu-Lehtinen PL, Huovinen R, et al. Adjuvant capecitabine, docetaxel, cyclophosphamide, and epirubicin for early breast cancer: final analysis of the randomized FinXX trial. J Clin Oncol. 2012;30:11–8.
32. Lindman H, Kellokumpu-Lehtinen P-L, Huovinen R, et al. Integration of capecitabine into anthracycline- and taxane-based adjuvant therapy for triple-negative early breast cancer: final subgroup analysis of the FinXX study. Cancer Res. 2010;70:96s.
33. Steger GG, Barrios C, O'Shaughnessy J, et al. Review of capecitabine for the treatment of triple-negative early breast cancer. Cancer Res. 2010;70:96s.
34. Kaufman PA, Awada A, Twelves C, et al. A phase III, open-label, randomized, multicenter study of eribulin mesylate versus capecitabine in patients with locally advanced or metastatic breast cancer previously treated with anthracyclines and taxanes. Cancer Res. 2012;72:S6-6.
35. Gluz O, Liedtke C, Gottschalk N, et al. Triple-negative breast cancer—current status and future directions. Ann Oncol. 2009;20:1913–27.
36. von Minckwitz G, Schneeweiss A, Loibl S, et al. Neoadjuvant carboplatin in patients with triple-negative and HER2-positive early breast cancer (GeparSixto; GBG 66): a randomised phase 2 trial. Lancet Oncol. 2014;15:747–56.

37. Von Minckwitz G, et al. Early survival analysis of the randomized phase II trial investigating the addition of carboplatin to neoadjuvant therapy for triple-negative and HER2-positive early breast cancer (GeparSixto). SABCS 2015; Abstract S2-04.
38. Sikov WM, Berry DA, Perou CM, et al. Impact of the addition of carboplatin and/or bevacizumab to neoadjuvant once-per-week paclitaxel followed by dose-dense doxorubicin and cyclophosphamide on pathologic complete response rates in stage II to III triple-negative breast cancer: CALGB 40603 (Alliance). J Clin Oncol. 2014.
39. Sikov WM, et al. Event-free and overall survival following neoadjuvant weekly paclitaxel and dose-dense AC +/- carboplatin and/or bevacizumab in triple-negative breast cancer: outcomes from CALGB 40603 (Alliance). SABCS 2015; Abstract S2-05.
40. Kennedy RD, Quinn JE, Mullan PB, et al. The role of BRCA1 in the cellular response to chemotherapy. J Natl Cancer Inst. 2004;96:1659–68.
41. Gluz O, Nitz U, Liedtke C, et al. Comparison of 12 weeks neoadjuvant nab-paclitaxel combined with carboplatinum vs. gemcitabine in triple-negative breast cancer: WSG-ADAPT TN randomized phase II trial SABCS 2015, S6-07.
42. Tutt A, Ellis P, Kilburn LS, et al. TNT: a randomized phase III trial of carboplatin (C) compared with docetaxel (D) for patients with metastatic or recurrent locally advanced triple negative or BRCA1/2 breast cancer (CRUK/07/012). San Antonio Breast Cancer Symp. 2014:S3-01.
43. Cameron D, Brown J, Dent R, et al. Adjuvant bevacizumab-containing therapy in triple-negative breast cancer (BEATRICE): primary results of a randomised, phase 3 trial. Lancet Oncol. 2013;14:933–42.
44. Bear HD, Tang G, Rastogi P, et al. The effect on overall and disease-free survival (OS & DFS) by adding bevacizumab and/or antimetabolites to standard neoadjuvant chemotherapy: NSABP protocol B-40. San Antonio Breast Cancer Symp. 2014:PD2-1.
45. Colleoni M, Viale G, Zahrieh D, et al. Expression of ER, PgR, Her1, Her2, and response: a study of preoperative chemotherapy. Ann Oncol. 2008;19:465–72.
46. Semiglazov VF, Semiglazov V, Ivanov V, et al. The relative efficacy of neoadjuvant endocrine therapy versus chemotherapy in postmenopausal women with ER-positive breast cancer. J Clin Oncol. 2004;23:7s.
47. Mustacchi G, Ceccherini R, Milani S, et al. Tamoxifen alone versus adjuvant tamoxifen for operable breast cancer of the elderly: long-term results of the phase III randomized controlled multicenter GRETA trial. Ann Oncol. 2003;14:414–20.
48. Classe JM, Bordes V, Campion L, Mignotte H, Dravet F, Leveque J, Sagan C, Dupre PF, Body G, Giard S. Sentinel lymph node biopsy after neoadjuvant chemotherapy for advanced breast cancer: results of Ganglion. J Clin Oncol. 2009;27(5):726–32.
49. Boughey JC, Suman VJ, Mittendorf EA. Sentinel lymph node surgery after neoadjuvant chemotherapy in patients with node positive breast cancer: the ACOSOG Z 1071 (Alliance) clinical trial. JAMA. 2013;310:1455–61.
50. Kuehn T, Bauerfeind I, Fehm T, et al. Sentinel-lymph-node biopsy in patients with breast cancer before and after neoadjuvant chemotherapy (SENTINA): a prospective, multicentre cohort study. Lancet Oncol. 2013;14:609–18.
51. McGuire SE, Gonzalez-Angulo AM, Huang EH, et al. Postmastectomy radiation improves the outcome of patients with locally advanced breast cancer who achieve a pathologic complete response to neoadjuvant chemotherapy. Int J Radiat Oncol Biol Phys. 2007;68(4):1004–9.

24 Metastatic Breast Cancer

Berta Sousa, Joana M. Ribeiro, Domen Ribnikar, and Fátima Cardoso

24.1 Introduction

24.1.1 Epidemiology

Breast cancer (BC) is the second most common cancer in the world and, by far, the most frequent cancer among women with an estimated 1.67 million new cancer cases diagnosed in 2012 (25 % of all cancers) [1]. Metastatic breast cancer (mBC) remains incurable, however, a greater knowledge regarding tumour biology together with clinical factors hold the promise of a better selection of therapy and a tailored approach. In the last decades improvements have been achieved in the treatment of mBC with 5 year survival rates for patients with stage IV at initial diagnosis rising from 17 % in 1975–1979 to 33 % in 2005–2011 [2]. According to SEER in 2015 the 5 year survival rate for mBC is around 25 % [3, 4].

24.1.2 New Biology Insights

In recent years it has become increasingly apparent that advanced tumours follow a branched, i.e. Darwinian evolutionary trajectory. Molecular analyses of metastatic breast cancer support this concept as illustrated by the well-known discordance rates in ER, PR and HER2 status between primary and metastatic tumours that approaches 16, 40 and 10 %, respectively [5].

There are well-characterised drivers for BC as ER, ERBB2, PIK3CA and AKT1 although currently the only targetable molecular alterations are ER and HER2, which are both prognostic and predictive factors [6, 7]. Studies that reported the genomic landscape of mBC have shown a higher incidence of TSC1/TSC2 [8], TP53, PIK3CA and GATA3 mutations [9]. One of the main genomic alterations in this setting that mediates endocrine resistance is ESR1 mutations that occur in 10–30 % of ER-positive mBC that are resistant to AI [9]. In the MOSCATO-01 trial [10] enrolling 700 patients with advanced-stage cancer of which 70 had mBC, alterations of the PTEN/PI3K/AKT and FGFR/FGF pathways were the two most frequently detected actionable pathways observed across all tumour types.

The prognostic factors commonly used in mBC are mostly clinically based and comprise *relapse-free interval*, *involved organ sites*, *tumour biology* and others individual factors as *weight loss*, *performance status* or *serum lactic dehydrogenase* (will be discussed later in this chapter). There has been an effort to find new prognostic or predictive factors that could better guide treatment. An intense research has been conducted in circulating tumour cells (CTCs). Studies have shown that the presence of CTCs, defined usually as ≥5/7.5 mL whole blood, represent an independent negative prognostic factor associated with worst PFS and OS [11]. Furthermore, the dynamic changes in CTCs over the course of treatment also seem to correlate with clinical outcome [12] although in the larger SWOG SO500 study no benefit in OS has been seen when treatment decisions were based on CTC dynamics [13]. In summary, prognostic value has been found with CTCs in mBC patients but its clinical used needs additional research.

Predictive factors in mBC are mainly tissue-based biomarkers and comprise the status of hormone receptors and HER2. As previously said, discordance between the primary and the metastatic specimen is frequently described and can be found in 16 % for ER status, 40 % for PR status

B. Sousa · J.M. Ribeiro · F. Cardoso (✉)
Breast Unit, Champalimaud Clinical Center, AV. Brasília S/n, Doca de Pedrouços, Lisbon, 1400-038, Portugal
e-mail: fatimacardoso@fundacaochampalimaud.pt

B. Sousa
e-mail: berta.sousa@fundacaochampalimaud.pt

J.M. Ribeiro
e-mail: joana.ribeiro@fundacaochampalimaud.pt

D. Ribnikar
Medical Oncology Department, Institute of Oncology Ljubljana, Zaloska cesta 2, Ljubljana, 1000, Slovenia
e-mail: dribnikar@onko-i.si

I. Jatoi and A. Rody (eds.), *Management of Breast Diseases*, DOI 10.1007/978-3-319-46356-8_24

and 10 % for HER2 status [14]. According to the ABC guidelines [15, 16] a biopsy of a metastatic lesion should be performed, if easily accessible, not only to confirm diagnosis (particularly when metastasis is diagnosed for the first time) but also for biological markers reassessment (ER and HER-2), at least once in the metastatic setting. In case of discordance, it is currently not clear which result should be used for treatment decision-making since evidence is lacking to determine whether changing anticancer treatment on the basis of change in receptor status affects clinical outcomes. However, most recommendations consider the use of targeted therapy (ET and/or anti-HER-2 therapy) when receptors are positive in at least one biopsy regardless of timing.

Serum tumour biomarkers (CEA, CA15-5, CA 27-29) are assays that detect circulating MUC-1 antigen in the peripheral blood and are used to evaluate response to treatment, particularly in patients with non-measurable metastatic disease. A change in tumour markers alone should not be used solely switch treatment. Serum tumour biomarkers should be used as adjunctive assessments to contribute to decisions regarding therapy [17].

Liquid biopsies, including circulating cell-free DNA (cfDNA), provide a new promising, non-invasive tool for diagnosis, prognosis and therapeutic response or resistance monitoring in breast cancer. Regarding mBC setting it as been suggested that the detection of ctDNA may have prognostic and predictive value and can be used as a highly specific and sensitive biomarker [18] and that serial measurement of ctDNA may be a robust and accurate biomarker for occult metastatic disease in patients diagnosed with primary breast cancer.

Genomic techniques allowing the molecular characterisation of breast cancer, using several technologies are being used to investigate the association between gene mutations and therapeutic response. This would allow the identification of candidates for specific mutation-driven treatments. Next generation sequencing (NGS) technologies provide a more complete view of the tumours molecular state and various platforms for NGS for breast cancer are now commercially available. Although they cannot be recommend for routine clinical use because there is a lack of data supporting benefit in guiding treatment decisions for patients with breast cancer. Genomic within the context of mBC holds the promise to improve patient outcomes mainly through (a) *identification of oncogenic drivers* that are potential targets of genomic driven drug development like PIK3CA mutations [19] FGFR1 amplifications [20], AKT1 mutations or EGFR amplifications [21]. These candidates have already been associated with an objective response when targeted clinically. Other important contribution would be the (b) *identification of genomic alterations responsible for secondary resistance*—like ESR1 or TSC1/2 mutations that could be potentially targeted by agents like ER degrading agent GDC 0810 [22] or mTOR inhibitors [23], respectively. Other applications would be the (c) *identification of DNA repair defects, mutational processes and defects in the DNA duplication mechanism* to identify tumours that might be sensitive to PARP inhibitors for exemple or (d) *mechanisms of immune escape at the individual level.*

24.2 The Role of Imaging, Nuclear Medicine, and Other Technology

FDG uptake has high positive predictive value for breast cancer and its main application is for whole-body staging namely detection of distant metastasis. Retrospectives studies repotted sensitivity and specificity rates (97.4 and 91.2 %, respectively) that compare favourably with the ones described for a combination of conventional techniques (85.9 and 67.3 %, respectively) [24]. In the metastatic setting FDG-PET may allow early identification of nonresponders in order to avoid futile chemotherapy. FDG-PET with the addition of CT, as in most PET-CT scanners, seems to be the most accurate method for bone staging since it combines the best performance for osteolytic lesions seen versus bone scan [25] whilst the addition of CT to PET reveals osteoblastic lesions that may not be metabolically active on FDG-PET alone. PET imaging of proliferation, angiogenesis, and DNA damage/repair offers the opportunity to detect changes in these fundamental aspects of tumour biology that precede size reduction and may allow an earlier evaluation of therapeutic efficacy. In breast cancer, most studies have focused on proliferation imaging mainly based on (18)F-labelled thymidine analogues or (18) F-fluoroestradiol (18)F-FES for ER+ or 68Ga-ABY-025 for HER2 positive breast cancer.

Several other imaging techniques, like computed tomography (CT) scan or magnetic resonance imaging (MRI) can also allow assessment of tumour response. Scintigraphic bone scan is helpful but can be misleading due to "healing flare". Healing flare is a spurious increase in radionuclide uptake because of reparative mineralisation around healing metastases. The phenomenon is typically seen between 2 weeks and 3 months following therapy, but can rarely be seen as late as 6 months after treatment [26].

24.3 Treatment

24.3.1 General Principles

The main goal of treatment in mBC is to extend survival and maintain optimal quality of life against treatment toxicities [15, 16]. This requires management by a multidisciplinary team due to the complexity of the decision-making and fast introduction of new treatment modalities. This team ideally should include medical, radiation and surgical oncologists, imaging experts, pathologists, psycho-oncologists, social workers; specialised breast nurses palliative care specialists and nutritionists [15, 16]. There is also evidence relating improved survival to management in specialised institutions [27].

The first step in order to manage treatment is to confirm the histology of disease and biomarker expression such as ER, PR and HER-2, usually provided from the primary and metastatic specimen. The biology of the disease is determinant to select the best systemic treatment among the wide range of options. ER is a predictive marker of response to endocrine therapy (ET) [28] which is the preferred treatment because of the excellent tolerability profile. HER2 positivity (HER2+) is a predictive marker for treatment with anti-HER2 agents [29], and suppression of the HER2 pathway should be maintained throughout the duration of active treatment.

After assessment of the biology of disease several factors will influence the initial therapeutic approach such as [15, 16]:

- *Previous therapies response obtained and their toxicities*: The knowledge of previous treatments and best response obtained gives us information about the possibility of established mechanisms of resistance. In ER+/HER2 negative disease definitions for primary and secondary ET have been established [16] although the precise mechanisms of this phenomenon are not completely clear (see Sect. 1.3.2). Predictors of poor response to chemotherapy are progression to previous CT regimens in the metastatic setting or relapse within 12 months of adjuvant chemotherapy [30–32]. There are also individual factors that can predispose for drug toxicity and this knowledge is important to guide treatment.
- *Interval for disease relapse or progression*: Longer disease-free survival usually is associated to a more indolent disease phenotype and can be managed with less aggressive treatments, while the opposite scenario is seen if the disease-free interval or time to progression is short [33, 34].
- *Tumour burden* is defined by the number and sites of metastases. Higher burden of disease usually correlates with a more aggressive phenotype [33]. This may imply a preference for therapies with higher efficacy, even if less tolerable, in order to manage special sites or to achieve a faster disease control.
- *Physiologic age; performance status; co-morbidities* will influence treatment choices as a prediction of drug tolerability. It is important to notice the work of the international society of geriatric oncology (SIOG) on geriatric assessment tools to help guiding treatment choices for this population [35].
- *Need for rapid disease/symptom control*; this demands treatments with higher response rates. The term visceral crisis means a rapid progression of disease associated with severe organ dysfunction assessed by signs and symptoms, laboratory studies and imaging. It must be differentiated from the presence of visceral metastasis.
- *Socio-economic, psychological factors, and patient preference*. It is important to involve patients and their caregivers in the decision-making process as this will allow better quality of life achievements.

There has been an effort to find out new predictive and prognostic factors in mBC, in order to better tailor individual treatment. At the moment, accepted prognostic factors are disease-free interval, number of metastatic sites (burden of disease), visceral disease involvement and biological markers. The intrinsic classification of breast cancer in Luminal type (A/B), Basal, and HER-2 enriched has prognostic impact in early breast cancer [36] and these molecular profiles seem to be preserved in the metastatic setting [37]. However, there is no additional information provided for the management of metastatic disease with the use of genomic profiles in this setting. Molecular classification of metastatic disease is more complex and the knowledge of molecular alterations is a matter of intensive research. Studies of CTC's in metastatic breast cancer have demonstrated potential use as a prognostic and predictive factor but are still not ready for clinical use [38].

Traditionally, chemotherapy (CT) has shown higher efficacy in terms of response rate in visceral disease versus bone involvement, ER negative and HER-2 positive disease [39]. Bone involvement only, although having lower response rates to CT, has longer survival compared to other sites of disease, which is in agreement with less severe disease [33, 40]. Low performance status, multiple disease sites as well as progression with prior chemotherapy for advanced disease are predictors of low response to additional CT [33, 40]. Some algorithms to determine response to CT have been developed, but are not used clinically due to the heterogeneity of patients. Some data correlates response to chemotherapy and higher proliferation rate assessed by ki-67 [41], S-phase fraction by flow cytometry [42] and lower response rates with gene expression of genes that mediate resistance: P-glycoprotein (gp170); drug efflux pump; mutated p53 gene [43]. However, they are not ready for clinical use.

The multiplicity of factors needed to be taken into account for treatment decision exemplifies the complexity of management of mBC. Treatment needs to be individualised as a consequence of new emerging technologies and heterogeneity among patients. As previously highlighted in this chapter, for the HER-2 positive disease, systemic treatments should always include an anti-HER2 agent in combination with chemotherapy or ET. CT is the only systemic treatment available for triple negative disease, and it needs to be considered in the ER+ population when there is progression to endocrine agents, suspicious of resistance to ET or a rapid disease progression. Local treatments also need to be considered individually and in the next sections the details about systemic treatment and local treatment will be discussed.

Response to treatment should be assessed to monitor efficacy and treatment duration. This assessment was already discussed in this chapter and just to emphasise that it should be individualised to the goals of treatment (e.g. symptom palliation or tumour response) and the characteristics of the disease.

24.3.2 Treatment of ER+HER2 Negative ABC

The ER+/HER2− disease represents 2/3 of breast cancers and is better characterised molecularly nowadays by the intrinsic subtype classification in Luminal A/B breast cancers [36]. Compared to Luminal A, Luminal B have lower expression levels of ER or estrogen-regulated genes, lower or no progesterone receptor (PR) expression, higher tumour grade, higher expression of proliferation-related genes and activation of growth factor receptor signalling pathways such as IGF-1R and PI3 K/AKT/mTOR [44]. These translate into a more aggressive phenotype and substantially worse outcomes for this subtype. Approximately 20–30 % of ER+/HER2 negative will relapse within 15 years, showing some form of resistance to ET [45]. In the mBC setting the differentiation between Luminal A/B is not used to guide treatment, but it is important to be familiar with possible mechanisms of resistance, which are similar to the molecular changes that differentiate Luminal A versus B disease [46].

Currently, ERα expression is the main biomarker for ET sensitivity. *Mechanisms of endocrine resistance* can be multiple and are being the focus of intensive research. They can involve alterations of the estrogen receptor itself, which is a nuclear receptor, such as loss of the receptor by epigenetic silencing or increase in function due to mutations in the estrogen receptor-related gene (ESR1). The most frequent are mutations in the LBD domain that confer a ligand independent expression of ERα, and are found in 15–20 % of metastatic sites specimens of previously treated patients with ET [47]. ERs regulate cell growth and differentiation activation by ligands, such as 17b-estradiol (E2) and by binding directly to DNA at the estrogen response elements (ERE) which activate the transcriptional process. The binding to DNA needs recruitment of coactivators, against corepressors, or DNA bound transcriptional factors. For instance, upregulation of coactivators such as activator protein 1 (AP1), specificity protein 1 (SP1) and of the transcriptional factor the nuclear factor-kB (NF-kB) is associated with endocrine resistance [48].

There is also a complex network of pathways related to receptor kinase signalling that cross-talk in a bidirectional way with the ER pathway (Fig. 24.1). These pathways also regulate processes such cell cycle, survival, metabolism, motility and genomic instability. Activation of the PI3K/AKT/mTOR or MAPK signalling pathway is possible mechanisms of endocrine resistance [46, 49]. Downstream effectors associated to activation of several membrane receptors kinases, such as EGFR, HER2, IGFR-1 also interplay with this network. Overexpression of these receptors may be responsible for endocrine resistance [46]. Alterations in cell cycle regulators such as the overexpression of cyclin D1 and MYC [50, 51] and RB inactivation [52], can also lead to endocrine resistance.

In conclusion, ER+ advanced breast cancer is characterised by the presence of some degree of endocrine resistance, for which the precise mechanisms is not completely understood but new data is emerging from molecular testing in tumour specimens. The terms primary resistance (or de novo) and secondary (or acquired resistance) have been used in clinical practice to refer to the disease that progresses rapidly to ET treatment in the first case and disease that responds initially and later progresses [16]. This classification is arbitrary but has been used in clinical trials of new agents for ER+/MBC disease. A commonly accepted definition of endocrine resistance is provided by the ESO-ESMO ABC international consensus guidelines: (a) De novo resistance: "relapse while on the first 2 years of adjuvant ET, or progressive disease within 6 months of starting first-line ET for MBC"; (b) Acquired resistance: "relapse while on ET after the first 2 years, or a relapse within 12 months of completing such therapy, or progressive disease at ≥6 months after initiating ET for MBC".

24.3.2.1 Endocrine Therapy

ET is the treatment of choice for ER+ mBC except in cases of visceral crisis, or proven resistance to ET. In these situations CT is indicated. There are different classes of agents in clinical use: (a) Selective estrogen modulators (SERM) which antagonise the ER—*Tamoxifen*; (b) ER down-regulators—*Fulvestrant*; (c) Aromatase inhibitors (AIs) which are selective inhibitors of aromatase activity—*Anastrozole*, *Letrozole*, *Exemestane*; (d) Synthetic analogues of gonadotropin releasing hormone (GnRH)—*Goserrelin*; (e) derivates of 17-OH Progesterone (Progestins)—Medroxyprogesterone, Megestrol (see Table 24.1).

Tamoxifen was the first endocrine agent used in the metastatic setting, with reported response rates of 34 % and

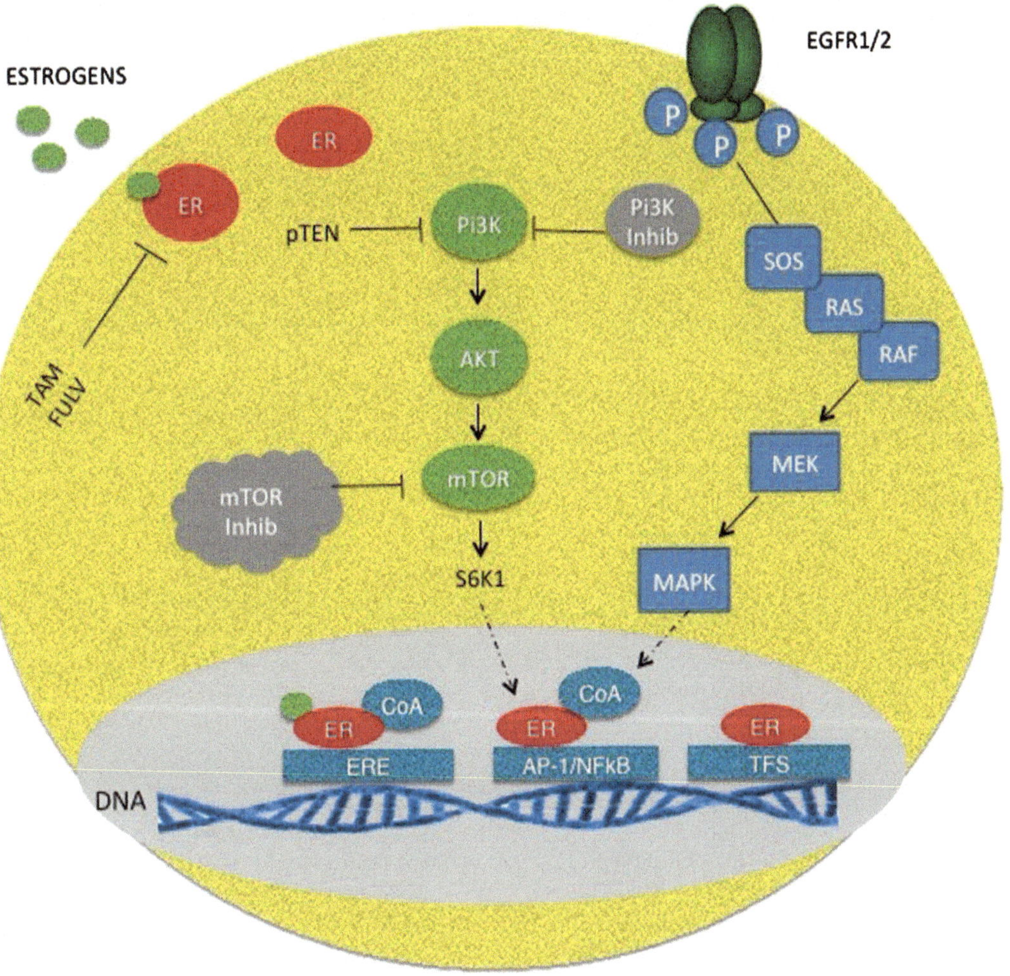

Fig. 24.1 Estrogen receptor cross-talk pathways. Estrogen receptor (ER) belongs to the nuclear transcription receptors family, which means that activation occurs throughout binding to oestrogens. This complex induces translocation to the nucleus, where DNA binding will activate transcription of genes involved in proliferation, apoptosis and angiogenesis. However, there is a cross-talk of ER with other receptors families, such as the HER family (human epidermal receptor), generating complex signalling pathways involving a variety of kinases, as illustrated in this figure in a simplified version. AP-1/NF-kB—transcription factors; AKT—protein kinase B; CoA—coactivator proteins ER—estrogen receptor; ERE—estrogen response elements; FULV—fulvestrant; Inhib—inhibitors; MAPK—mitogen-activated protein kinase; mTOR—mammalian target of rapamycin; PI3K—phosphatidylinositol 3-kinase; pTEN—phosphatase and tensin homolog; SOS-RAS.RAF-MEK—proteins of Ras pathway; S6K1—protein of mTOR pathway; TAM—tamoxifen; TFS—transcription factors

stable disease for at least 6 months in 19 % [53]. AIs were later introduced in the clinic [54] and several studies in metastatic disease proved superiority to tamoxifen, specially in the first line setting. A meta-analysis [55] evaluating the use of these agents in comparison to tamoxifen and progestins, in first line or beyond, revealed an advantage in overall survival (HR = 0.87; CI: 0.82–0.93) for AIs. These results led to the use of these agents as standard first-line treatment for postmenopausal women with mBC, with similar effect found between different AIs [56–58]. For premenopausal women, AIs cannot be used alone because the aromatase enzyme in healthy ovaries is very sensitive to gonadotropins which will be increased under treatment with AIs throughout a negative feedback loop. Treatment options are Tamoxifen or AIs plus ovarian suppression (GnRH agonists) or ablation (oophorectomy or ovarian irradiation). The advantage for the combination of LHRH with ET was shown in a meta-analysis of tamoxifen plus LHRH studies with increase in OS (HR = 0.78, $p = 0.02$) and response rates (39 % versus 30 %) [59].

Fulvestrant is a ER antagonist that binds to ER, prevents dimerisation, and leads to rapid degradation of the receptor. It has been approved in MBC patients that progress or recur after prior anti-estrogen therapy with similar results to AIs after progression to several lines of treatment (Clinical benefit rate approximately 30 %) [60, 61]. A meta-analysis [62] of several studies did not show a difference between Fulvestrant and other ET agents in survival and time to

Table 24.1 Summary of phase III trials of endocrine therapy (ET) in mBC

Study arms/author/year	Population	ORR and/or CBR	TTP/PFS (months)	OS (months)
ANA versus TAM (Nabholtz et al. 2000) [192]	1st line ER status unknown $n = 353$	21 % versus 17 %, p = n.s. 59 % versus 46 %, $\mathbf{p = 0.005}$	11 m versus 5.6 m $\mathbf{p = 0.005}$	33 m versus 32 m p = n.s.
LET versus TAM (Mouridsen et al. 2001) [193]	1st line ER + (30 % of ER unknown) $n = 907$	32 % versus 21 %, $\mathbf{p = 0.0002}$ 50 versus 38 %, $\mathbf{p = 0.0004}$	9.4 m versus 6.0 m $\mathbf{p < 0.0001}$	34 m versus 32 m p = n.s.
EXE versus TAM (Paridaens et al. 2008) [194]	1st line/2nd line ER+ $n = 391$	46 % versus 31 %, OR = 1.85; $\mathbf{p = 0.005}$	9.9 m versus 5.8 m p = n.s.	37 m versus 47 m p = n.s.
Systematic review AIs (Riemsama et al. 2010) [195]	4 RCTs LET, EXE and ANA versus TAM $n = 2309$	LET benefit RR = 0.65, **95 % CI 0.52–0.82** EXE benefit RR = 0.68, **95 % CI 0.53–0.99** ANA no benefit	LET benefit **HR = 0.70, 95 % CI 0.60–0.82** EXE marginal benefit RR = 0.87, **95 % CI 0.70–1.08** ANA benefit HR 1.42, **95 % CI 1.15 to not reported**	No difference
FULV250 versus TAM (Howell et al. 2004) [196]	1st line ER+/unknown $n = 578$	31.6 % versus 33.9 %, OR = 0.87, p = n.s.	6.8 m versus 8.3 m HR = 1.18, 95 % CI 0.98–1.44 p = n.s.	36.8 m versus 38.7 m HR = 1.29, 95 % CI 1.01–1.64 $\mathbf{p = 0.04}$
FULV250 versus ANA (Osborne et al. 2003) [60]	1st line ER+ (<10 % ER unknown) $n = 400$	17.5 % versus 17.5 %, OR = 1.01, p = n.s	5.4 m versus 3.1 m HR = 0.96, 95 % CI 0.81–1.13 p = n.s.	Not reported
FULV250 versus EXE (Chia et al. 2008) [61]	Previously treated (60 % at least 2 prior lines) ER+/unknown $n = 693$	7.4 % versus 6.7 %, p = n.s 32.2 versus 31.5 %, p = n.s.	3.7 m versus 3.7 m p = n.s.	Not reported
FULV250 versus FULV500 (Di Leo 2010 and 2014) [63, 197]	1st line ER+ $n = 736$	9.1 % versus 10.2 %. OR = 0.94, p = n.s 45.6 % versus 39.6 % OR = 1.28, p = n.s	6.5 m versus 5.5 m HR = 0.80, 95 % CI 0.68–0.94 $\mathbf{p = 0.006}$	25.2 m versus 22.8 m HR = 0.81, 95 % CI 0.69–0.96 $\mathbf{p = 0.02}$
Combination ET				
ANA versus ANA+FULV250 (Metha et al. 2012) [66]	1st line ER+ (60 % ET naive) $n = 707$	22 % versus 27 %, p = n.s. 70 % versus 73 %, p = n.s.	13.5 m versus 15 m HR = 0.80, 95 % CI 0.68–0.94 $\mathbf{p = 0.007}$	41.3 m versus 47.7 m HR = 0.81, 95 % CI 0.65–1.00 $\mathbf{p = 0.05}$
ANA+FULV250 versus ANA +placebo (Bergh et al. 2010) [65]	1st line ER+ (1/3 ET naive) $n = 514$	33.6 % versus 31.8 %, p = n.s. 55.1 % versus 55 %, p = n.s.	10.8 versus 10.2 m HR = 0.99, 95 % CI 0.81–1.2, p = n.s.	37.8 m versus 38.2 m HR = 1.00, 95 % CI 0.76–1.32, p = n.s.
ANA+FULV250 versus FULV250 +placebo versus EXEMESTANE (Johnston et al. 2013) [67]	1st line/2nd line ER+ (30 % ET naive) $n = 723$	7 % versus 7 % versus 4 %, p = n.s.	4.4 m versus 4.8 m versus 3.4 m HR = 1.00, 95 % CI 0.83–1.21 p = n.s.	20.2 m versus 19.4 versus 21.6 m HR = 0.95, 95 % CI 0.76–1.17, p = n.s. HR = 0.84, 95 % CI 0.84–1.29, p = n.s.

(continued)

Table 24.1 (continued)

Study arms/author/year	Population	ORR and/or CBR	TTP/PFS (months)	OS (months)
ET and biologicals				
LET versus LET+Lap (Jonhston et al. 2009) [127]	1st line ER+/HER2+ $n = 219$	15 % versus 28 % OR = 0.4; p = n.s. 29 versus 48 % OR = 0.4, $\mathbf{p = 0.003}$	3 m versus 8 m HR = 0.71, 95 % CI 0.53–0.96 $\mathbf{p = 0.019}$	32.3 m versus 33.3 m HR = 0.74, 95 % CI 0.50–1.1, p = n.s
ANA versus ANA+Trast (Kaufman et al. 2009) [126]	1st line ER+/HER2+ $n = 103$	20.3 % versus 6.8 %, $\mathbf{p = 0.018}$ 27.9 % versus 42.7 %, $\mathbf{p = 0.026}$	4.8 m versus 2.4 m HR = 0.63, 95 % CI 0.47–0.84, $\mathbf{p = 0.0016}$	28.5 m versus 23.9 m, p = n.s.
LET versus LET+Bev (Martin et al. 2015) [198]	1st line ER+/HER2− $n = 380$	22 % versus 41 %; $\mathbf{p < 0.001}$ 67 % versus 77 %; $\mathbf{p = 0.041}$	14.4 m versus 19.3 m HR = 0.83, 95 % CI 0.65–1.06, p = n.s.	51.8 m versus 52.1 m HR = 0.87, 95 % CI 0.58–1.32, p = n.s.
EXE+Eve versus EXE (Baselga 2012; Piccart 2014) [70, 71]	Previously treated ER+ $n = 724$	9.5 % versus 0.4 % $\mathbf{p < 0.001}$	7.8 m versus 3.2 m HR = 0.45 95 % CI 0.38–0.54 $\mathbf{p < 0.001}$	31 m versus 26.6 m HR = 0.89, 95 % CI 0.73–1.10 p = n.s.
FULV500+Palbo versus FULV500 (Turner et al. 2015) [77]	Previously treated ER+ $n = 521$	10.4 % versus 6.3 % p = n.s. 34 % versus 19 % $\mathbf{p < 0.001}$	9.2 m versus 3.8 m HR = 0.42, 95 % CI 0.32–0.56 $\mathbf{p < 0.001}$	Not reported

AIs—aromatase inhibitors; ANA—anastrozole; Bev—bevacizumab; CBR—clinical benefit rate; Eve—everolimus; ET—endocrine therapy; EXE—exemestane; FULV250—fulvestrant 250 mg; FULV500—fulvestrant 500 mg; Lap—lapatinib; m—months; ORR—overall response rate; OS—overall survival; Palbo—palbociclib; PFS—progression free survival; RCTs—randomised controlled trials; TAM—tamoxifen; TTP—time to progression; Trast—trastuzumab

progression, but potential benefit if first line treatment, in patients less exposed to ET and if higher doses of Fulvestrant were used. Recently, a phase 3 study [63] has shown survival benefit for the high-dose regimens (500 mg IM day 0, 14, 28 and then monthly) in comparison with low dose ones (median OS was 26.4 months for Fulvestrant 500 mg and 22.3 months for 250 mg, HR = 0.81; 95 % CI 0.69–0.96). A randomised phase III trial, the FALCON trial (ClinicalTrials. gov identifier: NCT01602380) will answer the question of best sequence between AIs and fulvestrant and is comparing first line treatment with anastrozole to fulvestrant 500 mg. The design of this trial was based on the results of Fulvestrant First-Line Study Comparing Endocrine Treatments (FIRST), which was a phase II, randomised, open-label, comparing efficacy and safety of Fulvestrant versus Anastrozole [64]. Fulvestrant was associated with 34 % decrease in the risk of progression (TTP 23.4 months versus 13.1 months, HR 0.66; 95 % CI: 0.47–0.92) and an unplanned OS survival analysis has shown a superior benefit (54 versus 48 months, HR 0.70; 95 % CI: 0.50–0.98) that needs to be confirmed in the phase 3 study.

The different mechanism of action of the different ET agents has been the rational for *ET combination trials.* Three main studies (SWOG, FACT, SoFEA) [65–67] were conducted, mainly in first line setting, comparing AIs plus Fulvestrant versus AIs alone. Overall, there was no benefit for the combination, and only one study [66] (SWOG) did show some improvement in PFS from 13.5 to 15 months (HR = 0.8, 95 % CI: 0.68–0.94) but the majority of patients (60 %) in this trial were ET naïve.

24.3.2.2 Biological and Endocrine Resistance

In order to overcome endocrine resistance new agents have been developed. There are several signalling pathways involved in this process, being the PI3K pathway (Fig. 24.1) the most frequently altered in human tumours (45 % Luminal A and 29 % in Luminal B breast cancers) [68]. *The* ***mTOR inhibitors*** everolimus and temsirolimus were the first agents tested in this setting, after preclinical evidence of synergism between these agents and AIs [69]. The phase III trial BOLERO-2 [70, 71], tested the combination of exemestane and everolimus in patients progressing to letrozole or anastrozole and did show a significant increase in PFS of 4.6 months by local assessment and 6.9 months by investigator assessment (HR = 0.38, 95 % CI 0.31–0.48) but with no significant OS improvement. On the other hand, Temsirolimus combined with letrozole in first line setting [72] (HORIZON trial) did not show improved efficacy, probably because the population of this trial were mainly ET naïve patients (56 % patients did not receiving any prior ET), and so not representative of an endocrine resistant population. The results of a phase II study of Tamoxifen and

Everolimus are also are in accordance to this rational [73] where the combination of tamoxifen and Everolimus was associated to significant increase of 4 months in TTP, and mainly in the patients defined as secondary hormone resistance. mTOR inhibitors are associated with higher toxicity compared to ET alone and patients close monitoring is needed. Main side effects are stomatitis (59 %), rash (39 %), fatigue (37 %), anorexia (31 %), diarrhea (34 %); less frequent but clinically relevant are non-infectious pneumonitis (16 %) and hyperglycemia (14 %) [70, 74]. There has been an effort to find predictive biomarkers of response to these drugs but so far without success. A recent biomarker analysis from BOLERO-2 has shown that lower chromosomal instability was correlated with benefit from everolimus but PIK3CA mutations, FGFR1 and CCND1 ones were not predictive [75].

Cyclin-dependent kinases (CDKs) are main regulators of cell-cycle in mammalians by controlling checkpoints throughout G1 to G2 phase. CDK 4, 6, 10 and 11 have a direct role in cell cycle progression and became important targets for cancer control [38]. The new compounds ***CDK4 and CDK6 inhibitors*** are under clinical evaluation in breast cancer. Palbociclib (PD0332991) is an oral small molecule selective inhibitor CDK4/6 and was evaluated in a phase II randomised study (PALOMA-1) [76], where 165 postmenopausal patients received as first line treatment for mBC a combination of Palbociclib and Letrozole versus Letrozole alone. An important increase in PFS from 10.2 to 20.2 months was seen (HR = 0.48, CI 95 % = 0.31, 0.74) and based on this study the combination was given provisional approval by FDA in this population setting. In order to identify biomarkers of response, a cohort of patients with amplification of Cyclin D1 gene (CCND1) and p16 loss were compared to the wild type population, but unfortunately not found to be predictive of response. A phase 3 trial with same design as PALOMA-1 has finished accrued and will be published soon. Subsequently, the PALOMA-3 study [77] showed that the combination of Fulvestrant 500 mg and Palbociclib in previously treated patients was also superior to fulvestrant (significant improvement in PFS from 3.8 to 9.2 months, HR = 0.42, CI 95 % = 0.32, 0.56). In this study, 36 % of patients were heavily pre treated having more than three lines of therapy and premenopausal women (21 %) were also include but all treated with Goserrelin. The planned subgroup analysis also showed a benefit independently of sites of disease, sensitivity to prior therapies or menopausal status. The addition of cdk4/6 inhibitors led to higher toxicity as neutropenia (78.8 versus 3.5 %), fatigue (38 versus 27), but it is reassuring that the rate of febrile neutropenia was very low (0.6 % in both arms) [78]. Ongoing studies are assessing several cdk4/6 inhibitors in clinical trials in mBC, as well in the neoadjuvant and adjuvant setting. Several new agents such as histone deacetylase inhibitors [79] and PI3K inhibitors [80] are also been evaluated in several clinical trials.

In summary, the treatment of ER+ mBC patients includes several ET treatments options, being the choice of treatment dependent on the agent previously treated. There is no clear evidence for the optimal sequence of treatment. First line treatment options in patients that previously received adjuvant ET includes AI, Fulvestrant and Tamoxifen. After first line, options are fulvestrant plus Palbociclib, AI or Tam plus Everolimus, AI, Fulvestrant, Tamoxifen or Megestrol acetate. For premenopausal patient ovarian suppression/ablation combined with another agent is the preferred choice. The other agent may be Tamoxifen, AI, Fulvestrant or Fulvestrant and Palbociclib.

24.3.2.3 Chemotherapy

In ER+ disease CT is only indicated in cases of rapid disease progression, ET resistance or large tumour burden [15, 16]. The choice of CT should take in account the general health status, tumour burden, prior treatments and patients preferences, towards a personalised treatment approach. For patients CT naïve which represent only a minority of todays patients, anthracyclines or taxanes monotherapy, have similar efficacy [81] (RRs 33–38 %; median OS 19.2–19.8 months). Several other agents are currently approved in mBC such as capecitabine [82, 83], vinorelbine [84], eribulin [85], gemcitabine [86], platinum agents [87] or CMF [88]. The optimal sequence is currently unknown. If there is concern for cardiotoxicity pegylated liposomal doxorubicin [89] has shown similar efficacy to weekly doxorubicin (median OS 22 versus 21 months), but with less risk of cardiac injury (7 % versus 26 %), less alopecia (66 versus 20 %), less nausea (53 versus 37 %) and vomiting (31 versus 13 %). Sequential monotherapy should be the preferred choice. Combination CT does not provide and OS advantage and should be reserved for cases where rapid response is needed [84, 90].

24.3.3 Treatment of HER+ABC

The overexpression or gene amplification of HER2 is present in 20–25 % of breast tumours [91]. HER2 is a membrane tyrosine kinase receptor, belonging to the epidermal growth factor receptor (EGFR) family and overexpression leads to the activation of several downstream pathways involved in increased proliferation [92].

Traditionally, HER2+ mBC was associated with poor prognosis, but the development of anti-HER2 agents has changed this scenario. In fact, nowadays this subtype has the longer survival times achieved in the metastatic setting. A retrospective study, analysing 2091 patients from the MDACC [7] compared survival rates among three groups of patients receiving first line treatment: (1) HER-2+ disease and treated with trastuzumab; (2) HER-2+ disease and not treated with trastuzumab and (3) HER2 negative disease. Highest 1-year OS rates were seen in HER2+ patients treated with trastuzumab (86.6 %) and lowest in this subtype but not receiving anti-HER2 treatment (70.2 %). The ER+ population had an intermediate survival time (1 year OS of 75.1 %).

For activation of the HER2 pathway, HER2 receptor will create homodimers or heterodimers with other EGFR proteins, allowing the EGRF intracellular domains to be autophosphorylated and/or transphosphorylated with subsequent activation of the Ras/Raf/mitogen-activated protein kinase, the phosphoinositide 3-kinase/Akt, and the phospholipase Cγ (PLCγ)/protein kinase C (PKC) pathways [92, 93].

Trastuzumab is a monoclonal antibody that binds to the extracellular domain of HER-2 (sub-domain IV) and was the first HER-2 directed agent approved in MBC. The mechanism of action of trastuzumab is diverse: (1) HER-2 internalisation and degradation throughout activity of tyrosine kinase- ubiquitin ligase c-CBL [94]; (2) Antibody-dependent cellular cytotoxicity (ADCC) throughout activation of natural killer (NK) cells [95]; (3) inhibition of the MAPK and PI3K/Akt pathway leading to inhibition of cell growth.

Subsequent agents were developed, working as blockers of the receptor or/and inhibitors of the downstream signalling of the HER2 pathway. In clinical use are 3 agents: (a) ***Lapatinib***: tyrosine kinase inhibitor of EGFR1 and HER2; (b) ***Ado-trastuzumab emtansine*** (also known as T-DM1): antibody–drug conjugate that incorporates trastuzumab and a thioter linker that connects it to an antimicrotubule agent, DM1 and (c) ***Pertuzumab***: like trastuzumab is a monoclonal antibody to the extracellular domain of HER-2, but that blocks a different site which is the binding domain (sub-domain II), preventing HER2 dimerization as an additional effect to trastuzumab (Fig. 24.1).

There is large amount of evidence to guide first line treatment in this population but the same is not truth when disease progresses. The best sequence of anti-HER2 agents is still an open question, since information regarding treatment efficacy after progression to several anti-HER2 agents, mainly the new ones, is not yet available. The current results of several trials are at least a confirmation of effectiveness of sustained suppression of the HER2 pathway throughout the lifetime of the patient.

24.3.3.1 First-Line Therapy (See Table 24.2)

Combination of CT and trastuzumab has shown higher efficacy compared to CT alone [29, 96–101]. The first main study conducted by Slamon et al. [29], evaluated 469 patients receiving AC (doxorubicin plus cyclophosphamide) or 3 weekly Paclitaxel (if previous treated or with anthracyclines) as first line treatment for mBC with or without Trastuzumab. Response rate (RR) was increased from 32 to 50 % ($p < 0.001$) and OS from 20.3 to 25 months ($p = 0.046$). Main secondary side effect was cardiac dysfunction, more prevalent and severe if anthracyclines were

Table 24.2 Combination of CT and anti-HER2 agents in mBC—main phase III trials

Study arms/author/year	Population	ORR and/or CBR	TTP/PFS	OS
First line treatment CT and trastuzumab				
Trast+CTp versus CT (Slamon et al. 2001) [29]	1st line HER2+ $n = 469$	32 % versus 50 %, $\mathbf{p < 0.0001}$	7.4 m versus 4.6 m RR 0.51, 95 % CI 0.41–0.81 $\mathbf{p < 0.0001}$	25 m versus 20.3 m RR 0.80, 95 % CI 0.64–1.00 $\mathbf{p = 0.046}$
Trast+PAC+CARBO versus Trast+PAC (Neyland et al. 2006) [98]	1st line HER2+ $n = 196$	52 % versus 36 %, $\mathbf{p = 0.004}$	10.7 m versus 7.1 m HR 0.66, 95 % CI 0.59–0.73 $\mathbf{p = 0.03}$	35.7 m versus 32.2 m HR 0.9 p = n.s.
Trast+VINO versus Trast+TAX (Burstein et al. 2007) [97]	1st line HER2+ $n = 81$ * early terminated (poor accrual)	51 % versus 40 %, p = n.s	8.5 m versus 6 m, p = n.s.	Not reported
Trast+VINO versus Trast +DOC (Andersson et al. 2011) [100]	1st line HER2+ $n = 284$	59.3 % versus 59.3 %, p = n.s	12.4 m versus 15.3 m HR 0.94, 95 % CI 0.71–1.25, p = n.s.	35.7 m versus 38.8 m HR = 1.01, 95 % CI 0.71–1.42, p = n.s.
Trast+TAX+CARBO versus Trast+TAX (Valero et al. 2011) [101]	1st line HER2+ $n = 263$	72 % versus 72 %, p = n.s	11.1 m versus 10.4 HR = 0.91, 95 % CI 0.69–1.20 p = n.s.	37.1 m versus 37.4 m HR = 1.0, 95 % CI 0.75–1.35 p = n.s.

(continued)

Table 24.2 (continued)

Study arms/author/year	Population	ORR and/or CBR	TTP/PFS	OS
First line treatment CT and other anti-HER2 agents				
Trast+DOC+Plac versus Trast+DOC+Pert (Baselga 2012) [111]	1st line HER2+ n = 808	69.3 % versus 80.2 %, p = 0.001	12.4 m versus 18.5 m HR = 0.62, 95 % CI 0.51–0.75, $\boldsymbol{p}$ **< 0.0001**	37.6 m versus not reported HR = 0.66, 95 % CI 0.52–0.84 $\boldsymbol{p}$ **= 0.0008**
TAX+Lap versus TAX+Trast (Gelmon et al. 2015) [117]	1st line HER2+ n = 652	54 % versus 55 %, p = n.s. 75.8 % versus 75.9 %, p = n.s.	9.0 m versus 11.3 m HR = 1.37, 95 % CI 1.13–1.65, $\boldsymbol{p}$ **= 0.001**	37.8 m versus 38.2 m HR = 1.00, 95 % CI 0.76–1.32, p = n.s.
Trast+TAX versus T-DM1 versus TDM1+PAC (Ellis et al. 2015) [114]	1st line HER2+ n = 365	67.9 % versus 59.7 % versus 64.2 %	***Trast+TAX versus T-DM1*** 13.7 m versus 14.1 m HR = 0.91, 95 % CI 0.73–1.13; p = n.s. ***Trast+TAX versus T-DM1+PAC*** 13.7 m versus 15.2 m HR = 0.87, 95 % CI 0.69–1.08; p = n.s. ***T-DM1 versus T-DM1 +PAC*** 14.1 m versus 15.2 m HR = 0.91, 95 % CI 0.73–1.13, p = n.s.	Not reported
Second line treatment and beyond				
CAP+Lap versus CAP (Geyer et al. 2006 and Cameron et al. 2010) [115]	Previously treated HER2+ n = 324	22 % versus 14 %, p = 0.009 27 % versus 18 %	8.4 m versus 4.4 m HR = 0.49, 95 % CI 0.34–0.74, $\boldsymbol{p}$ **= <0.001**	18.7 m versus 16.1 m HR = 0.87, 95 % CI 0.71–1.08, p = n.s.
Trast+Lap versus Lap (Blackwell et al. 2010) [124]	Previously treated HER2+ n = 296	10.3 % versus 6.9 %, p = n.s. 24.7 % versus 12.4 % $\boldsymbol{p}$ **= 0.01**	12 wks versus 8.1 wks HR = 0.73, 95 % CI 0.57–0.93, $\boldsymbol{p}$ **= 0.008**	9.7 m versus 7.9 m HR = 0.75, 95 % CI 0.53–1.07, p = n.s.
T-DM1 versus CAP+Lap (Verma et al. 2012) [120]	Previously treated HER2+ n = 991	43.6 % versus 30.8 %, $\boldsymbol{p}$ **= <0.001**	9.4 m versus 5.8 m HR = 0.66, 95 % CI 0.56–0.77 $\boldsymbol{p}$ **= <0.001**	30.9 m versus 25.1 m HR = 0.68, 95 % CI 0.55–0.85, $\boldsymbol{p}$ **= <0.001**
T-DM1 versus physician's choice (Krop et al. 2014; Wildiers et al. 2015) [122, 123]	Previously treated anti-HER2 ER+/HER2+ n = 602	31 % versus 9 %, $\boldsymbol{p}$ **= <0.001**	6.2 m versus 3.3 m HR = 0.52, 95 % CI 0.36–0.82, $\boldsymbol{p}$ **= 0.0016**	22.7 m versus 15.8 m HR = 0.68, 95 % CI 0.54–0.85, $\boldsymbol{p}$ **= 0.007**

CARBO—carboplatin; CAP—capecitabine; CTp—chemotherapy by protocol (Docetaxel or AC); DOC—Docetaxel; Lap—lapatinib; m—month; ORR—overall response rate; OS—overall survival; PAC—paclitaxel; Per—pertuzumab; PFS—progression free survival; TTP—time to progression; Trast—trastuzumab; TAX—taxane; T-DM1—trastuzumab emtansine; wks—weeks

combined to Trastuzumab with a frequency rate of 27 %, compared to 8 % if AC alone, 13 % if Paclitaxel plus trastuzumab and 1 % if Paclitaxel alone. Trastuzumab was approved for use in the metastatic setting in 1998. Other CT agents as Docetaxel, weekly Paclitaxel and Vinorelbine have been tested in this setting with equivalent efficacy. Docetaxel is globally less tolerated, with higher risk of neutropenia/leucopenia, infection, neuropathy, nail changes and edema [97, 100]. Compared to taxanes, Vinorelbine [97, 100] was better tolerated and with similar efficacy, only associated with anemia and neutropenia and hence less recommended to patients with cytopenias mainly secondary to bone marrow involvement. In this case, weekly paclitaxel is the preferred regimen.

Combination CT associated with trastuzumab has also been tested with platins and taxanes [98, 101–103], but no OS survival benefit was seen, but mainly a significant and meaningful increase in response rates at the cost of higher toxicity, mainly hematologic. These regimens should be considered when fast control of the disease is needed.

There has been a continuing effort to develop new anti-HER2 agents, with the aim to increase survival times, which are still modest, and to overcome resistance to trastuzumab treatment, as some patients do not respond initially to this drug (<35 %) [104, 105]. *Pertuzumab* was recently developed and the rational for combination with trastuzumab was based on their complementary mechanism of action by blocking different site domains of HER2. Phase I/II studies proved synergy and efficacy for the combination [106–108] leading to a phase III study—Cleopatra trial. This included 808 HER2+ mBC patients who were randomised to first line treatment with a combination of pertuzumab, trastuzumab and docetaxel or the same chemotherapy with trastuzumab alone. A benefit was seen of PFS by 6.3 months (HR 0.68 CI95 % 0.58–0.80) and a substantial benefit in OS by 15.7 months (40.8 months–56.5 months, HR 0.68, CI 95 % 0.56–0.84) which is rarely seen in mBC [109, 110]. Importantly, the population of this study included mainly trastuzumab naïve patients, with only 10 % receiving this treatment previously, and is not therefore representative of the majority of the mBC HER-2 population in daily clinic nowadays. In addition all patients included in the Cleopatra trial that received previous trastuzumab had a treatment free interval of at least 12 months. Undoubtedly, for untreated patients, the preferred first-line regimen is Docetaxel, Pertuzumab and Trastuzumab, being already approved for this setting. It's not clear yet if patients previously treated with trastuzumab derive the same amount of benefit and the optimal treatment of early relapses (≦12 months after or during Trastuzumab) is still unknown.

The cytotoxic component is discontinued after achieving best response to treatment (usually after 6–8 cycles) [111] and the monoclonal antibodies should be continued. If the tumour is ER+ it is recommended to add ET as maintenance therapy.

The dual HER2 blockade with Trastuzumab and Pertuzumab was associated with some increase in toxicity. Grade 3 toxicities described were neutropenia (40 versus 46.2 %), febrile neutropenia (7.6 % versus 13.8 %) and diarrhea (9.3 versus 5.1 %) but there were no differences in deaths due to febrile neutropenia or infection. Subsequently a phase II study [112] evaluated the efficacy and safety for the combination of weekly Paclitaxel (80 mg m^2) with 3 weekly Trastuzumab and Pertuzumab in 69 patients on first line (74 %) or second-line therapy (26 %). Median PFS in the update analysis was 19.5 months (95 % CI, 14–26 months), and at 1 year overall PFS was 70 % (95 % CI, 56–79 %), being higher in the first line setting compared to previously treated patients. The toxicity profile favours Paclitaxel, with no cases of febrile neutropenia or symptomatic left ventricular systolic dysfunction, being an option for patients not tolerating docetaxel. Combinations of dual blockade with Vinorelbine have also been reported and compare favourably; efficacy results are awaited [113].

The Marianne study was recently presented [114] and this was an important study, including 1095 patients that compared taxanes plus Trastuzumab to T-DM1 and T-DM1 plus pertuzumab. Non-inferiority was achieved between arms but superiority was not proven. Median PFS was similar in the three arms being 13.7 months, 14.1 months and 15.2 months, respectively. More details from this study are awaited in the full publication, and raise the question if the dual blocked in first line setting is preferred to Trastuzumab-based regimens.

24.3.3.2 Second-Line Therapy (See Table 24.2)

The first new anti-HER 2 agent approved in this setting was Lapatinib. In HER2+ mBC patients, previously receiving anthracyclines, taxanes and Trastuzumab, the addition of Lapatinib to Capecitabine [115, 116], compared to capecitabine alone, doubled TTP from 4.4 months to 8.4 months (HR = 0.49, 95 %: CI 0.34–0.71). Main additional side effect for the combination was diarrhea. This study led to the approval of this agent in this setting, but mainly what it did confirm was benefit of maintaining suppression of HER2 pathway, as two subsequent studies proved superiority of trastuzumab in this setting.

The MA.31 trial [117] randomised 636 mBC patients to first line therapy with taxanes for at least 24 weeks, with Trastuzumab or Lapatinib. Taxanes could be weekly Paclitaxel or 3 weekly Docetaxel. PFS was significantly superior in Trastuzumab arm, 11.4 months versus 8.8 months (HR = 1.37, 95 %CI 1.13–1.65) and also more deaths occurred in the Lapatinib arm (HR = 1.37, 95 % CI 1.13–1.65). The aim of the second study, CEREBEL trial [118] was to evaluate a potential benefit for first line capecitabine and lapatinib versus the combination with trastuzumab in preventing brain relapse as first relapse, based on previous studies as the Landscape trial [119]. The study was prematurely closed with 540 patients because of very low brain events. There was no statistical significance difference on the incidence of brain metastases in both arms (3 % in lapatinib arm versus 5 % in trastuzumab arm, $p = 0.360$), but PFS and OS were longer in trastuzumab arm, 2 and 5 months, respectively (HR for PFS, 1.30; 95 % CI, 1.04–1.64; HR for OS, 1.34; 95 % CI, 0.95–1.64).

In both trials [117, 118], toxicity in the lapatinib arm was associated with higher incidence of diarrhea, rash, nausea and hyperbilirrubinemia, being only better to trastuzumab for lower incidence of LVEF decrease.

The antibody–drug conjugate T-DM1 was later introduced and tested in second and subsequent lines of treatment against Capecitabine plus Lapatinib in the EMILIA study [120]. Primary endpoints were PFS, OS and safety, and 991 patients were included. It was shown an increase in OS of nearly 5 months (30.9 versus 25.1 meses, HR 0.68, CI 95 % 0.55–0.85) as well as increase in PFS of 3.2 months (HR 0.65, CI 95 % 0.55–0.77) together with less toxicity (grade ¾ events 57 % versus 41 %). TDM1 was only associated with more thrombocytopenia and increase in transaminases but higher occurrence of diarrhea, nausea, vomiting, hand–foot syndrome was seen in the Capecitabine and Lapatinib arm. The benefit of T-DM1 was seen irrespective of the lines of treatment received and also in patients progressing less than 6 months of completing trastuzumab in the adjuvante or neoadjuvant setting. For this reason the ASCO guidelines [121] recommend T-DM1 in first line setting if short disease-free interval.

24.3.3.3 Progression Beyond Second Line Therapy

Based on EMILIA study [120] T-DM1 is an option for third-line therapy, although previous treatment with Lapatinib was an exclusion criterion in this trial. The need for further evidence in previously treated HER2+ mBC patients with several anti-HER2 and CT agents was the context for the TH3RESA trial [122]. This was a phase 3 randomised study were patients must have received at least two lines of therapy, including a taxane in any setting, and were randomised to TDM1 versus physician choice. The majority of patients received Trastuzumab and CT (68 %), Trastuzumab +Lapatinib (10 %), Trastuzumab+ET (2 %) and Lapatinib +Capecitabine (3 %). There was a significant increase in PFS from 3.3 to 6.2 months (HR 0.52, CI 95 % 0.42–0.66) and in the recent update analysis of median OS from 15.8 months to 22.7 months (HR 0.68, CI 95 % 0.54–0.85) despite a 45 % of cross-over rate. T-DM1 arm had better tolerability (grade 3 events 32 % versus 43 %) [122, 123].

Before results from T-DM1 were available, the combination of trastuzumab and lapatinib was assessed in clinical trials, with the rational for testing dual-blocking in heavily pretreated patients. This was the population of EGF104900 trial [124] were patients were randomised to trastuzumab plus lapatinib versus lapatinib alone after having received a median of three prior trastuzumab-containing regimens; 55 % of cross-over rate was seen. The dual blockade was associated with a significant increase in PFS which was the primary endpoint (11.1 versus 8.1 weeks, HR = 0.74; 95 % CI, 0.58–0.94), increased CBR (24.7 % versus 12.4 %; $p = 0.01$) and a significant 4.5-month median OS advantage (14 versus 9.5 months, HR, 0.74; 95 % CI, 0.57–0.97). The main side effect for the combination was diarrhea and the incidence of cardiac events were low (7.3 % in combination arm and 2.1 % in monotherapy). Multivariate analysis has shown as factors associated with improved survival ECOG 0, non-visceral disease and less than three metastatic sites and less time from initial diagnosis till assignment in the study, which means less duration of treatment for metastatic disease.

Good data on pertuzumab use following disease progression on trastuzumab or other agents is not yet available. Only phase 2 studies are reported [112] [109] and showed CBR of 50 % and median PFS of 5.5 months, with good tolerability. A second cohort evaluated pertuzumab in monotherapy, but showed no efficacy [125] with CBR of 3.4 % versus 10.3 % when trastuzumab was also received.

In patients progressing after several lines of treatment it is recommended to maintain trastuzumab and switch the cytotoxic treatment [16, 121].

24.3.3.4 Treatment of HER2+/HR+ Disease

In selected cases of ER+/HER2+ disease, such as indolent, low burden disease or contraindication for chemotherapy, first line treatment with ET and Trastuzumab or Lapatinib is an option. There are two main randomised trials assessing treatment with Anastrozole and Trastuzumab [126] or Letrozole plus Lapatinib [127] in this setting. There was a significant increase in PFS but with no increase in overall survival. Around 50 % of HER2+ patients are also ER+ and this subtype is well represented in the CT clinical. Due to the OS advantage in these trials, combination of an anti-HER2 agent with CT is also the preferred first line treatment for this population but in some selected cases ET can be used. Maintenance therapy with ET and anti-HER2 therapy is recommended after maximum response is obtained with CT [15, 16, 121].

24.3.3.5 Unanswered Questions for Management HER2 Positive Disease

There are no data for the optimal duration of anti-HER2 therapy in patients who achieve a complete remission.

New agents: Neratinib is a potent pan-tyrosine kinase inhibitor that has activity against HER1, HER2 and HER4. It has shown activity when combined to Capecitabine in previously treated patients with Trastuzumab (PFS 35.9–40.3 months) [128] but with high diarrhea rates that occurred in 88 % of patients. An ongoing phase 3 study (NALA; NCT 01808573) is assessing capecitabine plus Neratinib or Lapatinib in patients progressing after 2 lines of treatment for MBC with anti-Her2 agents. In previously untreated patients recently it was reported a phase 3 trial comparing Paclitaxel and Trastuzumab or Neratinib in first line setting ($N = 479$). There was no difference in PFS (HR = 1.02; 95 % CI, 0.81–1.27) but Neratinib was associated with grade 3 in 30.4 % of patients. A finding in this trial that needs further confirmation with additional studies is a lower incidence of central nervous system recurrences (relative risk, 0.48; 95 % CI, 0.29–0.79; $P = 0.002$) and longer time to central nervous system metastases (HR, 0.45; 95 % CI,

0.26–0.78; $P = 0.004$) in the Neratinib and Paclitaxel arm [129].

24.3.4 Treatment of Triple Negative ABC

Since triple negative breast cancer (TNBC) lack all the three targets, ER, PR and HER-2 receptors, chemotherapy represents the only approved treatment approach. Response to systemic therapy in metastatic TNBC lack durability and overall survival is worse compared to other subtypes [130]. As previously discussed sequential single-agent chemotherapy is the best approach and combination chemotherapy should be considered if an increase in response rates is a major goal. Although conventional taxanes can be used as first line therapy, it should be noticed that they are commonly prescribed in the adjuvant setting and should not be rechallenged in case of disease-free interval of less than 12 months [131]. The BRCA functional status may play an important role in both, taxanes—and platinum compounds—sensitivity [132].

Wysocky and colleagues [133] found there was higher incidence of primary resistance to docetaxel-based therapy among BRCA1-mutated TNBC patients. Available data of clinical activity of platinum compounds suggest a promising efficacy mainly in the neoadjuvant setting [134] but also in metastatic setting [135]. However, recent results of a phase III trial conducted in UK (TNT trial) [136] helped to clarify the benefit of platins. This study included 376 mBC patients with TNBC or carriers of BRCA1/2 mutations independently of the biologic subtype. Patients were randomised to first line treatment with Carboplatin (AUCx6) or docetaxel (100 mg/m^2) for 6–8 cycles or till progression. No difference in overall response rate (ORR), PFS or OS was seen between the two arms, proving evidence for no superiority of platins in triple negative phenotype. An analysis of the intrinsic subtype by PAM50 assay was also performed and again no benefit was seen for platins if basal-like subtype. However, patients with BRCA1 or two mutations ($n = 43$) experienced higher ORR (68 % with carboplatin versus 33.3 % with docetaxel) and PFS (6.8 months versus 4.8 months) being this population the one that benefits more from platins.

Due to overall poor response of advanced TNBC patients to standard chemotherapeutic agents there is an urgent need for developing new molecular-directed targeted therapies for this specific BC population. Since TNBC is generally a highly proliferative neoplasm that needs constant angiogenesis throughout all the phases of its development [137] it was expected higher efficacy of the anti-VEGF monoclonal antibody bevacizumab in this disease. The latter has been shown to increase ORR and PFS in patients with MBC when added to first-line chemotherapy in various randomised phase III trials [138–141] but no OS benefit and the toxicity was higher. No significant improvement of efficacy was seen in the triple negative population [142] either.

Poly (ADP-ribose) polymerase (PARP)s are a large family of multifunctional enzymes. PARP1 and PARP2 are involved in the mechanism of single-stranded DNA base excision repair by homologous recombination. In preclinical models PARP inhibition has selective anticancer activity in BRCA-1 and BRCA-2-deficient tumours with 100–1000 times greater killing power compared to BRCA-proficient cells [143]. PARP inhibitors are an attractive target for TNBC but the encouraging early studies with iniparib [144] were not confirmed in a phase III trial of unselected TNBC [145]. Another PARP inhibitor, olaparib, has recently also been shown to be ineffective in the treatment of unselected TNBC [146], therefore monotherapy with these agents is not recommended. Further trials are ongoing and evaluating treatment with PARP inhibitors in patients BRCA 1 or 2—deficient tumours. Ongoing clinical trials are exploring the role of other potential targeted agents in such as EGFR inhibitors, mTOR inhibitors, Src tyrosine kinase inhibitors, and immunotherapeutic approaches and non-steroidal anti-androgens, in this last case for TNBC with androgen receptor expression [147].

24.3.5 Treatment According to Special Sites

24.3.5.1 Bone Metastasis

General Recommendations

The management of bone metastasis should be discussed in a multidisciplinary team that include orthopedic and neuro-surgeons besides medical oncologists, radiation oncologists and palliative care specialists [148].

24.3.5.2 Systemic Therapy of Bone Metastases

A bone modifying agent (bisphosphonate or denosumab) should be routinely used in combination with other systemic therapies [15].

Bisphosphonates are pyrophosphate analogues and bind to the hydroxyapatite mineral bone matrix preventing osteoclasts activity through induction of osteoclast apoptosis and inhibition of osteoclast maturation and differentiation [149]. They may also have antitumor effects by inducing apoptosis, inhibiting angiogenesis and reducing levels of vascular endothelial growth factor (VEGF) [150]. They have shown significant efficacy in reducing skeletal-related events (SREs) and delaying time to first SREs onset [148, 150]. There are many bisphosphonates available, including clodronate, which is a second-generation bisphosphonate, pamidronate, which requests 2 h of infusion time; and third-generation aminobisphosphonates ibandronate and zoledronic acid (ZA).

The efficacy of ZA given intravenously was firstly tested in a placebo-controlled trial randomising patients with BC and bone metastases to receive either 4 mg of ZA every 4 weeks for 1 year or placebo [151]. There was a 39 % risk reduction of SREs in patients who received ZA compared to those who received placebo. Furthermore, ZA significantly delayed time to first SRE with similar safety profile to placebo. Head to head comparison was done between ZA and pamidronate in a large trial where 1648 patients with metastatic bone lesions from BC were randomised to receive either intravenous pamidronate 90 mg or intravenous ZA 4 or 8 mg every 3–4 weeks [152]. There was increased creatinine level observed in the 8 mg ZA arm, therefore only the 4 mg ZA arm was considered for final analysis. ZA was superior to pamidronate for the time to first SRE, skeletal morbidity rate and risk of skeletal complications in patients receiving ET but not chemotherapy [153].

The toxicity profile of bisphosphonates is generally favourable with exception of renal adverse effects. However, prolonged use of these bone modifying agents can induce bone turnover suppression which may, in combination with systemic chemotherapy, radiation therapy, steroid treatment or dental procedures, cause osteonecrosis of the jaw (ONJ) [154]. The most common site of ONJ is the mandible bone (65 %), followed by maxilla bone (26 %), or both (9 %).

There is recent evidence showing similar efficacy of biphosphonates administration every 3 months compared with every 4 weeks. The large CALGB trial (Alliance) [155] (n = 1822/BC 833) showed non-inferiority for every 3 months regimen compared to the monthly one. A second study, the OPTIMIZE-2 included 403 mBC patients with bone disease that have received 10–15 months of IV biphosphonates and then randomised between the two schedules of administration. Again similar efficacy was found in the less frequent schedule of administration (SREs, pain control), together with fewer side effects (no cases of ONJ) and is common current practice, mainly when high risk for biphosphonates side effects.

Denosumab is another bone modifying agent that has shown efficacy based on rapid suppression of bone turnover [156]. It is a fully human immunoglobulin-G2 (IgG2) monoclonal antibody against RANKL [157] and was compared to ZA in three phase III trials. In the largest trial conducted by Stopeck and colleagues [158] 2046 patients were randomised to receive either subcutaneous Denosumab 120 mg and intravenous placebo or intravenous ZA 4 mg (adjusted to creatinine clearance) and subcutaneous placebo every 4 weeks [158]. It was demonstrated that Denosumab significantly delayed time to first SRE (HR 0.82, p = 0.01). Both drugs, ZA and Denosumab, were well-tolerated. There were more renal adverse events with ZA compared to denosumab whereas hypocalcemia occurred more frequently with denosumab. ONJ was rare (1.4 % with ZA and 2.0 % with denosumab). In this study, denosumab was also shown to improve pain-prevention and pain control. In those patients who had mild or absent pain at baseline, a 4-month delay in progression to moderate or severe pain was observed with denosumab compared to ZA (9.7 months versus 5.8 months; p = 0.02). Moreover, denosumab was superior to ZA in reducing bone-related complications and maintaining quality of life of metastatic BC patients [159].

24.3.5.3 Locoregional Therapy of Bone Metastases

There are two main locoregional treatment strategies for bone metastases from breast cancer, palliative radiotherapy and surgical management, respectively.

Palliative radiotherapy has two major goals, to prevent SREs and palliate pain [160]. Around 75–80 % of patients who receive radiotherapy (RT) achieves a good response on pain control and need no further analgesics. RT has a direct cytotoxic effect on tumour cells that leads to tumour shrinkage, reduced tumour infiltration in the bone and tumour cytokine production that is involved in nociception. Furthermore, there is evidence of effect of ionising radiation on osteoclasts and RANK-RANKL regulator system producing analgesic effect [161].

Conventional fractionation usually involves daily fractions of 1.8–2 Gy (5 fractions per week), however, the total dose of RT depends on cancer radio sensitivity and tolerance of tissues being exposed to radiant beam [162]. Another two options for RT delivery are hyper fractionation and hypo-fractionation. In hyper-fractionated RT the total dose is divided into small doses and treatments are given more than once per day; in hypo-fractionated RT, on the other hand, the total dose is divided into large doses and treatments are given once a day or less often. In a randomised clinical trial evaluating the role of single fraction RT or multiple fractions of RT [163] 272 patients with bone metastases from BC were randomised to receive a single 8 Gy fraction or 20 Gy in 5 fractions. It was concluded that single fraction RT is not as effective as multiple fraction RT for neuropathic pain treatment but may be considered for patients in poor performance status and poor prognosis. Those patients with good long-term prognosis or favourable biology of metastatic BC might benefit from more complex RT techniques, such as stereotactic radiosurgery and intensity-modulated radiotherapy that can prevent possible long-term complications of RT [164].

Surgical stabilisation followed by RT is usually indicated if a fracture of a long bone is revealed or if there is a high risk of fracture [15, 16]. The optimal management of symptomatic spinal metastases is a combination of surgical and RT treatments [165]. As it was shown in a cohort of 87 patients with metastatic BC treated with aggressive decompression, advances in surgical techniques have allowed more effective stabilisation of the spine as well as neurological symptom control [166]. Aggressive surgical decompression proved to be effective in achieving a good pain control with preoperative pain levels, assessed with visual analogue scale (VAS), reducing from a median of 6 to a median of 2 after the intervention. In addition, 85 % of all the patients in the study improved their neurologic function at 1 year. In spite of these advantages of descompressive surgery combined with RT, there is still no clear consensus nor evidence-based guidelines about the indications for surgery and this treatment strategy remains palliative and it does not prolong survival [165].

24.3.5.4 Brain Metastasis

General Recommendations

Treatment strategy of brain metastases from BC should take in account: location, size and number of lesions, biology of the disease, severity of symptoms and patient performance status and comorbidity. For patients with a solitary metastasis and/or those whose single metastasis causing significant cerebral edema and/or have severe symptoms because of a mass effect, resection with or without postoperative radiotherapy (RT) should be considered [167]. The role of resection of a single brain metastasis was firstly defined in a small randomised trial, which demonstrated a significant improvement in overall survival (OS) from 15 to 40 weeks for patients randomly assigned to resection and whole-brain radiotherapy (WBRT) compared to RT alone [168]. Patients with multiple brain metastases should also be offered resection of a dominant metastatic deposit if causing neurologic deficits and/or significant vasogenic edema, especially if midline shift is present [169].

Systemic Therapy of Brain Metastases

The majority of systemic agents used nowadays for systemic treatment of metastatic BC are thought not to cross the intact blood-brain-barrier (BBB) in significant concentrations to be able to treat brain metastases. However, there is evidence that disruption of the BBB occurs with metastatic brain lesions and/or brain tumours and moderate effect with some targeted drugs has been also reported [170]. Since patients with HER-2 positive BC have higher incidence of brain metastases, a specific interest in this subset exists. Trastuzumab, a monoclonal antibody against HER-2 receptor, has been shown to cross a disrupted BBB and is associated with longer time to the development of brain metastases and longer survival after its diagnosis [171, 172]. There are currently ongoing trials evaluating the role of high-dose trastuzumab and Trastuzumab-emtansine (TDM-1) on HER-2 positive BC brain metastases [173]. Apart from monoclonal antibodies such as trastuzumab, small molecule inhibitors have also been used to target HER-2 positive tumours. Geyer et al. found that combination therapy of lapatinib, an inhibitor of HER-1 and HER-2 receptors, and capecitabine was superior to capecitabine alone for treatment of brain metastasis HER-2 positive BC patients previously exposed to trastuzumab [115]. The Landscape trial was a single arm phase II study evaluating 45 patients with brain metastasis not previously treated with WBRT, capecitabine or lapatinib (i.e. first line treatment) where the combination of capecitabine and lapatinib resulted in 65.9 % of partial responses [119].

Radiotherapy for Brain Metastases

WBRT is the standard of care for patients with multiple brain metastases and those with limited choice of systemic therapy options. The usual dosing and fractionation schedule range from 20 Gy in 5 fractions to 30 Gy in 10 fractions or up to 37.5 Gy in 15 fractions. A significant clinical response after WBRT has been correlated with reduced deterioration of neurocognitive function and improvement in certain domains [174]. Adding WBRT to surgery has been shown to improve local control of the disease, decrease failures within the brain elsewhere and reduce death from intracranial progression [175]. In case if there is no radiotherapy given after surgery the estimated local failure rate is as high as 45–60 % [176]. Possible short-term toxic effects of WBRT include otitis media, otitis externa, dermatitis and alopecia, while long-term ones include neurocognitive decline, decline in cerebellar function, cataracts and blindness [177]. A clinically significant reduction in early neurocognitive decline can be achieved with the use of intensity-modulated radiotherapy (IMRT) that reduces the dose to the bilateral hippocampi [178].

Radiosurgery or Stereotactic radiosurgery (SRS) may be used nowadays for patients with a large solitary brain metastasis receiving initial surgical resection, for those with more than one but limited number of brain metastasis and/or after failing WBRT. Most series have reported so far an excellent rate of local control with the use of SRS alone or in combination with WBRT [177, 179]. The recently published EORTC 22952 trial, reported that SRS alone produced a local control rate greater than surgery alone with a local control rate at 1 year of 69 % versus 41 % for surgery and it improved to 81 % when SRS was combined with WBRT [180]. The main advantage of SRS technique is a more favourable toxicity profile in comparison to WBRT. It causes less neurocognitive decline at 4 months postradiotherapy than SRS and WBRT together [181]. The only agent that has shown promise in preserving neurocognitive decline is memantine, an NDMA receptor agonist, which reduces hippocampal injury [182].

24.3.5.5 Liver Metastasis

Because of a lack of prospective randomised data for the management of liver metastases from BC, local therapy of liver metastases should only be considered in highly selected patients. Each case should be discussed with a multidisciplinary tumour board, before any decision is made. The best option is inclusion in a clinical trial, when available [15, 16].

Treatment will include systemic therapy (biologics, ET, chemotherapy), and in highly selected cases radio frequency ablation, stereotactic RT, cytoreductive surgery or chemo-embolization. This evidence comes only from reports on single institutional experiences, including small number of patients and old surgical and imagiology techniques [183]. Based on this data liver resection is best suitable if:

(a) referral to centres where large volume of hepatic resections are performed together with multidisciplinary management;
(b) patients have a good overall disease control with systemic therapy;
(c) patients with normal liver function (up to 70 % of the liver volume may be removed without risks of post-operative failure) [184];
(d) although the evidence is less clear in BC in comparison to colorectal cancer, similar principles of liver resection used for colorectal liver metastases may be applied: unilobar disease should be resected with hepatectomy; solitary lesion can be ablated with radio frequency or resected segmentally or non-anatomically; there is no clear evidence for liver resection in bilobar multiple metastases; isolated lung and bone metastasis should not be a contraindication for liver resection;
(e) incomplete resection (R1, R2) of BC liver metastasis as cytoreductive surgery is not proven to be beneficial.

In conclusion, it has been proposed that liver surgery may be considered as an additional treatment strategy to systemic therapy in highly selected BC patients including patients with low operative risk, feasibility of complete resection, no extrahepatic disease, except solitary bone and/or lung lesion that is controlled with RT and/or surgery and disease control with systemic therapy. It is urgent to evaluate which patients with liver involvement will benefit from local control in terms of survival.

24.4 Supportive Care and Survivorship Issues

Every patient with metastatic disease needs to be told by their treating oncologist that the disease is incurable but treatable and this should be explained to them respecting their privacy, culture and wishes mBC is highly heterogeneous and the psychosocial experience for women living with the disease can also be diverse [185]. Some women are diagnosed with primarily metastatic BC, others with relapsed disease are able to live many years on well-tolerated systemic treatments, and yet others live with more aggressive disease that requests several treatments in a short period of time. A major challenge of living with MBC is maintaining a balance between threatening thoughts, feelings and several lines of different treatments while pursuing a meaningful and rewarding life. An important psychological aspect of metastatic disease includes also major changes in life style as cancer and its treatment has an impact in the life of patients and their families.

There are many challenges for patients with MBC. These include managing physical symptoms and side effects (pain, fatigue), dealing with constant and/or changing treatment schedules, accepting stable disease as a desirable outcome of a specific therapy and importantly, accepting palliative care [186]. Psychological challenges consist of coping with uncertainty and unpredictable outcome of the disease, fearing dependency of others, maintaining valued life goals, fearing death and especially suffering. Special challenges are interpersonal ones that include three major components: having concerns for loved ones, feeling socially isolated and lacking emotional support, communicating with friends and family about the disease and death.

The two most common symptoms experienced by MBC patients are pain and fatigue. Patients with BC bone metastases can have severe pain and be limited in function as a result of extensive bone lesions and nerve entrapment syndromes. However, bone metastases are frequently very responsive to palliative radiotherapy and analgesics are very effective. Visceral involvement can also cause severe pain. Treatments by itself can have important side effects: taxanes can cause severe neuropathy and radiation can contribute to fibrosis and nerve entrapment. Since many patients living with mBC desire to keep on working, the compliance to opioid analgesics can be low in this cases, and compromise quality of life.

Fatigue is a complex symptom to manage as it is multifactorial and not completely understood being in part the result of pro-inflammatory cytokines release [187] by the disease and systemic therapies. Treatment strategies for cancer-related fatigue include physical activity, pharmacologic therapy and complementary techniques such as yoga and Tai chi.

Metastatic BC patients also experience clinically significant depression and anxiety [188]. Cancer-related distress is also increased after diagnosis of recurrent disease [189]. Although cancer-specific distress and general quality of life improve over the year after diagnosis, physical symptoms of the disease and functioning disabilities persist [190]. Factors and/or patients characteristics that are associated with poorer psychological adjustment in metastatic BC setting are younger age, low social support, more severe physical symptoms and denying of rational facts of long-term outcome of metastatic disease [191].

Clinical visits include the monitoring of disease status but also support to patients and relatives concerning psychological issues, job issues, specific side effects of treatment and managing the most common symptoms of advanced cancer (fatigue, pain, cognitive decline, etc.). Palliative and supportive care must be introduced early when the disease is disseminated and patient's preferences must be taken into consideration [15, 16]. Palliative care should be managed individually as well.

Importantly, patients must be encouraged to report their symptom severity and the burden and the impact of these symptoms on their quality of life. It is of great importance to collect these data systematically and integrate them in other clinical assessments that guide decision about treatment and care, using validated patient reported outcomes.

24.5 Future Perspectives

The knowledge of mBC treatment has evolved in recent years. Still there is an urgent need for development of research in several fields: new drugs and targets especially in the triple negative population; predictive markers of treatment response to best tailor treatment and improve quality of life; development of easy and accurate tools to assess quality of life.

The complexity of treatment requires an effort for constant education among physicians, patients and society for proper implementation of advanced breast cancer guidelines.

References

1. International Agency for Research on Cancer. Breast Cancer estimate incidence mapwiAfhgifPfsca.
2. Howlader N, Noone AM, Krapcho M, Miller D, Bishop K, Altekruse SF, Kosary CL, Yu M, Ruhl J, Tatalovich Z, Mariotto A, Lewis DR, Chen HS, Feuer EJ, Cronin KA, editors. SEER Cancer Statistics Review, 1975–2013, National Cancer Institute. Bethesda, MD. http://seer.cancer.gov/csr/1975_2013/.
3. Society. AC. Breast cancer facts and figures 2003–2004. Atlanta, GA: American Cancer Society; 2003.
4. Institute NC. SEER stat fact sheets: breast cancer. http://seer.cancer.gov/statfacts/html/breast.html. Accessed 31 July 2015.
5. Amir E, Clemons M, Purdie CA, Miller N, Quinlan P, Geddie W, et al. Tissue confirmation of disease recurrence in breast cancer patients: pooled analysis of multi-centre, multi-disciplinary prospective studies. Cancer Treat Rev. 2012;38(6):708–14.
6. Osborne CK. Tamoxifen in the treatment of breast cancer. N Engl J Med. 1998;339(22):1609–18.
7. Dawood S, Broglio K, Buzdar AU, Hortobagyi GN, Giordano SH. Prognosis of women with metastatic breast cancer by HER2 status and trastuzumab treatment: an institutional-based review. J Clin Oncol (Official Journal of the American Society of Clinical Oncology). 2010;28(1):92–8.
8. Characterization of metastatic breast cancer (mBC): and ancillary study of the SAFIR01 & MOSCATO trials [abstract]. Ann. Oncol. 25 aO.
9. Toy W, Shen Y, Won H, Green B, Sakr RA, Will M, et al. ESR1 ligand-binding domain mutations in hormone-resistant breast cancer. Nat Genet. 2013;45(12):1439–45.
10. Massard C. Enriching phase I trials with molecular alterations: interim analysis of 708 patients enrolled in the MOSCATO 01 trial [abstract]. In: 13th international congress on targeted anticancer therapies, Paris, France, aO3.7 (2015).
11. Bidard FC, Peeters DJ, Fehm T, Nole F, Gisbert-Criado R, Mavroudis D, et al. Clinical validity of circulating tumour cells in patients with metastatic breast cancer: a pooled analysis of individual patient data. Lancet Oncol. 2014;15(4):406–14.
12. Hayes DF, Cristofanilli M, Budd GT, Ellis MJ, Stopeck A, Miller MC, et al. Circulating tumor cells at each follow-up time point during therapy of metastatic breast cancer patients predict progression-free and overall survival. Clin Cancer Res (An Official Journal of the American Association for Cancer Research). 2006;12(14 Pt 1):4218–24.
13. Smerage JB, Barlow WE, Hortobagyi GN, Winer EP, Leyland-Jones B, Srkalovic G, et al. Circulating tumor cells and response to chemotherapy in metastatic breast cancer: SWOG S0500. J Clin Oncol (Official Journal of the American Society of Clinical Oncology). 2014;32(31):3483–9.
14. Amir E, Miller N, Geddie W, Freedman O, Kassam F, Simmons C, et al. Prospective study evaluating the impact of tissue confirmation of metastatic disease in patients with breast cancer. J Clin Oncol (Official Journal of the American Society of Clinical Oncology). 2012;30(6):587–92.
15. Cardoso F, Costa A, Norton L, Cameron D, Cufer T, Fallowfield L, et al. 1st international consensus guidelines for advanced breast cancer (ABC 1). Breast. 2012;21(3):242–52.
16. Cardoso F, Costa A, Norton L, Senkus E, Aapro M, Andre F, et al. ESO-ESMO 2nd international consensus guidelines for advanced breast cancer (ABC2)dagger. Ann Oncol (Official Journal of the European Society for Medical Oncology)/ESMO. 2014;25(10):1871–88.
17. Van Poznak C, Somerfield MR, Bast RC, Cristofanilli M, Goetz MP, Gonzalez-Angulo AM, et al. Use of biomarkers to guide decisions on systemic therapy for women with metastatic breast cancer: american society of clinical oncology clinical practice guideline. J Clin Oncol (Official Journal of the American Society of Clinical Oncology). 2015;33(24):2695–704.
18. Dawson SJ, Tsui DW, Murtaza M, Biggs H, Rueda OM, Chin SF, et al. Analysis of circulating tumor DNA to monitor metastatic breast cancer. N Engl J Med. 2013;368(13):1199–209.

19. Janku F, Wheler JJ, Westin SN, Moulder SL, Naing A, Tsimberidou AM, et al. PI3K/AKT/mTOR inhibitors in patients with breast and gynecologic malignancies harboring PIK3CA mutations. J Clin Oncol (Official Journal of the American Society of Clinical Oncology). 2012;30(8):777–82.
20. Andre F, Bachelot T, Campone M, Dalenc F, Perez-Garcia JM, Hurvitz SA, et al. Targeting FGFR with dovitinib (TKI258): preclinical and clinical data in breast cancer. Clin Cancer Res. 2013;19(13):3693–702.
21. Andre F, Bachelot T, Commo F, Campone M, Arnedos M, Dieras V, et al. Comparative genomic hybridisation array and DNA sequencing to direct treatment of metastatic breast cancer: a multicentre, prospective trial (SAFIR01/UNICANCER). Lancet Oncol. 2014;15(3):267–74.
22. Dickler M. A first-in-human phase I study to evaluate the oral selective oestrogen receptor degrader GDC-0810 (ARN-810) in postmenopausal women with oestrogen receptor+ HER2–, advanced/metastatic breast cancer. AACR [abstract CT231] (2015).
23. Arnedos M. Genomic and immune characterization of metastatic breast cancer (mBC): and ancillary study of the SAFIR01 & MOSCATO trials [abstract]. Ann Oncol. 2014;25:a351O.
24. Niikura N, Costelloe CM, Madewell JE, Hayashi N, Yu TK, Liu J, et al. FDG-PET/CT compared with conventional imaging in the detection of distant metastases of primary breast cancer. Oncologist. 2011;16(8):1111–9.
25. Nakai T, Okuyama C, Kubota T, Yamada K, Ushijima Y, Taniike K, et al. Pitfalls of FDG-PET for the diagnosis of osteoblastic bone metastases in patients with breast cancer. Eur J Nucl Med Mol Imaging. 2005;32(11):1253–8.
26. Janicek MJ, Hayes DF, Kaplan WD. Healing flare in skeletal metastases from breast cancer. Radiology. 1994;192(1):201–4.
27. Fiteni F, Villanueva C, Bazan F, Perrin S, Chaigneau L, Dobi E, et al. Long-term follow-up of patients with metastatic breast cancer treated by trastuzumab: impact of institutions. Breast. 2014;23(2):165–9.
28. Early Breast Cancer Trialists' Collaborative Group (EBCTCG). Relevance of breast cancer hormone receptors and other factors to the efficacy of adjuvant tamoxifen: patient-level meta-analysis of randomised trials. Lancet. 2011;378(9793):771–84.
29. Slamon DJ, Leyland-Jones B, Shak S, Fuchs H, Paton V, Bajamonde A, et al. Use of chemotherapy plus a monoclonal antibody against HER2 for metastatic breast cancer that overexpresses HER2. N Engl J Med. 2001;344(11):783–92.
30. Rabinovich M, Vallejo C, Bianco A, Perez J, Machiavelli M, Leone B, et al. Development and validation of prognostic models in metastatic breast cancer: a GOCS study. Oncology. 1992;49 (3):188–95.
31. Rahman ZU, Frye DK, Buzdar AU, Smith TL, Asmar L, Champlin RE, et al. Impact of selection process on response rate and long-term survival of potential high-dose chemotherapy candidates treated with standard-dose doxorubicin-containing chemotherapy in patients with metastatic breast cancer. J Clin Oncol (Official Journal of the American Society of Clinical Oncology). 1997;15(10):3171–7.
32. Yamamoto N, Watanabe T, Katsumata N, Omuro Y, Ando M, Fukuda H, et al. Construction and validation of a practical prognostic index for patients with metastatic breast cancer. J Clin Oncol (Official Journal of the American Society of Clinical Oncology). 1998;16(7):2401–8.
33. Hortobagyi GN, Smith TL, Legha SS, Swenerton KD, Gehan EA, Yap HY, et al. Multivariate analysis of prognostic factors in metastatic breast cancer. J Clin Oncol (Official Journal of the American Society of Clinical Oncology). 1983;1(12):776–86.
34. Regierer AC, Wolters R, Ufen MP, Weigel A, Novopashenny I, Kohne CH, et al. An internally and externally validated prognostic score for metastatic breast cancer: analysis of 2269 patients. Ann Oncol (Official Journal of the European Society for Medical Oncology)/ESMO. 2014;25(3):633–8.
35. Biganzoli L, Wildiers H, Oakman C, Marotti L, Loibl S, Kunkler I, et al. Management of elderly patients with breast cancer: updated recommendations of the International Society of Geriatric Oncology (SIOG) and European Society of Breast Cancer Specialists (EUSOMA). Lancet Oncol. 2012;13(4):e148–60.
36. Perou CM, Sorlie T, Eisen MB, van de Rijn M, Jeffrey SS, Rees CA, et al. Molecular portraits of human breast tumours. Nature. 2000;406(6797):747–52.
37. Weigelt B, Hu Z, He X, Livasy C, Carey LA, Ewend MG, et al. Molecular portraits and 70-gene prognosis signature are preserved throughout the metastatic process of breast cancer. Cancer Res. 2005;65(20):9155–8.
38. Sanchez-Martinez C, Gelbert LM, Lallena MJ, de Dios A. Cyclin dependent kinase (CDK) inhibitors as anticancer drugs. Bioorg Med Chem Lett. 2015;25(17):3420–35.
39. Wilcken N, Hornbuckle J, Ghersi D. Chemotherapy alone versus endocrine therapy alone for metastatic breast cancer. Cochrane Database Syst Rev. 2003;2:CD002747.
40. Largillier R, Ferrero JM, Doyen J, Barriere J, Namer M, Mari V, et al. Prognostic factors in 1038 women with metastatic breast cancer. Ann Oncol (Official Journal of the European Society for Medical Oncology)/ESMO. 2008;19(12):2012–9.
41. Amadori D, Volpi A, Maltoni R, Nanni O, Amaducci L, Amadori A, et al. Cell proliferation as a predictor of response to chemotherapy in metastatic breast cancer: a prospective study. Breast Cancer Res Treat. 1997;43(1):7–14.
42. Hatschek T, Carstensen J, Fagerberg G, Stal O, Grontoft O, Nordenskjold B. Influence of S-phase fraction on metastatic pattern and post-recurrence survival in a randomized mammography screening trial. Breast Cancer Res Treat. 1989;14(3):321–7.
43. Schrag D, Garewal HS, Burstein HJ, Samson DJ, Von Hoff DD, Somerfield MR, et al. American Society of Clinical Oncology Technology Assessment: chemotherapy sensitivity and resistance assays. J Clin Oncol (Official Journal of the American Society of Clinical Oncology). 2004;22(17):3631–8.
44. Ignatiadis M, Sotiriou C. Luminal breast cancer: from biology to treatment. Nat Rev Clin Oncol. 2013;10(9):494–506.
45. Early Breast Cancer Trialists' Collaborative G. Effects of chemotherapy and hormonal therapy for early breast cancer on recurrence and 15-year survival: an overview of the randomised trials. Lancet. 2005;365(9472):1687–717.
46. Clarke R, Tyson JJ, Dixon JM. Endocrine resistance in breast cancer—an overview and update. Mol Cell Endocrinol. 2015;418 (Pt 3):220–34.
47. Jeselsohn R, Buchwalter G, De Angelis C, Brown M, Schiff R. ESR1 mutations-a mechanism for acquired endocrine resistance in breast cancer. Nat Rev Clin Oncol. 2015;12(10):573–83.
48. Nardone A, De Angelis C, Trivedi MV, Osborne CK, Schiff R. The changing role of ER in endocrine resistance. Breast. 2015;24 (Suppl 2):S60–6.
49. Ciruelos Gil EM. Targeting the PI3 K/AKT/mTOR pathway in estrogen receptor-positive breast cancer. Cancer Treat Rev. 2014;40(7):862–71.
50. Butt AJ, McNeil CM, Musgrove EA, Sutherland RL. Downstream targets of growth factor and oestrogen signalling and endocrine resistance: the potential roles of c-Myc, cyclin D1 and cyclin E. Endocr Relat Cancer. 2005;12(Suppl 1):S47–59.

51. Caldon CE, Daly RJ, Sutherland RL, Musgrove EA. Cell cycle control in breast cancer cells. J Cell Biochem. 2006;97(2):261–74.
52. Miller TE, Ghoshal K, Ramaswamy B, Roy S, Datta J, Shapiro CL, et al. MicroRNA-221/222 confers tamoxifen resistance in breast cancer by targeting p27Kip1. J Biol Chem. 2008;283(44):29897–903.
53. Litherland S, Jackson IM. Antioestrogens in the management of hormone-dependent cancer. Cancer Treat Rev. 1988;15(3):183–94.
54. Baum M, Budzar AU, Cuzick J, Forbes J, Houghton JH, Klijn JG, et al. Anastrozole alone or in combination with tamoxifen versus tamoxifen alone for adjuvant treatment of postmenopausal women with early breast cancer: first results of the ATAC randomised trial. Lancet. 2002;359(9324):2131–9.
55. Mauri D, Pavlidis N, Polyzos NP, Ioannidis JP. Survival with aromatase inhibitors and inactivators versus standard hormonal therapy in advanced breast cancer: meta-analysis. J Natl Cancer Inst. 2006;98(18):1285–91.
56. Rose C, Vtoraya O, Pluzanska A, Davidson N, Gershanovich M, Thomas R, et al. An open randomised trial of second-line endocrine therapy in advanced breast cancer. Comparison of the aromatase inhibitors letrozole and anastrozole. Eur J Cancer. 2003;39(16):2318–27.
57. Campos SM, Guastalla JP, Subar M, Abreu P, Winer EP, Cameron DA. A comparative study of exemestane versus anastrozole in patients with postmenopausal breast cancer with visceral metastases. Clin Breast Cancer. 2009;9(1):39–44.
58. Dixon JM, Renshaw L, Langridge C, Young OE, McHugh M, Williams L, et al. Anastrozole and letrozole: an investigation and comparison of quality of life and tolerability. Breast Cancer Res Treat. 2011;125(3):741–9.
59. Klijn JG, Blamey RW, Boccardo F, Tominaga T, Duchateau L, Sylvester R, et al. Combined tamoxifen and luteinizing hormone-releasing hormone (LHRH) agonist versus LHRH agonist alone in premenopausal advanced breast cancer: a meta-analysis of four randomized trials. J Clin Oncol (Official Journal of the American Society of Clinical Oncology). 2001;19(2):343–53.
60. Osborne CK, Pippen J, Jones SE, Parker LM, Ellis M, Come S, et al. Double-blind, randomized trial comparing the efficacy and tolerability of fulvestrant versus anastrozole in postmenopausal women with advanced breast cancer progressing on prior endocrine therapy: results of a North American trial. J Clin Oncol (Official Journal of the American Society of Clinical Oncology). 2002;20(16):3386–95.
61. Chia S, Gradishar W, Mauriac L, Bines J, Amant F, Federico M, et al. Double-blind, randomized placebo controlled trial of fulvestrant compared with exemestane after prior nonsteroidal aromatase inhibitor therapy in postmenopausal women with hormone receptor-positive, advanced breast cancer: results from EFECT. J Clin Oncol (Official Journal of the American Society of Clinical Oncology). 2008;26(10):1664–70.
62. Al-Mubarak M, Sacher AG, Ocana A, Vera-Badillo F, Seruga B, Amir E. Fulvestrant for advanced breast cancer: a meta-analysis. Cancer Treat Rev. 2013;39(7):753–8.
63. Di Leo A, Jerusalem G, Petruzelka L, Torres R, Bondarenko IN, Khasanov R, et al. Final overall survival: fulvestrant 500 mg vesus 250 mg in the randomized CONFIRM trial. J Natl Cancer Inst. 2014;106(1):djt337.
64. Ellis MJ, Llombart-Cussac A, Feltl D, Dewar JA, Jasiowka M, Hewson N, et al. Fulvestrant 500 mg versus anastrozole 1 mg for the first-line treatment of advanced breast cancer: overall survival analysis from the phase II FIRST study. J Clin Oncol (Official Journal of the American Society of Clinical Oncology). 2015;33(32):3781–7.
65. Bergh J, Jonsson PE, Lidbrink EK, Trudeau M, Eiermann W, Brattstrom D, et al. FACT: an open-label randomized phase III study of fulvestrant and anastrozole in combination compared with anastrozole alone as first-line therapy for patients with receptor-positive postmenopausal breast cancer. J Clin Oncol (Official Journal of the American Society of Clinical Oncology). 2012;30(16):1919–25.
66. Mehta RS, Barlow WE, Albain KS, Vandenberg TA, Dakhil SR, Tirumali NR, et al. Combination anastrozole and fulvestrant in metastatic breast cancer. N Engl J Med. 2012;367(5):435–44.
67. Johnston SRD, Kilburn LS, Ellis P, Dodwell D, Cameron D, Hayward L, et al. Fulvestrant plus anastrozole or placebo versus exemestane alone after progression on non-steroidal aromatase inhibitors in postmenopausal patients with hormone-receptor-positive locally advanced or metastatic breast cancer (SoFEA): a composite, multicentre, phase 3 randomised trial. Lancet Oncol. 2013;14(10):989–98.
68. Cancer Genome Atlas N. Comprehensive molecular portraits of human breast tumours. Nature. 2012;490(7418):61–70.
69. Boulay A, Rudloff J, Ye J, Zumstein-Mecker S, O'Reilly T, Evans DB, et al. Dual inhibition of mTOR and estrogen receptor signaling in vitro induces cell death in models of breast cancer. Clin Cancer Res (An Official Journal of the American Association for Cancer Research). 2005;11(14):5319–28.
70. Baselga J, Campone M, Piccart M, Burris HA 3rd, Rugo HS, Sahmoud T, et al. Everolimus in postmenopausal hormone-receptor-positive advanced breast cancer. N Engl J Med. 2012;366(6):520–9.
71. Piccart M, Hortobagyi GN, Campone M, Pritchard KI, Lebrun F, Ito Y, et al. Everolimus plus exemestane for hormone-receptor-positive, human epidermal growth factor receptor-2-negative advanced breast cancer: overall survival results from BOLERO-2dagger. Ann Oncol (Official Journal of the European Society for Medical Oncology)/ESMO. 2014;25(12):2357–62.
72. Wolff AC, Lazar AA, Bondarenko I, Garin AM, Brincat S, Chow L, et al. Randomized phase III placebo-controlled trial of letrozole plus oral temsirolimus as first-line endocrine therapy in postmenopausal women with locally advanced or metastatic breast cancer. J Clin Oncol (Official Journal of the American Society of Clinical Oncology). 2013;31(2):195–202.
73. Bachelot T, Bourgier C, Cropet C, Ray-Coquard I, Ferrero JM, Freyer G, et al. Randomized phase II trial of everolimus in combination with tamoxifen in patients with hormone receptor-positive, human epidermal growth factor receptor 2-negative metastatic breast cancer with prior exposure to aromatase inhibitors: a GINECO study. J Clin Oncol. 2012;30(22):2718–24.
74. Aapro M, Andre F, Blackwell K, Calvo E, Jahanzeb M, Papazisis K, et al. Adverse event management in patients with advanced cancer receiving oral everolimus: focus on breast cancer. Ann Oncol (Official Journal of the European Society for Medical Oncology)/ESMO. 2014;25(4):763–73.
75. Hortobagyi GN, Chen D, Piccart M, Rugo HS, Burris HA 3rd, Pritchard KI, et al. Correlative analysis of genetic alterations and everolimus benefit in hormone receptor-positive, human epidermal growth factor receptor 2-negative advanced breast cancer: results from BOLERO-2. J Clin Oncol (Official Journal of the American Society of Clinical Oncology). 2016;34(5):419–26.
76. Finn RS, Crown JP, Lang I, Boer K, Bondarenko IM, Kulyk SO, et al. The cyclin-dependent kinase 4/6 inhibitor palbociclib in combination with letrozole versus letrozole alone as first-line treatment of oestrogen receptor-positive, HER2-negative, advanced breast cancer (PALOMA-1/TRIO-18): a randomised phase 2 study. Lancet Oncol. 2015;16(1):25–35.

77. Turner NC, Huang Bartlett C, Cristofanilli M. Palbociclib in hormone-receptor-positive advanced breast cancer. N Engl J Med. 2015;373(17):1672–3.
78. Turner NC, Ro J, Andre F, Loi S, Verma S, Iwata H, et al. Palbociclib in hormone-receptor-positive advanced breast cancer. N Engl J Med. 2015;373(3):209–19.
79. Munster PN, Thurn KT, Thomas S, Raha P, Lacevic M, Miller A, et al. A phase II study of the histone deacetylase inhibitor vorinostat combined with tamoxifen for the treatment of patients with hormone therapy-resistant breast cancer. Br J Cancer. 2011;104(12):1828–35.
80. Baselga J, Im S-A, Iwata H, Clemons M, Ito Y, Awada A, Chia S, Jagiello-Gruszfeld A, Pistilli B, Tseng L-M, Hurvitz S, Masuda N, Cortés J, De Laurentiis M, Arteaga CL, Jiang Z, Jonat W, Hachemi S, Le Mouhaër S, Di Tomaso E, Urban P, Massacesi C, Campone M. PIK3CA status in circulating tumor DNA (ctDNA) predicts efficacy of buparlisib (BUP) plus fulvestrant (FULV) in postmenopausal women with endocrine-resistant HR+/HER2− advanced breast cancer (BC): first results from the randomized, phase III BELLE-2 trial. Abstract S6-01. Presented at: San Antonio Breast Cancer Symposium; 8–12 Dec 2015.
81. Piccart-Gebhart MJ, Burzykowski T, Buyse M, Sledge G, Carmichael J, Luck HJ, et al. Taxanes alone or in combination with anthracyclines as first-line therapy of patients with metastatic breast cancer. J Clin Oncol (Official Journal of the American Society of Clinical Oncology). 2008;26(12):1980–6.
82. Fumoleau P, Largillier R, Clippe C, Dieras V, Orfeuvre H, Lesimple T, et al. Multicentre, phase II study evaluating capecitabine monotherapy in patients with anthracycline- and taxane-pretreated metastatic breast cancer. Euro J Cancer. 2004;40(4):536–42.
83. Kaufman PA, Awada A, Twelves C, Yelle L, Perez EA, Velikova G, et al. Phase III open-label randomized study of eribulin mesylate versus capecitabine in patients with locally advanced or metastatic breast cancer previously treated with an anthracycline and a taxane. J Clin Oncol (Official Journal of the American Society of Clinical Oncology). 2015;33(6):594–601.
84. Martin M, Ruiz A, Munoz M, Balil A, Garcia-Mata J, Calvo L, et al. Gemcitabine plus vinorelbine versus vinorelbine monotherapy in patients with metastatic breast cancer previously treated with anthracyclines and taxanes: final results of the phase III Spanish Breast Cancer Research Group (GEICAM) trial. Lancet Oncol. 2007;8(3):219–25.
85. Cortes J, O'Shaughnessy J, Loesch D, Blum JL, Vahdat LT, Petrakova K, et al. Eribulin monotherapy versus treatment of physician's choice in patients with metastatic breast cancer (EMBRACE): a phase 3 open-label randomised study. Lancet. 2011;377(9769):914–23.
86. Rha SY, Moon YH, Jeung HC, Kim YT, Sohn JH, Yang WI, et al. Gemcitabine monotherapy as salvage chemotherapy in heavily pretreated metastatic breast cancer. Breast Cancer Res Treat. 2005;90(3):215–21.
87. Carrick S, Ghersi D, Wilcken N, Simes J. Platinum containing regimens for metastatic breast cancer. Cochrane Database Syst Rev. 2004;2:CD003374.
88. Stockler MR, Harvey VJ, Francis PA, Byrne MJ, Ackland SP, Fitzharris B, et al. Capecitabine versus classical cyclophosphamide, methotrexate, and fluorouracil as first-line chemotherapy for advanced breast cancer. J Clin Oncol (Official Journal of the American Society of Clinical Oncology). 2011;29(34):4498–504.
89. O'Brien MER. Reduced cardiotoxicity and comparable efficacy in a phase III trial of pegylated liposomal doxorubicin HCl (CAELYXTM/Doxil") versus conventional doxorubicin for first-line treatment of metastatic breast cancer. Ann Oncol. 2004;15(3):440–9.
90. Cardoso F, Bedard PL, Winer EP, Pagani O, Senkus-Konefka E, Fallowfield LJ, et al. International guidelines for management of metastatic breast cancer: combination vs sequential single-agent chemotherapy. J Natl Cancer Inst. 2009;101(17):1174–81.
91. Slamon DJ, Clark GM, Wong SG, Levin WJ, Ullrich A, McGuire WL. Human breast cancer: correlation of relapse and survival with amplification of the HER-2/neu oncogene. Science. 1987;235(4785):177–82.
92. Browne BC, O'Brien N, Duffy MJ, Crown J, O'Donovan N. HER-2 signaling and inhibition in breast cancer. Curr Cancer Drug Targets. 2009;9(3):419–38.
93. Vu T, Claret FX. Trastuzumab: updated mechanisms of action and resistance in breast cancer. Front Oncol. 2012;2:62.
94. Klapper LN, Waterman H, Sela M, Yarden Y. Tumor-inhibitory antibodies to HER-2/ErbB-2 may act by recruiting c-Cbl and enhancing ubiquitination of HER-2. Cancer Res. 2000;60 (13):3384–8.
95. Arnould L, Gelly M, Penault-Llorca F, Benoit L, Bonnetain F, Migeon C, et al. Trastuzumab-based treatment of HER2-positive breast cancer: an antibody-dependent cellular cytotoxicity mechanism? Br J Cancer. 2006;94(2):259–67.
96. O'Shaughnessy J, Vukelja SJ, Marsland T, Kimmel G, Ratnam S, Pippen J. Phase II trial of gemcitabine plus trastuzumab in metastatic breast cancer patients previously treated with chemotherapy: preliminary results. Clin Breast Cancer. 2002;3 (Suppl 1):17–20.
97. Burstein HJ, Keshaviah A, Baron A, et al. Trastuzumab and vinorelbine or taxane chemotherapy for HER2+ metastatic breast cancer: the TRAVIOTA study. J Clin Oncol 2006;24:40s (Abstr 650).
98. Robert N, Leyland-Jones B, Asmar L, Belt R, Ilegbodu D, Loesch D, et al. Randomized phase III study of trastuzumab, paclitaxel, and carboplatin compared with trastuzumab and paclitaxel in women with HER-2-overexpressing metastatic breast cancer. J Clin Oncol (Official Journal of the American Society of Clinical Oncology). 2006;24(18):2786–92.
99. Seidman AD, Berry D, Cirrincione C, Harris L, Muss H, Marcom PK, et al. Randomized phase III trial of weekly compared with every-3-weeks paclitaxel for metastatic breast cancer, with trastuzumab for all HER-2 overexpressors and random assignment to trastuzumab or not in HER-2 nonoverexpressors: final results of Cancer and Leukemia Group B protocol 9840. J Clin Oncol (Official Journal of the American Society of Clinical Oncology). 2008;26(10):1642–9.
100. Andersson M, Lidbrink E, Bjerre K, Wist E, Enevoldsen K, Jensen AB, et al. Phase III randomized study comparing docetaxel plus trastuzumab with vinorelbine plus trastuzumab as first-line therapy of metastatic or locally advanced human epidermal growth factor receptor 2-positive breast cancer: the HERNATA study. J Clin Oncol (Official Journal of the American Society of Clinical Oncology). 2011;29(3):264–71.
101. Valero V, Forbes J, Pegram MD, Pienkowski T, Eiermann W, von Minckwitz G, et al. Multicenter phase III randomized trial comparing docetaxel and trastuzumab with docetaxel, carboplatin, and trastuzumab as first-line chemotherapy for patients with HER2-gene-amplified metastatic breast cancer (BCIRG 007 study): two highly active therapeutic regimens. J Clin Oncol (Official Journal of the American Society of Clinical Oncology). 2011;29(2):149–56.
102. Pegram MD, Pienkowski T, Northfelt DW, Eiermann W, Patel R, Fumoleau P, et al. Results of two open-label, multicenter phase II studies of docetaxel, platinum salts, and trastuzumab in

HER2-positive advanced breast cancer. J Natl Cancer Inst. 2004;96(10):759–69.
103. Perez EA, Suman VJ, Rowland KM, Ingle JN, Salim M, Loprinzi CL, et al. Two concurrent phase II trials of paclitaxel/carboplatin/trastuzumab (weekly or every-3-week schedule) as first-line therapy in women with HER2-overexpressing metastatic breast cancer: NCCTG study 983252. Clin Breast Cancer. 2005;6(5):425–32.
104. Wolff AC, Hammond ME, Schwartz JN, Hagerty KL, Allred DC, Cote RJ, et al. American Society of Clinical Oncology/College of American Pathologists guideline recommendations for human epidermal growth factor receptor 2 testing in breast cancer. J Clin Oncol. 2007;25(1):118–45.
105. Narayan M, Wilken JA, Harris LN, Baron AT, Kimbler KD, Maihle NJ. Trastuzumab-induced HER reprogramming in "resistant" breast carcinoma cells. Cancer Res. 2009;69(6):2191–4.
106. Portera CC, Walshe JM, Rosing DR, Denduluri N, Berman AW, Vatas U, et al. Cardiac toxicity and efficacy of trastuzumab combined with pertuzumab in patients with [corrected] human epidermal growth factor receptor 2-positive metastatic breast cancer. Clin Cancer Res (An Official Journal of the American Association for Cancer Research). 2008;14(9):2710–6.
107. Scheuer W, Friess T, Burtscher H, Bossenmaier B, Endl J, Hasmann M. Strongly enhanced antitumor activity of trastuzumab and pertuzumab combination treatment on HER2-positive human xenograft tumor models. Cancer Res. 2009;69(24):9330–6.
108. Baselga J, Gelmon KA, Verma S, Wardley A, Conte P, Miles D, et al. Phase II trial of pertuzumab and trastuzumab in patients with human epidermal growth factor receptor 2-positive metastatic breast cancer that progressed during prior trastuzumab therapy. J Clin Oncol (Official Journal of the American Society of Clinical Oncology). 2010;28(7):1138–44.
109. Baselga J, Cortes J, Kim SB, Im SA, Hegg R, Im YH, et al. Pertuzumab plus trastuzumab plus docetaxel for metastatic breast cancer. N Engl J Med. 2012;366(2):109–19.
110. Swain SM, Kim S-B, Cortés J, Ro J, Semiglazov V, Campone M, et al. Pertuzumab, trastuzumab, and docetaxel for HER2-positive metastatic breast cancer (CLEOPATRA study): overall survival results from a randomised, double-blind, placebo-controlled, phase 3 study. Lancet Oncol. 2013;14(6):461–71.
111. Baselga J, Swain SM. CLEOPATRA: a phase III evaluation of pertuzumab and trastuzumab for HER2-positive metastatic breast cancer. Clin Breast Cancer. 2010;10(6):489–91.
112. Dang C, Iyengar N, Datko F, D'Andrea G, Theodoulou M, Dickler M, et al. Phase II study of paclitaxel given once per week along with trastuzumab and pertuzumab in patients with human epidermal growth factor receptor 2-positive metastatic breast cancer. J Clin Oncol (Official Journal of the American Society of Clinical Oncology). 2015;33(5):442–7.
113. Perez EA, Lopez-Vega JM, Del Mastro L, Petit T, Mitchell L, Pelizon CH, Andersson M. A combination of pertuzumab, trastuzumab, and vinorelbine for first-line treatment of patients with HER2-positive metastatic breast cancer: An open-label, two-cohort, phase II study (VELVET). J Clin Oncol 2012;30 (suppl; abstr TPS653).
114. Ellis PA, Barrios CH, Eiermann W et al. Phase III, randomized study of trastuzumab emtansine (T-DM1)± pertuzumab (P) vs trastuzumab + taxane (HT) for first-line treatment of HER2-positive MBC: primary results from the MARIANNE study. J Clin Oncol 2015;33(suppl; abstr 507).
115. Geyer CE, Forster J, Lindquist D, Chan S, Romieu CG, Pienkowski T, et al. Lapatinib plus capecitabine for HER2-positive advanced breast cancer. N Engl J Med. 2006;355(26):2733–43.
116. Cameron D, Casey M, Oliva C, Newstat B, Imwalle B, Geyer CE. Lapatinib plus capecitabine in women with HER-2-positive advanced breast cancer: final survival analysis of a phase III randomized trial. Oncologist. 2010;15(9):924–34.
117. Gelmon KA, Boyle F, Kaufman B, et al. Open-label phase III randomized controlled trial comparing taxane-based chemotherapy with lapatinib or trastuzumab as first-line therapy for women with HER2-positive metastatic breast cancer: Interim analysis of NCIC CTG MA.31/GSK EGF 108919. ASCO Annual Meeting Abstract LBA671; 2012.
118. Pivot X, Manikhas A, Zurawski B, Chmielowska E, Karaszewska B, Allerton R, et al. CEREBEL (EGF111438): a phase III, randomized, open-label study of lapatinib plus capecitabine versus trastuzumab plus capecitabine in patients with human epidermal growth factor receptor 2-positive metastatic breast cancer. J Clin Oncol (Official Journal of the American Society of Clinical Oncology). 2015;33(14):1564–73.
119. Bachelot T, Romieu G, Campone M, Diéras V, Cropet C, Dalenc F, et al. Lapatinib plus capecitabine in patients with previously untreated brain metastases from HER2-positive metastatic breast cancer (LANDSCAPE): a single-group phase 2 study. Lancet Oncol. 2013;14(1):64–71.
120. Verma S, Miles D, Gianni L, Krop IE, Welslau M, Baselga J, et al. Trastuzumab emtansine for HER2-positive advanced breast cancer. N Engl J Med. 2012;367(19):1783–91.
121. Giordano SH, Temin S, Kirshner JJ, Chandarlapaty S, Crews JR, Davidson NE, et al. Systemic therapy for patients with advanced human epidermal growth factor receptor 2-positive breast cancer: American Society of Clinical Oncology clinical practice guideline. J Clin Oncol (Official Journal of the American Society of Clinical Oncology). 2014;32(19):2078–99.
122. Krop IE, Kim S-B, González-Martín A, LoRusso PM, Ferrero J-M, Smitt M, et al. Trastuzumab emtansine versus treatment of physician's choice for pretreated HER2-positive advanced breast cancer (TH3RESA): a randomised, open-label, phase 3 trial. Lancet Oncol. 2014;15(7):689–99.
123. Wildiers H, Kim S-B, Gonzalez-Martin A, LoRusso PM, Ferrero J-M, Yu R, Smitt M, Krop I. Trastuzumab emtansine improves overall survival versus treatment of physician's choice in patients with previously treated HER2-positive metastatic breast cancer: final overall survival results from the phase 3 TH3RESA study. SABCS 2015 Abstract S5-05.
124. Blackwell KL, Burstein HJ, Storniolo AM, Rugo HS, Sledge G, Aktan G, et al. Overall survival benefit with lapatinib in combination with trastuzumab for patients with human epidermal growth factor receptor 2-positive metastatic breast cancer: final results from the EGF104900 Study. J Clin Oncol (Official Journal of the American Society of Clinical Oncology). 2012;30 (21):2585–92.
125. Cortes J, Fumoleau P, Bianchi GV, Petrella TM, Gelmon K, Pivot X, et al. Pertuzumab monotherapy after trastuzumab-based treatment and subsequent reintroduction of trastuzumab: activity and tolerability in patients with advanced human epidermal growth factor receptor 2-positive breast cancer. J Clin Oncol (Official Journal of the American Society of Clinical Oncology). 2012;30(14):1594–600.
126. Kaufman B, Mackey JR, Clemens MR, Bapsy PP, Vaid A, Wardley A, et al. Trastuzumab plus anastrozole versus anastrozole alone for the treatment of postmenopausal women with human epidermal growth factor receptor 2-positive, hormone receptor-positive metastatic breast cancer: results from the randomized phase III TAnDEM study. J Clin Oncol (Official Journal of the American Society of Clinical Oncology). 2009;27 (33):5529–37.

127. Johnston S, Pippen J Jr, Pivot X, Lichinitser M, Sadeghi S, Dieras V, et al. Lapatinib combined with letrozole versus letrozole and placebo as first-line therapy for postmenopausal hormone receptor-positive metastatic breast cancer. J Clin Oncol (Official Journal of the American Society of Clinical Oncology). 2009;27(33):5538–46.
128. Burstein HJ, Sun Y, Dirix LY, Jiang Z, Paridaens R, Tan AR, et al. Neratinib, an irreversible ErbB receptor tyrosine kinase inhibitor, in patients with advanced ErbB2-positive breast cancer. J Clin Oncol (Official Journal of the American Society of Clinical Oncology). 2010;28(8):1301–7.
129. Awada A, Colomer R, Inoue K, Bondarenko I, Badwe RA, Demetriou G, et al. Neratinib plus paclitaxel vs trastuzumab plus paclitaxel in previously untreated metastatic ERBB2-positive breast cancer: the NEfERT-T randomized clinical trial. JAMA oncology. 2016.
130. Kennecke H, Yerushalmi R, Woods R, Cheang MC, Voduc D, Speers CH, et al. Metastatic behavior of breast cancer subtypes. J Clin Oncol (Official Journal of the American Society of Clinical Oncology). 2010;28(20):3271–7.
131. Isakoff SJ. Triple-negative breast cancer: role of specific chemotherapy agents. Cancer J. 2010;16(1):53–61.
132. Wahba HA, El-Hadaad HA. Current approaches in treatment of triple-negative breast cancer. Cancer Biol Med. 2015;12(2):106–16.
133. Wysocki PJ KK, Lamperska K, Zaluski J, Mackiewicz A. Primary resistance to docetaxel-based chemotherapy in metastatic breast cancer patients correlates with a high frequency of BRCA 1 mutations. Med Sci Monit. 2008;14:SC7–SC10.
134. Byrski T, Gronwald J, Huzarski T, Grzybowska E, Budryk M, Stawicka M, et al. Pathologic complete response rates in young women with BRCA1-positive breast cancers after neoadjuvant chemotherapy. J Clin Oncol (Official Journal of the American Society of Clinical Oncology). 2010;28(3):375–9.
135. Byrski T, Foszczynska-Kloda M, Huzarski T, Dent R, Gronwald J, Cybulski C et al. Cisplatin chemotherapy in the treatment of BRCA-1 positive metastatic breast cancer (MBC). J Clin Oncol 2009;27: abstr 1099.
136. Tutt A, Ellis P, Kilburn L, et al. Abstract S3-01: The TNT trial: a randomized phase III trial of carboplatin (C) compared with docetaxel (D) for patients with metastatic or recurrent locally advanced triple negative or BRCA1/2 breast cancer (CRUK/07/012). Cancer Res May 1, 2015 75; S3-01. hirty-Seventh Annual CTRC-AACR San Antonio Breast Cancer Symposium; 9–13 Dec 2014; San Antonio, TX.
137. Schneider BP, Miller KD. Angiogenesis of breast cancer. J Clin Oncol (Official Journal of the American Society of Clinical Oncology). 2005;23(8):1782–90.
138. Miller K, Wang M, Gralow J, Dickler M, Cobleigh M, Perez EA, et al. Paclitaxel plus bevacizumab versus paclitaxel alone for metastatic breast cancer. N Engl J Med. 2007;357(26):2666–76.
139. Miles DW, Chan A, Dirix LY, Cortes J, Pivot X, Tomczak P, et al. Phase III study of bevacizumab plus docetaxel compared with placebo plus docetaxel for the first-line treatment of human epidermal growth factor receptor 2-negative metastatic breast cancer. J Clin Oncol (Official Journal of the American Society of Clinical Oncology). 2010;28(20):3239–47.
140. Robert NJ, Dieras V, Glaspy J, Brufsky AM, Bondarenko I, Lipatov ON, et al. RIBBON-1: randomized, double-blind, placebo-controlled, phase III trial of chemotherapy with or without bevacizumab for first-line treatment of human epidermal growth factor receptor 2-negative, locally recurrent or metastatic breast cancer. J Clin Oncol. 2011;29(10):1252–60.
141. Rossari JR, Metzger-Filho O, Paesmans M, Saini KS, Gennari A, de Azambuja E, et al. Bevacizumab and breast cancer: a meta-analysis of first-line phase III studies and a critical reappraisal of available evidence. J Oncol. 2012;2012:417673.
142. O'Shaughnessy J, Miles D, Gray RJ, et al. A meta-analysis of overall survival data from three randomized trials of bevacizumab (BV) and first-line chemotherapy as treatment for patients with metastatic breast cancer (MBC). J Clin Oncol 2010;28:15s: Abstr 1005.
143. Farmer H, McCabe N, Lord CJ, Tutt AN, Johnson DA, Richardson TB, et al. Targeting the DNA repair defect in BRCA mutant cells as a therapeutic strategy. Nature. 2005;434 (7035):917–21.
144. O'Shaughnessy J, Osborne C, Pippen JE, Yoffe M, Patt D, Rocha C, et al. Iniparib plus chemotherapy in metastatic triple-negative breast cancer. N Engl J Med. 2011;364(3):205–14.
145. J. O'Shaughnessy LSS, M. A. Danso, H. S. Rugo, K. Miller, D. A. Yardley, R. W. Carlson, R. S. Finn, E. Charpentier, M. Freese, S. Gupta, A. Blackwood-Chirchir, E. P. Winer. A randomized phase III study of iniparib (BSI-201) in combination with gemcitabine/carboplatin (G/C) in metastatic triple-negative breast cancer (TNBC). J Clin Oncol. 2011;29(suppl; abstr 1007).
146. Gelmon KA, Hirte H, Robidoux A, et al. Can we define tumors that will respond to PARP inhibitors? A phase II correlative study of olaparib in advanced serous ovarian cancer and triple-negative breast cancer. J Clin Oncol. 2010;28(15 suppl):3002.
147. Kumar P, Aggarwal R. An overview of triple-negative breast cancer. Arch Gynecol Obstet. 2016;293(2):247–69.
148. Fontanella C, Fanotto V, Rihawi K, Aprile G, Puglisi F. Skeletal metastases from breast cancer: pathogenesis of bone tropism and treatment strategy. Clin Exp Metastasis. 2015;32(8):819–33.
149. Dunstan CR, Felsenberg D, Seibel MJ. Therapy insight: the risks and benefits of bisphosphonates for the treatment of tumor-induced bone disease. Nat Clin Pract Oncol. 2007;4 (1):42–55.
150. Coleman RE. Bisphosphonates in breast cancer. Ann Oncol (Official Journal of the European Society for Medical Oncology)/ ESMO. 2005;16(5):687–95.
151. Kohno N, Aogi K, Minami H, Nakamura S, Asaga T, Iino Y, et al. Zoledronic acid significantly reduces skeletal complications compared with placebo in Japanese women with bone metastases from breast cancer: a randomized, placebo-controlled trial. J Clin Oncol (Official Journal of the American Society of Clinical Oncology). 2005;23(15):3314–21.
152. Rosen LS, Gordon D, Kaminski M, Howell A, Belch A, Mackey J, et al. Zoledronic acid versus pamidronate in the treatment of skeletal metastases in patients with breast cancer or osteolytic lesions of multiple myeloma: a phase III, double-blind, comparative trial. Cancer J. 2001;7(5):377–87.
153. Lipton A, Small E, Saad F, Gleason D, Gordon D, Smith M, et al. The new bisphosphonate, Zometa (zoledronic acid), decreases skeletal complications in both osteolytic and osteoblastic lesions: a comparison to pamidronate. Cancer Inv. 2002;20(Suppl 2):45–54.
154. Bamias A, Kastritis E, Bamia C, Moulopoulos LA, Melakopoulos I, Bozas G, et al. Osteonecrosis of the jaw in cancer after treatment with bisphosphonates: incidence and risk factors. J Clin Oncol (Official Journal of the American Society of Clinical Oncology). 2005;23(34):8580–7.

155. Andrew Louis Himelstein RQ, Paul J. Novotny et al. CALGB 70604 (Alliance): a randomized phase III study of standard dosing vs. longer interval dosing of zoledronic acid in metastatic cancer. J Clin Oncol 2015;33(suppl; abstr 9501).
156. Body JJ, Facon T, Coleman RE, Lipton A, Geurs F, Fan M, et al. A study of the biological receptor activator of nuclear factor-kappaB ligand inhibitor, denosumab, in patients with multiple myeloma or bone metastases from breast cancer. Clin Cancer Res (An Official Journal of the American Association for Cancer Research). 2006;12(4):1221–8.
157. Brown JE, Coleman RE. Denosumab in patients with cancer-a surgical strike against the osteoclast. Nat Rev Clin Oncol. 2012;9 (2):110–8.
158. Stopeck AT, Lipton A, Body JJ, Steger GG, Tonkin K, de Boer RH, et al. Denosumab compared with zoledronic acid for the treatment of bone metastases in patients with advanced breast cancer: a randomized, double-blind study. J Clin Oncol (Official Journal of the American Society of Clinical Oncology). 2010;28 (35):5132–9.
159. Martin M, Bell R, Bourgeois H, Brufsky A, Diel I, Eniu A, et al. Bone-related complications and quality of life in advanced breast cancer: results from a randomized phase III trial of denosumab versus zoledronic acid. Clin Cancer Res. 2012;18(17):4841–9.
160. Chow E, Harris K, Fan G, Tsao M, Sze WM. Palliative radiotherapy trials for bone metastases: a systematic review. J Clin Oncol (Official Journal of the American Society of Clinical Oncology). 2007;25(11):1423–36.
161. Hoskin PJ, Stratford MR, Folkes LK, Regan J, Yarnold JR. Effect of local radiotherapy for bone pain on urinary markers of osteoclast activity. Lancet. 2000;355(9213):1428–9.
162. Beyzadeoglu M, Ozyigit G, Ebruli C. Basic radiation oncology. Heidelberg: Springer;2010.
163. Roos DE, Turner SL, O'Brien PC, Smith JG, Spry NA, Burmeister BH, et al. Randomized trial of 8 Gy in 1 versus 20 Gy in 5 fractions of radiotherapy for neuropathic pain due to bone metastases (Trans-Tasman Radiation Oncology Group, TROG 96.05). Radiother Oncol (Journal of the European Society for Therapeutic Radiology and Oncology). 2005;75(1):54–63.
164. Yamada Y, Bilsky MH, Lovelock DM, Venkatraman ES, Toner S, Johnson J, et al. High-dose, single-fraction image-guided intensity-modulated radiotherapy for metastatic spinal lesions. Int J Radiat Oncol Biol Phys. 2008;71(2):484–90.
165. Ju DG, Yurter A, Gokaslan ZL, Sciubba DM. Diagnosis and surgical management of breast cancer metastatic to the spine. World J Clin Oncol. 2014;5(3):263–71.
166. Shehadi JA, Sciubba DM, Suk I, Suki D, Maldaun MV, McCutcheon IE, et al. Surgical treatment strategies and outcome in patients with breast cancer metastatic to the spine: a review of 87 patients. Eur Spine J. 2007;16(8):1179–92.
167. Tsao MN, Rades D, Wirth A, Lo SS, Danielson BL, Gaspar LE, et al. Radiotherapeutic and surgical management for newly diagnosed brain metastasis(es): an American Society for Radiation Oncology evidence-based guideline. Pract Radiat Oncol. 2012;2(3):210–25.
168. Patchell RA, Tibbs PA, Walsh JW, Dempsey RJ, Maruyama Y, Kryscio RJ, et al. A randomized trial of surgery in the treatment of single metastases to the brain. N Engl J Med. 1990;322 (8):494–500.
169. National Comprehensive Cancer Network. Central nervous system cancers (version 1.2014). Available from: http://www.nccn.org.
170. Lesser GJ. Chemotherapy of cerebral metastases from solid tumors. Neurosurg Clin N Am. 1996;7(3):527–36.
171. Park YH, Park MJ, Ji SH, Yi SY, Lim DH, Nam DH, et al. Trastuzumab treatment improves brain metastasis outcomes through control and durable prolongation of systemic extracranial disease in HER2-overexpressing breast cancer patients. Br J Cancer. 2009;100(6):894–900.
172. Dijkers EC, Oude Munnink TH, Kosterink JG, Brouwers AH, Jager PL, de Jong JR, et al. Biodistribution of 89Zr-trastuzumab and PET imaging of HER2-positive lesions in patients with metastatic breast cancer. Clin Pharmacol Ther. 2010;87(5):586–92.
173. Willett A, Wilkinson JB, Shah C, Mehta MP. Management of solitary and multiple brain metastases from breast cancer. Indian J Med Paediatr Oncol (Official Journal of Indian Society of Medical & Paediatric Oncology). 2015;36(2):87–93.
174. Li J, Bentzen SM, Renschler M, Mehta MP. Regression after whole-brain radiation therapy for brain metastases correlates with survival and improved neurocognitive function. J Clin Oncol (Official Journal of the American Society of Clinical Oncology). 2007;25(10):1260–6.
175. Patchell RA, Tibbs PA, Regine WF, Dempsey RJ, Mohiuddin M, Kryscio RJ, et al. Postoperative radiotherapy in the treatment of single metastases to the brain: a randomized trial. JAMA. 1998;280(17):1485–9.
176. Andrews DW, Scott CB, Sperduto PW, Flanders AE, Gaspar LE, Schell MC, et al. Whole brain radiation therapy with or without stereotactic radiosurgery boost for patients with one to three brain metastases: phase III results of the RTOG 9508 randomised trial. Lancet. 2004;363(9422):1665–72.
177. Tomasello G, Bedard PL, de Azambuja E, Lossignol D, Devriendt D, Piccart-Gebhart MJ. Brain metastases in HER2-positive breast cancer: the evolving role of lapatinib. Crit Rev Oncol/Hematol. 2010;75(2):110–21.
178. Gondi V, Mehta M, Pugh S, Tome W, Kanner A, Caine C, et al. Memory preservation with conformal avoidance of the hippocampus during whole-brain radiotherapy (WBRT) for patients with brain metastases: primary endpoint results of RTOG 0933. Oral presentation at 2013 Annual Meeting of the American Society for Radiation Oncology (ASTRO), Atlanta, Georgia, 23 Sept 2013.
179. Kondziolka D, Patel A, Lunsford LD, Kassam A, Flickinger JC. Stereotactic radiosurgery plus whole brain radiotherapy versus radiotherapy alone for patients with multiple brain metastases. Int J Radiat Oncol Biol Phys. 1999;45(2):427–34.
180. Robbins JR, Ryu S, Kalkanis S, Cogan C, Rock J, Movsas B, et al. Radiosurgery to the surgical cavity as adjuvant therapy for resected brain metastasis. Neurosurgery. 2012;71(5):937–43.
181. Chang EL, Wefel JS, Hess KR, Allen PK, Lang FF, Kornguth DG, et al. Neurocognition in patients with brain metastases treated with radiosurgery or radiosurgery plus whole-brain irradiation: a randomised controlled trial. Lancet Oncol. 2009;10(11):1037–44.
182. Brown PD, Pugh S, Laack NN, Wefel JS, Khuntia D, Meyers C, et al. Memantine for the prevention of cognitive dysfunction in patients receiving whole-brain radiotherapy: a randomized, double-blind, placebo-controlled trial. Neuro-oncology. 2013;15 (10):1429–37.
183. Howlader M, Heaton N, Rela M. Resection of liver metastases from breast cancer: towards a management guideline. Int J Surg. 2011;9(4):285–91.
184. Kubota K, Makuuchi M, Kusaka K, Kobayashi T, Miki K, Hasegawa K, et al. Measurement of liver volume and hepatic functional reserve as a guide to decision-making in resectional surgery for hepatic tumors. Hepatology. 1997;26(5):1176–81.
185. Ganz PA, Stanton AL. Living with metastatic breast cancer. Adv Exp Med Biol. 2015;862:243–54.
186. Low CA BT, Stanton AL. Adaptation in the face of advanced cancer. In Feuerstein M, editors. Handbook of cancer survivorship. Heidelberg: Springer; 2007. p. 211–228.

187. de Raaf PJ, Sleijfer S, Lamers CH, Jager A, Gratama JW, van der Rijt CC. Inflammation and fatigue dimensions in advanced cancer patients and cancer survivors: an explorative study. Cancer. 2012;118(23):6005–11.
188. Okamura H, Watanabe T, Narabayashi M, Katsumata N, Ando M, Adachi I, et al. Psychological distress following first recurrence of disease in patients with breast cancer: prevalence and risk factors. Breast Cancer Res Treat. 2000;61(2):131–7.
189. Andersen BL, Shapiro CL, Farrar WB, Crespin T, Wells-Digregorio S. Psychological responses to cancer recurrence. Cancer. 2005;104(7):1540–7.
190. Yang HC, Thornton LM, Shapiro CL, Andersen BL. Surviving recurrence: psychological and quality-of-life recovery. Cancer. 2008;112(5):1178–87.
191. Yang HC, Brothers B, Andersen BL. Stress and quality of life in breast cancer recurrence: moderation or mediation of coping? Ann Behav Med. 2008;35:188–197.
192. Nabholtz JM, Buzdar A, Pollak M, Harwin W, Burton G, Mangalik A, et al. Anastrozole is superior to tamoxifen as first-line therapy for advanced breast cancer in postmenopausal women: results of a North American multicenter randomized trial. Arimidex Study Group. J Clin Oncol. 2000;18(22):3758–67.
193. Mouridsen H, Gershanovich M, Sun Y, Perez-Carrion R, Boni C, Monnier A, et al. Superior efficacy of letrozole versus tamoxifen as first-line therapy for postmenopausal women with advanced breast cancer: results of a phase III study of the International Letrozole Breast Cancer Group. J Clin Oncol (Official Journal of the American Society of Clinical Oncology). 2001;19(10):2596–606.
194. Paridaens RJ, Dirix LY, Beex LV, Nooij M, Cameron DA, Cufer T, et al. Phase III study comparing exemestane with tamoxifen as first-line hormonal treatment of metastatic breast cancer in postmenopausal women: the European Organisation for Research and Treatment of Cancer Breast Cancer Cooperative Group. J Clin Oncol (Official Journal of the American Society of Clinical Oncology). 2008;26(30):4883–90.
195. Riemsma R, Forbes CA, Kessels A, Lykopoulos K, Amonkar MM, Rea DW, et al. Systematic review of aromatase inhibitors in the first-line treatment for hormone sensitive advanced or metastatic breast cancer. Breast Cancer Res Treat. 2010;123(1):9–24.
196. Howell A, Robertson JF, Abram P, Lichinitser MR, Elledge R, Bajetta E, et al. Comparison fulvestrant versus tamoxifen for the treatment of advanced breast cancer in postmenopausal women previously untreated with endocrine therapy: a multinational, double-blind, randomized trial. J Clin Oncol (Official Journal of the American Society of Clinical Oncology). 2004;22(9): 1605–13.
197. Di Leo A, Jerusalem G, Petruzelka L, Torres R, Bondarenko IN, Khasanov R, et al. Results of the CONFIRM phase III trial comparing fulvestrant 250 mg with fulvestrant 500 mg in postmenopausal women with estrogen receptor-positive advanced breast cancer. J Clin Oncol (Official Journal of the American Society of Clinical Oncology). 2010;28(30):4594–600.
198. Martin M, Loibl S, von Minckwitz G, Morales S, Martinez N, Guerrero A, et al. Phase III trial evaluating the addition of bevacizumab to endocrine therapy as first-line treatment for advanced breast cancer: the letrozole/fulvestrant and avastin (LEA) study. J Clin Oncol (Official Journal of the American Society of Clinical Oncology). 2015;33(9):1045–52.

Estrogen and Breast Cancer in Postmenopausal Women: A Critical Review

25

Joseph Ragaz and Shayan Shakeraneh

25.1 Introduction

This two-part review focuses on the long-term results of the recently completed trials of hormone replacement therapy [HRT] conducted between 1993 and 2002 by the Women's Health Initiative Group [the WHI]. The WHI is a US Government-funded project coordinating four large randomized studies evaluating women's health. The main part of the WHI project involved two HRT randomized studies which evaluated multiple outcomes of women's health, based on large sample size, with excellent statistics and methodologies.

While both WHI HRT trials are described in detail, the chapter narrative is primarily focused on the WHI HRT trial 2, based on estrogen alone. This trial, randomizing postmenopausal women aged 50–79 between conjugated equine estrogen (CEE, Premarin) versus placebo, emerged unexpectedly, for the first time in the history of HRT research, with a statistically significant reduction of breast cancer rates. Particularly robust were reduced breast cancer rates among the majority of trial participants [i.e. > 70 %] at low risk for breast cancer, such as women with *no family history of breast cancer,* and or women *without a past history of benign breast disease* (Tables 25.1 and 25.2). The estrogen-associated improved *breast cancer outcomes* constitute a paradigm shift of a hormone associated for over a century with an established *increase* in breast carcinogenesis.

In addition to the surprising reduction of breast cancer rates, participants assigned to estrogen aged 50–59 also had a significant reduction of coronary heart events, mostly myocardial infarctions, and observed was also a statistically significant all-cause mortality reduction, likely a cumulative result of improvement of all the outcomes [1–3]. These gains, as will be seen, are all in addition to the well-known impact of estrogen on preservation of bone mass, related reduction of skeletal fractures, as well as the documented quality of life [QOL] benefits of symptoms related to menopause.

These observations caught by surprise most of the experts involved in HRT research, particularly as these estrogen-associated gains emerged in the wake of much publicized overall "HRT harm"—reported since 2002 from the first WHI HRT trial, based on the estrogen and medroxyprogesterone Provera combination.

These estrogen-alone associated benefits seen as particularly meaningful and statistically significant among young postmenopausal women, open the door yet again to the much debated potential of estrogen-based HRT towards primary prevention of multiple health outcomes affecting the process of aging—the highly disputed gains constituting, in the first place, the main objectives of the WHI research.

Despite these level 1 evidence gains of estrogen-alone based HRT, most clinical reviews, consensus statements, and guideline documents are thus far substantially guarded, with no efforts underway at the present time considering changes in estrogen guidelines. Moreover, many clinicians including most oncologists, are not aware of the details of these estrogen-associated benefits. It was felt, therefore, that a more detailed evidence-based review highlighting the actual data and their more transparent interpretation, would be timely and of interest to oncologists.

A part of our work includes the actual data overview and their long-term follow-up. Some of those include cardiac data and all-cause mortality outcomes discussed in more detail in the second part of this review [HRT chapter 2: Estrogen and Cardiac Events with All-Cause Mortality: A Critical Review]. These data clearly indicate that if estrogen-endorsing guidelines are implemented for women entering menopause more uniformly, tens of thousands of lives could be affected annually in the USA alone, leading to multimillion dollar cost savings as a result [4, 5].

J. Ragaz (✉)
School of Population and Public Health, University of British Columbia, 2770 Wembley Dr., North Vancouver, BC V5Z 3B6, Canada
e-mail: joseph.ragaz@ubc.ca

S. Shakeraneh
Infection Prevention and Control, Providence Health Care, 5th Floor, 1190 Hornby Street, Vancouver, BC V6Z 2K5, Canada
e-mail: shayans@interchange.ubc.ca

I. Jatoi and A. Rody (eds.), *Management of Breast Diseases*, DOI 10.1007/978-3-319-46356-8_25

The other part of the chapter will discuss the logistics of one of the most important questions emerging from the WHI HRT trials: why are we seeing so much difference between the two trials: a substantial positive cost/benefit-ratio seen in the estrogen-alone trial, versus so much harm in the E + P combination? These points raise the issues of methodology and possible biases within the two trials. One such issue discussed in more detail is the evidence for possible "harm" identified with Provera, the progestational part of the hormonal combination used along with estrogen in the first, but not in the second, WHI HRT trial.

The other issue is the potential bias emerging in the 1st WHI HRT trial [but not in the 2nd WHI HRT trial] related to the massive unblinding of over 44 % participants—women with uteruses who became symptomatic as a result of starting HRT, with vaginal spotting or bleeding. Informing them about their allocated treatment with HRT was of course a necessity, which nevertheless converted basically a double-blind randomized trial [of the WHI HRT trial 1] into an observational trial, with all the fallacies and potential inaccuracies of any observational study.

25.2 Background: WHI Trials

The Women's Health Initiative [WHI] HRT trials were planned in the early parts of the 1990s because of rising concerns that past HRT observational and case-control studies were based on a small patient sample size or on study results with pre-selected participants who could be in a better state of health than women not on HRT [6, 7]. In its entirety, the WHI enrolled during the 15 years of its active accrual more than 160,000 postmenopausal women aged 50–79 into two HRT and two dietary / vitamin prevention trials [see below], making the WHI trials largest U.S. prevention project of its kind, with a planned budget of $625 million, but exceeding by the time of its completion to $1 billion.

Table 25.1 WHI HRT trials: invasive breast cancer

Ages	E + P* [8506] (%)	Placebo* [8102] (%)	Difference N/100,000	HR	95 % CI	P value/*interaction 3 age categories
WHI HRT trial 1						
All	0.43	0.34	+90	**1.28**	1.11–1.48	<0.001
50–59	0.37	0.28	+90	1.34	1.03–1.75	
60–69	0.43	0.34	+90	1.27	1.02–1.57	**0.72*
70–79	0.53	0.42	+110	1.25	0.94–1.67	
WHI HRT trial 2						
All	0.28	0.35	−70	**0.79**	0.65–0.97	***0.02***
50–59	0.23	0.30	−70	0.76	0.52–1.11	
60–69	0.29	0.37	−80	0.78	0.58–1.05	*0.70*
70–79	0.31	0.36	−50	0.85	0.56–1.28	

*Cumulative annual incidence, in %
BOLD: statistical significance, <0.05

Table 25.2 Rates of invasive breast cancer, WHI 2nd trial [CEE vs placebo]

	CEE*	Placebo*	HR	95 % CI
A. Past benign breast disease				
No	0.23 %	0.39 %	**0.57**	0.41–0.78
Yes, 1 Biopsy	0.45 %	0.29 %	**1.60**	0.82–3.14
Yes, > 1 Biopsy	0.41 %	0.19 %	2.54	0.73–8.86
B. First degree relative with breast cancer [high family history of breast cancer]				
None	0.23 %	0.34 %	**0.68**	0.50–0.92
>1	0.41 %	0.19 %	2.54	0.73–8.86

Impact of prior breast cancer risk determined by (A) history of past benign breast disease, and (B) first degree relative with breast cancer [high family history of breast cancer]
*Cumulative annual incidence, in %
BOLD: statistical significance, <0.05
Source Data from Ragaz et al. [4] and Stefanick et al. [12]

The design of the WHI HRT trials was based on the hypothesis that HRT therapy would result in a decrease in coronary heart disease and osteoporosis-related fractures. As such, the primary outcome of interest was coronary heart disease, as this is a major cause of morbidity and mortality among women age >65, and because, at the time, no clinical trial had been undertaken to prove the cardioprotective effects of HRT from a randomized design. Due to the concern over the relationship between HRT and elevated breast cancer risk as observed largely in past observational trials, breast cancer was selected at the time of the WHI HRT trial planning, as the primary adverse outcome. Additional outcomes monitored, as secondary objectives, would include stroke, pulmonary embolism (PE), endometrial cancer, colorectal cancer, hip fracture, and death due to other causes [6, 7].

Overall, the ultimate WHI objectives were to determine from large randomized and observational trials the individual HRT, dietary and vitamin related outcomes, in order to influence particularly the clinical HRT practice, where HRT was, since the early 1980s, increasingly prescribed not only for palliation of menopausal symptoms but also to slow down aging-related chronic degenerative conditions, and improve all-cause mortality reduction [8–10].

25.2.1 WHI Trials: Design

Enrollment into the WHI began in 1993 and ended in 1998 with the first two of the trials focusing on the HRT. The four WHI randomized case-control clinical trials were:

1. **TRIAL ONE** (WHI HRT trial 1) involved hormone replacement therapy (HRT), testing in a double-blind randomized design among healthy women with intact uterus, the impact of Estrogen,—the Conjugated Equine Estrogen (CEE, Premarin, 0.625 mg/day-E) **plus** Progestin (medroxyprogesterone acetate, Provera 2.5 mg/day-P) *versus* a Placebo. Of all the 16,608 participants in this HRT trial, 8506 versus 8102 women were assigned to E + P versus placebo. Initially, all women were started on Premarin alone, but in view of the more evident benefit of progestin reducing rates of uterine cancer, Provera was added to Premarin, with both agents soon after formulated as a single tablet, the PremPro [Wyeth Industries]. Thus, a shift to PremPro became a guideline requirement in the WHI trial 1 *after* the first 331 [3.9 %] were randomized to Premarin alone [6].
2. **TRIAL TWO** was designed for women *without a* uterus and randomized the participating women to Estrogen alone [with Premarin] versus placebo, with the same objectives as TRIAL ONE. Altogether, 10,739 women were recruited to this trial, 5310 to Estrogen and 5429 to Placebo. Our review is focused on the outcomes of this particular trial [7].
3. **TRIAL THREE** tested low-fat diet against conventional diet for breast and colorectal cancer prevention, with 48,835 women randomized.
4. **TRIAL FOUR** tested the impact of calcium and vitamin D supplementation. Hip fractures were the designated primary outcome, with other fractures and colorectal cancer as secondary outcomes. In total, 36,282 women were recruited to this trial.

The WHI program also included an observational study (ObSt) that comprised an additional 93,676 postmenopausal women recruited from the same population base as the randomized trials. The ObSt is intended to provide additional knowledge about risk factors for a range of diseases, including cancer, cardiovascular disease, and fractures. It has an emphasis on biological markers of disease risk and on risk-factor changes as risk modifiers.

25.2.2 WHI HRT Trial 1: E + P versus Placebo

The July 17, 2002 JAMA article reported the results of the first WHI HRT trial—the Estrogen plus Progestin (E2 + Prog) versus placebo [6]. This trial was terminated unexpectedly in 2002, on the weight of interim data and the advice of the independent Data and Safety Monitoring Board, after a mean 5.2 years of follow-up, because of overall assessment of harms exceeding benefits for chronic disease prevention.

Specifically, taking all patients as randomized [ages 50–80], reported were increased rates of coronary heart disease [CHD, RR = 1.29; 95 % CI = 1.02–1.63]; breast cancer incidence [RR = 1.26, 95 % CI = 1.00–1.59]; strokes [RR = 1.41, 95 % CI = 1.07–1.85]; and pulmonary emboli [RR = 2.13; 95 % CI = 1.39–3.25]. For benefit, observed were improved rates of colorectal cancer [RR = 0.63, 95 % CI = 0.43–0.92]; endometrial cancer [RR = 0.83, 95 % CI = 0.47–1.47]; and hip fractures [RR = 0.66, 95 % CI = 0.45–0.98].

All-cause mortality was unaltered [RR = 0.98, 95 % CI = 0.82–1.18]. The Global Index, an interactive summary of harms and benefits, was increased by 15 % (HR = 1.15, 95 % CI = 0.95–1.39). At the time of the 2013 follow-up, however, none of the hazards, with the exception of breast cancer [RR = 1.28, 95 % CI = 1.11–1.48] and venous thrombosis [RR = 1.24, 95 % CI = 1.01–1.31], were increased with statistical significance.

Thus, authors concluded that for an average 5.2 years follow-up time:

1. Overall health risks of combined estrogen plus progestin exceeded benefits among healthy postmenopausal US women.

2. All-cause mortality was not different between the two groups.
3. The risk-benefit profile is not consistent with the requirements for an intervention for primary prevention of chronic diseases.

In the wake of these hazards, the HRT trial was terminated in May 31, 2002, prematurely, at mean follow-up of 5.2 years, with all participants informed about the results and about the allocated therapy.

However, overall since the trial started, 40.5 % of the E + P recipients had their randomized treatment unblinded, primarily due to vaginal bleeding [6, 11]. With the additionally reassigned estrogen-alone recipients to the E + P combination [3.9 %], the *total* unblinding rate of the E + P trial at the time of trial termination was 44.4 %, compared to 6.8 % of the placebo recipients. The significance of the unblinding will be discussed below.

25.2.3 WHI HRT Trial 2: Estrogen Alone versus Placebo—The First 2004 Data

Despite the early termination of the first WHI E + P trial, the second WHI E-alone trial continued after 2002. As in the first trial, of all participants, only less than one-third (30.8 %) were < 60 years of age; and over 47 % were past or current HRT users before enrolment.

While all participants had hysterectomy, approximately 40 % also had oophorectomy (39.5 % vs. 42 % in arm of CEE vs. Placebo, respectively). Overall, 86 % of all patients had no first-degree relative with breast cancer; and 74.5 % had no benign breast disease in the past. Both risk factors, as will be seen, emerged with statistical significance for reduced breast cancer rates. At the time of the trial termination, 1.9 % and 1.5 % of the E-alone and placebo recipients, respectively, had been unblinded.

At the time of the initial April 2004 JAMA publication of the WHI HRT trial 2 at the average follow-up duration 6.8 years, and taking *all* participants ages 50–80, the estimated hazard ratios for Coronary Heart Disease [CHD, mostly myocardial infarctions] showed a nonsignificant 9 % reduction of CHD [RR = 0.91, 95 % CI = 0.75–1.12]; reduced were rates of breast cancer [RR = 0.77, 95 % CI = 0.59–1.01]; and observed was a significant 39 % reduction of hip fractures [RR = 0.61, 95 % CI = 0.63–0.79]; with overall mortality unaltered [RR = 1.04, 95 % CI = 0.88–1.22].

There was a 34 % (nonsignificant) increase in pulmonary embolism; a significant 39 % increase in strokes [RR = 1.10–1.77], and a nonsignificant 8 % increase in colorectal cancer. Total death rate was increased marginally, by 4 % [RR = 1.04, 95 % CI = 0.88–1.22]; and Global Index was basically unaltered [RR = 1.04, 95 % CI = 0.88–1.22]. On account of these results, the second WHI trial on CEE alone versus placebo concluded that the use of CEE, in women after hysterectomy, after follow-up of 6.8 years:

A. increases the risk of strokes
B. decreases the risk of hip fracture
C. does not affect the CHD incidence
D. may lead to a possible reduction in breast cancer risk, requiring further investigation
E. The sum of combined events was equivalent in the CEE and placebo groups, indicating no overall benefit and no hazards

In the final 2004 conclusion of the WHI HRT trial 2 first report, as was the case with the 2002 JAMA report of the trial 1, the WHI authors stated that Estrogen alone with CEE "should not be recommended for chronic disease prevention in postmenopausal women [7]." As a result of these data and recommendations, with over 90 % of participants completing their prescribed interventions, the National Institutes of Health (NIH) decided in February 2004 to end the intervention phase of the second WHI HRT trial early, with results published in the April 14, 2004 issue of the Journal of American Medical Association [7].

25.2.4 Trial 2: Estrogen and Invasive Breast Cancer—WHI HRT Trial 2 Follow-up

The unexpected yet potentially most important aspect of the WHI's HRT trial 2 involved the strong indication for reduced breast cancer rates by estrogen alone (Tables 25.1 and 25.2) [7]. At the time of the first 2004 analysis, mean 6.8 years of follow-up, and taking all trial participants, the hazards for invasive breast cancer showed a 23 % reduction, approaching statistical significance (HR = 0.77, 95 % CI = 0.59–1.01) [7].

A second 2006 review [12], with median follow-up time of 7.1 years, confirmed again the breast cancer rates reduced by 20 % [HR = 0.80, 95 % CI = 0.62–1.04], but also emerged with important subset analyzes (Table 25.1): among the 75 % of the trial participants *without prior benign breast disease*, the breast cancer rate decrease was more substantial, with a statistically significant 43 % rate reduction [HR = 0.57, 95 % CI = 0.41–0.78].

Similarly, among the 85 % of participants *without a strong family history,* the breast cancer rate reduction was also more substantial [HR = 0.68, 95 % CI = 0.50–0.92]

(Table 25.2), with the evidence supporting estrogen reduction of breast cancer rates also seen from the analysis of women *without prior HRT* [HR = 0.65, 95 % CI = 0.46–0.92] (Table 25.2).

These breast cancer gains, observed quite unexpectedly, basically heralding the promising role of estrogen as a primary prevention—are highlighted in the publication only as "*...CEE alone...does not increase breast cancer incidence...*"

The next 2011 WHI HRT trial 2 update [1] shows, after a median follow-up of 11.8 years, continued breast cancer rate reductions associated with estrogen. Taking the whole population as randomized [intention to treat analysis], the study shows now, for the first time, a statistical significance to the 23 % reduction of new breast cancers for all women randomized to estrogen (HR = 0.77, 95 % CI = 0.62–0.95) [1].

Also, this time is identified among women aged 50–59 a significant 46 % *reduction of myocardial infarction* due to Estrogen [HR = 0.54, 95 % CI = 0.34–0.86], while no increases in strokes are seen, with resulting statistically significant 27 % *rate reductions of all-cause mortality* [HR = 0.73, 95 % CI = 0.53–1.00]. Similar to the prior WHI publications, these gains are articulated with ongoing caution, concluding, "among postmenopausal women with prior hysterectomy, the CEE [conjugated equine estrogen] was not associated with an increased or decreased risk of CHD...or total mortality." However, WHI indicates for the first time "*A decreased risk of breast cancer persisted.*"

Next, Chlebowski et al. [13] confirmed not only the significance to the 23 % reduction of breast cancer rates, but also, for the first time, a statistically significant 63 % *reduction of breast cancer mortality* due to estrogen. Also, when considering participants of any age and risk category, a more robust 33 % reduction of breast cancer incidence [p = 0.03] was seen in the "*adherence-adjusted*" analysis [i.e., "as treated"—not "as intended."]

Furthermore, a companion analysis of Anderson et al. [14] shows that "*fewer women diagnosed with breast cancer died in the estrogen group compared with the placebo group* [HR = 0.62, 95 % CI = 0.39–0.97, p = 0.04]" and that "*... of all the deaths, significantly less were due to breast cancer in the estrogen than in the placebo group* [HR = 0.37, 95 % CI = 0.13–0.91, p = 0.03]."

In other words, both the *all-cause mortality* among women developing primary breast cancer, and also *the breast cancer specific mortality* among all participants were significantly lower among the estrogen recipients. This update also confirms the original 2006 observations [15] for women ***without*** past benign breast disease and/or without strong family history deriving a substantially higher and statistically more significant breast cancer rate reductions, with tests for "interaction" statistically significant [for PBD, p = 0.01; for no FH, p = 0.02] (Table 25.2).

Lastly, Manson et al. summarized in 2013 [2] the HRT outcomes of both WHI HRT trials, separately for the times *during* the intervention phases, *post* intervention phase, and for the overall combined analysis, representing the cumulative follow-up. The breast cancer risk reduction in the overall cumulative follow-up associated with estrogen use remained statistically significant [HR = 0.79, 95 % CI = 0.65–0.97]. Part two of the second HRT review [Chapter 26] also discusses results of other end points including myocardial infarction, stroke, and overall all-cause mortality, showing significance for the substantial reduction of cardiac events and of all-cause mortality for women aged 50–59.

Until 2009, no serious attempts were made to highlight the clinical significance of the breast cancer rate reduction by estrogen alone, despite the fact that these data would complement the past well-documented responses to estrogen of patients with stage IV breast cancer (i.e., response rate of 25–30 % to stilboestrol or other estrogens) [15–18]. These stage IV breast cancer results were also matched in the 1970s [19] by estrogen in vitro data showing suppression of breast cancer cell growth in vitro—observations, which have been recently investigated with more vigor, partially the result of the new WHI trial 2 observations, in relation with estrogen-associated effect on either breast cancer cell apoptosis or stem cells [19–21]. Despite all these data, however, the WHI restricted in most of their past publications reporting the actual 21–43 % breast cancer rate reduction by estrogen a conclusion, repeatedly, as "estrogen does not seem to increase breast cancer rates".

Between 2009 and 2012, Ragaz et al. [4, 22, 23] reviewed all the WHI HRT trials published between 2004 and 2006 emphasizing a qualitatively different set of conclusions: estrogen actually confers a major breast cancer benefit, particularly relevant for the substantial subsets of population without a past history of benign disease, and/or those with an absent family history, with a statistically significant 32–43 % reduction of breast cancer rates (Table 25.2). As a result, the 2010 British Columbia team articulated a proposal, based on these results, of "Dual role of Estrogen in breast carcinogenesis"—namely that "***Exogenous*** *Estrogen is breast cancer protective while* ***Endogenous*** *Estrogen remains carcinogenic*", and thus "Exogenous *Estrogen deserves merits for chemoprevention*" [4].

Despite the strengths of the published data and of these observations, and the 2010 review of the "exogenous versus endogenous estrogen concept," majority of the physicians remain uninformed about these data, and no changes of guidelines followed. Thus, inevitably, a question yet to be answered is why is there virtually no publicity to these important results and why basically only few in the medical establishment and scientific lay public at large, know these new estrogen breast cancer developments?

One possibility, and a likely one, is that WHI group has not publicized these data adequately, due to its own massively negative first 2002–2004 reports related to the adverse outcome results of trial 1, putting actually a lid on appropriate public overview of these new intriguing and difficult to explain trial 2 breast cancer estrogen-alone data, which emerged so much in more favourably, and so soon afterwards. The other reason could be the general insecurity in explaining the highly unexpected, albeit paradigm-changing data. This latter cause is likely more difficult to handle due to the emerging issues related to Methodology, as discussed below.

25.2.5 WHI Trials: Methodology

As seen in this review, there are several HRT conclusions, which could be made with more confidence in 2016 than in 2004. For one, the estrogen-alone-based HRT emerged with a substantially more appealing cost/benefit ratio of many outcomes, most contributing cumulatively towards reducing all-cause mortality among young women. As seen, virtually all of these gains are greatly relevant towards potential primary prevention guidelines related to HRT based on estrogen.

In evaluating the WHI trials, there are, however, still many unanswered questions requiring clarification, one in particular is, why so much discrepancy between the seeming benefits observed in the trial 2, particularly among young women, versus so much more harm reported from the trial 1? Let us, therefore, hone in more closely and review thc possible reasons for these differences.

25.2.5.1 Provera—A New Carcinogen or the Methodology?

The high quality of the design and execution of all the WHI trials provided, virtually, an undisputed acceptance of the data from the initial WHI trial 1 as published in 2002, all enforced by the universally perceived intellectual and statistical excellence of the whole WHI team, all much helped by the WHI group's well-coordinated effective media blitz which followed the first 2002 publication of their trial 1.

The so much publicized WHI HRT trial 1 data showed that, when compared to placebo, there was basically a series of substantial harm of the E + P combination, much more than expected. These conclusions were rapidly accepted virtually by the entire North American and European Medical establishment.

Thus, without much surprise, the subsequent HRT policies resulted in the discontinuation of close to 70 % of HRT prescriptions between North America and Europe, compared to their use prior to 2002, and that was HRT-based *either on estrogen plus progestin, or estrogen alone*—despite the fact that the Estrogen-alone trial was not yet analyzed until 2004, and continued ongoing as a double-blind randomized trial.

In the subsequent follow-up, however, methodology issues were raised regarding some aspects of the WHI FRT 1st trial with E + P combination, despite the fact that soon after 2002, not only the medical, but also the political and societal reactions to this trial had already impacted minds of physicians and women. And the result: the most massive guideline change—discontinuation of over 60 % of HRT prescriptions had been implemented as a result of the WHI HRT trial 1 negative publicity, faster than ever recorded in the history of human medicine.

25.2.5.2 Methodology 1—Impact of Provera

The first issue deserving scrutiny is the medroxyprogesterone Provera. Could this progestational agent added to estrogen in the first WHI trial of E + P reduce the benefits seen with estrogen alone? The data indeed showed a 23–43 % breast cancer rate *reduction* due to estrogen alone in the HRT trial 2 [i.e. HR ranges = 0.77–0.57], contrasting sharply with a 25–28 % breast cancer rate *increase* with E + P [i.e., HR ranges = 1.25–1.28]. Then, there are other major gains seen with estrogen-alone trial—i.e., the 40 % reduction of MIs among younger women—but no such gains in the E + P trial. So, a legitimate question is asked: could the problem be with the medroxyprogesterone Provera, an agent which is nowadays, in any event, prescribed much less by the gynecological, anti-aging, or menopause-management practices, at least in North America? Could it be that adding "it"—the Provera rather than the "HRT entity"—be the main reason for more "HRT harm"—seen in the WHI HRT trial 1—with Provera basically erasing the estrogen-associated breast cancer and or cardiac benefits?

Some studies show Provera, in contrast to other more recent plant-based progesterones, to be a tissue irritant, with possible inflammatory and/or carcinogenic proprieties [24, 25]. Furthermore, medroxyprogesterone may play an important role in stimulating the proliferation of breast cancer cells, as shown in the MCF-7 experiments. Here, Neubauer et al. showed that medroxyprogesterone, but not estradiol, stimulated the growth of human breast cancer cells [26], with cells exposed to medroxyprogesterone, subsequently increasing the yield of progesterone receptors [PgRs]. The PgRs were later shown to be associated with enhanced sensitization to estradiol-mediated cell division, and thus the growth rate *increase* of the same cells which in the absence of progestin were not stimulated by estrogen alone, displaying basically, without the medroxyprogesterone, estradiol resistance [26].

Furthermore, Gurney and Nachtigal [27] showed that natural and synthetic estrogens would enhance pancreatic insulin response to glucose, i.e., increased peripheral insulin sensitivity to rising glucose levels—a process *reducing* breast carcinogenesis [28]. In contrast, adding progestins to estrogens *increased* peripheral insulin resistance and raised insulin levels, with related insulin growth factors [IGFs] increase, both part of a metabolic syndrome linked more firmly with *increased breast carcinogenesis* [29–32].

Thus, the adverse breast cancer impact of Provera could be the pivotal point explaining the contrary outcomes of estrogen-alone-based HRT compared to E + P.

The other point of methodology contention, which may clarify differences between the two WHI HRT trials, involves the impact of the *unblinding rates, substantially higher in the WHI HRT trial 1.*

25.2.5.3 Methodology 2—Impact of Unblinding

The WHI HRT trial 1 started as a study clearly fulfilling all the criteria of double-blind randomization. But as Shapiro et al. indicate in their detailed review [11], soon into the trial start, and as is case with most E + P combinations, women without hysterectomy [i.e., with uterus] started developing hormone-associated vaginal spotting, at times hemorrhage, and/or breast tenderness, breast swelling and/or lumpiness. Most of these women in the E + P group would demand more physician care to focus on their symptoms, and within 2–3 years, according to the actual WHI records, over 40 % of E + P trial 1 participants had to be unblinded as to the trial treatment allocation [6, 11].

This is in addition to the 335 women [3.7 %] unblinded already from the onset, those who started unopposed E, and were soon switched to PremPro, for a total of 44.4 % unblinding rates - versus a rate of 6.4 % in the placebo arm. This compares to the unblinding rates in the WHI HRT trial 2 [estrogen alone vs. placebo] of less than 2 %! [11].

Informing symptomatic women participating in a closely watched double-blind randomized trial about medications which likely induce the above symptoms is of course unavoidable and does constitute a nonnegotiable ethical conduct of any approved medical study. This feature alone would convert though, unwittingly, a double-blind randomized WHI HRT trial 1 into an observational study.

25.2.6 Could This Have Influenced the Results?

Despite the WHI HRT trial 1 data indicating comparable rates of the ***recorded*** screening mammography between E + T versus placebo [11, 13], it has been established reasonably well that women aware of hormone intake would be more actively screened outside the allocation by the trial—both by their physicians and with more mammograms [33]. Not only would they have more screening mammograms, but also these would be interpreted more vigilantly by radiographers. All these steps, quite natural consequences of dealing with emotionally symptomatic female population on HRT, could nevertheless provide spuriously higher breast cancer rates—in addition to the "lead type bias" typical for any mammography screened populations and for most observational studies [11, 33].

For all of the above reasons, a *seeming* association in the E + T trial with higher breast cancer rates may be due to this methodological bias rather than the HRT actual causation. This conclusion, therefore, lays the foundation for the second important paradigm emerging from this review: HRT with E + P may not necessarily be breast "carcinogenic," despite the higher breast cancer rates detected among women allocated to the HRT arm.

25.3 Conclusion

Only few subjects in the medical science moved in the last decades so visibly as HRT policies through more turbulent periods of acceptance and rejections, and then more acceptance and even more rejections, with past medical practice HRT guidelines fluctuating between the 1960s and 2000s substantially according to the pendulum swings of differing HRT practice guidelines.

This chapter makes several points, which may bring more clarity towards the ongoing confusion as to the cost/benefit of estrogen-based HRT to manage menopausal symptoms, and/or preventing conditions such as heart attacks, bone fractures, and unexpectedly, also possibly breast cancer.

The breast cancer reduction potential of HRT based on estrogen alone, as reviewed in this chapter, is truly paradigm changing, and may lead to further advances in basic science attempting to identify the mode of estrogen action in reducing breast carcinogenesis. However, even before the basic science will bring more universally accepted explanations for estrogen benefit, the onus is already at the present time on the opinion of leaders of clinical policies, in the domain of Public Health and prevention. This is becoming particularly compelling as if the WHI outcome data of HRT based on estrogen alone are indeed correct, then according to reasonable and transparent estimates, estrogen **if** started at young postmenopausal age <60, may avoid thousands of deaths annually if implemented in guidelines [5].

It is the hope of the authors that a more critical consensus of the presently publicized HRT narrative will emerge as a result of this and the next [Chapter 26] HRT reviews. However, it is also expressed that it may have to be the WHI group itself, who needs to publicize these data much more assertively, for a more universal acceptance, both by the bulk of the medical establishment and by the anxious consumers, the women themselves, who may benefit from estrogen-based HRT much more substantially than expected, and much more than presently appreciated.

References

1. LaCroix AZ, Chlebowski RT, Manson JE, et al. Health outcomes after stopping conjugated equine estrogens among postmenopausal women with prior hysterectomy: a randomized controlled trial. JAMA. 2011;305:1305–14.
2. Manson JE, Chlebowski RT, Stefanick ML, et al. Menopausal hormone therapy and health outcomes during the intervention and extended poststopping phases of the women's health initiative randomized trials. JAMA. 2013;310:1353–68.
3. Chlebowski RT, Rohan TE, Manson JE, et al. Breast cancer after use of estrogen plus progestin and estrogen alone: analyses of data from 2 women's health initiative randomized clinical trials. JAMA Oncol. 2015;1:296–305.
4. Ragaz J, Wilson K, Muraca G, Budlovsky J, Froehlich J. Dual estrogen effects on breast cancer: endogenous estrogen stimulates, exogenous estrogen protects. Further investigation of estrogen chemoprevention is warranted. Cancer Res. 2010;70.
5. Sarrel PM, Njike VY, Vinante V, Katz DL. The mortality toll of estrogen avoidance: an analysis of excess deaths among hysterectomized women aged 50 to 59 years. Am J Public Health. 2013;103:1583–8.
6. Rossouw JE, Anderson GL, Prentice RL, et al. Risks and benefits of estrogen plus progestin in healthy postmenopausal women: principal results From the women's health initiative randomized controlled trial. JAMA. 2002;288:321–33.
7. Anderson GL, Limacher M, Assaf AR, et al. Effects of conjugated equine estrogen in postmenopausal women with hysterectomy: the women's health initiative randomized controlled trial. JAMA. 2004;291:1701–12.
8. Grady D, Rubin SM, Petitti DB, et al. Hormone therapy to prevent disease and prolong life in postmenopausal women [see comments]. Ann Intern Med. 1992;117:1016–37.
9. Ragaz J, Coldman AJ. Age-matched all-cause mortality impact of hormone replacement therapy: applicability to breast cancer survivors. Breast Cancer Res Treat. 1999;57:30.
10. Grodstein F, Stampfer MJ, Colditz GA, et al. Postmenopausal hormone therapy and mortality. N Engl J Med. 1997;336:1769–75.
11. Shapiro S, Farmer RD, Mueck AO, Seaman H, Stevenson JC. Does hormone replacement therapy cause breast cancer? An application of causal principles to three studies: part 2. The women's health initiative: estrogen plus progestogen. J Fam Plann Reprod Health Care. 2011;37:165–72.
12. Stefanick ML, Anderson GL, Margolis KL, et al. Effects of conjugated equine estrogens on breast cancer and mammography screening in postmenopausal women with hysterectomy. JAMA. 2006;295:1647–57.
13. Chlebowski RT, Anderson GL. Changing concepts: menopausal hormone therapy and breast cancer. J Natl Cancer Inst. 2012;104:517–27.
14. Anderson GL, Chlebowski RT, Aragaki AK, et al. Conjugated equine oestrogen and breast cancer incidence and mortality in postmenopausal women with hysterectomy: extended follow-up of the women's health initiative randomised placebo-controlled trial. Lancet Oncol. 2012;13:476–86.
15. Haddow A, David A. Karnofsky memorial lecture. Thoughts on chemical therapy. Cancer. 1970;26:737–54.
16. Boyer MJ, Tattersall MH. Diethylstilbestrol revisited in advanced breast cancer management. Med Pediatr Oncol. 1990;18:317–20.
17. Ingle JN, Ahmann DL, Green SJ, et al. Randomized clinical trial of diethylstilbestrol versus tamoxifen in postmenopausal women with advanced breast cancer. N Engl J Med. 1981;304:16–21.
18. Peethambaram PP, Ingle JN, Suman VJ, Hartmann LC, Loprinzi CL. Randomized trial of diethylstilbestrol vs. tamoxifen in postmenopausal women with metastatic breast cancer. An updated analysis. Breast Cancer Res Treat. 1999;54:117–22.
19. Song RX, Mor G, Naftolin F, et al. Effect of long-term estrogen deprivation on apoptotic responses of breast cancer cells to 17beta-estradiol. J Natl Cancer Inst. 2001;93:1714–23.
20. Lewis-Wambi JS, Jordan VC. Estrogen regulation of apoptosis: how can one hormone stimulate and inhibit? Breast Cancer Res: BCR. 2009;11:206.
21. Simoes BM, Piva M, Iriondo O, et al. Effects of estrogen on the proportion of stem cells in the breast. Breast Cancer Res Treat. 2011;129:23–35.
22. Ragaz J, Le N, Budlovsky J, Spinelli J. Protective effect of estrogen (E2) and increased risk of E2 plus progestin (Prog) on breast cancer (BrCa). The 2009 review of the Women's Health Initiative (WHI) hormone replacement therapy (HRT) published trials. Cancer Res. 2009;2009:69.
23. Ragaz J, Wilson K, Shakeraneh J, Budlovsky J. Estrogen and avoidance of invasive breast cancer, coronary heart disease and all-cause mortality. Public health impact of estrogen guidelines for women entering menopause. Cancer Res. 2012;P4-13-04.
24. Campagnoli C, Biglia N, Cantamessa C, Lesca L, Sismondi P. HRT and breast cancer risk: a clue for interpreting the available data. Maturitas. 1999;33:185–90.
25. Heald A, Selby PL, White A, Gibson JM. Progestins abrogate estrogen-induced changes in the insulin-like growth factor axis. Am J Obstet Gynecol. 2000;183:593–600.
26. Neubauer H, Yang Y, Seeger H, et al. The presence of a membrane-bound progesterone receptor sensitizes the estradiol-induced effect on the proliferation of human breast cancer cells. Menopause (New York, NY) 2011;18:845–50.
27. Gurney EP, Nachtigall MJ, Nachtigall LE, Naftolin F. The Women's Health Initiative trial and related studies: 10 years later: a clinician's view. J Steroid Biochem Mol Biol. 2014;142:4–11.
28. Suba Z. Interplay between insulin resistance and estrogen deficiency as co- activators in carcinogenesis. Pathol Oncol Res. 2012;18:123–33.
29. Godsland IF, Gangar K, Walton C, et al. Insulin resistance, secretion, and elimination in postmenopausal women receiving oral or transdermal hormone replacement therapy. Metab Clin Exp. 1993;42:846–53.
30. Rushakoff RJ, Kalkhoff RK. Effects of pregnancy and sex steroid administration on skeletal muscle metabolism in the rat. Diabetes. 1981;30:545–50.
31. Pollak M. Insulin and insulin-like growth factor signalling in neoplasia. Nat Rev Cancer. 2008;8:915–28.
32. Goodwin PJ, Ennis M, Pritchard KI, et al. Fasting insulin and outcome in early-stage breast cancer: results of a prospective cohort study. J Clin Oncol (Official Journal of the American Society of Clinical Oncology). 2002;20:42–51.
33. Banks E, Beral V, Cameron R, et al. Comparison of various characteristics of women who do and do not attend for breast cancer screening. Breast Cancer Res: BCR. 2002;4:R1.

26 Estrogen and Cardiac Events with all-cause Mortality. A Critical Review

Joseph Ragaz and Shayan Shakeraneh

26.1 Introduction

To begin with, the Women's Health Initiative [WHI] trial Hormone replacement trial 1 [HRT trial 1] of E + P combination showed at the time of its first publication in 2002, for all participants aged 50–79, that when compared to placebo, the E + P arm had a 29 % statistically significant *increase* in cardiac events, including myocardial infarctions and cardiac deaths. In the subsequent follow-up, the hazards for cardiac events remained elevated, with statistically significant increase only for the age group of 70–79 years old (HR = 1.34, 95 % CI = 1.05–1.72 [1, 2]) (Table 26.1).

However, the cardiac outcomes for participants using conjugated equine estrogen [Premarin] versus placebo [WHI trial 2], were totally different (Table 26.1). When reported first in 2004, taking all ages, the cardiac events were actually reduced by 9 % [3], with a substantial difference among age groups: while among young women aged 50–59 years old, estrogen alone arm emerged with a statistically significant 40 % reduction of myocardial infarction rates, there was little cardiac rate reduction identified among more elderly women.

Thus, the WHI HRT trial results have raised, perhaps more than any other HRT research, several pivotal questions:

1. Should the estrogen-based HRT be considered for Public Health guidelines of primary coronary disease and myocardial infarction prevention, particularly in view of other estrogen alone-based HRT benefits [i.e., reduction of breast cancer, bone loss, and bone fractures; improved quality of life; no increase in strokes, venous thrombosis, etc.]?
2. Taking the WHI HRT results [but not necessarily other HRT research], is the cardioprotection of HRT limited to estrogen alone formulations, with progestins such as Provera reducing the cardiac benefits of estrogen; and a related question, is there a difference between the medroxyprogesterone Provera used as a progestin in the WHI HRT trial 1—seemingly abolishing the estrogen-associated cardioprotection—versus other types of progesterones in trials where no such negative association was seen?
3. And lastly, is the HRT-associated cardioprotection restricted to young women, confirming the "estrogen timing hypothesis", i.e., reduction of cardiac events only before the process of cardiac atherosclerosis had started now fully confirmed, or is further research into this particular questions still required?

We will first review the evidence from the 1990s and early 2000s examining the epidemiology of HRT-associated cardiac outcomes. This part will also include the biochemical mechanisms of estrogen action on cardiac vasculature, with the outcomes of some of the principal atherosclerosis "surrogates," most of whom also support the estrogen timing hypothesis. In the last part of the review, we will discuss the related issues such as alternative hormonal menopausal developments with agents such as tibolone and bazedoxifene, and briefly the HRT issues involving high risk population carriers with BRCA gene mutation.

26.2 Cardiac Events and the Timing Hypothesis

The observations that estrogen helps to reduce CVS disorders, especially cardiac events, are not new. Already In 1992 Grady et al. confirmed all-cause mortality reduction associated with HRT [4], mostly attributed to the reduction of cardiac events, and Ragaz and Coldman estimated in 1998 substantial cardiac mortality reduction due to estrogen-based HRT [5].

J. Ragaz (✉) · S. Shakeraneh
School of Population and Public Health, University of British Columbia, 2206 East Mall, Vancouver, BC V6T 1Z3, Canada
e-mail: joseph.ragaz@ubc.ca

S. Shakeraneh
e-mail: shayans@interchange.ubc.ca

I. Jatoi and A. Rody (eds.), *Management of Breast Diseases*, DOI 10.1007/978-3-319-46356-8_26

One of the largest observational studies in the pre-WHI era was the North American Nurses' Health Study, with follow-up from 1976 to 1996, analyzing 70,533 postmenopausal women taking HRT. The HRT users were compared to similarly matched general population women without HRT, the never-users [6, 7]. First, among users [Premarin, same agent and dose as used subsequently in the WHI trials], the coronary event hazards were reduced significantly by 39 % [HR = 0.61, 95 % CI: 0.52–0.71]. Of interest was that compared with never-users, the cardiac event rate reduction was similar among those taking a half the dose of Premarin, 0.3 mg daily [HR = 0.58, 95 % CI: 0.37–0.92; as those with a full does of 0.625 mg [HR = 0.54, 95 % CI: 0.44–0.67].

Importance of age and/or time since menopause at HRT start vis-à-vis cardiac outcomes is seen from the long-term follow-up of this study [8]. Compared to HRT nonusers, the reduction of coronary heart disease among HRT users was seen, but restricted to women starting HRT at the age near menopause, with a 28–34 % event reduction (for estrogen alone, HR = 0.66, 95 % CI: 0.54–0.80; for estrogen with progestin, HR = 0.72, 95 % CI: 0.56–0.92). Those women starting HRT >10 years after menopause had no obvious estrogen benefit (HR = 0.87, 95 % CI: 0.69–1.10 for estrogen alone; HR = 0.90, 95 % CI: 0.62–1.29 for estrogen with progestin) [8].

By 2004, Salpeter et al. published a meta-analysis of HRT mortality outcomes according to age [9]. Authors conducted a comprehensive search of MEDLINE, CINAHL [Cumulative Index to Nursing and Allied Health Literature], and EMBASE [Excerpta Medica database = biomedical and pharmacological database of published literature], to identify randomized controlled HRT trials from 1966 to September 2002. Outcomes were total deaths, or deaths due to cardiovascular disease, or cancer, separately for age <60 versus >60 years at HRT start. While the pooled data from 30 trials taking _all_ 26,708 participants showed no mortality reduction, the rates were reduced significantly among women age <60 [HR = 0.68, 95 % CI: 0.48–0.96]—versus no difference among women age >60 [HR = 1.03, 95 % CI: 0.90–1.18]. Similarly as all-cause mortality, shown was also interaction of Coronary Heart Disease and age at HRT start [10], confirming HRT significantly reducing CHD events _only_ among younger postmenopausal women [ages <60 vs. >60, HR = 0.68, 95 % CI: 0.48–0.96, vs. HR = 1.03, 95 % CI: 0.91–1.16].

One of the most recent studies designed to test the estrogen timing hypothesis prospectively is the Early versus Late Intervention Trial (the ELITE trial) [11, 12]. In this study, a total of 643 postmenopausal women were stratified according to time since menopause [<10 or ≥10 years], and randomly assigned to receive either oral 17β-estradiol plus progesterone vaginal gel [the HRT], or placebo (plus sequential placebo vaginal gel for women with a uterus). The primary outcome was carotid-artery intima–media thickness (CIMT) changes, with secondary outcome coronary atherosclerosis assessed by cardiac CT scans performed after the completion of the randomly assigned regimen.

When compared to the HRT group, the placebo-allocated women who were <6 years past menopause at randomization, had after a median of 5 years of follow-up, twice the mean CIMT thickness (increase by 0.0078 mm/year—vs. 0.0044 mm/year in the HRT group, P = 0.008). In contrast, in women >10 years past menopause at randomization, the rates of CIMT progression were similar between the placebo and HRT groups (0.0088 and 0.0100 mm/year, respectively [P = 0.29].

The Danish Osteoporosis Prevention Study (DOPS) [13] was also a prospective randomized trial of 1006 postmenopausal women who were, overall, much younger than women in other HRT trials [average 50 years old (range 45–58)]. The participants were randomized to oral 17b-estradiol plus sequential norethisterone acetate [the HRT] or to an untreated group. After _treatment of 10 years duration_, the women were followed for another 6 years for a total follow-up of 16 years. In the HRT group, compared to controls, the overall cardiac events [cardiac mortality, myocardial infarction or heart failure] were reduced significantly by 52 % (HR = 0.48, 95 % CI = 0.27–0.89). Also, the cardiac mortality, measured separately as a single outcome, was reduced significantly by 43 % (HR = 0.57, 95 % CI = 0.30–1.08). After a follow-up of 16 years, the cardiac events and total mortality among the HRT users still remained almost 40 % lower than among controls, with no statistically significant increase in rates of breast cancer, stroke, or venous thromboembolism. While this trial did not set to test an older age group, the rather impressive long-term cardiac benefits attest to a great HRT potential for primary cardiac prevention among young postmenopausal women. It remains to be shown whether the total HRT duration of 10 years, overall much longer than seen in the majority of HRT studies, or the actual selection of HRT agents as given in this particular trial, or the very young age of the trial population, are all independent factors responsible for these strong cardiac gains.

26.3 HRT Agent Selection and Cardiac Outcome

The clear cardiac outcome superiority between of the second WHI trial [E-alone] over the first one [E + P combination], brings inevitably into the discussion the possible role of individual agents—especially benefits of estrogen alone versus the possible abrogation of this benefit by the agents of the progestational group.

A possible interaction of estrogen with various progesterones, and the timing of HRT start vis-a-vis cardiac outcomes, was tested in a study from Finland [14]. This more complex observational trial evaluated estradiol alone-based HRT, with estradiol plus any of the five different types of progestins [medroxyprogesterone (Provera), norethisterone acetate, dihydrogesterone, other progestins, or tibolone. Altogether, 498,105 women who had used E-alone or any of the E + P combinations, were evaluated between 1994 and 2009. As was seen also in the above discussed studies, the risk of CHD death in hormone users was related to age, with significantly better outcomes for starting HRT at younger age [age <60 vs >60, CHD mortality ratio, HR = 0.53, 95 % CI = 0.47–0.59, vs. HR = 0.76, 95 % CI = 0.71–0.82]. The sub-analysis of estrogen combined with different progestational agents showed, when compared to nonusers, protective cardiac effects with _any_ of the HRT combinations. Although the best profile was seen with E + tibolone for age <60, with a surprising 77 % reduction of cardiac mortality rates [HR = 0.23, 95 % CI = 0.17 = 0.31], all E + P combinations when compared to nonusers were associated with a similar magnitude statistically significant cardiac event reduction. Also, relevant to the above cardiac rate differences between the WHI HRT trials 1 [E + P] versus 2 [E-alone], authors demonstrated no difference between estradiol alone versus HRT based on estradiol + medroxyprogesterone combinations [HR = 0.44, 95 % CI: 0.42–0.46, and HR = 0.46, 95 % CI: 0.43–0.49, respectively]. However, the authors emphasize that in the WHI HRT trial 1 E + P combination, where no cardiac benefits were seen, the HRT was based on CEE—the Conjugated Equine synthetic Estrogen [CEE]—while in their study from Finland, the estrogen was an Esterified Oral Estradiol [EE], and this EE combined with P is emerging with better and safer cardiac profile than the CEE + P combination used in the WHI or in the HERS trials.

Other studies of various estrogen subtypes arrived at similar conclusions, an issue of major practical value in regards to the choice of individual estrogenic HRT choices. The most convincing evidence comes from Smith et al. [15]. Already in 2004, authors evaluated the risk of venous thrombosis [VT] among HRT users, with either EE or CEE. Compared with nonuser, current HRT EE users had no VT increase [HR = 0.92; 95 % CI: 0.69–1.22]. In contrast, women currently taking CEE had an elevated VT risk [HR = 1.65; 95 % CI: 1.24–2.19]. When analyses were restricted to estrogen users without progestins, current CEE users had significantly higher rate of VT than current EE users (HR = 1.78; 95 % CI: 1.11–2.84). And importantly, among all estrogen users, concomitant progestin use was [YES!] associated with increased VT risk compared with estrogen alone (HR = 1.60; 95 % CI, 1.13–2.26).

In the 2014, update of the study [16] extended to also follow myocardial and stoke outcomes between CEE and EE among 384 postmenopausal women aged 30–79 years. In adjusted analyses, CEE use compared with EE use was again associated with an increased VT (HR = 2.08; 95 % CI: 1.02–4.27; P = 0.045) and an increased myocardial infarction risk [HR = 1.87; 95 % CI: 0.91–3.84; P = 0.09), but not with the risk of stroke risk (HR = 1.13; 95 % CI: 0.55–2.31; P = 0.74). Among 140 controls, CEE users compared with EE users had higher [endogenous] thrombin potential-based normalized activated protein C sensitivity ratios (P < 0.001), indicating a stronger clotting propensity. Thus, in summary their 2004 study identified CEE as used in the WHI trials—but not the EE—with a higher risk of VT, a risk that will be potentially enhanced by the use of progestin's, also as identified within the WHI trials 2 versus 1 [15]. Also their 2014 update confirmed the original observation, along with the possibility that CEE use was also associated with a higher risk of myocardial infarctions, and the differential clotting effects between CEE and EE are supported by biological data [16].

Similar observations regarding better cost and benefit ratio of oral estradiol versus CEE were made in the WHI observational study of Shufelt et al. [17]. This large trial was evaluating among the 93,676 postmenopausal women aged 50–79 years the HRTs with several types of estrogen formulations. In direct comparisons, _oral estradiol_ was associated with lower hazard ratios (HRs) for stroke than the CEE (HR = 0.64; 95 % CI: 0.40–1.02), and similarly, transdermal estradiol CHD compared to CEE was also associated with a lower risk of cardiac and stroke events (HR = 0.63; 95 % CI: 0.37–1.06).

26.4 The WHI HRT Trials and the Cardiac Outcomes

When early data emerged from the WHI HRT trial 2 heralding estrogen benefits in cardiac events [18, 19], the issue of its timing and the age at HRT start influencing the outcome was still not entirely clear, as the age subgroup analyses of the trial WHI 2nd HRT trial were not yet officially reported. Thus, Barret-Connors [20], expanding on the timing hypothesis, stipulated that while "*the timing hypothesis is plausible, the pre-specified subgroup analyses in both WHI trials showed no significant interaction with age or years since menopause.*"

One year later, however, in 2007, Manson et al. published for the first time the WHI coronary artery calcium [CAC] measurements from the WHI HRT trial 2, confirming a 40 % reduced CAC _only_ among young postmenopausal women aged 50–59, but not among more elderly women [18]. This was followed in 2007 by the WHI combined coronary heart disease analysis of both trials 1 and 2 [altogether 27,347 participants aged 50–79], set to explore the HRT and age interaction. For women with <10 years since menopause began, there was an early 24 % CHD reduction in the HRT group [HR = 0.76, 95 % CI = 0.50–1.16); for those 10–19 years from menopause, it was 1.10 (95 % CI: 0.84–1.45); and for those >20 years, 1.28 (95 % CI: 1.03–1.58) (*P* for trend = 0.02). Noted is however, that even when controlled for age, the best group age <60 in this combined analysis [E + P and E-alone groups] shows substantially less cardiac benefit than the hazards seen after E-alone from the trial 2 [HR = 0.54, see below].

Indeed, by 2011, La Croix et al. [21]. reported the Estrogen alone versus Placebo cardiac analyses, separately according to age (groups 50–59, vs. 60–69, and 70–79, Tables 26.1, 26.2 and 26.3). These showed among young women aged 50–59 a much more favorable cardiovascular HRT profile, with a 46 % statistically significant reduction of myocardial infarctions (HR = 0.54, 95 % CI: 0.34–0.86). Noted was importantly, virtually no change in the rates of strokes (HR = 1.09, 95 % CI = 0.65–1.83) [21] (Table 26.2) or venous thrombosis [HR = 0.71, 95 % CI = 0.40–1.26].

Also, confirmed was in this young age group, in similarity to the above observational studies, a 27 % all-cause mortality reduction [HR = 0.73, 95 % CI = 0.53–1.00]. None of these estrogen-associated benefits were seen, among women aged >60 [tests for interaction, MI, p = 0.007; all-cause mortality, p = 0.04] (Tables 26.1 and 26.3]. In this 2011 analysis, bone fractures were also reduced among all participants consistently, with trends for more protection among younger women (HR = 0.33, for the ages 60–69, vs. HR = 0.62, for ages 70–79). Also, as discussed in Chap. 23, reduced were also in the trial 2 the rates of breast cancer incidence and mortality, contributing toward all-cause mortality benefits of estrogen among women age <60.

These 2011 estrogen alone data were confirmed in the 2013 WHI update by Manson et al. [2], with identical test for interaction confirming estrogen association with a substantial and significant 40 % rate reduction of heart attacks among young women age <60 but not among more elderly women [p for interaction = 0.007] (Table 26.1).

As a summary of the WHI observations, in 20 [16, 22] Bassuk and Manson representing the definitive WHI trial 2 review of the issue, confirmed that "...*timing of HRT initiation affects the relation between the HRT and coronary risk*..." and that "*Estrogen may have a beneficial effect on the heart if started in early menopause, when a woman's arteries are likely to be relatively healthy, but a harmful effect if started in late menopause, when those arteries are more likely to show signs of atherosclerotic disease.*"

26.5 Estrogen and Biochemical Surrogates of Cardiac Events

With the estrogen cardiac effects basically restricted to primary prevention among younger postmenopausal women, the exploratory analyses of biochemical surrogates of estrogen action and age of women affecting cardiac activity are also of major interest [18, 23–26].

One of the most comprehensive analyses of these issues is the above discussed meta-analysis of Saltpetre et al. focusing on estrogen association with clinical and biochemical surrogates of coronary heart disease [9]. It showed among women <u>without diabetes</u> that HRT reduced not only abdominal fat, but also rates of new-onset diabetes [HR = 0.70, 95 % CI: 0.60–0.90]; and among women <u>with</u> prior diabetes, HRT reduced consistently and significantly the fasting glucose, as well as low-density/high-density lipoprotein-cholesterol ratio [by −15.7 %] and lipoprotein (a) [Lap(a)] [by −25.0 %], and plasminogen activator

Table 26.1 WHI HRT trials: myocardial infarction

Ages	Estrogen + Provera* [8506] (%)	Placebo* [8102] (%)	Difference N/100,000	HR	95 % CI	P value/*interaction 3 age categories
WHI HRT trial 1; According to Manson et.al. [2]						
All	0.39	0.34	+50	1.15	0.99–1.34	
50–59	0.21	0.17	+40	1.25	0.88–1.76	
60–69	0.36	0.36	0	0.99	0.80–1.24	*0.46
70–79	0.76	0.57	+190	1.34	1.05–1.72	
WHI HRT trial 2; According to La Croix [21]						
All	0.46	0.45	+10	1.01	0.85–1.20	
50–59	0.15	0.27	−120	0.54	0.34–0.86	
60–69	0.51	0.48	+30	1.05	0.82–1.35	*0.007
70–79	0.82	0.66	+160	1.23	0.92–1.65	

*Cumulative annual incidence, in %

Table 26.2 WHI HRT trials: strokes

Ages	Estrogen + Provera* [8506] (%)	Placebo* [8102] (%)	Difference N/100,000	HR	95 % CI	P value/*interaction 3 age categories
WHI HRT trial 1; According to Manson et.al. [2]						
All	0.37	0.32	+50	1.16	1.00–1.35	
50–59	0.15	0.10	+40	1.37	0.89–2.11	
60–69	0.36	0.32	+50	1.16	0.92–1.45	*0.40
70–79	0.79	0.72	+80	1.10	0.87–1.38	
WHI HRT trial 2; According to La Croix [21]						
All	0.42	0.36	+60	1.19	0.98–1.43	
50–59	0.16	0.15	−10	1.09	0.65–1.83	
60–69	0.46	0.36	+100	1.27	0.97–1.67	0.87
70–79	0.74	0.66	+80	1.13	0.84–1.53	

*Cumulative annual incidence, in %

Table 26.3 WHI HRT trials: all-cause mortality

Ages	Estrogen + Provera* [8506] (%)	Placebo* [8102] (%)	Difference N/100,000	HR	95 % CI	P value/*interaction 3 age categories
WHI HRT trial 1; According to Manson et.al. [2]						
All	0.98	0.99	−10	0.99	0.91–1.08	
50–59	0.39	0.44	−50	0.88	0.70–1.11	
60–69	0.07	0.97	−10	0.99	0.87–1.13	0.23
70–79	2.07	1.97	+90	1.04	0.91–1.20	
WHI HRT trial 2; According to La Croix [21]						
All	1.02	1.00	−20	1.02	0.91–1.15	
50–59	0.35	0.48	−130	0.73	0.53–1.00	
60–69	1.00	0.96	+40	1.04	0.88–1.24	0.04
70–79	2.02	1.83	+190	1.12	0.94–1.33	

*Cumulative annual incidence, in %

inhibitor-1 (−25.1 %) [9]. all well-known markers of increased cardiac atherosclerogenesis.

The WHI study of Bray et al. [23]. reported estrogen reducing rates of cardiac events *only* among those women with a favorable LDL/HDL cholesterol ratio of <2.5. In these low risk category women, estrogen also reduced the incident coronary heart disease by 40 %, whereas among women with a high LDL/HDL cholesterol ratio >2.5, estrogen therapy resulted in a 73 % higher risk [p for interaction, p = 0.002] [23]. In the *actual age analyses* of this study, the estrogen-associated hazards were reduced by over 40 % among women aged 50–59 regardless of the LDL/HDL cholesterol ratio, while no improvement was seen among elderly women [23].

The other cardiac surrogate study confirming the estrogen timing hypothesis is the WHI exploratory study of Manson et al., which showed essentially the same observations, with estrogen impacting on the reduction of coronary artery calcium [CAC] build-up only among young women aged 50–59 [18].

Similar conclusions measuring a different biomarker were reported by Mendelssohn et al. [25], with the significance of estrogen enhancing *nitric oxide synthesis* with vasodilatation of coronary arteries, and a related *decrease* in the inflammatory cell adhesion. As a result, the overall slowing of the atherosclerotic plaque formation was seen, but only in women with relatively healthy arteries. In those with more substantial atherosclerotic plaque formation—more likely elderly women—no such benefits were seen [25].

The last study to indicate a possibility of cardiac benefit of estrogen in young postmenopausal women comes from the Kronos Early Estrogen Prevention Study (KEEPS) [26]. The objective of this randomized trial of 734 women was to assess rates of atherosclerosis progression, by measuring differences in the carotid intima thickness. Estrogen was randomized versus placebo, and also oral estradiol was randomized versus transdermal estradiol. While there was, overall, very little atherosclerosis progression in these young newly menopausal women, an important trend emerged for less accumulation of coronary calcium in the estrogen than in the placebo arms. Also, with oral estradiol, there was a significant reduction in low-density lipoprotein (LDL), with increase in high-density lipoprotein (HDL) cholesterol, as well as a significant reduction in the triglycerides and C-reactive protein levels—all surrogate markers for increased coronary arterial disease. In addition, with the transdermal estradiol, there was a significant improvement in insulin resistance [26].

All these data, in summary, provide strong level of evidence for cardiac benefits of estrogen, with or without progesterone, and in particular, for the estrogen timing hypothesis. These, and all of the data discussed above, would also explain *a failure* of the much publicized 1998 HERS study set to examine the HRT impact in reducing rates of coronary heart disease among women with ***prior*** heart attack or angina pectoris [i.e., women with prior advanced abnormal cardiac vessel pathology, with preformed atherosclerogenic plaques at the time of HRT start], as would be the case with cardiac analyses in the WHI trials in women over the age of 60 [27].

These data also illustrate the expanded concept of the estrogen timing hypothesis: both the advanced age AND the advanced [vascular] pathology among young [and of course among elderly] women, would preclude estrogen cardiac benefit. These data indeed indicate, as a confirmation of the principle, that high risk women with an unfavorable lipid ratio [i.e., surrogates for abnormal cardiac vascular pathology] would have similar "resistance" to estrogen cardiac protection as elderly women [i.e., women with more advanced age-related cardiac vascular pathology]—both populations representing the "**failed candidates**" for estrogen *primary* cardiac prevention.

While other studies also confirm the estrogen benefits for cardiac events seen particularly among young women [11, 28, 29], unanswered question, for the time being, remains the long-term cardiac and CVS outcomes among women starting estrogen at a younger age e.g. <60 and continuing towards an elderly age (>70 or >80). In those women, benefits of primary estrogen cardiac prevention will in all likelihood also materialize, and perhaps to a much higher extent than what is seen with a mean of 5–7 years of estrogen intake starting at age <60, as seen in the past HRT trials including the WHI HRT studies. The above discussed Danish study with a mean 10 years estrogen duration [13], attests to the concept of the principle identifying somehow more robust cardiac benefits than seen in studies of long-term HRT duration.

While only future randomized trials designed with estrogen duration the main objective outcome may provide more direct answers, the evidence available thus far suggests that from the cardiac perspective, women in their 1960s and 1970s who already started estrogen at the age <60, are probably safe, and are likely to enjoy potentially a more profound cardiac benefit than that observed in younger women with estrogen intake similar to what was in the WHI trial 2 [i.e., HRT duration restricted to just over 5 years only].

As to the ideal formulation of HRT, the above review provides evidence level 1 for protective cardiac effect of estrogen, with a possibility of better cardiac profile with oral estradiol rather than conjugated equine estrogen. In similarity to the closing comments regarding HRT duration, these concepts while quite sensible need confirmation in dedicated randomized trials.

26.6 New HRT Developments

26.6.1 TIBOLONE and BAZEDOXIFEN; and What to Do with BRCA 1 and 2 Mutations?

Other than estrogen and/or progesterone-based HRT, what else is available for women entering menopause and what to do with very high risk women such as those with BRCA 1 or 2 gene mutations? At least two new developments look promising, Tibolone and bazedoxifene, and at least one study of BRCA carriers looks promising for premenopausal women after oophorectomy.

26.6.2 Tibolone

Tibolone is a steroid hormone derived from the Mexican yam, and has been introduced for the management of menopause in the late 1980s. Its use is prevalent in most regions of the world, with the exception of the United States. Tibolone and its metabolites have estrogenic, progestational, and weak androgenic actions [30, 31].

The data indicate tibolone's tissue selectivity, most likely action of tibolone's metabolites exhibiting variable hormonal activity in different target tissues. In this, tibolone differs from SERMs such as tamoxifen, which produce their tissue selectivity through modulation of the ER. Thus, tibolone has been described as a "selective tissue estrogenic activity regulator" (STEAR), and also as a "selective estrogen enzyme modulator (SEEM)."

Specifically, as a result of its selective estrogenic effect in different tissues, seen is increased bone density but absence of primary breast tissues carcinogenicity, and thus some evidence for reduced breast cancer rates. Also, tibolone has estrogen-like effects in the brain preventing menopause-related hot flushes. Also, as a result of its androgenic effect, seen are increased energy and libido levels in women suffering with postmenopausal symptoms; and as a result of its progestational effects, seen is, importantly, a virtual absence of endometrium stimulation, with no uterine cancer as a side effect, while menopausal effects are decreased. In this particular effect, tibolone differs from tamoxifen.

In a randomized, double-blind, placebo-controlled clinical trial of 4538 postmenopausal women, Cummings et al. showed that tibolone reduced the risk of vertebral fractures (HR = 0.55; 95 % CI = 0.41–0.74; P < 0.001), nonvertebral fractures (HR = 0.74; 95 % CI = 0.58–0.93; p = 0.01), and invasive breast cancer (HR = 0.31; 95 % CI = 0.10–0.96; p = 0.04). As a main side effect, tibolone was, however, associated with increased risk of stroke—that risk was seen, however, only in older postmenopausal women (HR = 2.19; 95 % CI = 1.14–4.23) [32].

Most placebo-controlled randomized trials confirm safety in regards to breast cancer rates in healthy women are treated with tibolone, and some studies actually show reduction of breast cancer rates—with evidence for tibolone *not* increasing breast density. However, in established invasive breast cancer and stage IV setting, there some evidence, that tibolone may interfere with the effectiveness of other breast cancer hormonal therapies—thus its use in stage IV breast cancer at the present time is contraindicated [33].

26.6.3 HRT and Breast Cancer Patients with BRCA Mutations

One of the key management issues regarding the premenopausal young BRCA positive breast cancer patients who undergo oophorectomy but no PROPHYLACTIC MASTECTOMY, is the breast cancer risk of the HRT, an approach clearly indicated in order to alleviate menopausal symptoms related premature ovarian ablation.

Pivotal in this are studies of Eisen et al. who evaluated the breast cancer impact of oophorectomy among BRCA 1/2 mutation carriers after oophorectomy, with or without HRT. First, the 2005 review of 1439 patients with breast cancer and 1866 matched controls derived from a registry of BRCA1 and BRCA2 carriers [no breast cancer] showed a significant reduction in breast cancer risk of 56 % for BRCA1 carriers (HR = 0.44; 95 % CI, 0.29–0.66); and of 46 % for BRCA2 carriers (HR = 0.57; 95 % CI, 0.28–1.15) [34].

The risk reduction was greater if the oophorectomy was performed before age 40 (HR = 0.36; 95 % CI: 0.20–0.64) than after age 40 (HR = 0.53; 95 % CI: 0.30–0.91). The protective effect was evident for 15 years post-oophorectomy (OR = 0.39; 95 % CI, 0.26–0.57) [34].

The other study by the same team had shown among 472 postmenopausal women with a BRCA1 mutation, that HRT use of estrogen alone after oophorectomy actually decreased the risk of breast cancer [35] (OR = 0.51; 95 % CI = 0.27–0.98; p = 0.04), with HRT use of estrogen plus progesterone was not statistically significant (OR = 0.66; 95 % CI = 0.34–1.27; p = 0.21) [35].

26.7 Conclusion

The two HRT chapters highlight one of the most important evolving paradigms of science: estrogen, historically and presently considered the main human ***breast carcinogen***, confers paradoxically and unexpectedly, a statistically significant ***reduction*** of invasive breast cancer rates [21]. As a result, the use of estrogen as part of HRT deserves serious merits for breast cancer prevention [36]. This is particularly important in view of the other estrogen-related outcomes: a significant reduction of coronary heart disease, and of all-cause mortality among women age <60, in addition to the well-documented reduction of bone loss, bone fractures and related bone fracture mortality [21].

These measurable outcomes are additional to the well-established estrogen-related quality of life improvements, due to reduction of menopausal symptoms, improved urogenital health, and also low energy states with depressions and insomnia.

So at the end of this review, one cannot but raise questions as to why are these gains virtually unknown outside a narrow circle of experts; and a related question, how come more is not done to advertise these issues more assertively? As seen from this review, data is here and data is clear, therefore, these are mostly logistical and policy issues rather than science itself. Thus, as a likely answer to these infrequently asked questions, the data showing estrogen benefit may need to be clarified and publicized perhaps with the same level of conviction that what was seen with the WHI directed publicity of their first 2002 JAMA publication of Estrogen + Provera versus Placebo, the WHI HRT trial 1.

References

1. Rossouw JE, Anderson GL, Prentice RL, et al. Risks and benefits of estrogen plus progestin in healthy postmenopausal women: principal results From the Women's Health Initiative randomized controlled trial. JAMA. 2002;288:321–33.

2. Manson JE, Chlebowski RT, Stefanick ML, et al. Menopausal hormone therapy and health outcomes during the intervention and extended poststopping phases of the women's health initiative randomized trials. JAMA. 2013;310:1353–68.
3. Anderson GL, Limacher M, Assaf AR, et al. Effects of conjugated equine estrogen in postmenopausal women with hysterectomy: the women's health initiative randomized controlled trial. JAMA. 2004;291:1701–12.
4. Grady D, Rubin SM, Petitti DB, et al. Hormone therapy to prevent disease and prolong life in postmenopausal women [see comments]. Ann Intern Med. 1992;117:1016–37.
5. Ragaz J, Coldman AJ. Age-matched all-cause mortality impact of hormone replacement therapy: applicability to breast cancer survivors. Breast Cancer Res Treat. 1999;57:30.
6. Grodstein F, Stampfer MJ, Manson JE, et al. Postmenopausal estrogen and progestin use and the risk of cardiovascular disease [see comments] [published erratum appears in N Engl J Med 1996 Oct 31;335(18):1406]. N Engl J Med. 1996;335:453–61.
7. Grodstein F, Manson JE, Colditz GA, Willett WC, Speizer FE, Stampfer MJ. A prospective, observational study of postmenopausal hormone therapy and primary prevention of cardiovascular disease. Ann Intern Med. 2000;133:933–41.
8. Grodstein F, Manson JE, Stampfer MJ. Hormone therapy and coronary heart disease: the role of time since menopause and age at hormone initiation. J Women's Health. 2002;2006(15):35–44.
9. Salpeter SR, Walsh JM, Ormiston TM, Greyber E, Buckley NS, Salpeter EE. Meta-analysis: effect of hormone-replacement therapy on components of the metabolic syndrome in postmenopausal women. Diabetes Obes Metab. 2006;8:538–54.
10. Salpeter SR, Walsh JM, Greyber E, Salpeter EE. Brief report: coronary heart disease events associated with hormone therapy in younger and older women. A meta-analysis. J Gen Intern Med. 2006;21:363–6.
11. Hodis HN, Mack WJ, Henderson VW, et al. Vascular effects of early versus late postmenopausal treatment with estradiol. N Engl J Med. 2016;374:1221–31.
12. Hodis HN, Mack WJ, Lobo RA, et al. Estrogen in the prevention of atherosclerosis. A randomized, double-blind, placebo-controlled trial. Ann Intern Med. 2001;135:939–53.
13. Schierbeck LL, Rejnmark L, Tofteng CL, et al. Effect of hormone replacement therapy on cardiovascular events in recently postmenopausal women: randomised trial. BMJ (Clinical Research ed). 2012;345:e6409.
14. Savolainen-Peltonen H, Tuomikoski P, Korhonen P, et al. Cardiac death risk in relation to the age at initiation or the progestin component of hormone therapies. J Clin Endocrinol Metab. 2016: jc20154149.
15. Smith NL, Heckbert SR, Lemaitre RN, et al. Esterified estrogens and conjugated equine estrogens and the risk of venous thrombosis. JAMA. 2004;292:1581–7.
16. Smith NL, Blondon M, Wiggins KL, et al. Lower risk of cardiovascular events in postmenopausal women taking oral estradiol compared with oral conjugated equine estrogens. JAMA Intern Med. 2014;174:25–31.
17. Shufelt CL, Merz CN, Prentice RL, et al. Hormone therapy dose, formulation, route of delivery, and risk of cardiovascular events in women: findings from the women's health initiative observational study. Menopause (New York, NY) 2014;21:260–6.
18. Manson JE, Allison MA, Rossouw JE, et al. Estrogen therapy and coronary-artery calcification. N Engl J Med. 2007;356:2591–602.
19. Manson JE. The 'timing hypothesis' for estrogen therapy in menopausal symptom management. Women's Health (London, England) 2015;11:437–40.
20. Barrett-Connor E. Hormones and heart disease in women: the timing hypothesis. Am J Epidemiol. 2007;166:506–10.
21. LaCroix AZ, Chlebowski RT, Manson JE, et al. Health outcomes after stopping conjugated equine estrogens among postmenopausal women with prior hysterectomy: a randomized controlled trial. JAMA. 2011;305:1305–14.
22. Bassuk SS, Manson JE. The timing hypothesis: do coronary risks of menopausal hormone therapy vary by age or time since menopause onset? Metab Clin Exp. 2016;65:794–803.
23. Bray PF, Larson JC, Lacroix AZ, et al. Usefulness of baseline lipids and C-reactive protein in women receiving menopausal hormone therapy as predictors of treatment-related coronary events. Am J Cardiol. 2008;101:1599–605.
24. Mendelsohn M, Lobo R. Cardiovascular health and the menopause—an approach for gynecologists: an overview. Climacteric: J Int Menopause Soc. 2006;9(Suppl 1):1–5.
25. Mendelsohn ME, Karas RH. Molecular and cellular basis of cardiovascular gender differences. Science (New York, NY). 2005;308:1583–7.
26. Manson JE. The Kronos early estrogen prevention study by Charlotte Barker. Women's Health (London, England) 2013;9:9–11.
27. Grady D, Applegate W, Bush T, Furberg C, Riggs B, Hulley SB. Heart and estrogen/progestin replacement study (HERS): design, methods, and baseline characteristics. Control Clin Trials. 1998;19:314–35.
28. Gurney EP, Nachtigall MJ, Nachtigall LE, Naftolin F. The women's health initiative trial and related studies: 10 years later: a clinician's view. J Steroid Biochem Mol Biol. 2014;142:4–11.
29. Stuenkel C, Barrett-Connor E. Hormone replacement therapy: where are we now? West J Med. 1999;171:27–30.
30. Kloosterboer HJ. Tibolone: a steroid with a tissue-specific mode of action. J Steroid Biochem Mol Biol. 2001;76:231–8.
31. Formoso G, Perrone E, Maltoni S, et al. Short and long term effects of tibolone in postmenopausal women. Cochrane Database Syst Rev. 2012;2:CD008536.
32. Cummings SR, Ettinger B, Delmas PD, et al. The effects of tibolone in older postmenopausal women. N Engl J Med. 2008;359:697–708.
33. Kenemans P, Bundred NJ, Foidart JM, et al. Safety and efficacy of tibolone in breast-cancer patients with vasomotor symptoms: a double-blind, randomised, non-inferiority trial. Lancet Oncol. 2009;10:135–46.
34. Eisen A, Lubinski J, Klijn J, et al. Breast cancer risk following bilateral oophorectomy in BRCA1 and BRCA2 mutation carriers: an international case-control study. J Clin Oncol: Official Journal of the American Society of Clinical Oncology. 2005;23:7491–6.
35. Eisen A, Lubinski J, Gronwald J, et al. Hormone therapy and the risk of breast cancer in BRCA1 mutation carriers. J Natl Cancer Inst. 2008;100:1361–7.
36. Ragaz J, Wilson K, Muraca G, Budlovsky J, Froehlich J. Dual estrogen effects on breast cancer: endogenous estrogen stimulates, exogenous estrogen protects. Further investigation of estrogen chemoprevention is warranted. Cancer Res. 2010;70.

27 Breast Diseases in Males

Darryl Schuitevoerder and John T. Vetto

27.1 The Male Breast

The male breast is normally a rudimentary structure composed of small ducts and fibrous tissue with variable amounts of periductal fat, identical histologically to the breast of prepubertal females [1]. In the absence of estrogenic stimulation, lobules are not seen. The incidence of absent breasts or nipples and of supernumerary nipples in males is identical to that in females [2]. Breast tissue in the male is normally confined to the area directly behind the areola; therefore, clinical breast examination (CBE) is very easy in males and usually can be performed with just one or two examining fingers.

27.2 Gynecomastia

Gynecomastia, the most common clinical and pathologic benign condition of the male breast [3], is defined as an enlargement of the ductal and fibrous stromal components and is clinically and histologically distinct from pseudogynecomastia, in which clinical breast enlargement is due to swelling of the surrounding subcutaneous fat [2]. True gynecomastia may range in size from a small retroareolar disc to enlargement that approximates that of an adult female breast [4]. Primary (idiopathic, physiologic) gynecomastia occurs in 30–70 % of male children and is thought to occur during developmental periods of relative estrogen excess or androgen deficiency [1]. Typically, it resolves spontaneously, and, in the presence of an otherwise normal history and physical examination (PE), it requires no specific workup or treatment unless it persists or is severe, in which case psychological counseling and/or surgery may be needed in selected cases [5–7].

Secondary (pathologic) gynecomastia can be due to a myriad of underlying conditions (Table 27.1) and medications (Table 27.2) [1–3, 5, 8–14]. Careful history and PE often disclose the underlying cause without the need for additional testing or sex-steroid chemistry panels, and treatment consists of correction of the underlying condition or discontinuation of the causative medication. Suspected cases of pathologic gynecomastia in pediatric patients should be referred to a pediatric endocrinologist [7]. Medical treatment of secondary gynecomastia, however, may not be necessary or even possible in situations in which the underlying condition is not correctable, the patient is asymptomatic, or the causative medication should not be discontinued.

In symptomatic patients, a variety of hormonal options are available (testosterone, clomiphene, tamoxifen, danazol), none of which have been studied in a systematic manner and some of which can be associated with significant side effects [5, 7]. Published indications for surgery include: failure of medical therapy; persistence despite 1 year of observation; progressive size, symptoms, or psychosocial issues; and persistence after puberty [15]. In our hands, surgical excision (by subcutaneous mastectomy, sparing the nipple) is often the treatment of choice because it is definitive (provided care is taken to remove all the enlarged tissue) and, in some cases, can be accomplished with the patient under local anesthesia and/or in an outpatient setting. One series found that surgery for gynecomastia is associated with low rates of atypical findings on final pathology (3 %) and need for revision (7 %) [16]. In a recent study from the Netherlands, Lapid et al. performed a retrospective review of 5113 breasts excised with the diagnosis of gynecomastia. The overall incidence of invasive carcinoma and carcinoma in situ in this population was 0.11 and 0.18 %, respectively [17]. Higher

D. Schuitevoerder
Department of Surgery, Oregon Health & Science University, 3181 S.W. Sam Jackson Park Road, L223, Portland, OR 97239, USA
e-mail: schuitev@ohsu.edu

J.T. Vetto (✉)
Department of Surgery, Division of Surgical Oncology, Oregon Health & Science University, 3181 S.W. Sam Jackson Park Road, L619, Portland, OR 97239, USA
e-mail: vettoj@ohsu.edu

I. Jatoi and A. Rody (eds.), *Management of Breast Diseases*, DOI 10.1007/978-3-319-46356-8_27

Table 27.1 Conditions associated with gynecomastia

Endocrine	Adrenal insufficiency Thyrotoxicosis Testicular failure
Genetic	Kleinfelter's syndrome
Liver	Chronic liver failure
Pulmonary	Bronchiectasis Chronic bronchitis Tuberculosis
Renal	Chronic renal failure
Neurologic	Transverse myelitis
Tumors	CNS, especially hypothalamus, pituitary Lung Testicular, especially seminomas, teratomas Prostate (related to therapy)
Others	Malnutrition Trauma

Table 27.2 Drugs associated with gynecomastia

Class	Drug
Antiandrogens	Cyproterone Flutamide
Antibiotics/antifungals	Griseofulvin Isoniazid Ketoconazole Metronidazole
Cardiovascular agents	Amiodarone Captopril Digitoxin Enalapril Methyldopa Nifedipine Reserpine Verapamil
Chemotherapeutics	(Especially) Cyclophosphamide Methotrexate
Diuretics	Thiazides Spironolactone
HIV medications Hormones	Efavirenz Androgens and anabolic steroids Chorionic gonadotropin hGH Estrogens and estrogen agonists
Illicit drugs/drugs of abuse	Alcohol Amphetamines Heroin LSD Marijuana Methadone
Psychoactive agents	Diazepine Haloperidol Phenothiazine Tricyclic antidepressants
Ulcer medications	Cimetidine Omeprazole Ranitidine
Others	Phenytoin Penicillamine

complication rates are associated with higher patient BMI and specimen weights [16].

Because secondary gynecomastia may be unilateral and painless in many cases [6, 15], the major clinical concern regarding this lesion is distinguishing it from breast cancer [5, 6, 8, 11]. This topic is discussed in detail subsequently (see "Differential Diagnosis of Breast Masses in Males" and "FNA-based Evaluation of Breast Masses in Males").

27.3 Other Benign Breast Conditions

A variety of benign conditions common to the female breast are also seen in males and, with the exception of gynecomastia, are similar in both genders in terms of presentation, histology, diagnosis, and treatment [3]. These are listed in Table 27.3 [18–42].

Another occasional exception is nipple discharge; benign milky discharge can occur in males (especially the colostrum-like "witch's milk" of male neonates [1]), and benign non-milky discharge is occasionally seen in males, but bloody discharge in a male is more commonly associated with malignancy than it is in females [43–45]. For example, in a review by Amoroso et al. of 42 cases of nipple discharge in males more than half (57 %) were associated with a clinical breast cancer [46]. This finding is supported by a retrospective review from Memorial Sloan-Kettering Cancer Center that showed that 57 % of male patients presenting with nipple discharge harbored underlying malignancy [47]. Accordingly, males presenting with nipple discharge should be considered as having carcinoma until proven otherwise; those in whom a cancer is not found can be evaluated and treated in a fashion similar to females (i.e., ductography and papilloma excision) [44]. In the afore mentioned study by Amoroso et al., of the discharges associated with benign conditions, all nonbloody discharges were due to gynecomastia (and had often been present for years), whereas bloody but benign discharges were due to papilloma [46]. Nipple discharge in males is also discussed throughout the sections that follow.

27.4 Breast Cancer in Males

Breast cancer in males (BCM) is one of the oldest diseases in recorded history. First reported in the Smith Papyrus, European reports date back to a 1307 case report by an English surgeon, John of Aderne. Subsequent case reports by Ambroise Pare and Fabrius Hildanus in the sixteenth and

Table 27.3 Benign breast conditions in males

		Refs.[a]
Benign solid tumors of the breast and connective tissue		
	Fibroadenoma	[25, 26]
	Fibromatosis	[29, 31, 32]
	Leiomyoma	[35, 40]
	Mesenchymoma	[3, 216]
	Myofibroblastoma	[27, 39, 215, 366]
	Papilloma, intracystic papilloma	[19, 36]
	Phyllodes tumor (benign)	[3]
	Juvenile papillomatosis	[367]
	Benign hemangiopericytoma	[217]
Benign solid tumors of the dermis/subcutis		
	Granular cell tumor	[42]
	Lipoma, lipoblastoma	[18]
	Pilomatrixoma	[41]
Infections/infestations	Sparganosis	[23]
	Tuberculosis	[20, 22, 30]
Inflammatory and autoimmune conditions		
	Granulomatous mastitis	[28]
	Lupus mastitis	[38]
	Nodular fasciitis	[24]
Vascular lesions	Cavernous hemangioma	[34, 37]
	Hemangioma	[21, 33]

[a]*Ref* reference number-see table of contents

seventeenth century, respectively, followed [8]. Periodic reporting continued in the latter half of the twentieth century, when large series began to appear [8, 48–58], leading to our current understanding of the disease.

Although only about 1 % of breast cancer occurs in men, this disease accounts for 0.14 % of all cancer deaths in males (approximately 440 cancer deaths in the United States per year) [59–61]. The widely held notion of BCM as a late-presenting disease with a dismal prognosis is largely a result of earlier [49, 50, 52, 53, 56, 58, 62–65] and even some more recent [54, 66, 67] series consisting mostly of patients presenting with advanced stage disease. Much of the previous data are flawed by single-institution experience, repeated reports from the same institutional series, small sample size, and failure to control for stage and patient age. The well-known tendency for this disease to present late, in older males (who already may possess comorbid conditions leading to subsequent death from noncancer causes), and to be associated with second cancers may explain in part the previously reported low crude survival for BCM. In a review of the Surveillance, Epidemiology and End Results (SEER) database spanning 1973–2004, 1001 of 4873 patients with BCM (21 %) had another non-breast primary cancer recorded in the database [68].

As discussed later, newer series [48, 55, 57, 69–72], including our own [9], refute this notion and indicate that breast cancer in men carries the same prognostic factors as the disease in women and that the stage-for-stage outcomes are also the same. A 2006 series from Japan noted that survival from breast cancer among men had improved in that country since 1980–1984, while it had been stable in females [73]. One recent U.S. study has actually shown that men with breast cancer had significantly better disease-specific survival than their female counterparts [74]. Further, a recent study from Sweden showed similar all-cause and disease-specific survival between BCM and breast cancer in females (BCF) [75]. This newer information leads to the question of whether breast cancer is the same or a different disease in men and women. This issue is also discussed later in this chapter, including a detailing of how breast cancer in men is similar to, and how it differs from BCF.

A grammatical note: Tumors do not possess gender; therefore, the term "male breast cancer" is not as correct as BCM or even "cancer of the male breast" [8]. Thus, throughout this chapter, the disease is referred to as BCM.

27.4.1 Global Distribution

In a meta-analysis, Sasco and colleagues determined that the BCM accounts for about 1 % of all breast cancer worldwide [76]. The global distribution of BCM is similar to that of BCF (i.e., BCM is very rare in areas with a low incidence of breast cancer in general), with a few exceptions. For example, BCM is common in Egypt, an area of relatively low BCF incidence, likely due to high rates of schistosomiasis-related liver failure [77]. In contrast, BCM rates are low and fairly even in European countries (1.5–3 per million) and reflect variances in the rates for BCF, with higher rates found in France, Hungary, Austria, and Scotland [78].

27.4.2 U.S. Incidence

The overall number of BCM cases continues to slowly rise, while the percentage of breast cancer occurring in males has remained relatively constant in the U.S. In 2012 there were 2125 cases of BCM (up from 2,030 in 2007 and 1300 cases in 1999), which represented 0.95 % of all breast cancers (down from 1.27 % in 2012, but up from 0.74 % in 1999) [79]. Older U.S. reports suggest that the incidence of BCM may be rising [80–82]. However, a more recent study using the NCI's SEER data demonstrated a decrease in breast cancer incidence and mortality, with these trends being greater for women than men [83].

There were an estimated 40,290 deaths (out of a total of 231,840 cases) from BCF and 440 deaths from BCM in 2015. Thus, the current likelihood of dying from BCF and from BCM are similar (17.4 and 18.7 %, respectively) [61]. These numbers support the previously mentioned reports of a prognosis for BCM which is comparable to BCF. As previously noted, these figures pertain to disease-specific survival; crude survival in BCM is lowered by comorbidities, especially in older men, and by higher risks of second malignancies in men with breast cancer, especially younger men, and especially second breast primaries [68, 84, 85].

27.4.3 Associated Factors and Conditions

Factors associated with the development of BCM (Table 27.4) include the following:

1. *Advanced age*. The annual incidence of BCM increases steadily (lacking the premenopausal peak seen in females) [61] between 35 years of age (0.1 case per 100,000 men) and 85 years of age (11.1 cases per 100,000) [77]. The mean age of diagnosis was 64.5 years in our series [9] and 61.8 years in the series by Borgen et al. [57] compared with 55.5 years for matched female breast cancer controls in that same study. The greatest incidence occurs 5–10 years later in males than in females; in a recent VA cooperative study, the mean age at diagnosis was 67 years for BCM and 57 years for BCF [86]. BCM is rarely found before the age of 26, although it has been reported in a 5-year-old boy [87].

Table 27.4 Factors associated with the development of BCM[a]

Age[b]
Black race
Prolonged heat exposure
Previous chest wall radiation
Positive family history for breast cancer (in male or female relatives)
BRCA mutations (especially BRCA2)
Environmental exposures
Conditions of relative hyperestrogeny
Testicular abnormalities
Exogenous estrogens
Obesity
Liver disease/alcohol abuse
Klinefelter's syndrome[c]
Prostate cancer and treatment for prostate cancer

[a]Direct causation has not been established for some factors
[b]Incidence of BCM is directly related to age
[c]Increases BCM risk by 50-fold

2. *Black race*. Several studies have shown a disproportionate number of cases of BCM in Blacks [86, 88, 89]. A large study of BCM in California revealed an age-adjusted incidence rate/100,000 men of 1.65 for Blacks versus 1.31 for Whites; BCM rates were lowest for Hispanics and Asians/Pacific Islanders (0.68 and 0.66, respectively). Age and stage at diagnosis in that study also differed by race, with Blacks more likely to be diagnosed at a younger age and more advanced stage ($P > 0.001$) [88]. At least one study has shown racial disparities in BCM treatment and outcome, with Black men less likely to undergo Medical Oncology consultation and chemotherapy, and experiencing a breast-cancer specific mortality ratio more than triple that of White men [90]. A more recent, albeit smaller, study also showed higher mortality rates in Blacks aged 18–64 with BCM when compared to Whites. However, when adjusted for insurance and income this difference was no longer significant, suggesting that this disparity in mortality may have more to do with socioeconomic status than Race itself [91].
3. *Prolonged heat exposure*, which may have a suppressive effect on testicular function [62, 92–95]. The role of electromagnetic field exposure remains controversial [8, 92, 93, 95, 96].
4. *Previous chest wall radiation*, especially radiation given for the treatment of childhood malignancies [97, 98]. Children treated for lymphoma are at particular risk, felt to be due to both chest wall radiation and altered gonadal function [99]. The risk for breast cancer after radiation appears to be similar for men and women, as is the indirect relationship between age of exposure and risk and the lag time between exposure and disease (12–36 years) [96, 100–103]. Accordingly, it is generally recommended that males with such exposure history should be carefully observed [76]. A statistically significant increase in BCM risk among Japanese atom bomb survivors has also been reported [104].
5. *Conditions of relative hyperestrogeny*. These conditions include testicular abnormalities, such as the sequelae of mumps infection and infectious orchitis/epididymitis [8, 92, 105, 106], undescended testes [76, 92, 105], orchiectomy, late puberty, infertility, male potential hypogonadism [62, 92, 107, 108], disorders that cause gynecomastia (gynecomastia itself is associated with up to 43 % of BCM cases, but there are no data for direct causation) [3, 52, 106], exogenous estrogen, obesity, liver disease (due to cirrhosis, bilharziasis, schistosomiasis, and chronic malnutrition) [76, 92, 97, 98, 106, 109], and Klinefelter's syndrome, which (despite its rarity) accounts for 3 % of BCM cases [110] and is associated with a 50-fold increased risk of BCM [111].
The risk of breast cancer in men with Klinefelter's syndrome is probably due in part to altered estrogen: testosterone/androgen ratios and the fact that these men actually develop hypertrophied breasts that contain both acini and lobules (the normal male breast does not contain lobules) [110, 112]. This histological event explains the fact that lobular carcinoma in men is rare and usually only associated with Klinefelter-related cases (see "Histologies" section to follow). Men with Kleinfelter's syndrome are also at higher risk for non-Hodgkin's lymphoma and lung cancer, and their mortality from BCM is particularly high if they have XXY mosaicism [113].
Both prostate cancer and prostate cancer treatment have been linked to BCM [92, 114, 115], presumably due to

both medical and surgical castration. However, this association is controversial; breast cancer is rarely reported among men receiving estrogens for prostate cancer, and malignant breast masses in these patients are more often metastatic deposits than BCM [116].
The preceding associations would lead one to the conclusion that BCM is caused by relative estrogen excess. Although breast cancer can be easily promoted in a number of animal species by hormone administration, clear data indicating causation in humans are lacking, probably because of the relative rarity of BCM and the corresponding small sample sizes in most studies. For example, reports of BCM and fibroadenomas among males taking estrogen for transsexual male-to-female surgery have been anecdotal only [117–119]. Furthermore, there have been three recent studies looking at the incidence of breast cancer in male-to-female transsexuals, none of which showed an increased incidence of breast cancer in this population [120–122]. Data from blood chemistry studies attempting to demonstrate hormonal differences among BCM patients compared with control subjects have been sparse and conflicting. Taken together, most studies show no difference in testosterone, estradiol, and luteinizing hormone levels [123, 124], whereas one study showed increased prolactin and follicle stimulating hormone levels in BCM patients compared with matched controls [125].

6. *Alcohol* taken in excess has been linked to BCM risk in some series [92, 95], but this may be linked to the previously mentioned risks of liver disease and relative hyperestrogeny. One European Case-Control Study found an odds ratio of 5.89 for alcohol intake >90 g/day, compared to light consumers (<15 g/day) [126]. The effect of dietary factors (meat, fruit, and vegetable consumption) is unproven [92, 127].
7. *Suspected* genetic factors include BRCA mutations (discussed below), androgen receptor (AR) gene mutations, CYP17 polymorphisms as well as several single nucleotide polymorphisms identified by genome wide association studies [128, 129], Cowden's syndrome, and CHEK2 mutations [92, 130], although data for this later factor is conflicting [127, 131].
8. *Environmental factors*: Isolated reports also suggest links between BCM and occupational exposure to gasoline and combustion products [92, 132, 133] as well as employment in blast furnaces, steel works, and rolling mills [134].

27.4.4 Family History and Genetics

A family history of breast cancer, in males or females, is present in about 30 % of cases of BCM [76], with 14 % reporting breast cancer in a first-degree relative in one series [135]. Whereas multiple cases of BCM within families have been reported [63, 136], it is rare; more typically (as one would expect from the rarity of BCM), the risk for BCM is associated with a history of BCF. The NIH—AARP Diet and Health data, showed that men who reported a first-degree relative with breast cancer had an increased risk of BCM with a relaitve risk of 1.92 [137]. Similarly, a family history of BCM imparts increased breast cancer risk to the female relatives [138, 139].

Taken together, this information suggests that (a) similar to the situation in BCF, most cases of BCM are "sporadic" (i.e., a specific gene mutation is not identified) and (b) a familial form of breast cancer exists in which both males and females show an increased risk for developing breast cancer [77]. Similar to BCF, studies reveal the association of BCM with a multitude of chromosomal and gene abnormalities [60, 111, 140], especially on the 13q chromosome [140]. The best characterized of these mutations are in the *BRCA2* gene; these mutations may be associated with up to 20 % of BCM cases (particularly in Jews, in whom up to 19 % carry BRCA2 germline mutations, compared to only 4 % of non-Jewish men) [141, 142]. However, they have a low penetrance; only one in seven *BRCA2* carriers has a family history of breast cancer [143, 144]. The usefulness of *BRCA2* testing for relatives of BCM patients is discussed later (see "Testing of Family Members").

Data regarding the association between BCM and *BRCA1* mutations, which are typically point mutations, is conflicting [143–145]. The importance of BRCA2 mutations, commonly genomic rearrangements, in BCM is also controversial and may be population dependent; one study from France recommended screening for BRCA2 genomic rearrangements [146], while studies from the U.S., Italy, and Finland found low rates and did not recommend such screening [131, 147, 148]. Specific mutations in BRCA2 leading to BCM have been identified, including founder mutations such as 8765delAG, 185delAG, and 6174delAT [142, 149, 150]. Again, however, the penetrance is relatively low, with the risk of developing BCM by age 70 reported at 7 % and 8.4 % by age 80 [151, 152].

A hereditary nonpolyposis colon cancer (HNPCC) kindred has been identified in which a male member had both an *MLH1* mutation and breast cancer, suggesting that BCM may be part of the HNPCC syndrome [153]. Loss of the Y chromosome and another 13q chromosomal abnormality, del q13 [25], have been recurrent findings in BCM patients [154]. An AR gene mutation has been found in BCM associated with Reifenstein syndrome (inherited androgen resistance) [155], but at least one report suggests no correlation between AR expression and either the clinicopathologic features or outcome for BCM [156]. Although *p53* mutation rates are similar for BCM and BCF (43 %) [157], BCM is rarely seen in Li-Fraumeni syndrome [157], probably because of the relative rarity of both BCM and this syndrome.

27.4.5 Histologies

Because the male breast contains only ductal tissue, most cases of BCM are ductal type, predominantly invasive ductal (85–90 % of most series [8], 79 % in our series [9]), with the remainder usually "pure" ductal carcinoma in situ (DCIS) or ductal variants [45, 97, 158–162]. Atypical ductal hyperplasia has also recently been described in men undergoing biopsy for presumed gynecomastia [163, 164]. All histologies of breast cancer have been encountered in males, including Paget disease (unilateral and bilateral, both alone and associated with either DCIS or invasive tumors) [161, 165–167], inflammatory carcinoma [168], cribriform carcinoma [169], mucinous cancers [170], and papillary cancers (both solid and cystic) [170–174]. "Pure" DCIS accounts for 5–15 % of BCM [8, 160, 162] and is less common among BCM compared with BCF cases, probably because of the higher detection rate of ductal neoplasms at the DCIS stage in females by screening mammography [58]. Interestingly, DCIS rates in males have been rising over the last 3 decades, suggesting earlier detection despite the fact that BCM is not a screened-for disease [162].

As expected, lobular cancers are extremely rare in men (who lack lobular tissue) and usually are not found at all in many series [57, 66, 170], including our own [9], but have been described in case reports [97, 175, 176] and in large data sets [55, 177]. As mentioned previously, this event probably occurs in diseases associated with the formation of lobules in the male breast, notably Klinefelter's syndrome [110]. BCM is bilateral at diagnosis in about 2 % of cases, similar to the incidence for BCF [159, 165].

Secretory carcinoma, a rare variant of breast cancer that is the most common type seen in children, has been reported in boys [178–180] and in a 51-year-old man [181]. Because of its rarity, neither the natural history of this tumor nor the optimal management is well established, although the tumor generally behaves in an indolent fashion and the prognosis appears to be good [180].

27.4.6 Tumor Biology

Most cases of BCM are estrogen receptor (ER) positive (65–96 % in recent studies [57, 66, 72, 97, 182, 183] and 85 % in our series [9]); therefore, a greater percentage of male patients will be treated with tamoxifen or will respond to hormonal manipulation than will female patients [182, 184, 185]. Similarly, BCM is more commonly progesterone receptor (PR) positive (68–93 %) [183, 186, 187], although Blacks and Hispanics [188] as well as BRCA2 mutation carriers [189] have been shown to have a lower proportion of PR positive tumors. The proportion of HER2 Neu positive BCM cases varies greatly in the literature with a reported incidence ranging from 1.7 to 55 % [188, 190–194], reflecting a large variance in detection methodology and cutoff points. HER2 overexpression has been associated with BRCA2-related BCM [195].

Unlike the situation for BCF, hormone receptor expression in BCM does not seem to correlate with histologic grade of the lesion, tumor stage, or lymph node status [77]. However, a recent population-based study from California of 606 BCM cases showed that younger patients had more HER2 positive disease ($p = 0.02$) [188]. Further, because the majority of BCM cases are hormone receptor positive and because of the rarity of this disease, it is still uncertain if hormone receptor positive tumors carry the same positive prognostic implication as BCF [196]. However, PR negative status has been shown to correlate with decreased survival on multivariable analysis [187, 197]. As opposed to ER expression in BCF, in which ER-β expression tends to be reduced, BCM seems to express high levels of both ER-α and ER-β [183].

AR expression has been reported in 39–87 % of BCMs and seems more common in tumors from older patients [183, 186]. The clinical importance for AR expression in BCM has not been clearly demonstrated [155, 156], although a recent report from China showed significantly worse outcomes and poor response to tamoxifen therapy in AR positive patients [198, 199]. The incidence of high-grade histology among BCM varies widely among series (20–73 %) [9, 66] but overall is probably similar to the incidence in BCF [57]. One study, however, reported proportionately more high-grade histology among a cohort of low stage BCM patients [200]. Additionally, a collaborative multicenter study found a positive association between high-grade tumors and BRCA2 [189]. Whereas most (but not all) [74] breast cancer tends to present at later stages in males than in females (due, in part to the low index of suspicion and lack of screening in males), the discrepancy in stage distribution, and thus the difference in overall prognosis between BCM and BCF is shrinking as more and more recent series are examined (discussed in more detail in the section on "Prognosis").

27.4.7 Staging

BCM is staged using the same TNM (tumor, nodes, metastases) staging system of the American Joint Committee on Cancer (AJCC) as for BCF [201].

27.4.8 Physical Findings

Because BCM is not a screened-for disease, it presents primarily (up to 79–85 % of cases) as a unilateral firm, painless, or minimally tender, subareolar mass [55, 71, 184] found on either self-examination or CBE. In our own series, 70 % of the men presented in this fashion [9]. Because the skin of the nipple is frequently involved, up to 25–30 % of cases are technically stage T4 [71]. The mass is often eccentric (i.e., not directly behind the nipple, especially when there is coexisting gynecomastia or other conditions of ductal hypertrophy), slightly irregular, and firm [77]. Whereas nipple discharge in females is usually nonbloody and associated with benign conditions, discharge in men is more often bloody and a sign of malignancy, including DCIS [43, 45, 46, 162]. Discharge cytology may be diagnostic, and bloody discharge in a male has an 80 % likelihood of indicating an underlying tumor [46].

27.4.9 Imaging

Mammography has a limited role in the diagnosis of BCM for a variety of reasons. First, it is a rare disease for which general population screening is unlikely to be cost-effective. Second, the breast is not significantly enlarged in most cases and is therefore difficult to image [8]. Finally, the utility of mammography for detecting BCM is questionable; although there are indeed characteristic mammographic features of BCM (especially eccentricity [202]), these features are not always present, or there is substantial overlap between these features and the mammographic appearance of benign lesions [203].

For example, suspicious microcalcifications were found in only four of 50 cases of BCM evaluated by mammography by Borgen and colleagues [135], and Cooper et al. [204] found no malignant findings among 263 mammograms in males obtained for abnormal findings on CBE, even among those cases found to be cancer on biopsy. In our diagnostic test study of breast masses in males (See "Fine-Needle Aspiration-Based Evaluation of Breast Masses in Males), mammography was found to add no additional diagnostic information to the combination of physical exam (PE) and fine-needle aspiration (FNA) [205].

Accordingly, despite the previously reported high sensitivity and negative predictive value (NPV) for BCM detection [206], recent studies have concluded that mammography adds little information to initial patient evaluation [207, 208]; in one study of men undergoing mammography to evaluate a dominant suspicious mass, only four cancers were found, and all were suspected on clinical exam [208]. However despite this, given the absence other screening modalities, some authors recommend yearly mammography for patients with a history of BCM or BRCA2 mutation [209].

Evidence on the use of PET/CT in BCM is sparse. However, a recent retrospective study reported a 100 % sensitivity and negative predictive value with the use of PET/CT to aid in initial staging, restaging, and to evaluate for response to treatment [210].

High-resolution Doppler ultrasound can be useful in men for differentiating benign from malignant lesions, guiding biopsy, and staging known cancers [202, 206, 211]. Although ductography is helpful in evaluating discharge in females, it has a limited role in men [8]. The role of technetium-99 sestamibi scanning for the detection of BCM is limited by false-positive results caused by gynecomastia, lymphoma, and other benign and malignant conditions; compounds other than methoxyisobutyl (MIBI) may provide more accurate results [212–214]. More recent nuclear medicine techniques, such as breast-specific gamma imaging, have not yet been evaluated in males to any significant extent.

27.5 Differential Diagnosis of Breast Masses in Males

The differential diagnosis of a breast lump in a male includes both BCM and a variety of benign conditions and benign tumors (Table 27.3) [1–3], including myofibroblastomas [27, 39, 87, 215] and mesenchymomas (also known as *hamartomas* or *angiolipomas*) [3, 216]. Juvenile papillomatosis ("Swiss cheese disease"), which presents as a localized palpable mass, was recently reported in the breasts of male infants. This lesion often is associated with a family history of breast cancer and coexists with malignancy in almost half of cases [179]. Hemangiopericytomas have also been described in the male breast [97, 217, 218]; these connective tissue tumors can range from benign to highly malignant. Similarly, both benign [3] and malignant [97, 219] phyllodes tumors have been described in males.

The differential diagnosis of a mass in the male breast includes other malignancies besides BCM (Table 27.5), most commonly, primary lymphomas (especially non-Hodgkin's B cell lymphomas, occasionally linked to HIV infection) [220–223], angiosarcomas [224, 225], and metastases from other primaries [226]. Aside from BCM, this latter group is perhaps the most common malignancy in the male breast, similar to the situation in females. These come from a variety of primary sites, which in men include prostate cancer [116], eccrine carcinomas [227], lung cancer [228], and especially melanomas, the most common source of metastases to the male breast (58 % in one series) [170]. Other malignant tumors described in the male breast in case

Table 27.5 Malignant breast conditions in males

	Refs.[a]
Breast cancer in males	
Invasive ductal	(Many)
Invasive lobular	[55, 97, 175, 176]
Ductal carcinoma in situ (DCIS)	[158–160, 162]
Paget's disease	[161, 165–167]
Inflammatory carcinoma	[168]
Cribriform carcinoma	[169]
Mucinous cancers	[170]
Papillary carcinoma (both solid and cystic)	[170–174]
Secretory	[178–181]
Primary lymphomas	[220–223]
Sarcomas	
Angiosarcomas	[115, 224, 225]
Phyllodes tumors (malignant)	[97, 219]
Hemangiopericytoma	[97, 217]
Other malignant primary tumors	
Merkle cell carcinoma	[229]
Invasive squamous cell cancer	[230]
Adenoid cystic carcinoma	[231]
Metastases from other primaries	
Prostate cancer	[116]
Eccrine carcinoma	[227]
Lung cancer	[228]
Melanoma	[170]

[a]*Ref* reference number-see table of contents

reports include Merkle cell carcinoma [229], invasive squamous cell cancer [230], and adenoid cystic carcinoma [231].

The major point on the differential for BCM is gynecomastia, which (unlike BCM) has a bimodal age distribution. At presentation, however, older patients with gynecomastia have a similar mean age as BCM patients, and as many as 80 % (63 % in our study) [9] do not have pain or tenderness [11]. Although gynecomastia is typically rubbery and less firm than BCM, this distinction is not always clear on PE, and (as noted earlier), mammograms that are negative or show gynecomastia do not necessarily rule out malignancy. Thus, in the older male patient who presents to a surgeon or breast clinic with a unilateral palpable breast mass, the main diagnostic task is to rule out BCM (rare, but often treatable for cure) while avoiding open biopsy if possible (unnecessary in asymptomatic benign lesions, which will constitute the majority of masses seen) [10, 12].

Patient history does not reliably distinguish between gynecomastia and BCM, for two important reasons. First, the incidence of use of medications known to be associated with gynecomastia (Table 27.2) has been found to be similar between patients with benign breast conditions and BCM [10]. Second, it is evident that some conditions (especially chronic liver diseases and Klinefelter's syndrome) are associated with the development of both gynecomastia and BCM (Tables 27.1 and 27.4) [9]. Indeed, gynecomastia is associated with BCM [158, 159, 164], but studies are divided as to whether it is causative [92, 95].

27.5.1 Fine-Needle Aspiration-Based Evaluation of Breast Masses in Males

As discussed in the prior section, a frequent diagnostic challenge is to distinguish between gynecomastia and malignancy, both of which can be either unilateral or bilateral [232]. In experienced hands, FNA can distinguish between gynecomastia and BCM with good reliability (Fig. 27.1) [233–236]. Sensitivity, specificity, and accuracy rates were 100 % in a study by Joshi and colleagues [237], and similar results were found in a more recent review from the Netherlands with sensitivity and specificity of FNA being 100 and 90.2 %, respectively [238]. There is a small

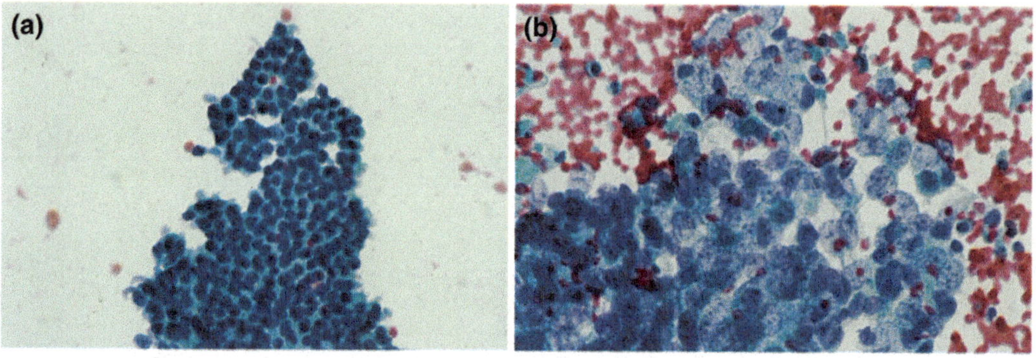

Fig. 27.1 Fine-needle aspiration can distinguish between gynecomastia and malignancy in the male breast. **a** Gynecomastia, demonstrating cohesive groups of ductal epithelial cells with small oval nuclei, scant cytoplasm with little variability in size and shape, and smooth nuclear contours; **b** Invasive ductal carcinoma, demonstrating a mitotic figure, hyperchromatic and pleomorphic nuclei. Diff-Quik staining, 40×

tendency in many reported series toward false-positive results, likely secondary to the high cellularity and epithelial hyperplasia commonly found in aspirates of gynecomastia [233]. Whereas some researchers believe that this "diagnostic dilemma" can be addressed only by routine open biopsy [10, 239], in our breast clinics we favor a multidisciplinary nonsurgical approach that combines PE with needle biopsy.

Because of our experience and success with FNA-based "triple testing" of palpable breast masses in female patients [240–242], we studied the accuracy and cost-effectiveness of the elements of the triple test (PE, FNA, and mammography) for the evaluation of breast masses in males. As noted previously, although some investigators advocate mammography for the evaluation of these lesions [11], experience is limited [10]. Its sensitivity is at best 88 % (i.e., no better than PE alone in ours and other studies) [205, 243], no benefit has been demonstrated for patients younger than 50 years of age [204], false-positive results are the rule with certain benign lesions such as gynecomastia [49] and epidermal cysts [12], published information on the relationship between calcifications and malignancy is conflicting [11, 97, 244], and its use for breast cancer detection in males is currently felt to be limited [202–204, 207, 208, 211]. Accordingly, we chose to study a diagnostic approach to palpable breast masses in males that used the combination of PE and FNA (PE+FNA) without mammography since we believed mammography would add only increased patient charges.

Indeed, in the 13 cases in our study where the referring provider had already ordered a mammogram, the test added no additional diagnostic information to that already provided by PE+FNA, nor did it change the clinical management of any case [205]. We do however recommend bilateral mammography as a preoperative test in cases where PE +FNA indicate the presence of a malignancy.

In our study, when both PE and FNA were benign, no cancers developed at the index sites during follow-up of these lesions (NPV and specificity 100 %). Open biopsy confirmed malignancy in all cases for which both tests were suspicious (positive predictive value [PPV] and sensitivity 100 %). In all seven cases where the tests were not in agreement, open biopsy was benign. In these cases, FNA (two false-positives) proved more accurate than PE (five false-positives). Overall the combination of PE+FNA avoided open biopsy in over half the cases, resulting in an average decrease in patient charges of $510 per case. We concluded that the combination of PE and FNA for the evaluation of breast masses in males is diagnostically accurate and results in a reduction in patient charges compared with routine open biopsy [205].

The nonoperative evaluation of breast masses in males can employ either cytology (FNA) or core biopsy, depending on which modality a given institution has more experience with. Whereas core needle biopsy is advocated for by many, we [205, 242, 244], like others [245–249], favor an FNA-based diagnostic scheme for the evaluation of breast masses in males because it is rapid and offers in-clinic results using Diff-Quik staining.

This approach, however, is associated with two caveats. First, lesions with concordant negative evaluations are followed clinically, resulting in a "true-negative" rate that is not based on pathology results. Although this method introduces potential error compared with routine open biopsy, in our study, no cancers were detected after up to 60 months of follow-up (which included eight subsequent open biopsies, all benign) [205]. This is consistent with the findings of a study by Somers et al. [250] which showed no tumors developing in female patients with concordant negative triple tests (TTs) after up to 74 months of follow-up. Second, concern may be expressed over the fate of lesions left unbiopsied and the potential effect this could have on patient care and potential charge reductions. The calculated reductions in our study took into account the "failure" rate for observation of benign concordant lesions that went on to undergo open biopsy anyway

(21 %) during the mean follow-up period [205]. This number is similar to the percentage of older male patients with benign breast conditions who present with pain or other symptoms prompting excision (20–34 %) as reported in ours and other series [9, 11]; in fact, we have not had any more "failures" with additional follow-up. Further, given the potential charge reduction of $510 per case with the use of PE+FNA, it would have taken the removal of all remaining observed lesion, plus one, to negate the observed cost-effectiveness of this diagnostic approach [205].

Other authors have looked at diagnostic test combinations for breast lesions in men. In a retrospective review from Italy of various combinations of PE, FNA, ultrasonography, and mammography, Ambrogetti et al. [243] found a sensitivity rate of 100 % for the combination of PE and mammography. We found the same sensitivity for PE+FNA and favor cytologic over mammographic information for the purposes of confidently reassuring patients that they do not need open biopsy and for avoiding disaster in centers where patients diagnosed clinically as having gynecomastia are treated by liposuction [16, 251]. Further, the information provided by FNA can be used to distinguish benign from malignant breast masses [252], primary breast cancers from metastases to the breast [253–255], and to determine grade and other tumor features prior to neoadjuvant therapy (especially by adding DNA image cytometry to cytologic evaluation of the material) [256]. The combination of history, PE, and mammography has also recently been advocated as being highly accurate for the evaluation of unilateral breast masses in males, but this conclusion was reached retrospectively, and without considering FNA in the analysis [257].

In summary, although open biopsy remains the gold standard for the evaluation of breast masses in men [3, 258], it is the most expensive choice, often unnecessary, and the use of FNA-based diagnosis can safely avoid it in most cases.

27.6 Breast Cancer in Males: Treatment and Outcomes

27.6.1 Surgery

Surgical excision is the mainstay for resectable BCM. For example, most (50 of 54, or 93 %) patients in our review had some type of primary surgical therapy (all three patients who presented with stage IV and one patient with stage IIIB disease did not) [9]. Although radical mastectomy (RM) was traditionally the treatment of choice because of the paucity of male breast tissue and the resultant proximity of these lesions to the chest wall, surgical therapy has evolved in both the United States and Europe toward more limited procedures. For example, a 30-year review of 170 cases treated at the National Cancer Institute of Italy in Milan noted a trend from RM to modified radical mastectomy (MRM) and, finally, total mastectomy (TM; for smaller and DCIS lesions) in the later period of the study [50]. A similar surgical trend was noted during approximately the same time period in the United States [135, 259], and more recent series report that RM is now used infrequently [9, 45, 57], probably because of the reported equivalent survival after MRM compared with RM [260] and the fact that most of these tumors do not invade beyond the pectoralis fascia and can be resected with limited in-continuity muscle excision when they do.

The National Cancer Data Base (NCDB) has reported on a large BCM treatment study in which the treatments received by 3627 matched pairs of BCM and BCF patients were compared. In this study, men were more likely to be treated with mastectomy than women (MRM, 65 % of men vs. 55.15 % of women; RM 2.5 % of men vs. 0.9 % of women; TM, 7.6 % of men vs. 3.4 % of women; $P < 0.001$) [261]. This is supported by a recent publication reviewing SEER data from 1973 to 2008 in which 87 % of BCM was treated with mastectomy compared to 38 % of BCF [262]. Although some studies advocate MRM or TM for men [71, 95, 263], others note the feasibility of breast conserving operations [264–266], and show that disease-specific survival is unaffected by type of surgery [267]. Others advocate for nipple sparing [268] if the lesions is eccentric. Using intraoperative sonography to augment breast conservation in men found to have occult cancers on workup of symptoms has also been reported [269].

Although two-level axillary dissection was the gold standard for pathologic staging of the clinically negative axilla in BCM, several reports and series have shown the utility and accuracy of sentinel lymph node biopsy (SLNB) in avoiding the need for routine axillary dissection for clinically node-negative cases [71, 95, 270–275]. Since at least half of BCM cases are node negative in large series [70], and in more recent series with more T1 lesions this number has increased to 55–80 % [270, 273, 274], this is important to consider. Similar to the experience in BCF, SLNB for BCM has been shown to be feasible and accurate; one difference is a higher rate of tumor in additional (non-sentinel) nodes in men compared to women [274].

These surgical trends have lead to a decrease in the magnitude and morbidity of breast operations in males.

Recommendations already exist for the treatment of DCIS in males with TM rather than MRM [276], and theoretically, one could extend current surgical recommendations for DCIS in females, such as the Van Nuys Prognostic Index (VNPI), [277] to males. Indeed, in our series of recently treated BCMs, five patients with stage T0 or small T1 disease ("minimal breast cancer") were treated with lumpectomy alone, with no local recurrences during the 4.5-year follow-up period [9]. Others have advocated for this limited approach [160], although some reports indicate that men with DCIS have high local failure rates and may still come to TM [158, 159].

Similar to the management of BCF, potentially curative operative therapy for BCM must be postponed or modified in the event of a concurrent immediately life-threatening condition. This judgment consideration is of particular importance in older men with frequent comorbid conditions. For example, a report from Japan documents a "two-stage" approach to BCM in a 61-year-old man suffering acutely from an aortic dissection. After successfully addressing the dissection, the surgeons removed the tumor with the patient under local anesthetic, completing a definitive breast procedure 1 month later [278].

27.6.2 Radiation

Radiation therapy (RT) has been applied inconsistently for the treatment of BCM in the past. For example, in large retrospective reviews such as the previously mentioned 1999 NCDB study, men were more likely to receive RT post-mastectomy than their matched female controls (men, 29 %; women, 11 %; $P < 0.041$) but were less likely to receive RT after lumpectomy (men, 54 %; women 68 %; $P < 0.001$) [261]. RT clearly reduces the reported 4–31 % postoperative loco-regional recurrence rate [8, 145, 279, 280], especially when the pectoralis muscle and chest wall are found to be involved at operation. As one would expect, adjuvant use of RT in this setting improves local control, but not disease-related survival [71, 279–281].

RT is often recommended after mastectomy for BCM [265, 279], where, as previously mentioned, it has been noted to be used more frequently post-mastectomy than in females [261, 281]. In fact, male gender was found to be an independent predictive factor for the use of post-mastectomy RT in a BC Cancer Agency review [282]. More recently, as noted in the prior section, RT has been used for breast preservation, especially in cases of DCIS [264, 265, 268, 269]. In fact, a review of BCM treated at Guys Hospital concluded that the indications for RT for BCM were similar to those for BCF [84]. Similarly, the BC Cancer Agency review concluded that men having mastectomy for breast cancer should receive adjuvant RT along guidelines similar to those for women, with the caveat that common indications for post-mastectomy RT (T4 lesions and extensive nodal involvement) may be more common in men [282].

27.6.3 Adjuvant Chemotherapy

Because of the rarity of BCM, the perceived role of tamoxifen as the cornerstone of adjuvant therapy, and the higher mean age of BCM patients (with attendant lower overall performance status), chemotherapy is less used for BCM than BCF, and therefore information on the use of adjuvant cytotoxic chemotherapy for BCM is sparse and mostly retrospective. In the NCDB study, men were less likely to receive chemotherapy than their matched female controls (men, 26.7 %; women, 40.6 %; $P < 0.001$) after any form of surgical therapy [261]. In a review of the 2004–05 SEER data, 37 % of invasive BCM cases were treated with chemotherapy [283].

Nonetheless, most series of BCM patients treated with chemotherapy report benefit [70, 95, 265, 284], particularly for groups at higher risk of disease-related death, such as younger patients with receptor-negative and node-positive disease [71, 90, 263]. In a combined experience from Memorial Sloan-Kettering Cancer Center and the Ochsner Clinic, Borgen et al. [135] found an 11 % reduction in distant relapse from adjuvant chemotherapy (from 57 to 46 %) for node-positive patients. Similarly, an improved 5-year survival rate (80 %) compared with stage-matched historical controls has been reported for a cohort of 24 node-positive patients treated with cytoxan-methotrexate-fluorouracil (CMF) [285].

The NCI MB-82 study prospectively treated 31 node-positive BCM patients with 12 cycles of CMF. Survival rates at 10, 15, and 20 years were 65, 52, and 42 %, respectively. The study was uncontrolled but the authors concluded that chemotherapy may produce a survival benefit [286]. Similar to the situation in BCF, some data in BCM also suggest a benefit of adjuvant chemotherapy for node-negative disease [287]. In the MD Anderson review adriamycin-based regimens were more commonly used (81 %) than CMF (16 %), and a decreased risk of death among patients receiving chemotherapy was also noted [70].

While adapted only gradually, the use of trastuzamab is now routine for the treatment of HER-2 positive BCM [288, 289]. Furthermore a recent phase II study showed good activity of Herceptin combined with bevacizumab, and capecitabine for metastatic or recurrent BCM [289, 290].

Interestingly, another prospective study of chemotherapy in BCM involved the use of high-dose chemotherapy and autotransplantation in 13 BCM patients; six had stage II disease, four were stage III, and three had metastatic disease. Of the 12 tumors tested for hormone receptors, all were positive. The median age at transplantation was 50 years. Five patients received cyclophosphamide, thiotepa, and carboplatin; the other eight patients received other alkylator-based regimens. There were no cases of nonengraftment and no treatment-related deaths. Three of the ten patients receiving autotransplantation for adjuvant therapy relapsed 3, 5, and 50 months post transplant and died of disease; the remaining patients were alive with no evidence of disease at the median follow-up time of 23 months (range,

6–30 months). Of the three men treated for metastatic disease, one progressed and the other two relapsed at 7 and 16 months post transplant [291]. However, at the present time autotransplantation for BCM is an unlikely option due to the negative results of prospective trials in BCF.

Other current chemotherapy treatment regimens used for BCM are based on the BCF literature and include various combinations of doxorubicin, cyclophosphamide, docetaxel, fluorouracil, epirubicin, and paclitaxel [292–296].

The use of primary systemic ("neoadjuvant") chemotherapy to "downsize" tumors and subsequently treat them with salvage mastectomy and/or chest wall radiation has been used for the treatment of locally advanced BCM with reported success [8, 70, 135]; 6 % of patients in the MD Anderson series were treated in this fashion. Unlike the situation in BCF, the goal of neoadjuvant therapy for BCM is to improve local control, rather than increase the use of breast conservation.

27.6.4 Hormone Therapy

Because up to 90 % of BCM cases are hormone receptor positive [95], hormone therapy is standard adjuvant therapy in men [71, 95, 196, 263], and is used more often than in women [86]. Tamoxifen is commonly accepted as first-line therapy for BCM [184, 185] and is often used alone, due in part to the older mean age and higher comorbidities of BCM patients. An early report of 1–2 years of adjuvant tamoxifen therapy in BCM patients revealed a 15 % improvement in 5 year overall survival (from 44 to 61 %) and a 28 % improvement in 5 year disease-free survival (from 28 to 56 %) [297]. The current recommendation is to use a standard 5-year tamoxifen course, although noncompliance with this regimen is higher in males than females (25 vs. 4 % in one series) [59]. The higher noncompliance rate with tamoxifen in BCM is associated with a greater frequency and severity of side effects in men, including (in descending order of frequency) decreased libido, weight gain, hot flashes, altered mood, and depression. This issue is highlighted by Xu et al. who looked at Tamoxifen compliance and impact on disease-free survival in 116 BCM patients. They found adherence rates of 65 % at one year, 46 % at two years, 29 % after three years, and 18 % in the fifth year. The 5 and 10 year disease-free survival was 95 and 73 % in the adherent group and 73 and 42 % in the noncompliant group, respectively, further underlining the significance of this issue [298].

Another antiestrogen, the pure ER antagonist fulvestrant, has been used for advanced BCM with reported success [299–301]. Aromatase inhibitors (AIs) have been found to produce effective suppression of estradiol levels in males and some reports have demonstrated objective responses in advanced BCM [302–304]. A recent study showed AIs to be inferior to tamoxifen as first-line endocrine therapy for non-metastatic BCM [305]. However, multiple current studies support the use of AIs as treatment for metastatic BCM [304, 306]. The role of gonadotropin-releasing hormone (GnRH) analogs in the management of metastatic BCM is uncertain [307], with recent studies conflicting as to whether combination with AIs confers benefit in this situstion [308, 309]. Further, another study suggests a GnRH analog added to AI therapy after detection of disease progression may provide benefit for metastatic BCM [310]. Interestingly, intratumoral aromatase has been found to be expressed in 27 % of breast tumors in males and to correlate with a more favorable histology and clinical outcome [311].

27.6.5 Palliative Therapy

As one would expect from the high rate of ER and PR expression in BCM, hormonal manipulation has been the cornerstone of the treatment of distant disease since its first description in 1942 by Farrow and Adair, who noted regression of metastatic BCM after orchiectomy [312]. Tamoxifen is the current mainstay of palliative hormonal therapy, with overall response rates of 70 % for receptor-positive tumors [184]. As indicated above, recent case reports suggest that patients with metastatic disease who relapse on tamoxifen probably should be treated with second-line hormonal therapy (similar to the situation for postmenopausal BCF patients) [299, 302, 303], with palliative chemotherapy reserved for nonresponders and receptor-negative tumors. Particularly advanced cases of BCM may metastasize to unusual locations, notably the eye [313–315], skin [316, 317], and mandibular region [318, 319], each demanding a tailored approach to palliation.

27.6.6 Prognostic Factors

Similar to BCF, the most significant prognostic factors for BCM are AJCC stage and its elements: tumor size and lymph node status [9, 45, 57, 70, 97, 320, 321]. Lymph node status seems to be particularly important [90, 320, 321]. This major similarity between BCF and BCM was first established in 1987, when Hultborn and colleagues demonstrated that among a group of 166 BCM patients age, tumor size, and lymph node status were the most important prognosticators by multivariate analysis [320]. In 1993, Guinee et al. reported that tumor size greater than 3 cm significantly impaired prognosis and that 5-year survival was directly related to the number of nodes involved: 55 % when four or more nodes were positive, 73 % for one to three positive nodes, and 90 % for node-negative patients (84 % at

10 years). Skin involvement, chest wall fixation, and tumor ulceration (all of which are more common in BCM than BCF) were not independently prognostic in their study [321].

Our group subsequently reported on a number of factors relating to disease-free survival. We examined the impact of several patient and tumor features, including the elements of TNM stage, tumor grade (low to intermediate vs. high), receptor status (positive vs. negative), personal or family history of breast cancer (positive vs. negative), age (younger or older than 60), and presentation (asymptomatic vs. pain and nipple discharge vs. painless mass) for prognostic impact in multivariate analysis using the Cox proportional hazards model [322]. Only AJCC stage and its components (tumor size, nodal status, and presence of metastases) correlated with survival [9].

We hypothesized that by controlling for the effect of age (by relating to disease-free rather than crude survival), age "dropped out" as significant, unlike earlier studies that used crude survival (see next section) [320]. Other recent multivariate analyses have come to similar conclusions [57, 71, 110, 323, 324], however recent studies have shown PR negative tumors to have a negative association with survival [187, 197]. As mentioned previously, a recent study by El-Tamer and colleagues actually found a better disease-specific survival for BCM compared to BCF because men were 4 times more likely than females to die of diseases other than their breast cancer [74]. Many of these diseases are second cancers—a recent study found that 12.5 % of men with breast cancer develop a second primary malignancy, particularly of the small intestine, rectum, pancreas, skin (non-melanoma), prostate, and lymphohematopoietic system [325]. BRCA2 (and to a lesser extent, BRCA1) mutations may explain the higher incidence of pancreatic and prostate cancers.

A study of fluorescence-activated cell sorting (FACS) analysis and Immunohistochemical (IHC) staining of BCM specimens found that both ER and HER2/neu expression were higher in BCM compared to BCF; 55 % of BCM specimens were found to have HER2/neu overexpression in this series [194]. This is contradicted by a more recent study in which only 17.2 % of the BCM cases had overexpression of HER2/neu, which was significantly lower than the rate of HER2/neu positivity in BCF ($p = 0.001$) [326]. This study also showed that HER2/neu overexpression carried a worse prognosis, although, as previously mentioned, the prognostic significance of hormone receptor positivity and HER2/neu overexpression in BCM is not entirely clear [77, 196, 326]. The aforementioned FACS analysis and IHC staining of BCM samples found that tumor expression of p53, ER, and cathepsin B correlated with better clinical outcome [194].

27.6.7 Prognosis: Are BCM and BCF "Different" Diseases? A Critical Appraisal of the Literature

In terms of prognosis, the essential question in BCM is whether or not the disease is biologically distinct from BCF. As mentioned previously, in part because BCM is a disease of older men (with, by definition, frequent comorbid conditions) who tend to present late (at a mean of 10.2 months in one series) [55], older series, which examined only crude (overall) survival (which does not control for age, stage, or comorbidity), reached the inevitable conclusion that it carries a worse prognosis than BCF [49, 50, 52, 56, 58, 62, 63, 65]. This concept also has been fostered by the occasional case report emphasizing widespread and unusual metastases in BCM patients [67, 313–319, 327–329], as well as more recent studies reporting only overall survival [71, 86]. By the early 1990s, however, some studies were reporting a worse prognosis only for men with positive nodes [52, 135]. These investigators hypothesized that because most cases of BCM were centrally located, node positivity was a worse sign than in cancers in women.

Subsequent series found similar survival between males and females afflicted with breast cancer when the cases in men were controlled for age and stage [55, 57, 330]. For example, Borgen et al., reviewing a 16-year, two-institution database, found similar AJCC stage-related survivals between 58 cases of BCM and matched BCF controls [57]. Donnegan et al. in an 18-institution review of 217 patients with BCM, also showed similar stage-related survival to cases of BCF, but they also found late presentation and advanced stage to be a common theme. The overall 10-year survival was low as a result of censored events (25 % of the patients in his series died during follow-up due to noncancer causes) [55]. As already mentioned, this phenomenon actually lead to better disease-specific survival in men compared to women in the study by El-Tamer et al. [74].

Accordingly, at our institution, we chose to study a more "recent" cohort of patients who presented mostly to multidisciplinary breast clinics for evaluation of their masses [9]. These factors may explain why [1] the mean tumor size in our series (2.7 cm) was smaller than that in even fairly recent reports [2, 49, 50, 52, 53, 56, 58, 71, 331] more than half (57 %) of our cases were early stage (AJCC stage groupings 0-IIA; half of tumors were stages T0 or T1 at presentation), and [3] 62 % were node negative (118 of 604 total lymph nodes removed [19.5 %] were pathologically positive for tumor). Whereas these figures are still higher than those for BCF, taken together with the literature as a whole, especially studies of BCM seen at different time frames [53], they do suggest a much called-for trend of increased awareness and

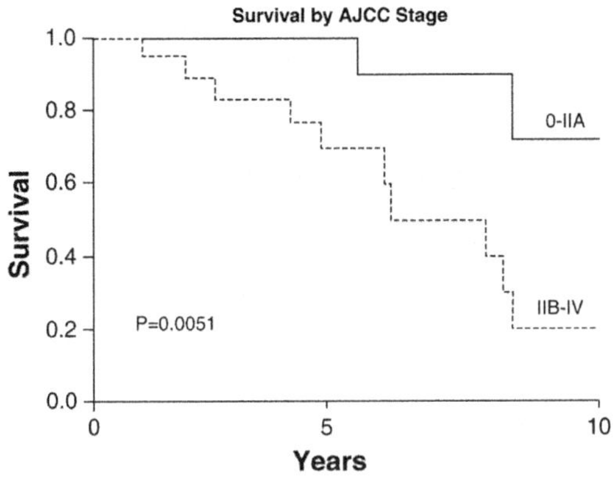

Fig. 27.2 Disease-free survival of males with breast cancer, by American Joint Committee on Cancer (AJCC) stages, for early (stage groupings I–IIA) and later (stage groups IIB–IV) disease, by the method of Kaplan and Meier. The curves are significantly different by the log-rank test (reprinted from Vetto et al. [9], Copyright 1999, with permission from Elsevier.)

earlier diagnosis [184, 330]. Some of the lower stages seen in our series may be attributable to our previously published standardized approach to breast masses in males, which involves a high index of suspicion combined with rapid and accurate evaluation of the mass in question by aspiration cytology (see "FNA-based diagnosis," above) [108, 205]. This approach has been used for the past 23 years at the institutions that contribute data to our studies.

We calculated disease-specific survival by the method of Kaplan and Meier, counting deaths from other causes as censored events [332] and comparing survival curves by log-rank analysis [333]. The overall 5-year disease-free survival for our entire patient group was 87 %, which is higher than that reported by series that included "older "data [70, 71]. As demonstrated in Fig. 27.2, 5- and 10-year disease-related survival rates were AJCC stage-related; 100 and 71 %, respectively, for early stage (stage groupings 0-IIA) disease, and 71 and 20 %, respectively for advanced stage (stage groupings IIB-IV) disease. This difference in survival was highly statistically significant by log-rank test ($P > 0.0051$).

Further, Table 27.6 lists the 5-year survivals of the patients in our study by the Surveillance, Epidemiology, and End Results (SEER) database staging system (localized, regionally metastatic, and distant disease), compared with published survival numbers by SEER stages for BCF during approximately the same time as our study [334]. As can be seen in the Table, the stage-related 5-year survivals for BCM and BCF were similar [9]. To reach this finding in our study, we needed to control only for stage, not age. However, it should be noted that the Kaplan–Meier method does somewhat control for age by censoring deaths from other causes.

The series from M.D Anderson also compared localized and regional disease in men and women and also found 5- and 10-year outcomes in men (localized: 86 and 75 % survival, respectively; regional: 70 and 43 % survivals, respectively) to be similar to those reported in women [70].

All existing data on BCM are marred by its retrospective, historical, and "patchy" nature. We applaud the Commission on Cancer for their efforts in performing a Patient Care Evaluation Study in BCM [184, 261] and also Memorial Sloan-Kettering Cancer Center's ongoing National Male Breast Cancer Registry (see section entitled "Tumor Registries" to follow).

Based on the trend we have seen in the literature (Fig. 27.3), including our own study [9], one wonders whether future data will show a further decrease in the presenting size and stage of BCM, with survival rates approaching those of BCF, without the necessity for even a stage correction. At present, this seems doubtful. Although the mean size of tumors in BCF cases is expected to decrease to below 1.0 cm in the next 10 years, such a trend for BCM is unlikely because this is an uncommon disease that is not screened for and therefore will continue to present in most cases as a palpable mass. Nonetheless, a high index of suspicion [184, 330] combined with a uniform approach to diagnosis [169] and education and screening of high-risk populations [97, 209] may bring about continued decreases in stage at presentation and attendant mortality.

For the present, one of the most important implications of the recent information suggesting that BCM is not a biologically more aggressive disease than the same condition in females is to emphasize to providers that BCM should be treated for cure in most cases. Similar to the situation in females, such treatment should include optimal (but not overly aggressive) local control [53, 264, 265, 268], adjuvant hormonal therapy for receptor-positive tumors (most breast tumors in men) [51, 70, 71, 95, 196, 200, 263], and consideration of adjuvant chemotherapy for high-risk patients [70, 95, 97, 265, 335].

Table 27.6 Five-year disease-free survival for breast cancer by surveillance, epidemiology, and end results (SEER) stages

SEER stage	Males[a] (%)	Females[b] (%)
Localized	100	97
Regional	81	78
Metastatic	33	22

[a]Data from Ref. [11]
[b]SEER data from Fritz [334]

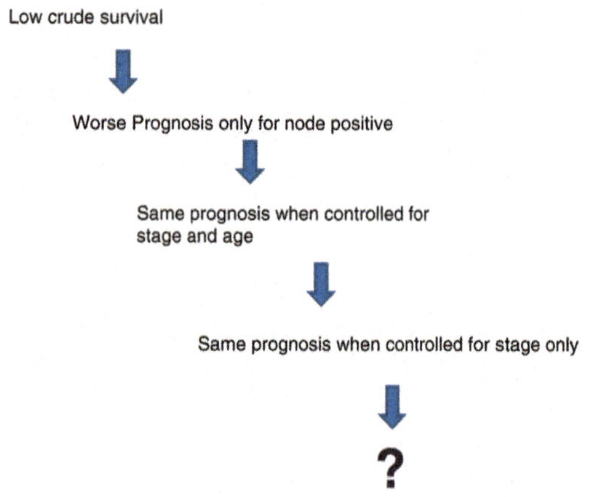

Fig. 27.3 Trends in the outcomes for breast cancer in males (BCM) compared to females, as reported in the literature (see text for details)

More recently, investigators have attempted to answer the question of whether or not BCM is a different disease from BCF by using biologic rather than descriptive data. On a cellular level, a recent report has catalogued four cases of CD34-positive BCM, suggesting the possible existence of a CD34-positive breast cancer stem cell, similar to the cancer stem cell postulated for BCF [336]. On a chromosomal level, Rudlowski et al. have reported a shared pattern of chromosomal imbalances between BCM and BCF, including +1q, −8p, +8q, −13q, +16p, −16q, +17q, and +20q, suggesting that similar genetic events may underlie the development and progression of breast cancer in both males and females [337]. Conversely, on a genetic level, a recent study found significant dissimilarities in DNA ploidy, p21, and p53 between clinically homogenous groups of BCM and BCF, suggesting somewhat distinct tumor oncogenesis [338]. Furthermore, a recent study from Sweden attempting to identify candidate driver genes of tumorigenesis compared 53 BCM to 359 BCF specimens. They found only two candidate driver genes in common between the male and female specimens, lending further credence to the argument that BCM and BCF differ at the genetic level [339]. Additionally, recent studies looking at the microRNA profile of BCM suggest differences in expression compared to BCF [340–342].

27.6.8 Similarities and Differences Between BCM and BCF: A Summary (Table 27.7)

Like BCF, BCM is most commonly of ductal histology [8, 9, 45, 97, 161], is associated with relative estrogen excess [8, 52, 56, 62, 76, 92, 98, 107, 108, 111], is staged by the TNM system [201], and is best treated by multimodal therapy (most often surgery followed by adjuvant therapy). Cases not resectable for cure can be treated by a combination of palliative therapies (surgery, chemotherapy, RT, or hormonal therapy). BCM and BCF appear to have similar prognostic factors [9, 45, 57, 70, 97, 320, 321] and similar stage-for-stage survival [9, 55, 57, 70, 330], especially if one controls for age and comorbid conditions. Like BCF, BCM appears to be mostly a singular event, with synchronous and metachronous tumors less common [343–346], although men do have a higher incidence of second non-breast primary tumors [325].

There are also several clear clinical differences between BCM and BCF. Besides the previously noted older mean age for BCM patients, this disease is by definition usually centrally located and often involves the nipple [97]. Accordingly, whereas nipple discharge in females is usually

Table 27.7 Comparison of BCM and females

Similarities	Differences
Associated factors Age Exposure to estrogens Chest wall radiation	Incidence, ability for early detection
Association with BRCA2 mutations	Association with BRCA1, other syndromes
Mostly ductal histologies	Incidence of lobular histology, pure DCIS
Usually solitary tumors	Most common location within the breast
Importance of physical examination (PE)	Role of mammography
Staging system	
Usefulness of FNA-based diagnosis	Differential diagnosis
Stage-for-stage treatment Central role of resection and sentinel node biopsy Importance of adjuvant hormonal therapy	
Main prognostic factors	Incidence of ER, PR expression
Stage-for-stage prognosis[a]	

FNA fine-needle aspiration
[a]When controlled for stage and comorbidities; see Fig. 27.2, Table 27.6, and text

nonbloody and associated with benign conditions, discharge in males is more often bloody and a sign of malignancy, including DCIS, and discharge cytology may be diagnostic [43, 45]. The vast majority of cases of BCM are hormone receptor positive (65–93 % in recent studies [57, 66, 70, 97] and 85 % in our series [9]). Thus, tamoxifen has become the mainstay of therapy for many patients [70, 71, 86, 95, 184, 185, 196, 263], although it may be associated with a greater frequency and severity of dose-limiting side effects in men than in women [59].

27.7 Breast Cancer Survivorship Issues in Males

27.7.1 Follow-Up

There are no recommendations for follow-up that are specific to BCM; rather, the same follow-up schedule used for BCF is generally recommended for BCM. For patients with invasive tumors, such schedules usually involve a history and PE (especially CBE) every 3 months for the first 2 years, then every 6 months for the next 2 years, and then yearly. This follow-up is based on the theory that 75 % of recurrences of breast cancer occur in the first 2 years and 10 % in the next 2-year period, with the recurrence rate leveling-off to approximately 1 % per year thereafter [347].

While PE is particularly important in male patients, the value of follow-up mammography for BCM has not been studied and would be expected to be lower than for BCF (see preceding discussion in section entitled "Diagnosis"). An American Society of Clinical Oncology consensus panel on breast cancer follow-up has not found clear efficacy of other tests, such as liver function tests, alkaline phosphatase level, and chest radiographs [348], although such tests are commonly ordered [347]. Both randomized and nonrandomized studies have demonstrated that more intensive tests for detecting recurrence, such as bone scans, computed tomography scans, and tumor markers, do not confer survival benefit and are best reserved for the detection of metastases in symptomatic patients [347, 349].

27.7.2 Testing of Family Members

There is a known association between BCM development and mutations in the BRCA genes; any BCM patient has a greater than 10 % risk of carrying a BRCA, (especially BRCA2) mutation, even in the absence of other first-degree relatives affected with breast, ovarian, or prostate cancer. Accordingly, current NCCN guidelines recommend testing men with BCM ("index relatives") for a BRCA mutation [350]. Nonetheless, it is important to remember that most cases of BCM are "sporadic" (i.e., not associated with known gene mutations) [351] and that BRCA2 gene mutations in men appear to have low penetrance in terms of actually causing the disease [143]; only 4–7 % of patients with BCM report having a first-degree relative of either sex with breast cancer. Penetrance does vary geographically; overall the risk of BCM among BRCA2 mutation carriers is only 6 %, while one series of BCM in Iceland found a rate of 40 % [350]. Also, it should be noted that a 6 % risk of BCM represents a 100-fold increase over population risk [350].

Because BCM is not usually a screened-for disease, the finding that a male individual in a BCM family is a mutation carrier gives little useful preventative information beyond emphasizing that PE and a low threshold for biopsy of any masses or areas of discharge should be a routine part of that person's regular medical care. Such increased awareness and measures may be instituted for these individuals even without genetic testing if the family history is concerning.

For female patients, however, the implications of discovering a BRCA mutation in a male index relative are much greater because such mutations confer on these persons a 56–87 % BCF risk by age 70 [352], a 2–12 % risk of contralateral BCF within 5 years of a diagnosis of BCF [353], and a 27 % ovarian cancer risk by age 70 [354]. In a study in Denmark, Storm and Olsen found female, but not male, offspring of BCM patients to have an increased relative risk (16.4) of breast cancer compared with the general population [355].

Accordingly, we would agree with the NCCN guidelines and with Diez and colleagues that "all new male cases of breast cancer should be regarded as being possibly inherited and should be fully investigated," especially if potential transmissions of BRCA2 mutations to female offspring are involved [350, 356].

Rarer but higher penetrance genetic events which have been associated with an increased risk of BCM include mutations in the PTEN tumor suppressor gene (Cowden's syndrome), AR gene, CHEK2 gene, and CYP17 (especially CYP17A1) polymorphisms [350]. As mentioned earlier, data for AR and CHEK2 is conflicting [92, 127, 156].

27.7.3 Tumor Registry

As mentioned previously, Memorial Sloan-Kettering Cancer Center has maintained a national registry of BCM cases (www.mskcc.org).

27.7.4 Psychological Issues/Resources/Support Groups

The often neglected psychological aspects of men having a "cancer of women" have only recently been recognized in the literature [357], In a phenomenological study from Liverpool investigators noted four key issues for BCM patients: living with the disease, concealment as a coping strategy, contested masculinity (which is worsened by the diminished libido effects and erectile dysfunction of tamoxifen), and interacting with health services geared toward treating breast cancer as a feminized illness [358]. Not surprisingly, investigators at Cardiff University found that a quarter of men with BCM experienced traumatic stress symptoms specific to their diagnosis, heightened by embarrassment, stigma, altered body image, and unmet informational needs in 56 % of patients surveyed, particularly for gender-specific information [359–361]. Furthermore, a recent population-based case-control study reported poorer life satisfaction, physical health, and more days in the last month when mental health was not good in BCM survivors compared to controls [362].

That said, at present gender-specific information on BCM is limited. However, because BCM is similar to BCF in terms of histology, prognostic factors, state-for-stage prognosis, and treatment recommendations, information regarding breast cancer in general is useful to male patients. The educational Web pages of national breast cancer awareness and support organizations such as the American Cancer Society (www.cancer.org), the National Cancer Institute (www.cancer.gov), the Susan G. Komen for the Cure Foundation (www.komen.org), as well as the internet resource www.breastcancer.org do contain fairly good sections on BCM.

Similarly, support groups for BCM are few. The Bridging the Gap Male Breast Cancer Awareness Group, a group formed in the Portland, Oregon area by BCM patients and their families, seeks to raise awareness of BCM to promote earlier diagnosis and treatment. The founders of this group wished to avoid the term *support*; hence, the members chose the term *awareness* instead. Information on this group can be obtained at www.breastfriends.com or by email to lagere@earthlink.net.

The John W. Nick Foundation is a not-for-profit private foundation headquartered in Vero Beach, Florida, founded in 1995 by Nancy Nick, with the help of her mother Patricia and son Adam, in memory of her father John Nick who died from breast cancer at the age of 58 in 1991. The mission of the foundation is to foster education regarding breast cancer in men, including risk, prevention, and treatment. The group has designed an awareness ribbon that is pink throughout (like the well-known ribbon) except for the right tip, which is blue, symbolizing the fact that breast cancer on occasion affects males as well. The foundation can be reached through its Web page at www.johnwnickfoundation.org.

There are very few books or articles available regarding BCM. Sadly, the book "The Warriors Way" by John Cope (Lake Oswego [OR]: Hearts that Care Publishing, 2000) has gone out of print since the author, a BCM patient, succumbed to a recurrence of his disease. Available references in print include:

1. Allen [363]. This is a BCM awareness article that focuses on various awareness and support efforts, especially on the part of a particular survivor, Dave Lyons, who is known to the author.
2. Parker and Parker [364]. A remarkably complete source book providing basic information on BCM and its treatment, medications and nutritional issues, resources and books, and legal and insurance information for patients.
3. Landay [365]. A valuable resource for all cancer survivors, regardless of diagnosis, gender, or age.

Acknowledgments The authors gratefully acknowledge the assistance of Si-Youl Jun, MD, Darius Paduch, MD, Heidi Eppich, and Richard Shih for their assistance in collection of the Oregon data on BCM; Waldemar Schmidt, MD, PhD, Rodney Pommier, MD, John DiTomasso, MD, Heidi Eppich, William Wood, MD, and Dane Moseson, MD, for their contribution to the diagnostic test data for the evaluation of breast masses in males; and Elsevier for granting permission to reprint parts of the resulting publications [9, 241]. The assistance of Irene Perez Vetto, RN, MN, ANP in reviewing and editing the manuscript is also gratefully acknowledged.

References

1. Ellis H. Anatomy of the breast. In: JH I, editor. Textbook of breast disease. St Louis: Mosby; 1992, p. 2.
2. LE Huhges MR, Webster DJT. Benign disorders and diseases of the breast: concepts and clinical management. London: Bailliere Tindall; 1989.
3. Rosen PPOH. Tumors of the mammary gland. Washington DC: Armed Forces Institute of Pathology; 1993.
4. Hall RAJ, Smart GA, et al. Fundamentals of clinical endocrinology. London: Pitman Medical; 1980.
5. Narula HS, Carlson HE. Gynecomastia. Endocrinol Metab Clin North Am. 2007;36(2):497–519.
6. Li RZ, Xia Z, Lin HH, et al. Childhood gynecomastia: a clinical analysis of 240 cases. Chin J Contemp Pediatr (Zhongguo dang dai er ke za zhi). 2007;9(5):404–6.
7. Cakan N, Kamat D. Gynecomastia: evaluation and treatment recommendations for primary care providers. Clin Pediatr. 2007;46(6):487–90.
8. Wilhelm MCLS, Wanebo HJ. Cancer of the male breast. In: Bland KICE, editor. The breast: comprehensive management of benign and malignant disease. Philadelphia: WB Saunders; 1998. p. 1416–20.

9. Vetto J, Jun SY, Paduch D, et al. Stages at presentation, prognostic factors, and outcome of breast cancer in males. Am J Surg. 1999;177(5):379–83.
10. O'Hanlon DM, Kent P, Kerin MJ, et al. Unilateral breast masses in men over 40: a diagnostic dilemma. Am J Surg. 1995;170 (1):24–6.
11. Chantra PK, So GJ, Wollman JS, et al. Mammography of the male breast. AJR Am J Roentgenol. 1995;164(4):853–8.
12. Braunstein GD. Gynecomastia. New Engl J Med. 1993;328 (7):490–5.
13. Johnson RE, Murad MH. Gynecomastia: pathophysiology, evaluation, and management. Mayo Clin Proc. 2009;84 (11):1010–5.
14. Deepinder F, Braunstein GD. Drug-induced gynecomastia: an evidence-based review. Expert Opin Drug Saf. 2012;11(5):779–95.
15. Abaci A, Buyukgebiz A. Gynecomastia: review. Pediatr Endocrinol Rev PER. 2007;5(1):489–99.
16. Handschin AE, Bietry D, Husler R, et al. Surgical management of gynecomastia—a 10-year analysis. World J Surg. 2008;32(1):38–44.
17. Lapid O, Jolink F, Meijer SL. Pathological findings in gynecomastia: analysis of 5113 breasts. Ann Plast Surg. 2015;74 (2):163–6.
18. Zani A, Cozzi DA, Uccini S, et al. Unusual breast enlargement in an infant: a case of breast lipoblastoma. Pediatr Surg Int. 2007;23 (4):361–3.
19. Yamamoto H, Okada Y, Taniguchi H, et al. Intracystic papilloma in the breast of a male given long-term phenothiazine therapy: a case report. Breast Cancer (Tokyo, Japan). 2006;13(1):84–8.
20. Winzer KJ, Menenakos C, Braumann C, et al. Breast mass due to pectoral muscle tuberculosis mimicking breast cancer in a male patient. Int J Infect Dis IJID (Official Publication of the International Society for Infectious Diseases). 2005;9(3):176–7.
21. Vourtsi A, Zervoudis S, Pafiti A, et al. Male breast hemangioma—a rare entity: a case report and review of the literature. Breast J. 2006;12(3):260–2.
22. Ursavas A, Ege E, Bilgen OF, et al. Breast and osteoarticular tuberculosis in a male patient. Diagn Microbiol Infect Dis. 2007;58(4):477–9.
23. Tung CC, Lin JW, Chou FF. Sparganosis in male breast. J Formos Med Assoc (Taiwan yi zhi). 2005;104(2):127–8.
24. Squillaci S, Tallarigo F, Patarino R, et al. Nodular fasciitis of the male breast: a case report. Int J Surg Pathol. 2007;15(1):69–72.
25. Sklair-Levy M, Sella T, Alweiss T, et al. Incidence and management of complex fibroadenomas. AJR Am J Roentgenol. 2008;190(1):214–8.
26. Shin SJ, Rosen PP. Bilateral presentation of fibroadenoma with digital fibroma-like inclusions in the male breast. Arch Pathol Lab Med. 2007;131(7):1126–9.
27. Sharma A, Sen AK, Chaturvedi NK, et al. Myofibroblastoma of male breast: a case report. Indian J Pathol Microbiol. 2007;50 (2):326–8.
28. Reddy KM, Meyer CE, Nakdjevani A, et al. Idiopathic granulomatous mastitis in the male breast. Breast J. 2005;11(1):73.
29. Meshikhes AW, Butt S, Al-Jaroof A, et al. Fibromatosis of the male breast. Breast J. 2005;11(4):294.
30. Marie I, Herve F, Robaday S, et al. Tuberculous myositis mimicking breast cancer. QJM (Journal of the Association of Physicians). 2007;100(1):59.
31. Macchetti AH, Marana HR, Ribeiro-Silva A, et al. Fibromatosis of the male breast: a case report with immunohistochemistry study and review of the literature. Clinics (Sao Paulo, Brazil). 2006;61(4):351–4.
32. Li A, Lui CY, Ying M, et al. Case of fibromatosis of male breast. Australas Radiol. 2007;51 Spec No.:B34–6.
33. Kondi-Pafitis A, Kairi-Vassilatou E, Grapsa D, et al. A large benign vascular neoplasm of the male breast. A case report and review of the literature. Eur J Gynaecol Oncol. 2005;26(4):454–6.
34. Kinoshita S, Kyoda S, Tsuboi K, et al. Huge cavernous hemangioma arising in a male breast. Breast Cancer (Tokyo, Japan). 2005;12(3):231–3.
35. Khachemoune A, Rodriguez C, Lyle S, et al. Genital leiomyoma: surgical excision for both diagnosis and treatment of a unilateral leiomyoma of the male nipple. Dermatol Online J. 2005;11(1):20.
36. Georgountzos V, Ioannidou-Mouzaka L, Tsouroulas M, et al. Benign intracystic papilloma in the male breast. Breast J. 2005;11 (5):361–2.
37. Franco RL, de Moraes Schenka NG, Schenka AA, et al. Cavernous hemangioma of the male breast. Breast J. 2005;11 (6):511–2.
38. Fernandez-Flores A, Crespo LG, Alonso S, et al. Lupus mastitis in the male breast mimicking inflammatory carcinoma. Breast J. 2006;12(3):272–3.
39. Desrosiers L, Rezk S, Larkin A, et al. Myofibroblastoma of the male breast: a rare entity of increasing frequency that can be diagnosed on needle core biopsy. Histopathology. 2007;51 (4):568–72.
40. Aranovich D, Kaminsky O, Schindel A. Retroareolar leiomyoma of the male breast. IMAJ (Israel Medical Association Journal). 2005;7(2):121–2.
41. Ali MZ, Ali FZ. Pilomatrixoma breast mimicking carcinoma. JCPSP (Journal of the College of Physicians and Surgeons-Pakistan). 2005;15(4):248–9.
42. Adeniran A, Al-Ahmadie H, Mahoney MC, et al. Granular cell tumor of the breast: a series of 17 cases and review of the literature. Breast J. 2004;10(6):528–31.
43. Lopez-Rios F, Vargas-Castrillon J, Gonzalez-Palacios F, et al. Breast carcinoma in situ in a male. Report of a case diagnosed by nipple discharge cytology. Acta Cytol. 1998;42(3):742–4.
44. Detraux P, Benmussa M, Tristant H, et al. Breast disease in the male: galactographic evaluation. Radiology. 1985;154(3):605–6.
45. Cutuli B, Dilhuydy JM, De Lafontan B, et al. Ductal carcinoma in situ of the male breast. Analysis of 31 cases. Eur J Cancer (Oxford, England: 1990). 1997;33(1):35–8.
46. Amoroso WL Jr, Robbins GF, Treves N. Serous and serosanguineous discharge from the male nipple. AMA Arch Surg. 1956;73(2):319–29.
47. Morrogh M, King TA. The significance of nipple discharge of the male breast. Breast J. 2009;15(6):632–8.
48. Vaizey C, Burke M, Lange M. Carcinoma of the male breast—a review of 91 patients from the Johannesburg Hospital breast clinics. S Afr J Surg (Suid-Afrikaanse tydskrif vir chirurgie). 1999;37(1):6–8.
49. Stierer M, Rosen H, Weitensfelder W, et al. Male breast cancer: Austrian experience. World J Surg. 1995;19(5):687–92 (discussion 92–3).
50. Salvadori B, Saccozzi R, Manzari A, et al. Prognosis of breast cancer in males: an analysis of 170 cases. Eur J Cancer (Oxford, England: 1990). 1994;30a(7):930–5.
51. Ribeiro G. Male breast carcinoma—a review of 301 cases from the Christie Hospital & Holt Radium Institute,Manchester. Br J Cancer. 1985;51(1):115–9.
52. Heller KS, Rosen PP, Schottenfeld D, et al. Male breast cancer: a clinicopathologic study of 97 cases. Ann Surg. 1978;188(1):60–5.

53. Gough DB, Donohue JH, Evans MM, et al. A 50-year experience of male breast cancer: is outcome changing? Surg Oncol. 1993;2 (6):325–33.
54. Goss PE, Reid C, Pintilie M, et al. Male breast carcinoma: a review of 229 patients who presented to the Princess Margaret hospital during 40 years: 1955–1996. Cancer. 1999;85(3):629–39.
55. Donegan WL, Redlich PN, Lang PJ, et al. Carcinoma of the breast in males: a multiinstitutional survey. Cancer. 1998;83 (3):498–509.
56. Cutuli B, Lacroze M, Dilhuydy JM, et al. Male breast cancer: results of the treatments and prognostic factors in 397 cases. Eur J Cancer (Oxford, England: 1990). 1995;31a(12):1960–4.
57. Borgen PI, Senie RT, McKinnon WM, et al. Carcinoma of the male breast: analysis of prognosis compared with matched female patients. Ann Surg Oncol. 1997;4(5):385–8.
58. Adami HO, Holmberg L, Malker B, et al. Long-term survival in 406 males with breast cancer. Br J Cancer. 1985;52(1):99–103.
59. Anelli TF, Anelli A, Tran KN, et al. Tamoxifen administration is associated with a high rate of treatment-limiting symptoms in male breast cancer patients. Cancer. 1994;74(1):74–7.
60. Teixeira MR, Pandis N, Dietrich CU, et al. Chromosome banding analysis of gynecomastias and breast carcinomas in men. Genes Chromosom Cancer. 1998;23(1):16–20.
61. Society AC. Current facts and figures 2015. Atlanta: 2015.
62. Thomas DB, Jimenez LM, McTiernan A, et al. Breast cancer in men: risk factors with hormonal implications. Am J Epidemiol. 1992;135(7):734–48.
63. Rosenblatt KA, Thomas DB, McTiernan A, et al. Breast cancer in men: aspects of familial aggregation. J Natl Cancer Inst. 1991;83 (12):849–54.
64. Demers PA, Thomas DB, Rosenblatt KA, et al. Occupational exposure to electromagnetic fields and breast cancer in men. Am J Epidemiol. 1991;134(4):340–7.
65. Anderson DE, Badzioch MD. Breast cancer risks in relatives of male breast cancer patients. J Natl Cancer Inst. 1992;84 (14):1114–7.
66. Willsher PC, Leach IH, Ellis IO, et al. Male breast cancer: pathological and immunohistochemical features. Anticancer Res. 1997;17(3c):2335–8.
67. Di Benedetto G, Pierangeli M, Bertani A. Carcinoma of the male breast: an underestimated killer. Plast Reconstr Surg. 1998;102 (3):696–700.
68. Wernberg JA, Yap J, Murekeyisoni C, et al. Multiple primary tumors in men with breast cancer diagnoses: a SEER database review. J Surg Oncol. 2009;99(1):16–9.
69. Hill TD, Khamis HJ, Tyczynski JE, et al. Comparison of male and female breast cancer incidence trends, tumor characteristics, and survival. Ann Epidemiol. 2005;15(10):773–80.
70. Giordano SH, Perkins GH, Broglio K, et al. Adjuvant systemic therapy for male breast carcinoma. Cancer. 2005;104(11):2359–64.
71. Cutuli B. Strategies in treating male breast cancer. Expert Opin Pharmacother. 2007;8(2):193–202.
72. Bradley KL, Tyldesley S, Speers CH, et al. Contemporary systemic therapy for male breast cancer. Clin Breast Cancer. 2014;14(1):31–9.
73. Ioka A, Tsukuma H, Ajiki W, et al. Survival of male breast cancer patients: a population-based study in Osaka, Japan. Jap J Clin Oncol. 2006;36(11):699–703.
74. El-Tamer MB, Komenaka IK, Troxel A, et al. Men with breast cancer have better disease-specific survival than women. Arch Surg (Chicago, Ill: 1960). 2004;139(10):1079–82.
75. Thalib L, Hall P. Survival of male breast cancer patients: population-based cohort study. Cancer Sci. 2009;100(2):292–5.
76. Sasco AJ, Lowenfels AB, Pasker-de Jong P. Review article: epidemiology of male breast cancer. A meta-analysis of published case-control studies and discussion of selected aetiological factors. Int J Cancer (Journal international du cancer). 1993;53 (4):538–49.
77. Mp M. Male breast cancer. In: Harris JRLM, Morrow M, et al., editors. Diseases of the breast. Philadelphia: Lipincott-Raven; 1996. p. 859–63.
78. La Vecchia C, Levi F, Lucchini F. Descriptive epidemiology of male breast cancer in Europe. Int J Cancer (Journal international du cancer). 1992;51(1):62–6.
79. Group USCSW. United states cancer statisitcs: 1999–2012 incidence and mortality web-based report 2015 [cited 2015 October 26th]. Available from: http://www.cdc.gov/uscs.
80. Stang A, Thomssen C. Decline in breast cancer incidence in the United States: what about male breast cancer? Breast Cancer Res Treat. 2008;112(3):595–6.
81. Hodgson NC, Button JH, Franceschi D, et al. Male breast cancer: is the incidence increasing? Ann Surg Oncol. 2004;11(8):751–5.
82. Male breast cancer rates rising. Health news (Waltham, Mass). 2004;10(8):13.
83. Anderson WF, Jatoi I, Tse J, et al. Male breast cancer: a population-based comparison with female breast cancer. J Clin Oncol (Official journal of the American Society of Clinical Oncology). 2010;28(2):232–9.
84. Satram-Hoang S, Ziogas A, Anton-Culver H. Risk of second primary cancer in men with breast cancer. BCR (Breast Cancer Research). 2007;9(1):R10.
85. Bagchi S. Men with breast cancer have high risk of second cancer. Lancet Oncol. 2007;8(3):198.
86. Nahleh ZA, Srikantiah R, Safa M, et al. Male breast cancer in the veterans affairs population: a comparative analysis. Cancer. 2007;109(8):1471–7.
87. Saltzstein EC, Tavaf AM, Latorraca R. Breast carcinoma in a young man. Arch Surg (Chicago, Ill: 1960). 1978;113(7):880–1.
88. O'Malley C, Shema S, White E, et al. Incidence of male breast cancer in california, 1988–2000: racial/ethnic variation in 1759 men. Breast Cancer Res Treat. 2005;93(2):145–50.
89. Goodman MT, Tung KH, Wilkens LR. Comparative epidemiology of breast cancer among men and women in the US, 1996 to 2000. CCC (Cancer Causes & Control). 2006;17(2):127–36.
90. Crew KD, Neugut AI, Wang X, et al. Racial disparities in treatment and survival of male breast cancer. J Clin Oncol (Official Journal of the American Society of Clinical Oncology). 2007;25(9):1089–98.
91. Sineshaw HM, Freedman RA, Ward EM, et al. Black/white disparities in receipt of treatment and survival among men with early-stage breast cancer. J Clin Oncol (Official Journal of the American Society of Clinical Oncology). 2015;33(21):2337–44.
92. Weiss JR, Moysich KB, Swede H. Epidemiology of male breast cancer. Cancer Epidemiol Biomarkers Prev (A Publication of the American Association for Cancer Research, cosponsored by the American Society of Preventive Oncology). 2005;14(1):20–6.
93. Rosenbaum PF, Vena JE, Zielezny MA, et al. Occupational exposures associated with male breast cancer. Am J Epidemiol. 1994;139(1):30–6.
94. Mabuchi K, Bross DS, Kessler II. Risk factors for male breast cancer. J Natl Cancer Inst. 1985;74(2):371–5.
95. Fentiman IS, Fourquet A, Hortobagyi GN. Male breast cancer. Lancet (London, England). 2006;367(9510):595–604.
96. Tynes T. Electromagnetic fields and male breast cancer. Biomed Pharmacother (Biomedecine & pharmacotherapie). 1993;47 (10):425–7.
97. Memon MA, Donohue JH. Male breast cancer. Br J Surg. 1997;84(4):433–5.

98. Hsing AW, McLaughlin JK, Cocco P, et al. Risk factors for male breast cancer (United States). CCC (Cancer Causes Control). 1998;9(3):269–75.
99. von der Weid NX. Adult life after surviving lymphoma in childhood. Support Care Cancer (Official Journal of the Multinational Association of Supportive Care in Cancer). 2008;16 (4):339–45.
100. Yahalom J, Petrek JA, Biddinger PW, et al. Breast cancer in patients irradiated for Hodgkin's disease: a clinical and pathologic analysis of 45 events in 37 patients. J Clin Oncol (Official Journal of the American Society of Clinical Oncology). 1992;10 (11):1674–81.
101. Hauser AR, Lerner IJ, King RA. Familial male breast cancer. Am J Med Genet. 1992;44(6):839–40.
102. Greene MH, Goedert JJ, Bech-Hansen NT, et al. Radiogenic male breast cancer with in vitro sensitivity to ionizing radiation and bleomycin. Cancer Invest. 1983;1(5):379–86.
103. Eldar S, Nash E, Abrahamson J. Radiation carcinogenesis in the male breast. Eur J Surg Oncol (The journal of the European Society of Surgical Oncology and the British Association of Surgical Oncology). 1989;15(3):274–8.
104. Ron E, Ikeda T, Preston DL, et al. Male breast cancer incidence among atomic bomb survivors. J Natl Cancer Inst. 2005;97 (8):603–5.
105. Brinton LA, Cook MB, McCormack V, et al. Anthropometric and hormonal risk factors for male breast cancer: male breast cancer pooling project results. J Natl Cancer Inst. 2014;106(3):djt465.
106. Brinton LA, Carreon JD, Gierach GL, et al. Etiologic factors for male breast cancer in the U.S. Veterans Affairs medical care system database. Breast Cancer Res Treat. 2010;119(1):185–92.
107. Hirose Y, Sasa M, Bando Y, et al. Bilateral male breast cancer with male potential hypogonadism. World J Surg Oncol. 2007;5:60.
108. Casagrande JT, Hanisch R, Pike MC, et al. A case-control study of male breast cancer. Cancer Res. 1988;48(5):1326–30.
109. Humphries MP, Jordan VC, Speirs V. Obesity and male breast cancer: provocative parallels? BMC Med. 2015;13:134.
110. Evans DB, Crichlow RW. Carcinoma of the male breast and Klinefelter's syndrome: is there an association? CA Cancer J Clin. 1987;37(4):246–51.
111. Hultborn R, Hanson C, Kopf I, et al. Prevalence of Klinefelter's syndrome in male breast cancer patients. Anticancer Res. 1997;17 (6d):4293–7.
112. Brinton LA. Breast cancer risk among patients with Klinefelter syndrome. Acta Paediatr (Oslo, Norway: 1992). 2011;100 (6):814–8.
113. Swerdlow AJ, Schoemaker MJ, Higgins CD, et al. Cancer incidence and mortality in men with Klinefelter syndrome: a cohort study. J Natl Cancer Inst. 2005;97(16):1204–10.
114. Yacoub J, Richardson C, Farmer M, et al. Male breast cancer during treatment with leuprolide for prostate cancer. Clin Adv Hematol Oncol H&O. 2007;5(7):555–6 (discussion 6–7).
115. Woo TC, Choo R, Chander S. An unusual case of concurrent breast and prostate cancer. Canad J Urol. 2004;11(5):2390–2.
116. Schlappack OK, Braun O, Maier U. Report of two cases of male breast cancer after prolonged estrogen treatment for prostatic carcinoma. Cancer Detect Prev. 1986;9(3–4):319–22.
117. Symmers WS. Carcinoma of breast in trans-sexual individuals after surgical and hormonal interference with the primary and secondary sex characteristics. Br Med J. 1968;2(5597):83–5.
118. Pritchard TJ, Pankowsky DA, Crowe JP, et al. Breast cancer in a male-to-female transsexual. A case report. JAMA. 1988;259 (15):2278–80.
119. Kanhai RC, Hage JJ, Bloemena E, et al. Mammary fibroadenoma in a male-to-female transsexual. Histopathology. 1999;35 (2):183–5.
120. Brown GR, Jones KT. Incidence of breast cancer in a cohort of 5,135 transgender veterans. Breast Cancer Res Treat. 2015;149 (1):191–8.
121. Asscheman H, Giltay EJ, Megens JA, et al. A long-term follow-up study of mortality in transsexuals receiving treatment with cross-sex hormones. Eur J Endocrinol Eur Fed Endocr Soc. 2011;164(4):635–42.
122. Gooren LJ, van Trotsenburg MA, Giltay EJ, et al. Breast cancer development in transsexual subjects receiving cross-sex hormone treatment. J Sex Med. 2013;10(12):3129–34.
123. Scheike O, Svenstrup B, Frandsen VA. Male breast cancer. II. Metabolism of oestradiol-17 beta in men with breast cancer. J Steroid Biochem. 1973;4(5):489–501.
124. Ballerini P, Recchione C, Cavalleri A, et al. Hormones in male breast cancer. Tumori. 1990;76(1):26–8.
125. Olsson H, Alm P, Aspegren K, et al. Increased plasma prolactin levels in a group of men with breast cancer—a preliminary study. Anticancer Res. 1990;10(1):59–62.
126. Guenel P, Cyr D, Sabroe S, et al. Alcohol drinking may increase risk of breast cancer in men: a European population-based case-control study. CCC (Cancer Causes Control). 2004;15 (6):571–80.
127. Rosenblatt KA, Thomas DB, Jimenez LM, et al. The relationship between diet and breast cancer in men (United States). CCC (Cancer Causes Control). 1999;10(2):107–13.
128. Orr N, Lemnrau A, Cooke R, et al. Genome-wide association study identifies a common variant in RAD51B associated with male breast cancer risk. Nat Genet. 2012;44(11):1182–4.
129. Orr N, Cooke R, Jones M, et al. Genetic variants at chromosomes 2q35, 5p12, 6q25.1, 10q26.13, and 16q12.1 influence the risk of breast cancer in men. PLoS Genet. 2011;7(9):e1002290.
130. Wasielewski M, den Bakker MA, van den Ouweland A, et al. CHEK2 1100delC and male breast cancer in the Netherlands. Breast Cancer Res Treat. 2009;116(2):397–400.
131. Falchetti M, Lupi R, Rizzolo P, et al. BRCA1/BRCA2 rearrangements and CHEK2 common mutations are infrequent in Italian male breast cancer cases. Breast Cancer Res Treat. 2008;110(1):161–7.
132. Hansen J. Elevated risk for male breast cancer after occupational exposure to gasoline and vehicular combustion products. Am J Ind Med. 2000;37(4):349–52.
133. Villeneuve S, Cyr D, Lynge E, et al. Occupation and occupational exposure to endocrine disrupting chemicals in male breast cancer: a case-control study in Europe. Occup Environ Med. 2010;67(12):837–44.
134. Cocco P, Figgs L, Dosemeci M, et al. Case-control study of occupational exposures and male breast cancer. Occup Environ Med. 1998;55(9):599–604.
135. Borgen PI, Wong GY, Vlamis V, et al. Current management of male breast cancer. A review of 104 cases. Annals of surgery. 1992;215(5):451–7 (discussion 7–9).
136. LaRaja RD, Pagnozzi JA, Rothenberg RE, et al. Carcinoma of the breast in three siblings. Cancer. 1985;55(11):2709–11.
137. Brinton LA, Richesson DA, Gierach GL, et al. Prospective evaluation of risk factors for male breast cancer. J Natl Cancer Inst. 2008;100(20):1477–81.
138. Olsson H, Andersson H, Johansson O, et al. Population-based cohort investigations of the risk for malignant tumors in first-degree relatives and wives of men with breast cancer. Cancer. 1993;71(4):1273–8.

139. Kozak FK, Hall JG, Baird PA. Familial breast cancer in males. A case report and review of the literature. Cancer. 1986;58(12):2736–9.
140. Wingren S, van den Heuvel A, Gentile M, et al. Frequent allelic losses on chromosome 13q in human male breast carcinomas. Eur J Cancer (Oxford, England: 1990). 1997;33(14):2393–6.
141. Rubinstein WS. Hereditary breast cancer in Jews. Fam Cancer. 2004;3(3–4):249–57.
142. Chodick G, Struewing JP, Ron E, et al. Similar prevalence of founder BRCA1 and BRCA2 mutations among Ashkenazi and non-Ashkenazi men with breast cancer: evidence from 261 cases in Israel, 1976–1999. Eur J Med Genet. 2008;51(2):141–7.
143. Haraldsson K, Loman N, Zhang QX, et al. BRCA2 germ-line mutations are frequent in male breast cancer patients without a family history of the disease. Cancer Res. 1998;58(7):1367–71.
144. Evans DG, Bulman M, Young K, et al. BRCA1/2 mutation analysis in male breast cancer families from North West England. Fam Cancer. 2008;7(2):113–7.
145. Stratton MR, Ford D, Neuhasen S, et al. Familial male breast cancer is not linked to the BRCA1 locus on chromosome 17q. Nat Genet. 1994;7(1):103–7.
146. Tournier I, Paillerets BB, Sobol H, et al. Significant contribution of germline BRCA2 rearrangements in male breast cancer families. Cancer Res. 2004;64(22):8143–7.
147. Tchou J, Ward MR, Volpe P, et al. Large genomic rearrangement in BRCA1 and BRCA2 and clinical characteristics of men with breast cancer in the United States. Clin Breast Cancer. 2007;7(8):627–33.
148. Karhu R, Laurila E, Kallioniemi A, et al. Large genomic BRCA2 rearrangements and male breast cancer. Cancer Detect Prev. 2006;30(6):530–4.
149. Palomba G, Cossu A, Friedman E, et al. Origin and distribution of the BRCA2-8765delAG mutation in breast cancer. BMC Cancer. 2007;7:132.
150. Miolo G, Puppa LD, Santarosa M, et al. Phenotypic features and genetic characterization of male breast cancer families: identification of two recurrent BRCA2 mutations in north-east of Italy. BMC Cancer. 2006;6:156.
151. Tai YC, Domchek S, Parmigiani G, et al. Breast cancer risk among male BRCA1 and BRCA2 mutation carriers. J Natl Cancer Inst. 2007;99(23):1811–4.
152. Evans DG, Susnerwala I, Dawson J, et al. Risk of breast cancer in male BRCA2 carriers. J Med Genet. 2010;47(10):710–1.
153. Boyd J, Rhei E, Federici MG, et al. Male breast cancer in the hereditary nonpolyposis colorectal cancer syndrome. Breast Cancer Res Treat. 1999;53(1):87–91.
154. Adeyinka A, Mertens F, Bondeson L, et al. Cytogenetic heterogeneity and clonal evolution in synchronous bilateral breast carcinomas and their lymph node metastases from a male patient without any detectable BRCA2 germline mutation. Cancer Genet Cytogenet. 2000;118(1):42–7.
155. Lobaccaro JM, Lumbroso S, Belon C, et al. Androgen receptor gene mutation in male breast cancer. Hum Mol Genet. 1993;2(11):1799–802.
156. Pich A, Margaria E, Chiusa L, et al. Androgen receptor expression in male breast carcinoma: lack of clinicopathological association. Br J Cancer. 1999;79(5–6):959–64.
157. Anelli A, Anelli TF, Youngson B, et al. Mutations of the p53 gene in male breast cancer. Cancer. 1995;75(9):2233–8.
158. Wadie GM, Banever GT, Moriarty KP, et al. Ductal carcinoma in situ in a 16-year-old adolescent boy with gynecomastia: a case report. J Pediatr Surg. 2005;40(8):1349–53.
159. Qureshi K, Athwal R, Cropp G, et al. Bilateral synchronous ductal carcinoma in situ in a young man: case report and review of the literature. Clin Breast Cancer. 2007;7(9):710–2.
160. Pappo I, Wasserman I, Halevy A. Ductal carcinoma in situ of the breast in men: a review. Clin Breast Cancer. 2005;6(4):310–4.
161. Kollmorgen DR, Varanasi JS, Edge SB, et al. Paget's disease of the breast: a 33-year experience. J Am Coll Surg. 1998;187(2):171–7.
162. Anderson WF, Devesa SS. In situ male breast carcinoma in the Surveillance, Epidemiology, and End Results database of the National Cancer Institute. Cancer. 2005;104(8):1733–41.
163. Prasad V, King JM, McLeay W, et al. Bilateral atypical ductal hyperplasia, an incidental finding in gynaecomastia—case report and literature review. Breast (Edinburgh, Scotland). 2005;14(4):317–21.
164. Hamady ZZ, Carder PJ, Brennan TG. Atypical ductal hyperplasia in male breast tissue with gynaecomastia. Histopathology. 2005;47(1):111–2.
165. Ucar AE, Korukluoglu B, Ergul E, et al. Bilateral Paget disease of the male nipple: first report. Breast (Edinburgh, Scotland). 2008;17(3):317–8.
166. Takeuchi T, Komatsuzaki M, Minesaki Y, et al. Paget's disease arising near a male areola without an underlying carcinoma. J Dermatol. 1999;26(4):248–52.
167. Bodnar M, Miller OF 3rd, Tyler W. Paget's disease of the male breast associated with intraductal carcinoma. J Am Acad Dermatol. 1999;40(5 Pt 2):829–31.
168. Choueiri MB, Otrock ZK, Tawil AN, et al. Inflammatory breast cancer in a male. NZ Med J. 2005;118(1218):U1566.
169. Nishimura R, Ohsumi S, Teramoto N, et al. Invasive cribriform carcinoma with extensive microcalcifications in the male breast. Breast Cancer (Tokyo, Japan). 2005;12(2):145–8.
170. Burga AM, Fadare O, Lininger RA, et al. Invasive carcinomas of the male breast: a morphologic study of the distribution of histologic subtypes and metastatic patterns in 778 cases. Virchows Archiv Int J Pathol. 2006;449(5):507–12.
171. Sinha S, Hughes RG, Ryley NG. Papillary carcinoma in a male breast cyst: a diagnostic challenge. Ann R Coll Surg Engl. 2006;88(5):W3–5.
172. Poultsidis AA, Kalra S, Bobrow L, et al. Intracystic papillary carcinoma; solid variant in a male breast—case report and review of the literature. J BUON (Official Journal of the Balkan Union of Oncology). 2002;7(2):157–9.
173. Erhan Y, Erhan Y, Zekioglu O. Pure invasive micropapillary carcinoma of the male breast: report of a rare case. Can J Surg (Journal canadien de chirurgie). 2005;48(2):156–7.
174. Degirmenci B, Gulhan S, Acar M, et al. Large cystic infiltrating ductal carcinoma in male breast. JCU (Journal of clinical ultrasound). 2007;35(2):102–4.
175. Mardi K, Sharma J. Invasive lobular carcinoma of male breast—a case report. Indian J Pathol Microbiol. 2006;49(2):272–4.
176. Erhan Y, Zekioglu O, Erhan Y. Invasive lobular carcinoma of the male breast. Can J Surg (Journal canadien de chirurgie). 2006;49(5):365–6.
177. Moten A, Obirieze A, Wilson LL. Characterizing lobular carcinoma of the male breast using the SEER database. J Surg Res. 2013;185(2):e71–6.
178. Yildirim E, Turhan N, Pak I, et al. Secretory breast carcinoma in a boy. Eur J Surg Oncol (The journal of the European Society of Surgical Oncology and the British Association of Surgical Oncology). 1999;25(1):98–9.
179. Titus J, Sillar RW, Fenton LE. Secretory breast carcinoma in a 9-year-old boy. Aus NZ J Surg. 2000;70(2):144–6.
180. Bhagwandeen BS, Fenton L. Secretory carcinoma of the breast in a nine year old boy. Pathology. 1999;31(2):166–8.
181. Kameyama K, Mukai M, Iri H, et al. Secretory carcinoma of the breast in a 51-year-old male. Pathol Int. 1998;48(12):994–7.

182. Winchester DJ. Male breast carcinoma: a multiinstitutional challenge. Cancer. 1998;83(3):399–400.
183. Murphy CE, Carder PJ, Lansdown MR, et al. Steroid hormone receptor expression in male breast cancer. Eur J Surg Oncol (The Journal of the European Society of Surgical Oncology and the British Association of Surgical Oncology). 2006;32(1):44–7.
184. Sandler B, Carman C, Perry RR. Cancer of the male breast. Am Surg. 1994;60(11):816–20.
185. Mercer RJ, Bryan RM, Bennett RC. Hormone receptors in male breast cancer. Aus NZ J Surg. 1984;54(3):215–8.
186. Munoz de Toro MM, Maffini MV, Kass L, et al. Proliferative activity and steroid hormone receptor status in male breast carcinoma. J Steroid Biochem Mol Biol. 1998;67(4):333–9.
187. Kornegoor R, Verschuur-Maes AH, Buerger H, et al. Immunophenotyping of male breast cancer. Histopathology. 2012;61(6):1145–55.
188. Chavez-Macgregor M, Clarke CA, Lichtensztajn D, et al. Male breast cancer according to tumor subtype and race: a population-based study. Cancer. 2013;119(9):1611–7.
189. Ottini L, Silvestri V, Rizzolo P, et al. Clinical and pathologic characteristics of BRCA-positive and BRCA-negative male breast cancer patients: results from a collaborative multicenter study in Italy. Breast Cancer Res Treat. 2012;134(1):411–8.
190. Korde LA, Zujewski JA, Kamin L, et al. Multidisciplinary meeting on male breast cancer: summary and research recommendations. J Clin Oncol (Official Journal of the American Society of Clinical Oncology). 2010;28(12):2114–22.
191. Bloom KJ, Govil H, Gattuso P, et al. Status of HER-2 in male and female breast carcinoma. Am J Surg. 2001;182(4):389–92.
192. Kornegoor R, Verschuur-Maes AH, Buerger H, et al. Molecular subtyping of male breast cancer by immunohistochemistry. Mod Pathol (An Official Journal of the United States and Canadian Academy of Pathology, Inc.). 2012;25(3):398–404.
193. Leach IH, Ellis IO, Elston CW. c-erb-B-2 expression in male breast carcinoma. J Clin Pathol. 1992;45(10):942.
194. Avisar E, McParland E, Dicostanzo D, et al. Prognostic factors in node-negative male breast cancer. Clin Breast Cancer. 2006;7 (4):331–5.
195. Ottini L, Rizzolo P, Zanna I, et al. BRCA1/BRCA2 mutation status and clinical-pathologic features of 108 male breast cancer cases from Tuscany: a population-based study in central Italy. Breast Cancer Res Treat. 2009;116(3):577–86.
196. Nahleh ZA. Hormonal therapy for male breast cancer: a different approach for a different disease. Cancer Treat Rev. 2006;32 (2):101–5.
197. Foerster R, Foerster FG, Wulff V, et al. Matched-pair analysis of patients with female and male breast cancer: a comparative analysis. BMC Cancer. 2011;11:335.
198. Wenhui Z, Shuo L, Dabei T, et al. Androgen receptor expression in male breast cancer predicts inferior outcome and poor response to tamoxifen treatment. Eur J Endocrinol/Eur Fed Endocr Soc. 2014;171(4):527–33.
199. Song YN, Geng JS, Liu T, et al. Long CAG repeat sequence and protein expression of androgen receptor considered as prognostic indicators in male breast carcinoma. PLoS ONE. 2012;7(12): e52271.
200. Wick MR, Sayadi H, Ritter JH, et al. Low-stage carcinoma of the male breast. A histologic, immunohistochemical, and flow cytometric comparison with localized female breast carcinoma. Am J Clin Pathol. 1999;111(1):59–69.
201. American joint committee on cancer staging manual. 7th ed. New York: Springer; 2010.
202. Chen L, Chantra PK, Larsen LH, et al. Imaging characteristics of malignant lesions of the male breast. Radiographics (A Review Publication of the Radiological Society of North America, Inc.). 2006;26(4):993–1006.
203. Appelbaum AH, Evans GF, Levy KR, et al. Mammographic appearances of male breast disease. Radiographics (A Review Publication of the Radiological Society of North America, Inc.). 1999;19(3):559–68.
204. Cooper RA, Gunter BA, Ramamurthy L. Mammography in men. Radiology. 1994;191(3):651–6.
205. Vetto J, Schmidt W, Pommier R, et al. Accurate and cost-effective evaluation of breast masses in males. Am J Surg. 1998;175(5):383–7.
206. Patterson SK, Helvie MA, Aziz K, et al. Outcome of men presenting with clinical breast problems: the role of mammography and ultrasound. Breast J. 2006;12(5):418–23.
207. Hines SL, Tan WW, Yasrebi M, et al. The role of mammography in male patients with breast symptoms. Mayo Clin Proc. 2007;82 (3):297–300.
208. Hanavadi S, Monypenny IJ, Mansel RE. Is mammography overused in male patients? Breast (Edinburgh, Scotland). 2006;15 (1):123–6.
209. Freedman BC, Keto J, Rosenbaum Smith SM. Screening mammography in men with BRCA mutations: is there a role? Breast J. 2012;18(1):73–5.
210. Groheux D, Hindie E, Marty M, et al. (1)(8)F-FDG-PET/CT in staging, restaging, and treatment response assessment of male breast cancer. Eur J Radiol. 2014;83(10):1925–33.
211. Caruso G, Ienzi R, Piovana G, et al. High-frequency ultrasound in the study of male breast palpable masses. Radiol Med (Torino). 2004;108(3):185–93.
212. Liu M, Husain SS, Hameer HR, et al. Detection of male breast cancer with Tc-99m methoxyisobutyl isonitrile. Clin Nucl Med. 1999;24(11):882–3.
213. Gellett LR, Farmer KD, Vivian GC. Tc-99m sestamibi uptake in a patient with gynecomastia: a potential pitfall in the diagnosis of breast cancer. Clin Nucl Med. 1999;24(6):466.
214. Du Y, Long Y, Ma R. Tc-99 m MIBI uptake by a male breast lymphoma accompanied by diffuse bone marrow metastases. Clin Nucl Med. 1999;24(6):454–5.
215. Eyden BP, Shanks JH, Ioachim E, et al. Myofibroblastoma of breast: evidence favoring smooth-muscle rather than myofibroblastic differentiation. Ultrastruct Pathol. 1999;23(4):249–57.
216. Chalkiadakis G, Petrakis I, Chrysos E, et al. A rare case of benign mesenchymoma of the breast in a man. Eur J Surg Oncol (The Journal of the European Society of Surgical Oncology and the British Association of Surgical Oncology). 1999;25(1):96–7.
217. Talwar S, Prasad N, Gandhi S, et al. Haemangiopericytoma of the adult male breast. Int J Clin Pract. 1999;53(6):485–6.
218. Wang CS, Li H, Gao CF, et al. Hemangiopericytoma of the adult male breast. Saudi Med J. 2011;32(11):1193–5.
219. Grabowski J, Salzstein SL, Sadler GR, et al. Malignant phyllodes tumors: a review of 752 cases. Am Surg. 2007;73(10):967–9.
220. Vignot S, Ledoussal V, Nodiot P, et al. Non-Hodgkin's lymphoma of the breast: a report of 19 cases and a review of the literature. Clin Lymphoma. 2005;6(1):37–42.
221. Mpallas G, Simatos G, Tasidou A, et al. Primary breast lymphoma in a male patient. Breast (Edinburgh, Scotland). 2004;13(5):436–8.
222. Kim SH, Ezekiel MP, Kim RY. Primary lymphoma of the breast: breast mass as an initial symptom. Am J Clin Oncol. 1999;22 (4):381–3.
223. Chanan-Khan A, Holkova B, Goldenberg AS, et al. Non-Hodgkin's lymphoma presenting as a breast mass in patients with HIV infection: a report of three cases. Leukemia Lymphoma. 2005;46(8):1189–93.

224. Wang ZS, Zhan N, Xiong CL, et al. Primary epithelioid angiosarcoma of the male breast: report of a case. Surg Today. 2007;37(9):782–6.
225. Fayette J, Martin E, Piperno-Neumann S, et al. Angiosarcomas, a heterogeneous group of sarcomas with specific behavior depending on primary site: a retrospective study of 161 cases. Ann Oncol (Official Journal of the European Society for Medical Oncology)/ESMO. 2007;18(12):2030–6.
226. Hachisuka A, Takahashi R, Nakagawa S, et al. Lung adenocarcinoma metastasis to the male breast: a case report. Kurume Med J. 2014;61(1–2):35–41.
227. McLean SR, Shousha S, Francis N, et al. Metastatic ductal eccrine adenocarcinoma masquerading as an invasive ductal carcinoma of the male breast. J Cutan Pathol. 2007;34(12):934–8.
228. Ucar N, Kurt OK, Alpar S, et al. Breast metastasis in a male patient with nonsmall cell lung carcinoma. South Med J. 2007;100(8):850–1.
229. Alzaraa A, Thomas GD, Vodovnik A, et al. Merkel cell carcinoma in a male breast: a case report. Breast J. 2007;13 (5):517–9.
230. Nair VJ, Kaushal V, Atri R. Pure squamous cell carcinoma of the breast presenting as a pyogenic abscess: a case report. Clin Breast Cancer. 2007;7(9):713–5.
231. Kshirsagar AY, Wader JV, Langade YB, et al. Adenoid cystic carcinoma of the male breast. Int Surg. 2006;91(4):234–6.
232. de Bree E, Tsagkatakis T, Kafousi M, et al. Breast enlargement in young men not always gynaecomastia: breast cancer in a 22-year-old man. ANZ J Surg. 2005;75(10):914–6.
233. Sneige N, Holder PD, Katz RL, et al. Fine-needle aspiration cytology of the male breast in a cancer center. Diagn Cytopathol. 1993;9(6):691–7.
234. Slavin JL, Baird LI. Fine needle aspiration cytology in male breast carcinoma. Pathology. 1996;28(2):122–4.
235. Gupta RK, Naran S, Dowle CS, et al. The diagnostic impact of needle aspiration cytology of the breast on clinical decision making with an emphasis on the aspiration cytodiagnosis of male breast masses. Diagn Cytopathol. 1991;7(6):637–9.
236. Das DK, Junaid TA, Mathews SB, et al. Fine needle aspiration cytology diagnosis of male breast lesions. A study of 185 cases. Acta Cytol. 1995;39(5):870–6.
237. Joshi A, Kapila K, Verma K. Fine needle aspiration cytology in the management of male breast masses. Nineteen years of experience. Acta Cytologica. 1999;43(3):334–8.
238. Wauters CA, Kooistra BW, de Kievit-van der Heijden IM, et al. Is cytology useful in the diagnostic workup of male breast lesions? A retrospective study over a 16-year period and review of the recent literature. Acta Cytologica. 2010;54(3):259–64.
239. Cooper RA, Ramamurthy L. Epidermal inclusion cysts in the male breast. Can Assoc Radiol J (Journal l'Association canadienne des radiologistes). 1996;47(2):92–3.
240. Vetto JT, Pommier RF, Schmidt WA, et al. Diagnosis of palpable breast lesions in younger women by the modified triple test is accurate and cost-effective. Arch Surg (Chicago, Ill: 1960). 1996;131(9):967–72 (discussion 72–4).
241. Vetto J, Pommier R, Schmidt W, et al. Use of the "triple test" for palpable breast lesions yields high diagnostic accuracy and cost savings. Am J Surg. 1995;169(5):519–22.
242. Morris A, Pommier RF, Schmidt WA, et al. Accurate evaluation of palpable breast masses by the triple test score. Archives of surgery (Chicago, Ill: 1960). 1998;133(9):930–4.
243. Ambrogetti D, Ciatto S, Catarzi S, et al. The combined diagnosis of male breast lesions: a review of a series of 748 consecutive cases. Radiol Med (Torino). 1996;91(4):356–9.
244. Tukel S, Ozcan H. Mammography in men with breast cancer: review of the mammographic findings in five cases. Australas Radiol. 1996;40(4):387–90.
245. Sneige N. Fine-needle aspiration of the breast: a review of 1,995 cases with emphasis on diagnostic pitfalls. Diagn Cytopathol. 1993;9(1):106–12.
246. Layfield LJ. Can fine-needle aspiration replace open biopsy in the diagnosis of palpable breast lesions? Am J Clin Pathol. 1992;98 (2):145–7.
247. Khalbuss WE, Ambaye A, Goodison S, et al. Papillary carcinoma of the breast in a male patient with a treated prostatic carcinoma diagnosed by fine-needle aspiration biopsy: a case report and review of the literature. Diagn Cytopathol. 2006;34(3):214–7.
248. Costa MJ, Tadros T, Hilton G, et al. Breast fine needle aspiration cytology. Utility as a screening tool for clinically palpable lesions. Acta Cytol. 1993;37(4):461–71.
249. Alenda C, Aranda FI, Segui FJ, et al. Secretory carcinoma of the male breast: correlation of aspiration cytology and pathology. Diagn Cytopathol. 2005;32(1):47–50.
250. Somers RG, Sandler GL, Kaplan MJ, et al. Palpable abnormalities of the breast not requiring excisional biopsy. Surg Gynecol Obstet. 1992;175(4):325–8.
251. Samdal F, Kleppe G, Amland PF, et al. Surgical treatment of gynaecomastia. Five years' experience with liposuction. Scand J Plast Reconstr Surg Hand Surg (Nordisk plastikkirurgisk forening [and] Nordisk klubb for handkirurgi). 1994;28(2):123–30.
252. McCluggage WG, Sloan S, Kenny BD, et al. Fine needle aspiration cytology (FNAC) of mammary granular cell tumour: a report of three cases. Cytopathol (Official Journal of the British Society for Clinical Cytology). 1999;10(6):383–9.
253. Shukla R, Pooja B, Radhika S, et al. Fine-needle aspiration cytology of extramammary neoplasms metastatic to the breast. Diagn Cytopathol. 2005;32(4):193–7.
254. Gupta RK. Immunoreactivity of prostate-specific antigen in male breast carcinomas: two examples of a diagnostic pitfall in discriminating a primary breast cancer from metastatic prostate carcinoma. Diagn Cytopathol. 1999;21(3):167–9.
255. Deshpande AH, Munshi MM, Lele VR, et al. Aspiration cytology of extramammary tumors metastatic to the breast. Diagn Cytopathol. 1999;21(5):319–23.
256. Dey P, Luthra UK, Prasad A, et al. Cytologic grading and DNA image cytometry of breast carcinoma on fine needle aspiration cytology smears. Anal Quant Cytol Histol/Int Acad Cytol [and] Am Soc Cytol. 1999;21(1):17–20.
257. Volpe CM, Raffetto JD, Collure DW, et al. Unilateral male breast masses: cancer risk and their evaluation and management. Am Surg. 1999;65(3):250–3.
258. Dershaw DD, Borgen PI, Deutch BM, et al. Mammographic findings in men with breast cancer. AJR Am J Roentgenol. 1993;160(2):267–70.
259. Kinne DHT. Male breast cancer. In: Harris JHS, Henderson IC, editors. Breast diseases. Philadelphia: Lippincott; 1991. p. 782–9.
260. Hodson GR, Urdaneta LF, Al-Jurf AS, et al. Male breast carcinoma. Am Surg. 1985;51(1):47–9.
261. Scott-Conner CE, Jochimsen PR, Menck HR, et al. An analysis of male and female breast cancer treatment and survival among demographically identical pairs of patients. Surgery. 1999;126 (4):775–80 (discussion 80–1).
262. Fields EC, DeWitt P, Fisher CM, et al. Management of male breast cancer in the United States: a surveillance, epidemiology and end results analysis. Int J Radiat Oncol Biol Phys. 2013;87 (4):747–52.
263. Rai B, Ghoshal S, Sharma SC. Breast cancer in males: a PGIMER experience. J Cancer Res Ther. 2005;1(1):31–3.

264. Golshan M, Rusby J, Dominguez F, et al. Breast conservation for male breast carcinoma. Breast (Edinburgh, Scotland). 2007;16 (6):653–6.
265. Czene K, Bergqvist J, Hall P, et al. How to treat male breast cancer. Breast (Edinburgh, Scotland). 2007;16(Suppl 2):S147–54.
266. Fogh S, Kachnic LA, Goldberg SI, et al. Localized therapy for male breast cancer: functional advantages with comparable outcomes using breast conservation. Clin Breast Cancer. 2013;13(5):344–9.
267. Cloyd JM, Hernandez-Boussard T, Wapnir IL. Outcomes of partial mastectomy in male breast cancer patients: analysis of SEER, 1983–2009. Ann Surg Oncol. 2013;20(5):1545–50.
268. Luini A, Gatti G, Brenelli F, et al. Male breast cancer in a young patient treated with nipple-sparing mastectomy: case report and review of the literature. Tumori. 2007;93(1):118–20.
269. Haid A, Knauer M, Dunzinger S, et al. Intra-operative sonography: a valuable aid during breast-conserving surgery for occult breast cancer. Ann Surg Oncol. 2007;14(11):3090–101.
270. Rusby JE, Smith BL, Dominguez FJ, et al. Sentinel lymph node biopsy in men with breast cancer: a report of 31 consecutive procedures and review of the literature. Clin Breast Cancer. 2006;7(5):406–10.
271. Intra M, Soteldo J, Bassani G. Sentinel lymph node biopsy in ductal carcinoma in situ of the male breast. Breast J. 2005;11 (2):154.
272. Hill AD, Borgen PI, Cody HS 3rd. Sentinel node biopsy in male breast cancer. Eur J Surg Oncol (The Journal of the European Society of Surgical Oncology and the British Association of Surgical Oncology). 1999;25(4):442–3.
273. Gentilini O, Chagas E, Zurrida S, et al. Sentinel lymph node biopsy in male patients with early breast cancer. Oncologist. 2007;12(5):512–5.
274. Boughey JC, Bedrosian I, Meric-Bernstam F, et al. Comparative analysis of sentinel lymph node operation in male and female breast cancer patients. J Am Coll Surg. 2006;203(4):475–80.
275. Flynn LW, Park J, Patil SM, et al. Sentinel lymph node biopsy is successful and accurate in male breast carcinoma. J Am Coll Surg. 2008;206(4):616–21.
276. Camus MG, Joshi MG, Mackarem G, et al. Ductal carcinoma in situ of the male breast. Cancer. 1994;74(4):1289–93.
277. Silverstein MJ, Craig PH, Lagios MD, et al. Developing a prognostic index for ductal carcinoma in situ of the breast. Are we there yet? Cancer. 1996;78(5):1138–40.
278. Uematsu M, Okada M, Ataka K. Two-step approach for the operation of male breast cancer: report of a case at high risk for surgery. Kobe J Med Sci. 1998;44(4):163–8.
279. Atahan L, Yildiz F, Selek U, et al. Postoperative radiotherapy in the treatment of male breast carcinoma: a single institute experience. J Natl Med Assoc. 2006;98(4):559–63.
280. Yu E, Suzuki H, Younus J, et al. The impact of post-mastectomy radiation therapy on male breast cancer patients–a case series. Int J Radiat Oncol Biol Phys. 2012;82(2):696–700.
281. Stranzl H, Mayer R, Quehenberger F, et al. Adjuvant radiotherapy in male breast cancer. Radiother Oncol (Journal of the European Society for Therapeutic Radiology and Oncology). 1999;53(1):29–35.
282. Csillag C. Radiotherapy after mastectomy more common in men. Lancet Oncol. 2005;6(8):547.
283. Harlan LC, Zujewski JA, Goodman MT, et al. Breast cancer in men in the United States: a population-based study of diagnosis, treatment, and survival. Cancer. 2010;116(15):3558–68.
284. Di Lauro L, Pizzuti L, Barba M, et al. Efficacy of chemotherapy in metastatic male breast cancer patients: a retrospective study. J Exp Clin Cancer Res. 2015;34:26.
285. Bagley CS, Wesley MN, Young RC, et al. Adjuvant chemotherapy in males with cancer of the breast. Am J Clin Oncol. 1987;10 (1):55–60.
286. Walshe JM, Berman AW, Vatas U, et al. A prospective study of adjuvant CMF in males with node positive breast cancer: 20-year follow-up. Breast Cancer Res Treat. 2007;103(2):177–83.
287. Jaiyesimi IA, Buzdar AU, Sahin AA, et al. Carcinoma of the male breast. Ann Intern Med. 1992;117(9):771–7.
288. Carmona-Bayonas A. Potential benefit of maintenance trastuzumab and anastrozole therapy in male advanced breast cancer. Breast (Edinburgh, Scotland). 2007;16(3):323–5.
289. Rugo HS, Brufsky AM, Ulcickas Yood M, et al. Racial disparities in treatment patterns and clinical outcomes in patients with HER2-positive metastatic breast cancer. Breast Cancer Res Treat. 2013;141(3):461–70.
290. Martin M, Makhson A, Gligorov J, et al. Phase II study of bevacizumab in combination with trastuzumab and capecitabine as first-line treatment for HER-2-positive locally recurrent or metastatic breast cancer. Oncologist. 2012;17(4):469–75.
291. McCarthy P, Hurd D, Rowlings P, et al. Autotransplants in men with breast cancer. ABMTR Breast Cancer Working Committee. Autologous blood and marrow transplant registry. Bone Marrow Transplant. 1999;24(4):365–8.
292. Tranum BL, McDonald B, Thigpen T, et al. Adriamycin combinations in advanced breast cancer. A Southwest Oncology Group Study. Cancer. 1982;49(5):835–9.
293. Tormey DC, Gelman R, Band PR, et al. Comparison of induction chemotherapies for metastatic breast cancer. An Eastern Cooperative Oncology Group Trial. Cancer. 1982;50(7):1235–44.
294. Misset JL, Dieras V, Gruia G, et al. Dose-finding study of docetaxel and doxorubicin in first-line treatment of patients with metastatic breast cancer. Ann Oncol (Official Journal of the European Society for Medical Oncology/ESMO. 1999;10 (5):553–60.
295. Jassem J, Pienkowski T, Pluzanska A, et al. Doxorubicin and paclitaxel versus fluorouracil, doxorubicin, and cyclophosphamide as first-line therapy for women with metastatic breast cancer: final results of a randomized phase III multicenter trial. J Clin Oncol (Official Journal of the American Society of Clinical Oncology). 2001;19(6):1707–15.
296. Buzdar AU, Kau SW, Smith TL, et al. Ten-year results of FAC adjuvant chemotherapy trial in breast cancer. Am J Clin Oncol. 1989;12(2):123–8.
297. Ribeiro G, Swindell R. Adjuvant tamoxifen for male breast cancer (MBC). Br J Cancer. 1992;65(2):252–4.
298. Xu S, Yang Y, Tao W, et al. Tamoxifen adherence and its relationship to mortality in 116 men with breast cancer. Breast Cancer Res Treat. 2012;136(2):495–502.
299. Agrawal A, Cheung KL, Robertson JF. Fulvestrant in advanced male breast cancer. Breast Cancer Res Treat. 2007;101(1):123.
300. Zagouri F, Sergentanis TN, Chrysikos D, et al. Fulvestrant and male breast cancer: a pooled analysis. Breast Cancer Res Treat. 2015;149(1):269–75.
301. de la Haba Rodriguez JR, Porras Quintela I, Pulido Cortijo G, et al. Fulvestrant in advanced male breast cancer. Ann Oncol (Official Journal of the European Society for Medical Oncology/ESMO). 2009;20(11):1896–7.
302. Zabolotny BP, Zalai CV, Meterissian SH. Successful use of letrozole in male breast cancer: a case report and review of hormonal therapy for male breast cancer. J Surg Oncol. 2005;90 (1):26–30.
303. Arriola E, Hui E, Dowsett M, et al. Aromatase inhibitors and male breast cancer. Clin Transl Oncol (Official Publication of the Federation of Spanish Oncology Societies and of the National Cancer Institute of Mexico). 2007;9(3):192–4.

304. Doyen J, Italiano A, Largillier R, et al. Aromatase inhibition in male breast cancer patients: biological and clinical implications. Ann Oncol (Official Journal of the European Society for Medical Oncology/ESMO). 2010;21(6):1243–5.
305. Eggemann H, Ignatov A, Smith BJ, et al. Adjuvant therapy with tamoxifen compared to aromatase inhibitors for 257 male breast cancer patients. Breast Cancer Res Treat. 2013;137(2):465–70.
306. Maugeri-Sacca M, Barba M, Vici P, et al. Aromatase inhibitors for metastatic male breast cancer: molecular, endocrine, and clinical considerations. Breast Cancer Res Treat. 2014;147 (2):227–35.
307. Soon Wong N, Seong Ooi W, Pritchard KI. Role of gonadotropin-releasing hormone analog in the management of male metastatic breast cancer is uncertain. J Clin Oncol (Official Journal of the American Society of Clinical Oncology). 2007;25 (24):3787.
308. Di Lauro L, Pizzuti L, Barba M, et al. Role of gonadotropin-releasing hormone analogues in metastatic male breast cancer: results from a pooled analysis. J Hematol Oncol. 2015;8:53.
309. Zagouri F, Sergentanis TN, Koutoulidis V, et al. Aromatase inhibitors with or without gonadotropin-releasing hormone analogue in metastatic male breast cancer: a case series. Br J Cancer. 2013;108(11):2259–63.
310. Di Lauro L, Vici P, Del Medico P, et al. Letrozole combined with gonadotropin-releasing hormone analog for metastatic male breast cancer. Breast Cancer Res Treat. 2013;141(1):119–23.
311. Dakin Hache K, Gray S, Barnes PJ, et al. Clinical and pathological correlations in male breast cancer: intratumoral aromatase expression via tissue microarray. Breast Cancer Res Treat. 2007;105(2):169–75.
312. Farrow JH, Adair FE. Effect of orchidectomy on skeletal metastases from cancer of the male breast. Science (New York, NY). 1942;95(2478):654.
313. Singh M, Kotagiri AK, Teimory M. Choroidal and optic disc metastases in a man with metachronous and metastatic breast carcinoma. Acta Ophthalmol Scand. 2007;85(6):688–9.
314. Lam A, Shields CL, Shields JA. Uveal metastases from breast carcinoma in three male patients. Ophthalmic Surg Lasers Imaging (The Official Journal of the International Society for Imaging in the Eye). 2006;37(4):320–3.
315. Cohen VM, Moosavi R, Hungerford JL. Tamoxifen-induced regression of a choroidal metastasis in a man. Arch Ophthalmol (Chicago, Ill: 1960). 2005;123(8):1153–4.
316. Karakuzu A, Koc M, Ozdemir S. Multiple cutaneous metastases from male breast carcinoma. J Am Acad Dermatol. 2006;55 (6):1101–2.
317. Ai-Ping F, Yue Q, Yan W. A case report of remote cutaneous metastasis from male breast carcinoma. Int J Dermatol. 2007;46 (7):738–9.
318. Kesting MR, Loeffelbein DJ, Holzle F, et al. Male breast cancer metastasis presenting as submandibular swelling. Auris Nasus Larynx. 2006;33(4):483–5.
319. Fontana S, Ghilardi R, Barbaglio A, et al. Male breast cancer with mandibular metastasis. A case report. Minerva Stomatol. 2007;56 (4):225–30.
320. Hultborn R, Friberg S, Hultborn KA, et al. Male breast carcinoma. II. A study of the total material reported to the Swedish Cancer Registry 1958–1967 with respect to treatment, prognostic factors and survival. Acta Oncol (Stockholm, Sweden). 1987;26(5):327–41.
321. Guinee VF, Olsson H, Moller T, et al. The prognosis of breast cancer in males. A report of 335 cases. Cancer. 1993;71(1):154–61.
322. Dr C. Regression models and life-tables. J R Stat Sac. 1972;4:187–220.
323. Hill A, Yagmur Y, Tran KN, et al. Localized male breast carcinoma and family history. An analysis of 142 patients. Cancer. 1999;86(5):821–5.
324. Hatschek T, Wingren S, Carstensen J, et al. DNA content and S-phase fraction in male breast carcinomas. Acta Oncol (Stockholm, Sweden). 1994;33(6):609–13.
325. Hemminki K, Scelo G, Boffetta P, et al. Second primary malignancies in patients with male breast cancer. Br J Cancer. 2005;92(7):1288–92.
326. Liu D, Xie G, Chen M. Clinicopathologic characteristics and survival of male breast cancer. Int J Clin Oncol. 2014;19(2):280–7.
327. Kreusel KM, Heimann H, Wiegel T, et al. Choroidal metastasis in men with metastatic breast cancer. Am J Ophthalmol. 1999;128 (2):253–5.
328. Kim JH, Benson PM, Beard JS, et al. Male breast carcinoma with extensive metastases to the skin. J Am Acad Dermatol. 1998;38(6 Pt 1):995–6.
329. Garcia GH, Weinberg DA, Glasgow BJ, et al. Carcinoma of the male breast metastatic to both orbits. Ophthalmic Plast Reconstr Surg. 1998;14(2):130–3.
330. Fullerton JT, Lantz J, Sadler GR. Breast cancer among men: raising awareness for primary prevention. J Am Acad Nurse Pract. 1997;9(5):211–6.
331. Malkin D. p53 and the Li-Fraumeni syndrome. Biochim Biophys Acta. 1994;1198(2–3):197–213.
332. Kaplan ELMP. Nonparametric estimation from incomplete observations. J Am Statist Sac. 1958;53:457–81.
333. Peto RPJ. Asymptomatically efficient rank invariant test procedures. J R Statist Sac. 1972;35:185–206.
334. Fritz A. SEER cancer statistics review, 1973–1995. Bethesda: NCI Cancer Statistics Brack; 1998.
335. Wagner JL, Thomas CR Jr, Koh WJ, et al. Carcinoma of the male breast: update 1994. Med Pediatr Oncol. 1995;24(2):123–32.
336. Milias S, Kalekou H, Bobos M, et al. Immunohistochemical investigation of CD34 antigen in male breast carcinoma. Clin Exp Med. 2007;7(3):122–6.
337. Rudlowski C, Schulten HJ, Golas MM, et al. Comparative genomic hybridization analysis on male breast cancer. Int J Cancer (Journal international du cancer). 2006;118(10):2455–60.
338. Andre S, Pinto AE, Laranjeira C, et al. Male and female breast cancer—differences in DNA ploidy, p21 and p53 expression reinforce the possibility of distinct pathways of oncogenesis. Pathobiol (Journal of Immunopathology, Molecular and Cellular Biology). 2007;74(6):323–7.
339. Johansson I, Ringner M, Hedenfalk I. The landscape of candidate driver genes differs between male and female breast cancer. PLoS ONE. 2013;8(10):e78299.
340. Pinto R, Pilato B, Ottini L, et al. Different methylation and microRNA expression pattern in male and female familial breast cancer. J Cell Physiol. 2013;228(6):1264–9.
341. Fassan M, Baffa R, Palazzo JP, et al. MicroRNA expression profiling of male breast cancer. BCR (Breast Cancer Research). 2009;11(4):R58.
342. Lehmann U, Streichert T, Otto B, et al. Identification of differentially expressed microRNAs in human male breast cancer. BMC Cancer. 2010;10:109.
343. Sosnovskikh I, Naninato P, Gatti G, et al. Synchronous bilateral breast cancer in men: a case report and review of the literature. Tumori. 2007;93(2):225–7.
344. Melenhorst J, van Berlo CL, Nijhuis PH. Simultaneous bilateral breast cancer in a male: a case report and review of the literature. Acta Chir Belg. 2005;105(5):531–2.

345. McQueen A, Cox J, Desai S, et al. Multifocal male breast cancer: a case report. Clin Breast Cancer. 2007;7(7):570–2.
346. Franceschini G, D'Alba P, Costantini M, et al. Synchronous bilateral breast carcinoma in a 50-year-old man with 45, X/46, XY mosaic karyotype: report of a case. Surg Today. 2006;36 (1):71–5.
347. Joseph E, Hyacinthe M, Lyman GH, et al. Evaluation of an intensive strategy for follow-up and surveillance of primary breast cancer. Ann Surg Oncol. 1998;5(6):522–8.
348. Recommended breast cancer surveillance guidelines. Am Soc Clin Oncol (Journal of clinical oncology: official journal of the American Society of Clinical Oncology). 1997;15(5):2149–56.
349. Impact of follow-up testing on survival and health-related quality of life in breast cancer patients. A multicenter randomized controlled trial. The GIVIO investigators. JAMA. 1994;271 (20):1587–92.
350. Nahleh Z, Girnius S. Male breast cancer: a gender issue. Nat Clin Pract Oncol. 2006;3(8):428–37.
351. Tirkkonen M, Kainu T, Loman N, et al. Somatic genetic alterations in BRCA2-associated and sporadic male breast cancer. Genes Chromosom Cancer. 1999;24(1):56–61.
352. Struewing JP, Hartge P, Wacholder S, et al. The risk of cancer associated with specific mutations of BRCA1 and BRCA2 among Ashkenazi Jews. New Engl J Med. 1997;336(20):1401–8.
353. Verhoog LC, Brekelmans CT, Seynaeve C, et al. Survival in hereditary breast cancer associated with germline mutations of BRCA2. J Clin Oncol (Official Journal of the American Society of Clinical Oncology). 1999;17(11):3396–402.
354. Ford D, Easton DF, Stratton M, et al. Genetic heterogeneity and penetrance analysis of the BRCA1 and BRCA2 genes in breast cancer families. The breast cancer linkage consortium. Am J Hum Genet. 1998;62(3):676–89.
355. Storm HH, Olsen J. Risk of breast cancer in offspring of male breast-cancer patients. Lancet (London, England). 1999;353 (9148):209.
356. Diez O, Cortes J, Domenech M, et al. BRCA2 germ-line mutations in Spanish male breast cancer patients. Ann Oncol (Official Journal of the European Society for Medical Oncology/ESMO). 2000;11(1):81–4.
357. Agrawal A, Ayantunde AA, Rampaul R, et al. Male breast cancer: a review of clinical management. Breast Cancer Res Treat. 2007;103(1):11–21.
358. Donovan T, Flynn M. What makes a man a man? The lived experience of male breast cancer. Cancer Nurs. 2007;30(6):464–70.
359. Iredale R, Williams B, Brain K, et al. The information needs of men with breast cancer. Br J Nurs (Mark Allen Publishing). 2007;16(9):540–4.
360. Iredale R, Brain K, Williams B, et al. The experiences of men with breast cancer in the United Kingdom. Eur J Cancer (Oxford, England: 1990). 2006;42(3):334–41.
361. Brain K, Williams B, Iredale R, et al. Psychological distress in men with breast cancer. J Clin Oncol (Official Journal of the American Society of Clinical Oncology). 2006;24(1):95–101.
362. Andrykowski MA. Physical and mental health status and health behaviors in male breast cancer survivors: a national, population-based, case-control study. Psycho-Oncology. 2012;21(9):927–34.
363. Allen T. This man survived breast cancer. Esquire. 2000:103–9.
364. Parker JN, Parker PM. The official patient's sourcebook on male breast cancer: a revised and updated directory for the internet age. San Diego: Icon Health; 2002.
365. David L. Be prepared: the complete financial, legal, and practical guide to living with cancer, HIV, and other life-challenging conditions. New York: Macmillan; 2000.
366. Vourtsi A, Kehagias D, Antoniou A, et al. Male breast myofibroblastoma and MR findings. J Comput Assist Tomogr. 1999;23(3):414–6.
367. Rice HE, Acosta A, Brown RL, et al. Juvenile papillomatosis of the breast in male infants: two case reports. Pediatr Surg Int. 2000;16(1–2):104–6.

Breast Cancer in the Older Adult 28

Emily J. Guerard, Madhuri V. Vithala, and Hyman B. Muss

28.1 Introduction and Epidemiology

Breast cancer is the most common cancer among 65 years and older women in the United States. The major risk factor for being diagnosed with breast cancer is increasing age. The median age of a new diagnosis of breast cancer is 61 years with more than half of the deaths from breast cancer occurring in women aged 65 years and older [1]. Nearly 90 % of woman diagnosed with breast cancer are surviving at least 5 years [1]; consequently, there are a substantial number of older breast cancer survivors. The incidence of cancer in older adults is expected to increase by 67 % by the year 2030, so there is now and will continue to be a need to better understand how to care for and treat older women with breast cancer [2]. The majority of older patients with breast cancer are diagnosed with Stage I or Stage II disease and survival for early stage disease is similar across age groups [3, 4]. About 10 % of older patients present with Stage III or Stage IV disease and some with unknown stage at diagnosis [5].

Older women with breast cancer are less likely to be managed according to guidelines [5, 6] and under treatment may result in poorer survival [7, 8]. Moreover, older women are less likely to be enrolled in clinical trials [9, 10] but when offered the opportunity are as likely to participate as younger patients—with about 50 % participation [11]. Barriers to trial participation include both physician bias about age and concerns regarding toxicity and patient and family bias that treatment is not worthwhile or too toxic [11, 12]. The objectives of this chapter are to review the clinical assessment of the older adult with breast cancer with a focus on the importance of comorbidity, prevention, screening, treatment of primary breast cancer, adjuvant systemic therapy, treatment of metastatic disease, and clinical trials.

E.J. Guerard (✉) · H.B. Muss
Medicine, Division of Hematology Oncology, University of North Carolina, 170 Manning Drive, Campus Box 7305, Chapel Hill, NC 27599, USA
e-mail: eguerard@unch.unc.edu

H.B. Muss
e-mail: hyman_muss@med.unc.edu

M.V. Vithala
Duke University, Durham Veteran Affairs, 508 Fulton St. (111G), Durham, NC 27705, USA
e-mail: madhuri.vithala@va.gov

28.2 Clinical Assessment of the Older Adult with Breast Cancer

Older adults are a heterogeneous population in regards to their overall health. Given this heterogeneity, estimating life expectancy should play a major role in decision making for older women with breast cancer. It has been estimated that at the age of 75, the top 25th percentile of women will live on average 17 years, the 50th percentile an average of 11.9 years, and lowest 25th percentile an average of 6.8 years [13]. Life expectancy is difficult to estimate during a routine oncologic assessment. Fortunately, there are several tools available to the oncologist to assist with estimating life expectancy. The easiest and most assessable tool is ePrognosis (www.ePrognosis.org). The ePrognosis website serves as a repository of published prognostic indices where busy clinicians can quickly access and obtain evidence-based information on a patient's estimated life expectancy. The Schonberg index is most commonly used for estimating 5-year mortality and the Lee index for 10-year mortality [14, 15]. Estimating a patient's life expectancy is important when considering the risk and benefits of adjuvant therapies.

Given the heterogeneity of older adults, an assessment of functional or physiologic age is also important as one cannot rely simply on chronologic age as a reliable estimate of a patient's functional status. The geriatric assessment (GA) gives the oncologist a tool to assess the functional age of older patients with breast and other cancers. The GA comprises an evaluation of physical function, instrumental activities of daily living, activities of daily living, falls, cognition, social support and activity, mental health, nutritional status, polypharmacy, and comorbid medical conditions. The Cancer and Aging Research Group (CARG) GA

I. Jatoi and A. Rody (eds.), *Management of Breast Diseases*, DOI 10.1007/978-3-319-46356-8_28

was developed specifically for patients with cancer and has proven feasibility in academic and community oncology clinics [16, 17]. The GA can accurately predict morbidity and mortality from cancer [18] and uncovers problems in patients with a provider-reported normal Karnofsky performance status (KPS) [19]. In addition, the GA has been shown to be predictive of chemotherapy toxicity in older adults with cancer [20, 21]. Although there is uncertainty as to whether information obtained from the GA can lead to interventions that improve survival, the GA can identify problems and provide appropriate interventions that maintain function and improve quality of life for older patients with cancer [22]. Recommendations for the use of the GA have been developed by the International Society of Geriatric Oncology (SIOG) and provide helpful guidelines for clinicians [23].

Concurrent with a breast cancer diagnosis, older women are also more likely to have other coexisting illness or "comorbidity" that can be captured during a GA. In one major study of comorbidity, 1800 postmenopausal women with breast cancer, diabetes, renal failure, stroke, liver disease, a previous malignant tumor, as well as smoking were significant predictors of shortened survival even when accounting for age and breast cancer stage [5]. All facets of breast cancer care may be effected by comorbid illness, including screening, pretreatment assessment, and the use of surgery, radiation, and adjuvant therapy. For example, in an observational study of 936 women, age 40–84 years with breast cancer, patients with three or more of seven selected comorbidities had a 20-fold higher rate of mortality from non-breast cancer causes and a fourfold higher rate of all-cause mortality when compared to those without any comorbid conditions. An early diagnosis of breast cancer in this study conferred no survival advantage in women with severe comorbidity [24]. These data suggest that older women with severe comorbidity are unlikely to derive a major benefit from adjuvant systemic therapy. Focusing on the assessment of functional or physiologic age as opposed to chronologic age will remind health care professionals that assessments such as the GA are an important factor in managing older patients with breast cancer.

28.3 Breast Cancer Prevention

Primary prevention of breast cancer requires modifying factors that are associated with an increase in risk. Obesity is a risk factor for breast cancer in older women [25] and may also be a predictor of breast cancer recurrence [26]. Although it is uncertain as to the value of weight reduction in reducing breast cancer risk, overweight elders might reduce cardiac as well as other non-breast cancer risk with weight reduction. Older women are less likely than younger patients to be carriers of the BRCA-1 and BRCA-2 genes, but a careful family history is mandatory for all patients with breast cancer, irrespective of age, as older women may be gene carriers resulting in important management and family considerations. Although the role of exercise is controversial as a risk reducing strategy for breast cancer in older women, it should be encouraged for its other major health benefits.

Chemoprevention of breast cancer with either tamoxifen, raloxifene, or an aromatase inhibitor is an effective risk reduction strategy in high risk women [27–29]. However, neither of these agents have been associated with improvements in survival and both are associated with increased risks of endometrial cancer and thromboembolism in older women. The benefits of tamoxifen use diminish with increasing age because older women have higher risks of mortality from competing causes, such as cardiovascular disease [30]. At present, only older women with an exceeding high risk for breast cancer should be considered for chemoprevention. Raloxifene may be a better choice than tamoxifen for these older patients as it is less likely to be associated with cataracts or thromboembolism [28]. If considering chemoprevention for older women, there should be a careful discussion with the patient about the risks, benefits, and alternatives of such therapy.

28.3.1 Screening

Mammographic screening has been shown to be effective in reducing breast cancer mortality in women aged between 40 and 74 years [31]. The sensitivity, specificity, and positive predictive value of mammography for detecting cancer increases with age as ductal tissue is replaced by fat resulting in an increase in the radiolucency of breast tissue. The evidence of the effectiveness of screening mammography in women age 75 years and older is limited and was recently summarized in a review by Walter et al. [32]. In one study of women of the age 80 years and older, those who obtained mammograms on a more regular basis were detected with lower stage breast cancer and had higher breast cancer-specific survival; however, deaths from other causes were also lower in women who received more frequent mammograms, suggesting a bias for mammography use among healthier older patients [33].

The precise age at which to discontinue screening mammography is uncertain. Older women face a higher probability of developing and dying of breast cancer but also many times have competing comorbidities that limit their life expectancy. The American Cancer Society recommends setting no upper age limit and the decision to stop regular screening mammograms should be individualized based on the patients overall health, longevity, and ability to undergo treatment if a breast cancer is diagnosed [34]. The U.S.

Preventive Services Task Force provides no recommendations for women over the age of 75 years as there is insufficient evidence to make a recommendation. In a recent review by Walter et al., the authors recommended to stop screening mammograms in women who have an estimated life expectancy of less than 10 years [32]. Life expectancy for older adults can be estimated using validated indices found on ePrognosis.org as described above. As prospective trials are unlikely to be performed in this older age group, the decision to stop screening mammograms will likely need to be individualized to each patient based on their estimated life expectancy, a discussion with the patient about their values/preferences and the risks and benefits to continued screening.

28.4 Treatment of Primary Breast Cancer

28.4.1 Surgery or Endocrine Therapy

Surgery is a cornerstone for the treatment of primary breast cancers. Older women in reasonable health tolerate surgery well and its safety is well established in older adults [35, 36]. Breast conserving therapy is now standard care for all patients with early stage breast cancer and should be offered irrespective of age. Body image is important in older women and they should be told about the effects mastectomy and breast conservation have on the body image. Older women should be offered breast conservation and or mastectomy with reconstruction similar to younger patients [37].

Primary endocrine therapy with tamoxifen or aromatase inhibitors (AIs) has been shown to be effective in controlling hormone receptor positive breast cancer in older women. Compared with endocrine therapy, surgery is associated with superior local control. Although endocrine therapy may result in local control for several years, the majority of patients are likely to have tumor progression after 5 years, resulting in the need for surgery. A Cochrane meta-analysis comparing surgery with endocrine therapy in women 70 years and older has confirmed the superiority of surgery for local control, but did not show a survival benefit [38]. At present, older women with surgically resectable tumors should be offered surgery. Patients who have a very limited life to expectancy, and with hormone receptor positive tumors, can be offered endocrine therapy with either tamoxifen or an aromatase inhibitor (AI).

28.4.2 Radiation Therapy

Radiation therapy after breast conservation surgery is the mainstay of treatment for patients with breast cancer. The Early Breast Cancer Trialists Collaborative Group (EBCTCG) overview showed that breast radiation after mastectomy reduced the risk of local recurrence regardless of tumor stage. In addition, this analysis showed that such radiation reduced 15-year mortality by 4–5 %. Mortality benefits from radiation were limited to women where radiation resulted in a 10 % or greater reduction in the 5-year local recurrence rate [39]. Importantly, a randomized trial of radiation plus tamoxifen versus tamoxifen alone after breast conservation surgery in women 70 years and older with node-negative, hormone receptor positive breast cancer 2 cm or less in diameter (T1) showed that the addition of radiation to lumpectomy and tamoxifen had no effect on overall survival [40]. Local recurrences were decreased in the radiation group (1 % radiotherapy (RT) group vs. 7 % lumpectomy alone) but mastectomy rates were similar (1 % RT vs. 3 % no RT) as some patients in the no RT group who had breast recurrence were able to be salvaged with repeat lumpectomy and breast radiation [40]. This trial focused on women with low risks for local-regional recurrence irrespective of the use of breast radiation, and the survival data was similar to the EBCTCG results. In addition, another study evaluated the importance of whole breast radiation therapy after breast conservation therapy in women over the age of 65 years with hormone receptor positive, node-negative breast cancer that was 3 cm of less in diameter. Patients were randomized to whole breast radiation plus hormonal therapy or hormonal therapy alone. After 5 years of follow-up, there were minor differences in the rate of local recurrences (4.1 % in no RT group vs. 1.3 % in RT group). There were no significant differences in regional recurrences or distant metastasis. In addition, there was no difference in 5-year overall survival [41]. In older women with small, node-negative breast cancers, breast radiation may be omitted without negative effects on overall survival as long as the patient is willing and able to take adjuvant hormonal therapy. The pros and cons of radiation in this setting should be carefully discussed with the patient. Older women tolerate breast and post-mastectomy radiation as well as younger women [42, 43]. Patients with a high risk for local recurrence should be considered for treatment especially if they have life expectancies exceeding 5 years. Partial breast radiation is also a good option for some elders as it may minimize treatment visits and reduce recurrence risk.

28.4.3 Management of the Axilla

A sentinel lymph node (SLN) biopsy is performed in patients with early stage breast cancer who are clinically and radiographically node-negative. Evidence supports that if the SLN biopsy is negative, then further axillary dissection is not required [44, 45]. For older women with major comorbid disease or frailty, detecting axillary node involvement is not likely to change management. For robust older women, however, knowing the tumor status of the axillary nodes will help in making more effective decisions about local and systemic therapies. An increasing body of data suggests that sentinel lymph node (SLN) biopsy is a safe and accurate method of evaluating the axillary nodes for metastasis, including older women. In one study of 241 patients 70 years and older, SLN was found to be a safe and accurate method of assessing axillary node status for elderly women with operable breast cancer less than 3 cm. At a median follow-up time of 30 months, no axillary recurrences were noted [46]. Axillary lymph node dissection in older patients should only be considered if there is clinical evidence of axillary node involvement. In this situation, axillary dissection plays a therapeutic as well as a staging role.

28.5 Adjuvant Systemic Therapy

28.5.1 Treatment Benefit

The overview of the EBCTCG includes 194 randomized trials of adjuvant therapy and showed that after 15 years of follow-up, 5 years of tamoxifen therapy in estrogen receptor (ER) positive patients reduced the annual breast cancer mortality rate by 31 % irrespective of age [47]. Moreover, about 6 months of an anthracycline-containing regimen reduced the annual breast cancer death rate by about 38 % in women younger than 50 years and by about 20 % in women 50–69 years. These reductions were seen irrespective of tamoxifen use [47]. Unfortunately, very few patients above 70 years were entered in these trials (only about 1200), precluding an accurate assessment of chemotherapy effects in women over the age of 70. Recommendations for systemic treatment are summarized in Table 28.1 and discussed in detail below.

28.5.2 Selecting Treatment

Studies from large databases such as the San Antonio and SEER programs show that older women are more likely to have favorable tumor characteristics when compared to younger patients [48, 49]. Diab et al. reported that in patients 55 years and older, there was an association between increasing age at diagnosis and the presence of more favorable tumor characteristics, including smaller tumor size, lower likelihood of being lymph node-negative, more tumors that express hormone receptors, lower proliferative rates, more diploidy, normal p53, and absence of the expression of epidermal growth factor receptor and HER-2 [48]. However, about 20–30 % of older patients have ER and progesterone receptor (PR) negative tumors, a phenotype that confers an increased risk for early recurrence [50, 51]. Similar results with less genetically aggressive tumor subtypes with increasing age have also been shown [51]. Infiltrating ductal carcinoma is the most common tumor histologic subtype, and more indolent subtypes such as mucinous and papillary carcinomas are also encountered more frequently in older age groups [52].

Selection of treatment depends on two main factors: (1) the patient's stage and the tumor's biologic characteristics (grade, hormone receptor, and HER-2 status) and (2) an assessment of the patient's functional or physiologic age. We suggest that for treatment selection, patients should be divided into three major subgroups: (1) ER and/or PR positive and HER-2 negative, (2) HER-2 positive (irrespective of ER and PR status), and (3) ER and PR-negative and

Table 28.1 Recommendations for adjuvant systemic therapy for women 70 years and older

Estrogen and/or progesterone receptor (PR) status	HER-2 status	Nodal status	Recommendations
Positive	Negative	Negative	Endocrine therapy for most OncotypeDX or other gene array testing to estimate possible chemotherapy benefit
		Positive	Endocrine therapy Consider OncotypeDx or other gene array testing to estimate possible chemotherapy benefit in patient with one to three positive lymph nodes Use calculators (see text) to calculate added value of chemotherapy in patients with 4 or more positive lymph nodes
Any	Positive	Any	Endocrine therapy for ER + or PR + and consider chemotherapy and trastuzumab for most
Both negative	Negative	Any	Consider chemotherapy for most. Use calculators to estimate value of different chemotherapy regimens

HER-2 negative (so called "triple-negative" breast cancer) groups. Estimates of recurrence and the benefits of both endocrine therapy and chemotherapy in these subgroups can be reasonably made using Adjuvant! (www.adjuvantonline.com) or Predict (http://www.predict.nhs.uk/predict.html). These programs can factor in age and expected life expectancy, and Adjuvant! can also calculate the effects of comorbidity on life expectancy. Unlike Adjuvant!, the Predict calculator allows for estimates of treatment benefit of trastuzumab for HER-2 positive patients. Caution is needed as these models have not been validated in older patients and Adjuvant! may overestimate the value of chemotherapy [53]. Recent reviews have provided excellent guidelines for the use of adjuvant therapy in older patients [54–56].

28.5.3 Treatment of Older Patients with Hormone Receptor Positive, HER-2 Negative Tumors

The vast majority of older adults with breast cancer have ER and/or PR positive, and HER-2 negative tumors, and comprise about 70 % of all new cases with invasive breast cancer. The majority of these patients will be node-negative. For these older patients with ER-positive, node-negative tumors that are 5 cm or less, the risk of metastases at 10 years can be accurately assessed using a 21 gene assay—OncotypeDx™ [57] (www.genomichealth.com). Adjuvant endocrine therapy with an AI or tamoxifen followed by and AI is appropriate for the majority of these patients, the exceptions being those with life spans less than 5 years or with small tumors with favorable tumor biology.

The AIs have been compared to tamoxifen using several randomized trial designs, including head-on comparisons, changing to an AI for 2–3 years after a 2–3 year period on tamoxifen, and comparing an AI with placebo after 5 years of tamoxifen. In aggregate, the AIs have been found to be superior to tamoxifen, decreasing breast cancer relapse rates by about 3–5 % [58, 59]. However, head-on trials comparing tamoxifen with an AI have not shown a benefit for initiating treatment with AIs, the largest trial showing almost identical mortality rates after 100 months of follow-up [60]. Tamoxifen followed by an AI is also worthy of consideration, with one trial showing a small but significant survival benefit using this strategy [61]. For those elders at high risk of recurrence who have had 5 years of tamoxifen, consideration of extended adjuvant therapy with an AI should be given [62, 63]. The ASCO guidelines suggest that AIs should be part of adjuvant endocrine therapy in post-menopausal patients should apply to older women as well [59]. A point in favor for the use of AIs when compared to tamoxifen is the more favorable toxicity profile of AIs in the older age group, especially the lack of an increased risk of thrombosis and endometrial cancer. In one trial comparing letrozole with placebo in elders who had 5 years of tamoxifen, no significant differences in toxicity were found between the AI and placebo [63]. Accelerated bone loss is a major concern for elders on AI therapy, and a baseline bone density prior to initiating AI should be done and patients managed according to accepted guidelines [64]. Adequate calcium intake and vitamin D supplementation should be considered in older women at risk for osteoporosis. AIs are considerably more expensive than tamoxifen and these issues should be discussed with patients before making a treatment decision.

There is little benefit of chemotherapy in elders with hormone receptor positive, HER-2 negative, and node-negative tumors. However, there are likely to be some patients in this group with node-negative tumors who might benefit from chemotherapy, and use of the 21 gene Oncotype™ assay can identify those women most likely to benefit. The role of chemotherapy for those with node-positive tumors is uncertain [65]. For those with node-positive tumors, estimates of the added value of chemotherapy can be calculated from Adjuvant! (www.adjuvantonline.com) or Predict (http://www.predict.nhs.uk/predict.html). An example of the benefits of treatment and the effects of comorbidity on outcome for patients with node-positive breast cancer calculated from Adjuvant! is shown in Table 28.2. The benefits of treatment in this example, especially chemotherapy, are small in patients with major comorbidity. In the overview, chemotherapy showed similar proportional reductions in relapse in ER-positive and ER-negative patients, but only after extended follow-up. Healthy elders with estimated survivals of more than 5–10 years might ultimately derive benefit from chemotherapy, and those at high risk for recurrence should be considered for such treatment. The use of non-anthracycline regimens such as docetaxel and cyclophosphamide is worth of consideration in this setting [66]. For those with positive nodes and at high risk, more aggressive, anthracycline and taxane-containing regimens might be considered, as similar benefits for more aggressive and compared to less aggressive chemotherapy have been shown for older as well as younger patients [67], although with greater risk for toxicity [68].

28.5.4 Treatment of Older Patients with HER-2 Positive Tumors

For older women with HER-2 positive breast cancer, the major consideration is the use of trastuzumab with chemotherapy. Several trials have shown that trastuzumab when added to chemotherapy causes a further 50 % proportional reduction in the risk of recurrence compared to chemotherapy alone [69–71]. Trastuzumab, although

Table 28.2 Estimation of treatment benefit and the effects of comorbidity on 10 year mortality for a 75-year-old woman with a 2 cm moderately differentiated hormone receptor positive, HER-2 negative infiltrating ductal cancer and four positive lymph nodes (calculated from adjuvantonline.com)

Comorbidity	Treatment	% alive at 10 years
None, excellent health	None[a]	53
	Endocrine therapy only[b]	61
	Endocrine + chemotherapy[c]	65
Average health for age[d]	None	41
	Endocrine therapy only	47
	Endocrine + chemotherapy	51
Major comorbidity[e]	None	14
	Endocrine therapy only	16
	Endocrine + chemotherapy	17

[a]Only surgery and/or radiation
[b]Tamoxifen or an aromatase inhibitor (AI)
[c]Chemotherapy is docetaxel and cyclophosphamide for 4 cycles
[d]From www.adjuvantonline.com
[e]At least one serious illness

generally well tolerated, is associated with an increased risk of cardiac toxicity that is age related [72]. Control of hypertension, if present, and optimal management of any preexisting cardiac disease should be obtained before initiating trastuzumab. Older women with HER-2 positive tumors should be offered trastuzumab but should be closely monitored for cardiac toxicity. In all older patients, the use of non-anthracycline regimens such a paclitaxel and trastuzumab for those with node-negative tumors up to 3 cm [73] or docetaxel, carboplatin, and trastuzumab for those with larger or node-positive tumors, should be considered [74]. The benefits of trastuzumab in older patients with small HER-2 positive, node-negative tumors (<1 cm) is uncertain and for those with short life expectancy treatment is not likely to be helpful.

28.5.5 Treatment of Older Patients with ER- and PR-Negative and HER-2 Negative Tumors

Older women with triple-negative breast cancer should be offered chemotherapy if they are in good health. Older women tolerate aggressive chemotherapy regimens almost as well as younger women [67]. An analysis of randomized trials of chemotherapy regimens in patients with node-positive tumors showed that more intensive, taxane-containing regimens were the most effective treatments in those with hormone receptor-negative tumors [75]. This analysis did not include HER-2 status but it is likely that most patients were HER-2 negative. A recent analysis of the EBCTG comparing chemotherapy or not in women with ER-poor tumors showed a 10-year reduction of 8 % in breast cancer mortality in women younger than 50 years and a reduction of 6 % in women 50–69 years [76]. Almost half of these patients received older chemotherapy regimens such as CMF (cyclophosphamide, methotrexate, and fluorouracil), and recent data would suggest that current regimens would substantially improve on these results [75]. It is likely that most of the women in this meta-analysis had HER-2 negative breast cancer, and thus would benefit from such treatment. Moreover, a randomized trial comparing capecitabine with standard chemotherapy (either CMF or doxorubicin and cyclophosphamide) showed superiority of standard treatment in improving both relapse-free and overall survival, with the major benefit being in hormone receptor-negative patients [77].

28.6 Treatment of Metastatic Disease

Metastatic breast cancer remains incurable. The goals of treatment of older women with metastatic breast cancer are the same as for younger women and include controlling the growth of cancer while maintaining the highest possible quality of life. For older women with hormone receptor positive breast cancer, different hormonal agents or hormonal agents and biologics should be tried until it is clear that metastases are refractory to endocrine therapy. Older patients with hormone receptor positive metastases may have previously had tamoxifen and/or an AI in the adjuvant setting. Those who have been off endocrine therapy for several years can be retreated with the same agent as used in the adjuvant setting, while those who develop metastases on an AI or tamoxifen can be treated with tamoxifen or an AI, respectively. For older patients with metastases resistant to both tamoxifen and AIs, trying a different AI, using a newer agent such as fulvestrant should be considered. Patients can also be retreated with agents that have been previously tried with an occasional response, provided there has been a reasonable period of time since use of the earlier agent. Using endocrine therapy until metastases are convincingly refractory to endocrine treatment allows for a delay in chemotherapy and maintenance of the highest quality of life before deciding on chemotherapeutic options [50]. Recently, the addition of palbociclib (a cyclin-dependent kinase 4 and 6 inhibitor) to endocrine therapy (letrozole first-line or fulvestrant second-line) in women who had relapsed or progressed on endocrine therapy alone showed an improvement in progression free survival when compared to endocrine therapy alone—20 months versus 10 months for the combination versus letrozole alone and 9.2 months versus 4 months for the combination versus fulvestrant alone [78, 79]. However, women over the age of 65 years only accounted for approximately 25 % of the study population and mature survival data are not yet available. Similarly for older women with tumor progression on a non-steroidal aromatase inhibitor (anastrozole or letrozole), the combination of everolimus and exemestane resulted in a marked improvement in progressions–free survival compared to exemestane alone (11 vs. 4 months) but with no improvement in overall survival [80]. The potential for increased toxicity of these biologic agents in older women remains unexplored.

Considerable debate persists as to whether to use combination or sequential single-agent chemotherapy in the treatment of metastatic breast cancer [81]. Retrospective reviews have shown that healthy older patients with metastatic breast cancer tolerate chemotherapy about as well as younger patients, including anthracycline-containing regimens [82, 83]. Sequential therapy with active single agents is generally associated with less toxicity and is more likely to maintain the highest quality of life and in our opinion remains the standard of care. Most combination chemotherapy regimens are likely to be more toxic than single agents but have higher response rates and longer times to progression than single agents; however, combination regimens have not been shown to be associated with improved survival [50]. We recommend starting with single agent therapy in most patients except those with rapidly progressive metastases or where even modest tumor progression will be life threatening. The exceptions are in women with HER-2 positive metastases where combinations of chemotherapy and trastuzumab can significantly prolong survival [84, 85]. Chemotherapy should be considered even in older adults with medical comorbidity; functional status and toxicity must be closely monitored during treatment in these patients. Recent reviews of the treatment of metastatic breast cancer in older women are available [86, 87]. In addition, calculators are available that can predict toxicity based on clinical and geriatric assessment-defined characteristics for older patients being considered for chemotherapy in both the adjuvant and metastatic setting [20, 21].

28.7 Clinical Trials

Older patients continue to be underrepresented in breast cancer clinical trials [10]. Available data suggest, however, that when offered trials, older and younger patients have similar rates of participation, approximating 50 % [11]. Healthy older women should be encouraged to participate in Phase II and III trials and efforts should be made to offer trials to such patients and encourage participation. Adding the GA as a part of these trials may also be of value in predicting treatment-related toxicity, and a short, mostly self-administered CGA instrument has shown to be feasible in the cooperative group setting [88]. Designing trials specifically for older breast cancer patients is another strategy to improve accrual. A recent ASCO statement was published on strategies/recommendations and action items to further enhance research for older adults with cancer [89].

28.8 Conclusions

Management of older adults with breast cancer is frequently challenging. Healthy or robust older adults with 5–10 more years of life expectancy should be managed like younger postmenopausal patients, including breast conservation therapy if technically feasible, and adjuvant systemic therapy. Comorbidity must be factored into treatment recommendations, especially for frail patients. A screening tool [90] or abbreviated GA should be used by oncologists identify problems that can lead to specific interventions to maintain function. Older patients with significant comorbid illness or frailty may require major modifications in treatment, including surgery and chemotherapy. Accrual of older adults into ongoing Phase II and Phase III trials should be encouraged and trials focusing on older women should be developed. Overcoming physician bias in breast cancer care of older patients, as well as offering older patients clinical trial participation remains a major problem. Educational efforts focused on breast cancer care in the older adult and directed at both patients and physicians need to be expanded. Since breast cancer is common among older women, having evidence-based practice to guide treatments is of great importance. The challenge of caring for older adults with cancer is a major national concern and all of us should strive to improve care for this expanding segment of the population [91].

References

1. Institute NC. SEER stat fact sheets: breast cancer 2015 [cited 2015 October 5]. Available from: http://seer.cancer.gov/statfacts/html/breast.html.
2. Smith BD, Smith GL, Hurria A, Hortobagyi GN, Buchholz TA. Future of cancer incidence in the United States: burdens upon an aging, changing nation. J Clin Oncol (Official Journal of the American Society of Clinical Oncology). 2009;27(17):2758–65.
3. Lyman GH, Lyman S, Balducci L, Kuderer N, Reintgen D, Cox C, et al. Age and the risk of breast cancer recurrence. Cancer Control: J Moffitt Cancer Center. 1996;3(5):421–7.
4. Masetti R, Antinori A, Terribile D, Marra A, Granone P, Magistrelli P, et al. Breast cancer in women 70 years of age or older. J Am Geriatr Soc. 1996;44(4):390–3.
5. Yancik R, Wesley MN, Ries LA, Havlik RJ, Edwards BK, Yates JW. Effect of age and comorbidity in postmenopausal breast cancer patients aged 55 years and older. JAMA. 2001;285(7):885–92.
6. Hebert-Croteau N, Brisson J, Latreille J, Blanchette C, Deschenes L. Compliance with consensus recommendations for the treatment of early stage breast carcinoma in elderly women. Cancer. 1999;85(5):1104–13.
7. Eaker S, Dickman PW, Bergkvist L, Holmberg L. Uppsala/Orebro breast cancer G. Differences in management of older women influence breast cancer survival: results from a population-based database in Sweden. PLoS Med. 2006;3(3):e25.
8. Hebert-Croteau N, Brisson J, Latreille J, Rivard M, Abdelaziz N, Martin G. Compliance with consensus recommendations for systemic therapy is associated with improved survival of women with node-negative breast cancer. J Clin Oncol (Official Journal of the American Society of Clinical Oncology). 2004;22(18):3685–93.
9. Hutchins LF, Unger JM, Crowley JJ, Coltman CA Jr, Albain KS. Underrepresentation of patients 65 years of age or older in cancer-treatment trials. N Engl J Med. 1999;341(27):2061–7.
10. Sateren WB, Trimble EL, Abrams J, Brawley O, Breen N, Ford L, et al. How sociodemographics, presence of oncology specialists, and hospital cancer programs affect accrual to cancer treatment trials. J Clin Oncol (Official Journal of the American Society of Clinical Oncology). 2002;20(8):2109–17.
11. Kemeny MM, Peterson BL, Kornblith AB, Muss HB, Wheeler J, Levine E, et al. Barriers to clinical trial participation by older women with breast cancer. J Clin Oncol (Official Journal of the American Society of Clinical Oncology). 2003;21(12):2268–75.
12. Trimble EL, Carter CL, Cain D, Freidlin B, Ungerleider RS, Friedman MA. Representation of older patients in cancer treatment trials. Cancer. 1994;74(7 Suppl):2208–14.
13. Walter LC, Covinsky KE. Cancer screening in elderly patients: a framework for individualized decision making. JAMA. 2001;285(21):2750–6.
14. Schonberg MA, Davis RB, McCarthy EP, Marcantonio ER. Index to predict 5-year mortality of community-dwelling adults aged 65 and older using data from the National Health Interview Survey. J Gen Intern Med. 2009;24(10):1115–22.
15. Cruz M, Covinsky K, Widera EW, Stijacic-Cenzer I, Lee SJ. Predicting 10-year mortality for older adults. JAMA. 2013;309(9):874–6.
16. Hurria A, Gupta S, Zauderer M, Zuckerman EL, Cohen HJ, Muss H, et al. Developing a cancer-specific geriatric assessment: a feasibility study. Cancer. 2005;104(9):1998–2005.
17. Williams GR, Deal AM, Jolly TA, Alston SM, Gordon BB, Dixon SA, et al. Feasibility of geriatric assessment in community oncology clinics. J Geriatr Oncol. 2014;5(3):245–51.
18. Extermann M, Hurria A. Comprehensive geriatric assessment for older patients with cancer. J Clin Oncol (Official Journal of the American Society of Clinical Oncology). 2007;25(14):1824–31.
19. Jolly TA, Deal AM, Nyrop KA, Williams GR, Pergolotti M, Wood WA, et al. Geriatric assessment-identified deficits in older cancer patients with normal performance status. Oncologist. 2015;20(4):379–85.
20. Hurria A, Togawa K, Mohile SG, Owusu C, Klepin HD, Gross CP, et al. Predicting chemotherapy toxicity in older adults with cancer: a prospective multicenter study. J Clin Oncol (Official Journal of the American Society of Clinical Oncology). 2011;29(25):3457–65.
21. Extermann M, Boler I, Reich RR, Lyman GH, Brown RH, DeFelice J, et al. Predicting the risk of chemotherapy toxicity in older patients: the chemotherapy risk assessment scale for high-age patients (CRASH) score. Cancer. 2012;118(13):3377–86.
22. Maas HA, Janssen-Heijnen ML, Rikkert MGO, Wymenga ANM. Comprehensive geriatric assessment and its clinical impact in oncology. Eur J cancer. 2007;43(15):2161–9.
23. Extermann M, Aapro M, Bernabei R, Cohen HJ, Droz JP, Lichtman S, et al. Use of comprehensive geriatric assessment in older cancer patients: recommendations from the task force on CGA of the International Society of Geriatric Oncology (SIOG). Crit Rev Oncol/Hematol. 2005;55(3):241–52.
24. Satariano WA, Ragland DR. The effect of comorbidity on 3-year survival of women with primary breast cancer. Ann Intern Med. 1994;120(2):104–10.
25. La Vecchia C, Negri E, Franceschi S, Talamini R, Bruzzi P, Palli D, et al. Body mass index and post-menopausal breast cancer: an age-specific analysis. Br J Cancer. 1997;75(3):441–4.
26. Senie RT, Rosen PP, Rhodes P, Lesser ML, Kinne DW. Obesity at diagnosis of breast carcinoma influences duration of disease-free survival. Ann Intern Med. 1992;116(1):26–32.
27. Fisher B, Costantino JP, Wickerham DL, Redmond CK, Kavanah M, Cronin WM, et al. Tamoxifen for prevention of breast cancer: report of the National Surgical Adjuvant Breast and Bowel Project P-1 Study. J Natl Cancer Inst. 1998;90(18):1371–88.
28. Vogel VG, Costantino JP, Wickerham DL, Cronin WM, Cecchini RS, Atkins JN, et al. Effects of tamoxifen vs raloxifene on the risk of developing invasive breast cancer and other disease outcomes: the NSABP Study of Tamoxifen and Raloxifene (STAR) P-2 trial. JAMA. 2006;295(23):2727–41.
29. Goss PE, Ingle JN, Ales-Martinez JE, Cheung AM, Chlebowski RT, Wactawski-Wende J, et al. Exemestane for breast-cancer prevention in postmenopausal women. N Engl J Med. 2011;364(25):2381–91.
30. Gail MH, Costantino JP, Bryant J, Croyle R, Freedman L, Helzlsouer K, et al. Weighing the risks and benefits of tamoxifen treatment for preventing breast cancer. J Natl Cancer Inst. 1999;91(21):1829–46.
31. Humphrey LL, Helfand M, Chan BK, Woolf SH. Breast cancer screening: a summary of the evidence for the U.S. preventive services task force. Ann Intern Med. 2002;137(5 Part 1):347–60.
32. Walter LC, Schonberg MA. Screening mammography in older women: a review. JAMA. 2014;311(13):1336–47.
33. Badgwell BD, Giordano SH, Duan ZZ, Fang S, Bedrosian I, Kuerer HM, et al. Mammography before diagnosis among women age 80 years and older with breast cancer. J Clin Oncol (Official

Journal of the American Society of Clinical Oncology). 2008;26 (15):2482–8.
34. Smith RA, Cokkinides V, Brooks D, Saslow D, Brawley OW. Cancer screening in the United States, 2010: a review of current American Cancer Society guidelines and issues in cancer screening. CA Cancer J Clin. 2010;60(2):99–119.
35. Audisio RA, Bozzetti F, Gennari R, Jaklitsch MT, Koperna T, Longo WE, et al. The surgical management of elderly cancer patients; recommendations of the SIOG surgical task force. Eur J Cancer. 2004;40(7):926–38.
36. Kemeny MM. Surgery in older patients. Semin Oncol. 2004;31 (2):175–84.
37. Figueiredo MI, Cullen J, Hwang YT, Rowland JH, Mandelblatt JS. Breast cancer treatment in older women: does getting what you want improve your long-term body image and mental health? J Clin Oncol (Official Journal of the American Society of Clinical Oncology). 2004;22(19):4002–9.
38. Hind D, Wyld L, Beverley CB, Reed MW. Surgery versus primary endocrine therapy for operable primary breast cancer in elderly women (70 years plus). Cochrane Database Syst Rev. 2006(1): CD004272.
39. Clarke M, Collins R, Darby S, Davies C, Elphinstone P, Evans V, et al. Effects of radiotherapy and of differences in the extent of surgery for early breast cancer on local recurrence and 15-year survival: an overview of the randomised trials. Lancet. 2005;366 (9503):2087–106.
40. Hughes KS, Schnaper LA, Berry D, Cirrincione C, McCormick B, Shank B, et al. Lumpectomy plus tamoxifen with or without irradiation in women 70 years of age or older with early breast cancer. N Engl J Med. 2004;351(10):971–7.
41. Kunkler IH, Williams LJ, Jack WJ, Cameron DA, Dixon JM, investigators PI. Breast-conserving surgery with or without irradiation in women aged 65 years or older with early breast cancer (PRIME II): a randomised controlled trial. Lancet Oncol. 2015;16(3):266–73.
42. VanderWalde N, Hebert B, Jones E, Muss H. The role of adjuvant radiation treatment in older women with early breast cancer. J Geriatr Oncol. 2013;4(4):402–12.
43. Wyckoff J, Greenberg H, Sanderson R, Wallach P, Balducci L. Breast irradiation in the older woman: a toxicity study. J Am Geriatr Soc. 1994;42(2):150–2.
44. Veronesi U, Paganelli G, Viale G, Luini A, Zurrida S, Galimberti V, et al. A randomized comparison of sentinel-node biopsy with routine axillary dissection in breast cancer. N Engl J Med. 2003;349(6):546–53.
45. Krag D, Weaver D, Ashikaga T, Moffat F, Klimberg VS, Shriver C, et al. The sentinel node in breast cancer–a multicenter validation study. N Engl J Med. 1998;339(14):941–6.
46. Gennari R, Rotmensz N, Perego E, dos Santos G, Veronesi U. Sentinel node biopsy in elderly breast cancer patients. Surg Oncol. 2004;13(4):193–6.
47. Early Breast Cancer Trialists' Collaborative. G. Effects of chemotherapy and hormonal therapy for early breast cancer on recurrence and 15-year survival: an overview of the randomised trials. Lancet Oncol. 2005;365:1687–717.
48. Diab SG, Elledge RM, Clark GM. Tumor characteristics and clinical outcome of elderly women with breast cancer. J Natl Cancer Inst. 2000;92(7):550–6.
49. Grann VR, Troxel AB, Zojwalla NJ, Jacobson JS, Hershman D, Neugut AI. Hormone receptor status and survival in a population-based cohort of patients with breast carcinoma. Cancer. 2005;103(11):2241–51.
50. Crivellari D, Aapro M, Leonard R, von Minckwitz G, Brain E, Goldhirsch A, et al. Breast cancer in the elderly. J Clin Oncol (Official Journal of the American Society of Clinical Oncology). 2007;25(14):1882–90.
51. Jenkins EO, Deal AM, Anders CK, Prat A, Perou CM, Carey LA, et al. Age-specific changes in intrinsic breast cancer subtypes: a focus on older women. Oncologist. 2014;19(10):1076–83.
52. Toikkanen S, Kujari H. Pure and mixed mucinous carcinomas of the breast: a clinicopathologic analysis of 61 cases with long-term follow-up. Hum Pathol. 1989;20(8):758–64.
53. de Glas NA, van de Water W, Engelhardt EG, Bastiaannet E, de Craen AJ, Kroep JR, et al. Validity of Adjuvant! Online program in older patients with breast cancer: a population-based study. Lancet Oncol. 2014;15(7):722–9.
54. Karuturi M, vanderWalde A, Muss HB. Approach and management of breast cancer in the elderly. Clin Geriatr Med. 2015; in press.
55. Biganzoli L, Wildiers H, Oakman C, Marotti L, Loibl S, Kunkler I, et al. Management of elderly patients with breast cancer: updated recommendations of the International Society of Geriatric Oncology (SIOG) and European Society of Breast Cancer Specialists (EUSOMA). Lancet Oncol. 2012;13(4):e148–60.
56. Williams GR, Jones E, Muss HB. Challenges in the treatment of older breast cancer patients. Hematol Oncol Clin North Am. 2013;27(4):785–804.
57. Paik S, Shak S, Tang G, Kim C, Baker J, Cronin M, et al. A multigene assay to predict recurrence of tamoxifen-treated, node-negative breast cancer. New Engl J Med. 2004;351 (27):2817–26.
58. Ingle JN. Endocrine therapy trials of aromatase inhibitors for breast cancer in the adjuvant and prevention settings. Clin Cancer Res (An Official Journal of the American Association for Cancer Research). 2005;11(2 Pt 2):900s–5s.
59. Winer EP, Hudis C, Burstein HJ, Wolff AC, Pritchard KI, Ingle JN, et al. American Society of Clinical Oncology technology assessment on the use of aromatase inhibitors as adjuvant therapy for postmenopausal women with hormone receptor-positive breast cancer: status report 2004. J Clin Oncol (Official Journal of the American Society of Clinical Oncology). 2005;23(3):619–29.
60. Arimidex TAoiCTG, Forbes JF, Cuzick J, Buzdar A, Howell A, Tobias JS, et al. Effect of anastrozole and tamoxifen as adjuvant treatment for early-stage breast cancer: 100-month analysis of the ATAC trial. Lancet Oncol. 2008;9(1):45–53.
61. Coombes RC, Kilburn LS, Snowdon CF, Paridaens R, Coleman RE, Jones SE, et al. Survival and safety of exemestane versus tamoxifen after 2–3 years' tamoxifen treatment (intergroup exemestane study): a randomised controlled trial. Lancet. 2007;369(9561):559–70.
62. Goss PE, Ingle JN, Martino S, Robert NJ, Muss HB, Piccart MJ, et al. Randomized trial of letrozole following tamoxifen as extended adjuvant therapy in receptor-positive breast cancer: updated findings from NCIC CTG MA.17. J Natl Cancer Inst. 2005;97(17):1262–71.
63. Muss HB, Tu D, Ingle JN, Martino S, Robert NJ, Pater JL, et al. Efficacy, toxicity, and quality of life in older women with early-stage breast cancer treated with letrozole or placebo after 5 years of tamoxifen: NCIC CTG intergroup trial MA.17. J Clin Oncol (Official Journal of the American Society of Clinical Oncology). 2008;26(12):1956–64.
64. Hillner BE, Ingle JN, Chlebowski RT, Gralow J, Yee GC, Janjan NA, et al. American Society of Clinical Oncology 2003 update on the role of bisphosphonates and bone health issues in women with breast cancer. J Clin Oncol (Official Journal of the American Society of Clinical Oncology). 2003;21(21):4042–57.
65. Giordano SH, Duan Z, Kuo YF, Hortobagyi GN, Goodwin JS. Use and outcomes of adjuvant chemotherapy in older women with

breast cancer. J Clin Oncol (Official Journal of the American Society of Clinical Oncology). 2006;24(18):2750–6.
66. Jones SE, Savin MA, Holmes FA, O'Shaughnessy JA, Blum JL, Vukelja S, et al. Phase III trial comparing doxorubicin plus cyclophosphamide with docetaxel plus cyclophosphamide as adjuvant therapy for operable breast cancer. J Clin Oncol (Official Journal of the American Society of Clinical Oncology). 2006;24 (34):5381–7.
67. Muss HB, Woolf S, Berry D, Cirrincione C, Weiss RB, Budman D, et al. Adjuvant chemotherapy in older and younger women with lymph node-positive breast cancer. JAMA. 2005;293(9):1073–81.
68. Muss HB, Berry DA, Cirrincione C, Budman DR, Henderson IC, Citron ML, et al. Toxicity of older and younger patients treated with adjuvant chemotherapy for node-positive breast cancer: the cancer and leukemia Group B experience. J Clin Oncol (Official Journal of the American Society of Clinical Oncology). 2007;25 (24):3699–704.
69. Hortobagyi GN. Trastuzumab in the treatment of breast cancer. New Engl J Med. 2005;353(16):1734–6.
70. Romond EH, Perez EA, Bryant J, Suman VJ, Geyer CE Jr, Davidson NE, et al. Trastuzumab plus adjuvant chemotherapy for operable HER2-positive breast cancer. New Engl J Med. 2005;353 (16):1673–84.
71. Piccart-Gebhart MJ, Procter M, Leyland-Jones B, Goldhirsch A, Untch M, Smith I, et al. Trastuzumab after adjuvant chemotherapy in HER2-positive breast cancer. New Engl J Med. 2005;353 (16):1659–72.
72. Telli ML, Hunt SA, Carlson RW, Guardino AE. Trastuzumab-related cardiotoxicity: calling into question the concept of reversibility. J Clin Oncol (Official Journal of the American Society of Clinical Oncology). 2007;25(23):3525–33.
73. Tolaney SM, Barry WT, Dang CT, Yardley DA, Moy B, Marcom PK, et al. Adjuvant paclitaxel and trastuzumab for node-negative, HER2-positive breast cancer. N Engl J Med. 2015;372(2):134–41.
74. Slamon D, Eiermann W, Robert N, et al. 2nd interim analysis phase III randomized trial comparing doxorubicin and cyclophosphamide followed by docetaxel with doxorubicin and cyclophosphamide followed by docetaxel and trastuzumab with docetaxel, carboplatin and trastuzumab in Her2neu positive early breast cancer patients. Br Ca Res Treat. 2006.
75. Berry DA, Cirrincione C, Henderson IC, Citron ML, Budman DR, Goldstein LJ, et al. Estrogen-receptor status and outcomes of modern chemotherapy for patients with node-positive breast cancer. JAMA. 2006;295(14):1658–67.
76. Early Breast Cancer Trialists' Collaborative G, Clarke M, Coates AS, Darby SC, Davies C, Gelber RD, et al. Adjuvant chemotherapy in oestrogen-receptor-poor breast cancer: patient-level meta-analysis of randomised trials. Lancet. 2008;371(9606):29–40.
77. Muss HB, Berry DA, Cirrincione CT, Theodoulou M, Mauer AM, Kornblith AB, et al. Adjuvant chemotherapy in older women with early-stage breast cancer. N Engl J Med. 2009;360(20):2055–65.
78. Turner NC, Ro J, Andre F, Loi S, Verma S, Iwata H, et al. Palbociclib in hormone-receptor-positive advanced breast cancer. N Engl J Med. 2015;373(3):209–19.
79. Finn RS, Crown JP, Lang I, Boer K, Bondarenko IM, Kulyk SO, et al. The cyclin-dependent kinase 4/6 inhibitor palbociclib in combination with letrozole versus letrozole alone as first-line treatment of oestrogen receptor-positive, HER2-negative, advanced breast cancer (PALOMA-1/TRIO-18): a randomised phase 2 study. Lancet Oncol. 2015;16(1):25–35.
80. Baselga J, Campone M, Piccart M, Burris HA, Rugo HS, Sahmoud T, et al. Everolimus in postmenopausal hormone-receptor–positive advanced breast cancer. N Engl J Med. 2012;366(6):520–9.
81. Miles D, von Minckwitz G, Seidman AD. Combination versus sequential single-agent therapy in metastatic breast cancer. Oncologist. 2002;7(Suppl 6):13–9.
82. Christman K, Muss HB, Case LD, Stanley V. Chemotherapy of metastatic breast cancer in the elderly. The Piedmont Oncology Association experience [see comment]. JAMA. 1992;268(1):57–62.
83. Ibrahim NK, Frye DK, Buzdar AU, Walters RS, Hortobagyi GN. Doxorubicin-based chemotherapy in elderly patients with metastatic breast cancer. Tolerance and outcome. Arch Intern Med. 1996;156(8):882–8.
84. Swain SM, Baselga J, Kim S-B, Ro J, Semiglazov V, Campone M, et al. Pertuzumab, Trastuzumab, and Docetaxel in HER2-Positive Metastatic Breast Cancer. N Engl J Med. 2015;372(8):724–34.
85. Slamon DJ, Leyland-Jones B, Shak S, Fuchs H, Paton V, Bajamonde A, et al. Use of chemotherapy plus a monoclonal antibody against HER2 for metastatic breast cancer that over expresses HER2. N Engl J Med. 2001;344(11):783–92.
86. Jolly T, Williams GR, Jones E, Muss HB. Treatment of metastatic breast cancer in women aged 65 years and older. Womens Health (Lond Engl). 2012;8(4):455–71.
87. van de Water W, Bastiaannet E, Egan KM, de Craen AJ, Westendorp RG, Balducci L, et al. Management of primary metastatic breast cancer in elderly patients-An international comparison of oncogeriatric versus standard care. J Geriatr Oncol. 2014;5(3):252–9.
88. Hurria A, Cirrincione CT, Muss HB, Kornblith AB, Barry W, Artz AS, et al. Implementing a geriatric assessment in cooperative group clinical cancer trials: CALGB 360401. J Clin Oncol (Official Journal of the American Society of Clinical Oncology). 2011;29 (10):1290–6.
89. Hurria A, Levit LA, Dale W, Mohile SG, Muss HB, Fehrenbacher L, et al. Improving the evidence base for treating older adults with cancer: American society of clinical oncology statement. J Clin Oncol (Official Journal of the American Society of Clinical Oncology). 2015;33(32):3826–33.
90. Min L, Yoon W, Mariano J, Wenger NS, Elliott MN, Kamberg C, et al. The vulnerable elders-13 survey predicts 5-year functional decline and mortality outcomes in older ambulatory care patients. J Am Geriatr Soc. 2009;57(11):2070–6.
91. Hurria A, Naylor M, Cohen HJ. Improving the quality of cancer care in an aging population: recommendations from an IOM report. JAMA. 2013;310(17):1795–6.

Breast Cancer in Younger Women

29

Manuela Rabaglio and Monica Castiglione

29.1 Introduction

The definition of "young" in the context of breast cancer differs considerably according to the analyzed topics, and according to the reporting people. In general, however, women are considered young if diagnosed with breast cancer before 40 years of age.

Breast cancer is very rare in young women. The estimated incidence is less than 0.2 per 100,000 women below the age of 20 years, increasing to 1.4 in women 20–24 years, 7.7 in women 25–29 years, and 25.5 in women 30–34 years old [1]. The report of a substantial increase in the incidence of breast cancer among women under the age of 40 in Geneva, during the 10 years period from 2002 to 2004 [2], were not confirmed by data from two other Swiss Cancer Registers [3] and a recent publication [4] showed for the period from 1996 to 2009 a modest increase of 1.8 % in Swiss women aged 20–39, which is in line with international studies [5–7] reporting an increase between 1 and 3 % in European and American women. In developed countries, breast cancer represents the main cause of death among women aged 15–49 years [8, 9].

Several authors have suggested that breast cancer in young women presents biological peculiarities compared with tumors in older women: a higher histological grade, no expression of estrogen receptors, and an aggressive growth pattern [10–15]. The prognosis and survival of young women with breast cancer remains a controversial issue, with several studies showing discordant results. A worse prognosis was shown by some [14, 16–22], whereas other studies have reported that age is not influencing disease-free or overall survival after adjustment for other prognostic factors [23–27].

Special care is needed when facing women below the age of 40 years. In particular, issues like fertility preservation and contraception, pregnancy after cancer or cancer during pregnancy, sexuality and body image, as well as familial, genetic, and career items are peculiar for young breast cancer patients. Younger women show greater psychological morbidity than older patients. This may be due to the fact that they face a severe disease and a burdensome treatment before they had the time and chance to achieve personal targets and purposes [28, 29].

29.2 Epidemiology

Data from the Surveillance, Epidemiology, and End Results (SEER) program of the United States show that 75 % of breast tumors occur in women aged >50 years, only 6.5 % in women aged <40 years, and a mere 0.6 % in women below 30 years. Nevertheless, invasive breast carcinoma is the most common cancer in young women in the US, with an estimated risk of 1 in 228 individuals developing the disease by age 40. In the age group below 35, the incidence is 1.8 % and the mortality is 6.4 % [1]. These epidemiological characteristics remain stable in the most recent published report that includes data from 1975 until 2012 [30]. Breast cancer is the leading cause of cancer death for women between 20 and 39 years old in the USA [31]. An analysis using data from nine registries of the SEER showed that the relationship between age and mortality is biphasic and for both N0 and N+ patients among the T1-2 group, the analysis suggested two age components. One component shows the natural linear increase of mortality with each year of age. The other component shows higher mortality in women diagnosed with breast cancer below 40 as compared to women around 50 years [32]. Data from Swedish breast cancer registers confirmed that younger women affected by

M. Rabaglio (✉)
Department of Medical Oncology,
University Hospital/Inselspital and IBCSG Coordinating Center,
Freiburgstrasse 4/ Effingerstrasse 40, 3010 Berne, Switzerland
e-mail: manuela.rabaglio@insel.ch

M. Castiglione
Coordinating Center, International Breast Cancer Study Group (IBCSG), Effingerstrasse 40, 3008 Berne, Switzerland
e-mail: monica.castiglione@bluewin.ch

I. Jatoi and A. Rody (eds.), *Management of Breast Diseases*, DOI 10.1007/978-3-319-46356-8_29

early breast cancer have higher mortality rates as compared to middle-aged women and that the risk of death was more pronounced in women with small tumors [33]. This study revealed that age at diagnosis is a strong predictor for local (LRFS) and distant recurrence-free survival (DRFS). This finding was confirmed also in a recent publication [34]: younger patients (<40) developed both local and distant recurrence more frequently than their older (>75) counterparts. However, during the first Advanced Breast Cancer conference (ABC1) in 2011 K. Gelmon presented data from the British Columbia Cancer Agency showing that after relapse, the outcome in young patients with advanced breast cancer is not worst or even slight better as in older patient, probably due to the higher treatment tolerance in young women.

29.3 Risk Factors/Prognosis

Several risk factors for the development of a breast cancer have been described in the past. Among them are familiarity, endocrine factors, obesity and physical activity, exposure to pesticides, and many more.

In several series, age remained independently prognostic when pathological variables were taken into account [14, 17, 35–37]. However, age-related worst outcome seems to be more evident in aggressive breast cancer patters, like Luminal B, triple-negative, or HER2 positive tumors [38, 39].

Women diagnosed with breast cancer at the age of <35 years are likely to have germline BRCA1 or BRCA2 mutations in up to 15–30 % of cases [40–43]. Typically, breast cancers occurring in BRCA-1 mutation carriers are high grade and have a high proliferation rate, with medullary or atypical medullary cancers being over-represented. In contrast, lobular cancers and extensive intraductal cancers are more frequent in women with germline BRCA-2 mutations [44, 45].

Family history of breast cancer and, in particular, mutation in BRCA1 gene seems to correlate with tumors of medullary subtypes. This was first suggested by Marcus based on the histological evaluation of 157 breast cancers from women whose families had shown evidence of genetic mutation in BRCA1 [46].

In a large analysis including 3345 patients who were aged ≤50 years at the time of breast cancer diagnosis, 7 % of patients had a BRCA1 mutation. However, BRCA1 carriers were significantly younger (mean age 41.9 vs. 44.1, $P < 0.001$), and had more ER-negative (84.1 % vs. 38.1 %, $P < 0.001$) and HER2-negative (93 % vs. 79 %, $P < 0.001$) tumors [47].

The data presented by Bernstein [48] show that among the endocrine factors influencing the occurrence of breast cancer, the use of oral contraceptives (OC) may represent an important issue in young women. Two studies conducted in Los Angeles County suggest that the relationship between oral contraceptives and breast cancer risk may have changed over time, possibly reflecting changes in pill formulation. The first study was a case-control study of women aged 37 years or younger that was completed in 1983 and showed that long-term use of combination-type OCs with a "high" content of the progestogen component before the age of 25 was associated with increased risk of breast cancer. In contrast, the use of combination-type OCs with a "low" progestogen component appears to increase breast cancer risk little or not at all [49]. Yet, in a subsequent case–control study of women diagnosed with breast cancer (1983–1989), risk was unrelated to oral contraceptive use [50]. In 1996, the Collaborative Group on Hormonal Factors in Breast Cancer published a reanalysis of data collected from 54 breast cancer studies conducted in 25 countries, which specifically gathered detailed information on oral contraceptive use [51]. In this report, a history of recent oral contraceptive use, rather than long duration of use, was related with increasing breast cancer risk. The effect of recent oral contraceptive use was the strongest among those women who first used oral contraceptives before the age of 20 years. In this pooled analysis, the breast cancers diagnosed among oral contraceptive users were at an earlier stage than those among women who had never used oral contraceptives. In individual epidemiologic studies, it was, albeit up to now, not possible to demonstrate an association between OC use and the risk of breast cancer.

In the Nurses' Health Study, after 36 years follow-up, all-cause mortality did not significantly differ between women who had ever used oral contraceptives and those who had never used OC. However, the association of oral contraceptive use with other causes of death including breast cancer was of borderline statistical significance [52]. In other studies as the Royal College of General Practitioners' study [53] and the one conducted by the Centers for Disease Control and Prevention, Atlanta, USA [54] no association between breast cancer mortality and the use of OC was found. In contrast in a recently published population-based, case-control study among women ages 20–44 residing in the Seattle-Puget Sound area from 2004 to 2010 suggests that current use of contemporary OC preparations for 5 years or longer confer an increased breast cancer risk [55]. The WECARE (Women's Environment, Cancer, and Radiation Epidemiology) study, a population-based, multicenter, case-control study of 708 women with asynchronous bilateral breast cancer and 1395 women with unilateral breast cancer, provided no strong evidence that use of oral contraceptives (OC) or postmenopausal hormones (PMH) increases the risk of a second cancer in the contralateral breast [56]. The role of OC in women with a familial predisposition to breast cancer is unclear and OCs may be associated with an increased risk of breast cancer in *BRCA1* mutation carriers, but data for *BRCA2* mutation carriers are limited [57]. *BRCA1* carriers who used OCs had a nonsignificant greater risk than nonusers (RR = 2.38; 95 % CI = 0.72–7.83). Total duration of OC use and at least 5 years of use before age 30 were associated with a nonsignificant increased risk among mutation carriers but not among non-carriers [58]. The IARC (International Agency for Research in Cancer) Working Group on the Evaluation of Carcinogenic Risks to Humans concluded, after review of available data, that there are increased risks for cancer of the breast in young women among current and recent users [59]. The Working Group noted that the preponderance of the evidence suggests that use of oral contraceptives is associated with an increased risk of breast cancer in carriers of *BRCA1* or *BRCA2* mutations. This association reflects a causal relationship, and then it could, at least in part, explain the observation summarized in the previous *IARC Monograph* that risk of breast cancer was increased in women under the age of 35 years who had begun using oral contraceptives at a young age and who were current or recent users.

Physical activity may positively influence the incidence of breast cancer, because of its potential effects on hormone profiles and weight gain. Strenuous physical activity is known to delay menarche and cause secondary amenorrhea and oligomenorrhea among woman athletes The analysis of data from the Nurses' Health Study II show no overall association between physical activity and risk of breast cancer among premenopausal women, but suggest that the effect of physical activity could be substantially modified by the underlying degree of adiposity [60].

Obesity in premenopausal women seems to be associated with a reduction of breast cancer risk in contrast to postmenopausal women. The results of a multi-ethnic, population-based case-control study conducted between 1995 and 2004 in the San Francisco Bay Area confirmed the findings of several previous reports. Increased body size was associated with decreased risk of hormone-sensitive breast cancer in premenopausal women [61]. The effect of obesity on the non-ovarian estrogen production is indeed the same in pre- and postmenopausal women, but this production adds only a small increment in the estrogen produced by the ovary during ovulatory menstrual cycles. Obese premenopausal women experience more anovulatory cycles with lower estrogen production than normal weight women, and this could explain the slightly decreased risk of breast cancer in the obese premenopausal women studies, premenopausal women with a BMI of 31 kg/m^2 or higher were 46 % less likely to develop breast cancer than those with a BMI <21 kg/m^2 [62].

It has been proposed that intrauterine exposure to high concentrations of both endogenous and exogenous estrogens during gestation will negatively influence a fetus's breast cancer risk in adult life, perhaps by influencing the number of and the degree of differentiation of breast stem cells. Fetal estrogen exposure could also increase the probability of gene mutations relevant to cancer development or alter the breast's sensitivity to hormones [63, 64]. Although not entirely consistent, some studies show that low birth weight translates into a lower breast cancer risk, as does experiencing preeclampsia in utero [65]. Birth order may also affect risk. Maternal estradiol levels are higher in the first than in the second pregnancy, but epidemiologic studies of birth order have not consistently shown that firstborn daughters have higher risk than those with higher birth order [66].

Excess breast cancer risk has been consistently observed in association with a variety of exposures to radiation, such as the Hiroshima or Nagasaki atomic explosions [67, 68], as well as after the Chernobyl accident [69–71] and radiotherapy treatments for medical conditions (e.g., Hodgkin's disease) in childhood or adolescence [72, 73]. Studies on survivors of the atomic bombing of Hiroshima and Nagasaki demonstrated that the carcinogenic effect of accidental radiation is highest when exposure occurs during childhood. Exposure at a younger age increases the subsequent risk of breast cancer to a greater degree, possibly because of the unopposed estrogen exposure, which occurs during adolescence, rendering undifferentiated breast cells maximally vulnerable to initiation by environmental carcinogens [74–76].

29.4 Diagnosis

The presentation of breast cancer in women under the age of 40 years may differ compared to older women. Due to lack of screening programs and to the insufficient imaging for their often dense breast, the majority of young women presents with symptoms or palpable mass [77–79]. Older women, on the other hand, are more likely to present with breast cancer detected by screening. Clinical and radiological examinations of the breast in younger women have a limited accuracy and may delay the diagnosis [13, 80]. The denser breast tissue limits the sensitivity on screening mammography and physical examination in asymptomatic women. The use of screening ultrasound in conjunction with mammography instead of breast palpation may increase the sensitivity of cancer detection from 75 to 97 % in this special population [81]. According to the guidelines of the American Cancer Society [82, 83] and of the European Society of Breast Cancer Specialists [84], screening MRI is recommended for women with an approximately 20–25 % or greater lifetime risk of breast cancer, including women with a strong family history of breast or ovarian cancer and women who were treated for Hodgkin's disease. For the other risk subgroups, including women with a personal history of breast cancer, carcinoma in situ, atypical hyperplasia, and extremely dense breasts on mammography, the available data are insufficient to recommend for or against MRI screening, and the decisions should be made on a case-by-case basis.

Breast cancer diagnosis in this young population tends to be delayed and the patients often have a longer history of palpable mass in the breast [85]. The delay is often caused by inadequate awareness of the disease among both patient and physician [79, 86].

The effectiveness of physical examination is lower in very young women, as they often have dense or nodular breast tissue that is subject to cyclical hormonal changes. Also, the accuracy of mammography is low in the young women with high breast gland density, with a sensitivity of only 62.9 % in women with extremely dense breasts [13, 80, 87, 88]. The use of breast MRI has shown higher sensitivity compared with mammography [89–91]. For this reason, MRI screening is recommended in women with higher breast cancer risk for genetic or other reasons [82, 84, 92]. In patients with breast cancer, there is little evidence that the use of preoperative MRI improves the outcome after breast-conserving surgery neither in term of local recurrence nor overall survival [93, 94]

29.5 Tumor Characteristics/Biology

Tumors in very young women show generally a more aggressive biological behavior leading to a worse prognosis. They are reported to be less differentiated, with higher proliferation fraction and more frequently lymphovascular invasion, extensive intraductal component, necrosis, overexpression of the HER-2 oncogene, absence of the estrogen receptor, and to show more frequently, an axillary nodal involvement than those in older females [13]. Results of the POSH (Prospective Study of Outcomes in Sporadic and Hereditary Breast Cancer) study, a large prospective observational study evaluating the pathological characteristics of 2956 breast cancer women under age 40, have recently been reported [95]. The majority had ductal histology (86.5 %) and grade III (58.9 %) tumors, 50.2 % had node-positive disease, and multifocality was observed in 27 % of patients. One-third of tumors were ER-negative and one-quarter were HER-2 positive. Similar results were showed in the first patients recorded in the Young Women's Breast Cancer Study [96], in particular high rates of lymphovascular invasion and lymphocytic infiltration were found.

A population-based study analyzing date from Californian women between 2005 and 2009 adds to the evidence that adolescent and young adult (AYA) women aged between 15 and 39 years with breast cancer have larger proportions of HR+/HER2+, HR−/HER2+, and triple-negative subtypes as compared with older women. Compared with White AYAs, Black and Hispanic women had lower incidence rates of HR+/HER2- cancer, whereas Black women had higher rates and Asians had lower rates of triple-negative breast cancer [97].

In addition to the classical immunohistochemistry, gene expression profiling has achieved growing value for the differentiation of breast cancer subtypes [98, 99]. Four main subtypes are recognized: luminal A, luminal B, HER-2 overexpressed, and basal-like. These subtypes correlate with classical classification and with clinical-pathological surrogates: luminal A-like (ER+ and PR+, low grade, and low proliferative rate), luminal B-like (ER+ and PR+, high proliferative rate), HER-2 positive (non-luminal), and triple-negative (ER-negative, PR-negative, and HER-2 negative).

The basal-like subtype refers to breast cancers with a gene expression profile resembling normal breast basal/myoepithelial cells, characterized by expression of basal cytokeratins (CK5/6, CK14, CK17), caveolin 1 and 2, cyclin-D1, vimentin and p-cadherin, and lack of expression of ER, PR, and HER2. About 71–91 % of the triple-negative breast cancers (TNBC) are basal-like subtype [100]. In addition TNBC have histologically and transcriptionally, similarities to BRCA1 associated breast cancer, suggesting a possible dysfunction in BRCA1 in this subset of sporadic cancers [101].

A large-scale genomic analysis illustrates that breast cancer arising in young women is characterized by less hormone sensitivity and higher HER-2/EGFR expression [102]. In the largest to date published study [15], patients younger than 40 had a significantly higher proportion of basal-like (34.3 %) and HER2+ tumors and were less likely to have luminal A breast cancer (17.2 %) as compared with others age groups.

In recent years genetic signature has been developed to predict the risk of recurrence [103] and the response to chemotherapy [104, 105]. Their definite relevance is not yet established, but they will probably become more important in the future. Two randomized clinical trials investigating the role of gene signature tools for the choice of adjuvant treatment have completed the patients' accrual: the TAILORx trial is comparing hormone therapy with or without combination chemotherapy in women who have undergone surgery for node-negative breast cancer. Patients are assigned to different treatment groups based on their risk of distant recurrence determined by Oncotype DX (21-gene panel) test [106]. The first results of the low-risk cohort of the TAILORx trial have recently been released [107]: in women with a recurrence score (RS) <11, at 5 years, the rate of invasive disease-free survival was 93.8 % (95 % confidence interval [CI], 92.4–94.9) and the rate of overall survival was 98.0 % (95 % CI, 97.1–98.6) with endocrine therapy alone. The MINDACT (Microarray In node-negative Disease may Avoid Chemotherapy) trial is a prospective, randomized study comparing the 70 gene signature developed in Amsterdam with the common clinical pathological criteria in selecting patients for adjuvant chemotherapy in node-negative (planned also for node-positive), hormone-sensitive breast cancer [108].

Prognostic genomic assays, like Oncotype DX, Mammaprint, PAM50, and Endopredict, were mostly developed using data in postmenopausal women. Nevertheless, the Dutch group [109] reported that 52/63 (82 %) young patients were classified as high risk on MammaPrint. The same findings were observed for Oncotype Dx, where the majority of patients under age 40 had a high-risk score (56 %) [110] and in a large cohort of women with ER-positive breast cancer Shak found that patients aged <40 years had higher average RS, lower ER expression, and higher expression of genes related to cell proliferation compared to older women. Immunohistochemical assays also showed higher Ki-67 expression in tumors from younger than older patients [111]. Moreover, a recent large study of 9321 ER-positive breast cancer patients showed that Ki-67 expression was inversely proportional to age at diagnosis and was significantly higher in tumors from patients aged <40 than in those aged ≥40 years [112].

29.6 Management/Treatment of Early Breast Cancer

29.6.1 Surgery (Breast-Conserving Versus Mastectomy)

Younger women show a higher incidence of local recurrences after mastectomy and after breast-conserving surgery [113].

A comparison of outcome after breast-conserving surgery (BCT) or mastectomy shows that patients younger than 35 years of age have a higher local relapse rate following less extensive surgery [114]. The data of two randomized clinical trials for stage I and II breast cancer patients were pooled and a total of 1772 patients (879 underwent breast-conserving surgery and 893 modified radical mastectomy) were analyzed. Age of 35 years or less and the presence of an extensive intraductal component were associated with an increased risk of local recurrence after breast-conserving therapy. Vascular invasion causes a higher risk of local recurrence after mastectomy as well as after breast-conserving therapy, and according to the author should therefore not be used as a criterion for the choice of surgical treatment. Jobsen [115] showed in a prospective cohort study of 1085 women with pathological T1 tumors treated with breast-conservative surgery, that the local recurrence-free survival (LRFS) was significantly different for the two age groups at 71 months follow-up: 89 % for women 40 years old or younger and 97.6 % for women aged more than 40 years. In a subset analysis, this significant adverse effect of young age on outcome appears to be limited to the node-negative patients and those with a positive family history. In order to analyze the possible prognostic differences between patients treated with mastectomy and breast-conserving surgery, Arriagada [116] and colleagues analyzed the characteristics and outcome of 2006 patients treated for relatively small breast cancer (<25 mm) and followed for a mean of 20 years: 717 were treated conservatively (lumpectomy and breast irradiation) and 1289 were treated with total mastectomy. Patients with negative nodes did not receive any systemic adjuvant treatment; for node-positive women, ovarian suppression was performed by radiotherapy in 26 % of the cases and chemotherapy or additive hormonal treatments were given in only 3 % of the patients. For women treated with mastectomy, histological grade and extensive axillary node involvement (10 nodes or more) were significant predictive factors for local relapse. Young age, however, was not a prognostic indicator for local recurrence. In contrast, for patients treated with a conservative approach, young age (≤40 years) was the main risk factor for local relapse. These younger patients had a fivefold increased risk of developing a breast recurrence compared with patients older than 60 years. Another cohort study analyzing data from the population-based Danish breast carcinoma database [117] focalized on 9285 premenopausal women with primary breast carcinoma who were below 50 years at diagnosis. No increased risk of death was observed among women who were treated by breast-conserving surgery compared with women who underwent radical mastectomy, regardless of age at diagnosis (<35 years, 35–39 years, 40–44 years, or 45–49 years), despite the increased risk of local recurrence among young women. A large, population-based analysis based on the Surveillance, Epidemiology, and End Results (SEER) database showed that in the 14,764 women aged 20–39 with early breast cancer included between 1990 and 2007 OS (hazard ratio [HR], 0.93; 95 % confidence interval [CI], 0.83e1.04; $p = 0.16$) and cause-specific survival (HR, 0.93; CI, 0.83e1.05; $p = 0.26$) were similar after mastectomy or BCT [118].

A recent meta-analysis including data of seven studies comparing OS between BCT and mastectomy for a total of 22,598 young patients (≤40 years) with T1–T2 N0–N + M0 breast cancer showed, after all the adjustments, including nodal status and tumor size, no difference in risk of death between the two groups (10 % not significant risk reduction in patients who underwent BCS compared to mastectomy; summary HR = 0.90; 95 %CI: 0.81–1.00 [119]. Achieving negative margins with "no tumor on ink" is an appropriate goal in breast-conserving surgery. Wider margins do not decrease recurrence rates [120–122].

During the last decade, a growing number of women with unilateral breast cancer in the US are choosing to undergo contralateral prophylactic mastectomy (CPM) even in the absence of known hereditary predisposition and despite no survival advantage. Furthermore, the risk of contralateral breast cancer in most women is relatively low and has been decreasing due to better adjuvant treatments [123]. Recently, an analysis of the California Cancer Registry data documented an increase in bilateral mastectomy rates among women of all ages; however, this trend was most pronounced in women diagnosed under the age 40: in 1998, 3.6 % of women under the age 40 underwent bilateral mastectomy, while in 2011, bilateral mastectomy represented 33 % [124].

29.6.2 Radiation

Local treatment involving radiation therapy after breast-conserving surgery has been shown to yield the same disease-free survival and overall survival as in women undergoing total mastectomy [125, 126]. In a first trial analyzing the role of radiation boost, patients with a microscopically complete excision received 50 Gy of radiation to the whole breast, and thereafter they were randomly assigned to receive either no further local treatment (2657 patients) or an additional localized dose of 16 Gy (2661 patients) [127]. Basal and HER-2 subtypes are significantly associated with higher rates of local recurrence, in particular, among younger women with pT1–T2 invasive breast cancer after BCT [128]. Young age is an independent risk factor for local recurrence [129] for both intraductal and invasive diseases [130]. Patients who are 40 years old or younger benefited most from the addition of the boost; at 5 years, their rate of local recurrence was 19.5 % with standard treatment and 10.2 % with additional radiation (hazard ratio, 0.46 [99 % confidence interval, 0.23–0.89]; $P = 0.002$). The EORTC "boost versus no boost" trial [131] showed that young patients need a 16 Gy boost after breast-conserving surgery to reduce effectively the local recurrence rate. 5.569 early stage breast cancer patients were entered in this large randomized trial. All patients underwent tumorectomy followed by whole breast irradiation with 50 Gy. Patients having a microscopically complete excision were randomized between receiving no boost or a 16 Gy boost, while patients with a microscopically residual disease were randomized between boost doses of 10 and 26 Gy. The boost significantly reduced the 5-year local recurrence rate from 7 to 4 % for patients with a complete excision ($P < 0.001$). No statistical differences in outcome have been shown between the complete (94 % of the women) and incomplete excision (6 %) groups. For patients 40 years of age or younger, the boost dose reduced the local recurrence rate from 20 to 10 % ($P = 0.002$). A recently published update of this trial showed that after a median follow-up period of 10.8 years, a boost dose of 16 Gy led to improved local control in all age groups, but no difference in survival could be observed. The absolute risk reduction at 10 years per age group was the largest in patients 40 years of age or younger, and severe fibrosis was statistically significantly increased in the boost group, with a 10-year rate of 4.4 % versus 1.6 % [132]. The ongoing "young boost" trial conducted by the EORTC will evaluate whether a higher boost dose will further reduce the risk of local recurrence with still acceptable cosmetic outcome and without long-term side effects [133]: patients aged 50 years or less will be randomized to receive 26 Gy boost versus 16 Gy to the tumor bed after breast-conserving therapy, following 50 Gy to the whole breast.

There is also increasing evidence that young women may benefit additionally from post-mastectomy breast irradiation in the setting of 1–3 positive axillary lymph nodes [134].

29.6.3 Chemotherapy

With adequate systemic treatment, the outcome of breast cancer in young women may approach the one reported for older women [135, 136]. There is no evidence for the use of specific chemotherapy for young women. In the last EBCTCG meta-analysis involving anthracycline and taxane-containing regimes, the proportional risk reduction was not generally influenced by age [137]. The addition of a taxane to an anthracycline-based regimen improves the DFS and OS of high-risk early breast cancer patients. The DFS benefit was independent of ER expression, degree of nodal involvement, type of taxane, age or menopausal status of patient, and administration schedule [138].

In patients with early breast cancer, chemotherapies are better tolerated and appear to be more effective on average in younger than in older patients [139]; however, single trials of adjuvant chemotherapy are generally not stratified by age and if stratified, the age cutoffs are set around the natural age of menopause. The difference in the efficacy may reflect the different distribution of ER-negative and ER-positive cancers in younger women [13, 136, 139, 140]. Patients with ER-negative tumors may yield a higher benefit from more intensive chemotherapies than patients with ER-positive breast cancer [141].

Timing of chemotherapy start may have relevance for young patients: an analysis of the International (Ludwig) Breast Cancer Study Group (IBCSG) Trial V at a median follow-up of 11 years suggested that early initiation (within 21 days from surgery) of adjuvant chemotherapy might improve outcome for premenopausal, node-positive patients whose tumors do not express estrogen receptors [142]. In contrast, clinical trials of the Danish Breast Cancer Cooperative Group could not show a survival benefit for early initiation of adjuvant chemotherapy within the first 2–3 months after surgery [143]. A retrospective review of the institutional database at The University of Texas MD Anderson Cancer Center showed that initiation of chemotherapy >61 days after surgery was associated with adverse outcomes in term of overall and disease-free survival in particular among patients with higher risk of recurrence (Stage III, HER2 positive, or triple-negative cancers) compared with those starting chemotherapy within 30 days after surgery [144].

A special issue is represented by the so-called triple-negative cancers (TNBC). This subgroup accounts for 15 % of all breast cancer and for an even higher percentage of breast cancer arising in premenopausal Hispanic, African, and African-American women. Histologically, these cancers are mostly infiltrating ductal carcinomas of high grade, poor tubule formation, and high mitotic count, with pushing border, central fibrosis, and lymphocytic infiltrate. However, the triple-negative IHC is found in several breast cancer types with different histologically features and sometime better clinical prognosis [145] as for example medullary, low-grade apocrine, secretory, adenocystic, or low-grade metaplastic carcinomas. The TNBC is resistant to anti-HER2 treatments and endocrine therapies. Potential targets for treatment development for this special group of breast cancers include surface receptors, such as epidermal growth factor receptors (EGFR) or c-KIT; protein kinase components of the mitogen activated protein (MAP)-kinase pathway; protein kinase components of the protein kinase B (Akt) pathway; induction of DNA damage by specific chemotherapy agents as these cancers might be more sensitive to agents that cause interstrand and double-stranded breaks like platin-containing compounds; and inhibition of already defective DNA repair, by poly ADP-ribose polymerase 1 (PARP1) inhibition [146]. In a population-based study using the California Cancer Registry data Bauer [147] showed that TNBC affects more frequently younger, non-Hispanic Black and Hispanic women in areas of low socioeconomic status. Regardless of stage at diagnosis, women with TNBC had poorer survival than those with other types of breast cancers. Within the population of TNBC, the patients whose cancer has the basal-like phenotype may have a particularly high probability of relapse [148]. The role and value of chemotherapy is clearly established in patients with ER-negative breast cancer. There are currently no data supporting the use of platinum in the adjuvant setting; however, in BRCA, mutation carrier's recent data—TNT trial—suggest advantage of platinum-based CT over taxane in first-line metastatic setting [149]. In patients with BRCA-associated triple-negative or endocrine-resistant metastatic breast cancer previously treated with an anthracycline and a taxane (in the adjuvant or metastatic setting), a platinum regimen may therefore be considered [150].

The EBCTCG meta-analysis [139] published 2005 provides a rationale for using adjuvant chemotherapy in young patient with ER-positive breast cancer, showing a reduction of the annual breast cancer death rate by about 38 %. Furthermore, the recently updated EBCTCG meta-analysis [137] shows that adding taxane to anthracycline may increase the benefit of adjuvant chemotherapy.

29.6.4 Endocrine Treatment

Since the St. Gallen consensus conference in 2005 [151], endocrine responsiveness has become the primary factor for the choice of the adjuvant treatment in breast cancer. This aspect was largely discussed and emphasized at the last meeting in 2015 [152]. According to the results of the Oxford meta-analysis [153], 5 years of treatment with tamoxifen halved the recurrence rate during years 0–4 and reduced it by a third during years 5–9 (with little further effect after year 10), so over all time periods the recurrence rate reduction averaged 39 %. The risk of death was reduced by 30 % at 15 years in women with ER-positive breast cancer. This effect was similar across all age groups and was not jeopardized by prior chemotherapy.

After the publication of the results of the ATLAS [154] and aTTom Trials, the updated ASCO Guidelines [155] recommended to consider the extension of the tamoxifen treatment to 10 years. In the ATLAS trial, the cumulative risk of death from breast cancer 15 years after diagnosis among women on tamoxifen for 10 years was 12.2 versus 15 % in women who stopped tamoxifen at 5 years, an absolute difference of 2.8 %.

Two randomized clinical trials confirmed the efficacy of tamoxifen treatment after anthracyclines-based adjuvant chemotherapy also in premenopausal women with estrogen receptor-positive disease, achieving an improvement of the disease-free survival of about 40 % [156, 157].

The suppression of ovarian function by oophorectomy, radiation therapy, or through gonadotropin-releasing hormone (GnRH) reduces the relative risk of recurrence by 17 % and the risk of death by 13 % in women younger than 40 years of age with an estrogen receptor-positive tumor, and the efficacy is larger if the suppression of the ovarian function (OFS) is not combined with adjuvant chemotherapy [139, 156]. This result is indeed expected as chemotherapy may frequently induce amenorrhea, in particular in older premenopausal women [158, 159]. Subgroup analysis of many randomized trials showed that goserelin after chemotherapy was only effective in women who did not experience ovarian failure with chemotherapy and in particular in patients younger than 40 years [157, 160].

Ovarian function suppression was at least as effective as CMF-based or anthracycline-based chemotherapy in some randomized clinical trials investigating suppression alone or in combination with tamoxifen [160–168].

In the metastatic setting, the combination of ovarian suppression and tamoxifen was shown to be superior to each single-agent treatment [169]. In the adjuvant setting, the ZIPP trial [170] showed a similar outcome for goserelin and tamoxifen, but the combination of both did not show a larger benefit.

The North American Intergroup trial 0142 [171] showed similar results and despite the fact that the statistical power was limited because the trial was closed early due to low accrual, the addition of ovarian ablation to tamoxifen did not result in an improved disease-free survival or overall survival but only in higher toxicity in terms of menopausal symptoms and sexual dysfunction. The SOFT trial (Suppression of Ovarian Function Trial) [172] was designed to evaluate whether OFS in combination with either tamoxifen or an AI (exemestane = E) added benefit compared to tamoxifen (T) alone. The results revealed that the lowest-risk women (e.g., those who did not receive chemotherapy) experienced outstanding outcomes, with 5-year breast cancer-free survival approximately equivalent between the three treatment arms (tamoxifen alone: 95.8 %; T+OFS: 95.1 %; E+OFS: 97.1 %). Among women who did receive chemotherapy and remained premenopausal, adding OFS to tamoxifen resulted in an absolute increase in 5-year breast cancer-free survival of 4.5 %. The benefit was even greater when comparing tamoxifen alone versus E+OFS, with a 5-year absolute increase in breast cancer-free and distant recurrence-free survival of 7.7 and 4.2 %, respectively. Subgroup analyses indicated that the greatest added benefit of OFS over tamoxifen alone was seen in the youngest women; among women younger than 35, 5-year breast cancer-free survival in the tamoxifen alone arm was 67.7 versus 78.9 % in T+OFS and 83.4 % in E+OFS with no clear survival advantage demonstrated to date. In the postmenopausal setting, the efficacy of the aromatase inhibitors (AI) is well established as shown in several randomized trials. AIs do not suppress the ovarian synthesis of estrogen and may even induce recovery of the ovarian function in premenopausal women amenorrhoeic after chemotherapy [173]. AIs were also shown to be useful in stimulating ovulation in the context of in vitro fertilization (IVF) [174, 175]. For all these reasons, their use in premenopausal patients is recommended only in combination with ovarian suppression.

Final results from the ABCSG-12 Trial, which compared the aromatase inhibitor, anastrozole, to tamoxifen among premenopausal women receiving OFS, revealed no difference in disease-free survival between the two arms, overall survival in the anastrozole arm was lower relative to the tamoxifen arm [176]. After a median follow-up of 8 years, overall survival for the entire study population, the majority of whom had not received chemotherapy, was 95.2 %. While the addition of zoledronic acid to OFS and endocrine therapy (ET) did not significantly improve disease-free in women aged 40 and younger, among women older than 40, both disease-free survival and overall survival were superior in the group randomized to zoledronic acid.

The TEXT [177] trial randomized premenopausal women receiving OFS to exemestane or tamoxifen. In contrast to the ABCSG 12 trial, women randomized to receive AI and OFS arm had significantly better disease-free survival compared to the tamoxifen and OFS arm, (HR: 0.72). Overall survival between the groups was not significantly different (HR: 1.14)

Data exist on the use of aromatase inhibitors in combination with ovarian function suppression in premenopausal women with advanced breast cancer. In a small study, including 16 patients [178], all previously treated with goserelin and tamoxifen, it has been shown that almost all benefited from the switch to anastrozole at progression. Another recently published trial evaluating 32 premenopausal women with T2–T4, N0–N2 breast cancer, who underwent neoadjuvant endocrine treatment with triptorelin and letrozole [179] showed that 16 patients had a response, 1 complete pathological response and 15 clinical and imaging partial responses.

The role of fulvestrant, a selective estrogen receptor downregulator has being investigated in at least one trial for premenopausal patients with advanced breast cancer: in 26 premenopausal women with hormone receptor-positive metastatic breast cancer the combination of fulvestrant 250 mg plus goserelin 3.6 mg appears to possess clinically meaningful activity [180]. To date, its use outside a clinical trial cannot be recommended in the adjuvant setting.

29.6.5 Targeted Treatment

An increasing number of compounds are being developed that target cellular mechanisms involved in the pathogenesis of breast cancer in a specific way. The rational use of such therapies should be based on the understanding of molecular pathways and on appropriate clinical trials with relevant endpoints.

29.6.5.1 Monoclonal Antibodies

Trastuzumab: The first widely used substance of this class was trastuzumab, a humanized monoclonal antibody, that binds to the extracellular segment of the HER2 receptor.

Cells treated with trastuzumab undergo arrest during the G1 phase of the cell cycle, therefore reducing their proliferative activity. It has been suggested that trastuzumab induces some of its effect by downregulation of HER2 leading to disruption of receptor dimerization and signaling through the downstream PI3K cascade. P27Kip1 is then not phosphorylated and is able to enter the nucleus and inhibit cdk2 activity, causing cell cycle arrest [181]. In addition, trastuzumab suppresses angiogenesis by both induction of antiangiogenic factors and repression of pro-angiogenic factors. It is thought that a contribution to the unregulated growth observed in cancer could be due to proteolytic cleavage of HER2 that results in the release of the extracellular domain. Trastuzumab has been shown to inhibit HER2 ectodomain cleavage in breast cancer cells [182].

Several clinical trials have shown that trastuzumab is effective as single substance and in combination with chemotherapy in the treatment of advanced [183] breast cancer overexpressing HER2. According to the results of five independent randomized studies, which enrolled in total 13.000 women in the adjuvant setting, trastuzumab combined with chemotherapy was able to reduce the risk of recurrence by at least one-third and in all but one studies [184], a reduction of the risk of death was also demonstrated [185–190]. Trastuzumab seems to be more effective when commenced concurrently with the taxane component of chemotherapy, as compared with sequential administration after completion of chemotherapy [191].

The HERA trial compared also a longer duration of trastuzumab (2 years vs. 1 year). After a median follow-up of 8 years, there were 367 DFS events in 1552 patients in the 1-year group and 367 events in 1553 patients in the 2 year group (HR 0.99, 95 % CI 0.85–1.14, $p = 0.86$) [190]. The administration of adjuvant trastuzumab for 2 years resulted in increased rate of Grade 3–4 adverse events and decrease in left ventricular ejection fraction (LVEF) during treatment as compared to the 1 year group. Trastuzumab-regimens shorter than 1 year have been assessed. The FinHER study randomized 232 women with early stage HER2-positive breast cancer after three cycles of docetaxel or vinorelbine, followed by three cycles of fluorouracil, epirubicin, and cyclophosphamide to receive 9 weekly trastuzumab infusions or not. In the final analysis after 62 months of medial follow-up, trastuzumab administration resulted in a trend towards improved distant DFS [192]. Based on the results of the FinHER trial, the PHARE trial explored the efficacy of shorter duration of adjuvant trastuzumab treatment. In total, 3.381 patients with HER2-positive early BC who had received at least four cycles of chemotherapy and up to 6 months of trastuzumab prior to randomization were randomized to continue trastuzumab for a total of 12 or to stop at 6 months [193]. The study did not meet the non-inferiority endpoint, and therefore the 6 months duration cannot be recommended. The administration of 1-year adjuvant trastuzumab concurrently to the taxane component of chemotherapy is considered as the standard of care [194]. A subgroup analysis of the HERA trial showed that patients under the age 35 have the same benefit from 1-year trastuzumab treatment as older ones [195].

Pertuzumab is a monoclonal inhibitor of the dimerization of the HER2 protein with the epidermal growth factor receptor (EGFR and HER1) and other pathways [196]. Its mode of action differs from trastuzumab and small molecule kinase inhibitors such as gefitinib. In the metastatic setting, the CLEOPATRA trial [197, 198] showed superior results, in terms of PFS (18.5 vs. 12.4 months) and 1-year survival (23.6 % vs. 17.2), of the triplet trastuzumab + pertuzumab + docetaxel compared to trastuzumab + docetaxel as first-line therapy. Currently, there is an ongoing randomized phase III study, the APHINITY trial, comparing the pertuzumab/trastuzumab doublet versus adjuvant trastuzumab single-agent, with the results of the primary endpoint analysis of iDFS expected during Q2 2016.

T-DM1 (Trastuzumab Emtansine) is an antibody–drug conjugate incorporating the human epidermal growth factor receptor 2 (HER2)–targeted antitumor properties of trastuzumab with the cytotoxic activity of the microtubule-inhibitory agent DM1. Trials in women with metastatic breast cancer have shown consistent and substantial benefits in terms of PFS and OS, both in the second line (vs. lapatinib + capecitabine, in the EMILIA trial) [199]; and beyond (vs. treatment of physician's choice, in the TH3RESA trial [200]). The KATHARINE study is a randomized phase III trial, currently evaluating the efficacy of T-DM1 versus trastuzumab in patients with residual disease following neoadjuvant chemotherapy and trastuzumab.

Bevacizumab is a monoclonal antibody directed against vascular endothelial growth factor (VEGF) that inhibits many functions of the VEGF. This compound was shown to be active as first-line treatment of metastatic breast cancer in combination with paclitaxel [201], but not in a later phase of the disease combined with capecitabine [202]. A randomized phase III trial compared bevacizumab and paclitaxel with paclitaxel alone as first-line therapy in 772 patients with metastatic disease. Paclitaxel plus bevacizumab significantly prolonged progression-free survival as compared with paclitaxel alone (median, 11.8 vs. 5.9 months; hazard ratio for progression, 0.60; $P < 0.001$) and increased the objective response rate (36.9 % vs. 21.2 %, $P < 0.001$). The overall survival rate, however, was similar in the two groups (median, 26.7 vs. 25.2 months; hazard ratio, 0.88; $P = 0.16$) [203]. The trial BEATRICE [204] randomized women with early stage triple-negative breast cancer to receive either chemotherapy followed by observation or the same chemotherapy combined with bevacizumab and followed by single-agent bevacizumab for 1 year. After a follow-up of median 31.5 months bevacizumab did not show any benefit in term of disease-free survival. HER2 overexpression has been associated with vascular endothelial growth factor (VEGF) upregulation and secretion in breast cancer cells, resulting in increased angiogenesis and metastatic dissemination of human HER2-overexpressing breast cancer cells. These findings led to clinical trials investigating the combination of bevacizumab and trastuzumab in the metastatic (AVAREL) and in the adjuvant (BETH) setting [205, 206]. Both showed no benefit in the addition of bevacizumab to trastuzumab.

29.6.5.2 Tyrosine Kinase Inhibitors

Lapatinib is an orally active dual kinase inhibitor that reversibly inhibits the HER1 and HER2 kinase activities; its activity seems to be limited to breast cancers with a strong expression of HER2 [207]. Preliminary results indicate that lapatinib is effective in the therapy of advanced HER2-positive breast cancer in combination with capecitabine after failure of anthracycline-, taxane- and trastuzumab-based therapy [208].

Patients with HER2-overexpressing breast cancer have been found to have a significantly higher risk of developing brain metastases [209–211]. Lapatinib, which is a small molecule capable of crossing the blood–brain barrier, has been used in clinical trials for the treatment of brain metastases. A phase-II trial using lapatinib in 39 patients, who developed brain metastases while receiving trastuzumab showed that one patient achieved a PR in the brain and seven patients (18 %) were progression free in both CNS and non-CNS sites at 16 weeks [212].

The use of lapatinib in the adjuvant therapy has been investigated in a randomized trial conducted by the BIG Group that compared lapatinib (L) with trastuzumab (T) as well as the sequential-(L+T) and combined (LT) treatment by lapatinib and trastuzumab (ALTTO) [213]. L+T showed a lower risk of a DFS event compared with T, and LT appeared non-inferior to T, but neither finding was statistically significant. The first DFS results of dual HER2 blockade in the adjuvant ALTTO trial at 4.5 years median follow-up are unexpected and surprising considering the effect shown by doubling the pCR rate with L+T versus T in the NeoALLTO trial.

Everolimus, another mTOR inhibitor, added to Exemestane in the metastastic setting showed a clinically meaningful and statistically significant improvement in the primary endpoint, PFS, but did not confer a statistically significant improvement in overall survival [214]. Two investigator-initiated studies are evaluating the role of everolimus in the adjuvant setting in women with poor prognosis, ER-positive and HER2-negative primary breast cancer (NCT01805271 and NCT01674140) [215].

Neratinib is an irreversible panHER tyrosine kinase inhibitor. The ExteNET study examined the advantage of extended adjuvant therapy with neratinib given orally for 1-year versus placebo in patients who had already completed adjuvant chemotherapy, as well as 12 months of adjuvant trastuzumab. Preliminary results announced in a press release indicate that neratinib improved DFS by 33 % compared with placebo (HR = 0.67; $p = 0.0046$) [216].

The molecular crosstalk between several receptor kinases and steroid hormone receptors is likely to be involved in the resistance to antiestrogens [16, 217]; thus, modifiers of these mechanisms will potentially improve the management of hormone-sensitive breast cancer patients [218–221].

29.6.5.3 PARP1 [Poly(ADP-Ribose) Polymerase-1]—Inhibitors

PARP1 activity is required for base-excision repair, a DNA damage repair pathway that recognizes and eliminates DNA bases damaged by oxidation in a process that occurs thousands of times during each normal cell cycle. In the absence of PARP1, oxidized bases accumulate eventually causing double-stranded DNA breaks. Normally, homologous recombination repairs these breaks, but should this mechanism be unavailable, as is the case when BRCA1 or BRCA2 is deficient or mutated, the cell dies [222]. Preclinical studies showed that inhibition of PARP would lead to selective and significant killing of *BRCA*-mutated cancer cells, a phenomenon described as synthetic lethality that is not observed in cells with intact BRCA function [223]. The oral PARP inhibitor olaparib in heavily pretreated ABC patients with BRCA mutations provides positive proof-of-concept of the efficacy and tolerability of this targeted approach [224, 225]. The OlympiA trial, a phase III clinical trial investigating the efficacy of a maintenance treatment with olaparib after completion of the (neo)-adjuvant chemotherapy is currently accruing (NCT02032823) [215]. Olaparib as well as other PARP inhibitors are being evaluated either alone, in combination with chemotherapy [226] or with other inhibitors [227] for BRCA deficient tumors in the adjuvant as well as the metastatic setting.

29.6.5.4 Vaccines and Immunotherapy

Active immunization by tumor antigens that are able to induce specific long-term antitumor immune responses is still an investigational approach in early and advanced breast cancer. Early data from clinical trials show some antitumor activity and low toxicity. Promising results have been reported from a small randomized clinical trial of active immunization with a vaccine targeting HER2 protein in 171 patients with early breast cancer: the vaccine significantly reduced the risk of recurrence without causing serious toxic effects. The clinical recurrence rate for the vaccinated patients was 5.6 % (5/90) compared to 14.8 % (12/81) for the observation patients ($p = 0.04$) at a median follow-up of 24 months [228]. The next generation of clinical studies will integrate breast cancer vaccines with standard therapies. The adjuvant setting is considered most promising as the immunosuppressive effect of bulky disease does not interfere with effective immune responses [229]. Multiple immunotherapy modalities are under investigation in patients with breast cancer. These include vaccine to enhance specific immune responses to tumor antigens such as WT-1, HER2 and NY-ESO-1, adoptive transfer of in vitro-expanded, naturally arising or genetically engineered tumor-specific lymphocytes, therapeutic administration of monoclonal antibodies to target and eliminate tumor cells, and inhibition of the molecular or cellular mediators of cancer-induced immunosuppression, such as CTLA-4, PD-1 or Treg cells [230].

29.7 Management/Treatment of Advanced Breast Cancer

As for early breast cancer, also in the metastatic setting, age alone should not be a reason to prescribe more aggressive therapy. Whenever feasible biopsy of the metastases should be performed for confirmation of the diagnosis and assessment of the biology [231], local treatment in case of isolated visceral metastasis [232] or oligometastatic presentation may be evaluated case by case. In young women with known endocrine responsive metastatic breast cancer, tamoxifen in combination with ovarian function suppression or ablation (OSF) remain the preferred treatment choice [233] unless rapid tumor shrinkage is needed. After progression on tamoxifen/OFS, treatment with aromatase inhibitor/OFS may be considered [146, 234]. There are only few data about the use of fulvestrant in premenopausal women [180]. Recently, its combination with the inhibitor of CDK4 and CDK6 palbociclib resulted in longer progression-free survival and a relatively higher quality of life than fulvestrant alone in patients with advanced hormone receptor-positive breast cancer that had progressed during prior endocrine therapy, regardless of the patient's menopausal status [235]. Based on the available data about chemotherapy, sequential monotherapy is recommended for metastatic breast cancer. However, doublets like docetaxel/capecitabine or paclitaxel/gemcitabine seem to prolong survival over monotherapy [236].

29.8 Side Effects of the Treatment

29.8.1 Surgery

Cellulitis or abscess of the breast occurs in 1–8 % of women undergoing breast-conserving surgery. In two separate reports, risk factors for breast cellulitis included drainage of a hematoma, postoperative ecchymosis, tumor stage, the volume of resected breast tissue, the number of breast seroma aspirations, breast and arm lymphedema, and removal of more than five axillary nodes [237, 238]. Cellulitis of the ipsilateral arm is a well-known complication in women who have undergone axillary lymph node dissection that typically occurs late after surgery [239]. In a retrospective analysis of 580 women treated for breast cancer between 1985 and 2004, it was shown that the overall incidence of delayed breast cellulitis (DBC) was 8 % and the median time to onset of DBC from the date of definitive surgery was 226 days [238].

Seroma formation occurs in almost all patients after mastectomy. In a prospective randomized trial, extensive axillary node involvement was the greatest predictor of prolonged lymphatic drainage need after mastectomy, followed by obesity and the performance of a surgical two-step procedure [240]. Sometimes patients describe a change in chest wall sensation after mastectomy reported as "phantom breast syndrome" [241]; it appears in short after mastectomy in almost 15 % of the patients [242]. Other neurological complications, in particular neuropathic pain, after surgery have been reported in about 30 % of the patients [243].

Differences in incidence of surgical side effects between younger and older women are not reported, and the frequency of adverse event and the cosmetic outcome are mostly related to the local situation (i.e., tumor extension in relation to the breast volume) and the surgical technique and not to age [244, 245].

29.8.2 Systemic Treatment

Side effects due to endocrine therapies are in general underestimated. In particular, tamoxifen treatment in premenopausal women is associated with a variety of symptoms, including vasomotor symptoms, vaginal complaints (dryness, itching, and discharge), decrease of libido, amenorrhea, insomnia,and mood disturbances, leading to significant restriction in the quality of life [246–249]. According to the recent results of the combined SOFT and TEXT analysis, women on tamoxifen plus OFS were more affected by hot flushes and sweats over 5 years than were those on exemestane plus OFS, although these symptoms improved during the course of treatment. Patients on exemestane plus OFS reported more vaginal dryness, greater loss of sexual interest, and difficulties becoming aroused than did patients on tamoxifen plus OFS; these differences persisted over time. In the SOFT, the SOFT trial, the global quality of life did not differ between treatment arms, women on tamoxifen and OFS reported more problems with vaginal dryness over the entire study period as well as short-term problems with hot flashes, sexual interest, and sleep, compared to women on tamoxifen alone. Among women who had received chemotherapy, the differences in symptom burden and changes in symptoms over time were attenuated [250]. Bone metabolism is highly affected by changes in ovarian function. An analysis of 89 women participating in the ZIPP trial showed that 2 years of ovarian ablation through goserelin treatment caused a significant reduction in bone mineral density, but there was a partial recovery from bone loss 1 year after cessation of treatment. The addition of tamoxifen seems to partially counteract the demineralizing effects of goserelin [251]. Tamoxifen alone, however, was associated with bone loss in patients who continued to menstruate after adjuvant chemotherapy [252]. Because of these variable treatment effects bone health has to be regularly checked in young women with breast cancer. In several reports, it has been shown that women undergoing oophorectomy before the onset of menopause had an increased risk of cognitive impairment, dementia, and even Parkinsonism [253, 254]. The impact of the estrogen deprivation on cognitive function in women treated with OFS for breast cancer is not yet exhaustively clarified. Cognitive function has been prospectively investigated in a subset of patients participating in the SOFT trial. This small longitudinal study was not able to provide evidence that the addition of OFS to oral adjuvant endocrine therapy affects cognitive function in a clinically meaningful way after 1 year of treatment [255]. It is well known that there is an increase in cardiovascular disease and cardiovascular risk factors after the menopause, but it is still unclear if this is related exclusively to the aging process or is primarily due to estrogen deprivation. No data are available about the long-term risk of cardiovascular events in young women treated with OFS. The short-term side effects of chemotherapy for early breast cancer in terms of gastrointestinal symptoms, bone marrow depression, and infection risk do mostly not differ in dependence of age, but chemotherapies are in general better tolerated by young women in terms of acute side effects [139]. A substantial portion of women treated with adjuvant chemotherapy, but particularly, premenopausal patients gain weight during treatment. On average, with CMF they gain 2–6 kg, less with AC [256]. The weight gain may be caused by reduced basal metabolic rate, increased food intake, diminished physical activity, and ovarian failure [257, 258]. The risk of chemotherapy-induced *amenorrhea and infertility* is lower in young premenopausal women [158, 259, 260], but menopausal symptoms induced by chemical castration and endocrine treatment have a high impact on the quality of life in younger women [261].

29.8.3 Radiation Therapy

The incidence of immediate skin reaction and subsequent telangiectasia was dramatically reduced with the use of modern equipment and smaller dose per fraction with consequent minimization of the radiotherapy dose delivered to the skin [262]. The data on effect of age on side effects of radiotherapy are inconsistent, and the effect of age seems to vary by site of irradiation [263]. In a report of 416 women followed between June 2003 and July 2005 for outcome and side effects of radiation therapy after breast-conserving surgery, increased age of the patient was a risk factor for the development of telangiectasia [264]. Another recent study conducted between 2006 and 2011 reported that after 50 Gy 3D radiotherapy to the whole breast acute skin toxicities (grade 2) was observed for larger breast volumes ($p = 0.004$), smoking during radiation therapy ($p = 0.064$), and absence of allergies ($p = 0.014$) as well as larger tumor size ($p = 0.009$) and antihormonal therapy ($p = 0.005$). Neither patient age, BMI, nor choice of chemotherapy showed any significant effect on higher grade toxicity [265].

Long-term side effects like *cardiac failure* are less frequently seen in young patients, but if present, their impact on quality of life and overall survival may be deleterious in young, otherwise healthy women [266–268].

Angiosarcomas arising in the irradiated breast are rare and represent about 1 % of all soft tissue sarcomas, but are being reported with increasing frequency over the past 20 years, as breast-conserving therapy combined with radiation therapy to the breast has replaced modified radical mastectomy as standard of care [269].

A special issue is represented by the risk of *lymphedema*. A prospective cohort trial in 666 women diagnosed with breast early breast cancer showed after a follow-up of 10.2 years that the oldest age group (60–64 years) had a lower risk of lymphedema than the youngest age group (35–44 years) (HR = 0.59, 95 % CI: 0.35–0.97) [270]. Young patients present frequently with more advanced disease, in part due to a later diagnosis. In addition, in young women there is a higher incidence of inflammatory breast cancer accompanied by extensive lymphovascular invasion and nodal involvement [271]. After breast-conserving surgery with radiation therapy, more breast edema is observed, and moreover, younger patients undergo fivefold more breast reconstructions, which may increase the risk of lymphedema [272]. Radiotherapy (particularly extensive in case of locally advanced disease) may also affect the lymphatic drainage of the limb, and this may have a greater impact in young women [273, 274].

29.9 Follow-up Recommendations and Survivors Care

Survival of patients with breast cancer has increased during the last decade, and therefore, more breast cancer survivors treated with surgery, irradiation, and adjuvant systemic therapy are in follow-up care. The most recent ASCO guidelines for follow-up of breast cancer survivors recommend annual mammography and more frequent medical history and physical examination to screen for new or locally relapsed breast cancers or symptoms of possible metastases or secondary malignancies, but no specific screening is recommended for occult metastatic disease in asymptomatic patients [275]. Although screening breast magnetic resonance imaging (MRI) seems to be more sensitive than conventional imaging at detecting breast cancer in high-risk women, there is no evidence that breast MRI improves outcomes when used as a breast cancer surveillance tool during routine follow-up in asymptomatic patients [84]. The decision to use breast MRI in high-risk patients should be made on an individual basis depending on the complexity of the clinical scenario.

The referral for genetic counseling is recommended for women who meet the criteria suggested by the Preventive Services Task Force and the National Comprehensive Cancer Network [276]. During follow-up, the consequences of premature menopause, other late side effects of antiestrogen therapy, and of other adjuvant therapies should be recognized and treated if indicated, but estrogen substitution therapy should possibly be avoided. Sexual dysfunction can be addressed through sexual counseling and vaginal dryness can frequently be sufficiently managed with non-hormonal preparations or with cautious use of estrogen ring preparations, recognizing that there is the potential for slight systemic absorption [277, 278]. The role of androgen treatment in this context is still controversial [279]. Beneficial effects of testosterone on libido and sexual function were reported in naturally or treatment-induced postmenopausal women, but no data are available about the safety profile of testosterone.

Bone mineral density should be assessed, adequate intake of calcium and vitamin D and regular weight-bearing exercise encouraged, and bisphosphonate treatment initiated, if indicated [280, 281].

29.10 Fertility Preservation

The increasing age at first and subsequent pregnancies in the western world and the improved survival for women diagnosed with breast cancer increases the relevance of fertility issues. Preserving fertility is frequently an important issue for younger female cancer survivors and their partners [282, 283]. In a web-based survey of 657 breast cancer patients, Partridge [284] showed fertility (after treatment) being a major concern for young women with breast cancer. In a longitudinal cohort study of 577 breast cancer patients, Ganz [285] showed that 20 % were planning or hoping to have children before the diagnosis of breast cancer. 11 % ($n = 61$) reported that they had considered getting pregnant since the breast cancer diagnosis. While 19 % of these 61 survivors reported that they were not planning a pregnancy due to physician's recommendation, 17 % said they were not planning a pregnancy because they were worried about the risk of relapse. Only 5 % of women reported a pregnancy and life birth after the breast cancer diagnosis. In a multicenter survey, Thewes [286] observed highest need in fertility-related information at the time of diagnosis and treatment decision. In later stages of treatment, menopause-related information was significantly more important. Little if any attention has been paid to fertility-related needs of partners. In a case-control study conducted in Israel [287], 30 breast cancer survivors and 13 husbands were compared to 29 healthy women and 15 husbands using qualitative questions and quantitative measures, including demographic and medical questionnaire. The experience of having breast cancer did not lower the overall positive motivation toward childbirth in this population. Initial concerns that fertility preservation interventions and/or a pregnancy might increase the risk of cancer recurrence in breast cancer and gynecological malignancies have not been confirmed to date. In 2013, the American Society of Clinical Oncology [288] recommended that involved physicians (e.g., oncologists) should discuss at the earliest point in time infertility as a potential risk of cancer treatment with patients and their partners. For patients at risk of infertility and interested in assessing their options of fertility preservation, earliest possible referral to appropriate specialists is suggested. Any decision about an appropriate therapy would ideally be supported by a team consisting of a gynecologist, a medical oncologist, a reproductive endocrinologist, and a psychosocial care provider. The decision-making should be based on agreed written protocols that can be shared with the patients and their families.

Ovagenesis begins at approximately 3 weeks after conception. At this time, the primordial germ cells, arising from the endodermal yolk sac, begin migration to the developing ovaries. The cells undergo progressive differentiation to become primary oocytes. After birth, no more primary oocytes develop. These oocytes remain in the prophase of the first meiotic division until puberty. A woman has 200,000 oocytes at puberty. This number decreases to about 400 at the time of menopause [289, 290]. Since many chemotherapy agents act on growing and dividing cells, both oocytes and ovarian follicles may be affected by chemotherapy.

The impact of adjuvant chemotherapy on ovarian function depends on the age of the woman, the class of drug used, and the duration of treatment. Review of the published data and some prospective studies showed that patients over 40 years have a greater risk of experiencing amenorrhea during treatment, and furthermore, the amenorrhea is less often reversible [158, 159, 291]. In a prospective trial assessing acute and long-term toxicity in 796 women treated between 1974 and 1982 with doxorubicin-containing post-operative adjuvant chemotherapy [261], 80 % of the pre-menopausal women reported amenorrhea. None of the patients under 30 years of age had menstrual abnormalities, whereas 96 % of those 40–49 years old developed amenorrhea. Amenorrhea was permanent for most women over 40, but for 50 % of patients under 40 years of age, it was reversible. In general, rates of both transient and prolonged amenorrhea are higher with CMF or CEF/CAF-type regimens as compared to AC [292, 293].

Even for younger women in whom ovarian activity resumes after chemotherapy, menopause tends to happen earlier, therefore shortening the window of opportunity for conception. Furthermore, the continuation or resumption of the menses is not always equivalent with fertility. After chemotherapy, the number of anovulatoric cycles is increased [294].

The management of gonadal toxicity due to adjuvant chemotherapy for breast cancer is complex and frequently difficult. It is therefore very important to consider the possibility of preventing ovarian failure and the therapeutic options available if infertility occurs before starting chemotherapy [295]. It has been postulated that suppression of germ cell stimulation may lead to protection of oocytes and ovarian follicles from the toxic effects of chemotherapy.

Ovarian suppression through gonadotropin-releasing hormone (GnRH) agonist or antagonist treatment during chemotherapy might be considered a reliable strategy not only to preserve ovarian function but also to increase the likelihood of becoming pregnant after the end of cytotoxic therapy [296]. The Southwest Oncology Group conducted a trial aimed at preventing early ovarian failure with GnRH agonists among women with hormone receptor-negative breast cancer who receive chemotherapy (IBCSG34/ Southwest Oncology Group 0230) [297]. Among 135 patients with complete primary endpoint data, the ovarian failure rate was 8 % in the goserelin group and 22 % in the chemotherapy-alone group (odds ratio, 0.30; 95 % confidence interval, 0.09–0.97; two-sided $P = 0.04$) Among the 218 patients who could be evaluated, pregnancy occurred in more women in the goserelin group than in the chemotherapy-alone group (21 % vs. 11 %, $P = 0.03$); women in the goserelin group also had improved disease-free survival ($P = 0.04$) and overall survival ($P = 0.05$). In contrast another randomized trial with a similar design, but using anthracycline-containing regimens (Zoladex Rescue of Ovarian Function [ZORO]/German Breast Group) [298] showed that premenopausal patients with breast cancer receiving goserelin simultaneously with neoadjuvant chemotherapy did not experience statistically significantly less amenorrhea 6 months after end of chemotherapy compared with those receiving chemotherapy alone. Small observational studies conducted in patients with Hogkin's disease also suggest that oral contraceptives may help preserve ovarian function when given during chemotherapy [299, 300]. Its use for preservation of fertility in patients with endocrine unresponsive breast cancer, however, remains controversial.

Embryo cryopreservation is considered an established fertility preservation method as it has routinely been used for storing surplus embryos after in vitro fertilization for infertility treatment. Because of lack of approval by health authorities and ethical bodies or insurance companies, this procedure is not available in all countries. Furthermore, a partner or sperm donor is required. This approach typically requires 2 weeks of ovarian stimulation with daily injections of follicle-stimulating hormone from the onset of menses, which may require a delay of 2–6 weeks in chemotherapy initiation. For women with hormone-sensitive tumors, alternative hormonal stimulation approaches such as letrozole or tamoxifen [174, 301, 302] have been used to theoretically reduce the potential risk of estrogen exposure. Short-term breast cancer recurrence rates after ovarian stimulation using letrozole or tamoxifen concurrent with follicle-stimulating hormone (FSH) administration have been compared to nonrandomized controls and no increase in cancer recurrence rates has been noted [174, 303]. Live birth rates after embryo cryopreservation and implantation depend on the patient's age and the total number of embryos available and may be lower than with fresh embryos. Embryo cryopreservation after ovarian stimulation with the letrozole and follicle-stimulating hormone protocol has been shown to preserves fertility in women with breast cancer and results in pregnancy rates comparable to those expected in a non-cancer population undergoing in vitro fertilization [304]. Seventeen of the thirty-three women attempting pregnancy had at least one child, translating into a fertility preservation rate of 51.5 % per attempting woman.

Oocyte cryopreservation is another option for fertility preservation, particularly in patients without a partner, or who have religious or ethical objections to embryo freezing.

Ovarian stimulation and harvesting requirements are identical to those of embryo cryopreservation, and thus this technique is associated with similar concerns regarding delays of therapy and potential risks of short-term exposure to high hormonal levels. As with embryo cryopreservation, letrozole or tamoxifen can be used. Preliminary study indicated that unfertilized oocytes are more prone to damage during cryopreservation procedures than embryos, and the overall pregnancy rates may be lower than with standard in vitro fertilization procedures [305]. However, recent reports showed that delivery rate using cryopreserved oocytes is comparable to conventional in vitro fertilization using fresh oocytes [306]. To date, more than 1000 births have been reported worldwide with this approach, and efforts to improve the efficiency of cryopreservation may further increase success rates [288, 307–309]. Oocyte collection has the advantage that it can be performed without ovarian stimulation ("natural cycle-IVF"), but the number of viable embryo yielded is extremely low [174, 303, 310] and this method remains experimental.

Ovarian tissue cryopreservation is an additional investigational method of fertility preservation and it has the advantage of requiring neither sperm donors nor ovarian stimulation. Ovarian tissue is removed laparoscopically and frozen. At a later time point, the ovarian tissue is thawed and reimplanted. Primordial follicles can be cryopreserved with great efficiency [311, 312], but because of the initial ischemia encountered after ovarian transplantation, a quarter or more of these follicles might be lost, as shown in xenografting studies [313]. The first ovarian transplant procedure was reported in 2000 [314]. Ovarian tissue can be transplanted orthotopically to pelvis or heterotopically to subcutaneous areas such as the forearm or lower abdomen, and initial studies reported restoration of ovarian endocrine function after both types of transplantation [314–318]. There have been 24 reports of live births after orthotopic ovarian transplantation in 60 cancer patients; more than 50 % of women were able to conceive naturally [319]. One concern with the reimplantation of ovarian tissue is the potential for reintroducing cancer cells. In patients without evidence of systemic metastasis, the likelihood of occult ovarian metastasis appears to be low [320, 321], and there are no reports of cancer recurrence after ovarian transplantation in a recent review of 60 cases [319].

The possibility that fertility preservation interventions and/or subsequent pregnancy may increase the risk of cancer recurrence is a concern for breast cancer patients and women with gynecologic malignancies. Several case-control and retrospective cohort studies have not shown a decrement in survival or an increase in risk of recurrence with pregnancy [322, 323]. While these data are reassuring, the studies are all limited by significant biases. After a feasibility assessment [324], the first international multicentric prospectively trial, investigating the safety and efficacy of an interruption of the adjuvant endocrine treatment to allow women to conceive (POSITIVE), has been started in 2014 and is currently accruing (NCT02308085).

29.11 Breast Cancer Associated with Pregnancy (Lactation)

Gestational or pregnancy-associated breast cancer is defined as a breast cancer that is diagnosed during pregnancy or in the first postpartum year, or at any time during lactation.

Breast cancer is the most common malignancy diagnosed during pregnancy, with an estimated 1 in 3000 to 1 in 10,000 deliveries being to pregnant breast cancer patients [325–327]. Between 0.2 and 3.8 % of breast cancers diagnosed in women under age 50 are detected during pregnancy or in the postpartum period [328]. In contrast, 10–20 % of breast cancers in women 30 years of age or younger are discovered during pregnancy or in the year following delivery [329]. Because the incidence of breast cancer increases with age, it has been hypothesized that the incidence of breast cancer diagnosed during pregnancy will increase as more women delay childbearing nowadays. Pregnancy itself may transiently increase an individual woman's risk of developing breast cancer, despite its long-term protective effect on the development of the disease. This was illustrated by three population-based series in which pregnancy was followed by a period of increased breast cancer risk lasting 3–10 years, which subsequently declined [330–332]. This observation has also been done for women with inherited BRCA2 mutations: the risk of breast cancer in the 2 years following a birth was 70 % higher for a BRCA2 carrier compared to nulliparous controls [333]. In addition, the data of three small studies show that women with a genetic predisposition to breast cancer seem to have an increased risk for pregnancy-related cancer. In a case-control study from Japan involving 343 women, a family history of breast cancer was three times more common among pregnant and lactating women with breast cancer than among controls [334]. Another small retrospective study found BRCA2 mutations in a significantly higher number of archival samples from women with pregnancy-associated breast cancer compared to samples from unmatched non-pregnant controls [335]. In a Swedish series of 302 women diagnosed with breast cancer before the age of 40 (47 from families with BRCA mutations), women with BRCA1 mutations were significantly more likely to develop breast cancer during pregnancy than those without inherited mutations [336]. Furthermore, in a matched case-control study comparing 1260 pairs of women with known BRCA mutations with and without breast cancer, increasing parity was associated with a higher risk of breast cancer before age 50 in BRCA2, but not in BRCA1 carriers [333].

Breast cancer occurring during pregnancy presents a challenging clinical situation for the mother, fetus, and treating clinicians because of the complex medical, ethical, and psychological problems arising in this situation. Breast cancer during pregnancy is often perceived as a situation that puts the life of the mother in conflict with that of her unborn child. However, limited data suggest that pregnancy termination does not improve the outcome for pregnant women with breast cancer. Pregnant women should be treated according to guidelines for non-pregnant patients, with some modification to protect the fetus [337–339]. Medical abortion is not usually recommended in cases of pregnancy-associated breast cancer, but may be considered during treatment planning, in particular in case of diagnosis in the first trimester. When considering management of the disease in this setting, there are two key issues: first, how the pregnancy affects the behavior of the cancer, and second, how the cancer and its treatment affect the pregnancy.

Making the diagnosis of breast cancer and performing a staging work-up is frequently more difficult due to the physiological changes in the breast that accompany pregnancy and lactation and the desire to limit radiation exposure to the unborn child.

Pregnant or postpartum women with breast cancer usually present similarly to non-pregnant women with a mass or thickening in the breast. Rarely, refusal by a nursing infant of a lactating breast that harbors an occult carcinoma has been described, and termed the milk rejection sign [340]. The physiologic changes in the breast occurring during pregnancy and lactation (engorgement, hypertrophy) make physical examination more challenging and interpretation of findings more difficult, and the density of the breast may limit the utility of mammography. The malignant mammography finding of clinical suspected breast cancer was histologically confirmed in about 78 % of the cases in a older report [341], and 86.7 % [342], respectively, 90 % [343] in two recent retrospective studies.

As a result, diagnostic delays of 2 months or longer are common in women with gestational breast cancer [344] and they adversely impact outcome, since even a 1 month delay in diagnosis can increase the risk of nodal involvement by 0.9–1.8 % [345]. Delay in diagnosis may be responsible, at least in part, for the larger size of tumors at diagnosis in pregnant women. At presentation, about 42 % of the patients are diagnosed with stage III or IV. A breast mass that persists for 2–4 weeks should always be investigated, although the majority (80 %) of breast biopsies performed in pregnant women will prove to be benign [346]. The result of a large meta-analysis involving 3628 cases and 37,100 controls, showed that patients with pregnancy associate breast cancer (BCP) had a significantly higher risk of death compared to those with non-pregnancy-related breast cancer and particularly those diagnosed shortly postpartum had a poor prognosis [347]. However a recently published multicentric cohort study comparing 311 women with BCP with 865 non-pregnant breast cancer patients showed similar OS for patients diagnosed with BCP compared with non-pregnant patients [348].

Mammography is not contraindicated in pregnancy, as the average glandular dose to the breast for a two view mammogram (200–400 mrad) provides a negligible radiation dose of 0.4 mrad to the fetus as long as abdominal shielding is used [349]. The sensitivity of the mammography is diminished by the increased water content, higher density, and loss of contrasting fat in the pregnant or lactating breast. In an early series, six of eight pregnant women with histologically documented breast cancer had falsely negative mammograms [350]. Somewhat better sensitivity rates, ranging from 63 to 78 %, are reported in more recent studies [334, 341–343, 351, 352].

Breast *sonography* is often the first diagnostic test performed to evaluate a breast mass in a pregnant woman. It can distinguish between solid and cystic breast masses in almost all cases without the risk of fetal radiation exposure. A focal solid mass is observed in the majority of cases of gestational breast cancer [334, 341, 342, 352], although in one report, two of the four malignant tumors had sonographic characteristics of a benign lesion [351]. If palpable nodes are present, axillary ultrasound and fine-needle aspiration (FNA) biopsy are important components of the initial staging evaluation.

Magnetic resonance imaging (MRI) has not been systematically studied for the diagnosis of breast masses in pregnant or lactating women. Although gadolinium-enhanced MRI appears to be more sensitive than mammography for detecting invasive breast cancer, particularly in women with dense breast tissue, the use of contrast agents such as gadolinium should be avoided during pregnancy. Gadolinium crosses the placenta, and has been associated with fetal abnormalities in rats [353, 354]. Other disadvantages of breast MRI include lack of specificity, inability to identify microcalcifications, high cost, and long examination times. MRI has been used for the diagnosis of metastases in women with newly diagnosed breast cancer during pregnancy. As long as contrast is avoided, there are no reported harmful effects from MR imaging to the pregnant woman or to the unborn child [349]. Nevertheless, some authorities recommend that all MRI scans be avoided in the first trimester [355].

There is minimal information regarding *positron emission tomography* (PET) in pregnancy. ^{18}F-FDG has been found to cross the placenta and to accumulate in fetal brain, heart, and bladder in a monkey study [356]. Healthy monkeys were born but the possibility of harms remains uncertain. The radiation dose to the uterus is 3.70–7.40 mGy, for the usual dose range of isotope injected. Recently, the case of a young woman treated for Hodgkin's disease was reported [357]. After 4 months of chemotherapy, a PET scan showed an unexplained hotspot in the right lower abdomen; 6 weeks later, the woman complained of abdominal distension and an ultrasound showed an unsuspected pregnancy with an estimated gestational age of 30 weeks. She delivered a girl by caesarian section without congenital abnormalities and at 6 years of age, she apparently has a normal development.

Although fine-needle aspiration can be used to clarify a breast mass in a pregnant patient, a core or excisional biopsy is often required for a definitive diagnosis of invasive cancer. Core, incisional or excisional biopsy can be performed relatively safely during pregnancy, preferably under local anesthesia [346]. During pregnancy and lactation, atypical cytomorphologic features are seen in normal breast tissue, and therefore interpretation of FNA samples needs special caution and accuracy [358–361]. To avoid misinterpretation and a false-negative result in doubtful cases, a second opinion slide review at a cancer center is recommended. The risk of false-positive results is negligible in the hands of experienced cytologists [338].

Because of the potential harms to the unborn child, staging procedures should be limited to a minimum. A fetal exposition to radiation doses of less than 0.1 Gy do not cause major damage, in particular in the third trimester of pregnancy, but in case of radiation above 2.5 Gy, malformations are likely and more that 30 Gy may cause abortion. The association of in utero diagnostic X-ray exposure with subsequent occurrence of childhood leukemia has been the subject of great controversy over the last 50 years. Combining the results of many case–control studies in different countries, a proportional increase in risk of about 40 % for malignancy, and in particular, for ALL in childhood after a radiographic examination of the abdomen in pregnant women has been reported in the year 1956 [362]. However, subsequent cohort investigations in the United Kingdom [363] and the United States [364] reported no increase in risk of childhood leukemia linked with maternal pelvimetry during pregnancy. In addition, risks of leukemia were not increased among offspring of Japanese atomic bomb survivors, who were pregnant at the time of the bombings [365] (Table 29.1).

Pregnant women with clinically positive nodes, T3 or T4 lesions, or suspicion for distant metastases should undergo a complete imaging evaluation of the most common sites for distant metastatic spread (lung, liver, and bone) like non-pregnant women. In contrast, women who are asymptomatic and have clinically node-negative, early stage breast cancer do not require formal evaluation since the incidence of unsuspected metastases is low [366]. There are no contraindications to chest radiography in pregnancy as long as abdominal shielding is used. However, the ability to evaluate the lower lung parenchyma is limited late in gestation when the gravid uterus is pressing against the diaphragm. Abdominal ultrasound is a safe procedure in pregnant women for the evaluation of liver metastases, but is significantly less sensitive than CT or MRI. CT scans are generally avoided during pregnancy because of the large cumulative radiation dose when multiple slices are obtained. MRI is preferred if further evaluation is required. MRI is also the safest and most sensitive way to scan the brain, although, as noted above, contrast agents such as gadolinium should be avoided during pregnancy. Radionuclide bone scans are reported to be safe during pregnancy but fetal exposure to radiation may result from proximity to radionuclides excreted into the maternal bladder; maternal hydration and frequent voiding can reduce this exposure but in general, bone scan procedures should better be avoided during pregnancy. MRI or plain skeletal radiographs, including spine or pelvis may be considered as alternative procedures. Alkaline phosphatase increases markedly during pregnancy due to placental production, and cannot be used as an indicator of bone metastases.

The safety of *surgery in pregnancy* was illustrated by a large retrospective study of 720,000 pregnant Swedish women in the 1970s and the 1980s. The rate of congenital malformations and unexplained stillbirths was similar between those women who underwent non-obstetric surgery requiring anesthesia (n = 5.405) and those who did not

Table 29.1 Fetal exposure by staging procedures

Investigation	Fetal dose (mGy)
Chest X-ray	<0.01
Thoracic CT scan	0.06 (max 0.96)
Abdominal CT scan	8 (max 49)
Pelvic CT scan	8 (max 79)
Bone scintigraphy	<4.5
FDG-PET	max 8

Source Data from International Commission on Radiological Protection ICRP. Pregnancy and medical radiation. *Ann ICRP*. 2000:30(1): iii–viii, 1–43

[367]. However, the rates of low birth weight infants (due to prematurity and growth retardation) and early neonatal death (death within 7 days of birth) were significantly increased in women who had had surgery. During surgery, the fetus is exposed to the transplacental effects of anesthetic agents. Commonly used anesthetics, including nitrous oxide, enflurane, barbiturates, and narcotics, have been extensively used safely in pregnancy.

Risks to the fetus during surgery are not just anesthetic related, but also include intraoperative complications, such as hypoxia and hypotension. Furthermore, decreased placental perfusion secondary to long-term positioning of the mother in the supine position is a mechanical problem in late pregnancy. Additionally, postoperative problems, such as fever, infections, gastrointestinal problems and changes in nutritional intake, thrombosis, and pulmonary embolus could have serious adverse effects on fetal well-being. However, anxieties about anesthesia during pregnancy are probably greater than the actual risks. Prophylactic treatments to improve fetal lung maturity should be administered where surgery carries a risk of precipitating premature delivery. Nonemergency surgery in pregnancy can be scheduled for the second trimester with the least risk of fetal harm, or of inducing abortion or premature labor.

Mastectomy with axillary lymph node dissection has been the most common breast surgery for stage I, II, and some stage III breast cancers when the patient wants to continue the pregnancy [329, 368]. A major advantage of mastectomy is the elimination of the need for breast radiation therapy. If breast reconstruction is desired, it should be delayed until after delivery. Mastectomy and *breast-conserving therapy* has been demonstrated to be equivalent in terms of disease-free and overall survival in non-pregnant women. Lumpectomy with axillary lymph node dissection is feasible and safe in the pregnant woman with breast cancer, and is reported to have no adverse impact on locoregional recurrence rates [369]. However, because of the need of subsequent radiation therapy to achieve optimal local control, this approach may be contraindicated in the early pregnancy [370]. Recently, a single-institution retrospective study evaluated treatment and biological features of 38 patients affected by BCP collected within the short period 7 years. Conservative surgery was performed in 15 of 21 patients during pregnancy with no local reappearance after a median follow-up of 24 months [371]. Neoadjuvant chemotherapy could be considered prior to definitive breast surgery for women with locally advanced disease at presentation or for the ones desiring breast conservation. In such cases, surgery could be performed later in the pregnancy or even postpartum.

Axillary dissection is an important component of therapy because nodal metastases are commonly detected in pregnancy-associated breast cancers, and nodal status affects the choice of adjuvant therapy. Sentinel lymph node (SLN) biopsy is being performed for axillary staging in non-pregnant patients with clinically node-negative early stage breast cancer. The safety and test performance of sentinel node biopsy during pregnancy has not been fully evaluated. Supravital dyes such as isosulfan blue dye should not be administered to pregnant women, because of the possible risk of anaphylactic shock [372, 373]. Some authors suggest that sentinel node biopsy is safe in pregnant patients with a minimal dose of 500–600 mCu using double filtered technetium sulfur colloid, but no supporting studies for this approach are available at the time being. Other investigators, by deriving estimates of absorbed dose at the level of epigastrium, umbilicus, and hypogastrium in non-pregnant women undergoing sentinel node biopsy for breast cancer, have concluded that expected levels of fetal exposure would be below the 50 mGy threshold absorbed dose for adverse effects [371, 374–377]. SNL appears to be safe and may be therefore offered to pregnant patients whenever it is indicated according to general rules [339].

The use of *radiation therapy* is generally avoided during pregnancy because of the risk of death, of teratogenicity to the fetus and induction of childhood malignancies and hematologic disorders [378, 379]. The amount of radiation to which the fetus is exposed depends upon the stage of pregnancy when therapeutic radiation is administered. Even with appropriate shielding, fetal exposure to therapeutic breast irradiation will increase as the fetus grows and moves closer to the diaphragm. The administration of 50 Gy external beam irradiation to the breast could result in a first trimester fetal dose of 0.04–0.15 Gy, or a third trimester dose as high as 2 Gy [380, 381]. Fetal malformations have been associated with doses of 0.1 Gy or more during the first trimester. Although there are several case reports of normal infants born after their mothers had been irradiated, including one exposed to 0.14–0.18 Gy in the third trimester, one exposed to 0.16 Gy at 24 weeks, and another exposed to 0.04 Gy in the first trimester, irradiation is generally avoided in pregnant women because absence of risk to the fetus cannot be guaranteed. In a multicenter, prospective case-control study involving 129 children, prenatally exposed to maternal cancer and cancer treatment, and their matched controls, the development of the 11 children who were exposed to radiotherapy did not differ significantly from that of children in the control group [382]. As RT is generally delayed in non-pregnant women for months until after completion of chemotherapy, it seems safe to delay it also in pregnant women until after delivery [383].

All *chemotherapy* agents used in the treatment of breast cancer are pregnancy category D, meaning that teratogenic effects have been observed in humans. However, the risk of spontaneous abortion, fetal death, and major malformations is highest when chemotherapy is administered in the first trimester. Outside that window, most reports show a safer profile [294, 384, 385]. In general, acute side effects of chemotherapy include spontaneous abortion, teratogenesis, organ toxicity, premature birth, and low birth weight. Delayed effects of antineoplastic agents can include carcinogenesis, sterility, slow physical or mental growth and development, and teratogenic effects in the offspring's of the exposed fetus. The teratogenic and mutagenic potentials of chemotherapy agents have been studied extensively in animals, although results cannot always be extrapolated across species. Additionally, other effects such as bone marrow suppression can result in serious problems, such as infection and bleeding in both the mother and the fetus. The gastrointestinal side effects of chemotherapy agents are also likely to be deleterious to both maternal and fetal well-being, but are difficult to quantify. Information on the effects of antineoplastic drugs administered during pregnancy has largely been derived from case reports, small case series, and collected reviews [327, 385–390]. The majority of these reports focused upon the frequency of spontaneous abortion and congenital malformations in infants exposed to chemotherapy in utero for a variety of malignancies. A review of 217 pregnant women treated with cytotoxic therapies for a variety of malignancies and other medical conditions published between 1983 and 1995 [391] reported 18 newborns with congenital abnormalities: two had chromosomal abnormalities, four were stillborn, and 15 spontaneous abortions were reported. Another review of literature published between 1976 and 2001 reported on 160 women treated with anthracyclines during pregnancy [385] and showed that the fetal outcome was frequently normal (73 %). The described abnormalities included malformations (3 %), fetal death (9 %), spontaneous abortion (3 %), fetal complications (8 %) and prematurity (6 %). Fetal death was often consecutive to maternal death due to progression of the underlying malignancy (40 %). An unfavorable fetal outcome was frequent in leukemia patients. In one of the first published review, the incidence of fetal malformations in 150 women given chemotherapy during the second or third trimesters of pregnancy was 1.3 % [384]. In a case-control study, women with gestational breast cancer were significantly more likely to have a premature infant than a control group matched for maternal age. The infants had a lower mean birth weight when compared to controls, which persisted after adjustment for gestational age [392]. This is the only consistent finding associated with antenatal chemotherapy in women with breast cancer [393, 394].

The experiences of the Royal Marsden Hospital [395], of the MD Anderson Cancer Center [396, 397] and the European Institute of Oncology [398, 399] were reported and they all confirmed the relative safety of adjuvant chemotherapy delivered during the second and third trimester of pregnancy.

The most commonly used regimen in pregnant women with breast cancer is doxorubicin combined with cyclophosphamide with or without fluorouracil (AC or FAC) [327, 386, 393, 396, 397]. The first report of the largest prospective single-arm study in 57 pregnant breast cancer patients treated with FAC in the adjuvant (n = 32) or neoadjuvant (n = 25) setting [396] showed that 40 women were alive and disease-free, three had recurrent breast cancer, 12 had died from breast cancer, one from other causes and one was lost to follow-up. Of the 25 patients who received neoadjuvant FAC, six had a pathologic complete response, while four had no tumor response to chemotherapy and eventually died of their disease. All 43 women who have delivered had live births. One child has a Down's syndrome and two have congenital anomalies (club foot; congenital bilateral ureteral reflux). The other children were healthy and those in school were doing well, although two had special educational needs. The authors concluded that breast cancer can be treated with FAC chemotherapy during the second and third trimesters without significant short-term complications for the children. They also commented that longer follow-up of the children in this cohort is needed to evaluate possible late side effects such as impaired cardiac function and fertility. A recently published update compared the outcome of 75 women undergoing chemotherapy for breast cancer during pregnancy between 1989 and 2009 with the outcome of non-pregnant patients treated during the same period at the same institution (M.D. Anderson Cancer Center): For patients who received chemotherapy during pregnancy, survival was comparable to—if not better than—that of non-pregnant women [400]. Whether in utero exposure to anthracyclines is cardiotoxic remains unknown. A single report in which fetal echocardiograms were performed every 2 weeks beginning at 24 weeks in a pregnant patient receiving doxorubicin and cyclophosphamide showed no abnormalities, even when postnatal echocardiograms were repeated at 2 years of age [401]. However, at least four cases of neonatal cardiac side effects have been reported after in utero exposure to anthracyclines, and there are several cases of in utero fetal death after exposure to idarubicin or epirubicin [394, 402–405]. Because of these reports, in the past, doxorubicin was preferred to idarubicin or epirubicin for use in pregnancy [393]. According to the data of later reports, epirubicin may be preferred to doxorubicin because of a better therapeutic index and fewer systemic and cardiac toxic effects [399, 406].

Chemotherapy should be ended/stopped 3–4 weeks before delivery to avoid transient neonatal myelosuppression and potential complications as sepsis, bleeding and death. At least one case report describes measurable tissue levels of anthracyclines in a stillborn whose mother had received doxorubicin shortly before delivery [407]. Furthermore, cyclophosphamide and doxorubicin can enter milk, therefore breastfeeding is contraindicated during chemotherapy.

Methotrexate should be avoided at all stages of pregnancy because of delayed elimination from sequestered spaces (such as amniotic fluid), as well as its abortive effect and teratogenic potential [384, 391].

The use of taxane (paclitaxel and docetaxel) in pregnancy has been described in several case reports for the treatment of breast cancer and ovarian cancer, suggesting short-term safety [394, 408–414]. A recent published review evidenced a favorable toxicity profile of taxanes during the second and third trimesters of pregnancy, supported by pharmacological evidence [415]. Furthermore, a retrospective study reporting the outcome of women receiving taxane during pregnancy and of their children concluded that taxane-based chemotherapy does not appear to increase the risk of fetal or maternal complications when compared with conventional chemotherapy [416].

No data are available on the safety of dose-dense anthracycline-containing regimens with or without taxanes, during pregnancy.

Trastuzumab has been administered in a few cases during pregnancy [417]. In five of the seven reported cases, trastuzumab was given in the metastatic setting. Reversible oligohydramnios/anhydramnios has been reported in five cases (one in association with reversible fetal renal failure) [417–421], while in two cases, no abnormality of the amniotic fluid was observed [422, 423]. Due to these observations, the use of trastuzumab during pregnancy requires ongoing monitoring of amniotic fluid volume and fetal renal status. Pregnancy occurred in 70 women participating in the HERA trial [424]: sixteen during trastuzumab treatment or within 3 months form discontinuation (group 1) 49 more than 3 months after discontinuation (group 2) and 9 in the control group (group 3). 25, respectively, 16 % of patients in groups 1 and 2 experienced spontaneous abortion, 2 congenital anomalies were reported, one in group 2 and one in group 3. No congenital anomalies were reported in those exposed to trastuzumab in utero. A recent meta-analysis included 18 reports of the use trastuzumab during pregnancy and 19 newborns [425]. Oligohydramnios and anhydramnios were the most frequent adverse effect (33 %), which was in general self-limiting when trastuzumab therapy was discontinued. However, most of the pregnancies ended prematurely and 4 of the newborns died as a result of complications of prematurity (mainly respiratory failure).

There is a single case report of exposure to lapatinib during pregnancy [426]. The patient was exposed to lapatinib for 11 weeks during the first and second trimester of pregnancy, she underwent an uncomplicated delivery of a healthy female infant, and the child was developmentally normal at 18 months of age.

The great majority of women with gestational breast cancer have ER-negative/PR-negative tumors, but patients with endocrine responsive breast cancer will be candidates for hormone therapy, either in the adjuvant setting or for the treatment of metastatic disease. The use of selective estrogen receptor modulators (SERMs) such as tamoxifen during pregnancy is generally avoided as these compounds have been associated with vaginal bleeding, spontaneous abortion, birth defects, and fetal death. Concerns about the use of tamoxifen in pregnancy are based on animal studies showing an increase in the incidence of abnormalities of the genital tract [427, 428] and irregular ossification of the ribs in rats [429]. In pregnant rats, tamoxifen has been associated with breast cancer in female offspring. About 50 cases of tamoxifen use during pregnancy are reported (reviewed in ref. [430]). Eight pregnancies resulted in early termination, 19 in healthy babies [431, 432], but 10 additional had fetal or neonatal disorders (two congenital craniofacial defects). Other rare abnormalities, such as Goldenhar's syndrome [433] and ambiguous genitalia [434] were also described. In addition, the long-term effects of tamoxifen, and whether it may increase gynecological cancers in daughters (as diethylstilbestrol does) are unknown. For women who require hormone therapy, the usual practice is to defer these agents until after delivery [435]. Data from the French National Cancer Centers (FNCLCC) showed that delayed adjuvant tamoxifen significantly improved overall survival, therefore delaying it in pregnant women seems an acceptable policy [436]. In this trial, women with early breast cancer were randomized to receive tamoxifen or placebo more than 2 years after completion of the primary treatment with surgery and chemotherapy.

Antiemetics, including promethazine (Phenergan), ondansetron [437], and droperidol combined with diphenhydramine or dexamethasone are often used to treat nausea and vomiting in pregnant women, and are generally considered safe. However, long-term dexamethasone therapy should be avoided, if possible, as chronic administration appears to increase the risk of preterm delivery due to premature rupture of membranes [438]. There may also be a slightly increased risk of oral clefts when the drugs are administered before 10 weeks of gestation [439, 440].

Although there are no randomized trials evaluating the use of granulocyte colony-stimulating factor (G-CSF) or granulocyte-macrophage colony-stimulating factor (GM-CSF) in pregnant women, these agents are safe in the treatment of neonatal neutropenia and/or sepsis [441, 442]. Safe use of G-CSF (and recombinant erythropoietin) in human pregnancy has been reported [443, 444]. Bisphosphonates should be deferred after delivery in view of their observed teratogenic impact in animals. Conversely, human reports regarding women exposed to bisphophonates before conception or during pregnancy did not demonstrate serious adverse effects either to fetuses or to the mothers. However, there are cases of shortened gestational age, low neonatal birth weight, and transient hypocalcaemia [445].

The timing of delivery should be carefully considered in relation to chemotherapy administration. Ideally, the delivery should occur following the mother's WBC nadir to reduce the risk of infectious complications and excess bleeding from thrombocytopenia. The child should be delivered after fetal pulmonary maturity and at 34 or more weeks of gestation, at which time morbidity is relatively low.

In summary, the management of pregnancy-related breast cancer should not differ from that of non-pregnant women, with the exception of some restriction in the use of staging procedures and chemotherapies to avoid fetal risk. Radiotherapy and endocrine treatment as well as the use of antibodies and newer substances should be postponed until after delivery.

29.12 Pregnancy After Breast Cancer

Cancer survivors are often fearful that their history of cancer or its treatment will have an adverse impact on their offspring by placing them at risk for malignancy, congenital anomalies, or impaired growth and development. They are also concerned about the risks of cancer recurrence, infertility, miscarriage, and achieving a successful pregnancy outcome.

Because of the lack of data concerning breast cancer survivors, reports about pregnancy outcomes in adult survivors of childhood and adolescent cancers provide additional information [446–450]. Overall observed rates of fetal malformations (ranging from 0 to 3 % minor congenital anomalies) are similar to the expected rates in offspring of the general population. Whether there are late cognitive or developmental abnormalities is not clear at the moment. It is encouraging that 42 children of 35 women treated for Hodgkin's disease have shown no unusual sequelae at a median follow-up time of 11 years. Concerns about an increased risk of cancer in the offspring may be relieved by data from the Five Center Study, showing that the risk of cancer in the offspring of chemotherapy-treated children and adolescents was not significantly greater than the risk observed in controls or in the general population [450].

The fear that pregnancy and all related hormonal changes subsequent to breast cancer treatment would result in activation of dormant micrometastases has not been substantiated in the literature, despite a clear link between female sex hormones and mammary carcinogenesis. The available clinical data did not show that women who became pregnant after a diagnosis of breast cancer have a worse outcome than those who did not [451, 452]. Published series have, in fact, shown either no impact on survival or a slightly protective effect when women deliver after breast cancer treatment [347, 453–455]. In a recent meta-analysis including 14 studies for a total of 1244 cases and 18'145 controls, women who got pregnant following breast cancer diagnosis had a 41 % reduced risk of death compared to women who did not get pregnant [PRR: 0.59 (90 % confidence interval (CI): 0.50–0.70)]. This difference was seen irrespective of the type of the study and particularly in women with history of node-negative disease. In a subgroup analysis, the outcome of women with history of breast cancer who became pregnant was compared to breast cancer patients who did not get pregnant and were known to be free of relapse. In this analysis, the authors did not find significant differences in survival between either group [PRR: 0.85; 95 % CI: 0.53–1.35] [452]. In another of these series, 94 women with early stage disease who became pregnant after breast cancer were compared to 188 breast cancer survivors without subsequent pregnancies matched for nodal status, tumor size, age, year of diagnosis, and duration of disease-free survival [322]. The risk ratio for death was significantly lower (0.44) for women who became pregnant subsequent to the diagnosis of breast cancer as compared to women with breast cancer who did not have a subsequent pregnancy. The Finnish Cancer Registry reported that among 2536 breast cancer patients under 40 years of age, 91 women delivered a child 10 months or more after the breast cancer diagnosis. The survival rates of these women were compared to controls with no deliveries matched for stage, age, and year of breast cancer diagnosis, and who had survived at least the interval between diagnosis and delivery of the case patient. The relative risk of death was 4.8 for the controls (95 % C.I. 2.2–10.3) compared to the women who had delivered a child, and survival rates at 10 years were significantly superior for the latter group (92 % vs. 60 %) [456]. Although these data could reflect selection bias, they are also consistent with a possible antitumor effect of the pregnancy. As the patients were matched for nodal status, tumor size and early stage disease, a "healthy mother effect" (only patients feeling well with a good prognosis conceive and therefore show improved survival) is unlikely to be the explanation for the findings. Other authors are more cautious in the interpretation of the available data and conclude that the effect of subsequent pregnancy on breast cancer prognosis and outcome is still unclear. The Danish Breast Cancer Cooperative Group [457] evaluated 5.725 women with primary breast cancer, aged 45 years or younger at the time of diagnosis. Among these women, only 173 became pregnant after breast cancer therapy. These women had a non-significantly reduced risk of death (relative risk 0.55, 95 % C.I. 0.28–1.06) when compared with controls, adjusting for age and tumor stage, who had not had a pregnancy.

There are only few data regarding the influence of the interval between breast cancer diagnosis and pregnancy on survival [456, 458]. In several studies, patients who delay pregnancy more than 2 years after breast cancer diagnosis experience an enhanced survival compared to patients with shorter diagnosis-to-pregnancy intervals (<6 months) [459, 460]. The survival advantage seen in patients with longer-delayed pregnancy is not necessarily caused by the longer disease-free survival before pregnancy [458]. Physicians generally advise women to wait for at least 2 years before attempting pregnancy. The primary reason for this recommendation is that most recurrences of breast cancer occur within the first 2 years after initial diagnosis and treatment.

There are few concerns with regard to treatment and conception. As an example, the half-life of methotrexate is approximately 8–15 h and it is retained for several weeks to months in the kidney and liver, respectively. Delaying conception at least 12 weeks after stopping methotrexate has been recommended [461].

Most women who have undergone irradiation for breast cancer are able to produce milk in the affected side, the amount being frequently less than that in a non-irradiated breast, particularly if the lumpectomy site was close to the areolar complex or transected many ducts [462, 463]. However, when breast milk is produced, breast feeding from the irradiated breast is often not advisable because of the difficulties for the treatment of a possible mastitis [464]. In a retrospective survey, 11 women who experienced 13 pregnancies after breast cancer treatment were interviewed [465]. All patients reported little or no swelling of the treated breast during pregnancy. After delivery, lactation from the treated breast was possible in four instances, absent in six, and pharmacologically suppressed in three. One patient successfully breast-fed from the treated breast for 4 months. In the majority of cases, breastfeeding from the untreated breast was successful.

Beside breast cancer and benign tumors, the majority of breast surgery is performed in a fertile age. Theoretically, reduction mammaplasty and augmentation should not impair the ability to nurse, as long as there is no free transplantation of the mamilla–areola complex or an ablation of the breast gland. The average frequency of nursing after reduction mammaplasty in five studies was about 31 % [466].

29.13 Psychosocial, Familial, and Professional Aspects

Younger women with breast cancer experience higher levels of anxiety and depression, more psychological and financial distress, and more problems related to their psychosocial roles than older women [247, 467]. The effects of a breast cancer diagnosis on interpersonal and family relations were assessed in a review of multiple studies. Age does not appear to have a direct relationship to husbands' adjustments, but younger husbands reported more problems carrying out domestic roles and a greater number of life stresses than older husbands. Studies on the impact of breast cancer on children are limited in number and scope but indicate that the effects of their mother's breast cancer vary according to the developmental level of the child [468]. A recent report based on the Basel Cancer Database analyzed an unselected, consecutive cohort of patients who were ≤40 years at breast cancer diagnosis [469]. Sixty patients had children at the time of diagnosis. About a third of the children whose mothers were diagnosed with breast cancer experienced the palliative situation and the death of their mother. A cross-sectional study used quantitative and qualitative methods to examine coping strategies used by 201 women who were aged 50 years or younger and were 6 months to 3.5 years after the diagnosis [29]. The coping strategies most frequently used were positive cognitive restructuring, wishful thinking, and making changes. For example, social support was helpful in dealing with anger or depression, whereas positive cognitive restructuring was more helpful for concerns about the future. Analyses also confirmed that most coping strategies cited in commonly administered coping scales were used frequently by these women. However, several other coping strategies were also deemed valuable, including engaging in physical activity, using meditations, and resting. These findings suggest that clinicians should identify patients' particular stressors and help with coping techniques targeting particular concerns.

In a survey conducted in 252 breast and endometrial cancer survivors, all women reported good adjustment to having had cancer, at an average of 3.7 years since treatment completion [470]. Most differences in psychosocial adjustment between the groups were small, but younger survivors reported significantly worse adaptation than older survivors, as measured by the hospital anxiety and depression scale (HADS, $p < 0.0001$), appearance-orientation scale (AOS, body image; $p = 0.02$), fear of recurrence ($p < 0.0001$), distress about long-term treatment-related cancer problems ($p = 0.01$), and number of sexual problems attributed to cancer ($p < 0.0001$).

To date, only sparse information about fertility-related psychosocial aspects in cancer patients is available. In general, healthy women with fertility problems seem to show a higher prevalence of negative emotions than women who conceived [471]. In cancer patients, fertility-related psychosocial issues/problems comprise uncertainty about the degree of damage and anxiety of potential side effects of treatment on pregnancy and offspring, as well as potential genetic inheritance of cancer risk [247, 472]. Nevertheless, the desire for pregnancy and motherhood is an important issue for many cancer patients [284]. First, investigations in this field show that breast cancer survivors who had successful pregnancies after treatment reported that it helped them to normalize their life and their transition to wellness, and having children improved their quality of life [473].

29.14 Conclusion

- Young women have, in general, more advanced and biological more aggressive cancer at presentation.
- The treatment of young breast cancer patients is not different from that in older women, with the exception of choice of the endocrine therapy and management of age-specific side effect (menopausal symptoms, sexual dysfunction, and social and emotional issues)
- Preserving fertility is frequently an important issue for younger female cancer survivors and their partners.
- Management of pregnancy-related breast cancer should not substantially differ from that of non-pregnant women.
- Pregnancy after breast cancer seems to be safe.
- Tailored long-term follow-up should be warranted.
- Younger women need special psychosocial support.

Breast cancer in young women is challenging in several aspects as medical, psychological, social issues, and the care for these patients need to take into account the peculiarities of this population.

References

1. Ries L, Melbert D, Krapcho M, Stinchcomb D, Howlader N, Horner M, et al. SEER Cancer Statistics Review, 1975–2005, National Cancer Institute. Bethesda, MD. http://seercancergov/csr/1975_2005/, based on Nov 2007 SEER data submission, posted to the SEER web site. 2008.
2. Bouchardy C, Fioretta G, Verkooijen HM, Vlastos G, Schaefer P, Delaloye JF, et al. Recent increase of breast cancer incidence among women under the age of forty. Br J Cancer. 2007;96(11):1743–6.
3. Levi F, Te VC, Maspoli M, Randimbison L, Bulliard JL, Vecchia CL. Trends in breast cancer incidence among women under the age of forty. Br J Cancer. 2007;97(7):1013–4.
4. Bodmer A, Feller A, Bordoni A, Bouchardy C, Dehler S, Ess S, et al. Breast cancer in younger women in Switzerland 1996–2009: a longitudinal population-based study. Breast. 2015;24(2):112–7.
5. Brinton LA, Sherman ME, Carreon JD, Anderson WF. Recent trends in breast cancer among younger women in the United States. J Natl Cancer Inst. 2008;100(22):1643–8.
6. Leclère B, Molinié F, Trétarre B, Stracci F, Daubisse-Marliac L, Colonna M. Trends in incidence of breast cancer among women under 40 in seven European countries: a GRELL cooperative study. Cancer Epidemiol. 2013;37(5):544–9.
7. Merlo DF, Ceppi M, Filiberti R, Bocchini V, Znaor A, Gamulin M, et al. Breast cancer incidence trends in European women aged 20–39 years at diagnosis. Breast Cancer Res Treat. 2012;134(1):363–70.
8. WHO. WHO World health organization.Mortality database. http://www-depdbiarcfr/who. Accessed 20 Nov 2007.
9. NBCC. NBCC, National Breast Cancer Coalition. Facts about breast cancer in the United States: Year 2007. http://wwwstopbreastcancerorg/bin/indexasp?Strid=427&depid=9&nid=2. Accessed 24 Nov 2007.
10. Albain KS, Allred DC, Clark GM. Breast cancer outcome and predictors of outcome: are there age differentials? J Natl Cancer Inst Monogr. 1994;16:35–42.
11. Althuis MD, Brogan DD, Coates RJ, Daling JR, Gammon MD, Malone KE, et al. Breast cancers among very young premenopausal women (United States). Cancer Causes Control. 2003;14(2):151–60.
12. Chung M, Chang HR, Bland KI, Wanebo HJ. Younger women with breast carcinoma have a poorer prognosis than older women. Cancer. 1996;77(1):97–103.
13. Colleoni M, Rotmensz N, Robertson C, Orlando L, Viale G, Renne G, et al. Very young women (<35 years) with operable breast cancer: features of disease at presentation. Ann Oncol. 2002;13(2):273–9.
14. Maggard MA, O'Connell JB, Lane KE, Liu JH, Etzioni DA, Ko CY. Do young breast cancer patients have worse outcomes? J Surg Res. 2003;113(1):109–13.
15. Azim HA Jr, Michiels S, Bedard PL, Singhal SK, Criscitiello C, Ignatiadis M, et al. Elucidating prognosis and biology of breast cancer arising in young women using gene expression profiling. Clin Cancer Res. 2012;18(5):1341–51.
16. Arpino G, Wiechmann L, Osborne CK, Schiff R. Crosstalk between the estrogen receptor and the HER tyrosine kinase receptor family: molecular Mechanism and Clinical Implications for Endocrine Therapy Resistance. Endocr Rev. 2008;29(2):217–33.
17. de la Rochefordiere A, Asselain B, Campana F, Scholl SM, Fenton J, Vilcoq JR, et al. Age as prognostic factor in premenopausal breast carcinoma. Lancet. 1993;341(8852):1039–43.
18. Lethaby AE, Mason BH, Holdaway IM, Kay RG. Age and ethnicity as prognostic factors influencing overall survival in breast cancer patients in the Auckland region. Auckland Breast Cancer Study Group. NZ Med J. 1992;105(947):485–8.
19. Nixon AJ, Neuberg D, Hayes DF, Gelman R, Connolly JL, Schnitt S, et al. Relationship of patient age to pathologic features of the tumor and prognosis for patients with stage I or II breast cancer. J Clin Oncol. 1994;12(5):888–94.
20. Swanson GM, Lin CS. Survival patterns among younger women with breast cancer: the effects of age, race, stage, and treatment. J Natl Cancer Inst Monogr. 1994;16:69–77.
21. Vanlemmens L, Hebbar M, Peyrat JP, Bonneterre J. Age as a prognostic factor in breast cancer. Anticancer Res. 1998;18(3B):1891–6.
22. Walker RA, Lees E, Webb MB, Dearing SJ. Breast carcinomas occurring in young women (<35 years) are different. Br J Cancer. 1996;74(11):1796–800.
23. Barchielli A, Balzi D. Age at diagnosis, extent of disease and breast cancer survival: a population-based study in Florence, Italy. Tumori. 2000;86(2):119–23.
24. Crowe JP Jr, Gordon NH, Shenk RR, Zollinger RM Jr, Brumberg DJ, Shuck JM. Age does not predict breast cancer outcome. Arch Surg. 1994;129(5):483–7 (discussion 7–8).
25. Gajdos C, Tartter PI, Bleiweiss IJ, Bodian C, Brower ST. Stage 0 to stage III breast cancer in young women. J Am Coll Surg. 2000;190(5):523–9.
26. Kroman N, Jensen MB, Wohlfahrt J, Mouridsen HT, Andersen PK, Melbye M. Factors influencing the effect of age on prognosis in breast cancer: population based study. BMJ. 2000;320(7233):474–8.

27. Richards MA, Gregory WM, Smith P, Millis RR, Fentiman IS, Rubens RD. Age as prognostic factor in premenopausal breast cancer. Lancet. 1993;341(8858):1484–5.
28. Howard-Anderson J, Ganz PA, Bower JE, Stanton AL. Quality of life, fertility concerns, and behavioral health outcomes in younger breast cancer survivors: a systematic review. J Natl Cancer Inst. 2012;104(5):386–405.
29. Manuel JC, Burwell SR, Crawford SL, Lawrence RH, Farmer DF, Hege A, et al. Younger women's perceptions of coping with breast cancer. Cancer Nurs. 2007;30(2):85–94.
30. Howlader N, Noone AM, Krapcho M, Garshell J, Miller D, Altekruse SF, Kosary CL, Yu M, Ruhl J, Tatalovich Z, Mariotto A, Lewis DR, Chen HS, Feuer EJ, Cronin KA (eds). SEER cancer statistics review, 1975–2012, National Cancer Institute. Bethesda, MD, http://seer.cancer.gov/csr/1975_2012/, based on Nov 2014 SEER data submission, posted to the SEER web site, Apr 2015. Available from: http://seer.cancer.gov/csr/1975_2012/.
31. Siegel R, Naishadham D, Jemal A. Cancer statistics, 2013. CA Cancer J Clin. 2013;63(1):11–30.
32. Tai P, Cserni G, Van De Steene J, Vlastos G, Voordeckers M, Royce M, et al. Modeling the effect of age in T1-2 breast cancer using the SEER database. BMC Cancer. 2005;5:130.
33. Fredholm H, Eaker S, Frisell J, Holmberg L, Fredriksson I, Lindman H. Breast cancer in young women: poor survival despite intensive treatment. PLoS ONE. 2009;4(11):e7695.
34. Rudra S, Yu DS, Yu ES, Switchenko JM, Mister D, Torres MA. Locoregional and distant recurrence patterns in young versus elderly women treated for breast cancer. Int J Breast Cancer. 2015;2015:213123.
35. Dubsky PC, Gnant MF, Taucher S, Roka S, Kandioler D, Pichler-Gebhard B, et al. Young age as an independent adverse prognostic factor in premenopausal patients with breast cancer. Clin Breast Cancer. 2002;3(1):65–72.
36. Han W, Kang SY. Korean Breast Cancer S. Relationship between age at diagnosis and outcome of premenopausal breast cancer: age less than 35 years is a reasonable cut-off for defining young age-onset breast cancer. Breast Cancer Res Treat. 2010;119 (1):193–200.
37. Kim K, Chie EK, Han W, Noh DY, Oh DY, Im SA, et al. Age <40 years is an independent prognostic factor predicting inferior overall survival in patients treated with breast conservative therapy. Breast J. 2011;17(1):75–8.
38. Cancello G, Maisonneuve P, Rotmensz N, Viale G, Mastropasqua MG, Pruneri G, et al. Prognosis and adjuvant treatment effects in selected breast cancer subtypes of very young women (<35 years) with operable breast cancer. Ann Oncol. 2010;21 (10):1974–81.
39. Zhu W, Perez EA, Hong R, Li Q, Xu B. Age-related disparity in immediate prognosis of patients with triple-negative breast cancer: a population-based study from seer cancer registries. PLoS ONE. 2015;10(5):e0128345.
40. Musolino A, Bella MA, Bortesi B, Michiara M, Naldi N, Zanelli P, et al. BRCA mutations, molecular markers, and clinical variables in early-onset breast cancer: a population-based study. Breast. 2007;16(3):280–92.
41. Peto J, Collins N, Barfoot R, Seal S, Warren W, Rahman N, et al. Prevalence of BRCA1 and BRCA2 gene mutations in patients with early-onset breast cancer. J Natl Cancer Inst. 1999;91 (11):943–9.
42. Robson M, Gilewski T, Haas B, Levin D, Borgen P, Rajan P, et al. BRCA-associated breast cancer in young women. J Clin Oncol. 1998;16(5):1642–9.
43. Turchetti D, Cortesi L, Federico M, Bertoni C, Mangone L, Ferrari S, et al. BRCA1 mutations and clinicopathological features in a sample of Italian women with early-onset breast cancer. Eur J Cancer. 2000;36(16):2083–9.
44. Armes JE, Trute L, White D, Southey MC, Hammet F, Tesoriero A, et al. Distinct molecular pathogeneses of early-onset breast cancers in BRCA1 and BRCA2 mutation carriers: a population-based study. Cancer Res. 1999;59(8):2011–7.
45. Fackenthal JD, Olopade OI. Breast cancer risk associated with BRCA1 and BRCA2 in diverse populations. Nat Rev Cancer. 2007;7(12):937–48.
46. Marcus JN, Watson P, Page DL, Narod SA, Lenoir GM, Tonin P, et al. Hereditary breast cancer: pathobiology, prognosis, and BRCA1 and BRCA2 gene linkage. Cancer. 1996;77(4):697–709.
47. Huzarski T, Byrski T, Gronwald J, Gorski B, Domagala P, Cybulski C, et al. Ten-year survival in patients with BRCA1-negative and BRCA1-positive breast cancer. J Clin Oncol. 2013;31(26):3191–6.
48. Bernstein L. Epidemiology of endocrine-related risk factors for breast cancer. J Mammary Gland Biol Neoplasia. 2002;7(1):3–15.
49. Pike MC, Henderson BE, Krailo MD, Duke A, Roy S. Breast cancer in young women and use of oral contraceptives: possible modifying effect of formulation and age at use. Lancet. 1983;2 (8356):926–30.
50. Ursin G, Ross RK, Sullivan-Halley J, Hanisch R, Henderson B, Bernstein L. Use of oral contraceptives and risk of breast cancer in young women. Breast Cancer Res Treat. 1998;50(2):175–84.
51. Cancer CGoHFiB. Breast cancer and hormonal contraceptives: collaborative reanalysis of individual data on 53 297 women with breast cancer and 100 239 women without breast cancer from 54 epidemiological studies. Collaborative Group on Hormonal Factors in Breast Cancer. Lancet. 1996;347(9017):1713–27.
52. Charlton BM, Rich-Edwards JW, Colditz GA, Missmer SA, Rosner BA, Hankinson SE, et al. Oral contraceptive use and mortality after 36 years of follow-up in the Nurses' health study: prospective cohort study. BMJ. 2014;349:g6356.
53. Hannaford PC, Selvaraj S, Elliott AM, Angus V, Iversen L, Lee AJ. Cancer risk among users of oral contraceptives: cohort data from the Royal College of General Practitioner's oral contraception study. BMJ. 2007;335(7621):651.
54. Marchbanks PA, McDonald JA, Wilson HG, Folger SG, Mandel MG, Daling JR, et al. Oral contraceptives and the risk of breast cancer. N Engl J Med. 2002;346(26):2025–32.
55. Beaber EF, Malone KE, Tang MT, Barlow WE, Porter PL, Daling JR, et al. Oral contraceptives and breast cancer risk overall and by molecular subtype among young women. Cancer Epidemiol Biomarkers Prev. 2014;23(5):755–64.
56. Figueiredo JC, Bernstein L, Capanu M, Malone KE, Lynch CF, Anton-Culver H, et al. Oral contraceptives, postmenopausal hormones, and risk of asynchronous bilateral breast cancer: the WECARE Study Group. J Clin Oncol. 2008;26(9):1411–8.
57. Bermejo-Pérez M, Márquez-Calderón S, Llanos-Méndez A. Effectiveness of preventive interventions in BRCA1/2 gene mutation carriers: a systematic review. Int J Cancer. 2007;121 (2):225–31.
58. Figueiredo JC, Haile RW, Bernstein L, Malone KE, Largent J, Langholz B, et al. Oral contraceptives and postmenopausal hormones and risk of contralateral breast cancer among BRCA1 and BRCA2 mutation carriers and noncarriers: the WECARE Study. Breast Cancer Res Treat. 2010;120(1):175–83.
59. Humans IWGotEoCRt. Pharmaceuticals. Volume 100 A. A review of human carcinogens. IARC Monogr Eval Carcinog Risks Hum. 2012;100(Pt A):1–401.
60. Colditz GA, Feskanich D, Chen WY, Hunter DJ, Willett WC. Physical activity and risk of breast cancer in premenopausal women. Br J Cancer. 2003;89(5):847–51.

61. John EM, Sangaramoorthy M, Hines LM, Stern MC, Baumgartner KB, Giuliano AR, et al. Overall and abdominal adiposity and premenopausal breast cancer risk among hispanic women: the breast cancer health disparities study. Cancer Epidemiol Biomarkers Prev. 2015;24(1):138–47.
62. van den Brandt PA, Spiegelman D, Yaun SS, Adami HO, Beeson L, Folsom AR, et al. Pooled analysis of prospective cohort studies on height, weight, and breast cancer risk. Am J Epidemiol. 2000;152(6):514–27.
63. Schernhammer ES. In-utero exposures and breast cancer risk: joint effect of estrogens and insulin-like growth factor? Cancer Causes Control. 2002;13(6):505–8.
64. Trichopoulos D. Hypothesis: does breast cancer originate in utero? Lancet. 1990;335(8695):939–40.
65. Michels KB, Trichopoulos D, Robins JM, Rosner BA, Manson JE, Hunter DJ, et al. Birthweight as a risk factor for breast cancer. Lancet. 1996;348(9041):1542–6.
66. Panagiotopoulou K, Katsouyanni K, Petridou E, Garas Y, Tzonou A, Trichopoulos D. Maternal age, parity, and pregnancy estrogens. Cancer Causes Control. 1990;1(2):119–24.
67. Carmichael A, Sami AS, Dixon JM. Breast cancer risk among the survivors of atomic bomb and patients exposed to therapeutic ionising radiation. Eur J Surg Oncol. 2003;29(5):475–9.
68. Land CE, Tokunaga M, Koyama K, Soda M, Preston DL, Nishimori I, et al. Incidence of female breast cancer among atomic bomb survivors, Hiroshima and Nagasaki, 1950–1990. Radiat Res. 2003;160(6):707–17.
69. Pukkala E, Kesminiene A, Poliakov S, Ryzhov A, Drozdovitch V, Kovgan L, et al. Breast cancer in Belarus and Ukraine after the Chernobyl accident. Int J Cancer. 2006;119(3):651–8.
70. Ogrodnik A, Hudon TW, Nadkarni PM, Chandawarkar RY. Radiation exposure and breast cancer: lessons from Chernobyl. Conn Med. 2013;77(4):227–34.
71. Prysyazhnyuk A, Gristchenko V, Fedorenko Z, Gulak L, Fuzik M, Slipenyuk K, et al. Twenty years after the Chernobyl accident: solid cancer incidence in various groups of the Ukrainian population. Radiat Environ Biophys. 2007;46(1): 43–51.
72. Guibout C, Adjadj E, Rubino C, Shamsaldin A, Grimaud E, Hawkins M, et al. Malignant breast tumors after radiotherapy for a first cancer during childhood. J Clin Oncol. 2005;23(1):197–204.
73. Kenney LB, Yasui Y, Inskip PD, Hammond S, Neglia JP, Mertens AC, et al. Breast cancer after childhood cancer: a report from the Childhood Cancer Survivor Study. Ann Intern Med. 2004;141(8):590–7.
74. Korenman SG. The endocrinology of breast cancer. Cancer. 1980;46(4 Suppl):874–8.
75. Ozasa K, Shimizu Y, Suyama A, Kasagi F, Soda M, Grant EJ, et al. Studies of the mortality of atomic bomb survivors, Report 14, 1950–2003: an overview of cancer and noncancer diseases. Radiat Res. 2012;177(3):229–43.
76. Little MP. Cancer and non-cancer effects in Japanese atomic bomb survivors. Journal of radiological protection: official journal of the Society for Radiological Protection. 2009;29(2a): A43–59.
77. Agnese DM, Yusuf F, Wilson JL, Shapiro CL, Lehman A, Burak WE Jr. Trends in breast cancer presentation and care according to age in a single institution. Am J Surg. 2004;188 (4):437–9.
78. Foxcroft LM, Evans EB, Porter AJ. The diagnosis of breast cancer in women younger than 40. Breast. 2004;13(4):297–306.
79. Ruddy KJ, Gelber S, Tamimi RM, Schapira L, Come SE, Meyer ME, et al. Breast cancer presentation and diagnostic delays in young women. Cancer. 2014;120(1):20–5.
80. Di Nubila B, Cassano E, Urban LABD, Fedele P, Abbate F, Maisonneuve P, et al. Radiological features and pathological-biological correlations in 348 women with breast cancer under 35 years old. Breast. 2006;15(6):744–53.
81. Kolb TM, Lichy J, Newhouse JH. Comparison of the performance of screening mammography, physical examination, and breast US and evaluation of factors that influence them: an analysis of 27,825 patient evaluations. Radiology. 2002;225 (1):165–75.
82. Saslow D, Boetes C, Burke W, Harms S, Leach MO, Lehman CD, et al. American Cancer Society guidelines for breast screening with MRI as an adjunct to mammography. CA Cancer J Clin. 2007;57(2):75–89.
83. Murphy CD, Lee JM, Drohan B, Euhus DM, Kopans DB, Gadd MA, et al. The American Cancer Society guidelines for breast screening with magnetic resonance imaging: an argument for genetic testing. Cancer. 2008;113(11):3116–20.
84. Sardanelli F, Boetes C, Borisch B, Decker T, Federico M, Gilbert FJ, et al. Magnetic resonance imaging of the breast: recommendations from the EUSOMA working group. Eur J Cancer. 2010;46(8):1296–316.
85. Ashley S, Royle GT, Corder A, Herbert A, Guyer PB, Rubin CM, et al. Clinical, radiological and cytological diagnosis of breast cancer in young women. Br J Surg. 1989;76(8):835–7.
86. Partridge AH, Hughes ME, Ottesen RA, Wong Y-N, Edge SB, Theriault RL, et al. The effect of age on delay in diagnosis and stage of breast cancer. Oncologist. 2012;17(6):775–82.
87. Ballard-Barbash R, Taplin SH, Yankaskas BC, Ernster VL, Rosenberg RD, Carney PA, et al. Breast cancer surveillance consortium: a national mammography screening and outcomes database. Am J Roentgenol. 1997;169(4):1001–8.
88. Buist DSM, Porter PL, Lehman C, Taplin SH, White E. Factors contributing to mammography failure in women aged 40–49 years. J Natl Cancer Inst. 2004;96(19):1432–40.
89. Sardanelli F, Giuseppetti GM, Panizza P, Bazzocchi M, Fausto A, Simonetti G, et al. Sensitivity of MRI versus mammography for detecting foci of multifocal, multicentric breast cancer in fatty and dense breasts using the whole-breast pathologic examination as a gold standard. Am J Roentgenol. 2004;183(4):1149–57.
90. Warner E, Messersmith H, Causer P, Eisen A, Shumak R, Plewes D. Systematic review: using magnetic resonance imaging to screen women at high risk for breast cancer. Ann Intern Med. 2008;148(9):671–9.
91. Kuhl CK, Schrading S, Leutner CC, Morakkabati-Spitz N, Wardelmann E, Fimmers R, et al. Mammography, breast ultrasound, and magnetic resonance imaging for surveillance of women at high familial risk for breast cancer. J Clin Oncol. 2005;23(33):8469–76.
92. Partridge AH, Pagani O, Abulkhair O, Aebi S, Amant F, Azim HA Jr, et al. First international consensus guidelines for breast cancer in young women (BCY1). Breast. 2014;23(3): 209–20.
93. Morrow M, Waters J, Morris E. MRI for breast cancer screening, diagnosis, and treatment. Lancet. 2011;378(9805):1804–11.
94. Houssami N, Turner R, Macaskill P, Turnbull LW, McCready DR, Tuttle TM, et al. An individual person data meta-analysis of preoperative magnetic resonance imaging and breast cancer recurrence. J Clin Oncol. 2014;32(5):392–401.
95. Copson E, Eccles B, Maishman T, Gerty S, Stanton L, Cutress RI, et al. Prospective observational study of breast cancer treatment outcomes for UK women aged 18–40 years at diagnosis: the POSH study. J Natl Cancer Inst. 2013;105 (13):978–88.
96. Collins LC, Marotti JD, Gelber S, Cole K, Ruddy K, Kereakoglow S, et al. Pathologic features and molecular

phenotype by patient age in a large cohort of young women with breast cancer. Breast Cancer Res Treat. 2012;131(3):1061–6.
97. Keegan TH, DeRouen MC, Press DJ, Kurian AW, Clarke CA. Occurrence of breast cancer subtypes in adolescent and young adult women. Breast Cancer Res. 2012;14(2):R55.
98. Perou CM, Sorlie T, Eisen MB, van de Rijn M, Jeffrey SS, Rees CA, et al. Molecular portraits of human breast tumours. Nature. 2000;406(6797):747–52.
99. Sorlie T, Perou CM, Tibshirani R, Aas T, Geisler S, Johnsen H, et al. Gene expression patterns of breast carcinomas distinguish tumor subclasses with clinical implications. Proc Natl Acad Sci USA. 2001;98(19):10869–74.
100. Kreike B, van Kouwenhove M, Horlings H, Weigelt B, Peterse H, Bartelink H, et al. Gene expression profiling and histopathological characterization of triple-negative/basal-like breast carcinomas. Breast Cancer Res. 2007;9(5):R65.
101. Turner N, Tutt A, Ashworth A. Hallmarks of 'BRCAness' in sporadic cancers. Nat Rev Cancer. 2004;4(10):814–9.
102. Anders CK, Hsu DS, Broadwater G, Acharya CR, Foekens JA, Zhang Y, et al. Young age at diagnosis correlates with worse prognosis and defines a subset of breast cancers with shared patterns of gene expression. J Clin Oncol. 2008;26(20):3324–30.
103. Glas AM, Floore A, Delahaye LJ, Witteveen AT, Pover RC, Bakx N, et al. Converting a breast cancer microarray signature into a high-throughput diagnostic test. BMC Genom. 2006;7:278.
104. Andre F, Pusztai L. Molecular classification of breast cancer: implications for selection of adjuvant chemotherapy. Nat Clin Pract. 2006;3(11):621–32.
105. Paik S, Tang G, Shak S, Kim C, Baker J, Kim W, et al. Gene expression and benefit of chemotherapy in women with node-negative, estrogen receptor-positive breast cancer. J Clin Oncol. 2006;24(23):3726–34.
106. Phase III Randomized Study of Adjuvant Combination Chemotherapy and Hormonal Therapy Versus Adjuvant Hormonal Therapy Alone in Women With Previously Resected Axillary Node-Negative Breast Cancer With Various Levels of Risk for Recurrence (TAILORx Trial).PDQ: NCT00310180.
107. Sparano JA, Gray RJ, Makower DF, Pritchard KI, Albain KS, Hayes DF, et al. Prospective validation of a 21-gene expression assay in breast cancer. N Engl J Med 2015.
108. MINDACT (Microarray In Node-negative Disease may Avoid Chemotherapy): A Prospective, Randomized Study Comparing the 70-Gene Signature With the Common Clinical-Pathological Criteria in Selecting Patients for Adjuvant Chemotherapy in Node-Negative Breast Cancer.PDQ: NCT00433589.
109. van de Vijver MJ, He YD, van't Veer LJ, Dai H, Hart AAM, Voskuil DW, et al. A gene-expression signature as a predictor of survival in breast cancer. N Engl J Med 2002;347(25): 1999–2009.
110. Paik S, Shak S, Tang G, Kim C, Baker J, Cronin M, et al. A multigene assay to predict recurrence of tamoxifen-treated, node-negative breast cancer. N Engl J Med. 2004;351(27): 2817–26.
111. Shak S. Quantitative gene expression analysis in a large cohort of estrogen-receptor positive breast cancers: characterization of the tumor profiles in younger patients (<40 yrs) and in older patients (>70 yrs) 33rd SABCC2010 Abstract #P3-10-01. 2010.
112. Kim J, Han W, Jung SY, Park YH, Moon HG, Ahn SK, et al. The value of Ki67 in very young women with hormone receptor-positive breast cancer: retrospective analysis of 9,321 korean women. Ann Surg Oncol. 2015;22(11):3481–8.
113. Kurtz JM, Jacquemier J, Amalric R, Brandone H, Ayme Y, Hans D, et al. Why are local recurrences after breast-conserving therapy more frequent in younger patients? J Clin Oncol. 1990;8 (4):591–8.
114. Voogd AC, Nielsen M, Peterse JL, Blichert-Toft M, Bartelink H, Overgaard M, et al. Differences in risk factors for local and distant recurrence after breast-conserving therapy or mastectomy for stage I and II breast cancer: pooled results of two large European randomized trials. J Clin Oncol. 2001;19(6):1688–97.
115. Jobsen JJ, van der Palen J, Meerwaldt JH. The impact of age on local control in women with pT1 breast cancer treated with conservative surgery and radiation therapy. Eur J Cancer. 2001;37(15):1820–7.
116. Arriagada R, Le MG, Contesso G, Guinebretiere JM, Rochard F, Spielmann M. Predictive factors for local recurrence in 2006 patients with surgically resected small breast cancer. Ann Oncol. 2002;13(9):1404–13.
117. Kroman N, Holtveg H, Wohlfahrt J, Jensen MB, Mouridsen HT, Blichert-Toft M, et al. Effect of breast-conserving therapy versus radical mastectomy on prognosis for young women with breast carcinoma. Cancer. 2004;100(4):688–93.
118. Mahmood U, Morris C, Neuner G, Koshy M, Kesmodel S, Buras R, et al. Similar survival with breast conservation therapy or mastectomy in the management of young women with early-stage breast cancer. Int J Radiat Oncol Biol Phys. 2012;83(5):1387–93.
119. Vila J, Gandini S, Gentilini O. Overall survival according to type of surgery in young (</=40 years) early breast cancer patients: a systematic meta-analysis comparing breast-conserving surgery versus mastectomy. Breast. 2015;24(3):175–81.
120. Adams BJ, Zoon CK, Stevenson C, Chitnavis P, Wolfe L, Bear HD. The role of margin status and reexcision in local recurrence following breast conservation surgery. Ann Surg Oncol. 2013;20(7):2250–5.
121. O'Kelly Priddy CM, Forte VA, Lang JE. The importance of surgical margins in breast cancer. J Surg Oncol. 2015.
122. Buchholz TA, Somerfield MR, Griggs JJ, El-Eid S, Hammond MEH, Lyman GH, et al. Margins for breast-conserving surgery with whole-breast irradiation in stage i and ii invasive breast cancer: American Society of Clinical Oncology Endorsement of the Society of Surgical Oncology/American Society for Radiation Oncology Consensus Guideline. J Clin Oncol. 2014;32 (14):1502–6.
123. Nichols HB, Berrington de Gonzalez A, Lacey JV Jr, Rosenberg PS, Anderson WF. Declining incidence of contralateral breast cancer in the United States from 1975 to 2006. J Clin Oncol. 2011;29(12):1564–9.
124. Kurian AW, Lichtensztajn DY, Keegan TH, Nelson DO, Clarke CA, Gomez SL. Use of and mortality after bilateral mastectomy compared with other surgical treatments for breast cancer in California, 1998–2011. JAMA. 2014;312(9):902–14.
125. Fisher B, Jeong JH, Anderson S, Bryant J, Fisher ER, Wolmark N. Twenty-five-year follow-up of a randomized trial comparing radical mastectomy, total mastectomy, and total mastectomy followed by irradiation. N Engl J Med. 2002;347 (8):567–75.
126. Veronesi U, Cascinelli N, Mariani L, Greco M, Saccozzi R, Luini A, et al. Twenty-year follow-up of a randomized study comparing breast-conserving surgery with radical mastectomy for early breast cancer. N Engl J Med. 2002;347(16):1227–32.
127. Bartelink H, Horiot JC, Poortmans P, Struikmans H, Van den Bogaert W, Barillot I, et al. Recurrence rates after treatment of breast cancer with standard radiotherapy with or without additional radiation. N Engl J Med. 2001;345(19):1378–87.
128. Hattangadi-Gluth JA, Wo JY, Nguyen PL, Abi Raad RF, Sreedhara M, Niemierko A, et al. Basal subtype of invasive breast cancer is associated with a higher risk of true recurrence after conventional breast-conserving therapy. Int J Radiat Oncol* Biol* Phys. 2012;82(3):1185–91.

129. (EBCTCG) EBCTCG. Effect of radiotherapy after breast-conserving surgery on 10-year recurrence and 15-year breast cancer death: meta-analysis of individual patient data for 10 801 women in 17 randomised trials. Lancet. 2011;378 (9804):1707–16.
130. Donker M, Litière S, Werutsky G, Julien J-P, Fentiman IS, Agresti R, et al. Breast-conserving treatment with or without radiotherapy in ductal carcinoma in situ: 15-year recurrence rates and outcome after a recurrence, from the EORTC 10853 randomized phase III trial. J Clin Oncol. 2013;31(32):4054–9.
131. Vrieling C, Collette L, Fourquet A, Hoogenraad WJ, Horiot JC, Jager JJ, et al. Can patient-, treatment- and pathology-related characteristics explain the high local recurrence rate following breast-conserving therapy in young patients? Eur J Cancer. 2003;39(7):932–44.
132. Bartelink H, Horiot J-C, Poortmans PM, Struikmans H, Van den Bogaert W, Fourquet A, et al. Impact of a higher radiation dose on local control and survival in breast-conserving therapy of early breast cancer: 10-year results of the randomized boost versus no boost EORTC 22881-10882 trial. J Clin Oncol. 2007;25 (22):3259–65.
133. Institute TNC. Radiation dose intensity study in breast cancer in young women. The Netherlands Cancer Institute. ClinicalTrials.-gov Identifier: NCT00212121.
134. Beadle BM, Woodward WA, Tucker SL, Outlaw ED, Allen PK, Oh JL, et al. Ten-year recurrence rates in young women with breast cancer by locoregional treatment approach. Int J Radiat Oncol* Biol* Phys. 2009;73(3):734–44.
135. Kroman N, Melbye M, Mouridsen HT. Prognostic influence of age at diagnosis in premenopausal breast cancer patients. Scand J Surg. 2002;91(3):305–8.
136. Rapiti E, Fioretta G, Verkooijen HM, Vlastos G, Schafer P, Sappino AP, et al. Survival of young and older breast cancer patients in Geneva from 1990 to 2001. Eur J Cancer. 2005;41 (10):1446–52.
137. Early Breast Cancer Trialists' Collaborative G, Peto R, Davies C, Godwin J, Gray R, Pan HC, et al. Comparisons between different polychemotherapy regimens for early breast cancer: meta-analyses of long-term outcome among 100,000 women in 123 randomised trials. Lancet. 2012;379(9814):432–44.
138. De Laurentiis M, Cancello G, D'Agostino D, Giuliano M, Giordano A, Montagna E, et al. Taxane-based combinations as adjuvant chemotherapy of early breast cancer: a meta-analysis of randomized trials. J Clin Oncol. 2008;26(1):44–53.
139. Early Breast Cancer Trialists' Collaborative Group (EBCTCG). Effects of chemotherapy and hormonal therapy for early breast cancer on recurrence and 15-year survival: an overview of the randomised trials. Lancet. 2005;365:1687–717.
140. Trialists' Collaborative Group. Polychemotherapy for early breast cancer: an overview of the randomised trials. Early breast cancer. Lancet. 1998;352(9132):930–42.
141. Berry DA, Cirrincione C, Henderson IC, Citron ML, Budman DR, Goldstein LJ, et al. Estrogen-receptor status and outcomes of modern chemotherapy for patients with node-positive breast cancer. JAMA. 2006;295(14):1658–67.
142. Colleoni M, Bonetti M, Coates AS, Castiglione-Gertsch M, Gelber RD, Price K, et al. Early start of adjuvant chemotherapy may improve treatment outcome for premenopausal breast cancer patients with tumors not expressing estrogen receptors. The International Breast Cancer Study Group. J Clin Oncol. 2000;18 (3):584–90.
143. Cold S, During M, Ewertz M, Knoop A, Moller S. Does timing of adjuvant chemotherapy influence the prognosis after early breast cancer? Results of the Danish Breast Cancer Cooperative Group (DBCG). Br J Cancer. 2005;93(6):627–32.
144. Gagliato Dde M, Gonzalez-Angulo AM, Lei X, Theriault RL, Giordano SH, Valero V, et al. Clinical impact of delaying initiation of adjuvant chemotherapy in patients with breast cancer. J Clin Oncol. 2014;32(8):735–44.
145. Oakman C, Viale G, Di Leo A. Management of triple negative breast cancer. Breast. 2010;19(5):312–21.
146. Cleator S, Heller W, Coombes RC. Triple-negative breast cancer: therapeutic options. Lancet Oncol. 2007;8(3):235–44.
147. Bauer KR, Brown M, Cress RD, Parise CA, Caggiano V. Descriptive analysis of estrogen receptor (ER)-negative, progesterone receptor (PR)-negative, and HER2-negative invasive breast cancer, the so-called triple-negative phenotype: a population-based study from the California cancer Registry. Cancer. 2007;109(9):1721–8.
148. Rakha EA, El-Sayed ME, Green AR, Lee AH, Robertson JF, Ellis IO. Prognostic markers in triple-negative breast cancer. Cancer. 2007;109(1):25–32.
149. Tutt A, Ellis P, Kilburn L, et al. The TNT trial: a randomized phase III trial of carboplatin (C) compared with docetaxel (D) for patients with metastatic or recurrent locally advanced triple negative or BRCA1/2 breast cancer (CRUK/07/012). Program and abstracts of the 2014 San Antonio Breast Cancer Symposium, 9–13 Dec 2014; San Antonio, Texas Abstract S3-01. 2014.
150. Metzger-Filho O, Tutt A, de Azambuja E, Saini KS, Viale G, Loi S, et al. Dissecting the heterogeneity of triple-negative breast cancer. J Clin Oncol. 2012;30(15):1879–87.
151. Goldhirsch A, Glick JH, Gelber RD, Coates AS, Thurlimann B, Senn HJ. Meeting highlights: international expert consensus on the primary therapy of early breast cancer 2005. Ann Oncol. 2005;16(10):1569–83.
152. Coates AS, Winer EP, Goldhirsch A, Gelber RD, Gnant M, Piccart-Gebhart M, et al. Tailoring therapies-improving the management of early breast cancer: St Gallen International Expert Consensus on the Primary Therapy of Early Breast Cancer 2015. Ann Oncol. 2015;26(8):1533–46.
153. Davies C, Godwin J, Gray R, Clarke M, Cutter D, Darby S, et al. Relevance of breast cancer hormone receptors and other factors to the efficacy of adjuvant tamoxifen: patient-level meta-analysis of randomised trials. Lancet. 2011;378(9793):771–84.
154. Davies C, Pan H, Godwin J, Gray R, Arriagada R, Raina V, et al. Long-term effects of continuing adjuvant tamoxifen to 10 years versus stopping at 5 years after diagnosis of oestrogen receptor-positive breast cancer: ATLAS, a randomised trial. Lancet. 2013;381(9869):805–16.
155. Burstein HJ, Temin S, Anderson H, Buchholz TA, Davidson NE, Gelmon KE, et al. Adjuvant endocrine therapy for women with hormone receptor-positive breast cancer: American Society of Clinical Oncology Clinical Practice Guideline focused update. J Clin Oncol. 2014;32(21):2255–69.
156. Arriagada R, Le MG, Spielmann M, Mauriac L, Bonneterre J, Namer M, et al. Randomized trial of adjuvant ovarian suppression in 926 premenopausal patients with early breast cancer treated with adjuvant chemotherapy. Ann Oncol. 2005;16 (3):389–96.
157. Davidson NE, O'Neill AM, Vukov AM, Osborne CK, Martino S, White DR, et al. Chemoendocrine therapy for premenopausal women with axillary lymph node-positive, steroid hormone receptor-positive breast cancer: results from INT 0101 (E5188). J Clin Oncol. 2005;23(25):5973–82.
158. Goodwin PJ, Ennis M, Pritchard KI, Trudeau M, Hood N. Risk of menopause during the first year after breast cancer diagnosis. J Clin Oncol. 1999;17(8):2365–70.
159. Petrek JA, Naughton MJ, Case LD, Paskett ED, Naftalis EZ, Singletary SE, et al. Incidence, time course, and determinants of

menstrual bleeding after breast cancer treatment: a prospective study. J Clin Oncol. 2006;24(7):1045–51.
160. Castiglione-Gertsch M, O'Neill A, Price KN, Goldhirsch A, Coates AS, Colleoni M, et al. Adjuvant chemotherapy followed by goserelin versus either modality alone for premenopausal lymph node-negative breast cancer: a randomized trial. J Natl Cancer Inst. 2003;95(24):1833–46.
161. Ejlertsen B, Mouridsen HT, Jensen MB, Bengtsson NO, Bergh J, Cold S, et al. Similar efficacy for ovarian ablation compared with cyclophosphamide, methotrexate, and fluorouracil: from a randomized comparison of premenopausal patients with node-positive, hormone receptor-positive breast cancer. J Clin Oncol. 2006;24(31):4956–62.
162. Jakesz R, Hausmaninger H, Kubista E, Gnant M, Menzel C, Bauernhofer T, et al. Randomized adjuvant trial of tamoxifen and goserelin versus cyclophosphamide, methotrexate, and fluorouracil: evidence for the superiority of treatment with endocrine blockade in premenopausal patients with hormone—responsive breast cancer—Austrian Breast and Colorectal Cancer Study Group Trial 5. J Clin Oncol. 2002;20(24):4621–7.
163. Jonat W, Kaufmann M, Sauerbrei W, Blamey R, Cuzick J, Namer M, et al. Goserelin versus cyclophosphamide, methotrexate, and fluorouracil as adjuvant therapy in premenopausal patients with node-positive breast cancer: The Zoladex Early Breast Cancer Research Association Study. J Clin Oncol. 2002;20(24):4628–35.
164. Roché H, Kerbrat P, Bonneterre J, Fargeot P, Fumoleau P, Monnier A, et al. Complete hormonal blockade versus epirubicin-based chemotherapy in premenopausal, one to three node-positive, and hormone-receptor positive, early breast cancer patients: 7-year follow-up results of French Adjuvant Study Group 06 randomised trial. Ann Oncol. 2006;17(8):1221–7.
165. Roché H, Mihura J, de Lafontan B, Reme-Saumon M, Martel P, Dubois J, et al. Castration and tamoxifen vs chemotherapy (FAC) for premenopausal, node and receptors positive breast cancer patients: a randomized trial with a 7 years follow-up. Proc Am Soc Clin Oncol. 1996;15:117.
166. Schmid P, Untch M, Kosse V, Bondar G, Vassiljev L, Tarutinov V, et al. Leuprorelin acetate every-3-months depot versus cyclophosphamide, methotrexate, and fluorouracil as adjuvant treatment in premenopausal patients with node-positive breast cancer: the TABLE study. J Clin Oncol. 2007;25(18):2509–15.
167. Scottish Cancer Trials Breast Group and ICRF Breast Unit. Adjuvant ovarian ablation versus CMF chemotherapy in premenopausal women with pathological stage II breast carcinoma: the Scottish trial. Lancet. 1993;341:1293–8.
168. von Minckwitz G, Graf E, Geberth M, Eiermann W, Jonat W, Conrad B, et al. CMF versus goserelin as adjuvant therapy for node-negative, hormone-receptor-positive breast cancer in premenopausal patients: a randomised trial (GABG trial IV-A-93). Eur J Cancer. 2006;42(12):1780–8.
169. Klijn JG, Blamey RW, Boccardo F, Tominaga T, Duchateau L, Sylvester R. Combined tamoxifen and luteinizing hormone-releasing hormone (LHRH) agonist versus LHRH agonist alone in premenopausal advanced breast cancer: a meta-analysis of four randomized trials. J Clin Oncol. 2001;19(2):343–53.
170. Baum M, Hackshaw A, Houghton J, Rutqvist Fornander T, Nordenskjold B, et al. Adjuvant goserelin in pre-menopausal patients with early breast cancer: results from the ZIPP study. Eur J Cancer. 2006;42(7):895–904.
171. Robert N, Wang M, Cella D, Martino S, Tripathy D, Ingle J, et al. Phase III comparison of tamoxifen versus tamoxifen with ovarian ablation in premenopausal women with axillary node-negative receptor-positive breast cancer <= 3 cm. Proc Am Soc Clin Oncol. 2003;22:5.
172. Francis PA, Regan MM, Fleming GF, Lang I, Ciruelos E, Bellet M, et al. Adjuvant ovarian suppression in premenopausal breast cancer. N Engl J Med. 2015;372(5):436–46.
173. Smith IE, Dowsett M, Yap YS, Walsh G, Lonning PE, Santen RJ, et al. Adjuvant aromatase inhibitors for early breast cancer after chemotherapy-induced amenorrhoea: caution and suggested guidelines. J Clin Oncol. 2006;24(16):2444–7.
174. Oktay K, Buyuk E, Libertella N, Akar M, Rosenwaks Z. Fertility preservation in breast cancer patients: a prospective controlled comparison of ovarian stimulation with tamoxifen and letrozole for embryo cryopreservation. J Clin Oncol. 2005;23(19): 4347–53.
175. Oktay K, Hourvitz A, Sahin G, Oktem O, Safro B, Cil A, et al. Letrozole reduces estrogen and gonadotropin exposure in women with breast cancer undergoing ovarian stimulation before chemotherapy. J Clin Endocrinol Metab. 2006;91(10):3885–90.
176. Gnant M, Mlineritsch B, Stoeger H, Luschin-Ebengreuth G, Knauer M, Moik M, et al. Zoledronic acid combined with adjuvant endocrine therapy of tamoxifen versus anastrozol plus ovarian function suppression in premenopausal early breast cancer: final analysis of the Austrian Breast and Colorectal Cancer Study Group Trial 12. Ann Oncol. 2015;26 (2):313–20.
177. Pagani O, Regan MM, Walley BA, Fleming GF, Colleoni M, Lang I, et al. Adjuvant exemestane with ovarian suppression in premenopausal breast cancer. N Engl J Med. 2014;371(2): 107–18.
178. Forward DP, Cheung KL, Jackson L, Robertson JF. Clinical and endocrine data for goserelin plus anastrozole as second-line endocrine therapy for premenopausal advanced breast cancer. Br J Cancer. 2004;90(3):590–4.
179. Torrisi R, Bagnardi V, Pruneri G, Ghisini R, Bottiglieri L, Magni E, et al. Antitumour and biological effects of letrozole and GnRH analogue as primary therapy in premenopausal women with ER and PgR positive locally advanced operable breast cancer. Br J Cancer. 2007;97(6):802–8.
180. Bartsch R, Bago-Horvath Z, Berghoff A, DeVries C, Pluschnig U, Dubsky P, et al. Ovarian function suppression and fulvestrant as endocrine therapy in premenopausal women with metastatic breast cancer. Eur J Cancer. 2012;48(13):1932–8.
181. Kute T, Lack CM, Willingham M, Bishwokama B, Williams H, Barrett K, et al. Development of Herceptin resistance in breast cancer cells. Cytometry Part A. 2004;57A(2):86–93.
182. Albanell J, Codony J, Rovira A, Mellado B, Gascon P. Mechanism of action of anti-HER2 monoclonal antibodies: scientific update on trastuzumab and 2C4. Adv Exp Med Biol. 2003;532:253–68.
183. Slamon DJ, Leyland-Jones B, Shak S, Fuchs H, Paton V, Bajamonde A, et al. Use of chemotherapy plus a monoclonal antibody against HER2 for metastatic breast cancer that overexpresses HER2. N Engl J Med. 2001;344(11):783–92.
184. Joensuu H, Kellokumpu-Lehtinen P-L, Bono P, Alanko T, Kataja V, Asola R, et al. Adjuvant docetaxel or vinorelbine with or without trastuzumab for breast cancer. N Engl J Med. 2006;354(8):809–20.
185. Piccart-Gebhart MJ, Procter M, Leyland-Jones B, Goldhirsch A, Untch M, Smith I, et al. Trastuzumab after adjuvant chemotherapy in HER2-positive breast cancer. N Engl J Med. 2005;353 (16):1659–72.
186. Robert N, Eiermann W, Pienkowski T, Crown J, Martin M, Pawlicki M, et al. BCIRG 006: Docetaxel and trastuzumab-based regimens improve DFS and OS over AC-T in node positive and high risk node negative HER2 positive early breast cancer patients: Quality of life (QOL) at 36 months follow-up. J Clin Oncol (ASCO Annual Meeting Proceedings Part I). 2007;25(June 20 Supplement):18S.

187. Romond EH, Perez EA, Bryant J, Suman VJ, Geyer CE Jr, Davidson NE, et al. Trastuzumab plus adjuvant chemotherapy for operable HER2-positive breast cancer. N Engl J Med. 2005;353 (16):1673–84.
188. Slamon D, Eiermann W, Robert N, Pienkowski T, Martin M, Press M, et al. Adjuvant trastuzumab in HER2-positive breast cancer. N Engl J Med. 2011;365(14):1273–83.
189. Smith I, Procter M, Gelber RD, Guillaume S, Feyereislova A, Dowsett M, et al. 2-year follow-up of trastuzumab after adjuvant chemotherapy in HER2-positive breast cancer: a randomised controlled trial. Lancet. 2007;369(9555):29–36.
190. Goldhirsch A, Gelber RD, Piccart-Gebhart MJ, de Azambuja E, Procter M, Suter TM, et al. 2 years versus 1 year of adjuvant trastuzumab for HER2-positive breast cancer (HERA): an open-label, randomised controlled trial. Lancet. 2013;382 (9897):1021–8.
191. Perez EA, Romond EH, Suman VJ, Jeong J-H, Davidson NE, Geyer CE, et al. Four-year follow-up of trastuzumab plus adjuvant chemotherapy for operable human epidermal growth factor receptor 2–positive breast cancer: joint analysis of data from NCCTG N9831 and NSABP B-31. J Clin Oncol. 2011;29 (25):3366–73.
192. Joensuu H, Bono P, Kataja V, Alanko T, Kokko R, Asola R, et al. Fluorouracil, epirubicin, and cyclophosphamide with either docetaxel or vinorelbine, with or without trastuzumab, as adjuvant treatments of breast cancer: final results of the FinHer trial. J Clin Oncol. 2009;27(34):5685–92.
193. Pivot X, Romieu G, Debled M, Pierga J-Y, Kerbrat P, Bachelot T, et al. 6 months versus 12 months of adjuvant trastuzumab for patients with HER2-positive early breast cancer (PHARE): a randomised phase 3 trial. Lancet Oncol. 2013;14(8):741–8.
194. Zardavas D, Fouad TM, Piccart M. Optimal adjuvant treatment for patients with HER2-positive breast cancer in 2015. Breast. 2015.
195. Partridge AH, Gelber S, Piccart-Gebhart MJ, Focant F, Scullion M, Holmes E, et al. Effect of age on breast cancer outcomes in women with human epidermal growth factor receptor 2-positive breast cancer: results from a herceptin adjuvant trial. J Clin Oncol. 2013;31(21):2692–8.
196. Agus DB, Gordon MS, Taylor C, Natale RB, Karlan B, Mendelson DS, et al. Phase I clinical study of pertuzumab, a novel HER dimerization inhibitor, in patients with advanced cancer. J Clin Oncol. 2005;23(11):2534–43.
197. Baselga J, Cortés J, Kim S-B, Im S-A, Hegg R, Im Y-H, et al. Pertuzumab plus trastuzumab plus docetaxel for metastatic breast cancer. N Engl J Med. 2012;366(2):109–19.
198. Swain SM, Kim SB, Cortés J, Ro J, Semiglazov V, Campone M, et al. Pertuzumab, trastuzumab, and docetaxel for HER2-positive metastatic breast cancer (CLEOPATRA study): overall survival results from a randomised, double-blind, placebo-controlled, phase 3 study. Lancet Oncol. 2013;14(6):461–71.
199. Verma S, Miles D, Gianni L, Krop IE, Welslau M, Baselga J, et al. Trastuzumab emtansine for HER2-positive advanced breast cancer. N Engl J Med. 2012;367(19):1783–91.
200. Krop IE, Kim SB, González-Martín A, LoRusso PM, Ferrero JM, Smitt M, et al. Trastuzumab emtansine versus treatment of physician's choice for pretreated HER2-positive advanced breast cancer (TH3RESA): a randomised, open-label, phase 3 trial. Lancet Oncol. 2014;15(7):689–99.
201. Miller K, Wang M, Gralow J, Dickler M, Cobleigh M, Perez E, et al. A randomized phase III trial of paclitaxel versus paclitaxel plus bevacizumab as first-line therapy for locally recurrent or metastatic breast cancer: a trial coordinated by the Eastern Cooperative Oncology Group (E2100). Breast Cancer Res Treat. 2005;94(Suppl 1):3.
202. Miller KD, Chap LI, Holmes FA, Cobleigh MA, Marcom PK, Fehrenbacher L, et al. Randomized phase III trial of capecitabine compared with bevacizumab plus capecitabine in patients with previously treated metastatic breast cancer. J Clin Oncol. 2005;23 (4):792–9.
203. Miller K, Wang M, Gralow J, Dickler M, Cobleigh M, Perez EA, et al. Paclitaxel plus bevacizumab versus paclitaxel alone for metastatic breast cancer. N Engl J Med. 2007;357(26):2666–76.
204. Cameron D, Brown J, Dent R, Jackisch C, Mackey J, Pivot X, et al. Adjuvant bevacizumab-containing therapy in triple-negative breast cancer (BEATRICE): primary results of a randomised, phase 3 trial. Lancet Oncol. 2013;14(10):933–42.
205. Gianni L, Romieu GH, Lichinitser M, Serrano SV, Mansutti M, Pivot X, et al. AVEREL: a randomized phase iii trial evaluating bevacizumab in combination with docetaxel and trastuzumab as first-line therapy for HER2-positive locally recurrent/metastatic breast cancer. J Clin Oncol. 2013;31(14):1719–25.
206. Slamon D, Swain S, Buyse M, Martin M, Geyer CE, Im YH, et al. BETH: a randomized phase III study evaluating adjuvant bevacizumab added to trastuzumab/chemotherapy for treatment of HER2þEarly breast Cancer. Presented at SABCS. 2013.
207. Spector NL, Xia W, Burris H 3rd, Hurwitz H, Dees EC, Dowlati A, et al. Study of the biologic effects of lapatinib, a reversible inhibitor of ErbB1 and ErbB2 tyrosine kinases, on tumor growth and survival pathways in patients with advanced malignancies. J Clin Oncol. 2005;23(11):2502–12.
208. Geyer CE, Forster J, Lindquist D, Chan S, Romieu CG, Pienkowski T, et al. Lapatinib plus capecitabine for HER2-positive advanced breast cancer. N Engl J Med. 2006;355(26):2733–43.
209. Bendell JC, Domchek SM, Burstein HJ, Harris L, Younger J, Kuter I, et al. Central nervous system metastases in women who receive trastuzumab-based therapy for metastatic breast carcinoma. Cancer. 2003;97(12):2972–7.
210. Clayton AJ, Danson S, Jolly S, Ryder WD, Burt PA, Stewart AL, et al. Incidence of cerebral metastases in patients treated with trastuzumab for metastatic breast cancer. Br J Cancer. 2004;91 (4):639–43.
211. Lin NU, Winer EP. Brain metastases: the HER2 paradigm. Clin Cancer Res. 2007;13(6):1648–55.
212. Lin NU, Carey LA, Liu MC, Younger J, Come SE, Ewend M, et al. Phase II trial of lapatinib for brain metastases in patients with human epidermal growth factor receptor 2—positive breast cancer. J Clin Oncol. 2008;26(12):1993–9.
213. Piccart-Gebhart MJ, Holmes AP, Baselga J, De Azambuja E, Dueck AC, Viale G, et al. First results from the phase III ALTTO trial (BIG 2-06; NCCTG [Alliance] N063D) comparing one year of anti-HER2 therapy with lapatinib alone (L), trastuzumab alone (T), their sequence (T → L), or their combination (T + L) in the adjuvant treatment of HER2-positive early breast cancer (EBC). ASCO Meeting Abstracts. 2014;32(18_suppl):LBA4.
214. Piccart M, Hortobagyi GN, Campone M, Pritchard KI, Lebrun F, Ito Y, et al. Everolimus plus exemestane for hormone-receptor-positive, human epidermal growth factor receptor-2-negative advanced breast cancer: overall survival results from BOLERO-2dagger. Ann Oncol. 2014;25(12):2357–62.
215. Health. UNIo. Available from: Clinicaltrials gov. Accessed 15 Oct 2015.
216. Puma Biotechnology I. Study in Women with Early Stage Breast Cancer (ExteNET). Available from: http://clinicaltrialsgov/show/NCT00878709. 2015.
217. Osborne CK, Shou J, Massarweh S, Schiff R. Crosstalk between estrogen receptor and growth factor receptor pathways as a cause for endocrine therapy resistance in breast cancer. Clin Cancer Res. 2005;11(2):865s–870.

218. Milano A, Dal Lago L, Sotiriou C, Piccart M, Cardoso F. What clinicians need to know about antioestrogen resistance in breast cancer therapy. Eur J Cancer. 2006;42(16):2692–705.
219. Zilli M, Grassadonia A, Tinari N, Di Giacobbe A, Gildetti S, Giampietro J, et al. Molecular mechanisms of endocrine resistance and their implication in the therapy of breast cancer. Biochimica et Biophysica Acta (BBA) Rev Cancer. 2009;1795 (1):62–81.
220. Giuliano M, Schiff R, Osborne CK, Trivedi MV. Biological mechanisms and clinical implications of endocrine resistance in breast cancer. Breast. 20(Supplement 3):S42–9.
221. Jordan VC, Obiorah I, Fan P, Kim HR, Ariazi E, Cunliffe H, et al. The St. Gallen Prize lecture 2011: evolution of long-term adjuvant anti-hormone therapy: consequences and opportunities. Breast. 2011;20(Supplement 3):S1–11.
222. Iglehart JD, Silver DP. Synthetic lethality—a new direction in cancer-drug development. N Engl J Med. 2009;361(2):189–91.
223. Farmer H, McCabe N, Lord CJ, Tutt AN, Johnson DA, Richardson TB, et al. Targeting the DNA repair defect in BRCA mutant cells as a therapeutic strategy. Nature. 2005;434 (7035):917–21.
224. Fong PC, Boss DS, Yap TA, Tutt A, Wu P, Mergui-Roelvink M, et al. Inhibition of poly(ADP-ribose) polymerase in tumors from BRCA mutation carriers. N Engl J Med. 2009;361(2):123–34.
225. Tutt A, Robson M, Garber JE, Domchek SM, Audeh MW, Weitzel JN, et al. Oral poly(ADP-ribose) polymerase inhibitor olaparib in patients with BRCA1 or BRCA2 mutations and advanced breast cancer: a proof-of-concept trial. Lancet. 2010;376(9737):235–44.
226. Dent RA, Lindeman GJ, Clemons M, Wildiers H, Chan A, McCarthy NJ, et al. Phase I trial of the oral PARP inhibitor olaparib in combination with paclitaxel for first- or second-line treatment of patients with metastatic triple-negative breast cancer. Breast Cancer Res. 2013;15(5):R88.
227. Matulonis U, Wulf GM, Birrer MJ, Westin SN, Quy P, Bell-McGuinn KM, Lasonde B, Whalen C, Aghajanian C, Solit DB, Mills GB, Cantley L, Winer EP. Phase I study of oral BKM120 and oral olaparib for high-grade serous ovarian cancer (HGSC) or triple-negative breast cancer (TNBC). J Clin Oncol. 2014;32:5s (suppl; abstr 2510).
228. Peoples G, Khoo S, Dehqanzada Z, Mittendorf E, Hueman M, Gurney J, et al. Combined clinical trial results of a HER2/neu (E75) vaccine for prevention of recurrence in high-risk breast cancer patients. Breast Cancer Res Treat. 2006;1:S6.
229. Curigliano G, Spitaleri G, Pietri E, Rescigno M, de Braud F, Cardillo A, et al. Breast cancer vaccines: a clinical reality or fairy tale? Ann Oncol. 2006;17(5):750–62.
230. Criscitiello C, Curigliano G. Immunotherapy of breast cancer. Progr Tumor Res. 2015;42:30–43.
231. Cardoso F, Loibl S, Pagani O, Graziottin A, Panizza P, Martincich L, et al. The European Society of breast cancer specialists recommendations for the management of young women with breast cancer. Eur J Cancer. 2012;48(18):3355–77.
232. Pagani O, Senkus E, Wood W, Colleoni M, Cufer T, Kyriakides S, et al. International guidelines for management of metastatic breast cancer: can metastatic breast cancer be cured? J Natl Cancer Inst. 2010;102(7):456–63.
233. Michaud LB, Jones KL, Buzdar AU. Combination endocrine therapy in the management of breast cancer. Oncologist. 2001;6 (6):538–46.
234. Carlson RW, Theriault R, Schurman CM, Rivera E, Chung CT, Phan SC, et al. Phase II trial of anastrozole plus goserelin in the treatment of hormone receptor-positive, metastatic carcinoma of the breast in premenopausal women. J Clin Oncol. 2010;28 (25):3917–21.
235. Turner NC, Ro J, André F, Loi S, Verma S, Iwata H, et al. Palbociclib in hormone-receptor-positive advanced breast cancer. N Engl J Med. 2015;373(3):209–19.
236. Cardoso F, Bedard PL, Winer EP, Pagani O, Senkus-Konefka E, Fallowfield LJ, et al. International guidelines for management of metastatic breast cancer: combination vs sequential single-agent chemotherapy. J Natl Cancer Inst. 2009;101(17):1174–81.
237. Brewer VH, Hahn KA, Rohrbach BW, Bell JL, Baddour LM. Risk factor analysis for breast cellulitis complicating breast conservation therapy. Clin Infect Dis. 2000;31(3):654–9.
238. Indelicato DJ, Grobmyer SR, Newlin H, Morris CG, Haigh LS, Copeland EM 3rd, et al. Delayed breast cellulitis: an evolving complication of breast conservation. Int J Radiat Oncol Biol Phys. 2006;66(5):1339–46.
239. Simon MS, Cody RL. Cellulitis after axillary lymph node dissection for carcinoma of the breast. Am J Med. 1992;93 (5):543–8.
240. Petrek JA, Peters MM, Nori S, Knauer C, Kinne DW, Rogatko A. Axillary lymphadenectomy. A prospective, randomized trial of 13 factors influencing drainage, including early or delayed arm mobilization. Arch Surg. 1990;125(3):378–82.
241. Jamison K, Wellisch DK, Katz RL, Pasnau RO. Phantom breast syndrome. Arch Surg. 1979;114(1):93–5.
242. Guerreiro Godoy MD, Pereira de Godoy AC, Matos MJ, Guimarães TD, Barufi S. Phantom breast syndrome in women after mastectomy. Breast J. 2013;19(3):349–50.
243. Pereira S, Fontes F, Sonin T, Dias T, Fragoso M, Castro-Lopes JM, et al. Neurological complications of breast cancer: a prospective cohort study. Breast. 2015;24(5):582–7.
244. Nesvold IL, Dahl AA, Lokkevik E, Marit Mengshoel A, Fossa SD. Arm and shoulder morbidity in breast cancer patients after breast-conserving therapy versus mastectomy. Acta Oncol. 2008;47(5):835–42.
245. Stubblefield MD, Keole N. Upper body pain and functional disorders in patients with breast cancer. PM&R. 2014;6(2): 170–83.
246. Ganz PA, Kwan L, Stanton AL, Krupnick JL, Rowland JH, Meyerowitz BE, et al. Quality of life at the end of primary treatment of breast cancer: first results from the moving beyond cancer randomized trial. J Natl Cancer Inst. 2004;96 (5):376–87.
247. Knobf MT. The influence of endocrine effects of adjuvant therapy on quality of life outcomes in younger breast cancer survivors. Oncologist. 2006;11(2):96–110.
248. Leining MG, Gelber S, Rosenberg R, Przypyszny M, Winer EP, Partridge AH. Menopausal-type symptoms in young breast cancer survivors. Ann Oncol. 2006;17(12):1777–82.
249. Mar Fan HG, Houede-Tchen N, Chemerynsky I, Yi QL, Xu W, Harvey B, et al. Menopausal symptoms in women undergoing chemotherapy-induced and natural menopause: a prospective controlled study. Ann Oncol. 2010;21(5):983–7.
250. Bernhard J, Luo W, Ribi K, Colleoni M, Burstein HJ, Tondini C, et al. Patient-reported outcomes with adjuvant exemestane versus tamoxifen in premenopausal women with early breast cancer undergoing ovarian suppression (TEXT and SOFT): a combined analysis of two phase 3 randomised trials. Lancet Oncol. 2015;16 (7):848–58.
251. Sverrisdottir A, Fornander T, Jacobsson H, von Schoultz E, Rutqvist LE. Bone mineral density among premenopausal women with early breast cancer in a randomized trial of adjuvant endocrine therapy. J Clin Oncol. 2004;22(18):3694–9.
252. Vehmanen L, Elomaa I, Blomqvist C, Saarto T. Tamoxifen treatment after adjuvant chemotherapy has opposite effects on bone mineral density in premenopausal patients depending on menstrual status. J Clin Oncol. 2006;24(4):675–80.

253. Rocca WA, Bower JH, Maraganore DM, Ahlskog JE, Grossardt BR, de Andrade M, et al. Increased risk of cognitive impairment or dementia in women who underwent oophorectomy before menopause. Neurology. 2007;69(11):1074–83.
254. Rocca WA, Bower JH, Maraganore DM, Ahlskog JE, Grossardt BR, de Andrade M, et al. Increased risk of parkinsonism in women who underwent oophorectomy before menopause. Neurology. 2008;70(3):200–9.
255. Phillips K, Feng Y, Ribi K, Bernhard J, Puglisi F, Bellet M, et al. Co-SOFT: the cognitive function sub-study of the suppression of ovarian function trial (soft). San Antonio Breast Cancer Symposium, 9–13 Dec 2014; Poster P1-12-01/Abstract 844.
256. Shapiro CL, Recht A. Side effects of adjuvant treatment of breast cancer. N Engl J Med. 2001;344(26):1997–2008.
257. Demark-Wahnefried W, Hars V, Conaway MR, Havlin K, Rimer BK, McElveen G, et al. Reduced rates of metabolism and decreased physical activity in breast cancer patients receiving adjuvant chemotherapy. Am J Clin Nutr. 1997;65(5):1495–501.
258. Demark-Wahnefried W, Winer EP, Rimer BK. Why women gain weight with adjuvant chemotherapy for breast cancer. J Clin Oncol. 1993;11(7):1418–29.
259. Bines J, Oleske DM, Cobleigh MA. Ovarian function in premenopausal women treated with adjuvant chemotherapy for breast cancer. J Clin Oncol. 1996;14(5):1718–29.
260. Del Mastro L, Venturini M, Sertoli MR, Rosso R. Amenorrhea induced by adjuvant chemotherapy in early breast cancer patients: prognostic role and clinical implications. Breast Cancer Res Treat. 1997;43(2):183–90.
261. Hortobagyi GN, Buzdar AU, Marcus CE, Smith TL. Immediate and long-term toxicity of adjuvant chemotherapy regimens containing doxorubicin in trials at M.D. Anderson Hospital and Tumor Institute. NCI Monogr. 1986;1:105–9.
262. Sainsbury JRC, Anderson TJ, Morgan DAL. ABC of breast diseases: breast cancer. BMJ. 2000;321(7263):745–50.
263. Bentzen S, Overgaard J. Patient-to-patient variability in the expression of radiation-induced normal tissue injury. Semin Radiat Oncol. 1994;4(2):68–80.
264. Lilla C, Ambrosone C, Kropp S, Helmbold I, Schmezer P, von Fournier D, et al. Predictive factors for late normal tissue complications following radiotherapy for breast cancer. Breast Cancer Res Treat. 2007;106(1):143–50.
265. Kraus-Tiefenbacher U, Sfintizky A, Welzel G, Simeonova A, Sperk E, Siebenlist K, et al. Factors of influence on acute skin toxicity of breast cancer patients treated with standard three-dimensional conformal radiotherapy (3D-CRT) after breast conserving surgery (BCS). Radiat Oncol (London, England). 2012;7:217.
266. Bird BRJH, Swain SM. Cardiac toxicity in breast cancer survivors: review of potential cardiac problems. Clin Cancer Res. 2008;14(1):14–24.
267. Jones LW, Haykowsky MJ, Swartz JJ, Douglas PS, Mackey JR. Early breast cancer therapy and cardiovascular injury. J Am Coll Cardiol. 2007;50(15):1435–41.
268. Perez EA, Suman VJ, Davidson NE, Kaufman PA, Martino S, Dakhil SR, et al. Effect of doxorubicin plus cyclophosphamide on left ventricular ejection fraction in patients with breast cancer in the North Central Cancer Treatment Group N9831 Intergroup Adjuvant Trial. J Clin Oncol. 2004;22(18):3700–4.
269. Monroe AT, Feigenberg SJ, Price Mendenhall N. Angiosarcoma after breast-conserving therapy. Cancer. 2003;97(8):1832–40.
270. Togawa K, Ma H, Sullivan-Halley J, Neuhouser ML, Imayama I, Baumgartner KB, et al. Risk factors for self-reported arm lymphedema among female breast cancer survivors: a prospective cohort study. Breast Cancer Res. 2014;16(4):414.
271. Osteen RT, Cady B, Friedman M, Kraybill W, Doggett S, Hussey D, et al. Patterns of care for younger women with breast cancer. J Natl Cancer Inst Monogr. 1994;16:43–6.
272. Pain SJ, Purushotham AD. Lymphoedema following surgery for breast cancer. Br J Surg. 2000;87(9):1128–41.
273. Perbeck L, Celebioglu F, Svensson L, Danielsson R. Lymph circulation in the breast after radiotherapy and breast conservation. Lymphology. 2006;39(1):33–40.
274. Senkus-Konefka E, Jassem J. Complications of breast-cancer radiotherapy. Clin Oncol (R Coll Radiol). 2006;18(3):229–35.
275. Khatcheressian JL, Hurley P, Bantug E, Esserman LJ, Grunfeld E, Halberg F, et al. Breast cancer follow-up and management after primary treatment: american society of clinical oncology clinical practice guideline update. J Clin Oncol. 2013;31(7):961–5.
276. Nelson HD, Fu R, Goddard K, Mitchell JP, Okinaka-Hu L, Pappas M, et al. U.S. Preventive Services Task Force evidence syntheses, formerly systematic evidence reviews. Risk assessment, genetic counseling, and genetic testing for BRCA-related cancer: systematic review to update the US preventive services Task Force Recommendation. Agency for Healthcare Research and Quality (US), Rockville (MD). 2013.
277. Roche N. Follow-up after treatment for breast cancer in young women. Breast. 2006;15(Suppl 2):S71–5.
278. Pruthi S, Simon JA, Early AP. Current overview of the management of urogenital atrophy in women with breast cancer. Breast J. 2011;17(4):403–8.
279. Krychman ML, Stelling CJ, Carter J, Hudis CA. A case series of androgen use in breast cancer survivors with sexual dysfunction. J Sex Med. 2007;4(6):1769–74.
280. Hayes DF. Follow-up of patients with early breast cancer. N Engl J Med. 2007;356(24):2505–13.
281. Hojan K, Milecki P, Molińska-Glura M, Roszak A, Leszczyński P. Effect of physical activity on bone strength and body composition in breast cancer premenopausal women during endocrine therapy. Eur J Phys Rehabil Med. 2013;49(3):331–9.
282. Schover LR. Psychosocial aspects of infertility and decisions about reproduction in young cancer survivors: a review. Med Pediatr Oncol. 1999;33(1):53–9.
283. Wenzel L, Dogan-Ates A, Habbal R, Berkowitz R, Goldstein DP, Bernstein M, et al. Defining and measuring reproductive concerns of female cancer survivors. J Natl Cancer Inst Monogr. 2005;34:94–8.
284. Partridge AH, Gelber S, Peppercorn J, Sampson E, Knudsen K, Laufer M, et al. Web-based survey of fertility issues in young women with breast cancer. J Clin Oncol. 2004;22(20):4174–83.
285. Ganz PA, Greendale GA, Petersen L, Kahn B, Bower JE. Breast cancer in younger women: reproductive and late health effects of treatment. J Clin Oncol. 2003;21(22):4184–93.
286. Thewes B, Meiser B, Taylor A, Phillips KA, Pendlebury S, Capp A, et al. Fertility- and menopause-related information needs of younger women with a diagnosis of early breast cancer. J Clin Oncol. 2005;23(22):5155–65.
287. Braun M, Hasson-Ohayon I, Perry S, Kaufman B, Uziely B. Motivation for giving birth after breast cancer. Psycho-Oncology. 2005;14(4):282–96.
288. Loren AW, Mangu PB, Beck LN, Brennan L, Magdalinski AJ, Partridge AH, et al. Fertility preservation for patients with cancer: American Society of Clinical Oncology clinical practice guideline update. J Clin Oncol. 2013;31(19):2500–10.
289. Coulam C. Neuroendocrinology and ovarian function. In: Scott JR, DiSaia PJ, Hammond CB, et al., editors. Danforth's obstetrics and gynecology. 6th ed. Philadelphia: Lippincott; 1990. p. 57–73.
290. Wallace WH, Kelsey TW. Human ovarian reserve from conception to the menopause. PLoS ONE. 2010;5(1):e8772.

291. Walshe JM, Denduluri N, Swain SM. Amenorrhea in premenopausal women after adjuvant chemotherapy for breast cancer. J Clin Oncol. 2006;24(36):5769–79.
292. Parulekar WR, Day AG, Ottaway JA, Shepherd LE, Trudeau ME, Bramwell V, et al. Incidence and prognostic impact of amenorrhea during adjuvant therapy in high-risk premenopausal breast cancer: analysis of a National Cancer Institute of Canada Clinical Trials Group Study–NCIC CTG MA.5. J Clin Oncol. 2005;23(25):6002–8.
293. Stearns V, Schneider B, Henry NL, Hayes DF, Flockhart DA. Breast cancer treatment and ovarian failure: risk factors and emerging genetic determinants. Nat Rev Cancer. 2006;6(11):886–93.
294. Sutton R, Buzdar AU, Hortobagyi GN. Pregnancy and offspring after adjuvant chemotherapy in breast cancer patients. Cancer. 1990;65(4):847–50.
295. Peccatori FA, Pup LD, Salvagno F, Guido M, Sarno MA, Revelli A, et al. Fertility preservation methods in breast cancer. Breast care (Basel, Switzerland). 2012;7(3):197–202.
296. Del Mastro L, Lambertini M. Temporary ovarian suppression with gonadotropin-releasing hormone agonist during chemotherapy for fertility preservation: toward the end of the debate? Oncologist. 2015.
297. Moore HC, Unger JM, Phillips KA, Boyle F, Hitre E, Porter D, et al. Goserelin for ovarian protection during breast-cancer adjuvant chemotherapy. N Engl J Med. 2015;372(10):923–32.
298. Gerber B, von Minckwitz G, Stehle H, Reimer T, Felberbaum R, Maass N, et al. Effect of luteinizing hormone-releasing hormone agonist on ovarian function after modern adjuvant breast cancer chemotherapy: the GBG 37 ZORO study. J Clin Oncol. 2011;29(17):2334–41.
299. Behringer K, Breuer K, Reineke T, May M, Nogova L, Klimm B, et al. Secondary amenorrhea after Hodgkin's lymphoma is influenced by age at treatment, stage of disease, chemotherapy regimen, and the use of oral contraceptives during therapy: a report from the German Hodgkin's Lymphoma Study Group. J Clin Oncol. 2005;23(30):7555–64.
300. Chapman RM, Sutcliffe SB. Protection of ovarian function by oral contraceptives in women receiving chemotherapy for Hodgkin's disease. Blood. 1981;58(4):849–51.
301. Azim A, Oktay K. Letrozole for ovulation induction and fertility preservation by embryo cryopreservation in young women with endometrial carcinoma. Fertil Steril. 2007;88(3):657–64.
302. Azim AA, Costantini-Ferrando M, Oktay K. Safety of fertility preservation by ovarian stimulation with letrozole and gonadotropins in patients with breast cancer: a prospective controlled study. J Clin Oncol. 2008;26(16):2630–5.
303. Oktay K. Further evidence on the safety and success of ovarian stimulation with letrozole and tamoxifen in breast cancer patients undergoing in vitro fertilization to cryopreserve their embryos for fertility preservation. J Clin Oncol. 2005;23(16):3858–9.
304. Oktay K, Turan V, Bedoschi G, Pacheco FS, Moy F. Fertility preservation success subsequent to concurrent aromatase inhibitor treatment and ovarian stimulation in women with breast cancer. J Clin Oncol. 2015;33(22):2424–9.
305. Oktay K, Cil AP, Bang H. Efficiency of oocyte cryopreservation: a meta-analysis. Fertil Steril. 2006;86(1):70–80.
306. Grifo JA, Noyes N. Delivery rate using cryopreserved oocytes is comparable to conventional in vitro fertilization using fresh oocytes: potential fertility preservation for female cancer patients. Fertil Steril. 2010;93(2):391–6.
307. Borini A, Bianchi V, Bonu MA, Sciajno R, Sereni E, Cattoli M, et al. Evidence-based clinical outcome of oocyte slow cooling. Reprod Biomed Online. 2007;15(2):175–81.
308. Kuwayama M. Highly efficient vitrification for cryopreservation of human oocytes and embryos: the Cryotop method. Theriogenology. 2007;67(1):73–80.
309. Noyes N, Porcu E, Borini A. Over 900 oocyte cryopreservation babies born with no apparent increase in congenital anomalies. Reprod Biomed Online. 2009;18(6):769–76.
310. von Wolff M, Nitzschke M, Stute P, Bitterlich N, Rohner S. Low-dosage clomiphene reduces premature ovulation rates and increases transfer rates in natural-cycle IVF. Reprod Biomed Online. 2014;29(2):209–15.
311. Meirow D, Baum M, Yaron R, Levron J, Hardan I, Schiff E, et al. Ovarian tissue cryopreservation in hematologic malignancy: ten years' experience. Leuk Lymphoma. 2007;48(8):1569–76.
312. Poirot C, Vacher-Lavenu MC, Helardot P, Guibert J, Brugieres L, Jouannet P. Human ovarian tissue cryopreservation: indications and feasibility. Human Reprod (Oxford, England). 2002;17(6):1447–52.
313. Newton H. The cryopreservation of ovarian tissue as a strategy for preserving the fertility of cancer patients. Human Reprod Update. 1998;4(3):237–47.
314. Oktay K, Karlikaya G. Ovarian function after transplantation of frozen, banked autologous ovarian tissue. N Engl J Med. 2000;342(25):1919.
315. Oktay K, Buyuk E, Rosenwaks Z, Rucinski J. A technique for transplantation of ovarian cortical strips to the forearm. Fertil Steril. 2003;80(1):193–8.
316. Oktay K, Buyuk E, Veeck L, Zaninovic N, Xu K, Takeuchi T, et al. Embryo development after heterotopic transplantation of cryopreserved ovarian tissue. Lancet. 2004;363(9412):837–40.
317. Radford JA, Lieberman BA, Brison DR, Smith AR, Critchlow JD, Russell SA, et al. Orthotopic reimplantation of cryopreserved ovarian cortical strips after high-dose chemotherapy for Hodgkin's lymphoma. Lancet. 2001;357(9263):1172–5.
318. Tryde Schmidt KL, Yding Andersen C, Starup J, Loft A, Byskov AG, Nyboe Andersen A. Orthotopic autotransplantation of cryopreserved ovarian tissue to a woman cured of cancer—follicular growth, steroid production and oocyte retrieval. Reprod Biomed Online. 2004;8(4):448–53.
319. Donnez J, Dolmans M-M, Pellicer A, Diaz-Garcia C, Sanchez Serrano M, Schmidt KT, et al. Restoration of ovarian activity and pregnancy after transplantation of cryopreserved ovarian tissue: a review of 60 cases of reimplantation. Fertil Steril. 2013;99(6):1503–13.
320. Kim SS, Radford J, Harris M, Varley J, Rutherford AJ, Lieberman B, et al. Ovarian tissue harvested from lymphoma patients to preserve fertility may be safe for autotransplantation. Human Reprod (Oxford, England). 2001;16(10):2056–60.
321. Sonmezer M, Shamonki MI, Oktay K. Ovarian tissue cryopreservation: benefits and risks. Cell Tissue Res. 2005;322(1):125–32.
322. Gelber S, Coates AS, Goldhirsch A, Castiglione-Gertsch M, Marini G, Lindtner J, et al. Effect of pregnancy on overall survival after the diagnosis of early-stage breast cancer. J Clin Oncol. 2001;19(6):1671–5.
323. Loibl S, Kohl J, Kaufmann M. Reproduction after breast cancer: what advice do we have for our patients? Zentralbl Gynakol. 2005;127(3):120–4.
324. Pagani O, Ruggeri M, Manunta S, Saunders C, Peccatori F, Cardoso F, et al. Pregnancy after breast cancer: are young patients willing to participate in clinical studies? Breast. 2015;24(3):201–7.
325. Antonelli NM, Dotters DJ, Katz VL, Kuller JA. Cancer in pregnancy: a review of the literature. Part II. Obstet Gynecol Survey. 1996;51(2):135–42.

326. Antonelli NM, Dotters DJ, Katz VL, Kuller JA. Cancer in pregnancy: a review of the literature. Part I. Obstet Gynecol Survey. 1996;51(2):125–34.
327. Berry DL, Theriault RL, Holmes FA, Parisi VM, Booser DJ, Singletary SE, et al. Management of breast cancer during pregnancy using a standardized protocol. J Clin Oncol. 1999;17 (3):855–61.
328. Wallack MK, Wolf JA Jr, Bedwinek J, Denes AE, Glasgow G, Kumar B, et al. Gestational carcinoma of the female breast. Curr Probl Cancer. 1983;7(9):1–58.
329. Anderson BO, Petrek JA, Byrd DR, Senie RT, Borgen PI. Pregnancy influences breast cancer stage at diagnosis in women 30 years of age and younger. Ann Surg Oncol. 1996;3(2): 204–11.
330. Albrektsen G, Heuch I, Kvale G. The short-term and long-term effect of a pregnancy on breast cancer risk: a prospective study of 802,457 parous Norwegian women. Br J Cancer. 1995;72 (2):480–4.
331. Lambe M, Hsieh C, Trichopoulos D, Ekbom A, Pavia M, Adami HO. Transient increase in the risk of breast cancer after giving birth. N Engl J Med. 1994;331(1):5–9.
332. Wohlfahrt J, Andersen PK, Mouridsen HT, Melbye M. Risk of late-stage breast cancer after a childbirth. Am J Epidemiol. 2001;153(11):1079–84.
333. Cullinane CA, Lubinski J, Neuhausen SL, Ghadirian P, Lynch HT, Isaacs C, et al. Effect of pregnancy as a risk factor for breast cancer in BRCA1/BRCA2 mutation carriers. Int J Cancer. 2005;117(6):988–91.
334. Ishida T, Yokoe T, Kasumi F, Sakamoto G, Makita M, Tominaga T, et al. Clinicopathologic characteristics and prognosis of breast cancer patients associated with pregnancy and lactation: analysis of case-control study in Japan. Jpn J Cancer Res. 1992;83(11):1143–9.
335. Shen T, Vortmeyer AO, Zhuang Z, Tavassoli FA. High frequency of allelic loss of BRCA2 gene in pregnancy-associated breast carcinoma. J Natl Cancer Inst. 1999;91(19):1686–7.
336. Johannsson O, Loman N, Borg A, Olsson H. Pregnancy-associated breast cancer in BRCA1 and BRCA2 germline mutation carriers. Lancet. 1998;352(9137):1359–60.
337. Amant F, Deckers S, Van Calsteren K, Loibl S, Halaska M, Brepoels L, et al. Breast cancer in pregnancy: recommendations of an international consensus meeting. Eur J Cancer. 2010;46 (18):3158–68.
338. Loibl S, von Minckwitz G, Gwyn K, Ellis P, Blohmer JU, Schlegelberger B, et al. Breast carcinoma during pregnancy. Cancer. 2006;106(2):237–46.
339. Loibl S, Schmidt A, Gentilini O, Kaufman B, Kuhl C, Denkert C, et al. Breast cancer diagnosed during pregnancy: adapting recent advances in breast cancer care for pregnant patients. JAMA oncology. 2015.
340. Saber A, Dardik H, Ibrahim IM, Wolodiger F. The milk rejection sign: a natural tumor marker. Am Surg. 1996;62(12):998–9.
341. Liberman L, Giess CS, Dershaw DD, Deutch BM, Petrek JA. Imaging of pregnancy-associated breast cancer. Radiology. 1994;191(1):245–8.
342. Ahn BY, Kim HH, Moon WK, Pisano ED, Kim HS, Cha ES, et al. Pregnancy- and lactation-associated breast cancer: mammographic and sonographic findings. J Ultrasound Med. 2003;22 (5):491–7; quiz 8–9.
343. Yang WT, Dryden MJ, Gwyn K, Whitman GJ, Theriault R. Imaging of breast cancer diagnosed and treated with chemotherapy during pregnancy. Radiology. 2006;239(1):52–60.
344. Barthelmes L, Davidson LA, Gaffney C, Gateley CA. Pregnancy and breast cancer. BMJ. 2005;330(7504):1375–8.
345. Nettleton J, Long J, Kuban D, Wu R, Shaefffer J, El-Mahdi A. Breast cancer during pregnancy: quantifying the risk of treatment delay. Obstet Gynecol. 1996;87(3):414–8.
346. Collins JC, Liao S, Wile AG. Surgical management of breast masses in pregnant women. J Reprod Med. 1995;40(11):785–8.
347. Azim HA Jr, Santoro L, Russell-Edu W, Pentheroudakis G, Pavlidis N, Peccatori FA. Prognosis of pregnancy-associated breast cancer: a meta-analysis of 30 studies. Cancer Treat Rev. 2012;38(7):834–42.
348. Amant F, von Minckwitz G, Han SN, Bontenbal M, Ring AE, Giermek J, et al. Prognosis of women with primary breast cancer diagnosed during pregnancy: results from an international collaborative study. J Clin Oncol. 2013;31(20):2532–9.
349. Nicklas AH, Baker ME. Imaging strategies in the pregnant cancer patient. Semin Oncol. 2000;27(6):623–32.
350. Max MH, Klamer TW. Pregnancy and breast cancer. South Med J. 1983;76(9):1088–90.
351. Samuels TH, Liu FF, Yaffe M, Haider M. Gestational breast cancer. Canadian Assoc Radiol J (Journal l'Association canadienne des radiologistes). 1998;49(3):172–80.
352. Vashi R, Hooley R, Butler R, Geisel J, Philpotts L. Breast imaging of the pregnant and lactating patient: physiologic changes and common benign entities. AJR. 2013;200(2):329–36.
353. Frank G, Shellock EK. Safety of magnetic resonance imaging contrast agents. J Magn Reson Imaging. 1999;10(3):477–84.
354. Shao-Pow Lin JJB. MR contrast agents: physical and pharmacologic basics. J Magn Reson Imaging. 2007;25(5):884–99.
355. Shellock FG, Crues JV. MR procedures: biologic effects, safety, and patient care. Radiology. 2004;232(3):635–52.
356. Benveniste H, Fowler JS, Rooney WD, Moller DH, Backus WW, Warner DA, et al. Maternal-fetal in vivo imaging: a combined PET and MRI study. J Nucl Med. 2003;44(9):1522–30.
357. ten Hove CH, Zijlstra-Baalbergen JM, Comans EI, van Elburg RM. An unusual hotspot in a young woman with Hodgkin's lymphoma. Haematologica. 2008;93(1):e14–5.
358. Bottles K, Taylor RN. Diagnosis of breast masses in pregnant and lactating women by aspiration cytology. Obstet Gynecol. 1985;66 (3 Suppl):76S–8S.
359. Mitre BK, Kanbour AI, Mauser N. Fine needle aspiration biopsy of breast carcinoma in pregnancy and lactation. Acta Cytol. 1997;41(4):1121–30.
360. Novotny DB, Maygarden SJ, Shermer RW, Frable WJ. Fine needle aspiration of benign and malignant breast masses associated with pregnancy. Acta Cytol. 1991;35(6):676–86.
361. Shannon J, Douglas-Jones AG, Dallimore NS. Conversion to core biopsy in preoperative diagnosis of breast lesions: is it justified by results? J Clin Pathol. 2001;54(10):762–5.
362. Stewart A, Webb K, Giles D. Malignant disease in childhood and diagnostic irradiation in utero. Lancet. 1956;2:447.
363. Court Brown WM, Doll R, Hill RB. Incidence of leukaemia after exposure to diagnostic radiation in utero. Br Med J. 1960;2 (5212):1539–45.
364. Diamond EL, Schmerler H, Lilienfeld AM. The relationship of intra-uterine radiation to subsequent mortality and development of leukemia in children. A prospective study. Am J Epidemiol. 1973;97(5):283–313.
365. Delongchamp RR, Mabuchi K, Yoshimoto Y, Preston DL. Cancer mortality among atomic bomb survivors exposed in utero or as young children, October 1950–May 1992. Radiat Res. 1997;147(3):385–95.
366. Puglisi F, Follador A, Minisini AM, Cardellino GG, Russo S, Andreetta C, et al. Baseline staging tests after a new diagnosis of breast cancer: further evidence of their limited indications. Ann Oncol. 2005;16(2):263–6.

367. Mazze RI, Kallen B. Reproductive outcome after anesthesia and operation during pregnancy: a registry study of 5405 cases. Am J Obstet Gynecol. 1989;161(5):1178–85.
368. Woo JC, Yu T, Hurd TC. Breast cancer in pregnancy: a literature review. Arch Surg. 2003;138(1):91–8 (discussion 9).
369. Kuerer HM, Gwyn K, Ames FC, Theriault RL. Conservative surgery and chemotherapy for breast carcinoma during pregnancy. Surgery. 2002;131(1):108–10.
370. Ruo Redda MG, Verna R, Guarneri A, Sannazzari GL. Timing of radiotherapy in breast cancer conserving treatment. Cancer Treat Rev. 2002;28(1):5–10.
371. Gentilini O, Masullo M, Rotmensz N, Peccatori F, Mazzarol G, Smeets A, et al. Breast cancer diagnosed during pregnancy and lactation: biological features and treatment options. Eur J Surg Oncol (EJSO). 2005;31(3):232–6.
372. Sprung J, Tully MJ, Ziser A. Anaphylactic reactions to isosulfan blue dye during sentinel node lymphadenectomy for breast cancer. Anesth Analg. 2003;96(4):1051–3.
373. Pruthi S, Haakenson C, Brost BC, Bryant K, Reid JM, Singh R, et al. Pharmacokinetics of methylene blue dye for lymphatic mapping in breast cancer-implications for use in pregnancy. Am J Surg. 2011;201(1):70–5.
374. Gentilini O, Cremonesi M, Trifiro G, Ferrari M, Baio SM, Caracciolo M, et al. Safety of sentinel node biopsy in pregnant patients with breast cancer. Ann Oncol. 2004;15(9):1348–51.
375. Keleher A, Wendt R 3rd, Delpassand E, Stachowiak AM, Kuerer HM. The safety of lymphatic mapping in pregnant breast cancer patients using Tc-99m sulfur colloid. Breast J. 2004;10 (6):492–5.
376. Pandit-Taskar N, Dauer LT, Montgomery L, St. Germain J, Zanzonico PB, Divgi CR. Organ and fetal absorbed dose estimates from 99mTc-sulfur colloid lymphoscintigraphy and sentinel node localization in breast cancer patients. J Nucl Med. 2006;47(7):1202–8.
377. Gropper AB, Calvillo KZ, Dominici L, Troyan S, Rhei E, Economy KE, et al. Sentinel lymph node biopsy in pregnant women with breast cancer. Ann Surg Oncol. 2014;21(8):2506–11.
378. Greskovich JF Jr, Macklis RM. Radiation therapy in pregnancy: risk calculation and risk minimization. Semin Oncol. 2000;27 (6):633–45.
379. Kal HB, Struikmans H. Radiotherapy during pregnancy: fact and fiction. Lancet Oncol. 2005;6(5):328–33.
380. Antypas C, Sandilos P, Kouvaris J, Balafouta E, Karinou E, Kollaros N, et al. Fetal dose evaluation during breast cancer radiotherapy. Int J Radiat Oncol Biol Phys. 1998;40(4):995–9.
381. Petrek JA. Breast cancer during pregnancy. Cancer. 1994;74(1 Suppl):518–27.
382. Amant F, Vandenbroucke T, Verheecke M, Fumagalli M, Halaska MJ, Boere I, et al. Pediatric outcome after maternal cancer diagnosed during pregnancy. N Engl J Med. 2015.
383. Huang J, Barbera L, Brouwers M, Browman G, Mackillop WJ. Does delay in starting treatment affect the outcomes of radiotherapy? A systematic review. J Clin Oncol. 2003;21 (3):555–63.
384. Doll DC, Ringenberg QS, Yarbro JW. Antineoplastic agents and pregnancy. Semin Oncol. 1989;16(5):337–46.
385. Germann N, Goffinet F, Goldwasser F. Anthracyclines during pregnancy: embryo-fetal outcome in 160 patients. Ann Oncol. 2004;15(1):146–50.
386. Byrd BF Jr, Bayer DS, Robertson JC, Stephenson SE Jr. Treatment of breast tumors associated with pregnancy and lactation. Ann Surg. 1962;155:940–7.
387. Murray CL, Reichert JA, Anderson J, Twiggs LB. Multimodal cancer therapy for breast cancer in the first trimester of pregnancy. A case report. JAMA. 1984;252(18):2607–8.
388. Turchi JJ, Villasis C. Anthracyclines in the treatment of malignancy in pregnancy. Cancer. 1988;61(3):435–40.
389. Wiebe VJ, Sipila PE. Pharmacology of antineoplastic agents in pregnancy. Crit Rev Oncol Hematol. 1994;16(2):75–112.
390. Williams SF, Schilsky RL. Antineoplastic drugs administered during pregnancy. Semin Oncol. 2000;27(6):618–22.
391. Ebert U, Loffler H, Kirch W. Cytotoxic therapy and pregnancy. Pharmacol Ther. 1997;74(2):207–20.
392. Zemlickis D, Lishner M, Degendorfer P, Panzarella T, Burke B, Sutcliffe SB, et al. Maternal and fetal outcome after breast cancer in pregnancy. Am J Obstet Gynecol. 1992;166(3):781–7.
393. Cardonick E, Iacobucci A. Use of chemotherapy during human pregnancy. Lancet Oncol. 2004;5(5):283–91.
394. Giacalone PL, Laffargue F, Benos P. Chemotherapy for breast carcinoma during pregnancy: a French national survey. Cancer. 1999;86(11):2266–72.
395. Ring AE, Smith IE, Jones A, Shannon C, Galani E, Ellis PA. Chemotherapy for breast cancer during pregnancy: an 18-year experience from five London teaching hospitals. J Clin Oncol. 2005;23(18):4192–7.
396. Hahn KM, Johnson PH, Gordon N, Kuerer H, Middleton L, Ramirez M, et al. Treatment of pregnant breast cancer patients and outcomes of children exposed to chemotherapy in utero. Cancer. 2006;107(6):1219–26.
397. Litton JK, Warneke CL, Hahn KM, Palla SL, Kuerer HM, Perkins GH, et al. Case control study of women treated with chemotherapy for breast cancer during pregnancy as compared with nonpregnant patients with breast cancer. Oncologist. 2013;18(4):369–76.
398. Gentilini O, Masullo M, Rotmensz N, Peccatori F, Mazzarol G, Smeets A, et al. Breast cancer diagnosed during pregnancy and lactation: biological features and treatment options. Eur J Surg Oncol. 2005;31(3):232–6.
399. Peccatori F, Martinelli G, Gentilini O, Goldhirsch A. Chemotherapy during pregnancy: what is really safe? Lancet Oncol. 2004;5 (7):398.
400. Litton JK, Warneke CL, Hahn KM, Palla SL, Kuerer HM, Perkins GH, et al. Case control study of women treated with chemotherapy for breast cancer during pregnancy as compared with nonpregnant patients with breast cancer. Oncologist. 2013;18(4):369–76.
401. Meyer-Wittkopf M, Barth H, Emons G, Schmidt S. Fetal cardiac effects of doxorubicin therapy for carcinoma of the breast during pregnancy: case report and review of the literature. Ultrasound Obstet Gynecol. 2001;18(1):62–6.
402. Achtari C, Hohlfeld P. Cardiotoxic transplacental effect of idarubicin administered during the second trimester of pregnancy. Am J Obstet Gynecol. 2000;183(2):511–2.
403. Peres RM, Sanseverino MT, Guimaraes JL, Coser V, Giuliani L, Moreira RK, et al. Assessment of fetal risk associated with exposure to cancer chemotherapy during pregnancy: a multicenter study. Braz J Med Biol Res. 2001;34(12):1551–9.
404. Reynoso EE, Huerta F. Acute leukemia and pregnancy—fatal fetal outcome after exposure to idarubicin during the second trimester. Acta Oncol. 1994;33(6):709–10.
405. Siu BL, Alonzo MR, Vargo TA, Fenrich AL. Transient dilated cardiomyopathy in a newborn exposed to idarubicin and all-trans-retinoic acid (ATRA) early in the second trimester of pregnancy. Int J Gynecol Cancer. 2002;12(4):399–402.
406. Eedarapalli P, Biswas N, Coleman M. Epirubicin for breast cancer during pregnancy: a case report. J Reprod Med. 2007;52 (8):730–2.
407. Karp GI, von Oeyen P, Valone F, Khetarpal VK, Israel M, Mayer RJ, et al. Doxorubicin in pregnancy: possible transplacental passage. Cancer Treat Rep. 1983;67(9):773–7.

408. De Santis M, Lucchese A, De Carolis S, Ferrazani S, Caruso A. Metastatic breast cancer in pregnancy: first case of chemotherapy with docetaxel. Eur J Cancer Care (Engl). 2000;9(4):235–7.
409. Gainford MC, Clemons M. Breast cancer in pregnancy: are taxanes safe? Clin Oncol (R Coll Radiol). 2006;18(2):159.
410. Gonzalez-Angulo AM, Walters RS, Carpenter RJ Jr, Ross MI, Perkins GH, Gwyn K, et al. Paclitaxel chemotherapy in a pregnant patient with bilateral breast cancer. Clin Breast Cancer. 2004;5(4):317–9.
411. Mendez LE, Mueller A, Salom E, Gonzalez-Quintero VH. Paclitaxel and carboplatin chemotherapy administered during pregnancy for advanced epithelial ovarian cancer. Obstet Gynecol. 2003;102(5 Pt 2):1200–2.
412. Nieto Y, Santisteban M, Aramendia JM, Fernandez-Hidalgo O, Garcia-Manero M, Lopez G. Docetaxel administered during pregnancy for inflammatory breast carcinoma. Clin Breast Cancer. 2006;6(6):533–4.
413. Potluri V, Lewis D, Burton GV. Chemotherapy with taxanes in breast cancer during pregnancy: case report and review of the literature. Clin Breast Cancer. 2006;7(2):167–70.
414. Sood AK, Shahin MS, Sorosky JI. Paclitaxel and platinum chemotherapy for ovarian carcinoma during pregnancy. Gynecol Oncol. 2001;83(3):599–600.
415. Mir O, Berveiller P, Goffinet F, Treluyer JM, Serreau R, Goldwasser F, et al. Taxanes for breast cancer during pregnancy: a systematic review. Ann Oncol. 2010;21(2):425–6.
416. Cardonick E, Bhat A, Gilmandyar D, Somer R. Maternal and fetal outcomes of taxane chemotherapy in breast and ovarian cancer during pregnancy: case series and review of the literature. Ann Oncol. 2012;23(12):3016–23.
417. Pant S, Landon MB, Blumenfeld M, Farrar W, Shapiro CL. Treatment of breast cancer with trastuzumab during pregnancy. J Clin Oncol. 2008;26(9):1567–9.
418. Bader AA, Schlembach D, Tamussino KF, Pristauz G, Petru E. Anhydramnios associated with administration of trastuzumab and paclitaxel for metastatic breast cancer during pregnancy. Lancet Oncol. 2007;8(1):79–81.
419. Fanale MA, Uyei AR, Theriault RL, Adam K, Thompson RA. Treatment of metastatic breast cancer with trastuzumab and vinorelbine during pregnancy. Clin Breast Cancer. 2005;6(4):354–6.
420. Sekar R, Stone PR. Trastuzumab use for metastatic breast cancer in pregnancy. Obstet Gynecol. 2007;110(2 Pt 2):507–10.
421. Watson WJ. Herceptin (trastuzumab) therapy during pregnancy: association with reversible anhydramnios. Obstet Gynecol. 2005;105(3):642–3.
422. Shrim A, Garcia-Bournissen F, Maxwell C, Farine D, Koren G. Favorable pregnancy outcome following Trastuzumab (Herceptin) use during pregnancy—case report and updated literature review. Reprod Toxicol (Elmsford, NY). 2007;23(4):611–3.
423. Waterston AM, Graham J. Effect of adjuvant trastuzumab on pregnancy. J Clin Oncol. 2006;24(2):321–2.
424. Azim HA Jr, Metzger-Filho O, de Azambuja E, Loibl S, Focant F, Gresko E, et al. Pregnancy occurring during or following adjuvant trastuzumab in patients enrolled in the HERA trial (BIG 01-01). Breast Cancer Res Treat. 2012;133(1):387–91.
425. Zagouri F, Sergentanis TN, Chrysikos D, Papadimitriou CA, Dimopoulos MA, Bartsch R. Trastuzumab administration during pregnancy: a systematic review and meta-analysis. Breast Cancer Res Treat. 2013;137(2):349–57.
426. Kelly H, Graham M, Humes E, Dorflinger LJ, Boggess KA, O'Neil BH, et al. Delivery of a healthy baby after first-trimester maternal exposure to lapatinib. Clin Breast Cancer. 2006;7(4):339–41.
427. Chamness GC, Bannayan GA, Landry LAJ, Sheridan PJ, McGuire WL. Abnormal reproductive development in rats after neonatally administered antiestrogen (Tamoxifen). Biol Reprod. 1979;21(5):1087–90.
428. Iguchi T, Hirokawa M, Takasugi N. Occurence of genital tract abnormalities and bladder hernia in female mice exposed neonatally to tamoxifen. Toxicology. 1986;42(1):1–11.
429. Tucker M, Adam H, Patterson J. Tamoxifen (Chap. 6). In: Laurence DR, McLean AEM, Wetherall M, editors.Safety testing of new drugs laboratory predictions and clinical performance. London: Academic Press; 1984. p. 125–61.
430. Barthelmes L, Gateley CA. Tamoxifen and pregnancy. Breast. 2004;13(6):446–51.
431. Andreadis C, Charalampidou M, Diamantopoulos N, Chouchos N, Mouratidou D. Combined chemotherapy and radiotherapy during conception and first two trimesters of gestation in a woman with metastatic breast cancer. Gynecol Oncol. 2004;95(1):252–5.
432. Isaacs RJ, Hunter W, Clark K. Tamoxifen as systemic treatment of advanced breast cancer during pregnancy–case report and literature review. Gynecol Oncol. 2001;80(3):405–8.
433. Cullins SL, Pridjian G, Sutherland CM. Goldenhar's syndrome associated with tamoxifen given to the mother during gestation. JAMA. 1994;271(24):1905–6.
434. Tewari K, Bonebrake RG, Asrat T, Shanberg AM. Ambiguous genitalia in infant exposed to tamoxifen in utero. Lancet. 1997;350(9072):183.
435. Goldhirsch A, Gelber RD. Life with consequences of breast cancer: pregnancy during and after endocrine therapies. Breast. 2004;13(6):443–5.
436. Delozier T, Switsers O, Genot JY, Ollivier JM, Hery M, Namer M, et al. Delayed adjuvant tamoxifen: ten-year results of a collaborative randomized controlled trial in early breast cancer (TAM-02 trial). Ann Oncol. 2000;11(5):515–9.
437. Einarson A, Maltepe C, Navioz Y, Kennedy D, Tan MP, Koren G. The safety of ondansetron for nausea and vomiting of pregnancy: a prospective comparative study. BJOG. 2004;111(9):940–3.
438. Cowchock S. Prevention of fetal death in the antiphospholipid antibody syndrome. Lupus. 1996;5(5):467–72.
439. Carmichael SL, Shaw GM. Maternal corticosteroid use and risk of selected congenital anomalies. Am J Med Genet. 1999;86(3):242–4.
440. Park-Wyllie L, Mazzotta P, Pastuszak A, Moretti ME, Beique L, Hunnisett L, et al. Birth defects after maternal exposure to corticosteroids: prospective cohort study and meta-analysis of epidemiological studies. Teratology. 2000;62(6):385–92.
441. Bilgin K, Yaramis A, Haspolat K, Tas MA, Gunbey S, Derman O. A randomized trial of granulocyte-macrophage colony-stimulating factor in neonates with sepsis and neutropenia. Pediatrics. 2001;107(1):36–41.
442. Schibler KR, Osborne KA, Leung LY, Le TV, Baker SI, Thompson DD. A randomized, placebo-controlled trial of granulocyte colony-stimulating factor administration to newborn infants with neutropenia and clinical signs of early-onset sepsis. Pediatrics. 1998;102(1 Pt 1):6–13.
443. Ghosh A, Ayers KJ. Darbepoetin alfa for treatment of anaemia in a case of chronic renal failure during pregnancy—case report. Clin Exp Obstet Gynecol. 2007;34(3):193–4.
444. Sangalli MR, Peek M, McDonald A. Prophylactic granulocyte colony-stimulating factor treatment for acquired chronic severe neutropenia in pregnancy. Aust NZ J Obstet Gynaecol. 2001;41(4):470–1.
445. Stathopoulos IP, Liakou CG, Katsalira A, Trovas G, Lyritis GG, Papaioannou NA, et al. The use of bisphosphonates in women

prior to or during pregnancy and lactation. Hormones (Athens, Greece). 2011;10(4):280–91.
446. Byrne J, Rasmussen SA, Steinhorn SC, Connelly RR, Myers MH, Lynch CF, et al. Genetic disease in offspring of long-term survivors of childhood and adolescent cancer. Am J Hum Genet. 1998;62(1):45–52.
447. Dodds L, Marrett LD, Tomkins DJ, Green B, Sherman G. Case-control study of congenital anomalies in children of cancer patients. BMJ. 1993;307(6897):164–8.
448. Edgar AB, Wallace WHB. Pregnancy in women who had cancer in childhood. Eur J Cancer. 2007;43(13):1890–4.
449. Li FP, Fine W, Jaffe N, Holmes GE, Holmes FF. Offspring of patients treated for cancer in childhood. J Natl Cancer Inst. 1979;62(5):1193–7.
450. Mulvihill JJ, Myers MH, Connelly RR, Byrne J, Austin DF, Bragg K, et al. Cancer in offspring of long-term survivors of childhood and adolescent cancer. Lancet. 1987;2(8563):813–7.
451. Mastro LD, Catzeddu T, Venturini M. Infertility and pregnancy after breast cancer: Current knowledge and future perspectives. Cancer Treat Rev. 2006;32(6):417–22.
452. Azim HA Jr, Santoro L, Pavlidis N, Gelber S, Kroman N, Azim H, et al. Safety of pregnancy following breast cancer diagnosis: a meta-analysis of 14 studies. Eur J Cancer. 2011;47(1):74–83.
453. Calhoun K, Hansen N. The effect of pregnancy on survival in women with a history of breast cancer. Breast Disease. 2005;23:81–6.
454. Blakely LJ, Buzdarm AU, Lozada JA, Shullaih SA, Hoy E, Smith TL, et al. Effects of pregnancy after treatment for breast carcinoma on survival and risk of recurrence. Cancer. 2004;100(3):465–9.
455. Raphael J, Trudeau ME, Chan K. Outcome of patients with pregnancy during or after breast cancer: a review of the recent literature. Curr Oncol. 2015;22:S8–18.
456. Sankila R, Heinavaara S, Hakulinen T. Survival of breast cancer patients after subsequent term pregnancy: "healthy mother effect". Am J Obstet Gynecol. 1994;170(3):818–23.
457. Kroman N, Jensen MB, Melbye M, Wohlfahrt J, Mouridsen HT. Should women be advised against pregnancy after breast-cancer treatment? Lancet. 1997;350(9074):319–22.
458. Harvey JC, Rosen PP, Ashikari R, Robbins GF, Kinne DW. The effect of pregnancy on the prognosis of carcinoma of the breast following radical mastectomy. Surg Gynecol Obstet. 1981;153(5):723–5.
459. Clark RM, Chua T. Breast cancer and pregnancy: the ultimate challenge. Clin Oncol (R Coll Radiol). 1989;1(1):11–8.
460. Mueller BA, Simon MS, Deapen D, Kamineni A, Malone KE, Daling JR. Childbearing and survival after breast carcinoma in young women. Cancer. 2003;98(6):1131–40.
461. Donnenfeld AE, Pastuszak A, Noah JS, Schick B, Rose NC, Koren G. Methotrexate exposure prior to and during pregnancy. Teratology. 1994;49(2):79–81.
462. Findlay PA, Gorrell CR, d'Angelo T, Glatstein E. Lactation after breast radiation. Int J Radiat Oncol Biol Phys. 1988;15(2):511–2.
463. Wobbes T. Effect of a breast saving procedure on lactation. Eur J Surg Acta Chir. 1996;162(5):419–20.
464. Hassey KM. Pregnancy and parenthood after treatment for breast cancer. Oncol Nurs Forum. 1988;15(4):439–44.
465. Higgins S, Haffty BG. Pregnancy and lactation after breast-conserving therapy for early stage breast cancer. Cancer. 1994;73(8):2175–80.
466. Zimpelmann A, Kaufmann M. Breastfeeding nursing after breast surgery. Zentralbl Gynakol. 2002;124(11):525–8.
467. Mor V, Malin M, Allen S. Age differences in the psychosocial problems encountered by breast cancer patients. J Natl Cancer Inst Monogr. 1994;16:191–7.
468. Northouse LL. Breast cancer in younger women: effects on interpersonal and family relations. J Natl Cancer Inst Monogr. 1994;16:183–90.
469. Guth U, Huang DJ, Alder J, Moffat R. Family ties: young breast cancer patients and their children. Swiss Med Wkly. 2015;145:w14163.
470. Kornblith AB, Powell M, Regan MM, Bennett S, Krasner C, Moy B, et al. Long-term psychosocial adjustment of older vs younger survivors of breast and endometrial cancer. Psycho-Oncology. 2007;16(10):895–903.
471. Oddens BJ, den Tonkelaar I, Nieuwenhuyse H. Psychosocial experiences in women facing fertility problems–a comparative survey. Human Reprod (Oxford, England). 1999;14(1):255–61.
472. Fertility preservation and reproduction in cancer patients. Fertil Steril. 2005;83(6):1622–8.
473. Dow KH. Having children after breast cancer. Cancer Pract. 1994;2(6):407–13.

30 Psychological Support for the Breast Cancer Patient

Donna B. Greenberg

A woman confronted by the diagnosis of breast cancer faces the challenges of a life-threatening illness. The seriousness of the diagnosis, the nature of treatment, and the natural history of illness defines the challenge to coping. Each woman looks to her physician first for clarification of the medical treatment. Since treatment often requires breast surgery, a combination of chemotherapy and radiation, and antiestrogen treatment that hastens menopause, the psychological effects are different for premenopausal women married with children, women concerned about their physical attractiveness, women who want to preserve fertility, and women concerned about the effect of the illness on their partners. The diagnosis has one meaning for a woman with a family history of breast cancer who suffered in her adolescence as her mother died of breast cancer, and another if she is married to a man who lost his mother to breast cancer.

The medical plan, as the first method of coping, clarifies the diagnosis and formulates a medical treatment to keep the threat of malignancy at bay. For each woman, the psychological challenge depends on psychiatric history, her other burdens, and her temperament [1]. Women tend, more than men, to seek and accept care for psychiatric and psychological needs, and psychiatry and psychology offer tools to help women cope as they go forward. The trained psychiatrist, psychologist, or social worker collaboratively bring to the bedside of women, technical skills in listening and the recognition of biological and psychological syndromes that simultaneously affect mood.

30.1 Anxiety at Diagnosis

Most women are quite alarmed when a mammogram is abnormal. Anxiety persists for several weeks even when the abnormality is a false positive. The more quickly the outcome is clarified, the better [2]. With a lump in the breast or an abnormal mammogram, the radiologist's and surgeon's effort to make the diagnosis can require several procedures with unclear answers or unclear margins. With each procedure, the patient continues to be anxious. Delays that are minor in a healthcare system are major for each woman's alarm system. A diagnosis of ductal carcinoma in situ (DCIS) or invasive cancer means that the woman may undergo a limited resection or mastectomy and consider breast reconstruction. Chemotherapy implies visible hair loss, fatigue, malaise, and menopausal symptoms. Antiestrogen medications augment menopausal symptoms. These treatments affect a woman's sexual confidence and fertility. She worries about babies not yet born, her children's risk of losing their mother, and the risk that the children themselves will be vulnerable to breast cancer.

A woman's capacity to ignore a breast lump, to deny the serious worry about cancer, and to delay bringing it to a doctor's attention has been associated with maladaptive coping skills. If a woman does not tell anyone about the lump, it is easier to suppress the worry, and that silence is a strong factor that predicts delay in diagnosis. Psychiatric history and poor social support explain delay in diagnosis in many but not all studies [3]. Other factors also contribute to delay: older age, fewer years of education, nonwhite ethnic origin, breast symptoms other than a lump, and not attributing breast symptoms to breast cancer.

30.2 Psychological Assessment

Once a diagnosis of breast cancer is made, we are often asked to consult on issues of decision-making, anxiety, depression, insomnia, fatigue, and adaptation. The first challenge is to hear the patient explain what the diagnosis means, what worries her, and what her burdens were before the diagnosis. Understanding her very individual considerations, age, and developmental challenges, and past psychiatric history, allows us to put in context any plan. Her

D.B. Greenberg (✉)
Department of Psychiatry, Harvard Medical School,
Massachusetts General Hospital, MGH Cancer Center, WRN 605,
55 Fruit St, Boston, MA 02114, USA
e-mail: dgreenberg@partners.org

I. Jatoi and A. Rody (eds.), *Management of Breast Diseases*, DOI 10.1007/978-3-319-46356-8_30

ability to cope is related to how recently she has become aware of the diagnosis and the urgency of medical treatment. Initial shock and denial give way, with the help of medical staff and other support, to recognition that there are some emergency issues and then a marathon of medical challenges. Sometimes, emotional issues are on the back burner until the medical challenges are met. Specific worries may relate to surgical procedures, radiation treatment, and changes in body image. Standard anticancer drugs like cyclophosphamide and doxorubicin cause catabolism, hair loss, weight gain, and fatigue. There is a prolonged focused period of treatment and partial disability. Taxanes like paclitaxel can also add neuropathic pain and numbness. Intermittent dexamethasone used to prevent hypersensitivity and vomiting has effects on mood, sleep, and weight. Depending on the patient's age, menopausal symptoms are temporary at first and then become permanent, sooner than would have occurred without treatment. Concerns about loss of control and the possibility of recurrence punctuate treatment and recovery.

30.3 Effect of Hormonal Treatment on Mood

The plan for hormonal treatment directly affects psychological status; as a woman tries to cope with serious illness, her emotions are modulated by estrogen deficiency. Women who are taking estrogen/progesterone hormone replacement usually stop abruptly at the time of diagnosis. Dysphoria, insomnia and hot flashes may also develop abruptly if the plan includes ovariectomy or leuprolide treatment. These changes come more gradually if adjuvant chemotherapy suppresses ovarian function and antiestrogen treatments are added later.

By the time women with estrogen-positive tumors are about to receive hormonal treatments—after completing surgery and/or chemotherapy, more than half have mood alterations, word finding problems and loss of libido. Tamoxifen or aromatase inhibitors are then added. In one study comparing exemestane and tamoxifen [4], exemestane caused more difficulty with sleep. Hot flashes increased in frequency for 3 months but decreased thereafter. On average, women who took tamoxifen had more hot flashes at 1 year than women on exemestane. There was no difference in mood alteration, impaired word finding, or low energy [5]. At 1 year, libido was worse with exemestane. Hot flashes tended to decrease with time with either tamoxifen or exemestane. Low energy was a problem for 75 % of women. For those intolerant to tamoxifen, letrozole or exemestane has been shown to improve side effects, including mood in the short term [6].

30.4 Adherence to Hormonal Medications

Most, but not all, women adhere to the prescribed many years of antiestrogen treatment; adherence reports vary widely. Because these medications are just pills, their critical role to prevent tumor recurrence is not always appreciated. Psychological support and clarification of the role of antiestrogen medications may be critical to disease outcome. Women tend to overestimate their faithfulness to a tamoxifen regimen [7]. In a study of a state insurance database of more than 2000 women, about 23 % of women taking tamoxifen failed to achieve optimal adherence of 80 % days covered by filled prescriptions. A five-year course was not completed by 31 % [8]. Overall, the likelihood that women would continue these treatments depends on whether they have a positive view of tamoxifen at the outset and an improving view as time goes on [9]. Women are more apt to persist in taking tamoxifen if they have more social support, if they feel they have had a role is decision-making, if a physician has input about the hormone prescription and if they are told the side effects in advance [10].

Many women with early-stage breast cancer who were prescribed an adjuvant aromatase inhibitor like anastrozole may also not take it faithfully. Mean adherence over the first 12 months of therapy ranged from 82–88 %; the mean adherence of anastrazole also decreased each year, dropping to 62–79 % in the third year [11]. Depression is associated with non-adherence to adjuvant endocrine therapy, especially in younger women [12].

30.5 Anxiety

While most patients are anxious about medical treatment, some patients have a history of anxiety disorder or phobia which quietly adds to the distress of treatment. Phobia of needles or claustrophobia during radiation treatment or magnetic resonance imaging can interfere with diagnosis and treatment. Some patients have a chronic tendency to expect the worst or to "catastrophize." They may always be preoccupied with planning the future and anticipating the next threat. Loss of control is a dominant theme. For those with anxiety disorder, higher levels of anxiety, panic attacks and phobias prior to breast cancer, anxiety already interferes with quality of life. During routine surveillance of a cancer patient, anxiety can begin a week or a month before each scan to check the status of the illness, so that there may be little peaceful time between tests. While every woman must face anxiety about new symptoms following diagnosis and seek reassurance from her physician, a subgroup may be preoccupied and unable to be reassured that new pains are not a signal of recurrent cancer. Generalized anxiety, panic disorder, or excessive worry about every physical symptom can be treated by medications and/or cognitive behavioral treatments specific for anxiety. Antidepressants, specific serotonin reuptake inhibitors, in particular, in low dose, can reduce the chronic level of anxiety. When anxiety is chronic, antidepressants are preferred over benzodiazepines. In addition, patients can learn strategies to reduce anxious thoughts about recurrence or medical complications by relaxation, distraction, thought stopping, substitution, or other techniques of cognitive treatments. Specific cognitive behavioral techniques have been developed for anxiety disorders, and these may be modified for the conditions of cancer treatment [13].

30.6 Sleep

Insomnia is a major complaint of women treated for breast cancer (Table 30.1). The alarm of a new diagnosis often disrupts sleep, especially in the first few months. Subsequently, the course of estrogen deficiency may intervene with nighttime hot flashes. Anxious worry about not falling asleep is a psychophysiologic cause of insomnia; anxiety about falling asleep can prevent falling asleep. For instance, the cascade of thoughts about sleep can follow from the desire to do everything on behalf of getting well. If a woman does not fall asleep, she fears she will not sleep well and will be damaging her effort against cancer. This assumption and the vicious cycle is a psychophysiologic cause of insomnia that can be treated with cognitive behavioral treatment [14]. Often, anxiety about falling asleep and sleep disorder predate breast cancer.

Several factors associated with chemotherapy can disrupt sleep. Women who have been taking benzodiazepines like lorazepam as a medication to facilitate chemotherapy and prevent nausea may have rebound insomnia when they stop hypnotics intermittently. Patients who take prochlorperazine for nausea may develop the extrapyramidal side effect, akathisia, or restless legs that prevent sleep. Because nausea is so common during chemotherapy, patients often fail to mention that they are using a phenothiazine like prochlorperazine, which can unexpectedly cause restlessness. Anticipatory anxiety associated with the next scan or the next chemotherapy treatment also prevents sleep. During chemotherapy, dexamethasone to prevent delayed nausea and vomiting or early emesis with chemotherapy is another cause of insomnia. Steroids are also added to prevent hypersensitivity to taxanes. Side effects of dexamathasone to prevent delayed nausea include insomnia, agitation, and depression post-cessation [15]. Caffeine, decongestants, and alcohol can also contribute to insomnia. Sleep-disordered breathing and sleep apnea must also be considered. Nocturnal oxygen desaturation may be a clue that a sleep study is needed [16–18].

Table 30.1 Causes of insomnia in breast cancer patients

New threat of diagnosis or recurrence
Estrogen deficiency with hot flashes
Worry about not falling asleep
Physiologic dependency on benzodiazepines
Side effects of antiemetic phenothiazines (akathisia)
Anticipatory anxiety about repeat scans
Dexamethasone treatment with chemotherapy
Caffeine, decongestants, alcohol
Sleep apnea

Insomnia is a feature of the estrogen deficiency. About 65 % of postmenopausal women treated for breast cancer have hot flashes. About three-quarters have hot flashes in the first 10 years after their last menstrual period, and half have hot flashes even later. These are more severe in younger tamoxifen users who had chemotherapy [19].

A hot flash begins with sweating, tachycardia, and increased peripheral blood flow. Evaporation of sweat may lead to cooling. Sometimes an aura of anxiety or thirst precedes the flash. The wave of heat spreads over the body, particularly the upper part. Menopausal women without breast cancer report trouble falling asleep, waking frequently at night, feeling unusually tired [20]. Savard found more wake time in the 10-min periods around hot flashes and more stage changes to lighter sleep in breast cancer survivors. Compared to nights without hot flashes, there was a lower percentage of stage II sleep and a longer rapid eye movement (REM) latency. Overall, hot flashes were found to be associated with less efficient, more disrupted sleep [21].

While menopausal women treated with estrogenic hormones sleep better, this option is not available to women with hormone-sensitive breast cancer. Antidepressants have been used as an alternative for vasomotor symptoms and sleep. Benefit has been documented for a number of antidepressants, both specific serotonin reuptake inhibitors: paroxetine [22], fluoxetine [23], and the specific serotonin norepinephrine reuptake inhibitor venlafaxine [24]. Serotonin mediation of hot flashes has been suggested. Gabapentin at 900 mg per day also reduces hot flashes in women with breast cancer [25]. Vasomotor symptoms and worse depressive symptoms were meaningful predictors of insomnia in women less than 4 years from stage I to IIIA breast cancer [26].

30.7 Cognitive Difficulties

Troubles with working memory and concentration are common complaints of patients who receive adjuvant chemotherapy for breast cancer. Specific neurocognitive deficits do not typically match subjective reports. One study showed that only about 20 % of breast cancer patients post-adjuvant treatment had elevated memory and/or executive function complaints that were significantly associated with domain-specific neuropsychological test performances and depressive symptoms [27]. Patients who are more distressed report more cognitive failures. In the acute setting, benzodiazepines, steroids, anticholinergic medications affect cognition and attention. The catabolism and fatigue, perhaps the inflammatory response, associated with chemotherapy further impairs function. In breast cancer as opposed to other tumors, the course of estrogen withdrawal also may add to cognitive dysfunction [28–30]. Broken sleep, anxiety, low mood, and the trauma of the diagnosis further contribute.

Talk of "chemobrain" leads women receiving adjuvant chemotherapy for breast cancer to worry about permanent cognitive dysfunction. A meta-analysis of studies of cognitive impairment associated with adjuvant chemotherapy in women with breast cancer reviewed 27 studies involving 1562 patients. In cross-sectional studies with varied methodological approaches, a significant association between adjuvant chemotherapy and subtle cognitive impairment held across studies; however, the level of cognitive impairment was not different between the group that received chemotherapy and the group that did not. For prospective studies, the reviewers found that cognitive function improved over time after receiving adjuvant chemotherapy [31]. It is reassuring to know that a Danish nationwide cohort of almost 1900 women treated for primary breast cancer found no differences in long-term subjective cognitive impairment at 7–9 years post-surgery between those who received systemic chemotherapy (CMF: cyclophosphamide, methotrexate, 5-fluorouracil or CEF: cyclophosphamide, epirubicin, 5-fluorouracil) and those that did not [32]. However, both neuropsychological testing studies and neuroimaging findings suggest that a small subset of women may have negative cognitive effects from treatment [33].

A clinical approach to cognitive impairment in breast cancer patients is to discontinue benzodiazepines, alcohol, and anticholinergic medications, to encourage the best sleep hygiene, and to optimize antidepressant treatment of major depressive disorder, Modafinil has shown some benefit for cognitive function in breast cancer survivors [34]. Methylphenidate 5 mg b.i.d did not show benefit in a randomized, placebo-controlled double-blind study in women undergoing adjuvant chemotherapy for early breast cancer [35]. Some preliminary work has suggested a role for donepezil in breast cancer survivors if cognitive impairment is a factor 1–5 years post-chemotherapy [36].

30.8 Overlap of Symptoms of Estrogen Deficiency and Depression

The diagnosis of clinical depression is complicated by the overlap of symptoms that make up the syndrome of major depressive disorder (MDD) and those symptoms associated with breast cancer treatment, but the psychological and biological stressors associated with treatment also make MDD more likely. Low mood, poor concentration, fatigue, insomnia, thoughts of death, and prominent anxiety often come with breast cancer treatment. Insomnia is a common symptom of MDD. Patients with MDD have trouble falling asleep and staying asleep [16]. They have less delta sleep, broken sleep, and alterations in timing, amount, and composition of REM sleep [17]. In addition to waking at night, the night is spent in dysphoria, anxiety, and hopelessness. In the setting of breast cancer, patients often attribute their unhappiness to the diagnosis of cancer and the natural concerns that come from the diagnosis. However, persistent insomnia, anhedonia, constant awareness of the diagnosis without the ability to concentrate on other things, or to enjoy what is normally enjoyed become markers for the syndrome of MDD. History of MDD and/or anxiety disorder, in other words, lifetime history, should add heavily to the assessment of the diagnosis. A history of anxiety disorder predisposes to depressive disorder.

As breast cancer treatment often moves a premenopausal or perimenopausal woman further toward menopause, dysphoria is often associated with menopausal symptoms. Independent of the psychological adjustment to breast cancer, some women are particularly sensitive to mood changes from female hormones. Postpartum or premenstrual changes have been linked with clinical mood syndromes that depend on the individual sensitivity of women to specific changes in female hormones [37]. Epidemiological studies have suggested that women approaching menopause are more at risk for MDD. Clinical depression has been associated with the transition to menopause [38]. Schmidt found a 14-fold increased risk for depressive symptoms in the 2 years surrounding menopause compared to the time of regular cycles. Irritability, nervousness, and frequent mood changes are common in the transition [39]. Both antidepressants and hormones ameliorate the symptoms. In one study in women without breast cancer, aged 40–60, who were perimenopausal or menopausal, escitalopram as well as estrogen/progesterone improved sleep and vasomotor symptoms, but escitalopram had a better effect on depressive mood [40, 41]. Other antidepressants also benefit mood in menopausal women; these include mirtazapine, fluoxetine, citalopram, paroxetine, and venlafaxine.

Clinical depression is more common with surgical menopause, suggesting that the risk of depression is greater with sudden cessation of estrogen. In breast cancer patients, this would occur with ovariectomy, leuprolide treatment, or abrupt cessation of hormone replacement treatment.

30.9 Fatigue

Fatigue may come from treatment side effects, MDD or both. Treatment for breast cancer, particularly with adjuvant chemotherapy, is itself fatiguing. Fatigue is related to the catabolic effects of treatment and associated inflammatory response, loss of estrogenic hormones, sleep impairment, and stress. The majority of women undergoing adjuvant chemotherapy, who have cancer-related fatigue, do not have clinical depression [42]. The diagnosis of MDD was established in only 17 % of those who met a case definition of cancer-related fatigue. Past history of clinical depression and prevalence and incidence of cancer-related fatigue were significantly related to the diagnosis of depression at post-treatment assessment. In the 6 months after treatment, those who tend to catastrophize and those who weigh more are more fatigued [43].

A minority of breast cancer patients report fatigue and impairment comparable to that seen in women with chronic fatigue syndrome. These women tend to score higher on measures of depression, interpersonal sensitivity, and obsessive-compulsive behavior [44]. Fatigue correlates strongly with self-reported neuropsychological function but not with objective neuropsychological function in a laboratory setting [45].

Persistent fatigue is a marker for women who tend to feel overwhelmed. High anxiety, high impairment in role function, and low sense of control over fatigue symptoms at baseline assessment are associated with persistent fatigue [46]. Women who experience depressive symptoms in the first years after diagnosis are at risk for long-term fatigue regardless of how tired they were at the outset [47].

The best treatment for MDD is critical for those with persistent cancer-related fatigue. In addition to antidepressant medication, cognitive behavioral treatment and graded exercise, which has been important in the treatment of chronic fatigue syndrome, might also be important for the subset of breast cancer patients with persistent fatigue and comorbid depressive disorder [48]. Cognitive behavioral techniques and programs of energy conservation have been used for cancer-related fatigue [49, 50]. Exercise programs and mind–body interventions like yoga have also been studied [51].

30.10 Prevalence of Major Depressive Disorder in Breast Cancer Patients

A recent review of the prevalence of MDD in breast cancer patients estimated 10–25 %, but came to the conclusion that the precise rate is difficult to determine because of the use of symptom screening tools, the different causes of similar symptoms, and the rare use of Diagnostic Statistical Manual case definition in previous studies [52]. Lifetime history of affective disorder becomes an important factor in diagnosis.

In Denmark, where there is both a psychiatric registry and tumor registry, between 1970 and 1993, breast cancer patients had a significantly increased incidence of psychiatric admission with affective disorders and anxiety disorders compared to other women [53]. The risk of nonnatural mortality was increased in the first year after diagnosis [54]. Suicide risk tended to increase with depression and age. An international population-based study of more than 700,000 women found that the suicide risk remained elevated among women diagnosed between 1990 and 2001 and throughout follow-up. It was highest among black women [55].

30.11 Treatment

For women who have MDD, particularly if they have a history of previous episodes of MDD, antidepressant medications are the standard of treatment. (Tables 30.2 and 30.3) These drugs may have additional benefit for cognitive, sleep, fatigue, and vasomotor symptoms, as already noted. Antidepressant medications have not been associated with increased risk of breast cancer in epidemiological studies [56, 57]. In general, there is no a priori reason to pick one antidepressant over another except to take advantage of the side-effect profile or to reduce side effects in a given patient. If the patient is taking tamoxifen, CYP 2D6 inhibition may lower the effective level of tamoxifen metabolites [58]. Whether this interaction is clinically meaningful is still unclear [58–61]. In that context, for instance, citalopram, escitalopram, or venlafaxine may be preferred.

Combination of antidepressant medication with tailored psychotherapy has a better outcome. Antidepressants are

Table 30.2 Syndromes treated by antidepressant medication

Panic disorder
Anxiety disorder with preoccupation about somatic symptoms
Hot flashes
Generalized anxiety disorder
Perimenopausal mood disorder
Major depressive disorder (MDD)

Table 30.3 Antidepressant medications

	Starting dose	Maintenance dose
Citalopram (Celexa)	10 mg/day	20–40 mg/day
Escitalopram (Lexapro)	5–10 mg/day	10–20 mg/day
Sertraline (Zoloft)	25–50 mg/day	50–150 mg/day
Mirtazapine (Remeron)	15 mg h	15–45 h sedating, weight gain
Venlafaxine (Effexor)	37.5 mg/day	75–300 mg/day XR is daily
Wellbutrin[a]	75 mg/day	150 SR b.i.d. or 300 XL
[a]Duloxetine	30 mg/day	60 mg q.d.
[a]Fluoxetine	10 mg/day	20–60 mg/day
[a]Paroxetine	10 mg/day	20–60 mg/day

[a]Consider 2D6 inhibition as a factor that may affect tamoxifen metabolism

often all the more effective for clinical depression when combined with cognitive behavioral treatment or other psychotherapy in patients without cancer [62].

In those women who have cancer, even those not clinically depressed, psychosocial interventions focused on the challenge of the cancer itself—group therapy, cognitive behavioral therapy, supportive-expressive formats, relaxation techniques, and individual therapy—can reduce distress and increase coping [63, 64]. Psychological interventions for women with non-metastatic breast cancer [65] and metastatic cancer [66] have been reviewed by the Cochrane collaboration. For non-metastatic breast cancer, cognitive behavioral therapy (CBT) was the most common intervention (24 of 28 studies). CBT was delivered individually, in couples, or in groups and reduced anxiety and mood disturbance. Effects on survival were uncertain. Some of the benefits of interventions like cognitive behavioral stress management for patients with non-metastatic breast cancer early in treatment may last up to 15 years later [67].

For women with metastatic breast cancer, the Cochrane review looked at 10 studies involving almost 1400 women, three with CBT and four with supportive-expressive therapy, mostly group treatments. Benefits were found for some psychological variables. Group psychosocial interventions per se were not found to increase survival [68–72].

Group-based cognitive behavioral stress management has also reduced depressive symptoms in patients who do not have breast cancer but feel that they are at greater risk for the diagnosis because of family history [73].

Formal talking therapies have strengthened a woman's feeling of control and reduced vulnerability and distress as she faces the uncertainty of cancer. With group and individual treatment, she is less alone. She may be more able to confront the existential plight and the difficult practical challenges that come with negotiating progressive illness. Education and support offer tools for expressing her wishes, using energy wisely, and living fully on her own terms. Social skills like ability to speak effectively with family and medical staff can improve. How to live with the change in breasts, how to grapple with dating and options for having children, worries about genetics of the cancer are topics within psychotherapy. Women may seek advice on their role as parents and how to discuss their illness with their children [74]; and practical and emotional concerns about their sexual relationships can be heard.

30.12 Patients with Psychotic Illness

There is no increased risk of breast cancer in patients with schizophrenia or bipolar disorder [75]; however, patients with psychosis often present with more advanced disease, after insufficient screening and little medical care [76]. Follow through with treatment is more variable.

Although psychosis is treated with dopamine blocking agents that may be associated with elevated prolactin levels, concern about prolactin level should not stand in the way of optimal treatment of a psychotic disorder. Some have worried that a rise in prolactin would add risk of cancer progression in breast cancer patients, but a recent review of preclinical and clinical evidence did not find support for this hypothetical concern [77].

Thoughtful communication with a woman with psychosis may take more time, and the psychiatric team may be critical for engaging the patient. Her particular delusions may affect her ability to comply with treatment. Many patients with psychoses have difficulty with abstract thinking. Explanations should be concrete. These patients may not trust family or physicians and may be more sensitive to feeling controlled. They may have more difficulty with simple decisions. Each decision should be made with respect, with alternatives of no treatment, with short deadlines to decision. When the patient's own executive function is impaired, thinking through in advance a plan to sustain adherence both to psychiatric and medical treatment is all the more important. Collaboration between psychiatrist and oncologist should be explicit.

30.13 Conclusion

Expert care means that each woman has the opportunity to be heard, to grapple with the existential plight, and to have syndromes of psychiatric diagnosis treated. Full treatment of MDD and anxiety disorder should also help to alleviate symptoms of hot flashes, insomnia, and fatigue. Antidepressant medications should be used methodically. Since response may take several weeks, how long the patient has taken a specific dose of antidepressant should be noted. If a benefit does not occur after 1 or 2 months, the regimen should be adjusted. In those women taking tamoxifen, antidepressant medications with less cytochrome P450 2D6 inhibition would be the first choice.

Expert psychopharmacological care should be augmented by appropriate cognitive behavioral, individual, or group treatments. For those who do not require the best specific treatments for psychiatric syndromes, coping strategies are strengthened by access to psychoeducation, relaxation, and expert group or individual interventions tailored to the treatments for best cancer care.

MDD is a relapsing syndrome with grave morbidity and mortality that must occur in some women who are treated for breast cancer [78]. Without breast cancer, it has a lifetime prevalence of 16.2 % and 12-month prevalence of 6.6 % in adults, more common in women than men, with a risk ratio of 1.7–1.0 over a lifetime [79]. Risk factors include personal or family history of depressive disorder, prior suicide attempts, lack of social supports, stressful life events, and current substance abuse. It is worth taking note of these risk factors when considering which women with breast cancer need surveillance for depression. We are bound to treat what is serious and treatable. Screening for depressive symptoms, for instance, with the Patient Health Questionnaire (PHQ-9), calls attention to the possibility of depression even when patients are quiet about their symptoms. The screen begins a discussion that can lead to appropriate treatment and better quality of life. Collaborative care programs in cancer centers that screen for depression, treat and assess outcome so that depression does not compromise oncological treatment in cancer patients have made a difference proven in multiple controlled studies [80].

Most patients with breast cancer do not develop MDD, but the adjustment to the diagnosis, hormonal changes associated with menopause and further antiestrogen treatments cause dysphoria, sleep disruption, fatigue, poor concentration, and anxiety. Some women are more susceptible to these hormonal changes than others. Some women have a history anxiety disorder that adds to their difficulty coping with medical illness. Psychosocial interventions help patients to adjust to the uncertainty of cancer, the loss of fertility, and body image. The best psychosocial interventions for breast cancer patients should include optimal treatment for MDD.

References

1. Brunault P, Champagne A-L, Huguet G, et al. Major depressive disorder, personality disorders, and coping strategies are independent risk factors for lower quality of life in non-metastatic breast cancer patients. Psycho-Oncology. 2015;. doi:10.1002/pon.3947.
2. Barton MB, Morley DS, Moore S, Allen JD, Kleinman KP, Emmons KM, Fletcher SW. Decreasing women's anxieties after abnormal mammograms: a controlled trial. J Natl Cancer Inst. 2004;96:529–38.
3. Ramirez AJ, Westcombe AM, Burgess CC, Sutton S, Littlejohns P, Richards MA. Factors predicting delayed presentation of symptomatic breast cancer: a systematic review. Lancet. 1999;353:1127–31.
4. Jones SE, Cantrell J, Vukelja S, Pippen J, O'Shaughnessy J, et al. Comparison of menopausal symptoms during the first year of adjuvant therapy with either exemestane or tamoxifen in early breast cancer: report of a tamoxifen exemestane adjuvant multi-center trial substudy. J Clin Oncol. 2007;25:4765–71.
5. Fallowfield L, Cella D, Cuzick J, et al. Quality of life of postmenopausal women in the Arimidex, Tamoxifen, Alone or in combination (ATAC) adjuvant breast trial. J Clin Oncol. 2004;22:4261–71.
6. Thomas R, Williams M, Marshall C, Walker L. Switching to letrozole or exemestane improves hot flushes, mood and quality of life in tamoxifen intolerant women. Brit J Cancer. 2008;98: 1494–9.
7. Waterhouse DM, Calzone KA, Mele C, Brenner DE. Adherence to oral tamoxifen: a comparison of patient selfreport, pill counts, and microelectronic monitoring. J Clin Oncol. 1993;11:1189–97.
8. Partridge AH, Wang PS, Winer EP, et al. Nonadherence to adjuvant tamoxifen therapy in women with primary breast cancer. J Clin Oncol. 2003;21:602–6.
9. Lash TL, Fox MP, Westrup JL, Fink AK, Silliman RA. Adherence to tamoxifen over the five-year course. Breast Cancer Res Treat. 2006;99:215–20.
10. Kahn KL, Schneider EC, Malin J, Adams JL, Epstein AM. Patient-centered experiences in breast cancer: predicting long-term adherence to tamoxifen use. Med Care. 2007;45:431–9.
11. Partridge AH, LaFountain A, Mayer E, Taylor BS, Winer E, Asnis-Alibozek A. Adherence to initial adjuvant anastrozole therapy among women with early stage breast cancer. J Clin Oncol. 2008;26:556–62.
12. Mausbach BT, Schwab RB, Irwin SA. Depression as a predictor of adherence to adjuvant endocrine therapy (AET) in women with breast cancer: a systematic review and meta-analysis. Breast Cancer Res Treat. 2015;152:239–46.
13. Greer JA, Park ER, Prigerson HG, Safren SA. Tailoring cognitive-behavioral therapy to treat anxiety comorbid with advanced cancer. J Cogn Psychother. 2010;24:294–313.
14. Johnson JA, Rash JA, Campbell TS, et al. A systematic review and meta-analysis of randomized controlled trials of cognitive behavior therapy for insomnia (CBT-I) in cancer survivors. Sleep Med Rev. 2015;27:20–8. doi:10.1016/j.smrv.2015.07.001.
15. Grunberg SM. Antiemetic activity of corticosteroids in patients receiving cancer chemotherapy: dosing, efficacy, and tolerability analysis. Ann Oncol. 2007;18:233–40.
16. Buysse DJ, Reynolds DC III, Hauri PJ, et al. Diagnostic concordance for DSM IV sleep disorders: a report from the APA/NIMH DSV-IV field trial. Am J Psychiatry. 1994;151: 1351–60.
17. Benca RM, Obermeyer WH, Thisted RA, et al. Sleep and psychiatric disorders: a meta-analysis. Arch Gen Psychiatry. 1992;49:651–68.
18. Weilburg JB, Stakes JW, Roth T. Sleep disorders. In: Stern TA, Rosenbaum JF, Fava M, Biederman J. Rauch SL, editors. Comprehensive Clinical Psychiatry. Mosby Elsevier; 2008. p. 285–99.
19. Carpenter JS, Andrykowski MA, Cordova M, Cunningham L, Studts J, McGrath P, Kenady D, Sloan D, Munn R. Hot flashes in postmenopausal women treated for breast carcinoma: prevalence,

severity, correlates, management, and relation to quality of life. Cancer. 1998;82:1682–91.

20. Kronenberg F. Hot flashes: phenomenology, quality of life, and search for treatment options. Exp Gerontol. 1994;29:319–36.
21. Savard J, Davidson JR, Ivers H, Quesnel C, Rioux D, Dupere V, Lanier M, Smard S, Morin CM. The association between nocturnal hot flashes and sleep in breast cancer survivors. J Pain Sympt Manage. 2004;27:513–22.
22. Stearns V, Beebe KL, Lyengar M, Dube E. Paroxetine controlled release in the treatment of menopausal hot flashes: a randomized controlled trial. JAMA. 2003;289:2827–34.
23. Loprinzi CL, Sloan JA, Perez EA, Quella SK, Stella PJ, Mailliard JA, et al. Phase III evaluation of fluoxetine for treatment of hot flashes. J Clin Oncol. 2002;20:1578–83.
24. Loprinzi CL, Kugler JW, Sloan JA, Mailliard JA, et al. Venlafaxine in management of hot flashes in survivors of breast cancer: a randomized controlled trial. Lancet. 2000;356:2059–63.
25. Pandya KJ, Morrow GR, Roscoe JA, Zhao H, et al. Gabapentin for hot flashes in 420 women with breast cancer: a randomized double-blind placebo-controlled trial. Lancet. 2005;366:818–24.
26. Bardwell WA, Profant J, Casden DR, Dimsdale JE, Ancoli-Israel S, Natarajan L, Rock CL, Pierce JP. The relative importance of specific risk factors for insomnia in women treated for early stage breast cancer. Psychooncology. 2008;17:9–18.
27. Ganz PA, Kwan L, Castellon SA, Oppenheim A, et al. Cognitive complaints after breast cancer treatments: examining the relationship with neuropsyhological test performance. J Nat Cancer Inst. 2013;105:791–801.
28. Jenkins V, Shilling V, Deutsch G, et al. A 3-year prospective study of the effects of adjuvant treatments on cognition in women with early stage breast cancer. Br J Cancer. 2006;94:828–34.
29. Joffee H, Hall JE, Gruber S, et al. Estrogen therapy selectively enhances prefrontal cognitive processes: a randomized, double-blind, placebo-controlled study with functional magnetic resonance imaging in premenopausal and recently postmenopausal women. Menopause. 2006;12:411–22.
30. Silverman DH, Dy CJ, Castellon S, Lai J, Pio BS, Abraham L, Waddell K, Petersen L, Phelps ME, Ganz PA. Altered frontocortical cerebellar and basal ganglia activity in adjuvant treated breast cancer survivors 5–10 years after chemotherapy. Breast Cancer Res Treat. 2007;103:303–11.
31. Ono M, Ogilvie JM, Wilson JS, et al. A meta-analysis of cognitive impairment and decline associated with adjuvant chemotherapy in women with breast cancer. Front Oncol. 2015;5:1–19. doi:10.3389/fonc.2015.00059.
32. Amidi A, Christensen S, Mehlsen M, et al. Long-term subjective cognitive functioning following adjuvant systemic treatment: 7–9 years follow-up of a nationwide cohort of women treated for primary breast cancer. Brit J Cancer. 2015;113:794–801.
33. Bower JE. Behavioral symptoms in breasst cancer patients and survivors: fatigue, insomnia, depression, and cognitive disturbance. J Clin Oncol. 2008;26:768–77.
34. Kohli S, Fisher SG, Tra Y et al. The effect of modafinil on cognitive function in breast cancer survivors. 2009;115:2605–16.
35. Mar Fan HG, Clemons M, Xu W, et al. A randomized, placebo-controlled, double-blind trial of the effects of d-methylphenidate on fatigue and cognitive dysfunction in women undergoing adjuvant chemotherapy for breast cancer. Support Care Cancer. 2008;16(577–583):34.
36. Lawrence JA, Griffin L, Balcueva EP et al. A study of donepezil in female breast cancer survivors with self-reported cognitive dysfunction 1 to 5 years following adjuvant chemotherapy. J Cancer Surviv. 2015 (epub ahead of print).
37. Schmidt P, Nieman LK, Danaceau MA, Adamas LF, Rubinow DR. Differential behavioral effects of gonadal steroids in women with and in those without premenstrual syndrome. N Engl J Med. 1998;338:209–16.
38. Cohen LS, Soares CN, Otto MW, Vitonis AF, Harlow BL. Risk for new onset of depression during the menopausal transition: the Harvard study of moods and cycles. Arch Gen Psychiatry. 2006;63:385–90.
39. Schmidt PJ, Haq N, Rubinow MD, David R. A longitudinal evaluation of the relationship between reproductive status and mood in perimenopausal women. Am J Psychiatry. 2004;161:2238–44.
40. Soares CN, Helga A, Joffe H, Bankier B, Cassano P, Petrillo LF, Cohen LS. Escitalopram versus ethyinyl estradiol and norethindrone acetate for symptomatic peri- and postmenopausal women: impact on depression, vasomotor symptoms, sleep, and quality of life. Menopause. 2006;13:780–6.
41. Soares CN, Almeida OP, Joffe H, Cohen LS. Efficacy of estradiol for the treatment of depressive disorders in perimenopausal women: a double-blind, randomized, placebocontrolled trial. Arch Gen Psychiatry. 2001;58:529–34.
42. Andrykowski MA, Schmidt JE, Salsman JM, Beacham AO, Jacobsen P. Use of a case definition approach to identify cancer-related fatigue in women undergoing adjuvant therapy for breast cancer. J Clin Oncol. 2005;23:6613–22.
43. Donovan KA, Small BJ, Andrykowski MA, Munster P, Jacobesen PB. From: Utility of a cognitive-behavioral model to predict fatigue following breast cancer treatment. Health Psychol. 2007;26:464–72.
44. Servaes P, Verhagen S, Bleijenberg G. Determinants of chronic fatigue in disease-free breast cancer patients: a cross-sectional study. Ann Oncol. 2002;13:589–98.
45. Servaes P, Verhagen CA, Bleijenberg G. Relations between fatigue, neuropsychological functioning and physical activity after treatment for breast carcinoma. Cancer. 2002;95:2017–26.
46. Servaes PM, Gielissen MF, Verhagen S, Bleijenberg G. The course of severe fatigue in disease-free breast cancer patients: a longitudinal study. Psycho Onology. 2007;16:787–95.
47. Bower JE, Ganz PA, Desmond KA, Bernards C, Rowland JH, Meyerowitz BE, Belin TR. Fatigue in long-term breast carcinoma survivors: a longitudinal investigation. Cancer. 2006;106:751–8.
48. Sharpe M, Hawton K, Simpkin S, Surawy C, Hackmann A, Klimes I, Peto T, Warrel D, Seagroatt V. Cognitive behaviour therapy for chronic fatigue syndrome: a randomized controlled trial. Br Med J. 1996;312:22–6.
49. Gielissen MF, Verhagn S, Witjes F, Bleijenberg G. Effects of cognitive behavioral therapy in severely fatigued disease-free cancer patients compared with patients waiting for cognitive behavioral therapy: a randomized controlled trial. J Clin Oncol. 2006;42:4882–7.
50. Barsevick AM, Dudley W, Beck S, et al. A randomzied clinical trial of energy conservation for patients with cancerrelated fatigue. Cancer. 2000;100:1302–10.
51. Bower JE. Cancer-related fatigue: mechanisms, risk factors, and treatments. Nat Rev Clin Oncol. 2014;11:597–609.
52. Fann JR, Thomas-Rich AM, Katon WJ, Cowley D, Pepping M, McGregor BA, Gralow J. Major depression after breast cancer: a review of epidemiology and treatment. Gen Hosp Psychiatry. 2008;30:112–26.
53. Hjerl K, Andersen EW, Keiding N, Mortensen PB, Jorgensen T. Increased incidence of affective disorders, anxiety disorders, and non-natural mortality in women after breast cancer diagnosis: a nation-wide cohort study in Denmark. Acta Psychiatr Scand. 2002;105:258–64.
54. Yousaf U, Christensen M-LM, Engholm G, Storm HH. Suicides among Danish cancer patients 1971–1999. Br J Cancer. 2005;92:995–1000.

55. Schairer C, Brown LM, Chen BE, Howard R, Lynch CF, et al. Suicide after breast cancer: an international population based study of 723810 women. J Natl Cancer Inst. 2006;98:1416–9.
56. Gonzalez-Perez A, Rodriquez LAG. Breast cancer risk among users of antidepressant medications. Epidemiology. 2005;16:101–5.
57. Haque R, Enger SM, Chen W, Petitti DB. Breast cancer risk in a large cohort of female antidepressant medication users. Cancer Lett. 2004;221:61–5.
58. Jin Y, Desta Z, Stearns V, Ward B, Ho H, Lee KH, et al. CYP2D6 genotype, antidepressant use, and tamoxifen metabolism during adjuvant breast cancer treatment. J Natl Cancer Inst. 2005;97:30–9.
59. Lim HS, Lee HJ, Lee KS, Lee ES, Jang IJ, Ro J. Clinical implications of CYP2D6 genotypes predictive of tamoxifen pharmacokinetics in metastatic breast cancer. J Clin Oncol. 2007;25:3837–45.
60. Goetz MP, Knox SK, Suman VJ, Safgren SL, Ames MM, Visscher DW, et al. The impact of cytochrome P450 2D6 metabolism in women receiving adjuvant tamoxifen. Breast Cancer Res Treat. 2007;101:1213–21.
61. Ratliff B, Dietze EC, Bean GR, Moore C, Wanto S, Seewaldt VL. Correspondence: Re: active tamoxifen metabolite plasma concentrations after coadministration of tamoxifen and the selective serotonin reuptake inhibitor paroxetine. J Natl Cancer Inst. 2004;96:883.
62. Keller MB, McCullough JP, Klein DN, Arnow B, Dunner DL, Gelenberg AJ, et al. A comparison of nefazadone, the cognitive behavioral—analysis system of psychotherapy, and their combination for the treatment of chronic depression. N Engl J Med. 2000;342:1462–70.
63. Fawzy FI, Fawzy NW, Arndt LA, et al. Critical review of psychosocial interventions in cancer care. Arch Gen Psychiatry. 1995;52:100–13.
64. Leubbert K, Dahme B, Hasenbring M. The effectiveness of relaxation training in reducing treatment-related symptoms and improving emotional adjustment in acute non-surgical cancer treatment: a meta-analytic review. Psycho Oncol. 2001;10:490–502.
65. Jassim GA, Whitford DL, Hickey A, Carter B. Psychological interventions for women with non-metastatic breast cancer. Cochrane Databases of Systematic Reviews: CD 008729; 2015.
66. Mustafa M, Carson-Stevens A, Gillespie D, Edwards AGK. Psychological interventions for women with metastatic breast cancer. Cochrane Database of Systematic Reviews CD004253; 2013.
67. Stagle JM, Bouchard LC, Lechner SC, et al. Long-term psychological benefits of cognitive-behavioral stress management for women with breast cancer: 11-year follow-up of a randomized controlled trial. Cancer. 2015;121:1873–81.
68. Spiegel D, Butler LD, Giese-Davis J, Koopman C, Miller E, et al. Effects of supportive-expressive group therapy on survival of patients with metastatic breast cancer. Cancer. 2007;110:1130–8.
69. Kissane DW, Li Y. Effects of supportive-expressive group therapy on survival of patients with metastatic breast cancer: a randomized controlled trial. Cancer. 2008;112:443–4.
70. Kissane D, Grabsch B, Clarke DM, et al. Supportive-expressive group therapy for women with metastatic breast cancer: survival and psychosocial outcome from a randomized controlled trial. Psychooncology. 2007;16:277–86.
71. Classen PJ, Butler LD, Koopman C, et al. Supportive-expressive group therapy and distress in patients with meta-static breast cancer: a randomized clinical intervention trail. Arch Gen Psychiatry. 2001;58:494–501.
72. Goodwin PJ, Leszcz M, Ennis M et al. The effect of group psychosocial support on survival in metastatic breast cancer. N Engl J Med. 2001;345:1719–26.
73. McGregor BA, Dolan ED, Murphy KM, et al. Cognitive behavioral stress management for healthy women at risk for breast cancer: a novel application of a proven intervention. Ann Behav Med. 2015;49:873–84.
74. Rauch P, Muriel AC. Raising an emotionally healthy child when a parent is sick. Boston: McGraw Hill; 2005.
75. Hippisley-Cox J, Vinogradova Y, Coupland C, Parker C. Risk of malignancy in patients with schizophrenia or bipolar disorder: nested case-control study. Arch Gen Psychiatry. 2007;64:1368–76.
76. Irwin KE, Henderson DC, Knight HP, Pirl WF. Cancer care for individuals with schizophrenia. Cancer. 2014;120:323–34.
77. Froes Brandao DF, Strasser-Weippi K, Goss PE. Prolactin and breast cancer: the need to avoid undertreatment of serious psychiatric illnesses in breast cancer patients: a review. Cancer Oct 12, 2015. doi:10.1002/cncr.29714.
78. Greenberg DB. Barriers to the treatment of depression in cancer patients. J Natl Cancer Inst Monogr. 2004;32:127–35.
79. Kessler RC, Berglund P, Bemler O, Jin R, Koretz D, Merkangas KR, et al. The epidemiology of major depressive disorder. JAMA. 2003;289:3095–105.
80. Fann JR, Ell K, Sharpe M. Integrating psychosocial care into cancer services. J Clin Oncol. 2012;30:1178–86.

31 Management of the Patient with a Genetic Predisposition for Breast Cancer

Sarah Colonna and Amanda Gammon

31.1 Hereditary Breast Cancer

Women who have close relatives with breast cancer have an increased risk of developing breast cancer themselves. Familial clustering of breast cancer may occur for several reasons. Breast cancer is a common disease, and clustering may be coincidental. Shared environmental or lifestyle factors may result in multiple cases of breast cancer within a family, particularly among siblings. Genetic risk factors are also known to explain some familial breast cancer clustering. While there has been a significant increase in genetics knowledge since *BRCA1* and *BRCA2* were identified over 25 years ago with additional genes now known to be associated with breast cancer risk, a large proportion of the family histories of breast cancer remain unexplained by current genetic testing. The ways we assess patients for hereditary breast cancer risk and the scope of genetic testing available have changed dramatically in the last few years. Understanding both the improvements and limitations of hereditary cancer assessment are crucial to provide appropriate risk management recommendations for patients. This chapter will review the basics of cancer genetics, outline selected genes associated with hereditary breast cancer, and discuss the importance of the family and personal history in identifying those who may have an inherited predisposition to breast cancer. Models for assessing the risk of developing cancer and of having a genetic predisposition to cancer will be described. Management of individuals at increased risk of breast cancer will be discussed, including genetic counseling and testing, interpretation of results, and options for modifying risk in those with a family history of breast cancer, with or without an identifiable gene mutation.

31.1.1 Somatic and Germline Genetics

All cancer is genetic; that is, all cancer is caused by the accumulation of genetic mutations in a specific cell line. Infrequently, cancer can be the result of a gene mutation that was inherited or occurred very shortly after conception (i.e. the mutation is present in every cell of the body). These types of mutations are called *germline* mutations. It is estimated that 5–10 % of all breast cancer cases are due to an inherited genetic factor that confers a high breast cancer risk [1]. Families with an inherited predisposition to cancer usually have more cases of cancer than would be expected by chance; cancer in several generations and cancer at earlier ages than are typical. Genetic testing for hereditary cancer predisposition most often requires a blood or buccal sample from the patient and looks for germline mutations. *Somatic* mutations typically occur during a person's lifetime and are thus not present in every cell in the person's body. Most tests that examine the genetics of a tumor are looking specifically for somatic mutations—mutations that are present in the cells that became cancerous but are typically not present in the rest of their cells (such as their germline (egg or sperm) cells). The purpose of these tests is not to identify hereditary cancer predispositions but to identify mutations within the tumor that could be potential therapeutic targets. However, if a patient has a germline mutation predisposing her to develop cancer, it should in theory be present in all of her cells, including their tumor cells. Some patients have first come to attention for hereditary cancer assessment due to an unexpected mutation identified in their tumor that was later determined to be germline [2]. On the other hand, due to differences in sequencing techniques and mutation reporting between tumor and germline genetic tests and the genetic alterations inherent in tumor formation, it is possible that a patient may have a germline mutation that is not

S. Colonna (✉)
Oncology, Huntsman Cancer Institute, 2000 Circle of Hope, Salt Lake City, UT 84112-5550, USA
e-mail: sarah.colonna@hci.utah.edu

A. Gammon
High Risk Cancer Research, Huntsman Cancer Institute, 2000 Circle of Hope, Rm#1148, Salt Lake City, UT 84112, USA
e-mail: amanda.gammon@hci.utah.edu

I. Jatoi and A. Rody (eds.), *Management of Breast Diseases*, DOI 10.1007/978-3-319-46356-8_31

detected/reported on tumor sequencing. If a patient is appropriate for hereditary cancer evaluation, she should be referred for genetic counseling and germline mutation testing, regardless of the tumor sequencing results. Also, if a mutation is detected in a patient's tumor and there is concern that the mutation may be germline, she should be referred for genetic counseling and germline mutation testing [2].

31.2 Genes Associated with Hereditary Breast Cancer

There are numerous genes that, when mutated in the germline, confer a significant risk for cancer, including several that increase the risk for breast cancer. Mutations in some genes confer high risks for breast cancer (defined here as causing over a fourfold increase in lifetime female breast cancer risk). More genes have been identified in the past 10 years whose mutations confer a more moderate increase in breast cancer risk (often defined as conferring at least a twofold increase in breast cancer risk). As of yet, there is no strict consensus on what constitutes a "high" versus "moderate" breast cancer risk, but similar cutoffs have been used in recent research and reviews [3]. We have divided these genes into these two risk categories to highlight differences in the assessment and management of mutations carriers. Table 31.1 identifies the genes whose mutations confer a high breast cancer risk while Table 31.2 provides an overview of genes associated with moderate risk. Other genetic changes, such as SNPs (single-nucleotide polymorphisims) have been associated with smaller alterations in breast cancer risk [4]. It is unclear how or whether an individual's breast cancer screening should be altered on the presence of an individual SNP. However, current research is exploring the incorporation of SNP data into comprehensive breast cancer risk assessment (including breast density and other risk factors) called a polygenic risk score [4, 5]. Clinical incorporation of polygenic risk scores may provide future refinement to currently available risk assessment techniques.

Most germline mutations that predispose to breast cancer are inherited in an autosomal dominant fashion, such that a mutation from either parent increases the risk for cancer. Spontaneous mutations are rare. Therefore, if an individual has a mutation, one of the parents is almost always a carrier, and siblings and children are each at 50 % risk of inheriting the familial mutation. Most of the genes are tumor suppressor genes which, when working properly, reduce the risk of developing cancer. When mutated, however, the protective function is lost and the risk of cancer is increased.

The risk for the development of cancer associated with mutations in these genes varies depending on the specific gene and the population analyzed. Early studies, which evaluated families based on a clinical ascertainment of four or more breast cancers, suggested a higher penetrance [6] than subsequent studies in families with a more modest family history [7]. Population-based studies test all individuals diagnosed with breast cancer for gene mutations, without regard to family history. In these studies, the risk for cancer in relatives is still lower [8]. It is likely that modifying genes or environmental factors affect penetrance from family to family.

Table 31.1 Hereditary breast cancer predispositions: high-risk

Gene (condition)	Approximate lifetime breast cancer risk for women	Other cancer risks and features
BRCA1 (Hereditary breast and ovarian cancer syndrome)	50–80 %	Cancers: ovary, prostate
BRCA2 (Hereditary breast and ovarian cancer syndrome)	50–80 %	Cancers: ovary, breast cancer in males, prostate, melanoma, pancreas
PTEN (Cowden syndrome)	25–50 %	Cancers: endometrial, thyroid (nonmedullary), colon, urinary tract Other features: macrocephaly, colon polyps (hamartomas, ganglioneuromas, juvenile polyps), skin lesions
CDH1 (Hereditary diffuse gastric cancer)	39–52 % (lobular breast cancer)	Cancers: gastric cancer (diffuse type); unclear if colon cancer risk is also increased
STK11 (Peutz-Jeghers syndrome)	45 %	Cancers: pancreas, colon, ovary, cervix, lung Other features: abnormal melanin deposits (lips, buccal mucosa, fingers, etc.)
TP53 (Li-Fraumeni syndrome)	High, but unclear due to rarity and high risks for many forms of cancer	Cancers: brain, adrenal cortex, sarcomas, leukemia, lung, GI tract; women have over a 90 % lifetime risk to develop cancer of some type
PALB2	35–60 %	Unclear if risk also increased for pancreatic cancer, ovarian, male breast cancer, or prostate cancer

Table 31.2 Moderate-risk genes

Gene	Approximate lifetime breast cancer risk for women (%)	Other cancer risks and features
ATM	30–40	Possible association with pancreatic cancer. Biallelic mutations cause ataxia-telangiectasia syndrome
CHEK2	20–45	Moderate colon cancer risk. Other moderate cancer risks possible (prostate, male breast cancer, etc.) Common founder mutation in Northern European ancestry = 1100delC
NBN	23	Unclear if other cancer risks present. Common founder mutation in Slavic population = c.657del5. Biallelic mutations cause Nijmegen breakage syndrome

Clinic-based ascertainment may select for families in which there is not only a gene mutation conferring breast cancer risk, but other genetic or environmental factors at play.

31.2.1 Hereditary Breast Cancer Predispositions: High-Risk

Table 31.1 summarizes the genes whose mutations confer high risks for breast cancer. Besides conferring a high risk for breast cancer, the majority of these gene mutations confer high risks for other forms of cancer. Most of these genes were associated with cancer risk over 20 years ago, so extensive research and clinical management recommendations are available [9].

The most common cause of hereditary breast cancer remains mutations in *BRCA1* or *BRCA2* which cause Hereditary Breast and Ovarian Cancer syndrome. A *BRCA1* or *BRCA2* mutation is found in approximately 1 in 300 to 1 in 800 Caucasians and about 1 in 40 individuals of Ashkenazi Jewish ancestry [8–10]. The rate in other ethnic groups is not well defined, although specific founder mutations have been identified in many countries, including the Netherlands [11] and Iceland [12]. *BRCA1* and *BRCA2* mutations are associated with a lifetime risk for female breast cancer of about 50–80 % in women [6, 13–15]. The lifetime risk for ovarian cancer in women is approximately 40–60 % with a *BRCA1* mutation and 20–30 % with a BRCA2 mutation [6, 13–15]. Men with *BRCA1* or *BRCA2* mutations also have an increased risk for breast cancer (up to 7 % lifetime risk with *BRCA2*; less with *BRCA1*) [16]. *BRCA1*-associated cancers are typically high grade, often with medullary features, usually estrogen and progesterone receptor negative, and do not overexpress HER2/neu (so-called "triple negative" breast cancer) [17]. *BRCA2*-associated breast cancers are generally estrogen receptor positive and of no specific histologic type [18, 19]. The ovarian cancers in *BRCA* mutation carriers are epithelial in origin and usually of serous histology [20, 21]. Fallopian tube cancers and primary peritoneal cancers are also prevalent; there is some evidence that the ovarian cancers associated with *BRCA1/2* mutations may originate in the fallopian tubes [22, 23].

Mutations in the *BRCA1* and *BRCA2* genes confer risks for cancers other than breast and ovarian. *BRCA2* mutations are associated with an increased risk of melanoma, pancreatic cancer, and prostate cancer [6, 24, 25]. Prostate cancer occurring in both *BRCA1* and *BRCA2* mutation carriers may be more aggressive than prostate cancers in the general population [26–28]. While very rare, biallelic mutations in *BRCA2* (i.e., a mutation on both the maternal and paternal alleles of the gene) are known to cause Fanconi Anemia; this occurs with biallelic mutations of many of the genes in the same pathway as *BRCA2* [29].

Cowden syndrome is caused by a mutation in the *PTEN* gene. It is often first recognized because of skin lesions and intestinal hamartomas [30], but is also associated with an increased risk of early-onset breast cancer that ranges from 25 to 50 %; newer studies indicate the lifetime risk may be higher than 50 % [31]. Besides breast cancer, nonmedullary thyroid cancer, endometrial cancer, colon, renal cancer, and possibly melanoma are increased [31, 32]. Benign findings that occur frequently include benign thyroid disease, trichilemmomas, which are flesh-colored bumps on the face and tongue, and macrocephaly above the 97th percentile [33].

Li-Fraumeni syndrome is a rare disorder caused by a mutation in *TP53*, the "guardian of the genome," that prevents cells with DNA damage from proceeding through the cell cycle. Somatic mutations in *TP53* are found in about half of all cancers. When present as a germline mutation, risk for cancer is extremely high [34, 35]. Approximately 50 % of individuals with mutations have developed cancer by age 30, and the prevalence by age 70 is 90 % [36]. Osteosarcomas, soft tissue sarcomas, brain tumors, leukemia and adrenal cortical carcinomas are the characteristic tumors, with breast cancer found in 25 % of those who do not die of childhood tumors [37]. Breast cancer tends to occur very early, often in the 20s. Virtually every other solid tumor is also found at very early ages in this population, with multiple primary tumors found in 57 % in a 30-year follow-up study [38]. New screening protocols have been created to address the multi-system cancer risks associated with Li-Fraumeni syndrome, incorporating brain and whole body MRI, in addition to mammogram and breast MRI, colonoscopy, and dermatology exams [39].

Peutz–Jeghers syndrome is caused by mutations in *STK11*. It is usually diagnosed based on distinctive hamartomatous polyps [40] and the presence of benign pigmented spots on the lips and buccal mucosa. The lifetime risk for cancer is up to 80 % in these families, with breast cancer being the most common at around 45 % [41–43].

Historically, mutations in *CDH1* have been associated with Hereditary Diffuse Gastric Cancer and confer a very high lifetime risk (67–83 %) for gastric cancer [9, 44]. Due to limitations in endoscopic surveillance, prophylactic gastrectomy is recommended for CDH1 mutation carriers in their early 20s [45]. Women with *CDH1* mutations also have between a 39 and 52 % lifetime risk for lobular breast cancer [9, 44]. With the advent of multigene testing for hereditary breast cancer risk, increasing numbers of individuals have been identified with *CDH1* mutations with no known family history of gastric cancer. This creates a dilemma for appropriate gastric cancer risk assessment and management as these families may not have the same high gastric cancer risks [46].

PALB2 was first identified in 2006 [47]. Recent studies have indicated that women with a *PALB2* mutation have a similar breast cancer risk to women with a *BRCA2* mutation [48]. The strength of an individual's family history of breast cancer appears to have a bearing on the degree of cancer risk conferred by a *PALB2* mutation [48]. *PALB2* mutations also appear to be associated with moderately increased risk for pancreatic cancer, although further research is needed to delineate this [49]. Currently, it is unclear if mutations in *PALB2* increase the risks for other cancers, such as male breast and ovarian [48]. Like with *BRCA2* mutations, biallelic *PALB2* mutations are known to cause Fanconi Anemia [50].

31.2.2 Hereditary Breast Cancer Predispositions: Moderate-Risk

Table 31.2 summarizes information on three genes whose mutations confer moderately increased breast cancer risks. For *ATM, CHEK2, and NBN* mutation carriers, NCCN (National Comprehensive Cancer Network) has made management recommendations [9]. Breast cancer risk management guidelines have also recently been released for individuals with mutations in *NF1* (which causes Neurofibromatosis Type 1); these are not reviewed here as many individuals with *NF1* mutations are identified through pediatric genetics evaluation [9]. Many more genes are suspected of conferring similar (or slightly lower) breast cancer risks; however, consensus management guidelines do not yet exist for mutation carriers [3]. Testing of these genes is often included on commercially available multigene tests, which can create difficulties for clinicians and patients in interpreting the results and determining clinical utility.

Biallelic mutations in *ATM* have been known for many years to cause the neurodegenerative disorder, Ataxia-telangiectasia [51]. Increasing numbers of studies have found that women with a monoallelic mutation of ATM have a two-threefold increase in breast cancer risk [52]. However, individuals with a missense mutation in certain key functional domains of *ATM* may have significantly higher breast cancer risks [53]. Carriers of one *ATM* mutation may also have a moderately increased risk for pancreatic cancer, but this and any other potential cancer risks require further definition [54].

The majority of data available on *CHEK2* mutation cancer risks stems from a common founder mutation (1100delC) present in 0.5–1.3 % of individuals of Northern European descent [55, 56]. The female breast cancer risk conferred by this mutation is estimated to be approximately threefold, but like mutations in *PALB2*, *ATM*, and *NBN* the exact magnitude can vary depending on a person's family history of breast cancer [55]. *CHEK2* mutations appear to predispose primarily to estrogen receptor positive breast cancers [55]. Other pathogenic mutations in *CHEK2* beyond 1100delC are expected to confer similar breast cancer risks. The risks for other cancers are still being delineated, although moderately increased risks for multiple other cancers (including colon and prostate) have been indicated in some studies [57].

Like *CHEK2*, *NBN* also has a common founder mutation, c.657del5, in the Slavic population [58]. This monoallelic mutation appears to confer a 2.7 fold increase in female breast cancer risk [3, 58]. As is the case with both *ATM* and *CHEK2*, some missense mutations in NBN appear to confer similar or greater breast cancer risks than truncating mutations [58]. Individuals with biallelic NBN mutations have a condition called Nijmegen breakage syndrome, which is characterized by microcephaly, cognitive impairment, immunodeficiency and increased cancer risks [59].

31.3 Identification of Individuals at Increased Risk for Breast Cancer

31.3.1 Family History

A woman's risk of developing breast cancer is strongly related to the number of affected relatives, their genetic proximity, and ages at which they were diagnosed. Collecting an accurate family history is the single most cost-effective approach to identifying individuals with hereditary breast cancer [60]. A three-generation family history should be collected on individuals who have a suspected predisposition to cancer and should include all first-degree relatives (children, siblings, parents) and second-degree relatives (uncles and aunts, nieces and nephews, grandparents), as well as more distant relatives who have cancer [61]. For each family member, essential information includes current age or age and cause of death, medical history including types of cancer and age of onset, ethnicity/country of origin, and other syndrome-specific features, for example multiple gastrointestinal polyps. A graphic representation of the family history using recognized pedigree nomenclature outlined in Fig. 31.1 allows assessment of inheritance patterns and permits this information to be communicated to other clinicians and to patients in a clear and consistent manner [62].

The cancer pedigree should include at least the number and gender of individuals in each generation, whether affected with cancer or not, so the ratio of affected to unaffected family members can be incorporated into the assessment. A common breast cancer genetic myth is that "you don't have to worry about breast cancer on your father's side of the family." It is essential to collect *both* maternal and paternal histories of cancer, since germline mutations are equally likely to be inherited paternally as maternally.

Knowledge of breast cancer in first-degree relatives is generally accurate [63], but is less reliable in more distant relatives [64, 65]. Knowledge of cancers in other organs is often less precise. Gastric cancer and ovarian cancer may both be reported as "stomach cancer," and cervical, uterine, and ovarian all reported as "female cancer." Ovarian cysts may also be misreported as cancer. Questioning the patient about outcomes may be helpful in determining the accuracy of the diagnosis. For example, a report of a relative with long-term survival after a diagnosis of "ovarian cancer" or "pancreatic cancer" should raise questions about the accuracy of the diagnosis since these cancers have low long-term survival rates. Family medical histories are dynamic, and it is important to remind the patient that if additional cases of cancer are diagnosed or discovered, they should recontact the provider because the new information may alter the risk calculation and subsequently alter recommendations for risk management [66].

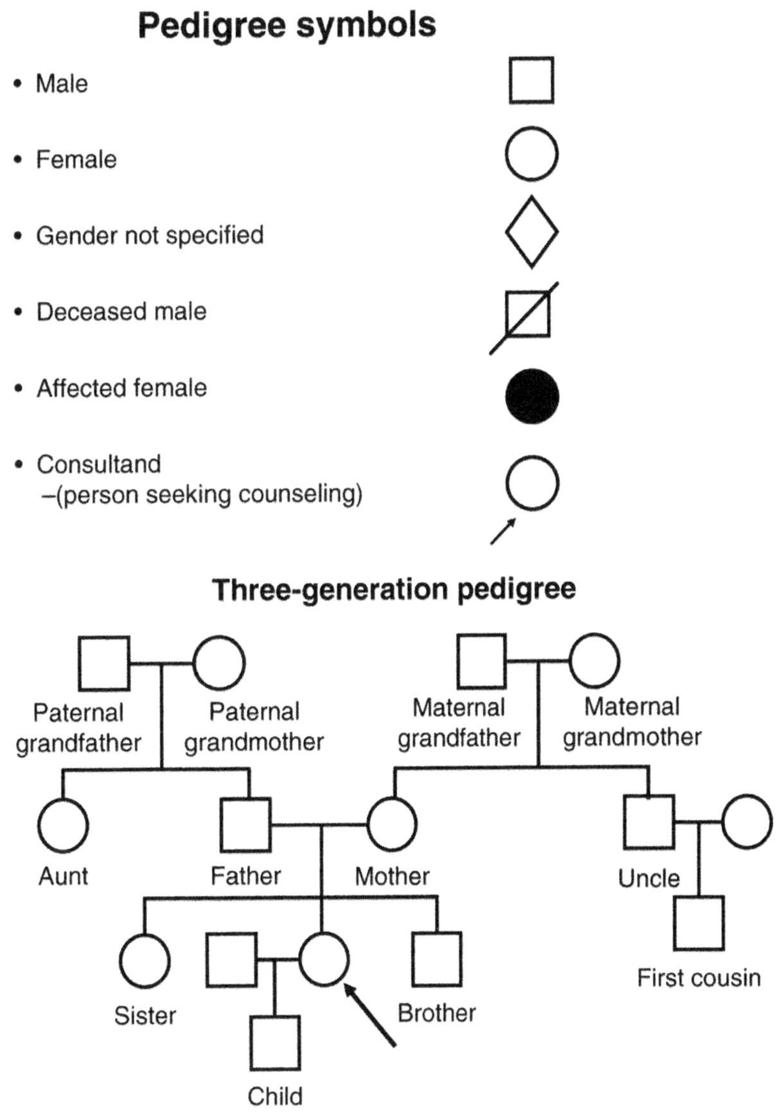

Fig. 31.1 Pedigree symbols and structure (represented by two slides). By using recognized pedigree nomenclature and structure, family history information can be communicated to other clinicians and patients in a clear and concise manner

Taking a detailed family history takes time. Some centers use a questionnaire that can be mailed prior to an appointment or completed in a waiting room. Several web-based questionnaires in both English and Spanish are readily available from resources such as the Centers for Disease Control and Prevention (http://www.hhs.gov/familyhistory/). Some centers utilize software such as Hughes Risk Apps (http://www.hughesriskapps.com/riskclinic.php) or Progeny (http://www.progenygenetics.com/) to create digital pedigrees. In some cases, small family size, adoption, and misidentified paternity complicate the analysis of a family history [67]. Despite these difficulties, obtaining an accurate family history reduces the likelihood of either overlooking the possibility of a hereditary cancer syndrome, which in turn leads to lost opportunities for cancer risk management and risk reduction in the patient as well as extended family members; or of inappropriately performing genetic testing. After obtaining an initial family history, referral to a cancer genetic service may be the most appropriate way to obtain a complete family history and risk assessment.

31.3.2 Personal Health History

In addition to information about the extended family, a cancer risk assessment includes a personal health history. The presence of cancer, cancer site, age of onset, the existence of multiple primaries or bilaterality, history of previous biopsies and whether the biopsy showed proliferative breast disease are important. Hormone-related factors such as age at menarche, nulliparity or age at first birth, number of pregnancies, duration of breast-feeding, age of menopause, and exogenous hormone use (oral contraception, hormone replacement therapy) also have an impact on the risk of developing cancer. Diet and exercise play a significant role in the development of breast cancer, not least of which is the impact of obesity on the increased rate of breast cancer in postmenopausal women [68]. Alcohol ingestion is also positively associated with breast cancer [69, 70]. Mammographic breast density is a recognized risk factor for breast cancer, and may be more strongly correlated with a risk for the development of breast cancer than any factors except for age, gender, and the presence of a breast cancer predisposition gene mutation [71]. Finally, radiation exposure, particularly during childhood and adolescence, increases the risk of breast, thyroid and other cancers [72]. Radiation was commonly administered in the 1940s through early 1970s for acne vulgaris, tinea capitis, hemangiomas, and enlargement of the tonsils or thymus, as well for Hodgkin's disease and other malignancies [72, 73]. The identification of a woman with both breast and thyroid cancer may suggest Cowden's syndrome, but in the presence of a history of radiation therapy, an environmental cause would be far more likely than an inherited one.

31.4 Risk Assessment

Two different but related risks are important to the individual patient: the risk of developing breast cancer, and the risk of carrying a mutation in a breast cancer predisposition gene.

Communication of risk requires an understanding of ways to present risk, the various models used to assess risk, the manner in which numbers can be interpreted, and the factors that are necessary to put them into context of the patient's perception of risk. Most women with a family history of breast cancer significantly overestimate their risk [74].

31.4.1 Absolute Risk

An absolute risk is the probability of an event occurring during a specific interval. For example, a well-known risk figure associated with breast cancer is 12 %, a cumulative incidence statistic, which means that about one in eight women in the general population will develop breast cancer at some point in her lifetime. Unless she has a breast cancer predisposition gene mutation, a woman who is presenting for risk assessment at age 30 has an absolute risk of developing breast cancer in the next 5 years of about 0.1 %, or one in a thousand, far less than the 12 % lifetime statistic [75].

31.4.2 Relative Risk

Most population-based studies of familial cancer report absolute risk, which compares the frequency of cancers within affected families to the frequencies expected in the general population. An observed-to-expected ratio (odds ratio) is used to quantify the risk [76] based on the particular environmental factor (parity, oral contraceptive use, diet, pesticide exposure) or the genetic proximity of an affected relative (sister, mother, aunt, grandmother). The risk is typically described as x-fold over that of the general population, such as a twofold risk for women with a sister diagnosed with postmenopausal breast cancer [77]. The degree of risk is influenced by the closeness of the relative and the age of diagnosis of breast cancer [77]. This may also be reported as a percent increase. Hormone replacement therapy may confer a relative risk of 1.2, for example, which is accurately reported as a 20 % increase in the risk. That concept is not always well-understood by patients who are confused and call their doctors wondering if their risk has increased from 12 to 32 % by their use of postmenopausal hormone replacement therapy, when a 1.2 relative risk has only increased their risk from 12 to 14 %.

31.4.3 Predicting Development of Breast Cancer: Gail Model and Claus Tables

Several mathematical models have been developed to estimate the risk of developing breast cancer. The Gail model computes individualized absolute risk in women receiving routine mammograms [78]. It uses six specific risk factors (age at evaluation, age at menarche, age at first live birth, number of prior breast biopsies, presence of proliferative breast disease on biopsy, and number of first degree relatives with breast cancer) to estimate 5-year and lifetime risk [79]. Although the model is a useful tool for defining risk estimates in the general population, it has several limitations in the context of a high-risk setting. It does not address the risk for women under age 35 or for those who are not undergoing regular mammograms. Most relevant to a high-risk population, the Gail model includes only first-degree relatives and therefore does not include paternal history, nor does it include a family history of ovarian cancer or age of onset of cancers. Therefore, it is not an appropriate model to assess risk for women in families with a known or suspected inherited cancer predisposition gene mutation.

The Claus tables [80] were subsequently developed based solely on family relationships and are more appropriate for estimating risk in women with a family history of breast cancer. This model includes first-and second-degree relatives and can be used to estimate cumulative risk over 10-year intervals. It includes relatives in only one lineage (either maternal or paternal) but not both. The model uses a single locus dominant genetic assumption, but those cases are limited to only about 5–10 % of breast cancers.

31.4.4 Models for Predicting Presence of a Gene Mutation and Cancer Development: BRCAPro, BOADICEA, and Tyrer-Cuzick

The most significant risk for breast cancer, except for gender and age, is the presence or absence of a specific germline mutation. Therefore, an important step in the risk assessment is to determine the likelihood that the family has a recognizable genetic mutation, as outlined in Tables 31.1 and 31.2 and discussed above. *BRCA1/2* gene mutations are the most prevalent of the genetic breast cancer predispositions. Due to this, most models currently available assess for BRCA1/2 mutation risk only and do not calculate a person's chance of having a mutation in another breast cancer predisposition gene.

The most commonly used model in the U.S. is BRCAPro, which includes age-specific cancer as well as positive and negative family history information of both first-and second-degree relatives from both sides of the family [81–83]. The information is then evaluated using a Bayesian approach to calculate carrier probabilities. Free registration for online access to this model is available at https://www4.utsouthwestern.edu/breasthealth/cagene/ as part of the CancerGene software package.

Another model, used widely in the U.K. and Australia, is BOADICEA (Breast and Ovarian Analysis of Disease Incidence and Carrier Estimation Algorithm), which was developed based on segregation analysis of breast and ovarian cancer [84]. Recent updates have added risk assessment for mutations in *CHEK2, ATM,* and *PALB2*—currently BOADICEA is the only model that provides specific risk estimates for mutations in these genes [85]. A user-friendly web-based program (http://www.srl.cam.ac.uk/genepi/boadicea_home.html) is available.

31.5 Genetic Testing

Genetic testing for a hereditary breast cancer risk has become increasingly complicated with the introduction of multigene tests [3]. Next-generation sequencing technology has greatly reduced the cost of genetic testing and allows for numerous genes to be analyzed in a single test. However, testing a mixture of genes associated with high or moderate breast cancer risks complicates the interpretation of results. Not all genes currently analyzed on commercially available tests have consensus guidelines for management of mutation carriers. Increasing the number of genes tested also increases the chance that a variant of uncertain significance will be detected. While comprehensive genetic testing is now easier to obtain than ever before for patients, thought and caution must still be exercised in identifying the best testing candidate in the family and in the results interpretation. Depending on the circumstances of testing, a negative (normal) test does not always lower the risk for breast cancer and should not always be considered "good news." Many families deemed to be appropriate for genetic testing have a sufficiently strong family history that warrants enhanced screening, even if no mutation is found [9]. Patients seek genetic testing for many reasons and the impact of the test result—whether positive, negative, or uninformative—on psychological health, social relationships and medical care needs to be explored prior to testing [86]. In addition, the test result has implications not only for the individual being tested, but for family members. As such, there is an ethical requirement to inform family members, and a strategy for doing so must be developed. Due to the complexities of genetic testing and the significant implications of the test results on patients and their family members, referral to a genetic professional can be very beneficial and is recommended by multiple organizations (NCCN, ACS, etc.). A list of genetic counselors can be found at http://www.nsgc.org or a cancer center can be located at the National Cancer Institute's website (http://www.cancer.gov/search/geneticsservices/). While more clinics and hospitals employ genetic counselors than ever before, genetic counseling services are also being made available by telemedicine or telephone to increase accessibility [87].

In general, referral for genetic testing is appropriate for an individual diagnosed with breast cancer at/under age 45, bilateral breast cancer, male breast cancer, or both breast and ovarian cancer. Families with two or more individuals with breast cancer under age 50, breast cancer under age 50 and ovarian cancer at any age, or three or more individuals with breast or pancreatic cancer at any age are also appropriate for genetic counseling and testing [9]. Some families have fewer cases of cancer but have a small number of women, or have related cancers such as pancreatic cancer, advanced prostate cancer, or melanoma. These may also be appropriated for genetic testing [67]. New data suggests that individuals of known Ashkenazi Jewish ancestry may consider testing for the three common *BRCA1/2* founder mutations regardless of reported personal or family history of cancer [88]. Ideally, the first person to receive genetic testing in a family should be someone affected with cancer, because if there is a mutation in the family, that person is more likely to carry the mutation than unaffected individuals. If a mutation is identified, testing for that specific gene mutation can then be performed in relatives, both male and female, based on the inheritance pattern of the particular gene. Testing for a known familial mutation is currently cheaper than full sequencing/deletion duplication testing of a gene, so if a mutation has already been identified in a family, it is typically most appropriate and cost-effective to only test relatives for the known mutation.

If a mutation is identified in a family, it is ideal from a scientific and psychosocial perspective to test other branches of the family, starting with the oldest generation alive. For example, rather than testing all cousins of a mutation carrier, testing aunts and uncles provides information for their descendants. If a parent has a mutation, all children, regardless of their cancer status, become testing candidates; if there is no mutation, subsequent generations do not need to be tested. From a psychosocial perspective, there are also advantages to testing a member of the oldest generation first, because it is often easier to share information from a parent to a child than from a child to a parent [89].

Since the 2013 Supreme Court decision regarding gene patenting, multiple laboratories in the U.S. offer genetic testing for hereditary breast cancer predispositions [3]. Testing can include *BRCA1/2* only or multiple genes associated with high and moderate breast cancer risks on a single test. The number of genes tested, as well as testing methodologies, variant classification methods, cost/billing, and financial assistance programs for patients vary between laboratories. A resource to help identify available laboratories for other cancer-related germline tests is GeneTests (www.genetests.org), available free of charge. This website, developed by the University of Washington, Seattle with funding from the National Library of Medicine and Maternal and Child Health Bureau, is an information resource that includes a directory of clinical and research laboratories that offer specific medical genetic tests.

31.5.1 Genetic Counseling

Prior to having a specimen obtained for genetic testing, genetic counseling is recommended and is now required in some cases to obtain insurance coverage for testing [9]. The purpose of genetic counseling is twofold: to provide genetic education and address psychosocial concerns. During a genetic counseling appointment, an individual will receive information on cancer etiology and a detailed risk assessment based on their personal and family history. The person's risk to develop cancer (or another cancer) and the chance to have an identifiable mutation in a cancer predisposition gene will be explored. A discussion will be had regarding the implications of genetic testing for both the individual and their family.

Genetic counseling involves interactive discussion about what the individual is hoping to learn from their risk assessment and what actions they are interested in pursuing (genetic testing, screening, cancer risk reduction). Many individuals have high expectations of what genetic testing can tell them about their cancer risks, when the reality may be quite different [90]. A frank discussion of the benefits and limitations of genetic testing is crucial to facilitating fully informed consent prior to pursuing genetic testing. A tailored plan is created with the patient for their cancer screening and risk reduction, regardless of whether or not they elect to pursue genetic testing. If the individual elects to pursue genetic testing, the genetic counselor can help coordinate this and create a plan for discussion of results.

Individuals differ in their belief on whether the identification of a mutation is good or bad news. For a woman with breast cancer, having a mutation may be good news in that it explains the etiology of her cancer. On the other hand, an unaffected woman who is the only one of her four sisters without a mutation may experience survivor guilt and see her result as bad news. Exploring the potential reactions to test results is an important part of the pretest session.

The genetic counseling process provides individuals the chance to express their interests and concerns about genetic testing. Some individuals are hesitant to consider genetic counseling and testing because of concerns regarding genetic discrimination [91]. Both federal and state laws have been passed that protect genetic privacy. In May 2008, the

Genetic Information Nondiscrimination Act was signed into law, and went into effect in May 2009 related to health insurance and in November 2009 related to workplace issues [92]. Through these laws, most individuals in the U.S. are protected from genetic discrimination as it relates to health insurance and employment. Currently, most individuals are not protected from potential genetic discrimination regarding life or disability insurance. However, while life insurance policies may inquire about genetic disorders within a family, they are more likely to inquire generally about family history (i.e., if a family history of cancer exists, etc.). Individuals with a personal or family history of cancer are already at risk to experience life or disability insurance discrimination based on family history whether or not they undergo genetic testing, which may put the potential risks of discrimination on the basis of genetic test results into perspective. Although the consequences of genetic discrimination may be significant, there are few documented cases of such discrimination, and the risk is likely to continue to diminish as genetic testing for adult conditions becomes more common. Other individuals elect not to pursue genetic testing due to financial cost. This barrier is diminishing with decreasing testing costs and financial assistance provided by many laboratories. Whether or not a person would alter their medical management on the basis of genetic test results and whether the person has any living relatives who would benefit from the information also plays a role in genetic testing decisions.

Most hereditary breast cancer predispositions (with the exception of Li-Fraumeni syndrome and some features of Cowden syndrome) are adult-onset. In the absence of documented medical benefit, offering genetic testing to minors for an adult-onset condition may compromise the autonomy of the child. Psychological consequences could include stigmatization of the child, or viewing the child as fragile [93, 94]. Due to these concerns, genetic testing for adult onset conditions is not recommended for minors. Most parents do discuss their genetic test results with their children in an age appropriate manner [95]. This can help children understand the screening/risk reduction measures their parent may be undertaking and help prepare them for their own future health decisions. Genetic counselors can assist individuals with strategies for disclosing their genetic test results to children and extended family members. They can also connect families with support, research, and educational resources on a local or national scale.

31.5.2 Interpretation of Test Results

Three basic categories of results are possible from genetic testing: positive, negative, or variant of uncertain significance. Oftentimes, the word "mutation" was used to connote a pathogenic (i.e., damaging) genetic change, where the word "variant" designated a genetic change of indeterminate consequence. While we have used this terminology throughout the chapter due to its persistence in common usage, genetics nomenclature has shifted to using the term "variant" for any genetic change to provide consistency [96]. In this section, we will use the term "variant" as recommended to highlight how genetic test results are currently reported in clinical practice. A positive test result indicates that an individual has a variant that increases the risk of developing breast cancer, as well as other cancers or benign conditions associated with that mutation. This result also means that other family members are candidates for genetic testing. On a test report, a positive result will usually be listed as a "pathogenic" or "deleterious" variant (or mutation). Variants that are considered "likely pathogenic/deleterious" should be considered a positive test result for clinical management purposes [97].

A negative test result means that no variants were detected that were either uncertain or pathogenic. The significance of a negative test result depends on whether or not there is a known pathogenic variant in the family. If the pathogenic variant in the family is already identified, this result is a true-negative test result and means (with greater than 99 % accuracy) that the patient did not inherit that variant. In a family carrying a pathogenic variant that confers high cancer risks, a true-negative test result typically means the individual would have a risk of developing cancer similar to the risk of a person in the general population. This may not hold true if the pathogenic variant in the family confers moderate cancer risks. In many families, a pathogenic variant conferring moderate cancer risks does not track with all of the relevant cancer diagnoses in the family. Thus some of the familial cancer risk may not be explained by the moderate risk pathogenic variant. Management recommendations for true negative individuals from families with a pathogenic mutation conferring moderate cancer risks are still being determined and should take into consideration personal and family history factors. In both types of families, management recommendations should incorporate other risk factors for breast cancer, including those assessed by the Gail model as well as breast density and family history of breast cancer on the other side of the family.

The predictive value of a negative test in an individual diagnosed with the cancer of interest is lower if the patient is the first one in the family being offered testing. There are a number of possible explanations for a negative test result in this case, including the possibility that the cancers in the family are not due to an inherited gene mutation but rather chance occurrences; that limitations of the technology do not allow a variant to be identified; that the variant is in a gene different from the one analyzed; or that the susceptibility gene that is predisposing to cancer in that family has not yet been discovered. Another possibility is that there is a familial gene variant accounting for the apparent increase in breast cancer; but that the individual tested does not have the mutation. In the presence of a striking family history, it may be appropriate to offer testing to a second affected family member. A result of "likely benign" or "likely polymorphism" is also clinically considered negative results [97].

A negative test result in an unaffected individual from a family that has not been previously tested provides limited information to the individual. Recommendations for risk management for this woman should be based on the family history [98].

Identification of a "variant of uncertain significance" means a genetic change has been found that may or may not increase the risk of cancer [97]. These results are common on multigene tests [3]. As more research is completed, most of these will be reclassified as either benign or pathogenic variants. Until the variant is reclassified, families with variants of uncertain significance should be managed based on family history. Unless testing is done for research purposes in an attempt to clarify the significance of the variant, testing other family members for the variant is typically discouraged since no clinically relevant interpretation can be derived from the result at this time. While standards for variant classification exist, laboratories may utilize different cutoffs from one another when determining when a variant would be considered benign, uncertain, or pathogenic [97]. This creates situations where one laboratory may call a variant uncertain while another laboratory calls the same variant pathogenic. Understandably, these varying interpretations create significant distress for clinicians and families. There is an increasing push for genetic laboratories to share data with the research community in anonymized public databases to facilitate resolution of these discrepancies. One such database, created by the NCBI, is ClinVar (http://www.clinvar.com/). Through this database, information on specific variants and their classification by submitting genetic laboratories can be reviewed. For clinicians, assessing the robustness of a genetic testing laboratory's variant classification system and commitment to research has become an increasing decision-point when choosing a laboratory for clinical use.

31.6 Medical Management of Breast Cancer Risk

Recommendations for medical management of individuals at increased risk for developing breast cancer, either because of family history or because of the presence of a known gene mutation, are based often on consensus and clinical judgment rather than randomized clinical studies [9]. Although the details vary, risk reduction options generally include enhanced screening, chemoprevention and surgical risk reduction.

31.6.1 Screening for Breast Cancer in Men

Men with a breast cancer predisposition gene mutation should be instructed remain aware of any changes in breast tissue and undergo clinical breast exam annually or semi-annually. Baseline mammogram may be considered in the presence of gynecomastia [9]. Although men with a BRCA mutation have a much higher risk of breast cancer than the general male population, it is less than half the risk for women in the general population, so routine imaging with mammograms or MRI is not currently part of the screening protocol in most centers.

31.6.2 Medical Management of a Woman with no Identifiable Mutation

Women without an identifiable mutation, who have a family history that includes only breast cancer, will have a risk of developing breast cancer based on empiric personal and family history data, such as that obtained from the a risk prediction model, or available literature [77]. In these families, first- and second-degree relatives of women with breast cancer should initiate annual mammograms 5–10 years before the earliest diagnosis in the family or age 40, whichever is youngest, but not before age 30. For women with a lifetime risk of breast cancer over 20 % (with most of the risk from family history), following a discussion about the increased risk of false positives, breast MRI should be offered annually for screening until their lifetime risk is beneath 20 % [9] In addition, since mammographic breast density (heterogeneously dense or extremely dense) makes interpretation of mammograms more difficult and also increases the risk of developing breast cancer [71], breast MRI may be an appropriate complement to mammogram in women with dense breasts and a family history of breast cancer, even if the risk does not reach 20 % by available mathematical models [98, 99]. In addition, chemoprevention or risk-reducing mastectomy, as discussed below, may be appropriate for some of these women [100]. Since the risk of ovarian cancer is not appreciably increased in breast-only histories, ovarian screening is not recommended.

31.6.3 Medical Management of High Risk Gene Mutation Carriers

The options for management include surveillance, chemoprevention and risk-reducing surgery. Most data come from carriers of mutations in *BRCA1* and *BRCA2,* but are generally appropriately applied to those with Cowden, Peutz-Jeghers, and Li-Fraumeni syndromes, and *PALB2* mutations except as noted. Each high risk mutation signifies other cancer risks in addition to breast cancer and screening for each individual cancer must be considered separately. Those other cancer risks are briefly described in Table 31.1 The efficacy of various options in reducing mortality is still being defined, and enrollment of high-risk subjects into research resources and clinical trials should be encouraged.

31.6.4 Medical Management of Moderate Risk Gene Mutation Carriers

Many new breast cancer predisposing mutations (Table 31.2) in genes such as *CHEK2* and *ATM* have been identified, and most of these increase the risk of breast cancer by 2-4-fold [3]. The long-term risks from these mutations are still being clearly refined, but many of these mutations increase a woman's risk of breast cancer above 20 % for her lifetime, and annual breast MRI in addition to annual mammogram is recommended. Women with these moderate risk mutations are not known to be at increased risk for ovarian cancer at this time, so risk reducing bilateral salpingo-oophorectomy (RRBSO) is not warranted. Additionally, the lifetime risks associated with moderate risk mutations are often not high enough to warrant risk reducing mastectomy, since most of these women will never develop breast cancer [9]. However some families with moderate risk mutations may have a more significant history of breast cancer than expected; in these families, risk-reducing mastectomy may be considered on a case-by-case basis [9]. Thus, consultation with a genetic counselor for these emerging mutations is strongly recommended and cautious decision making is required about risk reducing surgeries.

31.6.5 Screening for Breast Cancer in Women

In the general population, mammographic screening for breast cancer in women over age 50 has been proven to be effective in reducing breast cancer mortality. Screening between the ages 40 and 49 is controversial but generally recommended [101, 102]. Women with identifiable moderate and high risk mutations should undergo annual breast MRI and annual mammogram [9]. A randomized trial of MRI compared to mammogram among high risk women demonstrated the superiority of MRI with a sensitivity of 86 % compared to 18 % for mammogram, and that MRI diagnosed breast cancer at an earlier stage of breast cancer than with mammogram alone [103]. These factors act as a surrogate for the likely survival benefit of breast MRI given enough follow-up time. Breast MRI has lower specificity, resulting in a higher proportion of false positives, which is why women should be at a significant lifetime risk of breast cancer to warrant its use.

The age at screening initiation varies based on the yearly risks associated with each specific mutation (Table 31.3). Since breast cancer may occur earlier in women with Li-Fraumeni syndrome, screening begins at age 20–25 [9, 38]. For women with *BRCA1* or *BRCA2* mutation, annual breast MRI should begin at age 25. An observational study noted that women with BRCA mutations receiving mammograms before age 30 were at higher risk for breast cancer, presumably from radiation exposure, thus breast MRI is utilized exclusively among high risk women younger than 30 [104]. For women with a *PALB2* mutation, initiating screening at approximately age 30 is reasonable, based on available literature [9, 48]. Although *CDH1* and *PTEN* are high risk mutations, breast cancer risk increases at an older age, thus screening initiation is recommended at age 30–35 in carriers [9, 45]. The exact recommended age to initiate breast cancer screening for women with moderate risk mutations such as *ATM, CHEK2, and NBN* is still being determined, but starting around age 40 would be reasonable as this is when the breast cancer risk appears to start rising in carriers [9, 52, 55]. And for all mutation carriers, breast cancer screening should begin 5–10 years earlier than the earliest breast cancer that occurred in a close relative, if this would make screening start at an earlier age than the age ranges given above [9]. Breast MRI should be performed in a center that has a dedicated breast coil, experience in interpreting breast MRI and the ability to perform MRI-directed breast biopsies. Most centers alternate mammograms and MRI evaluations so that women receive some type of imaging every 6 months [105].

Although there is no proof that patient self-breast awareness or clinical breast examination reduces mortality from breast cancer in women either with or without a genetic predisposition to breast cancer, they are recommended components of screening for breast cancer [106]. The current recommendation is that women remain aware of any changes in their breasts and that clinical breast exam be performed bi-annually starting at age 25 (or earlier with Li-Fraumeni syndrome) for women at increased breast cancer risk [9]. The usefulness of clinical breast examination is related to the amount of time spent on the exam, and is most beneficial among women who do not have access to breast imaging [107]. In general, examination of both breasts should take approximately 3 min [108].

Table 31.3 Risk management according to breast cancer predisposing mutation

	BRCA1 BRCA2	TP53	PALB2	PTEN CDH1	ATM CHEK2 NBN
Age to start breast MRI	25	20–25	30	30–35	40
Age to start mammogram	30	30	30	30–35	40
Consider chemoprevention	Yes	Yes	Yes	Yes	Yes
Consider RRM	Yes	Yes	Yes	Yes	In some families
Consider RRSO	Yes	No	No	No	No

31.6.6 Chemoprevention for Breast Cancer

Tamoxifen is a selective estrogen receptor modulator that has been used since 1977 for treatment of breast cancer, both as adjuvant therapy and treatment of advanced disease. Women treated with tamoxifen were found to have a reduction in the incidence of contralateral breast cancer. This observation led to studies of tamoxifen as a breast cancer chemoprevention agent in women who were at high risk but did not have breast cancer. The largest such study, conducted by the National Surgical Adjuvant Breast and Bowel Project, demonstrated approximately a 50 % risk reduction in incidence of both invasive and in situ breast cancer in women who had an *a priori* 5-year risk of 1.7 % or greater as calculated by the Gail model [100, 109]. In observational studies, tamoxifen reduced breast cancer risk by 62 % among women with BRCA2 mutations; however, there is debate whether it is as effective among women with BRCA1 mutations [110, 111]. Only estrogen receptor-positive cancers are reduced with tamoxifen. There was no difference in the number of estrogen receptor-negative cancers [109]. Tamoxifen is associated with a doubling of the risk of endometrial cancer (from one to two cases per 1000 women per year) and a tripling of risk of pulmonary embolism (from 0.23 to 0.69 per 1000 women per year), both primarily in postmenopausal women. A second study, The Study of Tamoxifen and Raloxifene (STAR) demonstrated that raloxifene, another selective estrogen receptor modulator, provided benefits similar to tamoxifen in reducing the risk of invasive breast cancer, although in situ cancer was not reduced [112]. Exemestane and anastrazole, aromatase inhibitors have been shown to reduce the risk of breast cancer similarly to tamoxifen, however there are not long-term data yet. Aromatase inhibitors have never been compared directly with SERM's, and they increase the risk of osteoporosis, making the use of aromatase inhibitors as prevention agents more problematic [113, 114].

The use of chemoprevention agents in women with gene mutations is not well studied [111], however prospective observational data show that women with BRCA1/2 mutations who were treated adjuvantly with tamoxifen for breast cancer yielded about a 50 % reduction in the risk of a second breast cancer in the contralateral unaffected breast. In women with a family history of breast cancer but without an identifiable breast cancer predisposition gene mutation, either tamoxifen or raloxifene is recommended if the risk by the Gail model is over 1.7 %. Women with a family history of breast cancer, but no affected first-degree relatives, or women with dense breast tissue, may have a calculated risk lower than 1.7 %, but chemoprevention may still be appropriate.

31.6.7 Risk-Reducing Salpingo-Oophorectomy

Risk of ovarian cancer is greatly increased in families with *BRCA1* and *BRCA2* mutations, at about 40 % in *BRCA1* mutation carriers and 10–30 % in *BRCA2* mutation carriers. Risk reducing salpingo-oophorectomy (RRSO) is estimated to reduce the risk of ovarian cancer by 80–90 % [115], although there is still a risk of primary peritoneal carcinoma, which has the same microscopic appearance and biology as epithelial ovarian cancer [116]. The clinical issues in women contemplating RRSO include the appropriate age to undergo the procedure, the extent of the surgery, and the use of hormone replacement therapy [117].

The age-specific risk of ovarian cancer in mutation carriers increases sharply after age 40, although the risk per year is still low at that age. If risk-reducing surgery is to be performed, it is reasonable to consider this between age 35 and 40. Healthy women in their 70s may still accrue a benefit from this procedure, although the absolute benefit decreases with age. Meta-analyses of RRSO among women with BRCA revealed a 50 % reduction in breast cancer incidence [118]. Breast cancer risk reduction is observed even in women who take hormone replacement therapy after surgery.

RRSO in mutation carriers should be performed by a gynecologic oncologist or other surgeon experienced in performing oophorectomy for risk reduction in high-risk women. The ovaries should be multiple-sectioned, and examined by an experienced pathologist. The fallopian tubes should be removed and carefully examined since tubal carcinomas are increased in mutation carriers. The role of hysterectomy is less clear, as there seems to be no increased risk of endometrial cancer associated with *BRCA* mutations. Adding hysterectomy to RRSO increases per-operative risks and time to recovery slightly, however, women who wish to take tamoxifen may choose to undergo hysterectomy in order to reduce the risk of tamoxifen-associated endometrial hyperplasia [119]. Women who are planning to take estrogen may also choose hysterectomy to avoid the need for progestins. If hysterectomy would require an open procedure and tamoxifen or estrogen are not planned, it is reasonable to perform salpingo-oophorectomy alone.

The use of estrogen following RRSO is a subject of debate with no evidence that it increases the risk of breast cancer among women with BRCA mutations. RRSO in young women has been associated with increased mortality due to cardiovascular and bone effects of estrogen depletion, thus estrogen replacement therapy should therefore be strongly considered in younger premenopausal women undergoing risk-reducing oophorectomy [111, 117, 120]. Particularly if estrogen is used without progestin, breast cancer risk is still reduced after oophorectomy. One reasonable approach is to use estrogen (with progestin-containing IUD in women with a uterus) from the time of oophorectomy until around age 45–50, and then consider tamoxifen for 5 years. In general, women with a personal history of breast cancer should not take estrogen, and this decision should be made in consultation with the woman's oncologist.

31.6.8 Risk-Reducing Mastectomy

The most effective means of reducing the risk of breast cancer is with bilateral mastectomy. Since mastectomy has significant morbidity, including surgical risks and loss of sensation, options for reconstruction, the small risk of developing breast cancer in residual breast tissue, and the possibility of finding unsuspected cancer, only women at high lifetime risk (i.e., at least 30 %) of breast cancer should be offered this intervention. The seminal manuscript studied 639 women with a family history of breast cancer and found a 90 % reduction in breast cancer incidence compared with the incidence in sisters of women who did not have such surgery [121], and subsequent studies have confirmed the efficacy of this option [122, 123]. Mutation status among women in the seminal study was not known, but the reduction of risk was seen both in those with a moderate family history as well as those with a strong family history suggestive of a genetic predisposition. Most women in this series underwent subcutaneous mastectomy, a procedure that preserves the nipple-areolar complex and therefore leaves more breast tissue than a total mastectomy [124]. Options for risk-reducing mastectomy include total mastectomy, which removes the nipple-areolar complex, or total skin-sparing mastectomy in which the nipple is retained. If the latter procedure is performed, surgeons should remove as much breast tissue as possible from the underside of the nipple. A preoperative breast MRI should be performed since identifying an unsuspected cancer may alter the type of surgery that is performed, and specifically allows for cancer staging with a sentinel node biopsy.

Risk-reducing mastectomy is appropriate for some women and not for others, based primarily on the women's own beliefs and values. Many women are clear that identification of a high risk mutation would lead them to choose immediate mastectomy, and others are equally clear about their wish to avoid the procedure. For those who are undecided, several principles may assist in making a decision about this procedure.

- Prior diagnosis of breast cancer. Because not all women with breast cancer predisposition gene mutations develop breast cancer at all, some may wish to defer risk-reducing mastectomy until they are diagnosed with breast cancer, and then undergo therapeutic mastectomy on the affected side and contralateral risk-reducing mastectomy. The development of breast cancer in a woman with a *BRCA* gene mutation increases the 5-year risk of a contralateral breast cancer to around 20 %, and many women choose bilateral mastectomy at the time of diagnosis. However, most women will have a significantly greater risk of mortality from a prior breast cancer than from a breast cancer that has yet to be discovered, and the prognosis of the prior (or current) cancer should be considered in making this decision. The short- to intermediate-term risk of cancer recurrence in women with high-risk disease may be substantially higher than the risk of developing a second primary tumor. However, women with higher-risk cancers may be more likely to request bilateral mastectomy (or contralateral prophylactic mastectomy), and even if this does not improve prognosis, the procedure may provide sufficient peace of mind to be warranted.
- Risk of developing breast cancer. Most women who should consider risk-reducing mastectomy have high risk gene mutations, however given the expansion of panel testing, some women with moderate risk genes may now be considering mastectomy. Women may also wish to undergo mastectomy because of a combination of family history and personal risk factors defined by Gail [100], such as the need for prior breast biopsies based on suspicious mammograms or breast exams, and the presence of proliferative breast disease. Assuring that the woman understands her age-specific risks, as well as her lifetime risks, is also important. Although the lifetime risk of

developing breast cancer may be, for example, 70 %, a 50-year old woman has a risk that is less than that since she has already lived past some of that risk. Describing risk in quantifiable terms per year (usually around 0.5–1.5 % per year for women with mutations) may be helpful. Some women wish to undergo mastectomy because of an inflated sense of the risk of cancer, in which differentiating the age-specific and lifetime risk is useful.

- Ease of cancer detection. Breast cancer may be more or less difficult to detect, depending on the density of breast tissue on physical exam and imaging [71]. Detection is much easier in women with fatty-replaced breasts than in women with extremely dense breasts. Women may choose mastectomy over screening if screening tools are less likely to detect cancer at an early stage.
- Chemoprevention options. Risk reduction with tamoxifen or raloxifene may be an option instead of mastectomy. The degree of risk reduction in mutation carriers has not been evaluated in prospective trials, but is certainly less than with prophylactic mastectomy. Nevertheless, this option should be discussed.
- Psychological factors. Women consider prophylactic mastectomy for many reasons. For some, the family culture is to have risk-reducing surgery, and the pressure to undergo the procedure may be significant. These women should be supported if they wish to have surveillance alone. Other women have cared for family members with terminal cancer and may wish to spare their own families. Some fear developing cancer or are extremely anxious about screening, and the probability of early detection is not reassuring. All these issues should be explored in depth. Counseling or grief therapy may be appropriate in some cases. There is no absolute medical indication for this procedure, and the final decision about risk-reducing surgery is always therefore a psychological one.

31.6.9 Medical Management of Mutation Carriers Diagnosed with Breast Cancer

BRCA gene mutations have little influence on the management of breast cancer aside from decisions about breast surgery. Many women with mutations choose bilateral mastectomy if a unilateral cancer is found in order to reduce the substantial risk of developing a contralateral breast cancer. Lumpectomy with radiation therapy, however, has been demonstrated to provide good control of cancer with no increase in the risk of ipsilateral breast tumor recurrence [124].

Women who are newly diagnosed with breast cancer and judged to be testing candidates because of family history, age, or ethnicity are often required to make decisions about testing and cancer treatment simultaneously. Unless surgical treatment of the cancer itself is impacted by mutation status, there is little reason to perform testing in a woman who is not able to make a thoughtful decision about undergoing testing in a rushed situation. Test results are usually available within 2 weeks, although larger multigene panels may take longer. The major impact of genetic testing usually surgical treatment and not systemic treatment, however the use of platinum chemotherapy and PARP inhibitors to treat BRCA associated breast cancer is being investigated [125, 126]. Women with breast cancer who would choose lumpectomy over mastectomy if no mutation was found, can undergo lumpectomy, proceed with chemotherapy, and then make the decision to undergo mastectomy or post lumpectomy radiation, depending on the result of the genetic test.

31.7 Information for Extended Family Members

Although the focus of this chapter is the patient who presents with concerns about her particular family history, genetic testing is different from other medical testing in that it has implications for extended family members. Most obviously, a woman with an identifiable mutation has the chance of passing that mutation to her children, and since she almost certainly inherited it from a parent, her siblings also have a 50 % chance of having the mutation. However, extended family members can also be at risk for having the mutation, and several mechanisms, such as model letters, can be provided to patients to help them communicate with the appropriate testing candidates. Studies reveal that the majority of women share their mutation status with their families, especially with those members they believe are also at risk [127–129].

Women who do not have mutations can also provide useful information to extended family members [130]. In the case of individuals who are members of a family in which there is a known mutation, the children would have a risk of developing cancer similar to others in the general population. However, if the individual is a member of a family in which there is not a known mutation, the empiric risk information would be relevant to children, siblings, and possibly extended family members. Typically, the responsibility to share the implications of this information is given to the patient, after appropriate education, to preserve patient confidentiality.

31.8 In Summary

As the public becomes more aware of and informed about the genetics of breast cancer, there will be an increasing demand for genetic counseling and clinical testing. Whether as part of a comprehensive clinical breast cancer clinic or as a primary practitioner's service, families at increased risk of breast cancer will be identified and should be offered appropriate services. A variety of resources from both the oncology and genetic communities are available to provide specialized care to women and their families who need genetic counseling, result interpretation, or psychological support related to testing and subsequent management decisions (Table 31.4). The future of genetic testing will be a team effort, involving the primary care physician, the cancer center and the cancer genetic service, whether it is obtaining a family and personal health history to determine the magnitude of risk, conducting genetic counseling and/or testing, or facilitating long-term medical management of the patient and her extended family members.

Table 31.4 Additional resources: websites

Facing our risks of cancer empowered (FORCE): www.facingourrisk.org. This website is a resource for individuals and families who have a strong family history of breast cancers or are carriers of a mutation that confers an increased risk of developing cancer. General information, chat rooms, a blog, and discussion board are available online, while a national meeting in May of each year allows participants to gather, and local chapters are developing in several states
National society of genetic counselors: www.nsgc.org. This site is the resource for the genetic counseling profession and contains a search function to assist consumers and professionals in finding local genetic counseling services
National institutes of health: http://www.cancer.gov/search/geneticsservices/. Cancer Net PDQ contains information about cancer, clinical trials and providers of cancer genetic services
National comprehensive cancer network: www.nccn.org. National comprehensive cancer network (NCCN) is an alliance of cancer centers and was established in 1995 to provide state-of-the-art guidelines in cancer prevention, screening, diagnosis, and treatment through excellence in basic and clinical research. This site contains practice guidelines for identification and management of genetically high-risk patients Stanford Medicine Decision Tool for Women with BRCA Mutations. http://brcatool.stanford.edu/brca.html This decision support tool is designed for joint use by women with BRCA mutations and their health care providers, to guide management of cancer risks

References

1. Lynch HT, Lynch JF. Breast cancer genetics in an oncology clinic: 328 consecutive patients. Cancer Genet Cytogenet. 1986;22(4):369–71.
2. Jain R, et al. The relevance of hereditary cancer risks to precision oncology: what should providers consider when conducting tumor genomic profiling? J Natl Compr Canc Netw. 2016;14(6):795–806.
3. Easton DF, et al. Gene-panel sequencing and the prediction of breast-cancer risk. N Engl J Med. 2015;372(23):2243–57.
4. Mavaddat N et al. Prediction of breast cancer risk based on profiling with common genetic variants. J Natl Cancer Inst. 2015;107(5).
5. Evans DG, et al. Assessing individual breast cancer risk within the U.K. National Health Service Breast Screening Program: a new paradigm for cancer prevention. Cancer Prevent Res. 2012;5(7):943–51.
6. Ford D, et al. Risks of cancer in BRCA1-mutation carriers. Breast cancer linkage consortium. Lancet. 1994;343(8899):692–5.
7. Frank TS, et al. Sequence analysis of BRCA1 and BRCA2: correlation of mutations with family history and ovarian cancer risk. J Clin Oncol. 1998;16(7):2417–25.
8. Ford D, Easton DF, Peto J. Estimates of the gene frequency of BRCA1 and its contribution to breast and ovarian cancer incidence. Am J Hum Genet. 1995;57(6):1457–62.
9. National Comprehensive Cancer Network. NCCN Clinical Practice Guidelines in Oncology: Genetic/Familial High-Risk Assessment: Breast and Ovarian. V.1.2017. 2016.
10. Metcalfe KA, et al. Screening for founder mutations in BRCA1 and BRCA2 in unselected Jewish women. J Clin Oncol. 2010;28(3):387–91.
11. Petrij-Bosch A, et al. BRCA1 genomic deletions are major founder mutations in Dutch breast cancer patients. Nat Genet. 1997;17(3):341–5.
12. Johannesdottir G, et al. High prevalence of the 999del5 mutation in Icelandic breast and ovarian cancer patients. Cancer Res. 1996;56(16):3663–5.
13. Mavaddat N. Cancer risks for BRCA1 and BRCA2 mutation carriers: results from prospective analysis of EMBRACE. 2013;105(11):812–22.
14. Chen S, Parmigiani G. Meta-analysis of BRCA1 and BRCA2 penetrance. J Clin Oncol. 2007;25(11):1329–33.
15. Antoniou A, et al. Average risks of breast and ovarian cancer associated with BRCA1 or BRCA2 mutations detected in case series unselected for family history: a combined analysis of 22 studies. Am J Hum Genet. 2003;72(5):1117–30.
16. Liede A, Karlan BY, Narod SA. Cancer risks for male carriers of germline mutations in BRCA1 or BRCA2: a review of the literature. J Clin Oncol. 2004;22(4):735–42.
17. Schneider BP, et al. Triple-negative breast cancer: risk factors to potential targets. Clin Cancer Res. 2008;14(24):8010–8.
18. Lakhani SR, et al. The pathology of familial breast cancer: predictive value of immunohistochemical markers estrogen receptor, progesterone receptor, HER-2, and p53 in patients with mutations in BRCA1 and BRCA2. J Clin Oncol. 2002;20(9):2310–8.
19. Bane AL, et al. BRCA2 mutation-associated breast cancers exhibit a distinguishing phenotype based on morphology and molecular profiles from tissue microarrays. Am J Surg Pathol. 2007;31(1):121–8.
20. Lu KH, et al. Occult ovarian tumors in women with BRCA1 or BRCA2 mutations undergoing prophylactic oophorectomy. J Clin Oncol. 2000;18(14):2728–32.

21. Sherman ME, et al. Histopathologic features of ovaries at increased risk for carcinoma. A case-control analysis. Int J Gynecol Pathol. 1999;18(2):151–7.
22. Levine DA, et al. Fallopian tube and primary peritoneal carcinomas associated with BRCA mutations. J Clin Oncol. 2003;21(22):4222–7.
23. Harmsen MG, et al. Early salpingectomy (TUbectomy) with delayed oophorectomy to improve quality of life as alternative for risk-reducing salpingo-oophorectomy in BRCA1/2 mutation carriers (TUBA study): a prospective non-randomized multicentre study. BMC Cancer. 2015;15:593.
24. Anon (1999) Cancer risks in BRCA2 mutation carriers. The breast cancer linkage consortium. J Natl Cancer Inst. 1999;91 (15):1310–6.
25. Domchek SM, Weber BL. Clinical management of BRCA1 and BRCA2 mutation carriers. Oncogene. 2006;25(43):5825–31.
26. Agalliu I, et al. Associations of high-grade prostate cancer with BRCA1 and BRCA2 founder mutations. Clin Cancer Res. 2009;15(3):1112–20.
27. Narod SA, et al. Rapid progression of prostate cancer in men with a BRCA2 mutation. Br J Cancer. 2008;99(2):371–4.
28. Castro E, et al. Germline BRCA mutations are associated with higher risk of nodal involvement, distant metastasis, and poor survival outcomes in prostate cancer. J Clin Oncol. 2013;31 (14):1748–57.
29. Howlett NG, et al. Biallelic inactivation of BRCA2 in Fanconi anemia. Science. 2002;297(5581):606–9.
30. Schreibman IR, et al. The hamartomatous polyposis syndromes: a clinical and molecular review. Am J Gastroenterol. 2005;100 (2):476–90.
31. Pilarski R, et al. Cowden syndrome and the PTEN hamartoma tumor syndrome: systematic review and revised diagnostic criteria. J Natl Cancer Inst. 2013;105(21):1607–16.
32. Tan MH, et al. Lifetime cancer risks in individuals with germline PTEN mutations. Clin Cancer Res. 2012;18(2):400–7.
33. Pilarski R, Eng C. Will the real Cowden syndrome please stand up (again)? Expanding mutational and clinical spectra of the PTEN hamartoma tumor syndrome. J Med Genet. 2004;41 (5):323–6.
34. Olivier M, et al. Li-Fraumeni and related syndromes: correlation between tumor type, family structure, and TP53 genotype. Cancer Res. 2003;63(20):6643–50.
35. Varley JM. Germline TP53 mutations and Li-Fraumeni syndrome. Hum Mutat. 2003;21(3):313–20.
36. Lustbader ED, et al. Segregation analysis of cancer in families of childhood soft tissue sarcoma patients. Am J Hum Genet. 1992;51(2):344–56.
37. Birch JM, et al. Relative frequency and morphology of cancers in carriers of germline TP53 mutations. Oncogene. 2001;20 (34):4621–8.
38. Hisada M, et al. Multiple primary cancers in families with Li-Fraumeni syndrome. J Natl Cancer Inst. 1998;90(8):606–11.
39. Villani A, et al. Biochemical and imaging surveillance in germline TP53 mutation carriers with Li-Fraumeni syndrome: a prospective observational study. Lancet Oncol. 2011;12(6):559–67.
40. Giardiello FM, et al. Increased risk of cancer in the Peutz-Jeghers syndrome. N Engl J Med. 1987;316(24):1511–4.
41. Hearle N, et al. Frequency and spectrum of cancers in the Peutz-Jeghers syndrome. Clin Cancer Res. 2006;12(10):3209–15.
42. Mehenni H, et al. Cancer risks in LKB1 germline mutation carriers. Gut. 2006;55(7):984–90.
43. Giardiello FM, Trimbath JD. Peutz-Jeghers syndrome and management recommendations. Clin Gastroenterol Hepatol. 2006;4(4):408–15.
44. Hansford S et al. Hereditary diffuse gastric cancer syndrome: CDH1 mutations and beyond. JAMA Oncol. 2015;1(1):23–32.
45. van der Post RS, et al. Hereditary diffuse gastric cancer: updated clinical guidelines with an emphasis on germline CDH1 mutation carriers. J Med Genet. 2015;52(6):361–74.
46. Petridis C, et al. Germline CDH1 mutations in lobular carcinoma in situ. Br J Cancer. 2014;110(4):1053–7.
47. Xia B, et al. Control of BRCA2 cellular and clinical functions by a nuclear partner, PALB2. Mol Cell. 2006;22(6):719–29.
48. Antoniou AC, et al. Breast-cancer risk in families with mutations in PALB2. N Engl J Med. 2014;371(6):497–506.
49. Schneider R, et al. German national case collection for familial pancreatic cancer (FaPaCa): 10 years experience. Fam Cancer. 2011;10(2):323–30.
50. Tischkowitz M, et al. PALB2/FANCN: recombining cancer and Fanconi Anemia. Cancer Res. 2010;70(19):7353–9.
51. Geoffroy-Perez B, et al. Cancer risk in heterozygotes for ataxia-telangiectasia. Int J Cancer. 2001;93(2):288–93.
52. Marabelli M, Cheng SC, Parmigiani G. Penetrance of ATM gene mutations in breast cancer: a meta-analysis of different measures of risk. Genet Epidemiol. 2016;40(5):425–31.
53. Tavtigian S, et al. Rare, evolutionarily unlikely missense substitutions in ATM confer increased risk of breast cancer. Am J Hum Genet. 2009;85(4):427–46.
54. Roberts NJ, et al. ATM mutations in hereditary pancreatic cancer. Cancer Discov. 2012;2(1):41–6.
55. Schmidt MK et al. Age- and tumor subtype-specific breast cancer risk estimates for CHEK2*1100delC Carriers. J Clin Oncol. 2016; Epub ahead of print: June 6, 2016.
56. Weischer M, et al. CHEK2*1100delC genotyping for clinical assessment of breast cancer risk: meta-analysis of 26,000 patient cases and 27,000 controls. J Clin Oncol. 2008;26(4):542–8.
57. Cybulski C, et al. CHEK2 is a multiorgan cancer susceptibility gene. Am J Hum Genet. 2008;75(6):1131–5.
58. Damiola F, et al. Rare key functional domain missense substitutions in MRE11A, RAD50, and NBN contribute to breast cancer susceptibilty: results from a breast cancer family registry case-control mutation screening study. Breast Cancer Res. 2014;16(3):R58.
59. Ito A, et al. Expression of full-length NBS1 protein restores normal radiation responses in cells from Nijmegen breakage syndrome patients. Biochem Biophys Res Commun. 1999;265 (3):716–21.
60. Bennett IC, Gattas M, Teh BT. The management of familial breast cancer. Breast. 2000;9(5):247–63.
61. Hoskins KF, et al. Assessment and counseling for women with a family history of breast cancer. A guide for clinicians. JAMA. 1995;273(7):577–85.
62. Bennett RL, et al. Standardized human pedigree nomenclature: update and assessment of the recommendations of the National Society of Genetic Counselors. J Genet Couns. 2008;17(5):424–33.
63. Schneider KA, et al. Accuracy of cancer family histories: comparison of two breast cancer syndromes. Genet Test. 2004;8(3):222–8.
64. Kerber RA, Slattery ML. Comparison of self-reported and database-linked family history of cancer data in a casecontrol study. Am J Epidemiol. 1997;146(3):244–8.
65. Ziogas A, Anton-Culver H. Validation of family history data in cancer family registries. Am J Prev Med. 2003;24(2):190–8.
66. Acheson LS, et al. Family history-taking in community family practice: implications for genetic screening. Genet Med. 2000;2 (3):180–5.
67. Weitzel JN, et al. Limited family structure and BRCA gene mutation status in single cases of breast cancer. JAMA. 2007;297 (23):2587–95.

68. Calle EE, et al. Overweight, obesity, and mortality from cancer in a prospectively studied cohort of U.S. adults. N Engl J Med. 2003;348(17):1625–38.
69. Boffetta P, Hashibe M. Alcohol and cancer. Lancet Oncol. 2006;7 (2):149–56.
70. Boffetta P, et al. The burden of cancer attributable to alcohol drinking. Int J Cancer. 2006;119(4):884–7.
71. Boyd NF, et al. Mammographic density and the risk and detection of breast cancer. N Engl J Med. 2007;356(3):227–36.
72. Zheng T, et al. Radiation exposure from diagnostic and therapeutic treatments and risk of breast cancer. Eur J Cancer Prev. 2002;11(3):229–35.
73. El-Gamal H, Bennett RG. Increased breast cancer risk after radiotherapy for acne among women with skin cancer. J Am Acad Dermatol. 2006;55(6):981–9.
74. Hopwood P, et al. Do women understand the odds? Risk perceptions and recall of risk information in women with a family history of breast cancer. Community Genet. 2003;6(4):214–23.
75. Woloshin S, Schwartz LM, Welch HG. Risk charts: putting cancer in context. J Natl Cancer Inst. 2002;94(11):799–804.
76. Prasad K, et al. Tips for teachers of evidence-based medicine: understanding odds ratios and their relationship to risk ratios. J Gen Intern Med. 2008;23(5):635–40.
77. Slattery ML, Kerber RA. A comprehensive evaluation of family history and breast cancer risk; the Utah Population Database. JAMA. 1993;270:1563.
78. Gail MH, Benichou J. Validation studies on a model for breast cancer risk. J Natl Cancer Inst. 1994;86(8):573–5.
79. Rockhill B, et al. Validation of the Gail et al model of breast cancer risk prediction and implications for chemoprevention. J Natl Cancer Inst. 2001;93(5):358–66.
80. Claus EB, et al. The genetic attributable risk of breast and ovarian cancer. Cancer. 1996;77(11):2318–24.
81. Berry DA, et al. BRCAPRO validation, sensitivity of genetic testing of BRCA1/BRCA2, and prevalence of other breast cancer susceptibility genes. J Clin Oncol. 2002;20(11):2701–12.
82. Gilpin CA, Carson N, Hunter AG. A preliminary validation of a family history assessment form to select women at risk for breast or ovarian cancer for referral to a genetics center. Clin Genet. 2000;58(4):299–308.
83. Parmigiani G, Berry D, Aguilar O. Determining carrier probabilities for breast cancer-susceptibility genes BRCA1 and BRCA2. Am J Hum Genet. 1998;62(1):145–58.
84. Antoniou AC, et al. BRCA1 and BRCA2 mutation predictions using the BOADICEA and BRCAPRO models and penetrance estimation in high-risk French-Canadian families. Breast Cancer Res. 2006;8(1):R3.
85. Lee AJ et al. Incorporating truncating variants in PALB2, CHEK2, and ATM into the BOADICEA breast cancer risk model. Genet in Med. 2016; Epub April 14, 2016.
86. Trepanier A, et al. Genetic cancer risk assessment and counseling: recommendations of the National Society of Genetic Counselors. J Genet Couns. 2004;13(2):83–114.
87. Kinney AY. Expanding access to BRCA1/2 genetic counseling with telephone delivery: a cluster randomized trial. J Natl Cancer Inst. 2014;106(12).
88. Gabai-Kapara E. Population-based screening for breast and ovarian cancer risk due to BRCA1 and BRCA2. Proc Natl Acad Sci USA. 2014;111(39):14205–10.
89. Claes E, et al. Communication with close and distant relatives in the context of genetic testing for hereditary breast and ovarian cancer in cancer patients. Am J Med Genet A. 2003;116(1):11–9.
90. Press N, et al. Women's interest in genetic testing for breast cancer susceptibility may be based on unreasonable expectations. Am J Med Genet. 2001;99:99–110.
91. Hudson KL, et al. Genetic discrimination and health insurance: an urgent need for reform. Science. 1995;270(5235):391–3.
92. Hudson KL, Holohan MK, Collins FS. Keeping pace with the times–the genetic information nondiscrimination act of 2008. N Engl J Med. 2008;358(25):2661–3.
93. Bradbury AR, et al. How often do BRCA mutation carriers tell their young children of the family's risk for cancer? A study of parental disclosure of BRCA mutations to minors and young adults. J Clin Oncol. 2007;25(24):3705–11.
94. Bradbury AR, et al. Should genetic testing for BRCA1/2 be permitted for minors? Opinions of BRCA mutation carriers and their adult offspring. Am J Med Genet C Semin Med Genet. 2008;148C(1):70–7.
95. Bradbury AR et al. When parents disclose BRCA1/2 test results: their communication and perceptions of offspring response. 2012;118(13):3417–25.
96. den Dunnen JT, et al. HGVS recommendations for description of sequence variants: 2016 Update. Hum Mutat. 2016;37(6):564–9.
97. Plon S, et al. Sequence variant classification and reporting: recommendations for improving the interpretation of cancer susceptibility genetic test results. Hum Mutat. 2008;29(11):1282–91.
98. Warner E, et al. Surveillance of BRCA1 and BRCA2 mutation carriers with magnetic resonance imaging, ultrasound, mammography, and clinical breast examination. JAMA. 2004;292 (11):1317–25.
99. Plevritis SK, et al. Cost-effectiveness of screening BRCA1/2 mutation carriers with breast magnetic resonance imaging. JAMA. 2006;295(20):2374–84.
100. Gail MH, et al. Weighing the risks and benefits of tamoxifen treatment for preventing breast cancer. J Natl Cancer Inst. 1999;91(21):1829–46.
101. Hendrick RE, et al. Benefit of screening mammography in women aged 40–49: a new meta-analysis of randomized controlled trials. J Natl Cancer Inst Monogr. 1997;22:87–92.
102. Moss SM, et al. Effect of mammographic screening from age 40 years on breast cancer mortality at 10 years' follow-up: a randomized controlled trial. Lancet. 2006;368(9552):2053–60.
103. Passaperuma K, et al. Long-term results of screening with magnetic resonance imaging in women with BRCA mutations. Br J Cancer. 2012;107:24–30.
104. Pijpe A, et al. Exposure to diagnostic radiation and risk of breast cancer among carriers of BRCA1/2 mutations: retrospective cohort study (GENE-RAD-RISK). BMJ. 2012;345:e5660.
105. Lowry KP, et al. Annual screening strategies in BRCA1 and BRCA2 gene mutation carriers: a comparative effectiveness analysis. Cancer. 2012;118:2021–30.
106. Baxter N. Preventive health care, 2001 update: should women be routinely taught breast self-examination to screen for breast cancer? CMAJ. 2001;164(13):1837–46.
107. Saslow D, et al. Clinical Breast Examination: Practical Recommendations for Optimizing Performance and Reporting. CA Cancer J Clin. 2004;54:327–44.
108. Gaskie S, Nashelsky J. Clinical inquires. Are breast self-exams or clinical exams effective for screening breast cancer. J Fam Pract. 2005;54(9):803–4.
109. Fisher B, et al. Tamoxifen for prevention of breast cancer: report of the National Surgical Adjuvant Breast and Bowel Project P-1 Study. J Natl Cancer Inst. 1998;90(18):1371–88.
110. Gronwald J, et al. Tamoxifen and contralateral breast cancer in BRCA1 and BRCA2 carriers: an update. Int J Cancer. 2006;118:2281–4.
111. King MC, et al. Tamoxifen and breast cancer incidence among women with inherited mutations in BRCA1 and BRCA2: National Surgical Adjuvant Breast and Bowel Project

(NSABP-P1) breast cancer prevention trial. JAMA. 2001;286:2251–6.
112. Vogel VG, et al. Effects of tamoxifen vs raloxifene on the risk of developing invasive breast cancer and other disease outcomes: the NSABP Study of Tamoxifen and Raloxifene (STAR) P-2 trial. JAMA. 2006;295(23):2727–41.
113. Cuzick J, et al. Anastrozole for prevention of breast cancer in high-risk postmenopausal women (IBIS-II): an international, double-blind, randomised placebo-controlled trial. Lancet. 2014;383:1041–8.
114. Goss PE, et al. Exemestane for breast-cancer prevention in postmenopausal women. N Engl J Med. 2011;364:2381–91.
115. Kauff ND, et al. Risk-reducing salpingo-oophorectomy for the prevention of BRCA1- and BRCA2-associated breast and gynecologic cancer: a multicenter, prospective study. J Clin Oncol. 2008;26(8):1331–7.
116. Greene MH et al. A prospective study of risk-reducing salpingo-oophorectomy and longitudinal CA-125 screening among women at increased genetic risk of ovarian cancer: design Prev. 2008;17(3):594–604.
117. Rebbeck TR, et al. Effect of short-term hormone replacement therapy on breast cancer risk reduction after bilateral prophylactic oophorectomy in BRCA1 and BRCA2 mutation carriers: the PROSE study group. J Clin Oncol. 2005;23(31):7804–10.
118. Rebbeck TR, Kauff ND, Domchek SM. Meta-analysis of risk reduction estimates associated with risk-reducing salpingo-oophorectomy in BRCA1 or BRCA2 mutation carriers. J Natl Cancer Inst. 2009;101:80–7.
119. Gabriel CA, et al. Use of total abdominal hysterectomy and hormone replacement therapy in BRCA1 and BRCA2 mutation carriers undergoing risk-reducing salpingo-oophorectomy. Fam Cancer. 2009;8(1):23–8.
120. Rebbeck TR, et al. Effect of short-term hormone replacement therapy on breast cancer risk reduction after bilateral prophylactic oophorectomy in BRCA1 and BRCA2 mutation carriers: the PROSE study group. J Clin Oncol. 2005;23(31):7804–10.
121. Hartmann LC, et al. Efficacy of bilateral prophylactic mastectomy in women with a family history of breast cancer. N Engl J Med. 1999;340(2):77–84.
122. Hartmann LC, Degnim A, Schaid DJ. Prophylactic mastectomy for BRCA1/2 carriers: progress and more questions. J Clin Oncol. 2004;22(6):981–3.
123. Rebbeck TR, et al. Bilateral prophylactic mastectomy reduces breast cancer risk in BRCA1 and BRCA2 mutation carriers: the PROSE study group. J Clin Oncol. 2004;22(6):1055–62.
124. Clarke M. Early Breast Cancer Trialists' Collaborative Group (EBCTCG). Effects of radiotherapy and of differences in the extent of surgery for early breast cancer on local recurrence and 15-year survival: an overview of the randomised trials. Lancet. 2005;366(9503):2087–106.
125. Valsecchi ME, et al. Role of carboplatin in the treatment of triple negative early-stage breast cancer. Rev Recent Clin Trials. 2015;10(2):101–10.
126. Livraghi L, Garber JE. PARP inhibitors in the management of breast cancer: current data and future prospects. BMC Med. 2015;13:188.
127. Patenaude AF, et al. Sharing BRCA1/2 test results with first-degree relatives: factors predicting who women tell. J Clin Oncol. 2006;24(4):700–6.
128. MacDonald DJ, et al. Selection of family members for communication of cancer risk and barriers to this communication before and after genetic cancer risk assessment. Genet Med. 2007;9(5):275–82.
129. McGivern B, et al. Family communication about positive BRCA1 and BRCA2 genetic test results. Genet Med. 2004;6(6):503–9.
130. Forrest LE, et al. Increased genetic counseling support improves communication of genetic information in families. Genet Med. 2008;10(3):167–72.

32 Chemoprevention of Breast Cancer

Jack Cuzick

32.1 Chemoprevention of Breast Cancer[1]

Prospects for the prevention of breast cancer have never been greater. We are beginning to find the lifestyle factors that can reduce the risk for women of average risk, and targeted chemoprevention for high-risk women is developing on a number of fronts. Likewise the need for prevention has never been greater. There are 1.2 million new cases of breast cancer worldwide every year, which far exceeds the number of any other cancers, with cervix now being a distant second at about 400,000 [1]. Not only is breast cancer the commonest cancer in women, but it is also rapidly increasing, especially in the developing world.

While population-based programmes, based on reducing obesity and increasing exercise, are likely to be effective for breast cancer [2, 3] just as they have been for heart disease (Fig. 32.1). However, as in cardiovascular disease, targeting individuals at increased risk is likely to be a key part of an effective overall policy. Over the last 50 years cardiac deaths have been reduced by more than 50 % in the US and death from strokes has been reduced by more than two-thirds (Fig. 32.1). Much of this can be attributed to the identification of high-risk individuals by measuring blood pressure and cholesterol levels, and offering them targeted preventive treatment. This is not yet widely done for any cancer, but breast cancer is leading the way, and we now have some important risk factors/biomarkers with a high population attributable risk, which can be used to identify high-risk women. While risk factors only identify individuals most likely to develop a disease, a key requirement for a biomarker is that it responds to treatment in a way that predicts quantitatively the extent of risk reduction for an individual. At present, we have only candidate biomarkers for a few cancers, notably breast cancer and prostate cancer. Mammographic density is the most promising biomarker for breast cancer, and more than 40 studies that date back to the original work by Wolfe [4] have shown an increased risk for women with radiographically dense breasts [5]. Since then other researchers [6] have shown that quantification of the proportional area of the breast that is covered by mammographic dense tissue is the best measure available. We can expect further improvements in measurement of density through the use of computerised assessments, volume measurement, and identification of other radiologic features, such as diffuse disease versus nodular pattern, or structured densities. However, even using current techniques breast density is a common, readily measurable factor that indicates an appreciable increase in risk in both premenopausal and postmenopausal women [7, 8]. Although much remains to be learned about how changes in density affect risk, the fact that breast density is reduced by tamoxifen [9] and increased by hormone-replacement therapy [10] suggests that we might be able to predict the effect on risk from modification of breast density.

32.2 Chemoprevention Agents

32.2.1 Tamoxifen

Tamoxifen was first shown to prevent new contralateral tumours in women with breast cancer in 1985 [11]. This, plus supporting animal studies [12], led to the proposal to use this drug in primary prevention of high-risk women [13]. Four prevention trials have now been completed (Table 32.1). The combined results of these trials [14] indicated that about half of oestrogen receptor positive tumours can be prevented with 5 years of prophylactic tamoxifen (Fig. 32.2a), but this agent

[1]Chapter reproduced from Cuzick J. Chemoprevention of breast cancer. Breast Cancer. 2008;15(1):10–6 with kind permission of Springer Science + Business Media.

J. Cuzick (✉)
Wolfson Institute of Preventive Medicine, Queen Mary University of London, Centre for Cancer Prevention, Charterhouse Square, London, EC1M 6BQ, UK
e-mail: j.cuzick@qmul.ac.uk

I. Jatoi and A. Rody (eds.), *Management of Breast Diseases*, DOI 10.1007/978-3-319-46356-8_32

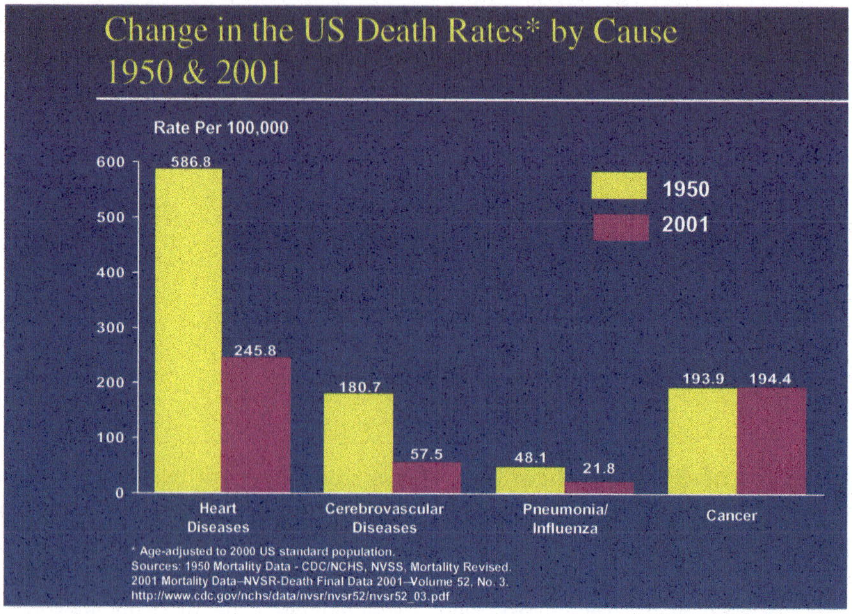

Fig. 32.1 Change in the US death rates by cause, 1950 and 2001. Note age-adjusted to 2000 US standard population. *Sources* 1950 Mortality Data—CDC/NCHS, NVSS, mortality revised. 2001 Mortality Data-NVSR-Death Final Data 2001-Volume 52, No. 3 http://www.cdc.gov/nchs/data/nvsr52/nvsr52_03.pdf

has no impact on oestrogen receptor negative women (Fig. 32.2b). Overall this amounts to a 38 % reduction in the risk of breast cancer.

On the other hand, there were two major side effects of tamoxifen—increases in endometrial cancer, and venous thromboembolic events during the active treatment phase. The former is increased about 21/2-fold whereas the latter is approximately doubled. In simple terms giving 5 years of tamoxifen to 1000 women aged 50 at double the population risk would lead to 11 fewer breast cancers, six additional deep vein thromboses and three extra endometrial cancers in the first five years of follow-up (Table 32.2). Given that breast cancer is the most serious of these events, the balance appears reasonably favourable.

However, a key question will be the extent to which benefits and side effects extend beyond the 5 year treatment period. Recent reports [15, 16] show that the benefits extend well beyond the active treatment period, but the side effects largely do not. In particular in years 5–10, after 5 years if tamoxifen in the IBIS-I trial, the risk of new ER-positive breast cancer was reduced by 44 %.

In addition, endometrial cancer and thromboembolic events were not in excess after completion of treatment. Thus one can expect that another 11 cancers will be prevented in this period and there will be no additional major side effects, so that the 10 year risk-benefit ratio will be substantially improved over the 5 year estimate currently available. Furthermore, as there was no diminution of benefit even at year

Table 32.1 Breast cancer prevention trials using tamoxifen

Trial (Entry dates)	Population	Number randomised	Agents (vs. placebo) and daily dose (mg)	Intended duration of treatment (years)
Royal Marsden (1986–1996)	High-risk	2471	Tamoxifen 20	5–8
	Family history			
NSABP-P1 (1992–1997)	High-risk women	13,388	Tamoxifen 20	5
	>1.6 % 5 years risk			
Italian (1992–1997)	Normal risk	5408	Tamoxifen 20	5
	Hysterectomy			
IBIS-I (1992–2001)	>twofold relative risk	7139	Tamoxifen 20	5
Adjuvant overview (1976–1995)	Women with ER + operable breast cancer in 11 trials	~15,000	Tamoxifen 20–40 with or without chemotherapy in both arms	3 or more (average ~5)

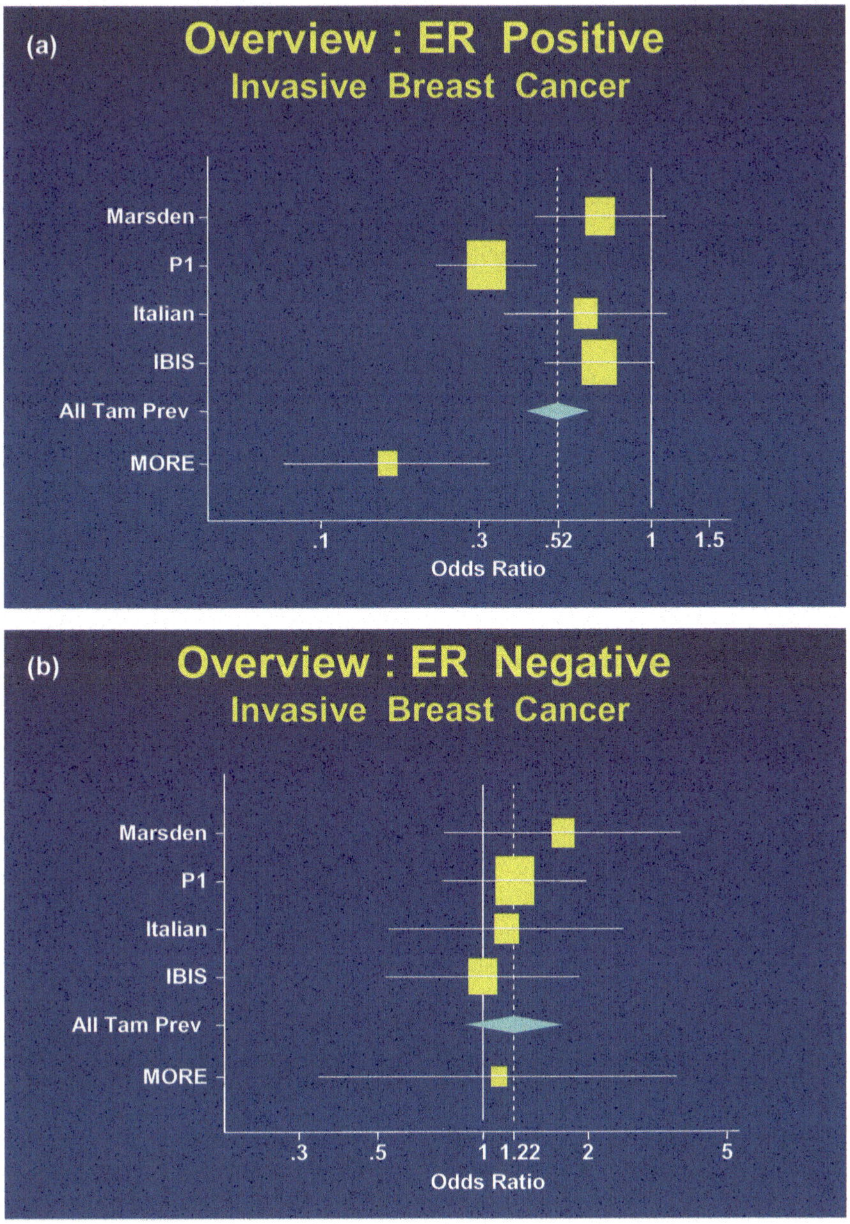

Fig. 32.2 **a** Overview of impact of tamoxifen in prevention trials for ER-positive invasive breast cancer. **b** Overview of impact of tamoxifen in prevention trials for ER-negative invasive breast cancer

Table 32.2 Predicted outcome in 1000 women aged 50 at high-risk of breast cancer followed for 5 or 10 years

	Follow-up period (years)	No treatment	Tamoxifen for 5 years
Breast cancer	5	30	19
	10	60	38
VTE	5	6	12
	10	12	18
Endometrial cancer	5	2	5
	10	5	8

Table 32.3 Prevention trials using raloxifene

Trial (Entry dates)	Population	Number randomised	Agents (vs. placebo) and daily dose (mg)	Intended duration of treatment (years)
MORE (1994–1999)	Normal risk	7705	Raloxifene 60 or 120 (3 arm)	4
	Postmenopausal women with osteoporosis			
CORE (2000–2004)	Normal risk	4011	Raloxifene 60	Additional 4
	Postmenopausal women with osteoporosis			
RUTH (1998–2000)	Postmenopausal women ≥55 years with CHD or risk factors	10,101	Raloxifene 60	5
STAR (2001–2005)	High-risk postmenopausal women >1.6 % 5 years breast cancer risk	19,747	Raloxifene 60 versus tamoxifen (20)	5

10, the benefits could persist even longer, making tamoxifen chemoprevention even more attractive, especially for women in the late premenopausal years, where life-expectancy is long. Raloxifene four trials have reported on the use of raloxifene for breast cancer prevention (Table 32.3). Two independent parts of the MORE/CORE trial have reported on the reduction of breast cancer in osteoporotic women. The original intent of this trial was to reduce bone fracture rates [17]. After 4 years of treatment a 65 % reduction in all breast cancer was found in the MORE segment [18]. This led to another 4 years of blinded treatment in the CORE study, where breast cancer was the primary endpoint. Results here were also very favourable with a 50 % reduction in breast cancer [19]. Raloxifene appears to be associated with some increase of thromboembolic complications, as with tamoxifen, but it does not stimulate the endometrium, so that there are no excess of endometrial cancers or other gynaecologic problems.

The RUTH study, which is evaluating the impact of raloxifene on cardiovascular endpoints in 10,101 women at increased risk of cardiovascular events [20] found reductions in breast cancer similar in size to that seen for tamoxifen in other studies. Also the STAR trial comparing raloxifene directly to tamoxifen in 19,747 women at high-risk for breast cancer recently found similar efficacy for the two drugs, but fewer gynaecologic and thromboembolic side effects with raloxifene [21]. Based on these results, one can safely anticipate that raloxifene will become a useful part of the armitarium for preventing postmenopausal breast cancer.

32.2.2 Aromatase Inhibitors

32.2.2.1 Efficacy

Most of what we know about the potential use of AIs in prevention derives from adjuvant studies in women with early breast cancer, where the development of isolated contralateral tumours as a first event is a good model for prevention of new tumours in healthy women. This has proved a reliable source for estimating the qualitative effects of tamoxifen in prevention, both in terms of major side effects, and in terms of efficacy. This approach has generally been more reliable than animal models or observational epidemiologic studies, although randomised intervention studies in the prevention setting remain essential for directly quantifying effectiveness in this setting and balancing risks and benefits.

To date, eight different adjuvant trials have reported on the use of three different AIs for postmenopausal women with breast cancer [22–29]. In these trials, adjuvant AIs have been found effective in three clinical settings, as initial treatment, after 2–3 years of tamoxifen, or as extended treatment after 5 years of tamoxifen.

In these trials, a consistent reduction in the rates of contralateral breast cancer has been observed in the group receiving the AI (Fig. 32.3). For example, in the ATAC trial, the number of contralateral breast cancers was reduced from 59 in the tamoxifen arm to 35 on anastrozole, a 42 % reduction (95 % CI, 12–62 %; $P = 0.01$). A larger reduction of 53 % (95 % CI, 27–71 %; $P = 0.001$) was seen in the hormone receptor-positive patients [22]. Tamoxifen itself is known to reduce the incidence of contralateral tumours by 46 % in women with mostly ER-positive primary tumours, suggesting that the overall reduction of receptor-positive breast cancer associated with anastrozole compared to no treatment may be around 70–80 %. Information on the receptor status of the second cancers in this trial is not yet available, but one would expect the preventive effect to be restricted to ER-positive contralateral tumours, and to be greater for this group than for new breast tumours overall.

32.2.2.2 Side Effects

The profound oestrogen depletion associated with AIs produces a new state of human existence, and this is bound to have other effects beyond those related to breast

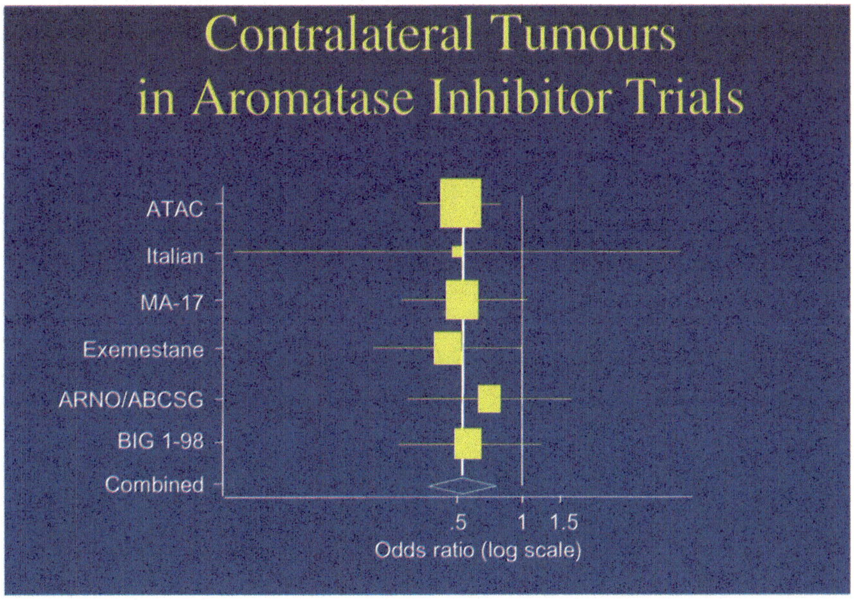

Fig. 32.3 Contralateral tumours in aromatase inhibitor trials. Combined odds ratio is 0.53 (95 % CI [0.41, 0.68])

carcinogenesis. These effects can most reliably be studied in prevention trials where a placebo is employed, allowing a direct determination of the effect of the AI. There are suggestions from adjuvant trials comparing AIs to tamoxifen, that AIs may also reduce endometrial cancer and cerebrovascular events to below baseline rates, but full evaluation is difficult because there is no untreated comparison group. Bone loss leading to increased fracture rates appear to be the most serious side effect of AIs, and methods for combating them will be essential if these drugs are to be used prophylactically [30]. Generally similar side-effect profiles are seen for all AIs and the results for anastrozole from the ATAC trial are shown in Tables 32.4 and 32.5.

32.3 Prevention Trials

Two primary prevention trials using AIs are currently in progress. One uses anastrozole while the other uses exemestane.

32.3.1 International Breast Cancer Intervention Study-II

The international breast cancer intervention (IBIS)-II trial began in February 2003 and is comparing anastrozole to placebo on 6000 postmenopausal women at increased risk of

Table 32.4 ATAC: predefined adverse events. From [22]

	Completion analysis (%)		*P* value
	A	*T*	
Hot flushes	35.7	40.9	<0.0001
Vaginal bleeding	5.4	10.2	<0.0001
Vaginal discharge	3.5	13.2	<0.0001
Endometrial cancer[a]	0.2	0.8	0.02
Ischaemic cerebrovascular event	2.0	2.8	0.03
Venous thromboembolic events	2.8	4.5	0.0004
Deep venous thromboembolic events	1.6	2.4	0.02
Joint symptoms	35.6	29.4	<0.0001
Total fractures[b]	11.0	7.7	<0.0001

Adverse events on treatment or within 14 days of discontinuation
[a]Excludes patients with prior hysterectomy and includes on- and off-therapy AEs
[b]Fractures occurring at anytime prior to recurrence (includes patients no longer receiving treatment)

Table 32.5 Non-predefined adverse events during treatment or within 14 days of discontinuation. From [31]

	Treatment first received (n [%])		Odds ratio[a] (99 % CI)	P value
	Anastrozole (n = 3092)	Tamoxifen (n = 3094)		
Hypertension	402 (13)	349 (11)	1.18 (0.96–1.44)	0.04
Diarrhoea	265 (9)	216 (7)	1.25 (0.98–1.60)	0.02
Dry mouth	113 (4)	73 (2)	1.57 (1.06–2.32)	0.003[b]
Reduction in libido	39 (1)	12 (<1)	3.28 (1.4–7.7)	0.0001[b]
Dyspareunia	28 (1)	9 (<1)	3.13 (1.16–8.42)	0.002[b]
Gynaecological events[c]	95 (3)	324 (10)	0.27 (0.20–0.37)	<0.0001
Hysterectomy[d]	30 (1)	115 (5)	0.25 (0.15–0.43)	<0.0001
Vaginal moniliasis	38 (1)	136 (4)	0.27 (0.17–0.44)	<0.0001
Urinary incontinence	74 (2)	133 (4)	0.55 (0.37–0.80)	<0.0001
Urinary-tract infection	244 (8)	313 (10)	0.76 (0.60–0.96)	0.002
Osteopenia or osteoporosis	325 (11)	226 (7)	1.49 (1.18–1.88)	<0.0001[b]
Muscle cramps	132 (4)	235 (8)	0.54 (0.41–0.72)	<0.0001
Carpal-tunnel syndrome	78 (3)	22 (1)	3.61 (1.93–6.75)	<0.0001[b]
Paresthaesia	215 (7)	145 (5)	1.52 (1.14–2.02)	0.0001[b]
Thrombocytopenia	13 (<1)	28 (1)	0.46 (0.19–1.10)	0.03
Anaemia	113 (4)	159 (5)	0.70 (0.51–0.97)	0.005
Nail disorder	54 (2)	92 (3)	0.58 (0.37–0.91)	0.002
Fungal infection	23 (1)	45 (1)	0.51 (0.26–0.99)	0.01
Increase in alkaline phosphatase	55 (2)	8 (< 1)	6.99 (2.63–18.56)	<0.0001[b]
Hypercholesterolaemia	278 (9)	108 (3)	2.73 (2.02–3.69)	<0.0001[b]

[a]Refers to anastrozole versus tamoxifen
[b]Favours tamoxifen
[c]Includes endometrial hyperplasia, endometrial neoplasia, cervical neoplasm, and enlarged uterine fibroids
[d]Recorded in 2229 patients assigned anastrozole and 2236 assigned tamoxifen (excluding those with hysterectomy at baseline)

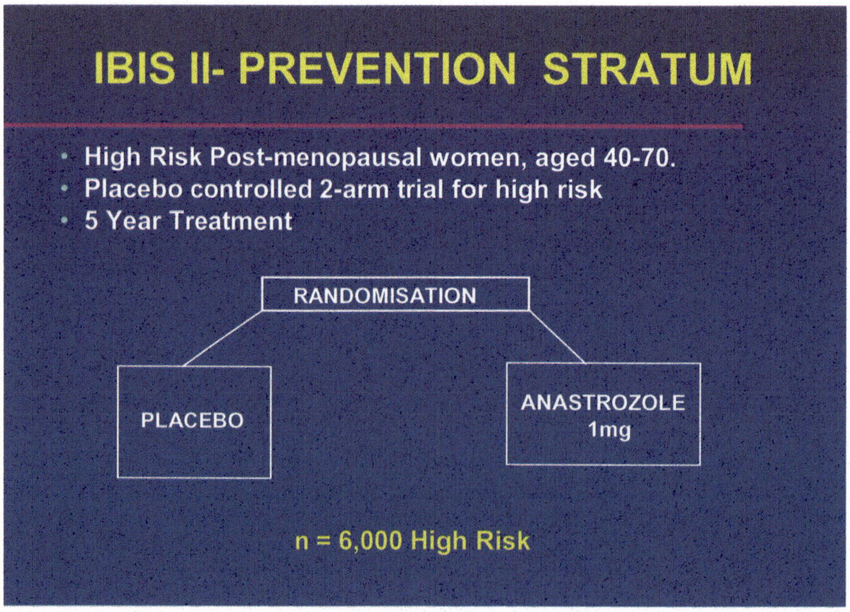

Fig. 32.4 IBIS II: prevention stratum

breast cancer (Fig. 32.4). This study is still open to recruitment. Entry criteria are similar to IBIS-I, except that only postmenopausal women are eligible and women with mammographic density covering at least 50 % of the mammogram, are also eligible. A parallel study of anastrozole versus tamoxifen in 4000 postmenopausal women with locally resected ER-positive DCIS is also being conducted as part of this activity.

32.3.2 Map.3

Another prevention trial with AIs is currently underway using exemestane. This trial sponsored by the NCIC-Clinical Trials Group compares exemestane for 5 years placebo in 3000 postmenopausal women at increased risk. Risk factors needed for eligibility include a Gail score >1.66, age >60 years, prior atypical ductal or lobular hyperplasia, or DCIS treated with mastectomy.

32.3.3 New Agents

Several lines of investigation for improved agents are underway. One approach is to search for SERMs that have an even more favourable profile that raloxifene, which still has thromboembolic concerns and leads to vasomotor symptoms such as hot flushes and night sweats. However, its lack of gynaecologic symptoms has stimulated the search for a perfect SERM which would be anti-oestrogenic for the breast, endometrium, and lipid profile, but have oestrogenic effects on bones and brain (vasomotor symptoms). Two compounds have completed stage III human testing, arzoxifene and lasofoxifene, and several more are in early development.

Oestrogen receptor negative tumours remain a challenge for prevention, and new targets will be needed to prevent these tumours. There is interest in EGFR blockers [gefitinib (sp.)] and agents targeting HER2 such as trastuzamab, and joint blockers of both targets (lapatinib), but these current agents are too toxic for prevention. NSAIDs [32, 33], COX-2 inhibitors [34, 35], retinoids, rexinoids [36], and statins [37–39] may also protect against both receptor positive and receptor negative tumours, but only results from observational studies or adjuvant studies or trials with other primary endpoints are available at the moment, and the results still have inconsistencies.

32.4 Conclusions

Approaches to prevent receptor positive are well established, and the challenge now is to reduce side effects and find agents with very favourable benefit to risk ratios. Raloxifene achieves a better side-effect profile than tamoxifen, but the efficacy is similar. The AIs hold promise for greater efficacy and fewer, but different side effects from SERMs. Unfortunately, a direct comparison of raloxifene versus letrozole in the NSABP P-4 trials looks unlikely to be funded, so decisions about which to use will have to be based on indirect comparisons of the other trials looking at AIs or SERMs separately. The side effect profiles will be critical in determining which to use both overall and for individual patients.

Good biomarkers will greatly accelerate our ability to evaluate new agents, and breast density is currently the most attractive candidate. However, its ability to predict the degree of risk reduction still needs validation and good serum markers are still awaited. The prevention of oestrogen receptor negative breast cancer remains an unmet challenge, but new agents offer an approach to preventing these cancers as well.

References

1. Parkin DM, Bray F, Ferlay J, et al. Global Cancer Statistics, 2002. CA Cancer J Clin. 2005;55(2):74–108.
2. Bernstein L, Patel AV, Ursin G, et al. Lifetime recreational exercise activity and breast cancer risk among black women and white women. J Natl Cancer Inst. 2005;97(22):1671–9.
3. Eliassen AH, Colditz GA, Rosner B, Willett WC, Hankinson SE. Adult weight change and risk of postmenopausal breast cancer. JAMA. 2006;296(2):193–201.
4. Wolfe JN. Risk for breast cancer development determined by mammographic parenchymal pattern. Cancer. 1976;37:2486–92.
5. Warner E, Lockwood G, Tritchler D, Boyd NF. The risk of breast cancer associated with mammographic parenchymal patterns: a meta-analysis of the published literature to examine the effect of method of classification. Cancer Detect Prev. 1992;16(1):67–72.
6. Brisson J, Diorio C, Masse B. Wolfe's parenchymal pattern and percentage of the breast with mammographic densities: redundant or complementary classifications? Cancer Epidemiol Biomarkers Prev. 2003;12(8):728–32.
7. Boyd NF, Byng R, Jong E. Quantitative classification of mammographic densities and breast cancer risk: results from the Canadian national breast screening study. J Natl Cancer Inst. 1995;87:670–5.
8. Boyd NF, Guo H, Martin LJ, et al. Mammographic density and the risk and detection of breast cancer. N Engl J Med. 2007;356(3):227–36.
9. Cuzick J, Warwick J, Pinney E, et al. Tamoxifen and breast density in women at increased risk of breast cancer. J Natl Cancer Inst. 2004;96(8):621–8.
10. Greendale GA, Reboussin BA, Slone S, et al. Postmenopausal hormone therapy and change in mammographic density. J Natl Cancer Inst. 2003;95:30–7.
11. Cuzick J, Baum M. Tamoxifen and contralateral breast cancer. Lancet. 1985;2(8449):282.
12. Jordan C. Tamoxifen for the prevention of breast cancer. In: DeVita, et al editors. Cancer prevention. 1990. p. 1–12.
13. Cuzick J, Wang DY, Bulbrook RD. The prevention of breast cancer. Lancet. 1986;2(8472):83–6.
14. Cuzick J, Powles T, Veronesi U, et al. Overview of the main outcomes in breast cancer prevention trials. Lancet. 2003;361(9354):296–300.

15. Cuzick J, Forbes JF, Sestak I, Cawthorn S, Hamed H, Holli K, Howell A. Long-term results of tamoxifen prophylaxis for breast cancer—96-month follow-up of the randomized IBIS-I trial. J Natl Cancer Inst. 2007;99:272–82.
16. Powles TJ, Ashley S, Tidy A, Smith IE, Dowsett M. Twenty-year follow-up of the Royal Marsden randomized, double-blinded tamoxifen breast cancer prevention trial. J Natl Cancer Inst. 2007;99(4):283–90.
17. Ettinger B, Black DM, Mitlak BH, et al. Reduction of vertebral fracture risk in postmenopausal women with osteoporosis treated with raloxifene: results from a 3-year randomized clinical trial. Multiple Outcomes of Raloxifene Evaluation (MORE) investigators. JAMA. 1999;282(7):637–45.
18. Cummings SR, Eckert S, Krueger KA, Grady D, Powles TJ, Cauley JA, Norton L, Nickelsen T, Bjarnason NH, Morrow M, Lippman ME, Black D, Glusman JE, Costa A, Jordan VC. The effect of raloxifene on risk of breast cancer in postmenopausal women: results from the MORE randomized trial. Multiple Outcomes of Raloxifene Evaluation. JAMA. 1999;281(23):2189–97.
19. Martino S, Cauley JA, Barrett-Connor E, Powles TJ, Mershon J, Disch D, Secrest RJ, Cummings SR. CORE Investigators. Continuing outcomes relevant to Evista: breast cancer incidence in postmenopausal osteoporotic women in a randomized trial of raloxifene. J Natl Cancer Inst. 2004;96(23):1751–61.
20. Barrett-Connor E, Mosca L, Collins P, et al. Effects of raloxifene on cardiovascular events and breast cancer in postmenopausal women. N Engl J Med. 2006;355(2):125–37.
21. Vogel VG, Costantino JP, Wickerham DL, Cronin WM, Cecchini RS, Atkins JN, Bevers TB, Fehrenbacher L, Pajon ER Jr, Wade JL 3rd, Robidoux A, Margolese RG, James J, Lippman SM, Runowicz CD, Ganz PA, Reis SE, McCaskill-Stevens W, Ford LG, Jordan VC. Wolmark N; National Surgical Adjuvant Breast and Bowel Project (NSABP). Effects of tamoxifen vs. raloxifene on the risk of developing invasive breast cancer and other disease outcomes: the NSABP Study of Tamoxifen and Raloxifene (STAR) P-2 trial. JAMA. 2006;295(23):2727–41.
22. ATAC Trialists' Group. Results of the ATAC (Arimidex, Tamoxifen Alone or in Combination) trial after completion of 5 years' adjuvant treatment for breast cancer. Lancet. 2005;365 (9453):60–2.
23. Boccardo F, Rubagotti A, Puntoni M, et al. Switching to anastrozole versus continued tamoxifen treatment of early breast cancer: preliminary results of the Italian Tamoxifen Anastrozole Trial. J Clin Orthod. 2005;23(22):5138–47.
24. Coates AS, Keshaviah A, Thurlimann B, et al. Five years of letrozole compared with tamoxifen as initial adjuvant therapy for postmenopausal women with endocrine-responsive early breast cancer: update of study BIG 1–98. J Clin Oncol. 2007;25(5):486–92.
25. Coombes RC, Kilburn LS, Snowdon CF, Paridaens R, Coleman RE, Jones SE, Jassem J, Van de Velde CJ, Delozier T, Alvarez I, Del Mastro L, Ortmann O, Diedrich K, Coates AS, Bajetta E, Holmberg SB, Dodwell D, Mickiewicz E, Andersen J, Lonning PE, Cocconi G, Forbes J, Castiglione M, Stuart N, Stewart A, Fallowfield LJ, Bertelli G, Hall E, Bogle RG, Carpentieri M, Colajori E, Subar M, Ireland E, Bliss JM; Intergroup Exemestane Study. Survival and safety of exemestane versus tamoxifen after 2–3 years' tamoxifen treatment (Intergroup Exemestane Study): a randomised controlled trial. Lancet. 2007;369(9561):559–70.
26. Goss, et al. A randomized trial of letrozole in postmenopausal women after five years of tamoxifen therapy for early-stage breast cancer. N Engl J Med. 2003;349:1793–802.
27. Jakesz R, Jonat W, Gnant M, et al. Switching postmenopausal women with endocrine-responsive early breast cancer to anastrozole after 2 years' adjuvant tamoxifen: combined results of ABCSG Trial 8 and ARNO 95 trial. Lancet. 2005;366(9484):455–62.
28. Jakesz R, Samonigg H, Greil R, et al. Extended adjuvant treatment with anastrozole: results from the Austrian Breast and Colorectal Cancer Study Group Trial 6a (ABCSG-6a). Proc Am Soc Clin Oncol. 2005;23:10 s abstract 527.
29. Mamounas E, Jeong J-H, Wickerham DL, et al. Benefit from exemestane (EXE) as extended adjuvant therapy after 5 years of tamoxifen (TAM): Intent-to-treat analysis of NSABP B-33. abstract for the San Antonio breast cancer symposium, December 2006.
30. Eastell R, Hannon RA, Cuzick J, et al. Effect of an Aromatase inhibitor on bmd and bone turnover markers: 2-year results of the Anastrozole, Tamoxifen, Alone or in Combination (ATAC) trial. J Bone Miner Res. 2006;21(8):1215–23.
31. The ATAC Trialists' Group, Buzdar A, Howell A, Cuzick J, Wale C, Distler W, Hoctin-Boes G, Houghton J, Locker GY, Nabholtz JM. Comprehensive side-effect profile of anastrozole and tamoxifen as adjuvant treatment for early-stage breast cancer: long-term safety analysis of the ATAC trial. Lancet Oncol. 2006;7 (8):633–43.
32. Rahme E, Ghosn J, Dasgupta K, et al. Association between frequent use of nonsteroidal anti-inflammatory drugs and breast cancer. BMC Cancer. 2005;5:159.
33. Swede H, Mirand AL, Menezes RJ, et al. Association of regular aspirin use and breast cancer risk. Oncology. 2005;68(1):40–7.
34. Harris RE, Beebe-Donk J, Alshafie GA. Reduction in the risk of human breast cancer by selective cyclooxygenase-2 (COX-2) inhibitors. BMC Cancer. 2006;6:27.
35. Mazhar D, Ang R, Waxman J. COX inhibitors and breast cancer. Br J Cancer. 2006;94:346–50.
36. Wu K, Zhang Y, Xu XC, et al. The retinoid X receptor-selective retinoid, LGD1069, prevents the development of estrogen receptor-negative mammary tumors in transgenic mice. Cancer Res. 2002;62(22):6376–80.
37. Bonovas S, Filioussi K, Tsavaris N, et al. Use of statins and breast cancer: a meta-analysis of seven randomized clinical trials and nine observational studies. J Clin Oncol. 2005;23(34):8606–12.
38. Cauley JA, Zmuda JM, Lui LY, et al. Lipid-lowering drug use and breast cancer in older women: a prospective study. J Womens Health (Larchmt). 2003;12(8):749–56.
39. Eliassen AH, Colditz GA, Rosner B, et al. Serum lipids, lipid-lowering drugs, and the risk of breast cancer. Arch Intern Med. 2005;165(19):2264–71.

Design, Implementation, and Interpretation of Clinical Trials

33

Carol K. Redmond and Jong-Hyeon Jeong

33.1 Introduction

The findings from Phase III randomized clinical trials (RCTs) conducted since the 1950s have led to major advances in the clinical treatment and prevention of breast cancer. The impact of these clinical trials is best evaluated by examining the substantial decline in mortality attributed to breast cancer in countries that have accepted and applied the results from Phase III clinical trials in the broader clinical setting [1]. Concomitant with the wider acceptance of the merits of RCTs for testing new therapeutic interventions, there have been important developments in the biostatistical methods utilized in RCTs that reflect recognition of the integral role of statistical science in clinical research.

The purpose of this chapter is to summarize salient features of the design, conduct, and analysis of modern cancer clinical trials, particularly those in breast cancer. The emphasis is on concepts and methods that are deemed essential for assuring that clinical trials incorporate optimal scientific, clinical, statistical, ethical, and practical considerations from the time an idea for an RCT surfaces until the results are reported. Within this chapter we illustrate major design considerations and issues that have arisen in breast cancer clinical trials based on our experience with landmark trials of the National Surgical Adjuvant Project for Breast and Bowel Cancers (NSABP), as well as, when appropriate, citing examples from other clinical trial groups that have made substantive contributions in the development of clinical trial methodology. Our focus is on fundamental principles that are essential for conducting RCTs and methods that are most relevant for multicenter RCTs. In order to have the material serve as a practical guide for clinical and basic scientists, we have minimized the use of statistical notation and technical jargon. For readers who may desire more statistical details on particular concepts or methods, the references with each topic should prove useful. In addition, two papers by Peto et al. [2, 3] provide a particularly insightful introduction to fundamental concepts in the design and conduct of cancer RCTs.

33.1.1 Highlights in the Evolution of Clinical Trials

Inherent in the experimental design of a clinical trial is the notion of a comparative (control) group against which a new intervention is tested. The earliest appreciation of the importance of a controlled clinical trial is generally credited to Daniel (in the Book of Daniel, Chap. 1: Verses 12–15) in the Old Testament of the Bible [4]. Daniel believed that he and his fellow Israelites would be defiled by consuming the food and wine provided by the Babylonian king, Nebuchadnezzar. He requested that the Israelites receive only pulse (leguminous plants, such as peas or beans) and water for 10 days, following which their "countenances" were to be compared to the "countenances" of those men who ate the king's diet. The conclusion of the trial, as reported in the Book of Daniel is:

> And at the end of 10 days their countenances appeared fairer, and they were fatter in the flesh, than all the youths that did eat of the king's food (Daniel 1:15).

In the fourteenth century, Petrarch, who was skeptical of the clinical approaches of the time, wrote a letter to Boccaccio, in which he envisioned a comparative trial of two equal-sized groups of men with similar age, environment, lifestyle, and temperament, and who had developed the same disease within the same time frame. The group assigned to the current physicians' "prescriptions" would then be compared to those taking no medicine to evaluate who "escapes" the disease. In his hypothetical trial Petrarch states: "I have no doubt as to which half would escape." [5].

An inadvertent clinical trial occurred in 1537 when the surgeon, Ambroise Paré, resorted to the application of a

C.K. Redmond · J.-H. Jeong (✉)
Department of Biostatistics, University of Pittsburgh,
310 Parran Hall, 130 DeSoto Street, Pittsburgh, PA 15261, USA
e-mail: jjeong@pitt.edu

I. Jatoi and A. Rody (eds.), *Management of Breast Diseases*, DOI 10.1007/978-3-319-46356-8_33

digestive concoction of egg yolks, rose oil, and turpentine to wounds received during battle when the usual treatment consisting of pouring boiling oil over wounds was in short supply [6]. He employed what he regarded was likely to be an ineffective therapy, but to his surprise he observed that:

> Those to whom I applied the digestive medicament feeling but little pain, their wounds neither swollen nor inflamed, and having slept through the night. The others to whom I had applied the boiling oil were feverish and with much pain and swelling about their wounds (Translation in [7]).

Based on his clinical impressions, Paré decided to abandon the standard treatment in favor of more humane approaches to treating battle wounds.

Paré's description of his findings does not include a statistical summary of how many soldiers received each of the two treatments or whether there were any soldiers who did not show a better result with the new therapy. However, Paré's personal observations on an unspecified number of wounded soldiers were dramatic enough to convince him to change his clinical approach to treating battle wounds at a time prior to the development of formal statistical methods.

In the eighteenth century, Lind [8] carried out his now famous clinical trial of six dietary treatments on seamen suffering from scurvy. He conducted a trial of 12 seamen with scurvy whose "cases were as similar as I could make them," in which two of the men received two oranges and one lemon daily. Therefore, the original evidence for the use of citrus fruit in the prevention and treatment of scurvy, which was shown many years later to be a sequelae of vitamin C deficient diets during long sea voyages, was based on a sample size of two men.

Whether "numerical methods" had an essential role in evaluating the effectiveness of treatments became a topic for debate in the mid-1800s. In his *Essay on Clinical Instruction* published in 1834, P.C.A. Louis, a noted physician and pathologist, strongly recommended the use of the numerical method in clinical research, while acknowledging the difficulties in implementation:

> The only reproach which can be made to the numerical method … is that it offers real difficulties in its execution. It neither can, or ought to be applied to other than exact observations, and these are not common; and on the other hand, this method requires much more labour and time than the most distinguished members of our profession can dedicate to it [9].

Louis's enthusiasm for the use of statistics in evaluating therapeutic interventions was not necessarily shared by other physicians. F.J. Double, in an article entitled "The inapplicability of statistics to the practice of medicine," which appeared in the London Medical Gazette, stated:

> Individuality is an invariant element in pathology…. Numerical and statistical calculations, open to many sources of fallacy, are in no degree applicable to therapeutics [10].

In his response entitled "The applicability of statistics to the practice of medicine," which was published in the same issue of the London Medical Gazette, P.C.A. Louis stated:

> A therapeutic agent cannot be employed with any discrimination or probability of success in a given case, unless its general efficacy, in analogous cases, has been previously ascertained; therefore, I conceive that without the aid of medical statistics nothing like real medical science is possible [9].

An invaluable contribution to the development of clinical trial methodology was the concept of randomization among treatments, which Sir Ronald A. Fisher introduced in agricultural experiments [11, 12]. As initially applied in clinical trials, patients were split into groups depending on the number of treatments and then the groups were randomly allocated to a particular treatment. However, statisticians soon noted that allocation of individuals between treatments was better because the replication afforded the opportunity to calculate an error term. A number of early clinical trials used a systematic allocation approach, such as alternately assigning patients between a control and experimental treatment, but this method has a potential for bias since the treatment assignments can be predicted prior to entry of the patient into the clinical trial.

The Medical Research Council (MRC) Streptomycin Trial published in the *British Medical Journal* [13], which ushered in the modern era in clinical trial methods, is generally cited as the first example of a "properly randomized clinical trial [14]." In the MRC trial, patients were randomly allocated between treatments utilizing random sampling numbers. Sir A. Bradford Hill, the distinguished medical statistician, was recognized for his role in the conceptualization and conduct of this seminal trial. He did much to bring attention to the importance of assuring that sound scientific principles were incorporated into future clinical trials.

A bibliography and many original documents related to these and other early developments in clinical trials are available online through the James Lind Library at the University of Edinburgh. The Lind Library is a valuable annotated resource for individuals interested in the evolution of fundamental concepts in clinical trial methods.

33.1.2 History of Cancer Clinical Trial Cooperative Groups

The Cancer Cooperative Groups Program in the United States had its origin when Dr. Sidney Farber, Mrs. Albert Lasker, and others persuaded Congress to allocate an additional $5 million for the National Cancer Institute (NCI) to fund the Cancer Chemotherapy National Service Center (CCNSC). The NCI was fortunate to have several individuals with much foresight involved with planning for the new initiative. Foremost among these were Dr. Kenneth Endicott, Head, CCNSC, Dr. Gordon Zubrod, Clinical Director, National Cancer Institute, and Dr. Marvin Schneiderman, Chief, Biometrics Section, CCNSC. Their vision for the CCNSC was to form cooperative networks of institutions that had established clinical cancer research programs encompassing medical specialties such as medical oncology, radiation oncology, and surgical oncology, who in partnership with biostatisticians as full collaborators, would carry out controlled clinical trials to address important questions about cancer treatment. These outstanding NCI leaders were able to attract some of the most talented clinical researchers and statisticians of that era to organize and participate in the original cancer cooperative groups program. From the inception of CCNSC, the organizers recognized the need to establish, in conjunction with the formation of the clinical groups, Statistical Centers that would provide resources essential for the conduct of clinical trials that incorporate sound scientific principles. The earliest cancer clinical cooperative groups were organized according to geographic areas within the United States [15].

Several specialty cooperative groups also were initiated in the latter half of the 1950s as part of the CCNSC. Among these was the NSABP, a cancer clinical cooperative group of surgeons established in 1957 under the leadership of Dr. I.S. Ravdin, and dedicated to carrying out RCTs in patients with operable breast cancer. By 1960 there were nine funded NCI clinical cooperative groups. Eventually, in succeeding years, more than 30 clinical cooperative groups were formed, but due to consolidation and attrition, there are today only a handful of cancer clinical cooperative groups. The Veteran's Administration (VA) Cooperative Studies Program for VA Medical Centers, which was organized in 1945, expanded its scope considerably during the time when the CCNSC was being initiated by adapting approaches developed by the early NCI groups to accommodate the VA system [16]. Following the initiation of the cancer clinical cooperative groups in the United States, clinical collaborative groups with organizational structures similar to the CCNSC program were also established in Western Europe. For example, the European Organization for Research and Treatment of Cancer (EORTC), which is a cooperative endeavor among several European countries, was formally established in 1974 with assistance from several American statisticians and support from NCI [17].

The first trials conducted by these groups consisted of short-term chemotherapy trials in patients with advanced disease and utilized tumor response as the primary endpoint. In these early trials, patient follow-up was very short and mortality was not considered as the endpoint of choice. However, these trials advanced several essential features that provided a strong foundation for the cancer clinical trials that would follow the earliest endeavors. Each of the investigators participating in the original groups had to agree: (1) to follow a predefined common protocol that specified inclusion and exclusion criteria for patients who could be entered into the clinical trial; (2) that patients entered into the protocols would be randomly allocated among treatments using a proper randomization procedure in order to provide unbiased comparisons; (3) to centralize clinical and pathologic data collection for quality control, monitoring, as well as a program for long-term follow-up; and (4) to centralize statistical analysis and collaborative reporting of the findings of the RCTs. These guiding principles remain as relevant today as they were in the initial founding of the clinical trials cooperative group program [18].

The concurrent establishment of ongoing Statistical Centers to collaborate with each of the cancer cooperative groups fostered: (1) major new and innovative developments in statistical methodology tailored to address questions relevant to cancer clinical trials; (2) access to and increased use of high speed computational facilities and creation of specialized software packages for database management and statistical analysis; and (3) creation of professional specialties, such as data managers, to support the collection, processing, and quality control of clinical trial data [19, 20].

33.2 Fundamental Features

33.2.1 Collaboration

Clinical trials involve collaborations among many disciplines, but a strong collaborative relationship between the lead clinical scientist and the primary biostatistician for a major trial is essential to ensure that an RCT adheres to the best scientific and ethical principles and methods throughout its course. At the inception of the modern era in RCTs, Hill [21] recognized the necessity for this ongoing collaboration:

> (T)he statistically designed clinical trial is above all a work of collaboration between the clinician and the statistician and that collaboration must prevail from start to finish [21].

Today the need for statistics and statisticians in modern clinical trial research is no longer a topic for debate, as it was in the time of P.C.A. Louis. There is an acceptance of the role of statistical methods and there are many fine examples of highly successful collaborations in breast cancer clinical trials. Unfortunately, there also is unevenness in the extent to which optimal statistical methods are evident in published clinical trial reports, indicating that there is still opportunity for improvement in the collaborations. Biostatisticians and clinical scientists have written extensively about how to foster collaborative relationships. However, collaboration in practice relies on a complex mixture of factors relating to the key investigators, which include not only academic qualifications and professional competencies, but also less easily defined factors such as leadership and management styles, effectiveness in communication in interdisciplinary settings, and mutual commitment to establishing working environments that encourage cross-disciplinary interactions.

There are numerous reasons why some trials fail to achieve the expectations of ongoing collaboration between the clinical specialists and the biostatisticians involved throughout the course of a clinical trial. One overarching reason may be that statistical concepts and issues utilized in the conduct of clinical trials are still not well understood by many nonstatisticians. Approaches considered essential by the statistician in order to have a statistically sound RCT may be regarded by clinical colleagues as being unnecessarily time-consuming, non-cost-effective, or simply irrelevant rather than fundamental for the scientific validity of the trial or to assure the quality of the data. In addition, some concepts that are promoted as important in clinical trials, for example, intention-to-treat analysis, are counterintuitive to nonstatistical scientists and may become contentious issues in specifying analytic methods and interpretation of clinical trials. There is a difference as well in how physicians and statisticians are trained to think. In medicine, emphasis is on the individual patient and tailoring a treatment prescription to a particular patient, as eloquently expressed by Double in the debate with P.C.A. Louis over 150 years ago. Whereas physicians evaluate the individual patient by a process of tests and clinical judgment that leads to a differential diagnosis and treatment, statisticians rely on summarizing groups of patients with certain characteristics in common in order to identify treatments that are useful on average for a specific group of patients.

Ellenberg [22] presents an excellent summary of the broad scope of biostatistical collaboration in medical research. Our collaborations in numerous NSABP cancer clinical trials lead us to the following recommendations for promoting collaborative relationships that produce RCTs of highest scientific quality.

First and foremost, key investigators in an RCT, including the primary trial biostatistician, should agree at the initiation to accept shared authority and responsibility for the scientific integrity of the research conducted. Biostatisticians who are content to be consulted to write the statistical considerations for a protocol that has already been drafted except for defining the statistical hypothesis to be tested, calculating the sample size, and outlining the analytic approaches to interim and final analysis are not full collaborators. Clinical scientists who visualize their interaction with the biostatistician as one in which the biostatistician provides sample size justifications, randomization scheme, and analytic plans when the protocol is designed and then has no major participation until it is time for the data analysis are not fulfilling the expectations associated with collaborative relationships in clinical trials. It may be difficult for busy investigators, including the primary biostatistician, to find the time for discussions during the initial conceptual phases in designing a protocol, but it is the most critical time for assuring that the design is scientifically sound and consistent with the best methodology currently available. Moreover, working together in drafting sections of a protocol, such as the statement of the primary aims of the study, definitions of study outcomes, and detailed follow-up schedules enables the primary biostatistician not only to have a more informed understanding of factors important for developing the statistical considerations section, but also provides opportunities to make a contribution to other sections that leads to more rigorous design overall.

Second, all key collaborators in a trial should meet together during the early phases of clinical trial planning and discuss the rationale and other major facets important for the study. In-person meetings are especially crucial during the preliminary phases of trial design in order to discuss and agree upon major elements important for the conduct of the trial. The biostatistician should enter into the discussions asking insightful questions of the investigators and be prepared to discuss at an appropriate time what the critical issues are from the statistical standpoint. These meetings are likely to be most productive when all parties have read the relevant background material, such as the reports of findings from the early phase trials in advance of the meetings.

Third, even though individual investigators will have assignments for drafting particular portions of the protocol for a clinical trial, all key collaborators, including the biostatistician, should review and agree on the entire final draft of the protocol, as well as substantive changes that are made subsequently during the conduct of the RCT. An analogous process should be followed when reports or publications of results are in preparation.

Finally, while the establishment of independent statistical and data coordinating centers, in conjunction with governance structures that facilitate shared authority and shared responsibilities in the conduct of RCTs, have done much to stimulate collaboration among clinical and statistical disciplines, the best collaborations depend also on interpersonal and work environment factors. Although it may be impossible to specify all the intangible factors that contribute to optimal collaborations, written protocols and publications serve as evidence post facto as to whether the RCT has been a joint intellectual research endeavor among the key investigators.

33.2.2 Phases in Development and Testing of New Drugs

For many years following their creation, the cancer cooperative groups defined three stages, referred to as Phases I, II, and III, necessary to evaluate new drugs in studies with human subjects [19]. The three phases develop evidence important for recommending a drug's use as a clinical treatment. Preclinical in vitro studies on parts of living organisms, such as tissue samples, and in vivo animal studies provide vital information on potential efficacy, likely toxicities, pharmacokinetics, and initial dose estimates that guide researchers in the design of the human studies. The objective of Phase I studies is to obtain data on dosing and safety concerns, with collection of preliminary data on biological activity against the disease. In contrast with many disease conditions, where Phase I studies may recruit healthy volunteers to test new drugs because they are anticipated to have limited toxicity, usually patients with advanced, end-stage cancer, are the participants in Phase I studies of new cancer drugs which tend to have greater toxicity. Phase I trials do not have control groups; the goal is to define an estimate of the maximum tolerated dose (MTD).

Following the completion of Phase I studies to establish a tolerable dose level for use in future trials, investigators recruit patients for Phase II trials that have as their primary objective to evaluate whether a drug shows sufficient promise of efficacy to move forward to testing in comparative trials against the current standard therapy. The earliest Phase II trials typically set some estimate of efficacy, based on clinical judgment and historical experience with current standard therapies, of what response rate is necessary for the drug to go forward to Phase III trials. Patients in Phase II trials are usually patients with metastatic disease and may have had extensive treatment with other drug regimens. The outcome used for the response rate usually is some early indicator that the drug is active against the metastases, such as the extent to which the tumor shrinks in size or disappears following administration of the test drug. Phase IIA designs, which test a single drug, may have one or multiple stages. The most popular design for Phase II trials is a two-stage design, in which drugs that demonstrate little or no activity against the tumor can be dropped earlier when fewer patients have been treated [23]. If a drug shows sufficient activity during the first stage, then additional patients are treated in order to obtain a sufficiently precise estimate of the response rate to use in the design of a Phase III trial. Phase IIB generally refers to trials in which one or more new treatments are compared to the standard therapy. Patients may be randomly allocated among the treatments. It is sometimes difficult to distinguish between a Phase IIB design and a Phase III trial other than the sample size is not adequate for testing with a definitive outcome. There are some Bayesian approaches to Phase I and Phase II trials that merit consideration [24, 25]. Some recently developed approaches for Phase II two-stage designs take into account both efficacy and safety outcomes jointly in deciding about early termination of the trial (see, e.g., [26]).

The Phase III trial entails comparisons of the promising new regimen to the best available standard therapy, and relies upon a more definitive outcome measure such as mortality. The participants in Phase III trials are generally those who have earlier stage disease or have not received prior treatment for advanced disease.

Scientific and statistical considerations for the design and conduct of each of the three stages in the development of new therapies are different. Table 33.1 summarizes some of the salient features of each of the phases. There has been a tendency, particularly in the design and conduct of Phase I and Phase II studies, to rely upon statistical methods established many years ago. Some newer methods, which have some attractive statistical properties, have been proposed and merit further evaluation in carefully monitored clinical trials in order to determine whether they will provide more optimal approaches for successful drug development. It is difficult to carry out new, more complex designs, in busy clinical settings, but some commitment of resources is merited if a new statistical approach has the potential to reduce the number of patients exposed to adverse risks and/or to be more cost effective than the classical methods. The types of therapies under development today, such as targeted therapies or vaccines, differ from the classical drug trials. Statisticians are active in developing methods that are tailored for these new therapies, although most of the published clinical trials do not yet incorporate these advances in statistical approaches.

In recent years, as regulatory agencies have moved to more rapid approval of drugs, there has been added a requirement for continuation of safety surveillance and technical support on the part of the drug company for a period following the approval for marketing of the drug. The collection of data on patients receiving the drug following approval by the regulatory body is referred to as a Phase IV trials or Postmarketing Surveillance Trial. These postmarketing studies have many serious limitations, which include lack of appropriate comparison groups to discriminate between adverse events associated with the disease condition or the drug and incomplete reporting of adverse events.

As an alternative to the phases in drug development discussed above, some statisticians prefer to refer to the stages as translational, treatment mechanism (TM), dose-finding (DF), dose-ranging, safety and activity (SA), comparative (CTE), and expanded safety (ES) ([27], Sect. 6.3, pp. 132–134).

Table 33.1 Summary of various phases of clinical trials on human subjects

	Phase 0	Phase I	Phase II	Phase III	Phase IV
Definition	First studies on human subjects to understand the path of a drug (small amount) in the body	Studies on clinical pharmacology and toxicity to establish a safe dose and schedule of drug administration	Initial clinical investigation for treatment effect and toxicity	Full-scale studies to determine efficacy of a new treatment, as well as to compare severity of side effects, relative to standard therapy	Final step for evaluating new therapies (postmarketing surveillance)
Outcome	Pharmacokinetics; Pharmacodynamics	MTD (maximum tolerated dose)	Proportion of patients responding; average blood or tissue levels of a drug	Time to events with possible censoring; toxicity grades from CTCAE (common terminology criteria for adverse events)	Proportion of patients experiencing long-term side effects such as cardiac toxicity
Sample size	10–15	20–50	50–100	Substantial number of patients from multicenter (several hundreds to several thousands)	Substantial number of patients from multicenter (several hundreds to several thousands)
Statistical methods	Exploratory analysis such as ranking the outcome measurements	CRM (continual reassessment method) [150];	Early stopping of ineffective therapies [151]; Two-stage design [23]	Kaplan–Meier method [83]; Log-rank test [80]; Cox's proportional hazards model [81]	Statistical inference based on, say, the proportion

33.2.3 Explanatory and Pragmatic Considerations

Different viewpoints frequently occur among key investigators regarding basic features that need to be specified when planning a clinical trial. For instance, a common clinical approach, analogous to what is done in laboratory experiments, is to minimize the heterogeneity among patients who are eligible for the RCT in order to limit the accrual to patients in whom it is believed that the experimental treatment is likely to be most beneficial. Other collaborators may advocate the use of the fewest possible eligibility criteria that are medically necessary for assuring known safety concerns in order to test the treatment on as heterogeneous a group of patients as possible, thereby increasing the generalizability of the trial results. These two approaches, referred to as explanatory and pragmatic, respectively, arise when the rationale for the trial includes a biological hypothesis that the researchers are interested in testing within the framework of the Phase III trial. Usually the biological hypothesis may already have been formulated based on findings from laboratory animal experiments or *translational* studies in humans. On the other hand, if the main stated objective of the clinical trial is to decide which treatment is better overall for patients rather than to test an underlying biological hypothesis, this leads to different design and analytic approaches. Schwartz and Lellouch [28] discussed the issues associated with these two philosophies toward designing clinical trials, and there have been numerous papers since their paper elaborating on the "explanatory" and "pragmatic" approaches to RCTs. Table 33.2 lists the contrasting features that are associated with these two different philosophical approaches to the design of RCTs.

Lellouch and Schwartz pointed out that, since RCTs involve human subjects, ethical, as well as statistical considerations, often lead to a pragmatic approach in the overall design. Ethical concerns (as discussed below) direct us to choose a design that will have the greatest potential for benefiting the patients who consent to participate in the trial and future patients to whom the treatment might be given. The pragmatic approach, which enhances the ability to generalize the findings of the trial to the broadest population of patients, is consistent with the rationale for carrying out large collaborative clinical trials that encompass many clinical centers.

Therefore, the stated primary aim of a Phase III study generally is a clinical, rather than a biological, hypothesis. When there is a biological hypothesis of interest, the use of a pragmatic design does not necessarily preclude obtaining valuable information relating to an explanatory hypothesis. Optimally designed clinical trials incorporate features that provide for obtaining scientifically valid information relating to biological questions of interest. Additional study aims can be formulated to evaluate the relationships between the treatment outcomes and host–tumor factors of interest, when ethical or other considerations do not preclude collecting measurements that are needed for testing the underlying

Table 33.2 Contrasting features of pragmatic and explanatory philosophies in RCTs

Pragmatic	Explanatory
Generalizability	Efficiency
Heterogeneity	Homogeneity
Broad entry criteria	Narrow entry criteria
Larger sample size	Smaller sample size
Real world	Laboratory
Equalized	Optimal
Treatment	Biology
Typical treatment effect	Maximal treatment effect
All patients randomized	Patients adhering to protocol
Unbiased	Potential for bias
Intention-to-treat (ITT)	Treated per protocol (TPP)
Decision	Understanding

Source Data from [27]

biological hypothesis. RCT designs that are pragmatic, but also have a biological rationale that can be tested, are more complex to design than those that simply provide a decision about treatment.

NSABP Protocol B-06, which was a randomized clinical trial consisting of three treatment groups that compared total mastectomy to lumpectomy (the control arm) to lumpectomy with or without postoperative radiation therapy, had major pragmatic and explanatory features to consider in the study design [29]. At the time of the initiation of the B-06 protocol in 1976, principles put forth by the distinguished surgeon, Dr. William Halstead, had dominated the approach for the treatment of primary operable breast cancer for more than 75 years. Surgeons considered the radical mastectomy, which consisted of removal of not only the breast but also regional axillary nodes and chest muscle, necessary in order to prevent the further spread of the cancer. The untested belief that the radical mastectomy would "cure" more patients with operable breast cancer was based on anatomical and mechanistic principles relating to how breast cancer metastasizes. However, long-term follow-up of women apparently cured of the primary breast cancer indicated that breast cancers continued to recur at distant body sites many years after the initial surgery. Laboratory studies, conducted during the 1960s, of how breast cancer metastasizes, as well as clinical observations on the history of the disease in women following surgery, indicated that there was not an orderly progression in the pattern of dissemination of tumor cells to distant parts of the body and that it was likely that clinically occult metastases have occurred in many women prior to the clinical detection of the primary breast cancer. Dr. Bernard Fisher, Group Chairman of the NSABP, proposed that these differing views relating to breast cancer metastases must be tested in a rigorous manner in a well-designed RCT. The appropriate outcome for comparing the biological hypothesis scientifically, as well as for the pragmatic aim of determining whether less surgery was equivalent to more extensive surgery, was survival. It is noteworthy that the outcome of interest in NSABP Protocol B-06 involved designing a trial to evaluate equivalence, rather than the more usual RCTs of drug therapies where the test question is whether the experimental drug is superior to the standard therapy. This chapter presents in subsequent sections some of the unique challenges that occurred in designing and conducting this paradigmatic surgical RCT.

Another example of a pragmatic trial incorporating seminal biological hypotheses is NSABP Protocol B-09. Protocol B-09 evaluated long-term administration of tamoxifen, an antiestrogenic drug, as adjunct therapy with chemotherapy for women with Stage II operable breast cancer. In the 1970s when NSABP Protocol B-09 was initiated, it was biologically and clinically important to assess the extent that responsiveness to tamoxifen therapy related to the quantitative levels of estrogen and progesterone receptors (ER and PR) in the primary tumor. In order to evaluate the role of these hormone receptors in a scientifically sound manner, determinations of the receptor values on tumor specimens from all patients entered into NSABP B-09 were made either at a central laboratory or at laboratories that had been approved based on their demonstrated capability to conduct the hormone receptor assays in a valid and reproducible manner. Two papers published 25 years ago in the *Journal of Clinical Oncology* were the first to conclusively demonstrate in unbiased comparisons from almost 2000 patients entered into NSABP B-09 [30, 31] that therapeutic response to tamoxifen was related to quantitative hormone levels. These articles, recently featured in an invited commentary in the *Journal of Clinical Oncology*, utilized statistical models to estimate the relationship between ER and PR levels and disease-free survival, while simultaneously controlling for other known prognostic factors [32]. Because there has been a requirement in all NSABP protocols for centralized review of histopathological features, the multivariable analyses also gave insights into the close correspondence between the degree of morphologic differentiation in tumors and the presence of hormone receptors.

In summary, as shown by the two examples above, optimally designed RCTs can achieve primary aims that encompass both explanatory and pragmatic aspects. Even if the findings of such trials are nonpositive with respect to the experimental therapy, the inclusion of the explanatory aim provides valuable biological insights that are useful in enhancing understanding of disease and/or treatment mechanisms.

33.2.4 Selection of the Primary Question for Investigation

The primary question that the trial will be designed to answer must be clearly stated from the outset in designing a clinical trial. While this may seem to be selfevident, it is imperative that the question be sufficiently important to utilize the time and resources of numerous professionals required to design and conduct the clinical trial, as well as justifying that human subjects take on risks or discomforts for uncertain clinical benefits to themselves or future individuals who may suffer from the same disease condition. It would seem that ongoing cancer cooperative groups need to be particularly vigilant in choosing research questions that are the most relevant, timely, and innovative rather than proposing trials that represent minor departures from previously conducted studies that have not resulted in major improvements in therapy. Most Phase III RCTs in breast cancer require 5 or more years devoted to recruitment and follow-up to complete the trial. There may be a plethora of questions available for further study, but questions, which if successfully answered, would have the most impact on curing or reducing morbidity from the disease should receive first consideration by experienced clinical trial investigators. The choice of a novel question that has a strong rationale for study usually requires a substantial amount of discussion among collaborators and time invested to develop a study plan that is scientifically sound, clinically feasible, and ethically appropriate. In Phase III studies there has to be sufficient background information available on safety concerns and potential for substantial efficacy to provide support for study on a large number of patients. From the statistician's perspective the question must be amenable to developing a testable statistical hypothesis, with sufficient information available to specify important statistical aspects of the study design, such as the primary outcome and sample size considerations.

The philosophy followed by the NSABP has been that the choice of the primary aim for a protocol should be formulated only after actively seeking the counsel of knowledgeable scientists from a variety of disciplines regarding questions that are believed to be the most likely to provide answers that have both clinical and biological importance for the treatment of breast cancer. While a small number of additional secondary aims can be incorporated, if they fit well with the primary study aim, a protocol with numerous secondary aims selected because of the interests of the investigators participating in the clinical trial is to be avoided as such "appeasement protocols" tend to divert attention and resources from the primary aim, lead to overly complex protocol designs that become difficult to follow in practice, and may jeopardize the completion of the trial [33].

33.3 Design Considerations

33.3.1 Assuring Precision and Eliminating Bias

Most clinical trials involve testing for treatment effects that are small or moderate in size. Two universal concerns that must be taken into account in such trials are how to avoid random errors and systematic errors. In order to obtain reliable estimates of treatment effects, it is necessary to control appropriately the extent of random variation present. Control of random error is achieved by assuring that a trial has an adequate sample size. Unfortunately, some previous RCTs in breast cancer have had inadequate sample sizes to identify small, but important, treatment effects on outcomes, such as mortality. Inadequate control of random error was a major problem in early trials of tamoxifen or chemotherapy carried out during the 1970s that were designed to consider whether systemic therapy prolonged disease-free survival. Although the trials showed large effects of systemic therapies in preventing recurrences, the sample sizes were inadequate to provide reliable results on mortality.

Systematic errors, which result in biased estimates of the treatment effect, may arise due to an improper study design or may be introduced during the course of the study due to unforeseen events that affect differential loss of data between treatment groups. An important tool available for avoiding moderate biases is randomization. Properly randomized trials that employ appropriate methods for analysis and emphasize the overall findings in the interpretation of the trial are utilizing the best approaches to prevent serious biases in the conclusions from the trial. Other important features that can reduce or eliminate systematic biases include:

(1) blinding of treatments; (2) centralized classification of endpoints using objectively defined criteria; and (3) minimizing exclusion of patients after randomization. Statistical bias inherent in some analytic methods frequently can be eliminated computationally or may be inconsequential relative to other sources of error. Systematic overviews of all relevant trials also are useful in preventing moderate biases since they prevent an overemphasis in the literature on the results of subjectively selected RCTs.

33.3.2 Defining Study Outcomes

The specific aims of the clinical trial determine the outcomes (also referred to as endpoints) that will be measured and analyzed. Although the stated objectives and specific aims of the clinical trial lead directly to the choice of an outcome in a general sense, defining the specific outcome, as it will be measured in the trial, is not always as straightforward. When using the classical frequentist approach to the statistical elements of design, the objective for the trial is usually restated in the form of a statistical hypothesis for testing. In order to specify a testable hypothesis, the outcome measure must be defined carefully with consideration given to its clinical relevance, objectivity, quantifiability, validity, and reproducibility. Typically, there may be a number of outcomes or interest, but in most Phase III studies there is a single primary outcome selected. Of course, there are occasions when there is more than one outcome that may be of major interest, leading to specification of more than one "primary" outcome, but the usual approach is to select the most meaningful clinical outcome as primary, and other important clinical outcomes as secondary. There are also trials in which a composite outcome may be constructed to accommodate a combination of outcomes as a single summary measure. Hard outcomes, such as mortality, are generally preferred for evaluating responses to treatment over "softer" outcomes such as tumor regression. In order to calculate the power of the study to detect a clinically important difference between treatments, it is necessary to select a single primary outcome measure; the power associated with the secondary outcomes then is a passive consequence of the sample size specified for the primary outcome. Piantadosi [27] gives an insightful discussion of issues associated with selection of the primary outcome.

Time-to-event Outcome: Since time-to-event outcomes, such as survival, disease-free survival, recurrence-free interval, progression-free interval, etc., are the most common outcomes used in breast cancer clinical therapeutic trials, it is worthwhile to discuss some of the considerations related to such measures. Time-to-event outcomes have become widely used, replacing binomial outcomes such as 5-year survival probability as a measure of response to therapy. There are two numerical values that must be specified for each subject's outcome for time-to-event at the time when an analysis is done.

First, there is a binary variable for each subject that indicates whether the person has experienced the event of interest. For example, if the outcome is survival, then each subject is classified as alive or dead at the time of the last recorded follow-up. Generally, there is an indicator variable coded as 0 (alive) or 1 (dead) associated with the vital status of each person at the end of follow-up. The second numerical value is the actual time from randomization (initial treatment) until death or, if not dead, time from randomization until the last follow-up time. Study subjects alive at the last regular follow-up scheduled time are generally referred to as censored. Some study subjects may not have continued under observation throughout the course of the study for various reasons, so there is not up-to-date information on their vital status.

Censoring: Statisticians distinguish between those who are administratively censored because of a planned analysis and those whose follow-up is delinquent, referring to the latter as "lost-to-follow-up." Since patients are generally accrued into a clinical trial over some period of time, often several years, until the requisite sample size is achieved and then followed for the outcome for some additional years, the censoring times will vary for patients who have not yet died. It is reasonable to assume that patients with short observation periods due to their late entries may have similar treatment response rates as those with longer follow-ups, whereas patients with shorter follow-up times due to some lack of compliance to the study (lost-to-follow-up) may not have responses that are independent of the study outcome, which could introduce a bias in the estimation of treatment effect. Study subjects who do not adhere to the follow-up schedule may also not have adhered to the treatment schedule when treatment consists of receiving therapy over time. There is also a particular concern if the loss rates differ between the treatment groups. If there are a substantial proportion of patients with incomplete observation times due to "lost-to-follow-up," then the analysis needs to take into account potential for bias in the treatment outcomes. Many sample size formulas have the capability to specify a rate of lost-to-follow-up in the calculation, but it is important in the design and conduct of the study that the proportion of losses be kept low in order to avoid the potential bias. Sections on sample size and analysis considerations below provide additional insights into issues that arise in defining outcome measures.

Surrogate Outcome: Because of the lengthy study period required to observe the primary outcomes of direct interest (death or recurrence) in early stage breast cancers, investigators may think of using a "surrogate" outcome that occurs earlier in the course of follow-up. Surrogate outcomes have considerable clinical appeal because they usually are associated with some biological change caused by the treatment that it is believed will eventually be reflected in the treatment effect on the longer term outcome. Moreover, surrogate outcomes, when valid and reliable, can lead to more efficient trials due to smaller sample size requirement, as well as shorter follow-up times to observe the surrogate outcome. Surrogate outcomes are commonly employed in the earliest phases of testing on humans. Unfortunately, surrogate outcomes often have serious limitations and uncertain validity in comparative trials so that statisticians will generally discourage their use in Phase III RCTs. Fleming and DeMets [34] provide an excellent overview of surrogate outcomes and the serious problems that can arise. It is often worthwhile, however, to consider including the surrogate outcome as a secondary explanatory aim in the Phase III trial, since the resulting information can be valuable for enhancing understanding of the biological role of the surrogate outcome in determining the definitive outcome of the trial.

33.3.3 Choice of Control Group

The design of clinical trials always involves decisions about the appropriate comparison against which the experimental intervention will be evaluated. The earliest phases of development in new therapies typically do not entail randomized control groups. As noted above, Phase IIA cancer trials do not have concurrent or randomized control groups incorporated in the design, but rather rely upon assumptions derived from historical experience with the standard therapies, to evaluate the probable efficacy of an experimental therapy.

Randomization serves several valuable purposes in assuring the scientific integrity of the clinical trial design. Randomization helps to distinguish between association, which is what is measured in observational studies, and causation so that differences in outcome between treatment groups can be attributed to the therapy. As noted earlier, randomization has a role in the elimination of bias in the treatment comparisons. When sample sizes are adequate, randomization tends to assure balance in the distributions of prognostic factors across the treatment groups. An important feature of randomization, that is not inherent in other methods such as statistical adjustment to control for potential confounding effects of imbalances in prognostic factors, is that randomization balances not only known prognostic factors, but also balances unknown (or unmeasured) prognostic factors. The balance on prognostic factors tends to improve with increasing sample size. Finally, random allocation of participants to treatment groups guarantees the validity of the statistical tests comparing the interventions. Although the focus in this chapter is on drawing inferences from clinical trials based on the classical frequentist methods of statistical design and analysis, it is worthy of mention that randomization is also relevant for the Bayesian and likelihood approaches. For example, in the Bayesian approach to analysis, randomization is necessary in order to assure the absence of confounding [35].

Although the majority of clinical trialists now accept the RCT as the gold standard for comparing a standard to an experimental therapy, some researchers have been proponents of the use of other comparison groups, such as historical or nonrandomized concurrent controls, as an alternative to randomization for many trials. They argue that there is no ethical dilemma in treating patients in a historically controlled trial (HCT) and that an HCT requires a smaller sample size. They generally rely on multivariable modeling to adjust for known prognostic variables to alleviate potential bias in comparisons.

Most Phase III breast cancer clinical trials seek to identify small or moderate differences between treatments. There are serious concerns about biases that may remain due to unknown or unmeasured prognostic factors associated with diseases, such as breast cancer, for which all factors associated with the clinical outcome are still not well understood. The philosophy that has guided the NSABP relating to randomization has been:

> When ethical issues do not preclude its use, the appropriate focus should be upon how the principles may be best utilized rather than upon what the alternative approaches to the randomized clinical trial might be [36].

The numerous examples in the literature of uncontrolled studies, studies with historical controls or nonrandomized concurrent controls that have created at times undue enthusiasm for treatments subsequently determined to be of little worth, provide a strong practical justification for randomization in clinical trials. When considering the value of RCTs, it is good to be aware of the lessons learned recently from the Women's Health Trial, in which the hormone replacement treatment (HRT) arm was discontinued early, due to the surprising result that there was a harmful cardiovascular effect of the treatment rather than the potentially strong benefit for heart disease, which was predicted based on the findings of earlier observational studies (WHI [37]).

33.3.4 Masking and Placebos

The rationale for masking is that the investigators, who recruit patients, administer treatments, or collect and evaluate data on outcomes, or the patients will not make judgments relating to the conduct of the study based on knowing the treatment received by individual patients. Among the numerous biases that masking helps to prevent are patient biases in reporting of subjective outcomes or side effects, physician bias in patient management, bias in evaluation of clinical response to treatment, bias in data management within the clinic, and bias in decisions related to interim monitoring of a trial.

Placebos are inactive chemical compounds formulated to resemble the active test drug in terms of taste, smell, and appearance that are given to patients allocated to the non-experimental therapy. Sometimes "sham" procedures that resemble the actual treatment are also done to disguise which patients receive test medical procedures. Approaches to assure masking can become quite elaborate; therefore, it is worthwhile to provide details of how masking was achieved for studies involving masking. Although ethical questions have been raised with the use of placebos, if the procedures employed include careful attention to details, such as when and how the patient will be unmasked and which investigators have access to unmasked data, these concerns can be largely addressed. Members of interim data monitoring committees (DMCs) should always retain the right to review unmasked data in masked trials, since their primary responsibility is to ensure the safety of the participants and cannot rely on statistical guidelines as the sole means of distinguishing benefit from harm. Another caution is that masking does not guard against biases important in equivalence trials, since masking cannot provide protection against concluding equivalence when actually one treatment is superior [38].

In the majority of breast cancer RCTs, it is not feasible to mask the clinical investigators who treat patients or the participants to the treatments that are being received, since they are of a disparate nature in terms of the administration or the adverse effects. However, there are some trials in which it is not only possible to mask the treatment allocation, but also is important to protect the scientific integrity of the trial from biases that may be introduced following randomization. The first NSABP trial of long-term chemotherapy (NSABP B-05) compared the oral drug, l-phenylalanine mustard (LPAM) to placebo in a double-blinded RCT. The blinding was useful in assuring that subjective side effects were reported in an unbiased fashion. During the design of Protocol B-14, which was the first NSABP RCT in women with pathologically Stage I breast cancer, the biostatisticians strongly recommended the use of a placebo so that the trial would be double-masked in evaluating patients' response to the drug tamoxifen. The trials of tamoxifen that had been conducted by other groups had generally had a control arm that had no further therapy following surgery for breast cancer. The primary reason for a placebo was a concern that there was a potential for patients to be crossed over to the tamoxifen group during the course of the study. The power of the study to identify a difference in survival could be seriously compromised if the "drop-ins" to the tamoxifen group were not kept to a minimum since the mortality difference predicted was relatively modest given the favorable prognosis of women eligible for the trial. The placebo encouraged investigators to adhere to the protocol and provided a means of monitoring carefully unmasking for non-protocol specified reasons. The masking proved to be very worthwhile also in assuring unbiased reporting of rare adverse effects, such as thromboembolic events, and subjective side effects, such as the frequency and severity of hot flashes, which are increased by tamoxifen, but which are common also in women who do not receive tamoxifen.

When it is not possible to mask the study interventions, it is still desirable to consider whether it is possible to mask the clinical staff who will assess the clinical outcome, particularly when the outcome is something other than overall survival. Another approach to maintain objectivity in determination of outcomes is to have a committee that reviews and classifies all outcome data without knowledge of the treatments that patients have received.

33.4 Sample Size and Study Power

33.4.1 Clinical Significance Versus Statistical Significance

Choice of the treatment effect (Δ) for the sample size calculation is a critical decision in the design of an RCT. This decision entails careful deliberation among the key investigators about what treatment effect would be sufficient to have a clinically important impact. It is necessary to keep in mind that the apparent treatment effect that is observed in the clinical trial will be less than what would be achievable in an idealized experiment because of issues related to patient adherence and follow-up. The clinical impact, if the experimental treatment is superior to the standard therapy, will therefore be less than the true efficacy of the treatment. While larger sample sizes will detect smaller differences as statistically significant, treatment effect sizes should be selected, based on consideration of the smallest clinically meaningful effect size. The choice of a clinically meaningful effect size, which is done collaboratively among investigators, is one of the most challenging issues in the design of an RCT. The biostatistician can facilitate the discussion about what constitutes a clinically meaningful difference by preparing tables that show the number of deaths or recurrences that will be prevented for treatment differences of various size for patients in the trial and when findings from the trial are generalized to similar patients in the general population. Ultimately, however, it is the clinical investigators who have the lead role and assist the statistician in making this decision. Once the choice is made, it will not only affect the total sample size needed, but also other factors, such as number of clinical sites needed, anticipated duration of recruitment, and total length of time to complete the clinical trial. It is not scientifically sound to design a trial in which the effect sizes anticipated are smaller than there is good statistical power to identify.

33.4.2 Statistical Significance and Study Power

The selection of values for the Type I (α) and Type II (β) error rates in sample size calculations for breast cancer treatment trials often relies upon conventions that have become established in medical research. Conventional values of 0.05 or 0.01 (two-sided) for a and 0.20 or 0.10 for b are selected most often as the error rates in comparative trials. While these values may be acceptable for many clinical trials, statistical considerations should explicitly address selection of their values as part of developing sample size considerations for a clinical trial. The choice of Type I and Type II error rates is an opportunity to weigh issues relating to risks and benefits of the control and experimental treatments. The balancing of benefits and risks in selection of error rates also depends upon whether the patients have advanced disease, early stage disease, or are healthy volunteers at increased risk of disease participating in a breast cancer prevention trial.

The question of when one-sided or two-sided Type I error rates are appropriate has also been a topic for some debate in the literature. When the standard therapy is a systemic therapy against which a new experimental therapy is to be compared, there is general agreement that the sample size and statistical test should use Type I error values corresponding to two-sided tests of the alternate hypothesis. When the standard group is a placebo or control arm that does not receive any drug, then some statisticians would favor a one-sided statistical hypothesis. When there is a placebo, the question is not which drug is better (two-sided) but rather whether the test drug is better than no drug. In the latter circumstance, it is still possible to use a lower, more stringent, α, such as 0.025 or 0.01, which in a practical sense obviates the argument over whether the test should be one- or two-sided.

33.4.3 Baseline Outcome Rates and Population Measures of Variability

Often one does not know precisely all the parameters needed in the equation for calculating sample size. There may be uncertainty about what the baseline outcomes will be in the group on standard therapy which will affect the sample size needed. The sample size formula also assumes that we know the value of the standard deviation (measure of variability) in the population, but frequently we can only approximate it from available preliminary data or sometimes can only guess at a likely range of values. Therefore, we may choose a range of values for the uncertain parameters and then using some conservative assumptions calculate a sample size that seems feasible and likely to achieve the scientific objectives of the study.

33.4.4 Sample Sizes for Other Common Experimental Designs

The sample size formula above was for a trial in which the hypothesis of interest was a test of the superiority of an experimental therapy as compared to the standard therapy. When the hypothesis is that the experimental therapy has an outcome that is similar to that of the standard therapy, i.e., equivalence trial, no difference must be defined by specifying the largest acceptable difference, say δ, as part of the null hypothesis. This specified difference plays a role in the *P*-value at the end of the trial and whether the nominal significance level is attained. Schumi and Wittes [39] provided detailed comparison among superiority, equivalence, and noninferiority tests, and discusses the related regulatory issues.

33.4.5 Time-to-Event Outcomes

The most common definitive outcomes in breast cancer clinical trials are time-to-event outcomes, such as survival or disease-free survival (DFS). For time-related outcomes, the power of the statistical tests is related to the number of events (deaths, recurrences) that have occurred at the time the analysis is performed rather than the number of patients that have been randomized. One simple approach to sample size calculations uses the ratio of the hazard (mortality) rates and assumes that the corresponding survival curves will follow an exponential curve, i.e., that the hazard rate is constant over time. If $\Delta = \lambda_1/\lambda_2$, where λ_1 and λ_2 are the hazard rates for the control and experimental groups, respectively, then the maximum likelihood estimates of λ will be the number of events observed divided by the total time followed (at risk). Using this method one can solve for the number of events needed for the trial given specified Type I and Type II error rates. The required number of events can be calculated from

$$d = \frac{(Z_{1-\alpha/2} + Z_{1-\beta})^2}{\pi(1-\pi)\theta^2},$$

where α is Type I error probability, $1 - \beta$ is power, θ is the log hazard ratio, and π is the fraction of patients assigned to the control group. Once the required number of evens is determined and the event rate in the control group and the feasible accrual rate are provided, the accrual and follow-up periods can be projected to reach the required number of events.

33.4.6 Sample Size Adjustments

Other more complex formulas that accommodate nonconstant hazard rates and adjust the treatment effect size projected for noncompliance (nonadherence to treatment allocation such as drop-ins or dropouts and losses to follow-up) or a phasing in of the treatment effect over time have been developed. Since the impact of noncompliance is to reduce the apparent treatment effect observed in the RCT, there is a need to inflate the sample size. Simple, conservative adjustment based on the proportion (p_m) of anticipated noncompliance is to use the factor $1/(1 - p_m)$. If p_m is 0.20, then sample size needs to be inflated by 56 % to maintain power. If noncompliance is as high as 0.30, then the sample size required is approximately doubled (2.04). Because of issues about bias associated with noncompliance, we try to reduce noncompliance as much as possible, but still need to take noncompliance into account in determining sample size [40].

Lakatos and Lan [41] have developed methods for sample size calculation utilizing the most common test for time-to-event outcomes, the log-rank statistic, and incorporating flexibility in the adjustment for nonuniform accrual patterns, nonconstant and nonproportional hazard rates, lags in treatment effects, loss to follow-up and dropouts. For a detailed presentation of sample size formulae and compendium of sample size tables, the book by Shuster [42] is a useful reference. Software is readily available for calculating sample sizes that take into account anticipated accrual patterns, more than two treatment groups, and adjustments for noncompliance and other factors to ensure that the trial will have adequate power. The statistical package, PASS, is a relatively inexpensive package for estimating sample sizes or study power for the majority of clinical trials (NCSS, PASS, and GESS, http://www.ncss.com). There are also numerous useful programs that can be downloaded freely from trustworthy Websites of clinical trial biostatisticians, such as the departmental Website of Biostatistics and Applied Mathematics, at MD Anderson Cancer Center (http://biostatistics.mdanderson.org/SoftwareDownload/) and the National Cancer Institute Website (http://www.cancer.gov/statistics/tools).

Further adjustment of sample size can be done to accommodate plans for interim data monitoring during the conduct of the trial based on group sequential designs. Such adjustments can be quite complex. EaST is a more sophisticated, albeit costly, software package that provides the capability to take into account the plans for interim monitoring of data (Cytel: Statistical Software and Services, http://www.cytel.com).

There is also freeware that can be found on various Websites for sample size calculations and simulating the outcomes of trials under varying assumptions about the design parameters.

33.5 Randomization Methods

The biostatistician works closely with the clinical investigators prior to the initiation of the clinical trial in specifying all aspects of the randomization process in order to ensure that the implementation proposed is appropriate and feasible. In addition, the process should be carefully documented thoroughly throughout the trial. Detailed written procedures of the process and training of all personnel involved in randomizing participants are important. It is also essential that procedures are in place for backing up randomization when computers fail. If the trial is blinded, there should be a well-defined plan that includes who has access to unblinded treatment allocations, how blinding is maintained, the indications for unblinding a participant, and who will be contacted to unblind (including a sequence of backup staff for times when the primary person is unavailable). Often, it is necessary to provide coverage for randomization and unblinding on a 7-day, 24-h basis. Although unblinding of patients in most RCTs is an uncommon, sporadic occurrence, NSABP has experience with rare events related to young children (or even on one occasion, the pet dog) who accidentally swallowed some of a patient's pills on a weekend evening with the consequence that there was a need to unblind immediately to determine whether the pills were a harmless placebo or active drug. All deviations from the randomization procedures and handling of voided randomizations or other violations should be documented fully for interim and final reporting of the trial findings.

Randomization should be centralized at a data coordinating center outside the clinical setting whenever feasible. The randomization list, if generated in advance of the trial, should be prepared by a qualified person (usually study biostatistician) who is not involved with recruitment or treatment of trial subjects. During the conduct of the study, the details of the generation of the randomization lists should not be disclosed to any of the clinical personnel involved with the trial participants. (Generally access to the randomization lists is restricted to only a few individuals who have a need to know for protection of subjects and to assure backup in the event that the biostatistician who generated the list is not available.)

Random allocation for all subjects is often done prior to the initiation of recruitment for early phase experiments of healthy volunteers, experiments with dietary manipulations, or vaccine trials with closed populations. Alternatively, random allocation may be done sequentially as the participants enter the trial. This approach is done in many Phase III cancer trials that have a prolonged recruitment period. In trials of operable breast cancer, participants are not known in advance and may not have been diagnosed with the condition until sometime during the course of the RCT. The randomization process may be stepwise. In some trials, randomization is done for groups of individuals (cluster or group randomization) rather than for each individual. Group randomization may be the method of choice when the intervention is administered in clinical settings to groups of patients, such as an educational program or a dietary intervention. Random allocation of the clusters makes this approach scientifically acceptable as long as the cluster remains the unit for statistical analysis.

Statisticians no longer rely upon tables of random numbers and preparation of sealed envelopes containing the treatment allocations that are opened in sequence at the clinical site when a patient agrees to participate in a clinical trial (as was done for the NSABP B-04 and B-06, the surgical RCTs conducted in the 1970s). Use of randomized assignments in sealed envelopes at clinical sites should be avoided. While this was a common method in the past for randomization, it is questionable, especially when the study is not blinded since the investigator can either deliberately or by mistake invalidate the randomization process. Further, with modern communication methods such as fax or Web-based randomization programs that permit the randomization to occur in real time (when no problems are identified following a check of the eligibility criteria prior to randomization), there is generally no justification for envelope randomization. Any new system for randomization should be fully pretested prior to the randomization of the first patient. Software for Web-based systems is now available, but it should be pretested in the actual context of the trial prior to adoption.

The random allocation should occur as close in time to the initiation of the intervention as practically feasible. Delays between randomization and initiation of therapy can increase the number of dropouts or subjects who do not receive the allocated therapy. Omitting from analysis the patients who do not receive the allocated therapy can lead to bias. Bias may not occur related to the delay if the treatments are blinded, but should be suspected in unblinded studies. To avoid bias associated with dropouts occurring following randomization, but before initiation of therapy, analysis should include outcomes for all participants as randomly allocated regardless of whether treatment was actually received, i.e., intention-to-treat.

Patients may be stratified into groups based on important prognostic factors and randomly allocated to treatment groups within the strata in order to ensure balance on critical prognostic factors. For example, in clinical trials of operable breast cancer, it is common to stratify on the number of positive axillary nodes because number of positive nodes is the strongest prognostic factor in determining outcomes such as disease-free survival and survival. Another prognostic factor of interest for stratification in trials of early stage breast cancer is the age of the patient at diagnosis, since outcomes differ by age group with younger (premenopausal) women tending to have more aggressive tumors that have a poorer outcome. It is desirable, as well in multicenter studies to balance treatment allocations by clinical site in the design, in order to assure that the numbers of patients allocated to each treatment group within centers are balanced overall, as well as at times of interim data analysis during the course of the RCT. In addition, there may be heterogeneity among the clinical centers, not only with respect to the patient prognostic factors, but also in the adherence rates to the study treatments and the follow-up of patients which make stratification or balancing on clinical centers.

The next step in the process is to create the randomization within each stratum. The random allocations may be generated in a number of ways. According to Wittes [34]: "The ideal device (for randomized allocation) is a perfectly unbiased coin tossed by an angel." A person tossing a coin is fallible and there may be problems with validating the process, such as filing to record all tosses if a particular toss does not agree with the desired treatment allocation. Random and "haphazard" treatment allocations are not the same. For example, assignment by alternating sequences of the treatment is not a proper method for random allocation although supporters of this method have argued that since patients enroll in a chance order, an alternating assignment of treatments to patients will result in groups roughly at equal risk. However, the person doing the randomization can influence which participants receive a specific therapy. Even when therapy is blinded using alternative sequences, one inadvertent unblinding of treatment reveals the entire sequence of treatment allocations (see [27], p. 335). Similarly, a scheme that allocates patients to different treatments based on alternating days has problems. Once clinical staff becomes aware of the sequence, they can control which patients are randomized to which therapy. This allocation procedure is especially subject to bias when used for nonemergency conditions. Under emergency conditions, if all patients are randomized, the bias issue may be minimal since treatment cannot be delayed until the next day. However, the statistical problem relating to the two outcomes still applies.

Most clinical trials today rely on computer generated treatment assignments. Computers generate "pseudorandom" numbers, not random numbers. The common algorithm for generating a pseudorandom sequence is the linear congruential method [43] which may lead to sequences that are serially correlated and have repetitive series if algorithm's parameters are not appropriately chosen. There is a need to choose a "good" random number generator and to evaluate the program thoroughly before initiating randomization and during the course of a large trial to ensure that the program is not looping back improperly and, therefore, generating repetitive sequences. Statistical tests should be performed to verify the validity of the randomization sequence. Proper randomization is one of the most crucial features in assuring the scientific integrity of an RCT. If it is discovered at the conclusion of a trial that there was a serious problem with the random allocation, the study can be criticized as invalid.

A simple randomized sequence has no memory of previous treatment assignments. However, it may have imbalance in the treatment assignments, which can be particularly problematic when number randomized is small or moderate in size. There is a nonnegligible probability of some imbalances between treatments and a small probability of serious imbalances. Imbalance increases the variance of the estimated treatment effect, but the amount of the increase will be slight if the imbalance is not severe. The treatment allocation may be relatively balanced and still have problems with imbalances in major prognostic factors.

To alleviate potential treatment imbalances that occur with simple randomization, statisticians will often employ a constrained randomization scheme that helps to assure balance in the numbers on each treatment. Random permuted blocks is a method of restricted randomization to ensure exactly equal treatment numbers at certain equally spaced points in the sequence of patient assignment. Block sizes are multiples of the number of treatment groups. For each block of patients, we use a different random ordering of the assignments for each treatment. For example, if there are two treatments and the designated block size is four, there will be six possible orderings of the treatments within a block. The randomization consists of selecting at random (with replacement) strings of the blocks. Sometimes treatment allocation sequences are generated with blocks of varying size to reduce the predictability of the sequence of treatments, but the block size should be relatively small to assure balancing of the treatments. Imbalances may still occur with this approach, the extent of imbalance is less due to the balance within blocks. The random permuted blocks is an appropriate randomization scheme in RCTs when there is an expectation of relatively large numbers accrued from each of the clinical center.

It is common in breast cancer treatment trials that there are many clinical centers, but the majority of centers may accrue only a small number of patients to the RCT. In order to assure that the numbers of patients are balanced by treatment and major prognostic factors, cancer biostatisticians have often preferred to use an adaptive (dynamic) method of allocating patients to treatments while controlling for balance on prespecified major prognostic factors. Efron [44] introduced the notion of "biased coin" randomization as a procedure to control imbalances. The implementation of this adaptive randomization approach that is most popular in cancer clinical trials is usually referred to as minimization method [45, 46].

33.5.1 An Example of Biased Coin Algorithm

The following is a specific example of the biased coin algorithm adopted by the National Adjuvant Breast and Bowel Project (NSABP).

1. Obtain the number of patients on each treatment arm for the current protocol at the current institution.
2. Calculate the difference in number of patients between the treatment arm(s) with the fewest number of patients (first group) and the treatment arm(s) with the highest number of patients. Define the second group as one including all the treatment arms that have the number of patients greater than the minimum.
3. If the difference is greater than two patients, then the treatment is then assigned with a g % ($g > 0.5$) probability that it will be a treatment from the first group, and a $(1 - g)$% probability that it will be a treatment from the second group. Within the groups, the probability for each treatment is evenly divided.

Example 1: Suppose an institution had the following patients currently:

Arm 1: 5 patients
Arm 2: 6 patients
Arm 3: 8 patients

The biggest difference in patients is three. Thus, assuming $\gamma = 70$, Group 1 will consist only of Arm 1 with 70 % probability, and Group 2 will consist of Arm 2 and Arm 3 with 30 % probability. Therefore, the probabilities for the individual treatment arms break down as follows:

Arm 1: 70 % probability of being the assigned treatment arm
Arm 2: 15 % probability of being the assigned treatment arm
Arm 3: 15 % probability of being the assigned treatment arm

4. If the difference in number of patients between the treatment arm(s) with the fewest number of patients and the treatment arm(s) with the highest number of patients is less than or equal to 2 then

Table 33.3 Example 2: protocol distribution of patients across three arms at the current stage

	Age	Nodal status	ER status
Arm 1	Younger: 5 patients Older: 4 patients	Negative: 4 patients Positive: 5 patients	Negative: 6 patients Positive: 3 patients
Arm 2	Younger: 4 patients Older: 4 patients	Negative: 5 patients Positive: 3 patients	Negative: 3 patients Positive: 5 patients
Arm 3	Younger: 4 patients Older: 4 patients	Negative: 5 patients Positive: 3 patients	Negative: 2 patients Positive: 6 patients

a. Calculate a score for each treatment arm by adding the number of patients on that arm on the current protocol at each of the patient's stratification levels multiplied by a preassigned weight for each stratum variable (see Example 2 below).
b. If all treatment arms have the same score, then generate a random number between 1 and the number of treatment arms on the current protocol and assign the treatment accordingly.
c. If all treatment arms do not have the same score, then divide the treatment arms into two groups, the first group consisting of all treatment arm(s) with the lowest score, and the second group containing all other treatment arms. Within the groups, the probability for each treatment is evenly divided.

Example 2: Suppose there are three stratification factors to be used for designing a new study; age (dichotomous), nodal status (negative, positive), and estrogen receptor (ER) (negative, positive). Suppose the protocol had the following distribution of patients across three arms at the current stage (Table 33.3).

Now suppose that the patient being randomized has these stratification levels as younger, node-negative, and ER-positive. Assuming that the weight given to each stratification variable is 1, the score for each treatment is shown below:

Score for Arm 1 = $(5 \times 1) + (4 \times 1) + (3 \times 1) = 12$,
Score for Arm 2 = $(4 \times 1) + (5 \times 1) + (5 \times 1) = 14$,
Score for Arm 3 = $(4 \times 1) + (5 \times 1) + (6 \times 1) = 15$.

So Group 1 would include only Arm 1 with 70 % probability and Group 2 would consist of Arm 2 and Arm 3 with 30 % probability. Therefore, the probabilities for the patient to be randomized to each arm break down as follows:

Arm 1: 70 % probability of being the assigned treatment arm
Arm 2: 15 % probability of being the assigned treatment arm
Arm 3: 15 % probability of being the assigned treatment arm

33.6 Ethical and Related Considerations

A fundamental responsibility of clinical trial researchers is to assure the conduct of RCTs that are ethical in all features from the design through the final closeout of the study. Ethical considerations are interwoven with many of the scientific facets involved with clinical trials. This section deals mainly with ethical concerns that predominate in the planning of an RCT as they relate to specific design elements. Although we do not present in detail the evolution of protections for human subjects in clinical research studies, all staff involved with the conduct of clinical trials should be knowledgeable about the background and content of major codes, laws, guidelines, and principles, such as the Nuremberg Code [47], Declaration of Helsinki [48], Belmont Principles [49], and regulations that pertain to national and international studies that conduct research with human participants. The elements of informed consent should also be familiar to all investigators and staff, not just those who are responsible for recruitment of subjects to clinical trials. The National Institutes of Health (NIH) and other funding bodies require training in the principles and legal requirements for research involving human subjects and Institutional Research Boards must approve research protocols and review adverse events on an annual basis.

Clinical thinking about an ethical requirement for signed informed consent of participants in clinical trials has changed greatly in many countries since the 1960s when, at a meeting of the Medical Research Council (MRC) to consider the legal and ethical concerns regarding RCTs, the attendees:

> ...decided that there was no obligation on the part of an investigator to inform a patient that he was participating in a trial. Particularly is this so in the trial of methods of treatment for desperate cases of advanced disease. If the trial is ethically the criteria outlined and if therefore the choice of treatments is really being made by the 'toss of a coin,' it is not to be considered to be the best part of doctoring to inform a patient so gravely ill that we do not know how to treat her, and that the choice of treatment is being so determined [50].

Zelen [51] proposed as a design for the RCT that, when a standard therapy is to be compared to a new experimental therapy, it is ethical to randomize and then seek informed consent only from the patients who are randomly allocated to the experimental therapy, since the patients allocated to the standard therapy would be treated in the same manner as if there had been no clinical trial. Although this design, sometimes referred to as the "informed consent" design, has generally been deemed as not ethical, it is worthy of mention because it stimulated consideration of the possibility of some modifications in the approach to obtaining informed consent such as the "prerandomization" approach employed in the NSABP Protocol B-06 lumpectomy trial, as discussed in more detail below.

Current procedures for ethical conduct of clinical trials incorporate two important protections for human subjects. Ethics Committees, or Institutional Review Boards (IRBs) as they are referred to in the United States, are independent bodies which must follow various legal and ethical requirements that protect human subjects in research studies. IRBs are charged with reviewing and approving protocols prior to implementation, annual review, and approval of study progress, as well as intervening substantive protocol changes. Unexpected adverse events occurring during the course of the trial are also reported to the IRB for their review and approval of actions taken.

With few exceptions, such as when the situation does not permit (e.g., heart or stroke victims requiring immediate emergency treatment) or in the case of minors or others unable to give informed consent, signed informed consent must be obtained from all subjects prior to enrolling them in a trial. Thus, the approach to clinical trials today strongly affirms that it is an ethical obligation of the investigators to obtain informed consent from *all* participants in a clinical trial. The informed consent process involves providing the potential participant with complete, accurate information on several aspects, including: (1) a clear statement that the participant is being requested to become a participant in a research study; (2) explanation of the purpose of the research and the procedures that will be followed in the study; (3) description of experimental procedures; (4) potential benefits for the participant; (5) expected risks and discomforts that are known or suspected; (6) alternative methods available for treatment of the disease; (7) anticipated duration of the study; (8) availability and willingness of the investigator to answer questions about the study; and (9) the right of the participant to withdraw consent at any time during the course of the trial without any adverse consequences affecting future treatment. The informed consent should be constructed in language that is informative and understandable to the populations from which the participants are to be recruited. In multicenter clinical trials, this may entail that the consent form is translated into several languages and written in clear simple words that the public can understand rather than technical or legalistic terms.

Although there is now general agreement that participants in clinical trials should be given complete information and the opportunity to consent voluntarily to become a part of a clinical trial, issues can still arise about the process used in obtaining informed consent, particularly in clinical trials where the patient must simultaneously cope with a serious newly diagnosed disease such as breast cancer. Signatures and initials on multiple pages of a consent form are not an adequate substitute for dedicated and knowledgeable clinical trial staff that spends time with potential participants discussing the study and answering their questions in words that they can understand. With respect to the implementation of these tremendous gains in the protections of human subject protections, we have expressed the following caution:

> ...There is no dichotomy of purpose between preservation of human rights and dignity and freedom of inquiry. There must be strict vigilance to ensure that there is no serious conflict between the forces defending subjects rights and those defending freedom of inquiry. In such a confrontation, once again, 'winners may become losers' [33]

NIH and FDA require interim data monitoring plans for protection of human subjects during the conduct of the trial. As discussed below in the section on interim data monitoring, most Phase III have independent data monitoring committees. In spite of the many formal procedures in place to protect human subjects who participate in RCTs, those who design and conduct the trials should give thoughtful attention to addressing ethical concerns that arise. As illustrated in the examples below, ethical issues that arise may be complex and there may be disparate viewpoints regarding what is an ethical solution.

To be ethical a study must be scientifically sound. Rutstein [52] summarized this principle well:

> It may be accepted as a maxim that a poorly or improperly designed study involving human subjects... is by definition unethical. Moreover when a study is in itself scientifically invalid, all other ethical considerations become irrelevant. There is no point in obtaining informed consent to perform a useless study [52].

Clinical trial investigators have an ethical obligation to: (1) ask relevant important clinical questions; (2) use the best possible research design and methods throughout the conduct of the trial; (3) assure that the projected sample size is adequate to achieve clinically meaningful findings; (4) obtain informed consent of all participants; (5) implement quality assurance, as appropriate, in protocol requirements and data collection; (6) monitor accumulating data during the course of trial to identify known, as well as unexpected, adverse events of treatment and early evidence of treatment benefit or harm; (7) analyze data relating to all patients entered into the RCT, i.e., follow "intention-to-treat" principle; and (8) publish and disseminate the findings at the conclusion of the trial.

Similarly, the research team at institutional sites needs to be trained by experienced trial leadership in their responsibilities for ethical and scientific conduct of the trial, which include: (1) careful evaluation of potential participants for protocol eligibility to minimize errors in subject recruitment; (2) explain the protocol appropriately and obtain informed consent of participants prior to entering them into the trial;

(3) be knowledgeable and comply with all protocol requirements relating to eligibility, treatment, and follow-up; (4) promote adherence of participants by providing high quality care and a supportive clinical environment; (5) submit complete, accurate data in a timely manner; (6) report serious adverse events immediately to the appropriate personnel and agencies, e.g., the Food and Drug Administration (FDA) for trials funded by or conducted in the United States; and (7) work collaboratively with the trial management staff to resolve problems that arise during the conduct of the trial.

33.6.1 Ethical Concerns Relating to Randomization

Until a drug has been established as efficacious and adequately safe, or ineffective with adequate safety, or simply ineffective, the principle of "equipoise" can apply to justify randomization, provided that the participant has been fully informed of potential benefits and risks and consents freely to participate. Thus, the participant accepts uncertainties about individual benefits and risks. There is a fragile balance between individual and collective ethics. Individual ethics involves considering what is best for the individual patient, whereas collective ethics entails consideration of advancements in medicine and public health through careful scientific experimentation.

Opponents of randomization contend that "equipoise" seldom applies by the time a Phase III trial is conducted because there is evidence from animal studies and Phase I/II trials indicating that the therapy is efficacious with an acceptable level of toxicity [53]. However, the rejection of the ethical nature of an RCT leads to acceptance of therapies with limited comparative evidence and/or further observational studies to establish effectiveness of therapy involving historical comparisons or concurrent nonrandomized controls [54].

Those of us who consider randomization the method of choice argue that without randomization there will be limited advancement of medical science. Those who strongly support randomization believe that there should be a global standard of evidence that is based on randomized controlled clinical trials. Random allocation of patients to treatment groups has become accepted as the "gold standard" by the majority of biomedical researchers. Most clinical trial statisticians are strong advocates for the use of RCTs.

Moreover, with respect to the issue about when patients should be offered the opportunity to participate in an RCT, we recommend that clinical investigators adopt the "uncertainty principle," which has been endorsed by many researchers as an ethical approach. The uncertainty principle states that randomization should be offered when both the physician and patient are uncertain which treatment is better for the patient. Using this as the guiding principle for randomization of a patient places the emphasis on the individual patient rather than a group of patients with particular prognostic factors, and is, thus, more consistent with the usual clinical approach. The drawback for some physicians is that they must be able to discuss uncertainties in medical practice with the patient.

33.6.2 Ethical Controversies in Randomization and NSABP Protocol B-06

NSABP Protocol B-06 had as its primary hypothesis that survival following conservative surgery (lumpectomy) is comparable to that following more extensive surgery (total mastectomy). There was much controversy surrounding the conduct of this clinical trial. Although the radical mastectomy was the standard therapy for operable breast cancer in the United States at the time this protocol was initiated, a small number of surgeons believed that a lumpectomy was indeed as good as a radical mastectomy. They envisioned no ethical dilemma with doing a lumpectomy on patients with early stage breast cancer in the absence of a definitive direct comparison with the standard operation. A second important therapeutic question incorporated in the lumpectomy trial was whether patients in whom the breast was spared should also receive radiation therapy for the control of local recurrences. The leadership of the NSABP and many NSABP clinical investigators believed fervently that the ethical approach to resolve these controversial clinical questions was to conduct a multicenter RCT that was scientifically well designed in all respects to test both the relevant clinical and biological hypotheses. Accordingly, they developed a protocol with three treatment groups (mastectomy, lumpectomy, and lumpectomy with radiation to the breast) for women diagnosed with operable breast cancer that was 4 cm. or less and whose tumors were amenable to a cosmetically acceptable result. Axillary dissection was done in all three treatment groups, primarily to obtain pathologic information on whether the axillary nodes contained tumor cell, which was necessary since at that time systemic therapy was given only to women with pathologically Stage II breast cancer.

NSABP Protocol B-06 opened for accrual in April 1976 utilizing an envelope randomization scheme with treatments balance achieved within an institution using a classic Greco-Latin square design. The investigators discussed the protocol with eligible patients prior to surgery and obtained informed consent in the conventional manner without knowledge of which treatment the patient would receive if she agreed to enter the trial. The adoption of a noncentralized randomization was due to the clinical practice at that time of doing the surgery for removal of the cancer with the initial biopsy to establish the diagnosis of breast cancer. (An analogous randomization process had been successfully employed in the predecessor surgical trial, NSABP Protocol B-04.) Following the biopsy and availability of immediate pathologic diagnosis of breast cancer by frozen section, the surgeon would have staff open the next envelope in the sequence available at the site and would proceed to carry out the operation specified. The NSABP utilized this conventional randomization scheme for Protocol B-06 until 1978, when, due to chronic low accrual to the Protocol B-06 that threatened the capability to complete this paradigm shifting trial, discussions evolved about whether modifications to the randomization could be made that would make the trial more acceptable to both physicians and patients. As noted above, Zelen [51] had proposed an approach in which randomization between a standard and experimental therapy would be done prior to seeking informed consent and only patients who were randomly allocated to the experimental therapy would be approached to obtain informed consent. We rejected the Zelen approach, since it was deemed unethical to enter any patient into a research protocol without properly informing her about her participation in the research. However, Zelen's paper stimulated considerations as to whether it might be possible to modify the conventional randomization to enhance the accrual rate in a manner that was ethical and did not seriously jeopardize the ability to answer the scientific questions.

Some idea of how different physicians rationalized the uncertainties in the surgical treatment of breast cancer existing at that time are reflected in comments to a survey querying reasons why surgeons did not consider participation in an RCT of mastectomy versus lumpectomy [55]. One surgeon, who performed radical mastectomies on his patients, stated: "I don't fear the remorse of removing a breast unnecessarily as I do the remorse of losing one patient unnecessarily because of the trial," whereas another surgeon, who was a proponent of segmental mastectomy (the term for lumpectomy used in Protocol B-06) said:

> "I have performed the segmental mastectomy over the past few years and have no reason to regret the surgery. If I honestly believe that there is no choice between the operations and that I do not know which is better, then why, obviously, should my patients subject themselves to the mutilating mastectomy [55]."

These two surgeons obviously could not ethically participate in an RCT to test different surgeries because of their strong clinical opinions favoring one or the other therapies. However, some surgeons, who participated in NSABP and believed that an RCT was both ethically and scientifically necessary to resolve the uncertainties associated with the surgical treatment of breast cancer, still had difficulties with recruiting patients to NSABP Protocol B-06. They did not feel comfortable with presenting a clinical trial in which the patient had to make a choice between two such disparate surgeries at a time when the patient did not have a definite cancer diagnosis and would undergo surgery not knowing whether she would have her breast removed or only a portion of the breast involved with tumor. These concerns of NSABP clinical investigators lead us to consider modifications to the randomization approach in Protocol B-06. Eventually, after much discussion and debate, both within and external to the NSABP, the decision was made to change from an envelope randomization to a centralized randomization and to adopt an approach to obtaining informed consent that enabled the surgeon to tell the patient which surgery she would have prior to the actual operation. This novel approach, which was named "prerandomization," was a compromise reached in order to alleviate ethical concerns of some investigators and at the same time preserve the ability of the trial to be completed in a manner that preserved its scientific objectives. Interestingly, there were also investigators who believed the conventional randomization was entirely ethical and continued to recruit patients to the trial using that approach even after the introduction of prerandomization.

There were a number of critical aspects in the procedures for the implementation of the prerandomization process to preserve the ethical and scientific integrity of the trial. First, patients entered into the trial had to have a known diagnosis of invasive breast cancer, which meant that a biopsy had to be done prior to and separate from the definitive surgery. The protocol was changed from the usual one stage procedure for diagnosis and definitive surgery that was done during that era to a two-stage procedure. Because it was essential to monitor that the randomization process was appropriately conducted, central randomization replaced randomization by envelopes at the institutions. Having established that a patient had operable invasive breast cancer and satisfied other protocol inclusion and exclusion criteria, the site investigator could initiate the randomization process by telephoning the NSABP Biostatistical Center at the time when the patient was scheduled for a visit to discuss the options available for further treatment. During the telephone call a checklist verifying eligibility, including that the diagnosis of invasive breast cancer had been made. Following verification of eligibility, the random treatment assignment for that patient was provided to the investigator. The second step was for the investigator to present the protocol to the patient, providing all the treatment options in detail including potential risks and benefits. If the patient was receptive to entering the clinical trial, the third step was an explanation that the treatments were assigned by chance. The patient was informed which of the treatments she would receive based on the random assignment already provided to the surgeon if she agreed to participate in the trial. The patient received the information about the randomly allocated treatment prior to signing of informed consent. All other elements of the informed consent process were unchanged.

In contrast to the approach proposed by Zelen [51], the NSABP approached all potential participants for informed consent. Because of the prerandomization, there were some patients, who when informed of the treatment allocation prior to signing informed consent, refused the treatment assignment. In order to be able to evaluate whether patients who agreed to the treatment allocation differed from those who refused on important prognostic factors, patients refusing the treatment allocation were asked for consent to clinical follow-up for study outcomes. Most patients refusing the randomly allocated treatment because of a preference for the alternative treatment agreed to be followed within the trial.

The prerandomization also generated debate based on both scientific and ethical grounds. A scientific concern is that it is less efficient than a conventional randomization approach. Because the trial now included patients who refused the allocated treatment, there was a need to reevaluate and increase the sample size to ensure that there would be adequate numbers entered who agreed to the random treatment allocation. Scientifically, prerandomization is inefficient relative to conventional randomization. An ethical concern is that knowledge of the treatment assignment before obtaining informed consent of the patient might lead a physician, who wishes to promote the acceptance rate, to tailor the presentation of the treatment options in a manner to influence the patient's decision.

Because the sample size inflation factor (>1) increases rapidly as the refusal rate increases, it was essential that the refusal rate be kept as low as possible. For example, if the refusal rate were 10, 20, or 30 %, then the corresponding sample size inflation factors would be around 1.6, 2.8, and 6.3, respectively. The accrual rate increased sufficiently following the initiation of prerandomization to complete accrual to the trial although the accrual was extended over more years than most NSABP trials. When the trial closed accrual in 1984, more than 2100 patients had been randomized in equal numbers to the three treatment groups. Of the 2105 patients enrolled in the Protocol B-06 trial who consented to be followed and had follow-up information, 172 (8.2 %) refused their assigned therapy. The refusal rates varied somewhat across the three treatment groups with 11.3 % of patients refusing allocated treatment in the total mastectomy group, 5.2 % refusing in the lumpectomy alone group, and 8.1 % in the lumpectomy plus radiation therapy group. The initial findings from the trial published in the *New England Journal of Medicine* in 1985 provided physicians and women for the first time scientific evidence indicating that survival was essentially equivalent for women receiving lumpectomy to those receiving a mastectomy [29]. These results have subsequently been confirmed through 8, 12, and 20 years of follow-up in subsequent publications in the NEJM [56–59].

There were no easy resolutions to the complex ethical considerations involved with Protocol B-06. There was an unfailing belief among the leadership and clinical investigators that Protocol B-06 was a crucial trial to complete regardless of difficulties and criticisms encountered. More than 2000 dedicated women were willing to commit to participate in a trial spanning almost a decade in spite of the ongoing controversies. Fortunately, with the changes made in the trial design, the original aims were fulfilled. In hindsight, one could pose a number of questions about the ethics of RCTs with highly controversial treatment options based on the experience with Protocol B-06. Are there circumstances where it is better to rely on "expert opinion" or choices favored by the popular media as an alternative to conducting a controversial RCT? Would the patients' or public's interest have been better served by discontinuing the trial because of too slow an accrual rate using conventional randomization and publishing the findings, albeit unreliable, based on an inadequate sample size? Would the patients' or public's interests have been better served to continue to accrue patients utilizing conventional randomization even if the trial was prolonged for several more years? The NSABP response to these questions is apparent in their commitment to complete the RCT and to modify the sequence of steps in their randomization. The conclusions from this trial lead to dramatic alterations in the treatment options available after 1985 to women diagnosed with operable invasive breast cancer. In this instance the prerandomization alleviated sufficiently some ethical concerns of patients and physicians and provided for a paradigm changing trial to be completed. In spite of the success with prerandomization in NSABP B-06, however, classical approaches to randomization and informed consent are the preferred methods.

Although there were more ethical issues associated with Protocol B-06 than there are with the typical RCT involving the comparisons of drug interventions, nonetheless investigators conducting major clinical trials can expect that they will be confronted with complex ethical issues. With close collaboration between the clinical scientists and the statisticians for the trial, often resolutions to ethical concerns can be found that still preserve the scientific integrity of the trial.

33.6.3 Data Integrity

The importance of ensuring the integrity of data collected in clinical trials cannot be overemphasized. While findings from laboratory studies are likely to be eventually challenged if subsequent experiments fail to reproduce the results, it is often infeasible and ethically questionable to consider independent replication of a clinical trial that has been very costly in money, time, and other resources. Therefore, for many reasons it is essential that an RCT provide convincing and credible evidence that can be relied upon for clinical implementation, as well as planning future RCT.

Clinical trials carried out by major cancer cooperative groups have in place many procedures for checking data submitted on an ongoing basis throughout the course of the clinical trial. However, it can be difficult to discriminate between errors in data generation or reporting, which can be prevalent due to misunderstanding or carelessness, and instances of sporadic data falsification or fabrication, which are relatively uncommon. Statistical procedures can be useful for detecting some forms of fraud (see, for example, [60]). Clinical settings are not always optimal for data quality endeavors since RCTs which take many years to conduct must deal with attrition in key staff and/or changes in dedication to the objectives of the RCT:

> It is infinitely more difficult to maintain a level of enthusiasm year after year so that data is collected as meticulously and as thoroughly at the fifth year of study, for example, as at the fifth week. It is the obligation of those who institute and carry out a trial, as well as those who participate, to develop and cooperate in mechanisms to ensure the integrity of the data. Such efforts should not be considered by the investigator as adversary or demonstrating lack of trust. Rather, they are to achieve impeccability ([33], p. 269).

In spite of dedicated commitment to the principles above, the NSABP had occasion during the 1990s to experience firsthand the devastating controversy that can arise when the principles of data integrity, as articulated above, were found to have been violated by Dr. Roger Poisson, a surgeon at St. Luc Hospital in Montreal. It is beyond the scope of this chapter to relate the chronology of events and give our perspectives on the impact of events following the discovery that Dr. Poisson had fabricated or falsified data relating to eligibility on about 7 % of the approximately 1500 patients that he had entered on 22 NSABP trials. The NSABP discovered the problem, the leadership reported it to the appropriate governmental agencies, and assisted throughout the lengthy 3-year governmental investigation that ensued. The NSABP also reanalyzed promptly all trials in which Dr. Poisson had randomized patients which resulted in findings that were nearly identical to those in publications and substantiated the validity of the original conclusions. Although the NSABP had provided convincing information to other academicians and governmental agencies that the findings from NSABP trials were not sensitive to the inclusion or exclusion of data on St. Luc patients, an article published in the Chicago Tribune in March 1994, raised controversies and spread doubt about the results of NSABP trials, especially Protocol B-06, the lumpectomy trial. Events subsequent to the media frenzy that ensued lead to government hearings and serious disruptions to completion of several major NSABP clinical trials, including the first large-scale prevention trial (NSABP P-01). Although eventually the NSABP was able to successfully complete the trials in progress at that time and to continue with its primary mission, the effect of the Poisson episode were profound, not just for NSABP and its leadership, but for all involved in clinical trials. For a more detailed account and insightful perspectives on the nature of what transpired and the consequences for RCTs, we refer the reader to the article by Peto et al. [61] and the discussion in [27] (pp. 553–560).

33.7 Conduct of the Clinical Trial

The written protocol for a clinical trial provides clinical investigators and other professional staff with important information relating to the rationale and conduct of the clinical trial. The protocol helps to assure that the staff at all clinical centers follow common procedures in carrying out the major features of the clinical trial. The protocol is the major document relied upon by review committees in decisions relating to approval and funding. It also contains information relied upon by Ethics Committees or IRBs to ensure that patients rights and safety are well protected, as well as guidance for independent Data Monitoring Committees (DMCs). Different organizations have developed their own preferred formats for the content of a clinical trial protocol, so that there is not one standardized template that can be recommended for breast cancer clinical trials ([27], pp. 160–164) outlines 29 items essential for most protocols describing RCTs and provides a brief discussion of the content for each item. The majority of features are universal within the protocols of all groups that carry out multicenter clinical trials, so that the novice clinical trialist can readily adapt a template in recent use by one of the major cancer cooperative clinical trial groups for the development of a planned RCT.

The protocol does not usually contain detailed information on the organizational structure, administrative procedures, or many of the technical processes relating to data collection, management, and quality control for a clinical trial. These aspects become part of a separate written document, often referred to as the Manual of Operations (MOP). The MOP serves an important role in assisting all trial personnel with conducting the protocol in a manner consistent with the intent of the protocol. A carefully detailed MOP serves a major purpose in assuring the soundness of the data derived in the conduct of the clinical trial. The study protocol and MOP, which may serve for numerous clinical trials conducted by the same cooperative group, require time-consuming careful, often tedious, attention to details by experienced staff. The preparation of these documents prior to implementing a clinical trial may take several months of effort if no prototype is available from a prior trial, but the time involved can help prevent problems during the course of the trial that would lead to substantial delays and changes in approach that can jeopardize the scientific integrity of the clinical trial. Meinert's book *Clinical Trials: Design, Conduct, and Analysis* [62] contains detailed guidance on practical day-to-day aspects of conducting RCTs. The checklists provided in the book can also be utilized when writing the protocol and MOP to ensure that the implementation of a trial is comprehensive in scope.

Over time many features of cancer clinical trials have tended to become standardized across the cooperative clinical trial groups in order to facilitate data completeness and quality, as well as to provide for consistency in comparisons of outcomes across clinical trials utilizing similar patient populations. The International Conference on Harmonization (ICH), which is a collaborative effort of the United States, the European Union, and Japan, has developed numerous useful guidelines that encompass general considerations for clinical trials (ICH E8), good clinical practices (ICH E6), choice of control groups (ICH E10), and sound statistical principles (ICH E9). All guidelines can be readily accessed through their Website (URL: http://www.ich.org). Trials of patients with advanced disease now generally rely on the RECIST criteria for assessing the responsiveness of tumors to treatment, duration of complete response, and duration of overall response [63].

33.7.1 Interim Data Monitoring

Well-defined plans for interim monitoring of data during the course of a clinical trial are essential for the conduct of clinical trials. The primary rationale for interim data monitoring relates to ethical concerns, but there are also scientific concerns that are a part of interim monitoring. Interim monitoring establishes a mechanism to terminate the trial early for several reasons, including: (1) undue serious toxicity occurs; (2) the benefit of the experimental therapy is clearly established; (3) it becomes apparent that there is little or no chance for a clinically important benefit to occur based on the data that have already been accumulated (futility); (4) findings from other clinical trials have affected the need for the ongoing trial; or (5) design or conduct issues have arisen that have compromised the scientific integrity of the trial.

Interim monitoring also serves a role in quality assurance and quality control of the data. There are many potential problems that can occur in data collection and conduct that only become manifest when there is ongoing review of the emerging data in a clinical trial. Incompleteness or inaccuracies in reporting of critical data items that are not identified during routine data editing often become manifest during interim data analyses. Corrective measures can then be undertaken so that the scientific integrity of the entire trial is not jeopardized.

Meinert [64] has listed four monitoring models, which he characterized as: (1) blissful ignorance (nobody looks); (2) ask the statistician (statistical stopping rules decision-making); (3) treater investigator monitoring (monitoring performed by the collective set of study investigators); and (4) watertight separation (monitoring entrusted to a committee independent of the trial investigators). The first model is ethically untenable for the vast majority of cancer clinical trials, since most treatments have the potential for serious adverse events. There are situations in which accrual and treatment may be completed over too short an interval of time to permit interim monitoring of outcomes that leads to an early termination of accrual or ineffective therapy, but these are rare exceptions. The majority of Phase III breast cancer RCTs have a few years of accrual that are followed by additional years of observation for study outcomes.

Both NIH and the FDA have policies relating to interim data monitoring in clinical trials. Since 1998 NIH has required that all clinical trials must have a written approved data and safety monitoring plan. All Phase III trials must have an independent Data Monitoring Committee (DMC). The FDA recommends an independent DMC for "Pivotal" Phase III trials and trials with mortality or irreversible morbidity outcomes.

An independent DMC consists of clinical and basic scientists from relevant disciplinary areas, epidemiologists, biostatisticians, and ethicists or consumer (patient) representatives who are not affiliated with the clinical trial or those individuals who are conducting the clinical trial. The DMC deals with the complex issue of how much evidence in support of the superiority (or inferiority) of one of the treatments should be allowed to accumulate before a trial is stopped and the findings reported. The role of the DMC is particularly challenging when there are multiple outcomes of major interest and/or serious known or potential acute or long-term adverse effects associated with treatment. Usually, the results of statistical tests, where the significance level has been appropriately adjusted for the multiple comparisons involved with interim looks at the data, provide guidance to the DMC in making decisions about whether a trial should continue or not. One objective is to permit early termination of a trial that has a beneficial effect by means of conservative stopping guidelines so that a trial will not stop prior to answering the primary study hypotheses. There are various organizational structures for DMCs, but usually the DMC has responsibilities to the participants in the trial, the study investigators, the sponsor, local IRBs, and regulatory agencies.

The DMC meeting to review interim data generally has four parts. There is an open session that is attended by the sponsor, the Principal Investigator and other key investigators involved with the conduct of the trial, the lead biostatistician for the trial and other Statistical and Data Coordinating Center staff. The trial investigators report on the status of the trial providing information on accrual, data submission, protocol adherence, and other aspects including any serious problems that may have been encountered. There are three practices followed relating to presentation of interim outcome data during the open session. One approach is to present no outcome data. A second approach is to present outcome data for the combined treatment groups. A third approach is to present the outcome data for the treatment groups but to mask the treatment assignments. The third approach may be problematic as differences in treatment begin to emerge during the course of interim monitoring if the behavior of trial investigators is affected by speculation about which treatment group is doing better. Therefore, our preference is not to show outcome data by treatment group, even if masking is maintained, during the open session of the DMC meeting. The second part of the DMC meeting is a closed session during which the DMC reviews unmasked data by treatment group. The trial biostatistician and a representative of the sponsor may be in attendance at the closed session, but typically the trial PI and other clinical investigators are not present for the closed session. Following its review of outcome data during a closed session, the DMC members meet in an executive session to develop their final recommendations based on their review of interim data and other information about the trial. (Sometimes, the formulation of recommendations may be done within the closed session if the DMC does not have major issues to address.) The DMC recommends one of the following options: (1) continue the trial as designed; or (2) continue the trial, but make modifications to the protocol or operational aspects to deal with safety concerns or other addressable problems; or (3) stop the trial. There are many factors that DMCs take into account in formulating recommendations, such as whether the trial is meeting accrual goals, comparability of treatment groups, protocol adherence, study outcomes, safety concerns, coherence of the emerging data and consistency of findings with those from other trials that are available, net benefit based on weighing the benefits and risks, clinical and public import of interim data, and statistical considerations.

The Book Data Monitoring Committees in Clinical Trials: A Practical Perspective by Ellenberg et al. [65] is a valuable nontechnical reference for researchers who would like to become more familiar with the role, responsibilities, and procedures for independent DMCs.

Usually the lead biostatistician for the trial, in consultation with the DMC, develops the detailed plan for interim data analysis. Important considerations include: (1) deciding which outcomes should be monitored; (2) determining how often interim outcome analysis should be performed; and (3) deciding which nonoutcome variables, such as compliance, acute toxicity, long-term adverse events, quality of life, etc., should be included in interim data analyses.

Statistical issues arise in interim data monitoring that relate to repeated significance testing. If the significance level (P-value) for each interim analysis is the same as the P-value for the final analysis, then the Type I error will increase with each analysis conducted. For example, if a significance level of 0.05 is used for each interim analysis, then by the fifth interim analysis, the true Type I error will be 0.14. If there are ten interim analyses, then the error will be 0.20 by the tenth analysis.

Statistical methods have been developed that adjust the Type I error for the number of interim analyses. The earliest approaches to adjusting for multiple tests were the sequential monitoring methods such as SPRT in which statistical testing is done after each study outcome occurs. These methods can be especially useful when the outcome can be evaluated within a short interval of observation following treatment. In most cancer trials, however, interim analysis is done based on group sequential designs that have been adapted to trials in which the outcomes are delayed. The book by Jennison and Turnbull [66] is an excellent resource on the most common statistical approaches to interim monitoring. A typical approach to group sequential monitoring is to monitor the primary outcome once or twice per year after some prespecified minimum number of outcomes has been reported. There is a significance level at each interim analysis determined such that the overall experimentwise Type I error will be maintained at the desired level, say, e.g., 0.05. The data monitoring plan specifies in advance the maximum number of planned interim analyses, which may be based on the projected amount of information (outcomes) projected or on the projected meeting schedule of the DMC.

Some common conventional monitoring techniques are: (1) Pocock's [67] approach, which specifies the same lower nominal significance level at each prespecified interim analysis and final analysis; (2) Haybittle [68] approach, which specifies the same lower nominal significance level at each prespecified interim analysis with the overall significance level at the final analysis; (3) O'Brien and Fleming [69] approach in which the nominal significance levels are lowest for the earliest prespecified interim analysis which increases toward the overall significance level at the final analysis; and (4) Lan and Demets [70] alpha-spending function approach, which provides flexibility in the number and timing of interim analyses. Bayesian methods have also been proposed for interim data monitoring of RCTs, although Bayesian approaches have not been as widely used as the frequentist methods presented above.

Specific methods have also been developed for data monitoring that can be utilized to evaluate when the DMC should consider stopping the trial because the interim outcome data show that it would be unlikely or impossible for the final analysis to have a statistically significant positive result. The statistical approaches for such futility analysis are stochastic curtailment or conditional power [71, 72]. For example, Wieand's et al. [72] proposed a futility stopping rule that the study be stopped if, at 50 % of the expected total information, the estimate of the treatment effect suggests the new therapy is worse than the standard treatment. Recently, a more flexible method has been proposed, which provides a trajectory of stopping boundary due to futility where the negative indication of the new therapy could be at an arbitrary total expectation information point, not affecting the overall Type I and Type II error probabilities [73]. For an unplanned futility analysis, the conditional probability that the test statistic would cross the critical value at the final analysis given the accumulated data can be calculated [74].

Often the statistical procedures for interim data monitoring are called stopping rules. However, most experienced biostatisticians and DMC members prefer to call them guidelines or flags that are used to inform the DMC about when there should be serious discussion of the emerging data relative to the continuation of the trial rather than as strict rules for when the trial should stop, since there are other important factors to consider in addition to the primary efficacy outcome when deciding where to stop a trial and report the findings. The usual statistical interim monitoring strategy will have stopping guidelines for primary efficacy outcomes and may have stopping guidelines for serious adverse outcomes, although the latter may also be monitored without any formal statistical testing relying on the expert judgment of the DMC about when to consider stopping a trial because of undue risk to participants. During its review of the interim analyses the DMC generally relies on ad hoc weighing of the findings for the different outcomes.

The NSABP Breast Cancer Prevention Trial (BCPT), which tested 5 years of tamoxifen versus placebo in double-blind RCT of more than 13,000 women at increased risk of breast cancer, adopted an innovative alternative approach to data monitoring when there are multiple outcomes in a clinical trial [75]. The BCPT, presented complex challenges for interim data monitoring due to the large number of outcomes, both beneficial and deleterious, that the DMC needed to consider in the interim data monitoring. The interim monitoring strategy that was developed incorporated both guidelines for individual outcomes and a composite global index that weighted the individual outcomes according to their life-threatening potential. This more comprehensive strategy which includes formal statistical considerations of net benefit for a treatment may also have advantages for data monitoring in cancer treatment trials.

As another more recent example, the NSABP B-31 study was an interesting phase III 2-stage randomized trial. It was designed to evaluate an incremental effect in overall survival (OS) of a trastuzumab (Herceptin) to a chemo regimen (AC → Taxol) among positive node and HER2 gene positive patients. Since there was strong evidence of cardiac toxicity due to Herceptin, the B-31 trial was planned as a two-stage study. In the first stage, 1000 patients were to be randomized to AC followed by Taxol (ACT) or AC followed by Taxol + Herceptin (ACTH) to compare the cardiac toxicities. If the observed difference in proportion of cardiac events would be less than 4 %, then the second stage would be initiated to accrue an additional 1700 patients for the efficacy analysis of Herceptin based on the OS endpoint. Three formal statistical comparisons were planned to assess excessive cardiotoxicity on the experimental arm.

To design the second stage of the study, it was assumed that the addition of Herceptin would reduce the annual mortality rate by 25 %. It was also assumed that 5 % of patients who were randomized to ACTH arm would fail to begin Herceptin, and an additional 10 % will discontinue their Herceptin therapy uniformly over the 1-year course. These noncompliance assumptions further attenuated the 25 % reduction to 22.8 %. To detect this reduction in mortality with 80 % power, using a two-sided 0.05-level log-rank test, would require that the number of deaths be 480. Thus, if 2700 patients were accrued over 4 years and 9 months, the number of required events would be reached approximately 2 years and 9 months after the closure of accrual, i.e., 7 years and 6 months after the initiation of the study. However, the accrual to this study has stopped early due to strong evidence of efficacy of Herceptin [76]. The cardiac toxicity of Herceptin was reported in Tan-Chiu et al. [77].

Four interim analyses were scheduled prior to the definitive analysis: after 96, 192, 288, and 384 deaths. Asymmetric stopping boundaries were employed based on the O'Brien-Harrington-Fleming method [78]. Because these analyses must be timed to coincide with the semiannual meetings of the NSABP Data Monitoring Committee (DMC), in practice, the numbers of events at each interim analysis usually differ slightly from the plan. If significant deviations were necessary, the nominal levels of significance were to be adjusted by alpha-spending [70].

The NSABP B-31 design did not have the futility [71, 72] component in it, but it would be informative for the Data Monitoring Committee to consider stopping a trial when there is a strong trend that patients in the experimental arm are doing worse than ones in the control arm. To include the futility component, at each interim analysis, consideration may be given to dropping the experimental arm if it is significantly worse than the control arm, e.g., if the estimated hazard ratio versus control exceeds 1, at a prespecified nominal level.

33.8 General Analysis Considerations

The statistical design considerations and operational definitions of the outcome guide the statistical analysis of the primary outcome of the clinical trial. The statistical considerations in the protocol specify the analytic strategy for the primary outcome and major secondary outcomes of the clinical trial.

In order to prevent biased treatment comparisons the primary analysis performed for the majority of trials is the "intention-to-treat (ITT)" analysis which should also be prespecified in the study protocol. Three fundamental principles apply to the ITT analysis. They are: (1) participants in intervention comparisons should be counted in their randomly allocated group; (2) all participants randomly allocated to the intervention group should be counted in the denominator for that treatment; and (3) all events should be included in the intervention comparison for the primary outcome measure. Even for RCTs in which the "Treated Per Protocol (TPP)" analysis has been specified as the primary analysis, as may be done in equivalence trials, there is a need to conduct the ITT analysis and compare the finding to that of the TPP to evaluate possible biases in the TPP analysis. The well-written protocol will contain sufficient information for ITT analysis and TPP analysis datasets.

If a RCT has been well designed and carefully conducted in accordance with a detailed protocol, then the analysis for the primary outcome is often straightforward, although attention to data quality control checks and simple tabular and graphical summaries are important during the preliminary analysis phase to guide specific details of the analysis. Frequently, data inconsistencies not identified during routine editing of the data forms will surface during the preliminary analytic process, particularly when the biostatistician begins looking at multiple cross-tabulations of variables of interest.

The practice of the NSABP Biostatistical Center has been to create analysis files containing all variables that will be analyzed for a specified data cutoff date. The file includes not only original values of variables, but also some variables that are formed by combining information from several variables on the original data forms to facilitate the primary analyses, such as creation of flags and follow-up times for time-to-event analyses, specification of cutoff values for forming categories of interest for continuous variables, transformed data values indicated for certain analyses, etc. These analysis files are helpful for the statistician during the original analysis, and also provide documentation for any subsequent validation of an analysis. A useful preliminary analytic technique is to compute event rates (hazard rates) or outcomes, such as hazard rates for time-to-event outcomes or proportion of events within each level of baseline covariates in order to screen for main prognostic effects and potential interactions of major covariates with the intervention. These screening tabulations provide information useful in developing appropriate strategies to deal with issues, such as colinearity, sparseness in some data categories, missing observations, and unusual combinations of variables in the distributions, in multivariable modeling. For readers who desire more guidance on how to approach preliminary data analyses, Pocock's book, *Clinical Trials: A Practical Approach*, especially Chaps. 13 and 14 [79], is a basic, easily understood reference.

Although the possible outcomes employed in clinical trials may encompass variables of all types, including continuous, binary, categorical, etc., the majority of major RCTs in breast cancer have a time-to-event outcome, such as overall survival or disease-free survival as the primary outcome.

The brief summary of methods in this chapter focuses on some of the relevant considerations for trials where the definitive outcome is analyzed as a time-to-event. There are numerous books and journal articles that provide comprehensive treatment of the theoretical and technical background needed for the conduct of such analyses, and numerous software packages that perform these analyses appropriately, including SAS (SAS Institute Inc., http://www.sas.com), STATA (StataCorp LP, http://www.stata.com), and R (R Core Team, http://www.R-project.org/). We summarize below several conceptual features of the techniques that are most commonly utilized in practice and provide a few illustrative examples of analytic approaches that have broad applicability in modern breast cancer clinical trials.

There is an extensive history of the evolution of methods for survival analysis, but, as noted earlier, the development of methodology employed in cancer trials analyzing event times was greatly stimulated by the establishment of the NCI Cooperative Group Program in the 1950s. The major analytic approaches developed from the late 1950s through the seminal papers by Peto and Peto [80, 81] provided the fundamental approaches that continue to be used in most clinical trials today for testing differences in survival curves and estimating treatment response.

Summarization of time-to-event data typically involves display of data for each treatment in life table format as well as calculation of a test statistic to determine whether the differences between the control group and the experimental group(s) are statistically significant. Two joint outcome variables are associated with each participant in the trial at the calendar date chosen as the cutoff for the analysis. In the simplest example, if the outcome of interest is mortality (and all individuals have been observed until death or the last protocol scheduled follow-up, if alive), then one calculates the observed survival time for each patient from the time of entry to the study using some suitable unit of observation time. For breast cancer clinical trials, it has been customary to use months as the time unit for survival curves. The second variable, referred to as a "dummy variable," is given a value of "0" or "1" depending on whether the patient was alive or dead at the time of last observation. Formally, the term censored is used for patients with a code "0" since if the observation time were extended indefinitely, all patients would eventually die. Since patients enter clinical trials over a period of time, often several years duration, at the time of analysis, patients may be censored administratively at various times due to the early termination of their observation time, but they can contribute to the denominator in calculating a death rate until the time when they are censored at which time they are taken out of the denominator in calculating subsequent event rates.

The classical paper by Cutler and Ederer [82] presents the method for computing the life table from grouped data, which is often denoted as an actuarial life table. The classical Kaplan and Meier [83] method for estimating life table survival utilizes the exact death and censoring times, resulting in the familiar step function graphs found in many publications, where the downward steps in the curve occur when there are deaths. The product-limit estimator for the Kaplan–Meier survival is

$$\widehat{S}(t_k) = \prod_{i=1}^{k} [1 - d_i/N_i]$$

with variance estimated as

$$\widehat{V}\{\widehat{S}(t_k)\} = \widehat{S}(t_k)^2 \sum\nolimits_{i=1}^{k} \{d_i/N_i(N_i - d_i)\},$$

where N_i is the number of individuals who are at risk at time t_i, d_i is the number of individuals who have an event at time t_i, and d_i/N_i is an estimate of the probability of an event at time t_i given survival to a point just prior to time t_i.

Statistical testing to compare the treatment groups is generally based on some version of the log-rank or a related test, as shown below for grouped data. It is convenient to consider the data as a sequence of 2 × 2 tables, in which each table displays, for control and experimental treatment groups, the number of events and censored observations for a particular ordered interval of time as follows:

$$\text{Group A} : d_{iA} n_{iA} - d_{iA}$$
$$\text{Group B} : d_{iB} n_{iB} - d_{iB}$$

where d_{iA} is the number of deaths in group A at failure time t_i, d_{iB} is the number of deaths in group B at failure time t_i, n_{iA} is the number of people at risk in group A at failure time t_i, and n_{iB} is the number of people at risk in group B at failure time t_i.

The test statistic $Z = (O_A - E_A)/\sqrt{V_A}$, where

$$O_A = \sum_i w_i d_{iA},$$

$$E_A = \sum_i w_i \frac{n_{iA} d_i}{n_i}, \quad d_i = d_{iA} + d_{iB}$$

$$V_A = \sum_i w_i^2 d_i \frac{(n_i - d_i) n_{iA} n_{iB}}{(n_i - 1) n_1^2},$$

can be shown to be approximately a normally distributed variable.

If $w_i = 1$, the test is the usual log-rank test statistic. (The log-rank test sometimes includes other designations in recognition of statisticians who developed the earliest versions of the test prior to the publication of the more theoretically motivated presentation in the classical paper by Peto and Peto [80]. For example, the modification of the Mantel and Haenszel [84] by Mantel [85] is a version of the log-rank test.) The log-rank test is known to be optimal when the ratio of event rates between two groups does not change over time. There are also alternative test statistics that can be chosen, which have been shown to be similar to the log-rank test, but with a different weighting factor. Perhaps, the best known alternative to the log-rank test is the version developed by Gehan [86], as a modification of the nonparametric Wilcoxon test to take censoring into account. The statistic above becomes the Gehan Wilcoxon test (also sometimes called Gehan Breslow test) when the weight, $w_i = n_i$ is used in the above formulae. Here the weight function depends on the size of the risk set, so that more weights are put on early differences than later ones. Alternatively, the statistic becomes the Tarone and Ware test [87] when $w_i = \sqrt{n_i}$. The latter two tests are reasonable alternatives to the log-rank for some trials, but it is important that the rationale and choice of the test statistic be a part of the written Statistical Considerations in the protocol. A general form of the weight function has been also proposed to detect both early differences and late differences depending on the parameter that is raised to the power of Kaplan–Meier estimates [88].

When stratified randomization has been used, then intervention effects should be summarized within strata and then a combined test across strata utilized when computing the test statistics. Properties of many tests and estimation procedures often depend on "large sample theory" to provide approximations, as well as often other assumptions relating to normality and equality of variances among the treatment groups. Software for exact statistical tests, such as XACT and LOGXACT, are also now available for testing when sample sizes are not sufficiently large for use of large sample theory (Cytel: Statistical Software and Services, www.cytel.com). Resampling methods can be used for obtaining standard errors or confidence intervals when exact inference is not available or assumptions are violated [89].

33.8.1 Modeling Treatment Effects with Multivariable Models

The major utility of modeling treatment effects often relates to the testing of prespecified biological hypotheses about the relationship between patient prognostic factors and outcome, such as in the NSABP trials relating hormone receptors to treatment effectiveness in the trials employing tamoxifen, or adjusting the treatment effect for selected patient prognostic factors. Generally, the log-rank analysis, as described above, appropriately taking into account any stratification variables, will be the primary analysis. However, there is often a desire to adjust other possibly continuous prognostic factors for any imbalances as a supportive analysis using multivariable models. There may also be an interest in examining whether there are any treatment interactions with selected prognostic factors. A well-written protocol will include discussion about the rationale for models and details of whether they will be utilized in testing prespecified hypotheses or for exploratory analyses. The Statistical Considerations should incorporate how the models will be estimated, what approaches will be utilized for evaluating fit, and details on how the experimental error will be controlled.

Evaluation of potential subgroups should be based on findings of interaction tests, preferably prespecified, not on findings in subgroup comparisons of treatment effects. Quantitative interactions in treatment effects with covariates are expected to occur frequently and are model dependent. Qualitative interactions of covariates with treatment effects, in which some patients have a positive response and other patients a negative treatment response, are not model dependent, but do not occur frequently in practice. Statisticians are generally very cautious in approaching subgroup analyses, particularly when hypotheses about interactions have not been specified in advance of the analysis.

The Cox proportional hazards model has become the most popular for modeling time-to-event data since the publication of the paper by Cox [81]. Prior to that time there were a number of parametric models based on distributions such as the exponential, Weibull, or logistic model (choosing a fixed binary outcome, e.g., 5-year survival), that incorporated prognostic factors as covariates. There are several reasons why the Cox model has nearly universal appeal to statisticians. The most important rationale for its use is that it is an extension of the log-rank test statistic. Briefly, if $\lambda_0(t)$ is the event rate in the control group, $\lambda_1(t)$ is the event rate in the experimental treatment group, and X_{ij} is the jth covariate for the ith patient, then

$$\lambda_1(t_i) = \lambda_0(t_i)\exp\left(\sum_{j=1}^{k}\beta_j x_{ij}\right).$$

The flexibility of this model is great since, unlike the earlier parametric models, the baseline event (or hazard) rate is arbitrary and can be separated from modeling of the covariates; therefore, the event rates in both groups may vary over time and only the "relative risk" (i.e., ratio of event rates) is assumed to be constant with time. In spite of its popularity, there are still circumstances in which the proportionality assumption is questionable or when other models may be preferred, such as when a mechanistic model is suggested based on an underlying biological rationale. The proportional hazards model can be used to compare treatment groups adjusting for covariates and to test for statistical interaction of treatment with specific covariates as an assist in identifying subgroups. Several NSABP Protocols have entailed extensive multivariable modeling to characterize interactions between prognostic factors and treatment outcome to test biological hypotheses. One notable example is NSABP Protocol B-09 in which an apparent qualitative interaction between hormone receptors and mortality emerged in multivariable modeling [90]. Although the subgroup analyses were anticipated at the time of protocol design, the qualitative nature of the interaction was unexpected, necessitating considerable additional analyses and cautious interpretation about whether the findings were a rare chance occurrence or could be attributable to the treatment. Interestingly, the findings also motivated the development of new methods for testing specifically for qualitative interaction [91].

Additional considerations apply in modeling variables that vary over time following randomization. Failure to recognize and/or analyze appropriately time-related variables has occurred and may have contributed to a confusing literature on some important questions in breast cancer clinical trials. In 1981 a paper in the *New England Journal of Medicine* presented an analysis of total dose of chemotherapy received by breast cancer patients in a clinical trial of chemotherapy versus control that concluded that the size of the treatment effect was related to the total amount of chemotherapy received over multiple courses of therapy [92]. Unfortunately, the statistical method employed did not take into account the time-related nature of the total dose received.

In order to receive a high total dose, patients had to survive free of recurrence for most of the time planned for courses of therapy. We published a commentary and showed results for patients receiving placebo in an NSABP trial, using the method apparently employed in the paper. We illustrated that the outcome and amount of drug were inextricably linked such that even patients who received more placebo did better than patients who received less placebo. When more appropriate methods, such as a Cox model with a time-varying covariate, were used, the apparent dose response for the placebo, as well as that for the chemotherapy treated patients, was no longer present [93]. A second example, where a time-varying covariate analysis provided useful insights into a biological hypothesis, was in the analysis of ipsilateral breast cancer reoccurrence in patients treated with or without irradiation to the breast following lumpectomy (NSABP Protocol B-06) [94].

33.8.2 Multiplicity Considerations

Issues of multiplicity which influence the validity of the statistical significance tests arise in many contexts in clinical trials. They are often an important concern in interpreting the statistical tests and estimated treatment effects properly. Some of the typical situations in which multiplicity can become problematic, if not recognized and properly addressed in the analyses, include more than two treatment groups, multiple outcome measures, measurements over time of the same outcome measure, subgroup analyses, and interim data analyses. One of the most common approaches in the past used to control the Type I error probability was the Bonferroni inequality in which the nominal significance level was divided by the number of statistical tests employed. The resulting value was then used for each of the pairwise statistical tests to preserve the overall experimental error at the desired significance level. More recent papers have shown that the Bonferroni approach is more conservative than desirable in most multiplicity testing situations. The papers by Hochberg [95] and Cook and Farewell [96] provide relevant discussion of multiplicity considerations and approaches useful for current clinical trials.

33.8.3 Analysis of Multiple Outcomes Under Competing Risks

In clinical trial data, one of the popular primary outcomes is disease-free survival (DFS), defined as any first events consisting of local, regional, or distant recurrence of the original cancer, a new cancer other than the original one, and deaths prior to any aforementioned diseases. However, investigators are often more interested in making statistical inference on a subset of those first events, which needs to be cast over the competing risks setting. For example, radiation oncologist may be only interested in looking at the local or regional recurrences, to investigate whether irradiation could help reducing the recurrence rate in local areas around the original cancer [97]. Also in breast cancer studies, investigators may be interested in knowing whether a new therapy could reduce the rate of breast cancer-related death alone in the presence of nonbreast cancer deaths.

33.8.3.1 One Sample Case

Investigators sometimes are interested in estimating proportions of cause-specific events in one group. For example, in the NSABP B-14 protocol that studied the efficacy of the hormonal therapy with tamoxifen, a serious side effect was endometrial cancer. Estimation of the proportion of the endometrial cancer in tamoxifen group in this case would require consideration of other events that may have precluded the event of interest, such as death prior to developing the endometrial cancer. Statistical inference on a subset of the DFS events is usually based on the cumulative proportion of the events of particular interest (cause-specific events). One possible, but misleading, approach would be to censor the other events of no interest at their event times and estimate the cumulative probability of cause-specific events using 1-Kaplan–Meier (1-KM) estimates. It is, however, well known that this approach overestimates the true probabilities [98–101]. One way of removing the bias is to use the cumulative incidence function [102]. Gooley et al. [103] nicely provide a more intuitive interpretation of the 1-Kaplan–Meier approach and the cumulative incidence function approach. Another naïve way of removing the bias would be to rearrange the observed survival data, pretending that the events of no interest had never happened [104], so that they are always in the risk sets at observed failure times. The following example compares the 1-KM and nonparametric cumulative incidence methods.

33.8.3.2 Comparing 1-KM Method and Nonparametric Cumulative Incidence Approach in NSABP B-04 Data

In this example, we use a dataset from one of the Phase III trials conducted by the NSABP (B-04 study). The NSABP B-04 study evaluated the endpoint of overall survival to investigate whether a less aggressive surgical procedure (total mastectomy) is equivalent to the traditional mastectomy. The patients in this trial have been followed more than 30 years for cancer recurrence and mortality, so the B-04 follow-up data are often viewed as a natural history in breast cancer mortality without any adjuvant therapy. Fisher et al. [58, 59] presented an analysis result of the 25-year follow-up data from the B-04 study.

A total of 1665 patients (1079 node-negative; 586 node-positive) were originally randomized to five treatment groups; three groups in node-negative (radical mastectomy, total mastectomy + irradiation, total mastectomy) and two groups in node-positive (radical mastectomy, total mastectomy + irradiation). A subset of 586 node-positive patients will be used in this example.

Investigators in breast cancer research are often interested in evaluating an effect of a therapeutic agent in terms of reducing breast-cancer-related deaths only, in the presence of other causes of deaths. In this analysis, we will define deaths following the breast cancer events to be breast-cancer-related deaths, and nonbreast-cancer-related deaths otherwise. Figure 33.1 shows the comparison between the two methods in terms of estimating the proportion of breast-cancer-related deaths as a function of time in the presence of competing nonbreast-cancer-related deaths (dashed line). As mentioned earlier, the estimated curve from the 1-KM approach (dotted line) tend to overestimate the proportion of breast-cancer-related deaths compared to one from the cumulative incidence approach (solid line).

There also have been efforts to parameterize the cumulative incidence function completely [105–107] or partially [108] using popular distributions such as exponential or (extended) Weibull distributions. The key idea in parameterizing the cumulative incidence function is that the overall events are partitioned into different types of cause-specific events under competing risks, so the maximum proportion of each type of cause-specific events is less than 1 (improper). When the parametric assumption is correct, the parametric approach provides more accurate results in terms of bias and variation of the estimator compared to the nonparametric methods [106, 108]. The major advantage of the nonparametric approach is no need for an assumption for the baseline distribution of true failure time distribution. Therefore, nonparametric approaches may merit the designing stage of a study under competing risks while parametric methods may provide more accurate inference for ad hoc analysis of competing risks data if the parametric assumption can be justified.

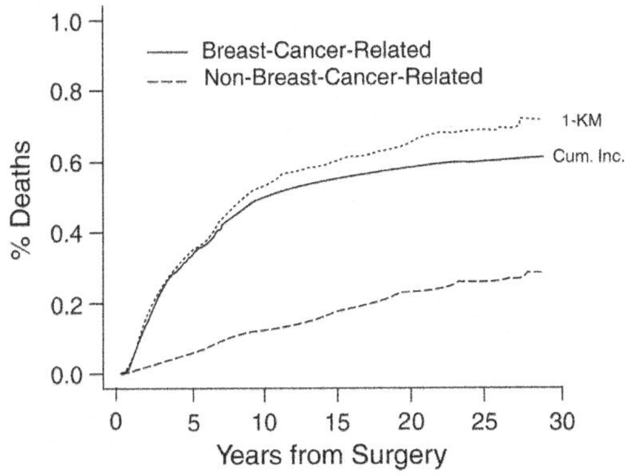

Fig. 33.1 Comparison of the 1-KM estimates and cumulative incidence estimates in NSABP B-04 data

33.8.3.3 Two-Sample Comparison

Investigators are often interested in comparing two or more failure time distributions with censoring under competing risks. For example, in randomized breast cancer studies, a new treatment may be given to one group of patients whereas the patients in the other group are on a conventional therapy or in placebo. The investigators may be interested in whether the new therapy delayed local or regional recurrences by comparing the cumulative probabilities of local or regional recurrences over time between the two groups. Pepe and Mori [101] proposed a two-sample test statistic for this type of comparison. Earlier Gray [104] proposed a (stratified) K-sample test statistic to compare the subdistribution cumulative probabilities, which has been implemented as a procedure *cuminc* in the *cmprsk* software package in R (http://www.r-project.org).

33.8.3.4 Regression on Cumulative Incidence Function

Regression model is useful in evaluating the effects of important prognostic factors in breast cancer on the subdistributions of cause-specific events, or evaluating interactions between treatment and prognostic factors. Fine and Gray [109] proposed a semiparametric proportional hazards model for subdistributions. This approach has been implemented as a function *crr* in the *cmprsk* software package in R. Jeong and Fine [110] proposed a parametric regression model on cumulative incidence function by assuming the Gompertz distribution [111, 112] for the baseline cumulative hazard function under the generalized odds rate model [113].

33.8.3.5 Design Under Competing Risks; Sample Size and Loss of Power

Recently, the primary endpoints in breast cancer clinical trials have been more specifically defined such as breast cancer recurrence [114]. In such designs, it would be more efficient to consider pattern of other competing events in the designing stage. Latouche et al. [115] provides a sample size formula under competing risks as

$$n = \frac{(u_{\alpha/2} + u_{\beta})^2}{(\ln \theta)p(1-p)\psi}.$$

In the formula above, p is the proportion of patients randomly allocated to the experimental group, the parameter θ is the subdistribution hazard ratio, and the parameter y controls the proportion of cause-specific events of interest. Thus the sample size will be affected by both the subdistribution hazard ratio and proportion of cause-specific events of interest. For example, if there is no other competing events such as in the DFS endpoint that typically includes any first event, the hazard ratio can be estimated from the previously observed distribution of DFS events, and ψ will be 1. However, if only a subdistribution of local or regional events is considered, $\psi < 1$ and the subdistribution hazard ratio will be affected by the pattern of other competing events. Even when it is assumed that the subdistribution hazard ratio in local or regional events and the hazard ratio in DFS are almost identical, a bigger sample size is still needed if $\psi < 1$, or in other words, the power will decrease if the sample size is calculated by assuming $\psi = 1$ in this case. In general, a substantial increase in sample size, or substantial loss of power, would be expected, if the absolute value of the hazard ratio in local or regional events is smaller than the hazard ratio in DFS *and* the proportion of cause-specific events is also small.

33.8.4 Building and Validating Prediction Models

After a clinical trial is conducted, it would be meaningful to build a prediction model to guide physicians how to treat their patients or design future studies. A simple example can be modeling the effects of patients' baseline characteristics on development of cardiac events, as in the NSABP B-31 study, such as congested heart failure or cardiac death in cardiotoxic treatment regimen [77]. In another example, a model can be built to predict the recurrence rate among tamoxifen-treated patients given information on their gene signatures [116]. A simplest approach would be to evaluate each gene effect on time-to-recurrence in the univariate Cox proportional hazards model (supervised) and select top genes to be included in the prediction model based on a stringent criterion such as the false discovery rate (FDR; [117, 118]) approach, adjusting for multiple comparisons. In case that the number of selected genes is large, a principal component regression modeling has been recently proposed to account for a possible correlation structure among genes [119]. After analyzing the multivariate Cox model including the final list of genes or principal components, a linear combination of the estimates of regression coefficients and covariate values from the analyzed cohort can be rescaled between 0 and 100 as a score. So when a patient visits a clinic, a score can be calculated based on the developed model to predict his/her recurrence probability, which might facilitate evaluation of risk/benefit aspects of a potentially toxic chemo- or hormonal therapy regimen.

Once a prediction model is built, it needs to be validated. The internal model validation process usually evaluates the abilities of calibration and discrimination of the developed model [120]. Both calibration and discrimination measure the degree of agreement between the predicted and observed outcomes. Specifically, calibration refers to bias. For example, if an *average* predicted probability of breast cancer recurrence in a group of patients is very close to the observed counterpart, the prediction model is considered to have good calibration ability. Discrimination measures the association at a more *individualized* level. For example, a commonly used quantity for evaluating the discrimination ability is so-called *C*-index [121], which measures the proportion of all possible usable pairs of patients in which the predictions and observed outcomes are concordant. For survival data, the usable pairs only include ones, at least one of whom has experienced an event. The *C*-index can be also interpreted as the area under the receiver operating characteristics (ROC) curve [122], ranging from 0.5 to 1 [123]. The *C*-index value closer to 1 would imply a better ability of discrimination of the model. Once a model is validated internally, including a bias correction step, the final model can be validated externally in a new data set collected from the similar population.

33.8.5 Interpretation

Interpretation of findings from RCTs should adhere to the ITT principle that guides the analysis of data. If randomized subjects are withdrawn from the analyses, there is a concern about the potential for biased results. Interpretation of the findings should always focus on the primary hypothesis tested with reliance on the overall estimated intervention effect and its confidence intervals. Adverse effects of treatment should also be discussed fully in a manner that elucidates the net benefit of the treatment. The CONSORT statements, which are referred to in Sect. 33.9, provide many additional insights into the appropriate manner to summarize and interpret the findings from RCTs.

Subgroup analyses have been an ongoing topic for debate in clinical trials methodology. Recent articles in clinical journals highlight the need for improvement in strategies for the conduct and reporting of subgroup analyses [124, 125]. Subgroup analyses of baseline characteristics should be limited in number, preferably prespecified, secondary to the overall study conclusion, and supported by formal statistical interaction tests. In other words, tests of significance within individual subgroups are not appropriate for deciding when to show individual subgroups. Issues of multiplicity of testing, as discussed in Sect. 33.8.2, are important to take into account. Subgroup analyses of post-randomization variables, such as adherence to protocol medication or intermediate disease markers, should be approached cautiously utilizing methods that have been developed for time-varying covariates or serial markers. Unless the RCT has been specifically designed to test variables such as total dose, dose intensity or dose timing, analyses of these factors should be interpreted as exploratory in nature. They may provide directions for hypotheses that are testable in future clinical trials. Subgroup findings other than those that have been predefined in the protocol should also be considered as hypothesis generating. At no stage in the analysis should the randomized treatment allocation be compromised.

33.9 Reporting and Publication

There has been a coordinated effort over the past 10 years to improve the quality of journal articles reporting the primary findings of RCTs. Most notable among these initiatives has been the Consolidated Standards of Reporting Trials (CONSORT) statement, which incorporates a systematic checklist recommended for structuring a publication that encompasses the contents of the title, abstract, introduction, methods, results, and discussion. The CONSORT statement also recommends inclusion of a flow chart that describes in detail the flow of patients in the trial from initial registration and randomization, as well as the reasons for attrition in the number of patients included in the analyses of the completed trial. Since publication of the original CONSORT statement which dealt with guidelines for parallel group trials, the CONSORT investigators have developed analogous guidelines for reporting noninferiority and equivalence trials [126, 127], cluster-randomized trials [128], nonpharmacologic treatments [129, 130], reporting results of harmful effects [131], and constructing informative abstracts [132, 133]. The CONSORT guidelines for parallel group designs have undergone some revisions since their original publication [134]; therefore, it is important to consult the most recent versions of the guidelines when preparing a paper for publication ([135–138]; and the Website http://www.consort-statement.org/) for the most recent versions of guidelines.

Following the publication of the original CONSORT guidelines several major journals, such as *Lancet* and the *New England Journal of Medicine*, require that papers reporting the findings of RCTs that are submitted for publication adhere to the CONSORT guidelines. Regardless of whether a specific journal requires following the CONSORT guideline, key investigators and biostatisticians who participate in the preparation of manuscripts should be familiar with the CONSORT statement and make every effort to adhere to the principles embodied in their conceptualization. Even for RCTs in which there are complex designs that may not conform exactly to the specific content provided in some of the CONSORT guidelines, they provide much useful guidance that can be adapted to enhance the quality of the manuscript.

33.10 Clinical Trial Overviews

The Early Breast Cancer Treatment Collaborative Group (EBCTCG), established by Sir Richard Peto, Oxford University, in the 1980s pools data from all known RCTs in order to determine which, if any, adjuvant therapies have an impact on survival. The first systematic overview demonstrated that there were indeed improvements in survival associated with systemic adjuvant tamoxifen and chemotherapy. The EBCTCG has continued to compile data from new RCTs and update follow-up information on all RCTs every 5 years. The papers from the EBCTCG, which synthesize, the worldwide data on various treatment questions, have been influential both in clinical practice and in providing information useful for designing new RCTs ([139–148]; Website, http://www.ctsu.ox.ac.uk/projects/ebctcg). The merits of the overviews depend upon having data from all properly randomized clinical trials that have followed all patients randomized for many years. Helpful guidelines are available for conducting overviews for researchers who wish to conduct formal statistical review of evidence from related RCTs [149].

Ultimately, the most convincing evidence on specific interventions comes from well-designed and conducted randomized trials on breast cancer that have sufficient numbers of patients to identify small to moderate sized differences in survival outcomes.

References

1. Peto R, Boreham J, Clarke M, Davies C, Beral V. UK and USA breast cancer deaths down 25 % in year 2000 at ages 20–69 years. Lancet. 2000;355(9217):1822.
2. Peto R, Pike MC, Armitage P, Breslow NE, Cox DR, Howard SV, et al. Design and analysis of randomized clinical trials requiring prolonged observation of each patient. I. Introduction and design. Br J Cancer. 1976;34(6):585–612.
3. Peto R, Pike MC, Armitage P, Breslow NE, Cox DR, Howard SV, et al. Design and analysis of randomized clinical trials requiring prolonged observation of each patient. II. Analysis and examples. Br J Cancer. 1977;35(1):1–39.
4. Lilienfeld AM. Ceteris paribus: the evolution of the clinical trial. Bull Hist Med. 1982;56:1–18.
5. Witkosky SJ. The evil that has been said of doctors: extracts from early writers. Trans. with Annotations by T.C. Minor, vol. 41/New Series 22. The Cincinnati Lancet-Clinic; 1889. p. 447–8.
6. Paré A. Les oeuvres de M. Ambroise Paré conseiller, et premier chirurgien du Roy avec les figures & portraicts tant de l'Anatomie que des instruments de Chirurgie, & de plusieurs Monstres. Paris: Gabriel Buon; 1575.
7. Bull JP. The historical development of clinical therapeutic clinical trials. J Chronic Dis. 1959;10:218–48.
8. Lind J. A treatise of the scurvy. In three parts. Containing an inquiry into the nature, causes and cure, of that disease. Together with a critical and chronological view of what has been published on the subject. Edinburgh: Printed by Sands, Murray and Cochran for A. Kincaid and A. Donaldson; 1753.

9. Louis PCA. The applicability of statistics to the practice of medicine. Lon Med Gaz. 1837;20:488–91.
10. Double M. The inapplicability of statistics to the practice of medicine. Lon Med Gaz. 1837.
11. Fisher RA. The arrangement of field experiments. J Ministry Agric. 1926;33:503–13.
12. Fisher RA, McKenzie WA. Studies in crop variation. II the manurial response of different potato varieties. J Agric Sci. 1923;13:315.
13. Medical Research Council. Streptomycin in Tuberculosis Trials Committee. Streptomycin treatment of pulmonary tuberculosis. Br Med J. 1948;2:769–83.
14. Armitage P. Trials and errors: the emergence of clinical statistics. J Roy Stat Soc Ser A. 1983;146:321–34.
15. Cancer Chemotherapy National Service Center. The national program of cancer chemotherapy research. Cancer Chemother Rep. 1960;1:5–34.
16. Henderson WG, Lavori PW, Peduzzi P, Collins JF, Sather MR, Feussner JR. Cooperative studies program, US Department of Veterans Affairs. In: Redmond CK, Colton T, editors. Biostatistics in clinical trials. Wiley; 2001. p. 99–115.
17. Sylvester R. European Organization for Research and Treatment of Cancer (EORTC). In: Redmond CK, Colton T, editors. Biostatistics in clinical trials. Wiley; 2001. p. 191.
18. Fisher B. NSABP and advances in the treatment of breast cancer. In: Redmond CK, Colton T, editors. Biostatistics in clinical trials. Wiley; 2001. p. 310–21.
19. Schneiderman MA, Gehan EA. History, early cancer and heart disease trials. In: Redmond CK, Colton T, editors. Biostatistics in clinical trials. Chichester: Wiley; 2001. p. 227–35.
20. Zelen M, Gehan E, Glidewell O. Biostatistics. In: Hoogstraten, editor. Cancer research: impact of the cooperative groups. Paris: Masson; 1980. p. 291–312.
21. Hill AB. The clinical trial III. In: Statistical methods in clinical and preventive medicine. London: E and S Livingstone; 1962. p. 291.
22. Ellenberg JH. Biostatistical collaboration in medical research. Biometrics. 1990;46:1–32.
23. Simon R. Optimal two-stage designs for phase II clinical trials. Control Clin Trials. 1989;10:1–10.
24. Thall PF, Simon R. Practical Bayesian guidelines for phase IIB clinical trials. Biometrics. 1994;50:337–49.
25. Thall PF, Simon R. A Bayesian approach to establishing sample size and monitoring criterion for phase II clinical trials. Control Clin Trials. 1994;15:463–81.
26. Bryant J, Day R. Incorporating toxicity considerations into the design of two-stage phase II clinical trials. Biometrics. 1995;51:1372–83.
27. Piantadosi S. Clinical trials: a methodologic perspective, 2nd edn. Wiley-Interscience; 2005.
28. Schwartz D, Lellouch J. Explanatory and pragmatic attitudes in therapeutic trials. J Chronic Dis. 1967;20:637–48.
29. Fisher B, Bauer M, Margolese R, Poisson R, Pilch Y, Redmond C, et al. Five-year results of a randomized clinical trial comparing total mastectomy and segmental mastectomy with or without radiation in the treatment of breast cancer. N Engl J Med. 1985;312:665–73.
30. Fisher B, Redmond C, Brown A, Wickerham DL, Wolmark N, Allegra J, Escher G, Lippman M, Savlov E, Wittliff J, et al. Influence of tumor estrogen and progesterone receptor levels on the response to tamoxifen and chemotherapy in primary breast cancer. J Clin Oncol. 1983;1(4):227–41.
31. Fisher B, Wickerham DL, Brown A, Redmond CK. Breast cancer estrogen and progesterone receptor values: their distribution, degree of concordance, and relation to number of positive axillary nodes. J Clin Oncol. 1983;1(6):349–58.
32. Fisher B, Redmond CK, Fisher ER. Evolution of knowledge related to breast cancer heterogeneity: a 25-year retrospective. J Clin Oncol. 2008;26:2068–71.
33. Redmond CK, Fisher B. Design of the controlled clinical trial. In: Pilch YF, editor. Surgical oncology. McGraw-Hill; 1984. p. 254–72.
34. Fleming TR, DeMets DL. Surrogate endpoints in clinical trials: are we being misled? Ann Int Med. 1996;125:605–13.
35. Wittes J. Randomized treatment allocation. In: Redmond CK, Colton T, editors. Biostatistics in clinical trials. Wiley; 2001. p. 384–92.
36. Rockette HE, Redmond CK, Fisher B. Impact of randomized clinical trials on therapy of primary breast cancer: the NSABP overview. Control Clin Trials. 1982;3:209–25.
37. Investigators Writing Group WHI. Risks and benefits of estrogen plus progesterone in healthy postmenopausal women. J Am Med Assoc. 2002;288:321–33.
38. Day SJ. Blinding or masking. In: Redmond CK, Colton T, editors. Biostatistics in clinical trials. Wiley; 2001.
39. Schumi J, Wittes JT. Through the looking glass: understanding non-inferiority. Trials. 2011;12:106. http://www.trialsjournal.com/content/12/1/106.
40. Latakos E. Sample size determination. In: Colton T, Redmond CK, editors. Biostatistics in clinical trials. Wiley; 2001.
41. Lakatos E, Lan KKG. A comparison of sample size methods for the logrank statistic. Stat Med. 1992;11:179–91.
42. Shuster JJ. CRC handbook of sample size guidelines for clinical trials. Boca Raton, FL: CRC Press; 1990.
43. Press WH, Teukolsky SA, Vetterling WT, Flannery BP. Numerical recipes in C: the art of scientific computing. 2nd ed. Cambridge: Cambridge University Press; 1992.
44. Efron B. Forcing a sequential experiment to be balanced. Biometrika. 1971;58:403–17.
45. Begg CB, Iglewicz BA. A treatment allocation procedure for sequential clinical trial. Biometrics. 1980;36:81–90.
46. Pocock SJ, Simon R. Sequential treatment assignment with balancing for prognostic factors in the controlled clinical trial. Biometrics. 1975;31:103–15.
47. Cancer Chemotherapy National Service Center. The Nuremberg code, 1947. Br Med J. 1996;313:1449.
48. World Medical Association. Declaration of Helsinki (1964, 1975, 1983, 1989, 1996). Br Med J. 1996;313:1449–50.
49. National Commission for Protection of Human Subjects of Biomedical and Behavioral Research. The Belmont Report: Ethical Principles and Guidelines for the Protection of Human Subjects of Research. Washington, DC: DHEW Publication Number (OS) 78-0012. Appendix I, DHEW Publication No. (OS) 78-0013; Appendix II, DHEW Publication No. (OS) 78-0014; 1978.
50. Hill AB. Medical ethics and controlled trials. Br Med J. 1963;1:1043.
51. Zelen M. A new design for randomized clinical trials. N Engl Med. 1979;300:1242.
52. Rutstein DR. Ethical aspects of human experimentation. Daedalus. J Am Acad Arts Sci. 1969; Spring:523.
53. Royall RM, Bartlett RH, Cornell RG. Ethics and statistics in randomized clinical trials. Stat Sci. 1991;6:52–88.
54. Byar DP. The use of data bases and historical controls in treatment comparisons. Recent Results Cancer Res. 1988;111:95–8.
55. Taylor KM, Margolese RG, Soskolne CL. Physicians' reasons for not entering eligible patients in a randomized clinical trial of surgery for breast cancer. N Engl J Med. 1984;310:1363–7.
56. Fisher B, Redmond C, Poisson R, Margolese R, Wolmark N, Wickerham DL, et al. Eight-year results of a randomized clinical trial comparing total mastectomy and lumpectomy with or

without irradiation in the treatment of breast cancer. N Engl J Med. 1989;320:822–8.
57. Fisher B, Anderson S, Redmond C, Wolmark N, Wickerham DL, Cronin W. Reanalysis and results after 12 years of follow-up in a randomized clinical trial comparing total mastectomy with lumpectomy with or without irradiation in the treatment of breast cancer. N Engl J Med. 1995;333(22):1456–61.
58. Fisher B, Anderson S, Bryant J, Margolese RG, Deutsch M, Fisher ER, Jeong JH, Wolmark N. Twenty-year follow-up of a randomized trial comparing total mastectomy, lumpectomy, and lumpectomy plus irradiation for the treatment of invasive breast cancer. N Engl J Med. 2002;347(16):1233–41.
59. Fisher B, Jeong J, Anderson S, et al. Twenty-five year findings from a randomized clinical trial comparing radical mastectomy with total mastectomy and with total mastectomy followed by radiation therapy. N Engl J Med. 2002;347:567–75.
60. Buyse M, Evans S. Fraud in clinical trails. In: Redmond C, Colton TE, editors. Biostatistics in clinical trials. Wiley; 2001. p. 200–8.
61. Peto R, Collins R, Sackett D, et al. The trials of Dr. Bernard Fisher: a European perspective on an American episode. Control Clin Trials. 1997;18:1–13.
62. Meinert CL. Clinical trials. Design, conduct and analysis. New York: Oxford University Press; 1985.
63. Therasse P, Arbuck SG, Eisenhauer EA, et al. New guidelines to evaluate the response to treatment in solid tumors. J Natl Cancer Inst. 2000;92:205–16.
64. Meinert CL. Workshop on interim data monitoring. Annual meeting of the society for clinical trials; 1996.
65. Ellenberg S, Fleming T, DeMets D. Data monitoring committees in clinical trials: a practical perspective. West Sussex, England: Wiley; 2002.
66. Jennison C, Turnbull BW. Group sequential methods with applications to clinical trials. Chapman & Hall/CRC; 2000.
67. Pocock SJ. Group sequential methods in the design and analysis of clinical trials. Biometrika. 1977;64:191–9.
68. Haybittle JL. Repeated assessment of results in clinical trials of cancer treatment. Br J Radiol. 1971;44:793–7.
69. O'Brien PC, Fleming TR. A multiple testing procedure for clinical trials. Biometrics. 1979;35:549–56.
70. Lan KG, Demets DL. Discrete sequential boundaries for clinical trials. Biometrika. 1983;70:659–63.
71. Pepe MS, Anderson GL. Two-stage experimental designs: early stopping with a negative result. J Roy Stat Soc Ser C (Appl Stat). 1992;41:181–90.
72. Wieand S, Schroeder G, O'Fallon JR. Stopping when the experimental regimen does not appear to help. Stat Med. 1994;13:1453–8.
73. Anderson JR, High R. Alternatives to the standard Fleming, Harrington, and O'Brien futility boundary. Clin Trials. 2011;8:270–6.
74. Proschan MA, Lan KKG, Wittes JT. Statistical monitoring of clinical trials: a unified approach. New York: Springer; 2006.
75. Redmond CK, Costantino JP, Colton T. Challenges in monitoring the breast cancer prevention trial. In: DeMets DL, Furberg CD, Friedman L, editors. Data monitoring in clinical trials: a case studies approach. Springer; 2006. p. 118–35.
76. Romond EH, Perez EA, Bryant J, et al. Trastuzumab plus adjuvant chemotherapy for operable HER2-positive breast cancer. N Engl J Med. 2005;353(16):1673–84.
77. Tan-Chiu E, Yothers G, Romond E, et al. Assessment of cardiac dysfunction in a randomized trial comparing doxorubicin and cyclophosphamide followed by paclitaxel, with or without trastuzumab as adjuvant therapy in node-positive, human epidermal growth factor receptor 2-overexpressing breast cancer: NSABP B-31. J Clin Oncol. 2005;23:7811–9.
78. Fleming TR, Harrington DP, O'Brien PC. Designs for group sequential tests. Control Clin Trials. 1984;5:348–61.
79. Pocock SJ. Clinical trials: a practical approach. New York: Wiley; 1983.
80. Peto R, Peto J. Asymptotically efficient rank invariant test procedures (with discussion). J Roy Stat Soc Ser A (Stat Soc). 1972;135:185–206.
81. Cox DR. Regression models and life-tables (with discussion). J Roy Stat Soc Ser B. 1972;34:187–202.
82. Cutler SJ, Ederer F. Maximum utilization of the life table method in analyzing survival. J Chronic Dis. 1958;8:699–712.
83. Kaplan EL, Meier P. Nonparametric estimator from incomplete observations. J Am Stat Assoc. 1958;53:457–81.
84. Mantel N, Haenszel W. Statistical aspects of the analysis of data from retrospective studies for disease. J Natl Cancer Inst. 1959;22:719–48.
85. Mantel N. Evaluation of survival data and two new rank order statistics arising in its consideration. Cancer Chemother Rep. 1967;50:163–70.
86. Gehan EA. A generalized two sample Wilcoxon statistic for comparing arbitrarily censored data. Biometrika. 1965;52:650–3.
87. Tarone RE, Ware J. On distribution free tests for equality of survival functions. Biometrika. 1977;64:156–60.
88. Fleming TR, Harrington DP. A class of hypothesis tests for one and two samples of censored survival data. Commun Stat. 1981;10:763–94.
89. Efron B. Bootstrap methods: another look at the jackknife. Ann Stat. 1979;7:1–26.
90. Fisher B, Redmond C, Brown A, et al. Treatment of primary breast cancer with chemotherapy and tamoxifen. N Engl J Med. 1981;305:1–6.
91. Gail M, Simon R. Testing for qualitative interactions between treatment effects and patient subsets. Biometrics. 1985;41:361–72.
92. Bonadonna G, Valagussa P. Dose-response effect of adjuvant chemotherapy in breast cancer. N Engl J Med. 1981;34:10–5.
93. Redmond C, Fisher B, Wieand HS. The methodologic dilemma in retrospectively correlating the amount of chemotherapy received in adjuvant therapy protocols with disease-free survival. Cancer Treat Rep. 1983;67:519–26.
94. Fisher B, Anderson S, Fisher ER, Redmond C, et al. Significance of ipsilateral breast tumor recurrence after lumpectomy. Lancet. 1991;338:327–31.
95. Hochberg Y. A sharper Bonferroni procedure for multiple tests of significance. Biometrika. 1988;75:800–2.
96. Cook RJ, Farewell VT. Multiplicity considerations in the design and analysis of clinical trials. J Roy Stat Soc Ser A. 1996;159:93–110.
97. Taghian A, Jeong J, Anderson S, et al. Pattern of loco-regional failure in patients with breast cancer treated by mastectomy and chemotherapy (+/− tamoxifen) without radiation: results from five NSABP randomized trials. J Clin Oncol. 2004;22:4247–54.
98. Gaynor JJ, Feuer EJ, Tan CC, et al. On the use of cause-specific failure and conditional failure probabilities: examples from clinical oncology data. J Am Stat Assoc. 1993;88:400–9.
99. Korn EL, Dorey FJ. Applications of crude incidence curves. Stat Med. 1992;11:813–29.
100. Lin DY. Non-parametric inference for cumulative incidence functions in competing risks studies. Stat Med. 1997;16:901–10.
101. Pepe MS, Mori M. Kaplan-Meier, marginal or conditional probability curves in summarizing competing risks failure time data? Stat Med. 1993;2:37–751.

102. Kalbfleisch JD, Prentice RL. The statistical analysis of failure time data. New York: Wiley; 1980.
103. Gooley TA, Leisenring W, Crowley J, et al. Estimation of failure probabilities in the presence of competing risks: new representations of old estimators. Stat Med. 1999;18:695–706.
104. Gray RJ. A class of K-sample tests for comparing the cumulative incidence of a competing risk. Ann Stat. 1988;16:1141–54.
105. Benichou J, Gail MH. Estimates of absolute cause-specific risk in cohort studies. Biometrics. 1990;46:813–26.
106. Jeong J. A new parametric distribution for modeling cumulative incidence function: application to breast cancer data. J Roy Stat Soc Ser A (Stat Soc). 2006;169:289–303.
107. Jeong J, Fine J. Direct parametric inference for cumulative incidence function. J Roy Stat Soc Ser C (Appl Stat). 2006;55:187–200.
108. Bryant J, Dignam JJ. Semiparametric models for cumulative incidence functions. Biometrics. 2004;60:182–90.
109. Fine JP, Gray RJ. A proportional hazards model for the sub-distribution of a competing risk. J Am Stat Assoc. 1999;94:496–509.
110. Jeong J, Fine J. Parametric regression on cumulative incidence function. Biostatistics. 2007;8:184–96.
111. Garg ML, Rao BR, Redmond CK. Maximum-likelihood estimation of the parameters of the Gompertz survival function. J Roy Stat Soc Ser C (Appl Stat). 1970;19:152–9.
112. Gompertz B. On the nature of the function expressive of the law of human mortality, and on the new mode of determining the value of life contingencies. Phil Trans Roy Soc London. 1825;115:513–80.
113. Dabrowska DM, Doksum KA. Estimation and testing in a two-sample generalized odds-rate model. J Am Stat Assoc. 1998;83:744–9.
114. Goss PE, Ingle JN, Martino S, et al. A randomized trial of letrozole in postmenopausal women after five years of tamoxifen therapy for early-stage breast cancer. N Engl J Med. 2003;349:1793–802.
115. Latouche A, Porcher R, Chevret S. Sample size formula for proportional hazards modeling of competing risks. Stat Med. 2004;23:3263–74.
116. Paik S, Shak S, Tang G, et al. A multigene assay to predict recurrence of tamoxifen-treated, node-negative breast cancer. N Engl J Med. 2004;351:2817–26.
117. Benjamini Y, Hochberg Y. Controlling the false discovery rate: a practical and powerful approach to multiple testing. J Roy Stat Soc Ser B. 1995;57:289–300.
118. Benjamini Y, Yekutieli D. The control of the false discovery rate in multiple testing under dependency. Ann Stat. 2001;29:1165–88.
119. Bair E, Tibshirani R. Semi-supervised methods to predict patient survival from gene expression data. PLoS Biol. 2004;2:511–22.
120. Harrell FE, Lee KL, Mark DB. Multivariable prognostic models: issues in developing models, evaluating assumptions and adequacy, and measuring and reducing errors. Stat Med. 1966;15:361–87.
121. Harrell FE, Califf RM, Pryor DB, Lee KL, Rosati RA. Evaluating the yield of medical tests. J Am Med Assoc. 1982;247:2543–6.
122. Hanley JA, McNeil BJ. The meaning and use of the area under the receiver operating characteristic (ROC) curve. Radiology. 1982;143:29–36.
123. Pencina MJ, D'Agostino RB. Overall C as a measure of discrimination in survival analysis: model specific population value and confidence interval estimation. Stat Med. 2004;23:2109–23.
124. Assmann SF, Pocock SJ, Enos LE, Kasten LE. Subgroup analyses and other misuses of baseline data in clinical trials. Lancet. 2000;355:1064–9.
125. Wang R, Lagakos SW, Ware JH, Hunter DJ, Drazen JM. Statistics in medicine—reporting of subgroup analyses in clinical trials. N Engl J Med. 2007;357:2189–94.
126. Elbourne DR, Altman DG, Pocock SJ, Evans SJW. Reporting of noninferiority and equivalence randomized trials: an extension of the CONSORT statement. J Am Med Assoc. 2006;295:1152–60.
127. Piaggio G, Elbourne DRY, Altman DG, Pocock SJ, Evans SJW. Reporting of noninferiority and equivalence randomized trials: an extension of the CONSORT statement. JAMA. 2006; 295:1152–60.
128. Campbell MK, Elbourne DR, Altman DG. CONSORT statement: extension to cluster randomised trials. Br Med J. 2004;328 (7441):702–8.
129. Boutron I, Moher D, Altman DG, Schulz K, Ravaud P, for the CONSORT group. Methods and processes of the CONSORT Group: example of an extension for trials assessing nonpharmacologic treatments. Ann Int Med. 2008:W60–W67.
130. Boutron I, Moher D, Altman DG, Schulz K, Ravaud P, for the CONSORT group. Extending the CONSORT statement to randomized trials of nonpharmacologic treatment: explanation and elaboration. Ann Int Med. 2008:295–309.
131. Ioannidis JP, Evans SJ, Gotzsche PC, O'Neil RT, Altman DG, Schulz K, Moher D. Better reporting of harms in randomized trials: an extension of the CONSORT statement. Ann Int Med. 2004;141:781–8.
132. Hopewell S, Clarke M, Moher D, Wager E, Middleton P, Altman DG, Schulz KF, The CONSORT Group. CONSORT for reporting randomized controlled trials in journal and conference abstracts: explanation and elaboration. PLoS Med. 2008;5(1):e20. doi:10.1371/journal.
133. Hopewell S, Clarke M, Moher D, Wager E, Middleton P, Altman DG, Schulz KF, The CONSORT Group. CONSORT for reporting randomised trials in journal and conference abstracts. Lancet. 2008;371:281–3.
134. Begg C, Cho M, Eastwood S, Horton R, Moher D, Olkin I, et al. Improving the quality of reports of randomized controlled trials: the CONSORT statement. J Am Med Assoc. 1996;276:637–9.
135. Altman DG, Schulz KF, Moher D, Egger M, Davidoff F, Elbourne D, et al. The revised CONSORT statement for reporting randomized trials: explanation and elaboration. Ann Int Med. 2001;134(8):663–94.
136. Moher D, Schulz KF, Altman DG. The CONSORT statement: revised recommendations for improving the quality of reports of parallel-group randomised trials. Lancet. 2001;357(9263):1191–4.
137. Moher D, Schulz KF, Altman D. The CONSORT statement: revised recommendations for improving the quality of reports of parallel-group randomized trials. J Am Med Assoc. 2001;285 (15):1987–91.
138. Moher D, Schulz KF, Altman DG. The CONSORT statement: revised recommendations for improving the quality of reports of parallel-group randomized trials. Ann Int Med. 2001;134(8): 657–62.
139. Early Breast Cancer Trialists' Collaborative Group. Effects of adjuvant tamoxifen and of cytotoxic therapy on mortality in early breast cancer: an overview of 61 randomized trials among 28,896 women. N Engl J Med. 1988;319:1681–91.
140. Early Breast Cancer Trialists' Collaborative Group. Treatment of early breast cancer, vol. I: Worldwide evidence 1985–1990. Oxford University Press; 1990.
141. Early Breast Cancer Trialists' Collaborative Group. Systemic treatment of early breast cancer by hormonal, cytotoxic, or immune therapy: 133 randomised trials involving 31,000 recurrences and 24,000 deaths among 75,000 women. Lancet. 1992;339:1–15 & 71–85.

142. Early Breast Cancer Trialists' Collaborative Group. Effects of radiotherapy and surgery in early breast cancer: an overview of the randomized trials. N Engl J Med. 1995;333:1444–55.
143. Early Breast Cancer Trialists' Collaborative Group. Ovarian ablation in early breast cancer: overview of the randomised trials. Lancet. 1996;348:1189–96.
144. Early Breast Cancer Trialists' Collaborative Group. Tamoxifen for early breast cancer: an overview of the randomised trials. Lancet. 1998;351:1451–67.
145. Early Breast Cancer Trialists' Collaborative Group. Polychemotherapy for early breast cancer: an overview of the randomised trials. Lancet. 1998;352:930–42.
146. Early Breast Cancer Trialists' Collaborative Group. Favourable and unfavourable effects on long-term survival of radiotherapy for early breast cancer: an overview of the randomised trials. Lancet. 2000;355:1757–70.
147. Early Breast Cancer Trialists' Collaborative Group (EBCTCG). Effects of chemotherapy and hormonal therapy for early breast cancer on recurrence and 15-year survival: an overview of the randomised trials. Lancet. 2005;365:1687–717.
148. Early Breast Cancer Trialists' Collaborative Group. Effects of radiotherapy and of differences in the extent of surgery for early breast cancer on local recurrence and on 15-year survival: an overview of the randomised trials. Lancet. 2005;366: 2087–106.
149. Moher D, Cook DJ, Eastwood S, Olkin I, Rennie D, Stroup, DF, for the QUOROM Group. Improving the quality of reports of meta-analyses of randomized controlled trials: the QUOROM statement. Lancet. 1999;354:1896–1900.
150. O'Quigley J, Pepe M, Fisher L. Continual reassessment method: a practical design for phase I clinical trials in cancer. Biometrics. 1990;46:33–48.
151. Gehan EA. The determination of the number of patients required in a preliminary and follow-up trial of a new chemotherapeutic agent. J Chronic Dis. 1961;13:346–53.

34 Structure of Breast Centers

David P. Winchester

34.1 Introduction

Evaluation and management of benign and malignant breast disease continue to be a major health problem in the United States. The American Cancer Society (ACS) estimated that there would be 231,840 female patients diagnosed with invasive breast cancer in the United States in 2015. In addition, the Society estimated that 60,290 women would be diagnosed with ductal carcinoma in situ [1].

The annual incidence of breast cancer in most developed countries can be accurately tracked through cancer registration systems. Contrariwise, there are no comprehensive databases to estimate the incidence of benign breast disease in the United States. This annual number likely runs in the millions. Countless patients seek evaluation and management of a broad spectrum of benign disease, which must be differentiated from breast cancer. The threat of breast cancer and broad media coverage combine to heighten the level of anxiety and concern among women with breast cancer symptoms and findings. These include breast pain, lumps, nipple discharge, the itching breast, mastitis, axillary node enlargement and abnormal imaging findings such as cystic and solid masses, the asymmetric density, microcalcifications, skin thickening, and enhancing lesions seen on breast MRI. Thus, millions of consistently anxious women around the world present with self-discovered findings or physician-detected abnormalities through physical exam or imaging studies. This places a significant burden on healthcare systems to conduct top quality, multidisciplinary evaluation and management in an optimally organized setting.

Silverstein recognized that the evaluation and management of breast patients was often fragmented, inefficient and time-consuming. He firmly believed that these patients should be promptly evaluated and test results communicated as quickly as possible. He also recognized the need to navigate patients through this complex environment. The result was the establishment of a multidisciplinary breast clinic at UCLA in 1973. Further refinements and philanthropic support led to the opening of the Van Nuys Breast Center, the first free-standing, multidisciplinary breast center in the United States [2]. Since that time, breast centers, hospital-based or free-standing, have rapidly proliferated.

D.P. Winchester (✉)
American College of Surgeons, 633 N Saint Clair Street, Chicago, IL 60611-3211, USA
e-mail: dwinchester@facs.org

34.2 The National Accreditation Program for Breast Centers

The American College of Surgeons has a long and distinguished history of accrediting and fostering clinical quality improvement programs in cancer, trauma, bariatrics, pediatric surgery, and the National Surgical Quality Improvement Program (NSQIP).

The American College of Surgeons was founded in 1913. Within 10 years, the first cancer registry in the United States was introduced and a cancer accreditation program took root. The Commission on Cancer, as presently constituted, consists of representatives from 56 national professional organizations committed to decreasing the morbidity and mortality of cancer patients through standard setting and the monitoring of outcomes. Thirty-six multidisciplinary standards must be met by accredited facilities verified at the time of triennial survey. Between 70–80 % of all newly diagnosed cancer patients in the United States are cared for in the Commission on Cancer-accredited programs. These 1500 centers are required to submit comprehensive data on all analytic cancer patients to the National Cancer Database (NCDB). The NCDB was initially organized in 1988 and now contains comprehensive information on over 34 million cancer patients. This has provided, through the years, a firm foundation for tracking patterns of care on a longitudinal basis and effecting change to keep pace with evidence-based changes in evaluation and management.

I. Jatoi and A. Rody (eds.), *Management of Breast Diseases*, DOI 10.1007/978-3-319-46356-8_34

The practice of medicine in the United States is undergoing transformation to a more transparent system of quality management and outcomes of cancer patients through accredited facilities and individual physician reporting. The large network of Commission on Cancer-accredited programs and the robust NCDB have formed an excellent framework to address these changes.

The idea of a National Accreditation Program for Breast Centers (NAPBC) was conceived in this transformational medical delivery system in the year 2005. The experience and success of the Commission on Cancer provided early guidelines for the NAPBC development. There was recognition, at the outset, that diseases of the breast, including breast cancer, required a multidisciplinary team for optimal patient evaluation and management. The Board of Regents of the American College of Surgeons approved seed funding in 2006 to support program development. A formal governing board of the NAPBC was organized and has been meeting regularly for the past 10 years. The board consists of representatives from 20 national, professional organizations (Table 34.1). In addition, six working committees were organized as outlined in Table 34.2. Thus, the NAPBC is an organization of organizations, housed and staffed at the American College of Surgeons national headquarters in Chicago but governed by the NAPBC board. The mission statement for this program states that "The NAPBC is a consortium of national, professional organizations dedicated to the improvement of the quality of care and monitoring of outcomes for patients with diseases of the breast." To meet this mission, five objectives were agreed upon (Table 34.3).

The original design of the NAPBC called for three categories of breast centers. The centers could be housed in a single geographic area or recognized as centers without walls as long as the breast center leadership had control of

Table 34.1 Member organizations

American board of surgery[a]
American Cancer Society (ACS) American College of Radiology Breast Imaging Commission (ACRBIC) American Cancer Radiology Imaging Network (ACRIN) American Institute for Radiologic Pathology (AIRP) American Society for Radiation Oncology (ASTRO)
American College of Surgeons
American Society of Plastic Surgeons (ASPS)
American Society of Breast Surgeons (ASBS)
American Society of Clinical Oncology (ASCO)
Association of Cancer Executives (ACE)
Association of Oncology Social Work (AOSW)
College of American Pathologists (CAP)
National Cancer Registrars Association (NCRA)
National Consortium of Breast Centers (NCBC) National Society of Genetic Counselors (NSGC)
Oncology Nursing Society (ONS) Society of Breast Imaging (SBI)
Society of Surgical Oncology (SSO)
Members-at-Large

[a]Liaison board membership

Table 34.2 NAPBC committees

Executive committee
Standards and Accreditation
International Committee
Education and dissemination Research Finance

Table 34.3 Mission objectives

Consensus development of standards for breast centers and a survey process to monitor compliance
Strengthen the scientific basis for improving quality care
Establish a national breast cancer database to effect quality improvement
Reduce the morbidity and mortality of breast cancer by improving access to screening and comprehensive care, promoting risk reduction and prevention and advocating for increased access and participation in clinical trials
Expand programs of quality improvement measurement and benchmark comparison

provided services. If provided services were not available on-site, referred services were required within reasonable distance for breast patients.

After 18 months of deliberation by the NAPBC board, there was consensus on the establishment of 28 standards for breast center accreditation.

In order to field test and validate center categories, components, standards, and the survey process, 18 voluntary pilot site surveys were conducted across the United States. Many lessons were learned. The 28 standards have undergone substantial revisions. Several deficiencies were encountered but appeared to be readily correctable through education. The structure of the centers confirmed the heterogeneous settings in which evaluation and management are conducted. A common model was community-based, consisting of private practitioners in general surgery, medical oncology, radiation oncology, radiology, and pathology working together to deliver high-quality evaluation and management of their patients. Some services, such as breast imaging, surgery, systemic therapy, and radiation therapy were provided on-site while other services, such as genetic counseling, plastic surgery, and survivorship programs were referred to nearby locales. Another common model encountered within or without walls was nonteaching hospitals or academic/teaching hospitals. In these settings, there were more provided services and fewer referred services. It was our observation that patients received excellent care, irrespective of the center model because they were afforded the full-range of services, whether provided or referred.

The experience of the pilot surveys led the NAPBC board to approve a single category for accreditation. The board reasoned that as long as breast patients were afforded the full-range of services for evaluation and management and all of the 28 standards were met, a single accreditation category would be inclusive rather than exclusive.

The NAPBC granted its first accreditation in the United States in December, 2008. The NAPBC has been widely regarded as a quality program improving outcomes and streamlining the evaluation and management of patients with breast disease. As of April, 2016 the NAPBC has accredited 650 programs. Many have undergone subsequent re-accreditation surveys, as the program works on a 3-year cycle. Attrition has been minimal.

There has been increasing interest in NAPBC international accreditation. Thirty-two breast centers in seventeen countries have requested information. The first international NAPBC accreditation was awarded in the Middle East in 2014. Two surveys are scheduled in Canada in 2016, as well as one in South Africa.

34.3 NAPBC Standards

The categories for standards include center leadership, clinical management, research, community outreach, professional education, and quality improvement.

34.4 Center Leadership

Purpose: The standard establishes the medical director and/or co-directors, or interdisciplinary steering committee as the Breast Program Leadership (BPL) responsible and accountable for breast center activities.

34.4.1 Level of Responsibility and Accountability

Standard 1.1 The organizational structure of the breast center gives the BPL responsibility and accountability for provided breast center services.

Leadership is the key element in an effective breast center and its success depends on effective BPL. The BPL is responsible for goal setting, as well as planning, initiating, implementing, evaluating, and improving all breast-related activities in the center.

The center or medical staff formally establishes the responsibility, accountability, and multidisciplinary membership required for the BPL to fulfill its role. The center documents the breast program leader's responsibility and accountability using a method appropriate to the center's organizational structure. Examples include, but are not limited to, the following:

- The center bylaws designate the breast program leader(s) as a subcommittee of the cancer committee in centers with CoC dual accreditation.
- Policies and procedures for the center define authority of the breast program leader(s).
- Policies and procedures for the medical staff define authority of the breast program leader.
- The medical staff bylaws designate the breast program leader(s) to be a standing committee with authority defined.

Other methods that are consistent with the center organization and operation are acceptable.

The BPL is responsible for an annual audit of the following:

- Interdisciplinary Breast Cancer Conference Activity (Standard 1.2)
- Breast Conservation Rate (Standard 2.3)
- Sentinel Lymph Node Biopsy Rate (Standard 2.4)
- Breast Cancer Staging (Standard 2.6)
- Needle Biopsy Rate (Standard 2.9)
- Radiation Oncology Quality Assurance (Standard 2.12)
- Support and Rehabilitation (Standard 2.15)
- Reconstructive Surgery Referral Rate (Standard 2.18)
- Breast Cancer Survivorship Care (Standard 2.20)
- Clinical Trial Accrual (Standard 3.2)
- Quality and Outcomes (Standard 6.1)
- Quality Improvement (Standard 6.2)

34.4.2 Cancer Conference

Standard 1.2 The BPL monitors and evaluates the interdisciplinary breast cancer conference frequency, multidisciplinary attendance, prospective case presentation and total case presentation annually, including AJCC staging and discussion of nationally accepted guidelines.

Conferences that include case presentations should be available to the entire medical staff and are the preferred format. Consultative services are optimal when physician representatives from diagnostic radiology, pathology (including AJCC staging), surgery, medical oncology, and radiation oncology participate in the breast conference.

Setting the Interdisciplinary Breast Conference frequency and format allow for prospective review of breast cancer cases and encourages multidisciplinary involvement in the care process. Breast cancer conferences are integral to improving the care of breast cancer patients by contributing to the patient management process and outcomes, and providing education to physicians and other staff in attendance. CME credit is recommended.

The Interdisciplinary Breast Conference is focused on treatment planning for newly diagnosed and recurrent breast cancer patients, and should include discussion of tumor stage and relevant, nationally accepted breast cancer patient care guidelines developed by national organizations. This conference should be designed for breast surgeons, medical oncologists, and radiation oncologists to provide a comprehensive update on new data and recent advances in surgery and systemic/local therapy that are critical to the optimal management of breast cancer patients. Radiologists and pathologists provide essential expertise in diagnosis. Nurses, fellows, and pharmacists in the oncology field are also invited to attend.

Conference frequency is dependent upon annual caseload. Depending on the analytic case volume, the conference should be held at least every two weeks or twice monthly to ensure timely prospective patient review. Centers with less than 100 cases per year can be included as part of the general cancer conference. 85 % of these cases must be presented prospectively. Centers with 100–250 annual cases must meet at least twice monthly. Weekly conferences are required with higher annual cases.

Prospective case reviews include, but are not limited to, the following:

- Imaging and pathology reviews.
- Newly diagnosed breast cancer and treatment not yet initiated.
- Newly diagnosed breast cancer and treatment initiated, but discussion and additional treatment is needed.
- Previously diagnosed, initial treatment completed, but discussion of adjuvant treatment or treatment recurrence or progression is needed.
- Previously diagnosed, and discussion of supportive or palliative care is needed.
- Consideration for clinical trials.

Monitoring of breast cancer conference activity by the BPL ensures that conferences provide consultative services for patients, as well as offer education to physicians and allied health professionals.

The surveyor attends a breast cancer conference to observe the multidisciplinary involvement in case discussions, at the time of survey.

34.4.3 Evaluation and Management Guidelines

Standard 1.3 The BPL identifies and references evidence-based breast care evaluation and management guidelines.

Patient management and treatment guidelines promote an organized approach to providing care. The BPL should review and adopt breast care evaluation and management guidelines developed by national organizations appropriate to the patients that are diagnosed and treated by the center. Examples of referencing these guidelines could include:

- PowerPoint presentations or handouts at cancer conferences or BPL meetings of relevant, nationally accepted breast care guidelines.

National organizations that have developed breast care guidelines include, but are not limited to, the following:

- American Cancer Society (ACS)
- American Society of Clinical Oncology (ASCO)
- American Society for Therapeutic Radiology and Oncology (ASTRO)
- National Quality Forum (NQF)
- National Comprehensive Cancer Network (NCCN)

Guidelines adopted by the BPL for use by the center are documented. This is in addition to patient management and treatment guidelines required by the NAPBC. The BPL establishes the concordance rate for adherence to adopted guidelines being used by the center, and monitors utilization through review of a random sample of cases for which these guidelines are applicable. The monitoring activity is reported to the BPL on a regular basis. The BPL addresses compliance levels that fall below the established concordance rates.

34.5 Clinical Management

Purpose: The standards identify the scope of clinical services needed to provide quality breast care to patients. The managing physician is essential to coordinating a multidisciplinary team approach to patient care.

34.5.1 Interdisciplinary Patient Management

Standard 2.2 A patient navigation process is in place to guide the patient with a breast abnormality through provided or referred services.

Breast cancer is a disease requiring interdisciplinary evaluation and management. The NAPBC has identified 17 components in the spectrum of breast cancer diagnosis, treatment, surveillance, and rehabilitation/support. These are described in the Appendix.

Standards 1.1, 1.2, and 2.1 are critical standards and must be met to be considered for NAPBC survey.

34.5.2 Patient Navigation

Standard 2.2 A patient navigation process is in place to guide the patient with a breast abnormality through provided or referred services.

The primary function of the patient navigation process is to coordinate services and guide patients through the health care system by assisting with access issues, identifying resources, providing educational materials, and developing relationships with service providers.

The patient navigation process should include a consistent care coordinator throughout the continuum of care able to assess the physical, psychological, and social needs of the patient. The results are enhanced patient outcomes, increased satisfaction, and reduced costs of care. This may involve different individuals at each point of care.

The following organizations provide patient navigation information and resources:

- American Cancer Society
- Patient Navigation in Cancer Care
- Educare
- Association of Community Cancer Centers
- Association of Oncology Social Work
- C-Change
- Harold P. Freeman Patient Navigation Institute
- National Consortium of Breast Centers
- Oncology Nursing Society

Qualifications of a patient navigator may include:

- Successful completion of a recognized patient navigator training program.
- Documentation of the requisite knowledge and skills from previous education and experience to provide patient navigation.

34.5.3 Breast Conservation

Standard 2.3 Breast-conserving surgery (BCS) is offered to appropriate patients with breast cancer. A target rate of 50 % of all eligible patients diagnosed with early stage breast cancer (Stages 0, I, II) are treated with BCS, and the BCS is evaluated annually by the BPL.

Breast-conserving surgery for patients with early stage breast cancer is a nationally accepted standard of care in appropriately selected patients. A target rate of 50 % may decrease in the future, as reported mastectomy rates are increasing.

34.5.4 Sentinel Node Biopsy

Standard 2.4 Axillary sentinel lymph node biopsy is considered or performed for patients with early stage breast cancer (Clinical Stage I, IIA, IIB) and compliance is evaluated annually by the BPL.

Patients currently considered candidates for sentinel lymph node biopsy include those with:

AJCC Stage I, IIA, and IIB invasive breast cancer with Clinical N0 disease, resectable, locally advanced, invasive breast cancer, either before or after, neoadjuvant systemic therapy, extensive DCIS requiring total mastectomy, with no suspicious axillary nodes, unilateral or bilateral prophylactic mastectomy and DCIS requiring wide excision in an anatomic location interfering with future node mapping, with no suspicious axillary nodes.

This technique most commonly utilizes a combination of radionuclide and blue dye, although some centers utilize radionuclide alone.

34.5.5 Breast Cancer Surveillance

Standard 2.5 A process is in place for assuring follow-up surveillance of breast cancer patients.

Follow-up surveillance includes history, clinical examination, upper extremity lymphedema measurements, and imaging studies. Frequency of follow-up will vary from patient to patient. Bone scan, PET scan, and other tests are the responsibility of the managing physician and are generally ordered for evaluation of symptoms or restaging.

Guidelines for follow-up surveillance are available at

- ASCO (www.asco.org)
- NCCN (www.nccn.org)

34.5.6 AJCC Staging

Standard 2.6 The BPL develops a process to monitor physician use of AJCC staging in treatment planning.

Proper staging of cancer allows the physician to determine appropriate treatment. Staging enables the reliable evaluation of treatment results and outcomes reported to various institutions on a local, regional, and national basis.

When using the AJCC system, either clinical or pathological staging is assigned to each primary. Both should be assigned and recorded in the medical record, if appropriate. Use the criteria for clinical and pathological staging outlined in the current edition of the *AJCC Cancer Staging Manual* [3] to determine the appropriate stage.

A designation of M_x makes the patient unstageable and this designation should not be used. The managing physician should designate whether the patient is M0 or M1.

The assignment of staging is most appropriate by the managing physician, who is ultimately responsible for planning the patient's treatment. The patient's managing physician evaluates all available staging information (X-rays, scans, laboratory tests, and operative and pathology reports), records the staging elements (TNM and Stage Group) in the medical record. Tumor registrars participate in documentation, if available.

34.5.7 Pathology Reports

Standard 2.7 The College of American Pathologists' (CAP) Cancer Committee guidelines are followed for all invasive breast cancers, including estrogen and progesterone receptors, and Her2 status for all invasive breast cancer patients. Estrogen receptor status is recommended for DCIS. Outside pathology is reviewed [4].

Patient management and treatment guidelines promote an organized approach to providing quality care. The NAPBC requires that 90 % of breast cancer pathology reports will contain the scientifically validated data elements outlined on the surgical case summary checklist of the (CAP) publication *Reporting on Cancer Specimens* [4]

- College of American Pathologists (CAP) synoptic reporting is required Imaging studies should be correlated with pathology when feasible

34.5.8 Diagnostic Imaging

Standard 2.8 Mammographic screening and diagnostic imaging, are conducted through Mammography Quality Standards Act (MQSA)-certified facilities.

Federal law mandates that mammography must be conducted and interpreted by a MQSA-certified radiologist.

MQSA information is available from:

- U.S. Food and Drug Administration (FDA)

ACR Guidelines for mammographic screening, diagnostic imaging, and breast MRI are available from:

- American College of Radiology
  - Guidelines for the Performance of Screening Mammography
  - Guidelines for the Performance of Diagnostic Mammography
  - Guidelines for the Performance of Magnetic Resonance Imaging (MRI) of the Breast

34.5.9 Needle Biopsy

Standard 2.9 Palpation-guided or image-guided needle biopsy is the initial diagnostic approach rather than open surgical biopsy.

Either fine needle aspiration for cytologic evaluation or core needle biopsy constitute the initial diagnostic approach for palpable or occult lesions. Open surgical biopsy as an initial approach should be avoided as it does not allow for treatment planning and is associated with a high re-excision rate. Compliance is reviewed annually with BPL.

34.5.10 Ultrasonography

Standard 2.10 Diagnostic ultrasound and/or ultrasound-guided needle biopsy are performed at an American College of Radiology (ACR) ultrasound-accredited facility or by an American Society of Breast Surgeon (ASBS)-Breast Ultrasound-certified surgeon.

34.5.11 Stereotactic Core Needle Biopsy

Standard 2.11 Stereotactic core needle biopsy is performed at an ACR accredited facility, or by surgeons under the standards and requirements developed by the ACR and the American College of Surgeons or by an American Society of Breast Surgeons (ASBS) Breast Procedure Program-certified surgeon.

34.5.12 Radiation Oncology

Standard 2.12 Radiation oncology treatment services are provided by or referred to board certified/eligible radiation oncologists. The center has been accredited either by the ACR, Radiation Oncology Practice Accreditation (ACR-ROPA), American Society for Radiation Oncology, Accreditation Program for Excellence (ASTRO-APEx) or the American College of Radiation Oncology (ACRO) or has a quality assurance program in place, and the breast quality measure endorsed by the National Quality Forum (NQF) for radiation.

34.5.13 Medical Oncology

Standard 2.13 Medical oncology treatment services are either provided by or referred to board certified/eligible medical oncologists, and the breast center quality measures endorsed by the NQF for medical oncology are utilized.

Standard 2.14 Nursing care is provided by or referred to nurses with specialized knowledge and skills in diseases of the breast. Nursing assessment and interventions are guided by evidence-based standards of practice and symptom management.

The complex needs of cancer patients and their families require specialized oncology nursing knowledge and skills to achieve optimal patient care outcomes. The oncology nurse is an integral member of the multidisciplinary breast team.

In larger centers, ONS-certified nurses are preferred. In smaller centers or private practice offices, ONS-certified nurses are optional, but nursing care should be provided by those with experience in breast diseases.

A clinical expert in oncology may include:

Oncology Nurse Practitioners (AOCNP) Oncology Clinical Nurse Specialist (AOCNS) Oncology Certified Nurse (OCN) Certified Breast Care Nurse (CBCN), defined as a nurse with documented knowledge and skills from previous education and experience in the care of women with breast disease.

34.5.14 Support and Rehabilitation

Standard 2.15 Support and rehabilitation services are provided or referred to clinicians with specialized knowledge of diseases of the breast.

Comprehensive breast cancer care is multidisciplinary and includes medical health professionals addressing patient needs identified along the breast cancer continuum from diagnosis through survivorship. Supportive services help patients and their families cope with the day-to-day details of a breast cancer diagnosis. These resources address emotional, physical, financial, and other needs of the breast cancer patient.

34.5.15 Genetic Evaluation and Management

Standard 2.16 High-risk counseling, genetic counseling, and testing services are provided or referred to a board certified/eligible genetic counselor.

Not all breast cancer patients will need to be referred to a cancer genetics professional. Genetic counseling is provided by: An American Board of Genetic Counseling professional (ABGC) An American College of Medical Genetics (ACMG) physician board certified in medical genetics. An advanced practice oncology nurse (APON) with specialized education in cancer genetics. A Genetics Clinical Nurse (GNCC) credentialed through the Genetics Nursing Credentialing Commission (GNCC). A board certified/eligible physician with expertise in medical genetics.

34.5.16 Educational Resources

Standard 2.17 Culturally appropriate educational resources are available for patients along with a process to provide them. The materials provided are appropriately adjusted for the patient population and reviewed annually.

Centers should provide patients with educational information covering the entire spectrum of evaluation and management of breast disease. Some centers have patient education libraries, while others provide printed materials that are either locally generated or provided by national organizations. Audiovisual education is a very effective delivery method.

34.5.17 Reconstructive Surgery

Standard 2.18 All appropriate patients undergoing mastectomy are offered a preoperative referral to a reconstructive/plastic surgeon. Reconstructive surgery is provided by or referred to a board certified/eligible reconstructive/plastic surgeon.

Patients undergoing mastectomy should be afforded a discussion on the options of breast reconstruction with a board certified/eligible plastic/reconstructive surgeon. There is an increasing trend in immediate breast reconstruction utilizing tissue expanders, implants, or autologous tissue transfer. Some patients may desire delayed reconstruction. Patients need to understand that breast reconstruction does not interfere with surveillance or detection of local recurrence.

34.5.18 Evaluation and Management of Benign Breast Disease

Standard 2.19 Evaluation and management of benign breast disease follows nationally recognized guidelines.

Benign breast disease is defined as breast findings found on clinical breast examination deemed non-suspicious by the examiner or a BIRADS category one or two on breast imaging.

If the mass is cystic and tender, needle aspiration may be done at the time or deferred until breast imaging is done. If ultrasound is available to the initial examining physician, confirmation of the cyst and complete aspiration with ultrasound guidance is preferred. Palpation-guided cyst aspiration is acceptable. The mass should completely resolve and follow-up options should be discussed. The fluid, if benign in appearance, should be discarded. Incomplete resolution of the mass and/or bloody fluid are indications for submission of the cyst fluid for cytologic evaluation.

A clinically benign, but solid mass requires additional evaluation. Mammography and ultrasound, unless recently performed, should be done to confirm the solid, but benign characteristics of the palpable mass. Office-based fine needle aspiration or core needle biopsy can be palpation and/or ultrasound -guided. Ultrasound-guided needle biopsy would be expected in a radiology department setting. If a benign diagnosis, without atypia, is confirmed, the patient may be observed or excisional biopsy performed, depending on circumstances and patient/physician preferences.

Occult, asymptomatic cysts, found with mammography/ultrasound require no intervention but thorough discussion with the patient. BIRADS 3 findings are usually managed with a 3–6 month imaging follow-up and clinical breast exam. This applies to both benign masses and micro calcifications.

Atypical ductal or lobular hyperplasia found on needle biopsy requires follow-up excisional biopsy to accurately define the lesion.

34.5.19 Breast Cancer Survivorship Care

Standard 2.20 A comprehensive breast cancer survivorship care process, including a survivorship care plan with accompanying treatment summary, is in place within six months of completing active treatment and no longer than one year from date of diagnosis. The survivorship care process is evaluated annually by the BPL.

34.6 Research

Purpose: The standards promote advancement in prevention, early diagnosis, and treatment through the provision of clinical trial information and patient accrual to breast cancer-related clinical trials and research protocols.

34.6.1 Clinical Trial Information

Standard 3.1 Information about the availability of breast cancer-related clinical trials is provided to patients through a formal mechanism.

By providing information about the availability of breast cancer-related clinical trials, the facility offers patients the opportunity to participate in the advancement of evidence-based medicine.

The following organizations offer patient information and resources related to clinical trials:

- American Cancer Society
- National Cancer Institute
- U.S. Food and Drug Administration
- CenterWatch
- Coalition of Cancer Cooperative Groups.

A formal process is in place to provide information about breast cancer-related clinical trials to patients seen at the center. Methods of providing information include, but are not limited to, the following:

- Access to the internet or Intranet search services through the patient library.
- Articles in facility newsletters.
- Pamphlets or brochures in patient waiting rooms or patient packets.
- Physician/nurse education.

34.6.2 Clinical Trial Accrual

Standard 3.2 Two percent (2 %) or more of eligible breast cancer patients are accrued to treatment-related breast cancer clinical trials and/or research protocols annually.

Clinical research advances science and ensures that patient care approaches the highest possible level of quality.

Facilities must accrue patients to breast cancer-related clinical research at the minimum percentage rate of 2 %. Patients eligible to meet this standard are those patients

- Seen at the center for diagnosis and/or treatment and placed on a clinical trial through the facility.
- Seen at the center for diagnosis and/or treatment and placed on a trial through the office of a staff physician.
- Seen at the center for diagnosis and/or treatment and placed on a trial through another facility.
- Seen at the center for any reason and placed on a prevention or breast cancer control trial.

Basic science, clinical, and prevention and control research is generally conducted in cancer centers supported by grants from the National Cancer Institute (NCI) or in academic health centers. Research in community hospitals typically involves therapeutic and nontherapeutic trials.

Treatment-related clinical trial groups include, but are not limited to, the following:

- NCI-sponsored programs such as the Community Clinical Oncology Program (CCOP).
- Cooperative trial groups such as the Alliance for Clinical Trials.
- University-related research.
- Pharmaceutical company research.
- Locally developed, peer-reviewed studies.

Cancer control research studies include, but are not limited to, the following:

- Primary prevention.
- Early Detection.
- Quality of life.
- Economics of care.

Centers participating in clinical research show that an independent review mechanism consistent with national standards is in place and used. Research projects involving participation by human subjects must be approved by an internal or external institutional review board (IRB). Patients participating in clinical trials must give their informed consent.

A study coordinator, data manager, or other clinical research professional is available to assist in enrolling patients, monitoring patient accrual, and identifying and providing information and/or education about new trials.

Patient accrual is monitored, and the results are documented.

Information about breast cancer clinical trials is available through the following:

- National Cancer Institute (NCI)

34.7 Community Outreach

Purpose: The standards ensure that breast cancer education, prevention, and early detection programs are provided on-site or coordinated with other facilities or local agencies targeted to the community and follow-up is provided to patients with positive findings.

34.7.1 Education, Prevention, and Early Detection Programs

Standard 4.1 Each year, two or more breast cancer education prevention and/or early detection programs are provided by the center or coordinated with other facilities or local agencies targeted to the community with expectations for follow-up of positive findings.

34.8 Professional Education

Purpose: The standard promotes increased knowledge of breast cancer program staff through participation in local, regional, or national educational activities.

34.8.1 Breast Program Staff Education

Standard 5.1 Professionally certified/credentialed members of the breast center participate in local (in addition to breast cancer conference attendance), state, regional, or national breast-specific educational programs annually.

The breast cancer care team members should include, but is not limited to, the following professionals:

- Radiologist
- Pathologist
- Surgeon
- Medical oncologist
- Radiation oncologist
- Genetic counselor
- Nursing staff
- Patient navigator
- Social worker
- Physical therapist
- Plastic reconstructive surgeon

34.9 Quality Improvement

Purpose: The standard ensures that breast services, care, and patient outcomes are continuously evaluated and improved.

34.9.1 Quality and Outcomes

Standard 6.1 Each year, the BPL conducts or participates in two or more center-specific studies that measure quality and/or outcomes and one or more of your physician members participate in their specialty-specific quality improvement program. The findings are communicated and discussed with the breast center staff, participants of the interdisciplinary conference, or the cancer committee, where applicable.

The annual evaluation of services and care provide a baseline to measure quality and an opportunity to correct or enhance patient outcomes. Quality improvement is a multidisciplinary effort and must include support and representation from all clinical, administrative, and patient perspectives. Successful participation in quality improvement programs/initiatives from other breast-related health care organizations can meet some, or all, of these quality and outcomes requirement to be an approved breast center. The following are examples of recommended quality improvement programs/initiatives:

- The ASBS Mastery of Breast Surgery Program
- The National Outcomes and Analysis Database Project of the ASBS—www.breastsurgeons.org [5]
- The Committee on Quality and Safety of the ASBS establishes standards for breast surgery quality—www.breastsurgeons.org [5]
- Participation in the National Consortium of Breast Centers' Quality Initiatives benchmarks available for performance comparison—www.breastcare.org [6]
- The NQFs breast cancer measures—www.quality-forum.org [7]
- The American College of Surgeons, Commission on Cancer, National Cancer Data Base breast cancer benchmarks—www.facs.org/cancer [8]

34.10 Survey Process

To facilitate a thorough and accurate evaluation of the breast center, the center must complete or update an online SAR. Each year, the facility is notified of the areas of the SAR requiring annual updates.

In addition to capturing information about breast center activity, the individuals responsible for completing portions of the SAR will perform a self-assessment and rate compliance with each standard using the Breast Center Standards Rating System.

The survey is conducted by one trained surveyor with a major interest in diseases of the breast. The survey requires approximately 5–6 h. Approximately 1 h is allotted for the surveyor to speak/meet with the breast center leadership and key staff responsible for various aspects of the program to assess compliance with each standard through review of the survey application. Two hours are allotted for the surveyor to review at least 20 charts containing information on patients diagnosed with breast cancer for AJCC staging and compliance with the CAP protocol for breast pathology reports, and ten charts containing information for patients diagnosed with benign breast disease. One hour is spent for the breast conference, with the remaining time allotted to touring the center and a summation with the breast center team.

34.11 Accreditation Awards

Accreditation decisions are based on consensus rating from the surveyor, NAPBC staff and Center Criteria and Approvals Process Committee. Table 34.4 describes the accreditation award matrix.

Appeals to the accreditation award are reviewed by the Center Criteria and Approvals Process Committee.

34.12 Accreditation Award Matrix

See Table 34.4

34.13 Benefits of Being a NAPBC-Accredited Center

Accreditation by the NAPBC offers many notable benefits that will enhance a breast center and its quality of patient care. NAPBC-accredited programs offer the following:

- A model for organizing and managing a breast center to ensure multidisciplinary, integrated, and comprehensive breast care services.
- Self-assessment of breast program performance based on recognized standards.
- Recognition by national healthcare organizations as having established performance measures for high-quality breast healthcare.
- Free marketing and national public exposure.
- Access to breast center comparison benchmark reports containing national aggregate data and individual facility data to assess patterns of care and outcomes relative to national norms.

From a patient's perspective, obtaining care at a NAPBC-accredited center ensures that one will receive the following:

- Quality care close to home.
- Comprehensive care offering a range of state-of-the-art services and equipment.
- A multidisciplinary, team approach to coordinate the best care and treatment options available.
- Access to breast cancer-related information, education, and support.
- Breast cancer data collection on quality indicators for all subspecialties involved in breast cancer diagnosis and treatment.
- Ongoing monitoring and improvements in care.
- Information about clinical trials and new treatment options.

Acknowledgments Much of the content of this chapter is derived from the NAPBC Standards Manual [9].

Appendix

- Imaging
  - Screening Mammography (Digital or Analog)
  - Diagnostic Mammography
  - Ultrasound
  - Breast MRI
- Needle Biopsy

Table 34.4 Accreditation award matrix

	Three-year/full accreditation	Three-year/provisional accreditation	Accreditation deferred
Twenty-eight Standards	Ninety percent or more of eligible standards are met. Full accreditation awarded with recommendation for improvement in any deficient standards within a 12-month period	Less than 90 % of eligible standards are met. Full accreditation withheld until correction of deficient standards is documented within a 12-month period	Less than 75 % of eligible standards are met. Full accreditation deferred until correction of deficient standards and resurvey in 12 months

  - Needle biopsy—palpable
  - Image guided—Stereotactic
  - Image guided—Ultrasound
  - Image guided—MRI (if available)
- Pathology
  - Report completeness/CAP protocols
  - Radiology-Pathology correlation
  - Prognostic and predictive indicators
  - Gene studies (if available)
- Interdisciplinary Conference
  - Pre-and Post-treatment interdisciplinary discussion
  - History and findings
  - Imaging studies
  - Pathology
- Patient Navigation
  - Facilitates navigation of patient through system
- Genetic Evaluation and Management
  - Risk assessment
  - Genetic counseling
  - Genetic testing
- Surgical Care
  - Surgical correlation with imaging/concordance
  - Preoperative planning after biopsy for surgical care
  - Breast biopsy: lumpectomy or mastectomy
  - Lymph node surgery: SNB/ALND
  - Post-initial surgical correlation/treatment planning
- Plastic Surgery Consultation/Treatment
  - Tissue expander/Implants
  - TRAM/Latissimus flaps
  - DIEP flap/free flaps (if available)
- Nursing
  - Nurses with specialized knowledge and skills in diseases of the breast
- Medical Oncology Consultation/Treatment
  - Hormone therapy
  - Chemotherapy
  - Biologics
  - Chemoprevention
- Radiation Oncology Consultation/Treatment
  - Whole breast irradiation with or without boost
  - Regional nodal irradiation
  - Partial breast irradiation treatment or protocols
  - Palliative radiation for bone or systemic metastasis
  - Stereotactic radiation for isolated or limited brain metastasis
- Data Management
  - Data collection and submission
- Research
  - Cooperative trials
  - Institutional original research
  - Industry sponsored trials
- Education, Support, and Rehabilitation
  - Education (nurse) along continuum of care (pre-treatment, during, post-treatment)
  - Psychosocial Support
    Individual Support
    Family Support
    Support Groups
  - Symptom management
  - Physical therapy (e.g., lymphedema management)
- Outreach and Education
  - Community education: at large (including low-income/medically underserved)
  - Patient education
  - Physician education
- Quality Improvement
  - Continuous quality improvement through annual studies
- Survivorship Program
  - Follow-up surveillance
  - Rehabilitation
  - Health promotion/risk reduction

References

1. American Cancer Society Cancer Facts and Figures 2015, Atlanta: American Cancer Society; 2015.
2. Silverstein MJ. The Van Nuys Breast Center. The first free-standing multidisciplinary breast center. Surg Oncol Clin North Am. 2003;9 (2):159–76.
3. AJCC. Cancer Staging Manual Seventh Edition. Springer, New York; 2010.
4. College of American Pathologists Reporting on Cancer Specimens, Northfield, IL 2005; 16.
5. American Society of Breast Surgeons [Internet]. Columbia, MD: The Society, c 2015 [cited 2016 May 13]. Guidelines and quality measures. Available from: http://www.breastsurgeons.org/new_layout/about/statements/#quality_measures.
6. Kaufman CS, Shockney L, Rabinowitz B, et al. National Quality Measures for Breast Centers (NQMBC): a robust quality tool: breast center quality measures. Ann Surg Oncol. 2010;17(2):377–85. doi:10.1245/s10434-009-0729-5 Epub 2009 Oct 16.
7. NQF Cancer Project Report from 2012 "Cancer endorsement summary." National Quality Forum. October 2012 [cited 2016 May 20]. Available from: http://www.qualityforum.org/WorkArea/linkit.aspx?LinkIdentifier=id&ItemID=72130.
8. The American College of Surgeons [Internet]. Chicago, IL; The College, c 1996–2016 [cited 2016 May 13]. National Cancer Data Base Breast Cancer Benchmarks. Available from: https://www.facs.org/quality-programs/cancer/ncdb/qualitytools.
9. National Accreditation Program for Breast Centers (NAPBC) Standards Manual, 2014 ed. American College of Surgeons, Chicago, IL; 2014.

Index

Note: Page numbers followed by "f" and "t" indicate figures and tables respectively

I. Jatoi and A. Rody (eds.), *Management of Breast Diseases*, DOI 10.1007/978-3-319-46356-8

F

G

H

I

Q

R

U

V

W

Z

Printed by Printforce, the Netherlands